The Textbook of Clinical Sexual Medicine

The Textbook of Clinical Sexual Medicine

Editor
Waguih William IsHak

Springer

Editor
Waguih William IsHak
Cedars-Sinai Department of Psychiatry and Behavioral Neurosciences
Cedars-Sinai Medical Center
Los Angeles, CA, USA

David Geffen School of Medicine at University of California Los Angeles (UCLA)
Los Angeles, CA, USA

ISBN 978-3-319-52538-9 ISBN 978-3-319-52539-6 (eBook)
DOI 10.1007/978-3-319-52539-6

Library of Congress Control Number: 2017934048

Printed on acid-free paper

This Springer imprint is published by Springer Nature
The registered company is Springer International Publishing AG
The registered company address is: Gewerbestrasse 11, 6330 Cham, Switzerland

To the love of my life, the incredibly amazing
Asbasia (Hanan) Mikhail-IsHak, M.D., F.A.C.E.P.,
and the fruits of our love William and Michael.

To the phenomenal father:

William Makram IsHak, M.D.
May he rest in peace.

To the remarkable mother:

Nawara Yacoub Dawoud-IsHak, M.D.

To the exceptional brother:

Rafik William IsHak, M.D., F.R.C.S.

To the loving parents-in-law:

Mr. Aboelkhair and Mrs. Aziza Mikhail.

To the wonderful brother and sister-in-law:

Dr. Albert Mikhail and Mrs. Lamia Maalouf.

For their inspiration, encouragement, and love.

Foreword

Cardiovascular health and sexual health have their roots in a healthy endothelium, the most important site of production of nitric oxide (NO) in blood vessels. Our discoveries of the fundamental roles of NO in regulating blood flow, blood pressure, and blood coagulation, as well as functioning as the principal neurotransmitter mediating erectile function, signaled the exploration of the role of NO in penile blood flow, leading to the application of the first oral agent to treat erectile dysfunction. This and other revolutionary contributions to the field in the past 25 years place clinicians at the optimal position to evaluate very carefully the impact of biological as well as psychosocial factors on sexual functioning in addition to integrating biological treatments and psychosocial approaches to improve sexual function and, hence, the quality of life.

The *Textbook of Clinical Sexual Medicine* utilizes the biopsychosocial approach to inform physicians, practitioners, residents, trainees, and students about the latest that science has to offer for the evaluation and treatment of sexual dysfunctions especially the utilization of the full armamentarium of assessment methods and treatment interventions in order to restore sexual health and enhance quality of life.

The discovery of the cardiovascular protective and blood flow regulatory actions of NO continues to give potential applications in aging, neurodegenerative disorders, and overall well-being. Therefore, despite the lack of instant gratification, I cannot stop getting excited about basic research, and I always look forward to the inevitable scientific discoveries and resulting vital contributions to humankind, leading us all on the road to wellness.

Louis J. Ignarro
Nobel Prize in Medicine, 1998

Preface

The purpose of this textbook is to arm the reader with practical knowledge in how to recognize, address, and treat most modern-time sexual medicine issues and complications. In the remote past, issues and complications arising from one's sexuality were considered taboo. Gradually, sexual medicine gained greater importance, as in our current world one's sexuality has become a vital aspect of human quality of life. Unfortunately, some individuals who suffered from sexual disorders were still at a loss because clinicians were not equipped with the most up-to-date treatment modalities and standards to care for such patients. With this textbook, physicians, practitioners, residents, trainees, and students alike will confidently learn about sexual medicine and be able to practically apply their knowledge toward real-world clinical problems.

This textbook is divided into three parts. Part I covers fundamental knowledge regarding the clinical approach to sexual medicine. Part II contains dedicated chapters to each sexual dysfunction. Classic disorders of desire, arousal, orgasm, and sexual pain are covered in two separate chapters for each disorder: an evaluation chapter and a treatment chapter. Evaluation chapters review the etiology, phenomenology, and the assessment tools for each sexual disorder so as to offer an in-depth understanding of each disorder. These chapters then lead to further chapters detailing the specific treatment for each of the sexual disorders discussed previously. Part III covers a fascinating range of topics associated with sex in general, from myths about sexual activity to sexual emergencies. Related topics such as paraphilias and gender identity disorders are beyond the scope of this book and are covered elsewhere by recent publications. The appendices include reference materials for the reader. Appendix I reviews the rating instruments used for sexual medicine and includes copies of the most cutting-edge measurement tools of sexual functioning provided by the US National Institute of Health known as the Patient-Reported Outcome Measurement Information System (PROMIS). Appendix II highlights the published evaluation and treatment algorithms for the most common sexual dysfunctions especially algorithms from the International Society of Sexual Medicine (ISSM). The acknowledgment section is a testimony to the generous and nurturing individuals for whom the editor is eternally grateful.

This volume also advances the critical need of the integration of the biological and psychological schools of thought by embedding the biopsychosocial approach in the everyday evaluation and treatment of sexual dysfunctions in individuals and couples. I truly hope that this textbook will provide you with the necessary tools you need to lead a productive and satisfying practice.

Los Angeles, California, USA — Waguih William IsHak

Acknowledgments

I am grateful for a long list of supportive and nurturing figures throughout my career, and it gives utmost pleasure to reacknowledge them in this volume. I begin with Virginia Sadock, M.D., who taught me most of what I know about this field; I have had the pleasure of outstanding supervision by Bertina Baer, L.C.S.W., Ph.D., working alongside of the exceptional co-therapist Laura Berman, L.C.S.W., Ph.D., co-teaching with the impressive teacher Uri Peles, M.D., discovering with the extraordinary inventor Daniel Berman, M.D., learning from the unique scientist Robert Pechnick, Ph.D., and the incredibly creative Robert Cohen, Ph.D., M.D. I am eternally indebted to Norman Sussman, M.D., for giving me the opportunity of a lifetime to train at NYU. I continue to value on daily basis the priceless mentorship of Benjamin Sadock, M.D., who showed me not only how to scientifically write and edit but also how to create; Carol Bernstein, M.D., who demonstrated to me how to move mountains (and move them swiftly!); Manuel Trujillo, M.D., who taught me how to stand for, defend, and materialize world-changing ideas; Brian Ladds, M.D., who shared with me, competently and generously, his savoir-faire (know-how) about science, management, and life issues; and Lloyd Sederer, M.D., who provided me graciously with invaluable guidance about book making in addition to precious career advice. I am appreciative of Itai Danovitch, M.D.'s sincere encouragement throughout the stages of this volume's development and genuine support of my professional involvements at Cedars-Sinai. I was inspired and given growth opportunities and learned a great deal from leaders, teachers, and friends over the years, and I gratefully acknowledge my debt to them, as they have contributed in a fundamental way (albeit indirectly) to the creation of this textbook.

I would like to express my gratitude to (chronologically):

William Makram IsHak, M.D.
Sir Magdi Yacoub, M.D., F.R.C.S.
Monsieur Nagy Habib
Director Youssef Chahine
Mr. Shafik Yacoub Dawoud
Mr. Nabil Morcos
George IsHak and Faten Morcos
Mr. Kamel Morcos
Mr. Ibrahim El-Betout
Dr. Montasser El-Ghoz
Dr. Mohsen El-Ghoz
Mr. Samy Abdelazim
Mr. Mohamed El-Masry
Mr. Abdou Raafat Awad
Mr. Ayman Rashad
Professor Ahmad Abouelmagd
Prof. Dr. Adel Fawzy
Dean Hashem Fouad
Professor Dr. Yehia El-Rakhawy
Dr. Salah Shaheen
Dr. Abdeen
Dr. Emad Hamdy Ghoz
Dr. Tarek Gawad
Dr. Abdelhameed Hashem
Dr. Nahed Khairy
Dr. Zeinab Nasser
Dr. Zakaria Halim
Dr. Samir Abouelmagd
Dr. Soad Moussa
Reda Girgis, M.D.
Ayman Tadros, M.D.
Dr. Nabil Raguai
Dr. Tamer Goueli
Dr. Mohamed Foda
Dr. Cherif Abdel-Al
Dr. Nehad El-Mekawy
Dr. Wael Gawad
Dr. Amr Wael Farag
Mrs. Mona Altrash
Dr. George Milad
Nancy Hanna, M.D.
Dr. Hussein Gohar
Dr. Hossam El-Gamal
Dr. Ayman Abdel-Halim
Dr. Adel Badr
Dr. Bassel Ebeid
Dr. Hala Fakhry
Dr. Amr El-Shabrawishy
Dr. Ashraf Ramadan
Dr. Khaled Massoud
Dr. Wael Sakr
Drs. Wael and Monda Kahil
Dr. Dalia Ismail

Dr. Mohamed Salah
Dr. Shamel Hashem
Professor Dr. Refaat Mahfouz
Professor Dr. Hassib El-Defrawi
Dr. Ahmad Abdallah
Dr. Yehia Gaafar
Hesham Shafik, M.D.
Manar ElBohy, M.D.
Dr. Mervat ElAdaros
Dr. Aref Khweiled
Dr. Manal Hassan
Dr. Mustafa Hassan
Dr. Sayed El-Refayi
Mrs. Olfat Allam
Dr. Ahmad Hussein
Ms. Mai El-Rakhawy
Ms. Eman Abdelatif Zaid
Ms. Marlene Sedky
Dr. Nabil El-Kot
Dr. Monsef Mahfouz
Mr. Mohamed Salama
Dr. Nagui Gamil
Dr. Liliane Helmy
Dr. Ibrahim
Dr. Salwa Girgis
Samy Rizk, M.D.
Mrs. Mary-Terez Rizk
Khaled Mohamed, M.D.
Doug Fogelman, M.D.
Jose DeAsis, M.D.
Holly Schwartz, M.D.
Samoon Ahmad, M.D.
Marylinn Markarian, M.D.
Peter Sass, M.D.
Stacey Lane, M.D.
Fidel Ventura, M.D.
Paulina Loo, M.D.
Antonio Abad, M.D.
Elyse Weiner, M.D.
Adarsh Gupta, M.D.
Ann Maloney, M.D.
John Heussy, M.D.
Robert Cancro, M.D.
Robert Delgado, M.D.
David Nardacci, M.D.
Zebulon Taintor, M.D.
Martin Kahn, M.D.
Richard Hanson, M.D.
Burt Angrist, M.D.
Eric Peselow, M.D.
Samuel Slipp, M.D.
Maged Habib, M.D.
Greg Alsip, M.D.
Bruce Rubenstein, M.D.
Cliff Feldman, M.D., J.D.
Gary Gosselin, M.D.
Phill Halamandaris, M.D.
Laura M. O'Brien, CSW
Mr. Kim Hopper
Eugene West, M.D.
Linda Carter, Ph.D.
Martha Scotzin, Ph.D.
Morton Rubinstein, M.D.
Leonard Adler, M.D.
Marc Waldman, M.D.
Howard Silbert, M.D.
Richard Oberfield, M.D.
Asher Aladjem, M.D.
Victor Schwatrz, M.D.
Myrl Manley, M.D.
Henry Weinstein, M.D.
Howard Welsh, M.D.
Murray Alpert, Ph.D.
George Nicklin, M.D.
Arthur Meyerson, M.D.
Mr. Ben Goldhagen
Mr. J.J. Larrea
Jean Endicott, Ph.D.
Mr. Frank Schorn
Peter Goertz, M.D.
Bruce Levine, M.D.
Tal Burt, M.D.
Michael Welner, M.D.
Henry Chung, M.D.
Laura Roberts, M.D.
Danni Michaeli, M.D.
Victor Rodack, M.D.
Julie Pierce, M.D.
Michelle Montemayor, M.D.
Michael Sobel, M.D.
Ayman Fanous, M.D.
Abdullah Hassan, M.D.
Manuel Santos, M.D.
Patrick Callahan, Ph.D.
Russell Lim, M.D.
A. John Rush, M.D.
Sherwyn Woods, M.D.
Shlomo Melmed, M.D.
Peter Panzarino, M.D.
Jeffrey Wilkins, M.D.
Syed Naqvi, M.D.
Russell Poland, Ph.D.
Thomas Trott, M.D., Ph.D.
Saul Brown, M.D.
Frank Williams, M.D.
Arnold Gilberg, M.D., Ph.D.
George Simpson, M.D.
Lev Gertsik, M.D.
Lawrence Gross, M.D.
Father Michael Gabriel
Ms. Yvonne Neely
Andrea Rogers, L.C.S.W.
Richard Rosenthal, M.D.
Mark Rapaport, M.D.
Thomas Rosko, M.D.
Daniel Winstead, M.D.
Jay Yew, M.D.
Ira Lesser, M.D.
Ernst Schwarz, M.D., Ph.D.
Anne Peters, M.D.
Louis Ignarro, Ph.D.
Irwin Goldstein, M.D.
Glenn Braunstein, M.D.
Margi Stuber, M.D.
Fawzy I. Fawzy, M.D.
Thomas Strouse, M.D.
Michael Gitlin, M.D.
Peter Whybrow, M.D.
Gail Wyatt, M.D.
Jennice Vilhauer, Ph.D.
Harold Young, L.C.S.W.
Father Cyril Gorgy
Ibrahim and Rose Hanna
Bill and Nevein Sayed
Remon and Jackie Hanna
Hany and Nancy Gobreial
Ned Cowen, M.D.
Raymond Lam, M.D.
Bruce Gewertz, M.D.
Mr. Thomas Gordon
James Mirocha, M.S.
Lee T. Miller, M.D.
Jonathan Hiatt, M.D.
LuAnn Wilkerson, Ed.D.
Edward Phillips, M.D.
Andrew Klein, M.D.
Ms. Anita Parsons
Evgeny Tsimerinov, M.D.
Ramin Gabbai, M.D.
Charles Louy, M.D.
Bradley Rosen, M.D.
Sami Maalouf, Ph.D.
Edward Feldman, M.D.
Stephen Pandol, M.D.
Gil Melmed, M.D.
Teryl Nuckols, M.D.
Brennan Spiegel, M.D.
William Sledge, M.D.
Li Cai, Ph.D.
George Awad, M.D.

I would like to especially thank Nadina Persaud, Michael D. Sova, Jessica Gonzalez, and the staff at Springer for their outstanding professional work and patience throughout the duration of this project.

This book is dedicated to the medical students, residents, and faculty at Cairo University School of Medicine, Dar El-Mokattum Milieu Therapy Hospital, New York University School of Medicine (NYU), Cedars-Sinai Medical Center, and the David Geffen School of Medicine at University of California at Los Angeles (UCLA).

Waguih William IsHak

Contents

Contributors

Albert Aboseif
University of Southern California, Western University of Health Sciences, Pomona, CA, USA

Violeta Sabina Niego Perestrelo de Alarcão
Instituto de Medicina Preventiva e Saúde Pública, Faculdade de Medicina, Universidade de Lisboa, Lisboa, Portugal

Luis Filipe de Almeida Roxo
Instituto de Medicina Preventiva e Saúde Preventiva, Lisboa, Portugal

Richard Balon
Department of Psychiatry and Behavioral Neurosciences, Wayne State University School of Medicine, Detroit, MI, USA; Department of Anesthesiology, Wayne State University School of Medicine, Detroit, MI, USA

Bret Becker
Department of Psychiatry, Wright State University Boonshoft School of Medicine, Dayton, OH, USA

Klaus M. Beier
Institut für Sexualwissenschaft und Sexualmedizin, Centrum Human- und Gesundheitswissenschaften, Charité – Universitätsmedizin Berlin, Berlin, Germany

Almaz Borjoev
Heart Institute, Southern California Hospital, Culver City, CA, USA

Andrea Bradford
Section of Gastroenterology and Hepatology, Baylor College of Medicine, Houston, TX, USA

Stuart Brody
Department of General Anthropology, Charles University, Prague, Czech Republic

Michael J. Butcher
Sexual Medicine Department, Park Nicollet/Health Partners, Saint Louis Park, MN, USA

Khushminder Chahal
Department of Psychiatry and Behavioral Neurosciences, Wayne State University, Detroit, MI, USA

Anjali Chandra
Heart Institute, Southern California Hospital, Culver City, CA, USA

Steven Clevenger
Western University of the Health Sciences, Pomona, CA, USA

Danielle M. Cohn
Department of Psychology, American University, Washington, DC, USA

Ahmed I. El-Sakka
Department of Urology, Suez Canal University, Ismailia, Egypt

Sallie M. Foley
Graduate School & Social Work, University of Michigan, Ann Arbor, MI, USA

Katerina A. Furman
Department of Psychology, University of California Berkeley, Berkeley, CA, USA

Dania Gambini
Department of Gynecology and Obstetrics, San Raffaele Hospital Milan, Milan, Italy

Irene María López García
Department of Obstetrics and Gynecology, University of Granada (Spain), Granada, Spain

Alessandra Graziottin
Gynecology and Medical Sexology, H. San Raffaele Resnati, Milano, Italy

Jared Matt Greenberg
Desert Pacific Mental Illness Research, Education, and Clinical Center, VA Greater Los Angeles Healthcare System and University of California, Los Angeles, Los Angeles, CA, USA

Tamara Grisales
Department of Obstetrics and Gynecology, University of California Los Angeles, Los Angeles, CA, USA

Nicolás Mendoza Ladrón de Guevara
Department of Obstetrics and Gynecology, University of Granada (Spain), Granada, Spain

Marika Hess
Spinal Cord Injury Medicine, VA Boston Healthcare System, West Roxbury, MA, USA

Trisha A. Hicks
Magee Rehablilitation Hospital, Philadelphia, PA, USA

Sigmund Hough
Department of Spinal Cord Injury Service, VA Boston Healthcare System/Harvard Medical School, West Roxbury, MA, USA

Waguih William IsHak
Cedars-Sinai Department of Psychiatry and Behavioral Neurosciences, Cedars-Sinai Medical Center, Los Angeles, CA, USA; David Geffen School of Medicine at University of California Los Angeles (UCLA), Los Angeles, CA, USA

Ezzat A. Ismail
Department of Urology, Suez Canal University, Ismailia, Egypt

Adriana Janicic
Department of Psychology, Pepperdine University, Los Angeles, CA, USA

Tae Y. Kim
Western University of Health Sciences, Pomona, CA, USA

Anna Klimowicz
Western University of Health Sciences, Pomona, CA, USA

Roy J. Levin
Independent Research Investigator, Sheffield, Yorkshire, England

Ronald William Lewis
Department of Surgery/Urology, Medical College of Georgia
at Augusta University, Augusta, GA, USA

Kurt K. Loewit
Klinik für Medizinische Psychologie und Psychotherapie, Arbeitsgruppe Sexualmedizin, Innsbruck, Austria

Erica Marchand
Center for Cancer Prevention and Control Research/Department
of Hematology and Oncology, UCLA, Los Angeles, CA, USA

Salome Masghati
Department of Obstetrics and Gynecology, White Memorial Hospital, Los Angeles, CA, USA

Barry McCarthy
American University, Washington, DC, USA

Cindy M. Meston
Department of Psychology, The University of Texas at Austin, Austin, TX, USA

Asbasia A. Mikhail
Department of Emergency Medicine, Huntington Memorial Hospital, Pasadena, CA, USA

Lancer Naghdechi
Western University of Health Sciences, Pomona, CA, USA

Prem K. Pahwa
Department Counseling, DePaul University, Chicago, IL, USA

Thomas Parisi
Western University of Health Sciences, Pomona, CA, USA

Robert N. Pechnick
Department of Pharmacology, Western University of Health Sciences, Pomona, CA, USA

Maria Manuela Peixoto
Psychotherapy and Psychopathology Research Unit from Research Center
on Psychology (CIPsi), School of Psychology, University of Minho, Braga, Portugal

Demetria Pizano
Department of Psychiatry and Behavioral Neurosciences, Cedars-Sinai Medical Center, Los Angeles, CA, USA

Lucy Postolov
Cedars-Sinai Medical Center, Los Angeles, CA, USA

Andrea Rapkin
Department of Obstetrics and Gynecology, University of California Los Angeles (UCLA), Los Angeles, CA, USA

Margaret Redelman
The Male Clinic, Woolloomooloo, NSW, Australia

David L. Rowland
Department of Psychology, Valparaiso University, Valparaiso, IN, USA

Ernst R. Schwarz
Heart Institute, Southern California Hospital, Culver City, CA, USA

Ege Can Serefoglu
Department of Urology, Bagcilar Training & Research Hospital, Bagcilar, Istanbul, Turkey

Kyle P. Smith
Semel Institute for Neuroscience and Human Behavior, University of California Los Angeles, Los Angeles, CA, USA

Amelia M. Stanton
Department of Psychology, The University of Texas at Austin, Austin, TX, USA

Alexander Joseph Steiner
Department of Psychiatry and Behavioral Neurosciences, Cedars-Sinai Medical Center, Los Angeles, CA, USA

Gabriel Tobia
Department of Psychiatry and Behavioral Neurosciences, Wayne State University, Detroit, MI, USA

Ana Virgolino
Instituto de Medicina Preventiva e Saúde Preventiva, Faculdade de Medicina, Universidade de Lisboa, Lisboa, Portugal

Marcel D. Waldinger
Department of Pharmacology and Physiology, Drexel University College of Medicine, Philadelphia, PA, USA;
Private practice in Psychiatry and Neurosexology, Amstelveen, The Netherlands

About the Editor

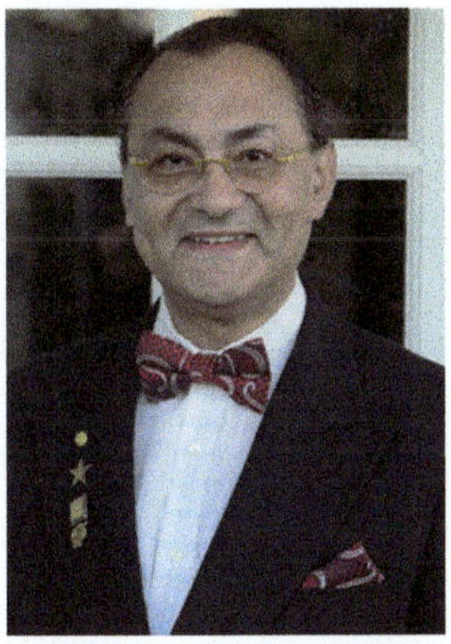

Waguih William IsHak has nearly 30 years of experience in psychiatry, psychotherapy, and psychopharmacology, with specific training and expertise in sexual medicine and outcome measurement in psychiatric disorders particularly depressive symptom severity, functioning, and quality of life. He is researching innovative ways to measure and improve the detection and treatment of depression in people seeking medical care, as a way to restore/maintain health in the population at large in order to remove behavioral barriers to wellness. Dr. IsHak has lectured and published on quality of life as a critical outcome measure of healthcare interventions, mood disorders especially depression, sexual medicine, and outcome measurement in psychiatry as well as computer applications in psychiatry. He was also the author and designer of Health Education Programs for the Public, including the Online Depression Screening Test (ODST), Online Screening for Anxiety (OSA), and Online Screening Tests for Sexual Disorders. He has edited and authored four books: this volume, the *Guidebook of Sexual Medicine* (A&W Publishing, 2008), *Outcome Measurement in Psychiatry: A Critical Review* (APPI, 2002), and *On Call Psychiatry* (WB Saunders, 2001). His articles have appeared in many prestigious journals, such as *JAMA Psychiatry*, *Journal of Clinical Psychiatry*, *Harvard Review of Psychiatry*, *Journal of Affective Disorders*, *Journal of Sexual Medicine*, *Journal of Graduate Medical Education*, and *Quality of Life Research*. He is a member of several professional societies, including the American Psychiatric Association, the American Association of Directors of Psychiatry Residency Training, and the International Society of Sexual Medicine. Dr. IsHak was awarded the 2002 and 2010 Golden Apple Teaching Award, Department of Psychiatry, Cedars-Sinai Medical Center; 2007 Outstanding Medical Student Teaching Award, Department of Psychiatry and Biobehavioral Science at UCLA; 2011 Excellence in Education Award, David Geffen School of Medicine at UCLA; 2012 Parker J. Palmer Courage to Teach Award, Accreditation Council for Graduate Medical Education; and 2012 Nancy Roeske Award for Excellence in Medical Student Education, American Psychiatric Association, and was elected to the Gold Humanism Honor Society in 2012. Dr. IsHak served as a Chief proctor and examiner for the American Board of Psychiatry and Neurology, Clinical professor of psychiatry at the David Geffen School of Medicine at UCLA Department of Psychiatry and Biobehavioral Sciences, and Distinguished fellow of the American Psychiatric Association.

Part I
Clinical Approaches in Sexual Medicine

1
Introduction to Sexual Medicine

Katerina A. Furman, Bret Becker, and Waguih William IsHak

Introduction

Kolodny, Masters, and Johnson coined the term sexual medicine in their well-known *Textbook of Sexual Medicine* [1]. Sexual medicine is the branch of medicine that focuses on the evaluation and treatment of sexual disorders, which have a high prevalence rate. Approximately 43% of women and 31% of men are affected by these disorders [2]. Today the field of sexual medicine continues to evolve. There have been recent changes in classification of disorders, advancements in pharmaceutical management, and improvement in behavioral therapies. This introductory chapter provides a concise review of relevant topics to sexual medicine including recent classification changes in the International Classification of Diseases, 10th edition (ICD-10) and Diagnostic and Statistical Manual of Mental Disorders 5th edition (DSM-5).

Milestones in Sexual Medicine

The ancient Egyptians illustrated sexual scenes in tomb carvings/painting, papyrus, and sculptures (Figure 1.1). The Turin Erotic Papyrus dating back to 1105BC depicted at least 12 sex positions (Figure 1.2).

One of the first sex manuals in history is the Kama Sutra, written in India, in second century BC. Techniques of sexual pleasure enhancement including positions are fully explained including the spiritual aspects. Some of the positions were carved inside the Mukteswar Temple in Bhubaneswar, India (Figure 1.3).

In 1896, Havelock Ellis, an English physician (Figure 1.4), published "Studies in the Psychology of Sex," discussing normal and abnormal sexuality. Around the same time, in 1898, Richard von Krafft-Ebing, a German psychiatrist (Figure 1.5), published in Latin a book called "Psychopathia Sexualis" (Figure 1.6), which is the first modern text on sexual disorders including the paraphilias. By 1918, Sigmund Freud (Figure 1.7), the founder of psychoanalysis, considered sexuality central to his psychoanalytic theory.

Early in the twentieth century, German physician Magnus Hirschfeld (Figure 1.8) founded the first sex-research institute in Germany. He conducted the first large-scale sex survey, collecting data from 10,000 men and women. He also initiated the first journal for publishing the results of sex studies. The Nazis destroyed most of his materials during World War II. In the early 1930s, American anthropologist Margaret Mead and British anthropologist Bronislav Malinowsky began studying sexual behavior in different cultures [3].

In the USA, Alfred Kinsey (Figure 1.9) published a survey of 18,000 subjects regarding sexual behaviors in 1947. William Masters and Virginia Johnson followed this survey with rigorous lab study of sexual encounters. Masters and Johnson developed key concepts in sexual medicine such the sexual response cycle, and developed an effective treatment technique for sexual dysfunction named sex therapy. Helen Singer Kaplan followed with a major expansion on training sex therapists, including desire in the sexual response cycle, and examining premature ejaculation from psychological as well as behavioral angles.

In 1981, Ronald Virag (Figure 1.10) discovered during a surgical procedure on the penis that papaverine caused an erection when injected into the penis. In 1983, Giles Brindley (Figure 1.11) gave his notorious AUA Lecture in Las Vegas when he had previously injected himself with a vasodilator, identified as phentolamine in some accounts and papaverine in others. The self-injection became later one of the most reliable interventions to produce an erection.

The National Health and Social Life Survey (NHSLS), also known as the Chicago Study or Chicago Survey, is a landmark epidemiological study of sexual function and dysfunction examining randomly selected 3432 subjects who underwent face-to-face surveys. This well-designed survey revealed that about 43% of women and 31% of men suffer from sexual dysfunction.

W.W. IsHak (ed.), *The Textbook of Clinical Sexual Medicine*, DOI 10.1007/978-3-319-52539-6_1

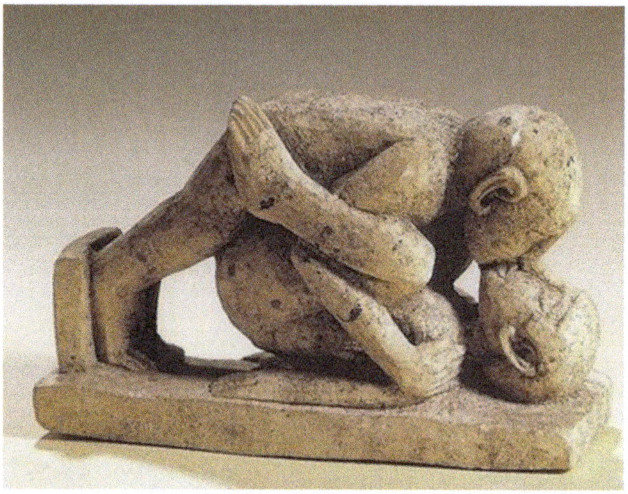

FIGURE 1-1. Small sculpture of a sexual scene [Reprinted from: https://commons.wikimedia.org/wiki/Category:Ancient_Egyptian_erotic_art#/media/File:Egypt-sex.jpg with permission from Creative Commons].

The most significant breakthrough was the identification of nitric oxide as the principal neurotransmitter responsible for the relaxation of the corpus cavernosum smooth muscle, by Louis Ignarro, Ph.D. in 1997, as a result of 2 decades of research. This discovery enabled the development of oral pharmacological agents for the treatment of erectile dysfunction. Dr. Ignarro (Figure 1.12) was awarded the Nobel Prize for this momentous discovery in 1998 [4].

The late 1990s brought more focus on women's sexual health, largely due to the efforts of Jennifer and Laura Berman, who were originally mentored by Irwin Goldstein at Boston University [5]. Rosemary Basson introduced the circular model of the sexual response cycle in women where arousal could overlap with desire. The current state of the field is an exciting one, with a plethora of biochemical and physical interventions, in addition to well-tested and effective psychosocial ones.

Classifications of Sexual Dysfunctions

There are several major classification systems of both male and female sexual dysfunction. One of the most common classifications is in the ICD-10: The International Classification of Diseases, 10th edition, which was published by the World Health Organization in 1992. The ICD-11 is expected to be published in 2017. The ICD codes disorders as either organic (physiologic) or non-organic (psychosomatic). Non-organic disorders may be intermittent and occur on a case-by-case basis. For example, a male who complains of erectile dysfunction (ED) but has a normal morning erection has a non-organic rather than organic cause of ED since there is no physiologic dysfunction. Non-organic disorders are those such as sexual aversion, sexual desire disorder, non-organic vaginismus, non-organic dyspareunia, and excessive sexual drive. Organic disorders have a physiological/somatic basis and include ED, vaginismus, and dyspareunia.

Another widely known system of classification for sexual dysfunction is the DSM-5: The Diagnostic and Statistical Manual of Mental Disorders (5th edition). The DSM has been widely used by the American Psychiatric Association to classify sexual disorders as well as other types of psychological conditions. The most recent edition has been published in May 2013 and contains several important changes including the criterion that nearly all sexual dysfunction diagnoses now require a minimum duration of 6 months as well as a frequency of 75–100% of the time. Additionally, many disorders are now listed as gender specific, and several of the female disorders are consolidated into single diagnoses. Additionally, a new group of criteria called "associated features" is introduced, dividing potential contributing factors of sexual dysfunction into five categories: (1) partner factors, (2) relationship factors, (3) individual vulnerability factors, (4) cultural factors, and (5) medical factors. Several disorders are deleted from the DSM such as male dyspareunia or sexual aversion disorder. Duration and frequency requirements are implemented to increase the validity and clinical usefulness of the manual to the psychiatric community [6].

Women and Sexual Medicine

In women, the most common cause of sexual dysfunction is vaginal dryness or failure of lubrication. Approximately 8–28% of sexually active women report lubrication difficulties, which can be attributed to pathologic/organic causes, psychogenic/non-organic causes, or estrogen deficiency [8].

Women's sexual function is a complex neuromuscular process. Along with hormonal changes, arousal is marked by blood volume and pressure changes in the clitoris and labia (Figures. 1.13 and 1.14). Irregularities in various psychological, hormonal, physiological, and environmental factors can account for female sexual dysfunction in a number of ways. Female sexual dysfunction can be characterized by sexual pain disorders, desire/arousal disorders, and orgasmic disorders [9].

The DSM-5 has eliminated and condensed the diagnoses of female sexual dysfunction from five disorders of desire, arousal, orgasm, vaginismus, and dyspareunia to three disorders [10]. Female hypoactive desire disorder is combined with arousal disorder to form female sexual interest/arousal disorder. This diagnosis is even less contingent upon physical stimuli and is characterized by persistent deficiency of sexual thoughts or desire for sexual activity [6]. Orgasmic disorder has remained unchanged. Vaginismus and dyspareunia are merged into genito-pelvic pain/penetration

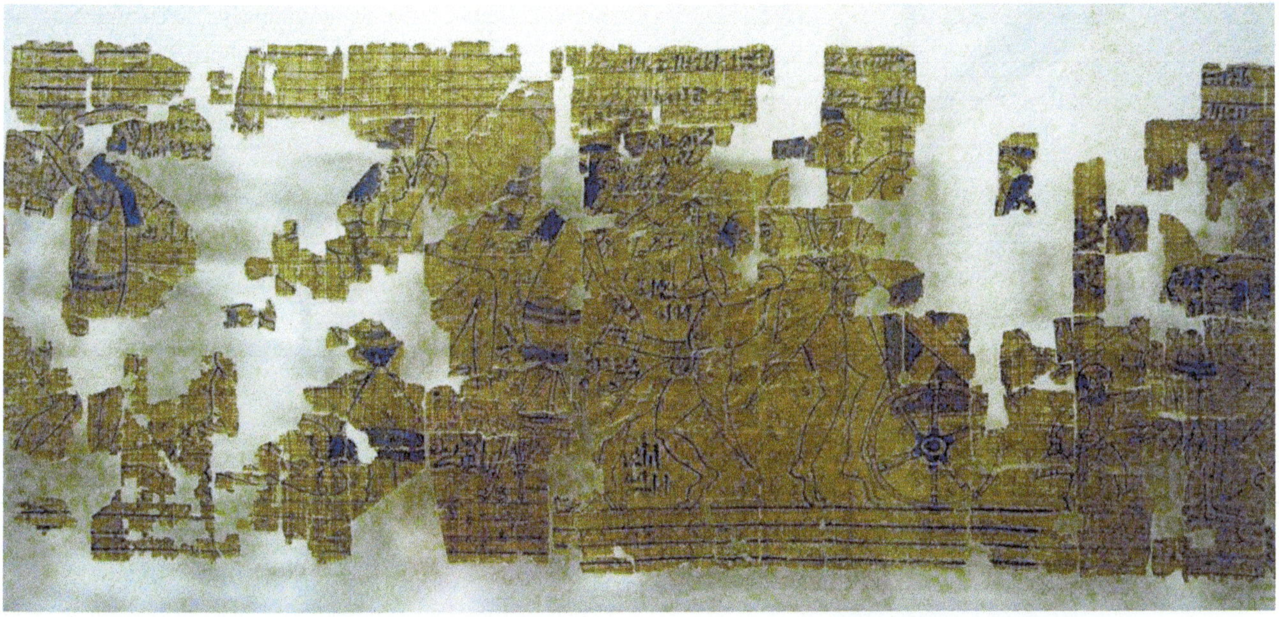

FIGURE 1-2. Turin erotic papyrus (damaged) [Reprinted from: https://commons.wikimedia.org/wiki/File:Turin_Erotic_Papyrus.jpg].

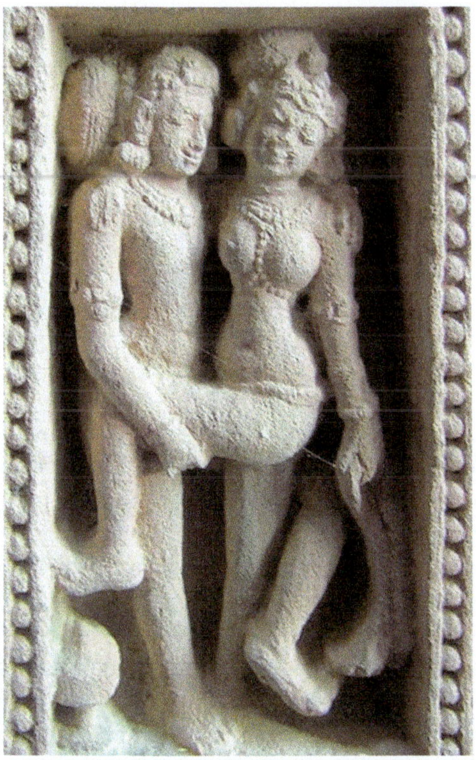

FIGURE 1-3. Kama Sutra [Reprinted from: https://commons.wikimedia.org/wiki/File:Mukteswar_temple.jpg with permission from Creative Commons].

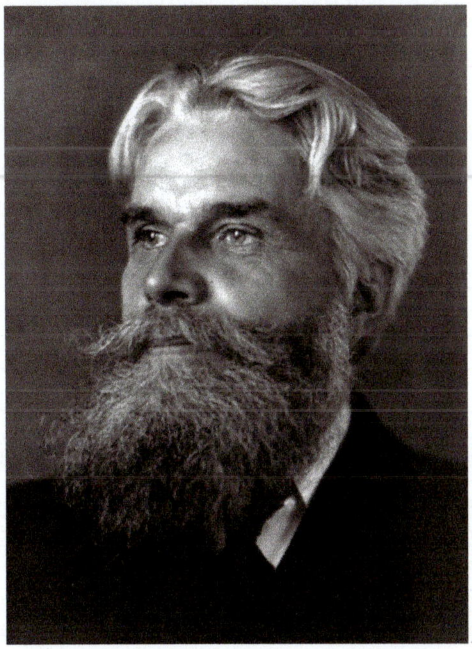

FIGURE 1-4. Havelock Ellis [Reprinted from: https://commons.wikimedia.org/wiki/File:Havelock_Ellis_cph.3b08675.jpg].

disorder, as it has been decided that the two disorders could not be reliably differentiated due to the lack of empirical evidence of vaginal muscle spasm and the overlap of fear of penetration [6].

There is epidemiological data indicating that 40–45% of women have at least one form of sexual dysfunction. The prevalence of women expressing low levels of sexual interest increases with age, with about 10% of women up to age 49, 22% of those ages 50–65, and 74% of 66–74 year olds expressing low levels of desire [11].

Such dysfunctions may be a lifelong problem or acquired later in life. Risk factors for decreased lubricative function,

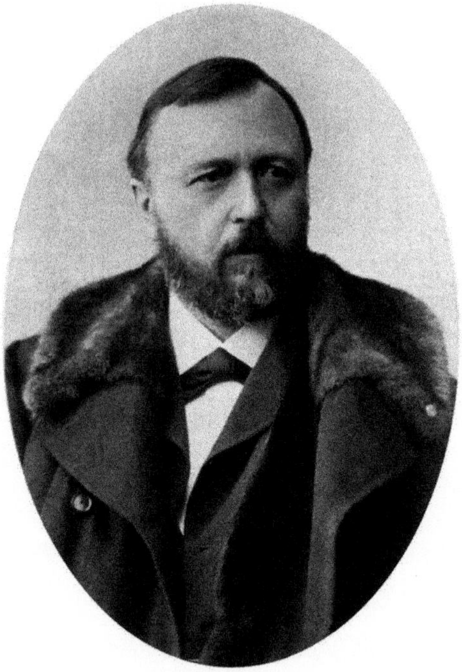

FIGURE 1-5. Richard von Krafft-Ebing [Reprinted from: https://en.wikipedia.org/wiki/Richard_von_Krafft-Ebing#/media/File:Richard_v._Krafft-Ebing.jpg].

anorgasmia, and other sexual disorders include but are not limited to age, sociocultural factors, alcohol use, prescription and non-prescription drug usage. Other factors that increase the risk of sexual dysfunction include medical conditions such as hypertension, certain hormone imbalances, urinary incontinence, cardiovascular disease, diabetes mellitus, and depression [11].

Female sexual interest/arousal disorder is described as significantly reduced interest in sexual activity, reduced or absent erotic thoughts, or reduced initiation or receptivity to sexual activity. As many as 75–100% of these women may experience diminished pleasure during sexual encounters, absent/reduced sexual arousal in response to internal or external cues, and reduced genital sensations during 75–100% of sexual encounters. Different cases have reported various duration of symptoms. Older women generally report less distress about low sexual desire than younger women, as sexual desire also decreases with age [11].

Female orgasmic disorder constitutes a marked delay, infrequency, or absence of orgasm, or it can be defined as a reduced intensity of orgasmic sensations. Orgasmic disorder must be accompanied by clinically significant distress and cannot be justified by significant interpersonal or contextual factors. Approximately 10% of women do not experience orgasm throughout their lifetime. Reported prevalence rates for female orgasmic disorder range widely from 10 to 42%, though only a small proportion of women also report associated distress [10].

Genito-pelvic pain/penetration disorder is defined as at least 6 months of persistent or recurrent difficulties with vaginal penetration; vulvovaginal or pelvic pain during intercourse attempts; fear or anxiety about vulvovaginal or pain before, during, or after vaginal penetration; or marked tensing of the pelvic floor muscles during attempted vaginal penetration. The disorder can range from complete inability to experience vaginal penetration to situational inability to experience penetration. Inadequate sexual education and/or religious rigidity have been common predisposing factors of genito-pelvic pain/penetration disorder. Many women with this diagnosis are also diagnosed with a comorbid condition such as endometriosis, pelvic inflammatory disease, lichen sclerosis, or vulvovaginal atrophy. There are no tools or diagnostic methods that can determine if the penetration disorder is primary or secondary [10]. However, comorbidity with other diagnoses is high, as well as with relationship distress. Often amending factors within the relationship such as increasing foreplay or addressing sexual dysfunction of a male partner may ameliorate a women's fear of and pain during penetration [10].

Men and Sexual Medicine

The penis, the primary organ responsible for male sexual function and reproduction, is composed of two functional compartments: the corpus cavernosum and the corpus spongiosum (Figures 1.15 and 1.16).

It is innervated by somatic and autonomic nerve fibers that provide the penis with sensory fibers and supply the perineal skeletal muscles with motor fibers. This autonomic innervation is both parasympathetic and sympathetic.

Norepinephrine is responsible for the regulation of the corpus cavernosum smooth muscle tone via the alpha-1 and alpha-2 adrenergic receptors. Other substances involved with the smooth muscle tone of the corpus cavernosum include endothelin-1, PGF-2a, thromboxane A-2, angiotensin II, and calcium [12]. The penis functions as part of the peripheral nervous system and is constantly modulated by sex steroid hormones as well as gonadal, adrenal, and neuroactive steroids that regulate the epithelium and vasculature.

Nitric oxide is believed to be the main vasoactive non-noradrenergic, non-cholinergic (NANC) neurotransmitter of erectile action. Penile nitric oxide synthase is fundamental to the cellular signaling of vascular tone in the corpus cavernosum, which is necessary to obtain an erection. NOS protein content showed a 55% decrease in castrated animals, proving its vital role in the physiological response to male sexual arousal and function [13].

Louis Ignarro's identification in 1997 of nitric oxide as the principal neurotransmitter responsible for the action of the smooth muscles of the corpus cavernosum enabled the development of oral pharmacological agents for erectile

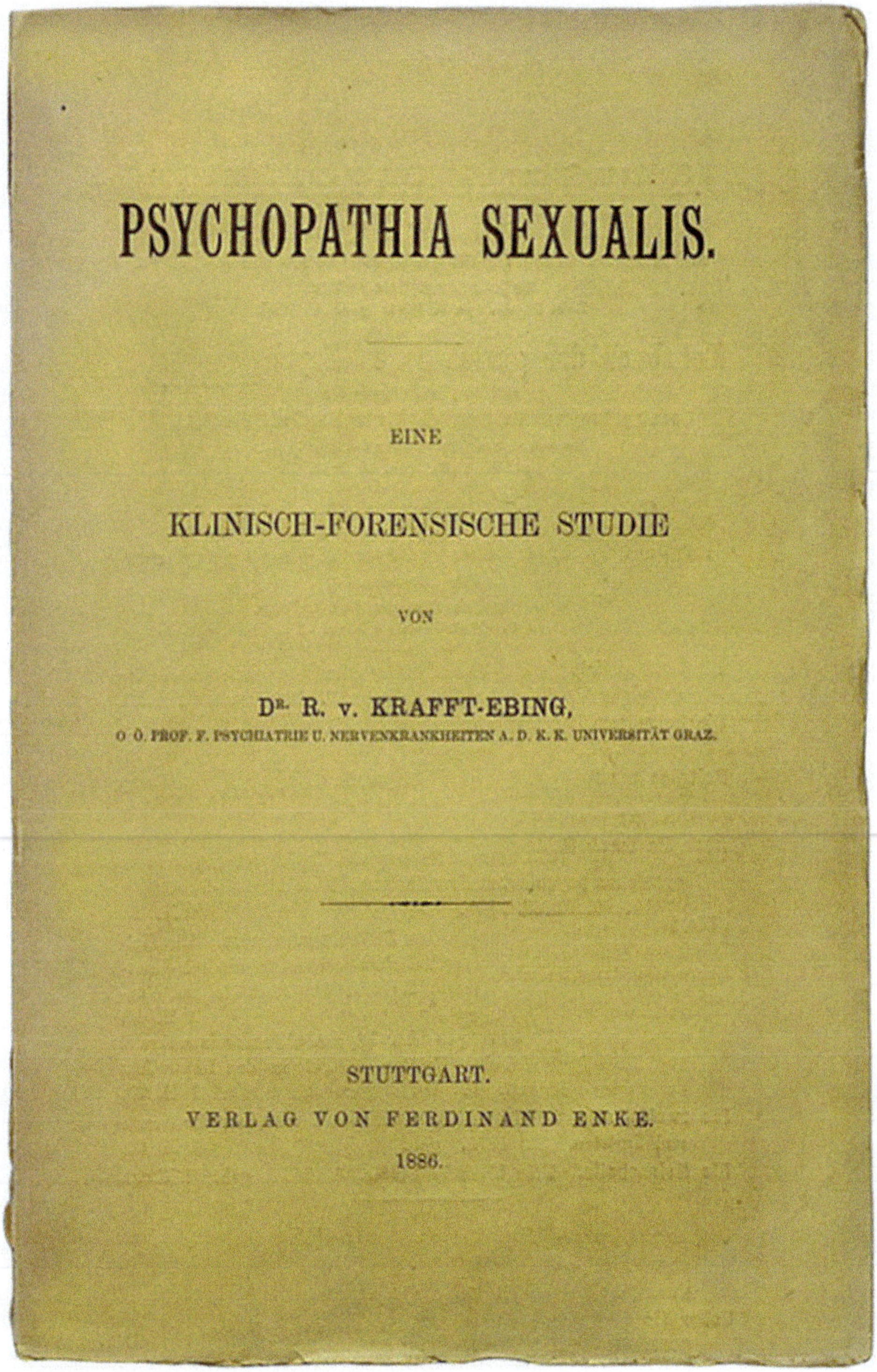

FIGURE 1-6. Krafft-Ebing's book [Reprinted from: https://en.wikipedia.org/wiki/Richard_von_Krafft-Ebing#/media/File:Krafft-Ebing_Psychopathia_sexualis_1886.jpg with permission from © Foto H.-P. Haack (H.-P. Haack)].

dysfunction [14]. Sildenafil (Viagra) was the accidental result of an experiment to find a treatment that would lower blood pressure in patients with angina in 1996. In 2008, sales of sildenafil had reached 1.5 billion dollars annually, with nine pills being dispensed every second. The further development of new drugs for both male and female sexual dysfunction is currently underway.

For men, sexual dysfunction includes male hypoactive sexual desire disorder, erectile disorder, premature ejaculation, and delayed ejaculation. Epidemiological data from the

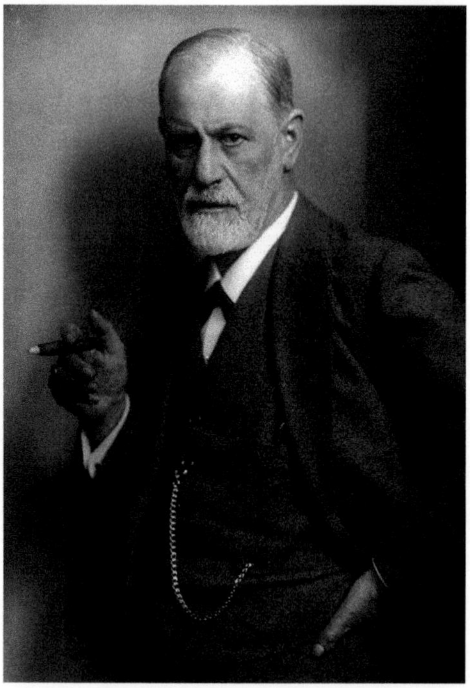

FIGURE 1-7. Sigmund Freud [Reprinted from: https://commons.wikimedia.org/wiki/File:Sigmund_Freud_LIFE.jpg].

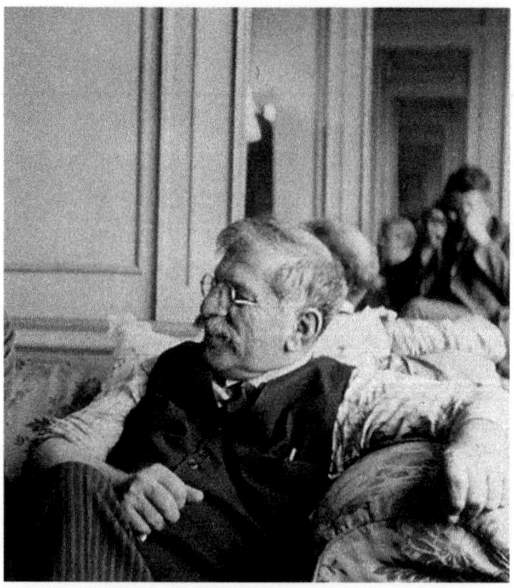

FIGURE 1-8. Magnus Hirschfeld [Reprinted from: https://wellcomeimages.org/indexplus/email/299273.html with permission from Creative Commons].

National Health and Social Life Survey indicate that 15% of all men experience low sexual desire, 31% of men between the ages of 18 and 59 years have significant sexual concerns or problems, and that one-third of men struggle with premature ejaculation [15]. According to the Florey Adelaide Male Ageing Study in Australia, 31.7% of men between the ages of 35 and 80 who were normal at baseline developed ED at a 5-year follow-up [16].

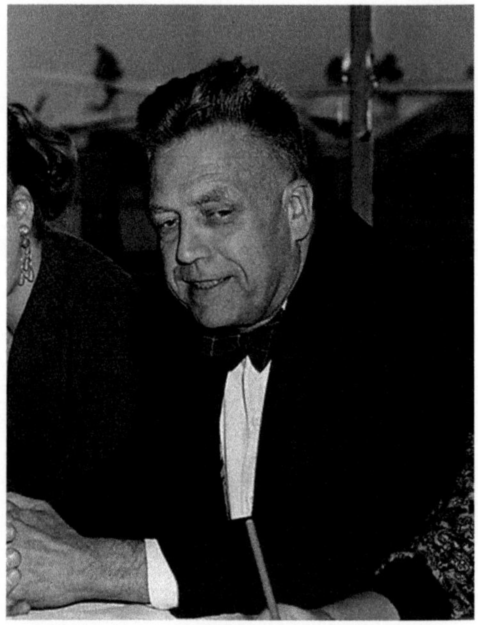

FIGURE 1-9. Alfred Kinsey [Reprinted from: https://commons.wikimedia.org/wiki/File:Alfred_Kinsey_1955.jpg].

Potential risk factors for male sexual dysfunction, primarily erectile disorder (ED), include age, obesity, metabolic syndrome, insulin-dependent diabetes mellitus, cardiovascular disease, hypertension, tobacco use, hyperprolactinemia, abnormal dehydroepiandrosterone sulfate levels, urinary tract diseases, surgery, trauma, spinal cord injury, endothelial dysfunction, other chronic diseases, as well as psychological and psychiatric factors [15].

The DSM-5 describes male hypoactive sexual desire disorder (HSDD) as persistently or recurrently deficient (or absent) sexual/erotic thoughts or fantasies and desire for sexual activity. The clinician should also take outside factors into account when diagnosing HSDD such as age, relationship status, medical record, and other sociocultural contexts of the patient's life. HSDD may be lifelong, acquired, generalized, situational, mild, moderate, or severe. Some associated features supporting the diagnosis of HSDD are erectile and/or ejaculatory concerns, as persistent difficulties with erection may cause a loss of interest in sexual activity for many men. Relationship-specific preferences should also be taken into account. For example, men are generally more likely to initiate sexual activity, though many men prefer their partner to initiate. In this case, their diagnosis would be dependent upon their lack of receptivity rather than their hesitance or failure to initiate sexual acts. Relationship status should also be taken into account in accordance with one's emotional and psychosocial attitude towards new sexual partners. The development and course of this disorder is contingent on the mere fact that the potency of sexual cues is known to decrease with age. Endocrine disorders such as

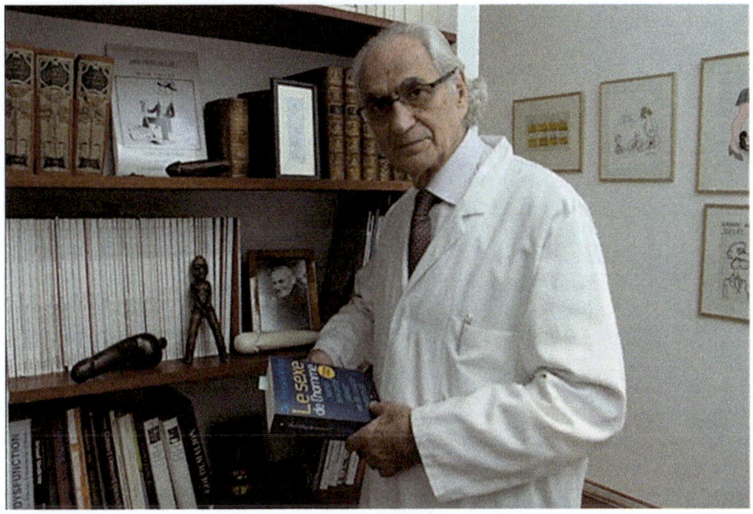

FIGURE 1-10. Ronald Virag [Reprinted from: https://commons.wikimedia.org/wiki/File:Dr._Ronald_Virag,_working.jpg with permission from Creative Commons].

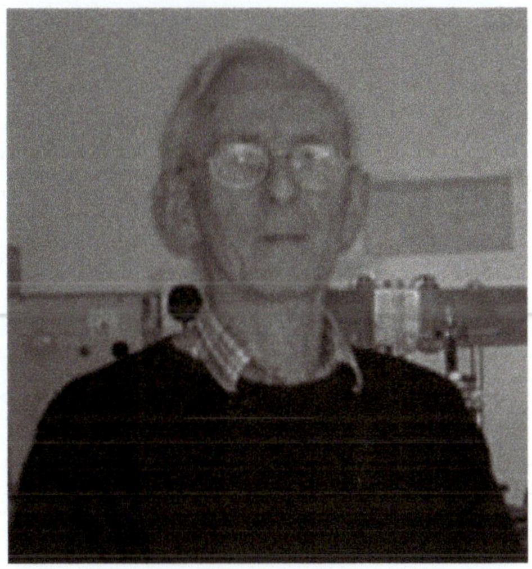

FIGURE 1-11. Giles Brindley [Reprinted from Goldstein, I.R.W.I.N., The Hour Lecture That Changed Sexual Medicine—The Giles Brindley Injection Story. Journal of Sexual Medicine 2012; 9(2): 337-342. with permission from Elsevier].

hyperprolactinemia (elevated levels of the protein prolactin) have been found to act as a significant risk factor for low levels of desire in males. Studies have also found higher prevalence of HSDD in hypogonadal men as well as a speculated critical threshold below which testosterone will affect sexual desire in men.

Erectile disorder can be defined as difficulty obtaining or maintaining an erection during sexual activity or a marked decrease in erectile rigidity. Symptoms must persist for a minimum of 6 months and, like most other disorders in the DSM, must cause clinically significant distress and not be explained by any other medical condition or substance. Many men with ED also suffer from low self-esteem and self-confidence, depressed affect, and a decreased sense of masculinity. As mentioned earlier, etiology, diagnosis, and potential treatments are dependent on the following five factors: (1) partner, (2) relationship, (3) individual vulnerability, (4) culture/religion, and (5) medical factors relevant to prognosis or treatment [10].

The DSM-5 classifies premature or early ejaculation as a persistent or recurrent pattern of ejaculation occurring during partnered sexual activity within approximately 1 min following vaginal penetration and before the individual wishes it on 75–100% of events of partnered activity. Symptoms must be present for at least 6 months and must cause clinically significant distress in the individual. The level of severity is established using the duration from vaginal penetration to ejaculation (severe = within 15 s, moderate = 15–30 s, and mild = 30–60 s).

The DSM-5 classifies delayed ejaculation as marked delay or infrequency/absence in ejaculation on 75–100% of events of partnered activity. Symptoms must be present for at

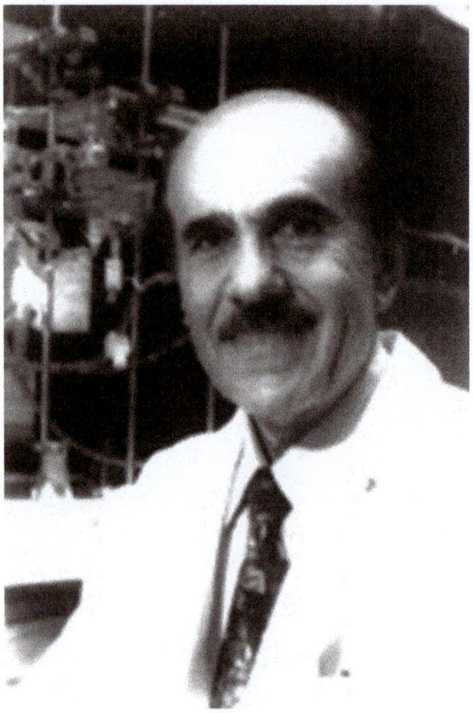

FIGURE 1-12. Louis Ignarro, Ph.D. [Reprinted from: https://sv.wikipedia.org/wiki/Fil:Louis_J._Ignarro_portrait.jpg].

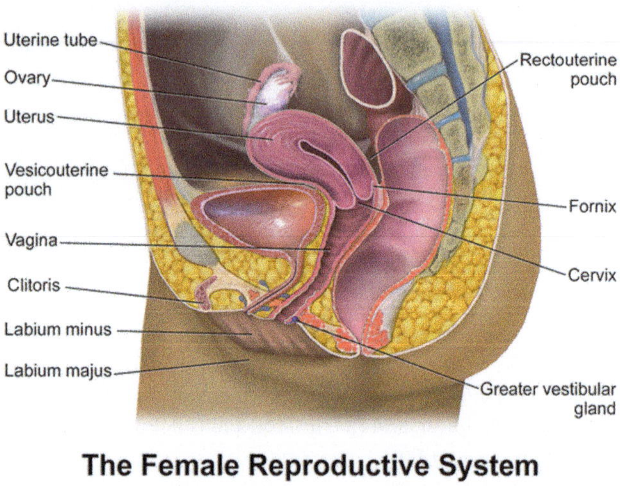

FIGURE 1-13. Female sexual and reproductive organs [Reprinted from https://commons.wikimedia.org/wiki/File:Blausen_0400_FemaleReproSystem_02.png with permission from Creative Commons].

least 6 months and must cause clinically significant distress in the individual. It is essential that the sexual dysfunction cannot be the result of a nonsexual mental disorder or other stressor or substance. Delayed ejaculation is specified as lifelong or acquired, generalized or situational, and mild or severe.

Treatments in Sexual Medicine

Treatment for sexual dysfunction may vary depending on the nature of the dysfunction, the patient, the desired outcome, and the physician. Some of the most commonly used pharmaceutical treatments are phosphodiesterase type 5 (PDE5) inhibitors. PDE5 inhibitors are primarily used to treat erectile disorder. They function by blocking the degradation of cyclic GMP in the smooth muscle cells of the blood vessels of the corpus cavernosum by cGMP-specific PDE5. Examples of common PDE5 inhibitor drugs are sildenafil (Viagra), tadalafil (Cialis), and vardenafil (Levitra).

Addressing biopsychosocial factors in behavioral therapy can also be a means of treating sexual dysfunction. Althof and Needle showed that "medical treatments are directed narrowly at a specific sexual dysfunction and fail to address the larger biopsychosocial issues" [17].

Sex therapy is a common strategy in treating sexual dysfunction. This consists of a form of psychotherapy administered by social workers, therapists, or physicians certified by the American Association of Sex Educators, Counselors and Therapists (AASECT). It is important to take into account the impact that mood disorders such as anxiety and depression can have on sexual functioning. In fact, mood and sexual disorders are often comorbid and share many of the same causes. Sex therapy has, in recent years, become an increasingly large part of treatment programs targeting sexual dysfunction. One form of treatment is an adaptation of the Masters and Johnson behavior modification style of therapy. It incorporates a masturbation desensitization program developed by LoPiccolo and Lobitz [11]. Many sex therapists suggest the use of sex toys, especially by women, in cases of sexual dysfunction in relationships. It is vital to focus mainly on the couple to improve sexual functioning and subsequent quality of life [14].

The Permission, Limited Information, Specific Suggestions, and Intensive Therapy (PLISSIT) model of sex therapy was introduced by American Psychologist Jack Annon in 1976. It provides a framework for therapists to intervene and treat patients for sexual dysfunction. Often times sexual problems are caused or worsened by guilt or anxiety about one's actions. This first step of the model merely gives the patient professional permission to do what he/she is doing (e.g., masturbation) in order to alleviate this unnecessary anguish. LI stands for limited information and means ensuring patients have sufficient anatomical and physiological information and expectations of themselves. The next step is SS, or specific suggestions, and includes many of the exercises of mutual pleasuring recommended by Masters and Johnson such as sensate focus and stop start. IT is the last step and is intensive therapy. It requires a long-term intervention to address complex underlying issues on an individual as well as partner level. [18]

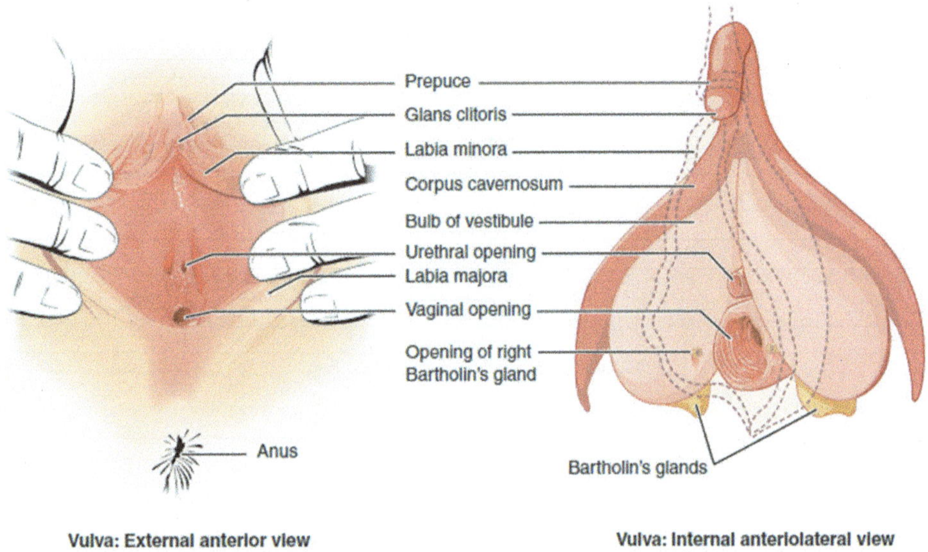

FIGURE 1-14. External female sexual organs [Reprinted from: https://commons.wikimedia.org/wiki/File:Figure_28_02_02.jpg with permission from Creative Commons].

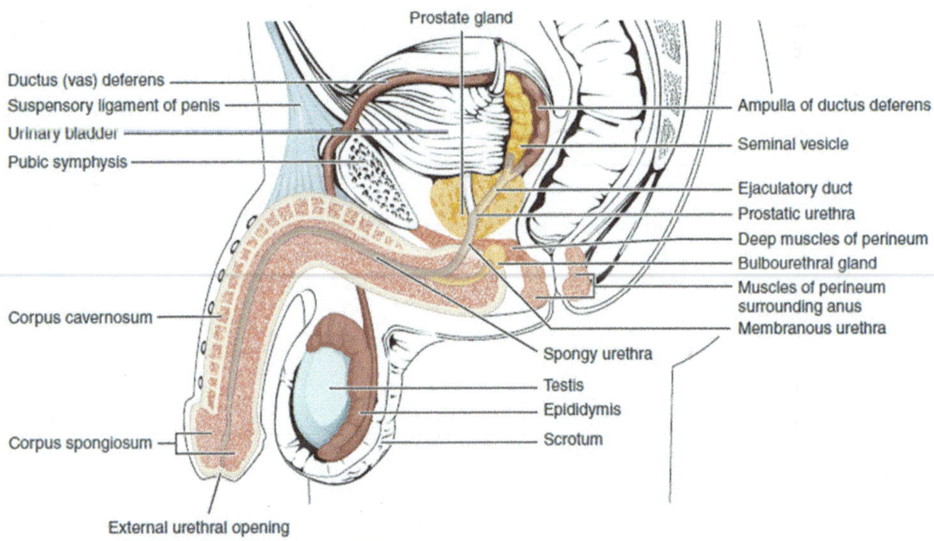

FIGURE 1-15. Male sexual and reproductive organs [Reprinted from: https://commons.wikimedia.org/wiki/File:Penis_lateral_cross_section.jpg with permission from Creative Commons].

The question remains unanswered as to what constitutes success for sex therapy as it is a lengthy process and outcomes vary on a case-by-case basis. Treatment can be extensive and must take into account the needs, flaws, and limitations of a sexual partner. A key step in treatment is the realization of "good-enough sex," or sex that realistically acknowledges that performance is variable and is vulnerable to both one's own and partner's current emotional and physical state [19]. Sex therapy is not focused on the frequency of sexual contact or changes in ejaculatory latency or coital orgasms, but rather emphasizes the patient's own report of enhanced sexual confidence, pleasure, or intimacy [19]. It is impossible to separate mind from body and it is paramount to recognize in treating sexual dysfunctions that these problems are most often a combination of physical and psychological factors. Therefore we must acknowledge that treatment should integrate a fusion of psychological, interpersonal, and pharmacological interventions [20].

Treatment specifically geared towards female sexual dysfunction has included hormone therapies, such as estrogen therapy, androgen therapy, flibanserin (Addyi), and oxytocin. Potential treatments that are currently being investigated are a synthetic steroid called Tibolone, phosphodiesterase inhibitors, and sildenafil (Viagra) [21]. It is important to note that flibanserin aims to treat a problem that exists on a continuum, therefore making it difficult to establish a clear-cut diagnosis. For many people who consider themselves asexual, absence of or diminished desire is considered a sexual orientation rather than a dysfunction. In addition, female sexual dysfunction is much less inconspicuous than male dysfunction, where the absence of arousal or orgasm is physically observable. The female sexual response

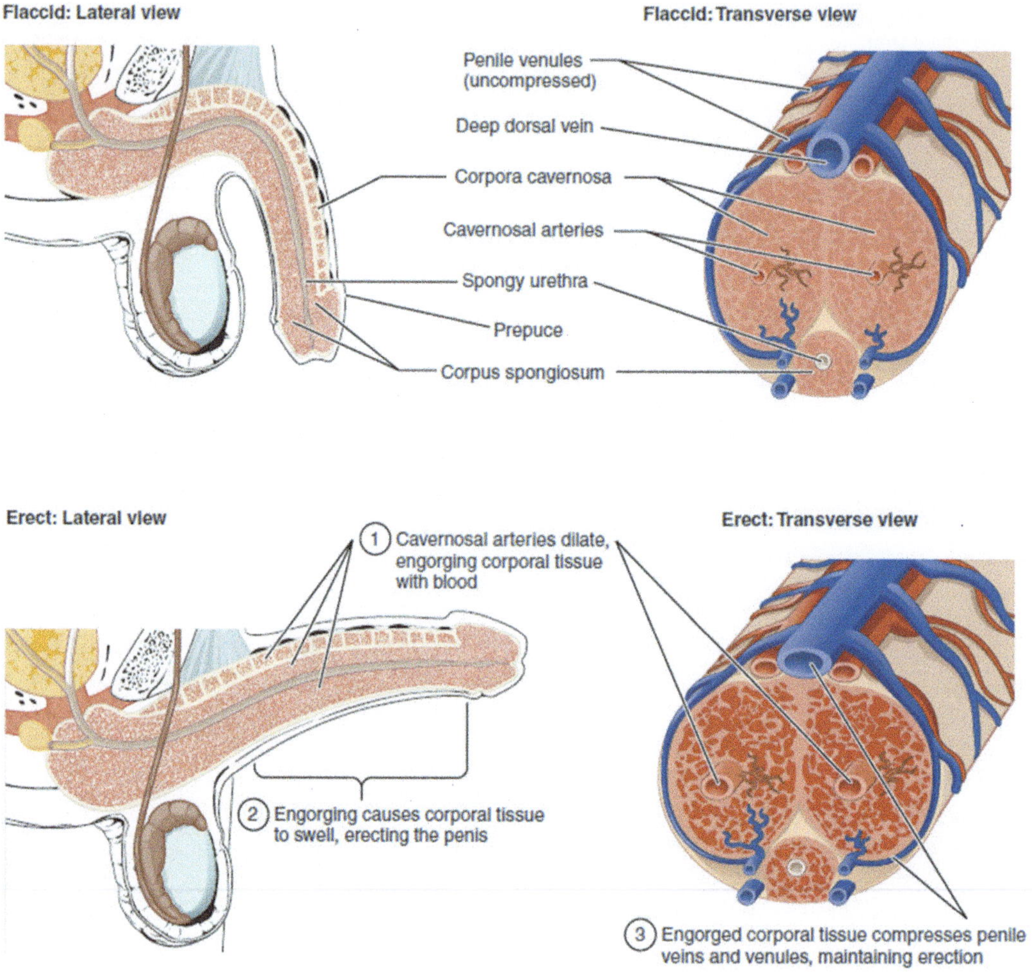

FIGURE 1-16. Penis, lateral view and cross section before and during erection [Reprinted from: https://pl.wikipedia.org/wiki/Zaburzenia_erekcji#/media/File:Figure_28_01_06.jpg. With permission from Creative Commons].

is not only more hidden but also more elusive and even taboo [22].

Estrogen and androgen hormonal therapy were both observed to have benefits on sexual function in females. One-fourth of menopausal women reported vulvovaginal atrophy and dyspareunia, symptoms which often lead to pain and decreased sexual interest, arousal, response. This then frequently leads to avoidance of sexual encounters [22]. The synthesis of estrogen within extragonadal compartments takes place during one's reproductive life as well as after menopause. Androgens are fundamental precursors in the biosynthesis of estrogens. Estrone sulfate is the most abundant estrogen in circulation in postmenopausal women at 10–24 times higher levels than estrone or estradiol. Estrone and estradiol are partly bound to sex hormone-binding globulin (SHBG) in their non-sulfate forms. Transdermal and oral estrogens increase sex hormone-binding globulin (SHBG) levels, and oral estrogen can lead to a clinically significant decrease in non-SHBG-bound sex steroids. Estradiol is most concentrated in the female brain in the hypothalamus and preoptic regions [23].

Topical estrogen therapy was reported by Santoro et al. to improve sexual function significantly in postmenopausal women with what was referred to by the DSM-IV as vulvovaginal atrophy (VVA) and dyspareunia. The topical treatment comes in various forms including creams, tablets, and rings. Vaginal topical estrogen treatment has been shown to improve vaginal lubrication and decrease dyspareunia [23].

Testosterone has also been demonstrated to have a role in treating sexual dysfunction in women. A testosterone patch has become a common treatment of hypoactive sexual desire disorder in surgically menopausal women with the intent to enhance female sexual motivation [23].

Oxytocin has been found in a large number of studies to have a positive impact on both the female and male sexual experience. Oxytocin is secreted by the pituitary gland during intimate physical contact, orgasm, and childbirth. It has been found to foster trust, cooperation, and openness, both in romantic relationships as well as in friendship and business. Oxytocin levels generally increase during arousal and peak during orgasm for both men and women. After an initial report of successful use of oxytocin in male anorgasmia, a 2014 study reported that oxytocin increased the intensity of orgasm and contentment after sexual intercourse [24]. The study administered intranasal oxytocin to 29 healthy heterosexual couples. Researchers then studied the acute effects on their sexual drive, arousal, orgasm, and refractory aspects of sexual behavior along with partner interactions. Biomarkers such as cortisol, alpha-amylase, and heart rate were monitored. Findings showed that while these effects were more pronounced in men, women also benefited from intranasal oxytocin doses. Women in the study reported feeling more relaxed in the context of their sexual experiences as well as an improved ability to share sexual desires or empathize with their partners. Intranasal oxytocin did not alter classical patterns of sexual function, but it did improve orgasmic and post-orgasmic sensation as well as partner interaction [25].

Several studies reveal that erection and orgasm in male rats are controlled by oxytocin as well as dopamine. For example, a study by Succu et al. shows that stimulation of dopamine receptors in the paraventricular nucleus of the hypothalamus of male rats induces penile erection and increases extracellular dopamine in the nucleus accumbens. More research is needed on effects of oxytocin and dopamine on female sexual function [26].

The FDA approved flibanserin (Addyi) in August 2015 to treat low sexual desire in premenopausal women. Flibanserin, colloquially known as the "female Viagra," is designed to treat female hypoactive sexual desire disorder. However, the two medications do not share a mechanism of action. While Viagra (sildenafil) acts by dilating blood vessels to increase blood flow, flibanserin raises levels of dopamine and norepinephrine while lowering levels of serotonin. This mechanism is thought to work because dopamine and norepinephrine are neurotransmitters involved with sexual excitement, but serotonin may contribute to sexual inhibition if these chemicals are out of balance. Flibanserin is generally prescribed to be taken once daily and the cost ranges anywhere from $400 to $800 per month [27].

Tibolone is a synthetic steroid used in Europe and Australia for treatment of postmenopausal osteoporosis. It mimics the activity of female sex hormones estrogen and progesterone and prevents dryness and soreness of the vaginal tissue. It has therefore been used to treat hypoactive sexual desire in menopausal women in other countries, but it is not approved by the FDA for use in the USA due to concerns of increased breast cancer risk [28].

Phosphodiesterase inhibitors are generally used to treat erectile disorder. These medications function by blocking the breakdown of cyclic guanosine monophosphate (cGMP) which results in vasodilation and prolongation of the mediators of blood flow such as nitric oxide. This means increased dilation of the veins, which allows for increased blood flow to the penis to obtain an erection. Phosphodiesterase inhibitors have been shown to elicit minor improvements in women with sexual dysfunction, though evidence is not strong enough to make generalized statements. PDE (phosphodiesterase) isoenzymes 4 (cAMP-PDE) and 5 (cGMP-PDE) were found in the human vagina. In addition, signals related to PDE10 and PDE11 were found in the epithelium and glandular-like structures [29]. Results indicated that PDE inhibitors could relax human vaginal tissue of the labia minora and increase levels of cGMP. This means that the pharmacological concept of PDE inhibition could be applicable to the treatment of symptoms of female sexual arousal disorder. PDE inhibitors have been used to treat erectile disorder since 1989, but the presence of cAMP-PDE type 4 and cGMP-PDE type 5 in vascular and nonvascular smooth muscle of the vaginal wall supports the hypothesis that the use of iso-enzyme-selective PDE inhibitors can lead to vaginal smooth muscle relaxation, thus improving hypoarousal. These findings also suggest a connection between the NO-cGMP pathway and control of the vaginal smooth muscle tone [30]. Ultimately this means that in addition to treating male erectile disorder, urinary incontinence, and lower urinary tract pathology, PDE-5 inhibitors may be a pharmacological treatment option for female arousal and orgasm disorders [27].

Sexual medicine is evolving, expanding, and advancing with recent strides in pharmacology, psychology, and relationship counseling. Recent changes in classification are changing the way we conceptualize and define sexual dysfunction. Combined with pharmaceutical advances, the available options for the management and treatment of sexual dysfunction continue to increase for both men and women. Evaluation of sexual dysfunction, however, begins with the understanding that the causes may be multifactorial (Figure 1.17). The biopsychosocial model ensures a comprehensive assessment of multiple factors (psychosocial, medical, and the effect of substances) (Figure 1.18) that can affect sexual functioning, so that the individual and/or the couple can benefit from different types of interventions, whether they are biological, psychosocial, or both [31].

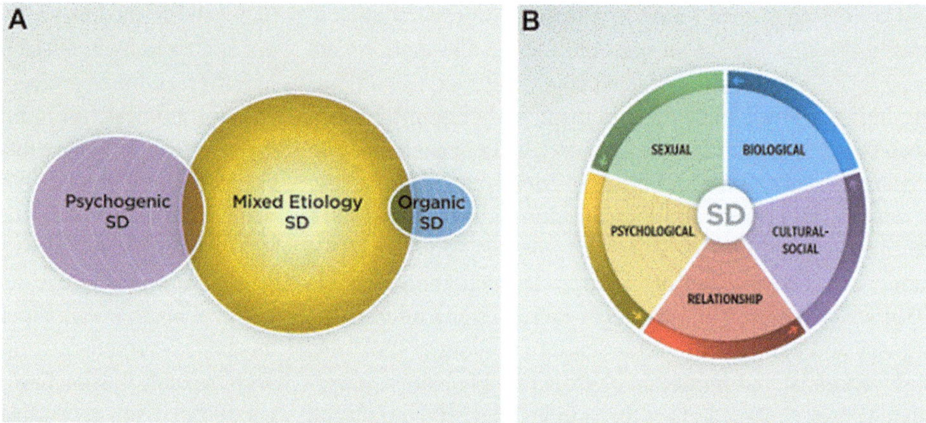

Panel A shows the previously held, traditional view of SD as psychogenic, organic, or mixed. Panel B shows the alternative, current view of SD as a multifactorial problem, with interacting contributing factors. Arrows around the periphery are intended to illustrate the dynamic, interactive potential among the different factors shown. SD=sexual dysfunction.

FIGURE 1-17. Traditional and alternative views of the factors contributing to sexual dysfunction [Reprinted from Hatzichristou D, Kirana PS, Banner L, Althof SE, Lonnee-Hoffmann RA, Dennerstein L, Rosen RC. Diagnosing Sexual Dysfunction in Men and Women: Sexual History Taking and the Role of Symptom Scales and Questionnaires. J Sex Med. 2016;13(8):1166–82 with permission from Elsevier].

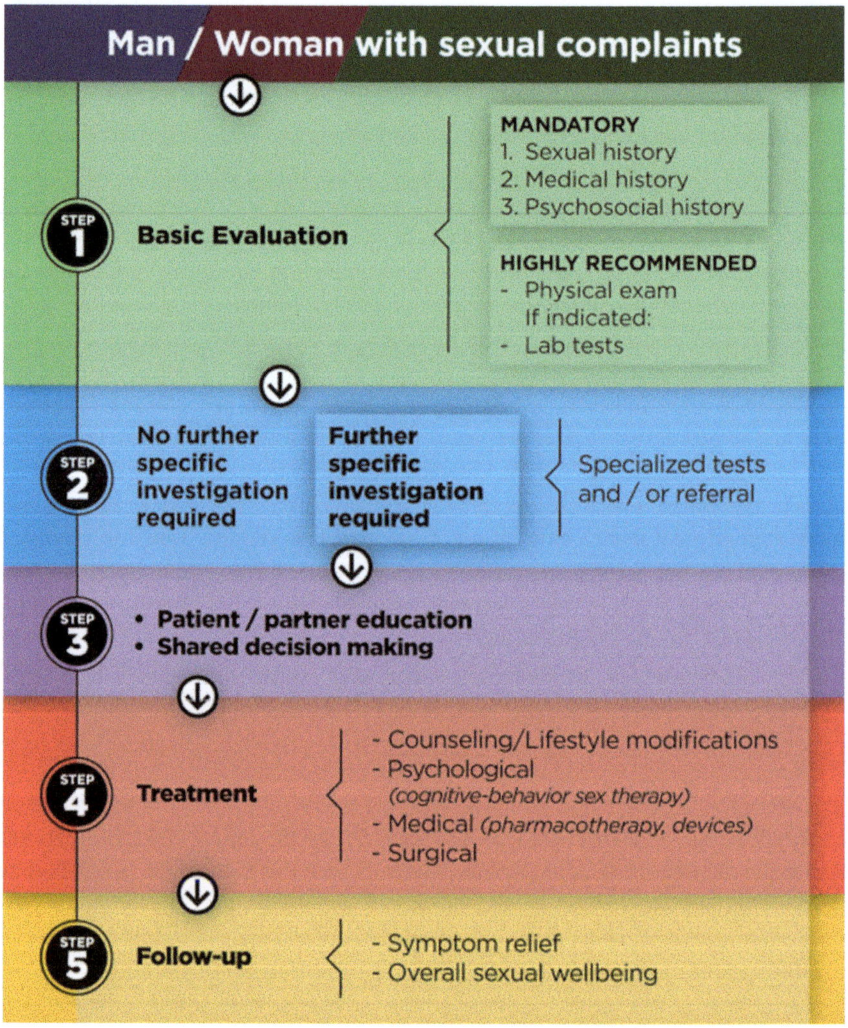

FIGURE 1-18. The revised international consultation on sexual medicine five-step algorithm for the management of sexual dysfunctions in men and women [Reprinted from Hatzichristou D, Kirana PS, Banner L, Althof SE, Lonnee-Hoffmann RA, Dennerstein L, Rosen RC. Diagnosing Sexual Dysfunction in Men and Women: Sexual History Taking and the Role of Symptom Scales and Questionnaires. J Sex Med. 2016;13(8):1166–82 with permission from Elsevier].

References

1. Kolodny RC, Masters WH, Johnson VE. Textbook of sexual medicine. Boston, MA: Little Brown; 1979.
2. Rosen RC. Prevalence and risk factors of sexual dysfunction in men and women. Curr Psychiatr Rep. 2000;2(3):189–95.
3. Sanders SA. Human sexuality in microsoft encarta online encyclopedia. http://encarta.msn.com. 2006.
4. Ignarro L. Nitric oxide: a unique endogenous signaling molecule in vascular biology. Nobel Lecture, December 8, 1998, posted in full text at http://nobelprize.org/nobel_prizes/medicine/laureates/1998/ignarro-lecture.pdf. 1998.
5. Berman J, Berman L, Bumiller E. For women only: a revolutionary guide to overcoming sexual dysfunction and reclaiming your sex life. New York, NY: Henry Holt Company; 2001.
6. IsHak WW, Tobia G. DSM-5 Changes in diagnostic criteria of sexual dysfunctions. Reprod Syst Sex Disord. 2013;2: 122. http://dx.doi.org/10.4172/2161-038X.1000122. Accessed 17 Sept 2016.
8. McCabe M, Sharlip I, Atalla E, Balon R, Fisher A, Laumann E, et al. Definitions of sexual dysfunctions in women and men: a consensus statement from the fourth international consultation on sexual medicine 2015. J Sex Med. 2016;13(2):135–43.
9. Allahdadi K, Tostes R, Webb R. Female sexual dysfunction: therapeutic options and experimental challenges. Cardiovasc Hematol Agents Med Chem. 2009;7(4):260–9.
10. American Psychiatric Association. Diagnostic and statistical manual of mental disorders. 5th ed. Arlington, VA: American Psychiatric Publishing; 2013.
11. Lewis RW, Fugl-Meyer KS, Bosch R, Fugl-Meyer AR, Laumann EO, Lizza E, Martin-Morales A. Epidemiology/risk factors of sexual dysfunction. J Sex Med. 2004;1(1):35–9.
12. Kandeel F. Male sexual function and its disorders: physiology, pathophysiology, clinical investigation, and treatment. Endocrine Rev. 2001;22(3):342–88.
13. Penson D. Adrenal control of erectile function and nitric oxide synthase in the rat penis. Endocrinology. 1997;138(9):3925–32.
14. IsHak WW. The guidebook of sexual medicine. Beverly Hills, CA: A&W Publishing; 2008.
15. Laumann EO, Paik A, Rosen RC. Sexual dysfunction in the United States: prevalence and predictors. JAMA. 1999;281:537–44.
16. McCabe MP, Sharlip ID, Lewis R, Atalla E, Balon R, Fisher AD, Laumann E, Lee SW, Segraves RT. Incidence and prevalence of sexual dysfunction in women and men: a consensus statement from the fourth international consultation on sexual medicine 2015. J Sex Med. 2016;13(2):144–52.
17. Althof SE, Needle RB. Psychological and interpersonal dimensions of sexual function and dysfunction in women: an update. Arab J Urol. 2013;11(3):299–304.
18. Crowe MRidley J. Therapy with couples. Oxford: Blackwell Scientific Publications; 1990.
19. Leiblum SPervin L. Principles and practice of sex therapy. New York: Guilford Press; 1980.
20. Assalian P. Psychological and interpersonal dimensions of sexual function and dysfunction [Internet]. Science Direct. 2016 [cited 25 Aug 2016]. http://dx.doi.org/10.1016/j.aju.2013.07.007.
21. Female Sexual Dysfunction Treatments and Drugs [Internet]. Mayo Clinic. 2016 [cited 1 Sept 2016]. http://www.mayoclinic.org/diseases-conditions/female-sexual-dysfunction/basics/treatment/con-20027721.
22. Goodchild van Hilten L. How labeling a drug "female Viagra" is misleading women [Internet]. Elsevier Connect. 2016 [cited 2 Sept 2016]. https://www.elsevier.com/connect/how-labeling-a-drug-female-viagra-is-misleading-women.
23. Santoro N, Worsley R, Miller K, Parish S, Davis S. Role of estrogens and estrogen-like compounds in female sexual function and dysfunction. J Sex Med. 2016;13(3):305–16.
24. IsHak W, Berman D, Peters A. Male anorgasmia treated with oxytocin. J Sex Med. 2008;5(4):1022–4.
25. Behnia B, Heinrichs M, Bergmann W, Jung S, Germann J, Schedlowski M, et al. Differential effects of intranasal oxytocin on sexual experiences and partner interactions in couples. Horm Behav. 2014;65(3):308–18.
26. Succu S, Sanna F, Melis T, Boi A, Argiolas A, Melis M. Stimulation of dopamine receptors in the paraventricular nucleus of the hypothalamus of male rats induces penile erection and increases extra-cellular dopamine in the nucleus accumbens: involvement of central oxytocin. Neuropharmacology. 2007;52(3): 1034–43.
27. What is flibanserin and how does it work? [Internet]. ISSM. 2016 [cited 2 Sept 2016]. http://www.issm.info/sexual-health-qa/what-is-flibanserin-and-how-does-it-work/.
28. Female sexual dysfunction treatments and drugs—Mayo Clinic [Internet]. Mayoclinic. 2016 [cited 20 Sept 2016]. http://www.mayoclinic.org/diseases-conditions/female-sexual-dysfunction/basics/treatment/con-20027721.
29. Ückert S, Oelke M, Albrecht K, Stief C, Jonas U, Hedlund P. Original research—basic science: immunohistochemical description of cyclic nucleotide phosphodiesterase (PDE) isoenzymes in the human labia minora. J Sex Med. 2011;4(3): 602–8.
30. Ückert S, Ehlers V, Nüser V, Oelke M, Kauffels W, Scheller F, et al. In vitro functional responses of isolated human vaginal tissue to selective phosphodiesterase inhibitors. World J Urol. 2005;23(6): 398–404.
31. IsHak WW, Mikhail AA, Amiri SR, Berman L, Vasa M. Sexual dysfunction. Focus. 2005;3:520–5.

2 The History of Modern Sexual Medicine

Ronald William Lewis

When asked to prepare this chapter I was honored, but faced a rather daunting task of developing a chapter on the history of sexual medicine of where to begin. I then decided that to me one of the turning points of the development of this area as more scientific in nature occurred with the publication of the seminal work of Kinsey [1], and Masters and Johnson [2, 3], where their close observation studies of couples sexual interactions and intense history gathering of these individuals began to take sexual activity out of the realm of mystery, interactive intrigue, and intense psychoanalysis necessary to provide relief for these couples. Thus I added the word "modern" to the title. As an example of getting back to some of our scientific roots I remember an example that Masters gave in a talk at Tulane while I was a medical student there in the mid 1960s of solving of a sexual dilemma for two Ph.D. individuals, who after seeing many specialists and both having what appeared to be super normal fertility potential as individuals were simply asked about their copulatory pattern in detail. They had been going to bed and "sleeping together" at the correct times but rather surprisingly naïve never actually having intercourse. What Dr. Masters stressed that he did not find this particularly unexpected in this highly educated but rather sexually uninformed couple but that they had found each other on the campus. I remembered this as an early lesson to me the importance of getting details on the history of any medical condition, particularly to those that involve sexual matters, without any preconceived notion of what the answer to such obvious question may reveal. Their infertility was promptly solved with just a mild intervention process.

As I also prepared to develop this chapter, I was reminded of a challenging but very fun educational activity of one of my undergraduate courses entitled History of Biology in which the professor had divided the centuries in six required times in which we as students were required to develop an essay during the semester of each of these periods expressing the conflict of either Mystery or Religion versus Scientific thought as it reflected on the culture of that particular time. What struck me for most of these time periods the dominant and accepted norms were often emanating from mystery or religion and the upstart scientific realm was often fighting an uphill battle. It is sometimes difficult to write as history such a new and continually developing field as sexual medicine since the field as a science is less than a century old. I will try to include what I think have been the most significant events that have driven this field into the more scientific realm that it has become today. Now, to quiet some potentially critical points of view, I by no means intend to indicate that sexual medicine disorders become science if only "medicalizing" the diagnosis and management of these distinct disorders as simple or isolated individual approaches is the determining factor that makes this field scientific. We all must never forget that most of sexual disorders or problems are not only a concern for the individual but also for a "partner(s) " as well and that we all who work in this area should be ever mindful of our inadequacies of truly dealing with this inter-active and intra-active nature of the management of sexual disorders. So even some of the magic of dealing with these problems prior to Masters and Johnson era still have a bearing of importance for us. I will try to highlight seminal scientific approaches in this young field as it occurred in time. I, by no means, have the ability to cite all of the important contributors in this field but have included those who have been dominant in pushing us into a more scientific field.

As we get into the modern history much of the early science centered on erectile dysfunction (ED) but other areas are highlighted in the chapter. Each major division indicated by bold title could possible lead to its on full chapter on the history so this is a very succinct attempt at history of sexual medicine in general. I have tried to select references that include many who have contributed to the field in their bibliographies which cite major contributors in the field.

W.W. IsHak (ed.), *The Textbook of Clinical Sexual Medicine*, DOI 10.1007/978-3-319-52539-6_2

Observational Studies Leading to Major Changes in the Therapeutic Approach to Sexual Disorders

Although the observations of Masters and Johnson [2, 3] gave a more documented and descriptive nature of sexual physiology it was followed soon by the realization that simple treatment behavioral modification did not work in all individuals because of the overlapping secondary individual and partner interactive processes playing a "resistant" to cure so therefore a new paradigm for therapy was developed that combined behavioral modification of sexual symptoms of classic therapy with brief, active psychodynamically oriented management of the patient's resistance [4]. A third seminal development in understanding human sexuality from a monistic process to the development of a triphasic paradigm was proposed by Dr. Kaplan in the late 1970s [5, 6]. Even this triphasic stepwise nature of sexual reactivity has been recently modified (see below). This triphasic nature of the sexual response moved the evaluation and treatment from a simple clinical entity to more complex interactions in the one individual to several interacting components but also to a series of interactions between the partner's sexual response as well. An example of the inadequacy of treating a man for ED without recognizing the patient's main problem may be hypoactive sexual desire, which if not addressed as well, would lead to therapeutic failure to treat the impotence [7]. Michael Perelmann about 7 years ago nicely summarized a new integrative approach to the management of sexual dysfunction [8].

A New Focus on Vascular Disorders of the Male Genitalia

At about the same time that this new focus on the diagnosis and therapy was occurring in the sexual therapist realm two studies emanated out of Europe focusing on recognition of possible vascular restoration occurring with pelvic vascular surgery for impotence [9]. The other publication was the elegant radiological evaluation of the intracoporeal and pelvic vasculature via specialized arteriography [10]. These caught the attention of two key clinical investigators at that time, Adrian Zorgniotti of New York City and Gorm Wagner of Denmark, who also had performed some elegant observational studies of physiological changes in the female genitalia and the male corpus cavernosum, to team as leaders in preparing a meeting in New York City in the fall of 1978 to discuss some of this new cutting edge treatment and evaluation of impotence which sequentially became the biennial meeting for at first impotence, then all of male sexual dysfunction to eventually sexual dysfunction in men and women under the current organization , the International Society for Sexual Medicine [11]. More detailed historical data regarding Dr. Zorgniotti can be found in Dr. Lizza's 2005 article [12]. At the 1978 meeting in New York City 188 revascularization procedures, mostly inferior epigastric artery to the corpus cavernosum (Michal I) were presented from 7 international sites with as high as 77% positive functional result [11]. The sophistication of presentations led to plans to address more science associated with penile erection and treatment of impotence at a second meeting in Monaco in 2 years in 1980. See Ref. [10] and the book that also was published on data from this initial 1978 meeting [11, 13]. By the time of the meeting in Monaco results of revascularization of the corpora cavernosa for impotence was reported from nine new centers in addition to Michal's group, most now using the Michal II, inferior epigastric artery anastomosis to the dorsal artery of the penis [11]. A unique revascularization procedure using the inferior epigastric artery to the deep artery of the corpora were also reported in a few cases from Latin America and the United States but long term follow up of these procedures and later reports of similar surgeries never appeared again. This revascularization group also included the first report of the Virag Technique of deep dorsal vein arterialization for vascular treatment of erectile dysfunction [11].

It is beyond the scope of this brief history of evolving sexual medicine to continue where this initial enthusiasm for penile revascularization treatment led but long term results were certainly mixed with major occlusion eventually for the revascularization arteries, probably due to some of the need for physiological runoff for successful revascularization and the non-physiologic connections such as to deep dorsa vein without runoff established to the corpora cavernosa itself or direct connection to the corpus cavernosa. Today only specific traumatic damaged pelvic internal pudendal arteries or the branches to the corpora verified by specific sophisticated pelvic arteriography (with ability to use the inferior epigastric artery as a donor artery to anastomotic vessels beyond the specific damage site such as dorsal arteries with definite branches to the corpus cavernosal deep artery serving as run-off vessels) should be the patient of choice for revascularization procedures. These are usually young patients with specific pelvic trauma. Certainly arterial damage is more generally small vessel disease in the corpora cavernosa itself now proved by more anatomical and physiological studies particularly in those patients with generalized vascular disease such as arteriosclerosis and microvascular injury in association with such diseases as diabetes mellitus (DM). This medical approach tended to blossom with overenthusiastic surgeons before some of the needed anatomical and physiological sciences of the corpus cavernosa were well understood.

The Ultimate Reconstructive Surviving Treatment of Erectile Dysfunction

Before the "new focus" on understanding the nature of the tissue of the penis erectile tissue and the 1978 awakening of alternative vascular repair for this disorder, a group of surgeons from various regions of the world had gradually developed the replacement of the physiologic process of erection with penile prostheses. This progressed from several types of artificial "os penis "devices being placed in the penis, but not into the corpora cavernosa itself, to intracavernous rigid and semirigid devices placement to various hydraulic intracavernosal prostheses. Semirigid, and two or three piece devices persevered to remain a major therapeutic success story of the treatment of ED. The reader of this historical piece is encouraged to read previous selected publications which well spell out this history of prosthetics for the treatment of ED [14]. One persistent characteristic of this modality is the constant nature of the surgeon and engineer to improve these devices to lessen mechanical wear, to develop infection resistant materials to aid in that devastating end point prevention, to improve the surgical techniques for placement of the devices, and to develop sophisticated salvage procedures when failure occurs. Key early pioneers in this field include Brantley Scott, William Furlow, Steve Wilson, Carl Montague, and Gerald Timms from Minnesota. At the second international meeting on impotence in Monaco in 1980, this area was highlighted in the program. A supplement to the Journal of Sexual Medicine in November, 2015 presents a review of historical papers with commentary in penile implant surgery [15]. Also another history review was published in sexual medicine reviews [16].

Intracavernosal Injection Therapy Treatment for ED

By the time of the 1982 third meeting on penile revascularization in Copenhagen, and certainly by the fourth meeting in Paris 1984, a new dominant therapy for ED was developing rapidly, injection of vasoactive agents into the corpus cavernosum [17, 18]. Another rich historic narrative on injection therapy from its beginnings can be found in a chapter from a Wagner and Kaplan 1993 publication [19]. Giles Brindley and Ronald Virag were the early pioneers in this field in 1982 and 1983 [17]. At first Virag proposed intracavernous injection therapy as an office procedure but auto-injection at home was proposed by Zorgniotti and LeFleur in a publication in 1985 [20]. At the fifth international meeting in Prague in 1986 the introduction of prosta glandin E-1 as the newest injection agent was made in laboratory and patient studies were presented from Singapore, Japan, and Vienna, Austria [17, 18]. A 3 year follow/up of 69 patients using self-injection of prostaglandin E1 was reported from Finland in 1999 [21]. In 1996 intraurethral prostaglandin E1 was approved but its efficacy was less than injection therapy [22].

One cannot discuss the history of injection therapy without citing a most seminal review article in the field by Junemann and Alken in 1989 [23]. The major agents used in diagnostic studies and therapy are two- or three-agent combinations using papaverine, phentolamine, or PGE-1 or using one of two FDA-approved PGE-1 agents alone [18]. Although a highly successful therapy for the treatment the invasive nature of the treatment is not well accepted by all patients and the long term dropout is still relative high. To demonstrate the rapid spread of this treatment for ED, at the 1984 meeting in Paris there were only five presentations dealing with intracavernous treatment for ED and in the subsequent 1986 and 1988 meetings there were over 45 presentations on the same subject [17]. Pharmacologic agent injection also became a major part of some of the diagnostic procedure as discussed below. The use of injection therapy for diagnosis, evaluation, and treatment of ED has been recently reviewed [24].

The Other Vascular Therapy for ED

By the time of the third and fourth meetings of the international group in Copenhagen in 1982 and Paris in 1984 some therapeutic and diagnostic studies stressing the veno-occlusive mechanism of erection were being addressed. Our group from Tulane University in New Orleans reported at the fourth international meeting in Paris in 1984 a dynamic corpus cavernosography [25]. We, in the introduction to that paper, discussed some of the early venous surgery for ED by Lowsley as early as 1953 and we presented some of our early vein surgery patients. We also credited early modern pioneers of venous surgery in the modern era, Ebbehof, Wagner, and Virag. In 1990 we presented an article on venous ligation surgery for venous leak in which we reviewed the earlier contributors and the then known results from around the world [26]. However long term results of this type of surgery were not sustained overtime mainly because it became apparent that veno-occlusive disorders were mostly the result of fibrotic changes in the sinuses of the corpora cavernosa and addressing the external veins would not change the lack of veno-occlusion which was dependent on total relaxation of the corpora sinuses. This type of surgery is now reserved for rare congenital venous defects in the wall of the corpora cavernosa and some rare cases of trauma or iatrogenic damage to the tunica albuginea.

The Other Early, But Less Sophisticated, Solution for ED

Another treatment for erectile dysfunction with origins predating the 1970 by patents but significant papers did not appear until 1986. Although not as sophisticated the modality still persists as an option for ED treatment. These were the vacuum erection deviceswhich history has been well described by this author in a previous publication [27]. Early pioneers and authors of papers in this field include Perry Nadig and Roy Witherington. Although a rather crude solution the noninvasive nature of the treatment persists and is highly successful for many couples. This solution works best when both partners truly accept this as their "best choice" for ED.

Anatomic and Physiologic Studies in the Development of the Science of Sexual Medicine

Following the first two meetings of what was to become the International Society of Sexual Medicine in Monaco in 1980 and Copenhagen in 1982 there was an emphasis to better understand the anatomy and physiology of the corpus cavernosa of the penis. It would be impossible, for it would result in a very long chapter in itself to recount all of the discoveries that emanated from the various laboratories around the world. In 2003, some of the key pharmacological and physiological studies were included in the 102 references from a book chapter by Tom Lue's group [28]. A very seminal work by deGroat and Steers outlining the key neurological pathways involved in the reproductive tract should be mentioned since that author was not included in the comprehensive list in the aforementioned bibliography in the Lue group article [29]. Another source of key historical participants in the basic research can be found in the basic science section of the textbook published in 2009 [30]. It would take myriads of pages and references to do the key basic science discoveries justice in this rather broad history perspective.

Suffice it to say, that all of this work described some of the central and spinal cord pathways involved in the initiation and maintenance of sexual activity. The anatomical studies clearly showed the vascular anatomy that fed the very "modified-capillary" connection between arteries and venous called cavernosal sinuses and the relaxation of these filled spaces to produce veno-occlusion dependent on an elastic and intact tunica albuginea. Most importantly the molecular nature of what happened to result in erection and detumescence led to an understanding of NOS and the initiation of Intracavernosal smooth muscle relaxation via nNOS release of nitric oxide with maintenance by shear force eNOS which resulted in relaxation of the smooth muscle of the sinus spaces, with intra chemical messengers through GAP junctions to produce a coordinated relaxation with calcium changes in the cell. Once a sympathetic release following orgasm, the mostly activated cyclic GMP dependent system was returned to a contracted state with key input from enzymes, primarily phosphodiesterase 5. The normal tonic contraction of the penis in the flaccid state was maintained by such systems as the Rho-kinase system.

Measuring the Problem: Development of Epidemiology

Understanding the incidence and prevalence and developing key definitions is crucial in understanding the nature of sexual disorders in the population. These areas are key to establishing this field as science. There have been four international consultations regarding sexual function, but the first focused only on males. In the second and third International Consultation in Paris in 2004 and 2009 and the fourth international consultation in Madrid in 2015 epidemiologic data for sexual disorders in men and women from data collected from the mid 1990s until the most recent time before the meeting were evaluated by the panels making up this committee. Articles which reference lists include the main contributors in the field were selected from the literature which met evidence-based criteria and the results are best summarized in four articles and one book chapter which the reader of this brief history are referred [31–35]. It is the epidemiological data that helps establish the now established fact that arterial erectile dysfunction can be a harbinger for cardiac arterial disease. Also the strong association with diseases such as diabetes mellitus has prompted myriads of anatomical, physiological, and molecular studies of this disease effect on the corpora tissue further clarifying treatment of this disorder.

History of Key Diagnostic Study Development in Sexual Medicine Science

At the first meeting on arterial revascularization the exquisite work of pelvic arteriography of Ginestie were presented without some of the modern sophisticated technical aspects of radiography [9]. We published an updated discussion of radiology of ED in 1990 from the Mayo Clinic group [36].

Erectile function during REM sleep was as a measurement of impotence was originally presented by Karacan in 1970 [37]. He was one of two featured guest contributors to the meeting in Monaco of the international group interested in ED which had convened in 1980 to further review corpora cavernosa revascularization. His early studies led to the development of the Rigiscan device which became an important diagnostic tool after this time [38]. After the development of color duplex Doppler studies of the corpora cavernosa the use of rigiscan diminished in importance but still remains an important part of evaluation of response to pharmaceutical agents in trial studies and some still think it crucial in the workup of ED. Using video sex stimulation erections and nocturnal erection measurement Slob et al. in 1990 reported their early result and follow-up with the use of penile vibration during the video sessions [39, 40].

Irwin Goldstein's group in Boston was a key contributor to development of dynamic cavernosometry and cavernosography as evaluation tools of the venous function of the corpora cavernosa. One of their key presentations appeared in 1987 [41].

After the development of injection agents, Tom Lue presented the concept of using penile color Doppler ultrasonography in 1985 [42]. At Mayo clinic in 1988–1999 a team of urology and radiology published several key papers on penile arteriography and the use of color Doppler ultrasonography [43–45]. In the AJR volume in 1989 in which the Quam article appeared [43] four other groups reported their early work on the use of color Doppler evaluation of impotence. Recently, in a paper by Sikka et al. standardization of color duplex Doppler studies was proposed [46].

As the field became more scientific there was a need for questionnaires to assess sexual disorders and two of the most successful validated instruments were the International Index of Sexual Functions (IIEF) and the Female Sexual Function Index (FSFI) first presented as publications in 1997 and 2000 [47, 48]. The design and development of such questionnaires is discussed in a book chapter in 2009 [49].

Major Breakthrough for Treatment of ED: Oral Pharmacotherapy

In March of 1998, sildenafil citrate, the first orally delivered selective PDE-5 inhibitor was approved by the United States Food and Drug Administration (FDA) for the treatment of ED. This class of drugs was an initial candidate antianginal agent but this medication and the many that came after it literally turned the tables on the management of ED because of its widespread effective use. An excellent reference of historical significance for the first 5 years of use of these compounds can be found in a book chapter by Harin Padma-Nathan [50]. In that same book put together by Dr. Gregory Broderick other chapters present more about this class of pharmaceuticals.

Other Than ED: The Science of Peyronie's Disease, Priapism, and Ejaculation Problems

Most of this discussion of the history of modern scientific sexual medicine has focused on ED but equally important for sexual disorders in men has been the science during the last years for understanding, diagnosing and treating other sexual problems in men. These areas include Peyronie's disease, priapism, and premature ejaculation.

In Peyronie's disease basic science studies have led to more scientific treatment of the local plaque prior to moving to the traditional surgical therapy of either plication procedures, excision of plaque with graft, or penile implant surgery [51, 52].

Priapism has been classified into ischemic or non-ischemic types and basic science studies have clarified some of the molecular changes in the cavernosal tissue such as changes in enzyme milieu in priapism associated with sickle cell disorders. An excellent review from Hellstrom's group includes priapism in males and females [53].

Premature ejaculation has been better defined, some central controls understood, and a more scientific approach to its management is now available. See the recent comprehensive review by Chris McMahon to view an historical summary of this disorder [54].

An excellent review of pathophysiology and management of delayed ejaculation has recently been published in 2016 [55].

In 1999, my colleague, Tom Mills and I reviewed the literature on the role of androgens in the maintenance of the erectile response citing in that article a number of studies [56]. Maggi's group in 2009 published an excellent review of the endocrinology of male sexual function [57]. Recently a process of care paper was published from the International Society for Sexual Medicine in their journal in 2015 [58]. From the fourth international consultation on sexual medicine a paper was published reviewing the literature supporting endocrinologic control of men's sexual desire and arousal/erection [59].

Catching Up: The Science of Sexual Medicine for Disorders in Women

At the International Meeting in Australia in 2000, it was recognized that the society needed to focus on the emerging science associated with women's sexual health, so for the first time a section of the program was entirely on women's sexual health issues. At the international meeting in Argentina in 2004 the organization changed its name to the current International Society for Sexual Medicine reflecting the need to focus on sexual medicine in both sexes. Soon after that the International Society for the Study of Women's Sexual Health was founded.

Some key papers that establish the science of sexual function and dysfunction in women are included in Refs. [60–67].

In fact, the first medication for a sexual dysfunction in women, flibanserin in premenopausal women, has recently been released [68, 69].

History of Sexual Medicine Science Drives Us to Optimal Treatment or We Are Not There Yet

The history of science of sexual medicine is not over and is not stagnant. Gene therapy and regenerative medicine developments to prevent damage to crucial sexual tissue or treat specific disorders such as ED are already developing. Penile transplant surgery is being pursued as a real possibility. Transgender medicine is now developing into a more stable scientific identity. As more understanding of the brain and mid-brain science of sex is understood perhaps designed medication to affect these areas may become reasonable. Finally, we can never stress enough, the importance of treating the couple for sexual disorders for epidemiologic data clearly shows this and the interaction between sexual partners is as paramount as treating individual disorders. History moves on.

References

1. Kinsey AC, Pomeroy WB, Martin CE, Gebhard PH. Sexual behavior in the human male. Philadelphia, PA: WB Saunders; 1948.
2. Masters WB, Johnson VE. The human sexual response. Boston: Little, Brown, and Co.; 1966.
3. Masters WB, Johnson VE. Human sexual inadequacy. Boston: Little, Brown, and Co.; 1970.
4. Kaplan HS. The new sexual therapy. New York: Brunner/Mazel; 1974.
5. Kaplan HS. Hypoactive sexual desire. J Sex Marital Ther 3(1):1977.
6. Kaplan HS. Disorders of sexual desires. New York: Brunner/Mazel; 1979.
7. Wagner G, Kaplan HS. The new injection treatment for impotence. New York: Brunner/Mazel; 1993.
8. Perelmann MA. Integrated sex therapy: a psychosocial-cultural perspective intergrading behavioral, cognitive, and medical approaches. In: Carson CC, Kirby RS, Goldstein I, Wyllie MG, editors. Textbook of erectile dysfunction. New York, NY: Informa Healthcare; 2009. p. 61–71.
9. Michal V, Viramar R, Pospichal J, Hejhal L. Arterial epigastricocavernous anastomosis for the treatment of sexual impotence. World J Surg. 1977;1:515–9.
10. Gineste JF, Romieu A. Radiologic exploration of impotence. The Hague, The Netherlands: Martinus Nijhoff; 1978.
11. Lewis RW, Wagner G. History of the International Society for Sexual Medicine (ISSM)—the beginnings. J Sex Med. 2008;5:740–5.
12. Lizza EF. History-Adrian Walton Zorgniotti (1925-1994): renaissance urologist. J Sex Med. 2005;2:272–7.
13. Zorgniotti AW and Rossi G, editors. Vasculogenic impotence. Proceedings of the first international conference on corpus cavernosum revascularization. Springfield, IL: Charles C. Thomas Publisher; 1980.
14. Mulcahy JJ. The development of modern penile implants. Sex Med Rev. 2016;4:177–89.
15. Multiple Authors. Contemporary review of historical papers in penile implant surgery. J Sex Med. 2015;12(Suppl 7):413–68.
16. Trost L, Hellstrom WJG. History, contemporary outcomes and future of penile prostheses: a review of the literature. Sex Med Rev. 2013;3:150–63.
17. Lewis RW. The international society for sexual medicine: a rich history and a bright future. Sex Med Rev. 2013;1:65–75.
18. Lewis RW. In: Paulson DF, editor. The pharmacologic erection in the impotent man: problems in urology. Philadelphia: J.P. Lippincott; 1991. p. 541–58.
19. Wagner G. The development of injection therapy. In: Wagner G, Kaplan HS, editors. The new injection treatment for impotence. New York: Brunner/Mazel; 1993. p. 18–29.
20. Zorgniotti A, Lefleur RS. Auto-injection of the corpus cavernosum with a vaso-active drug combination for vasculogenic impotence. J Urol. 1985;133:39–41.
21. Kunelius P, Lukkarinen O. Intracavernous self-injection of prostaglandin E1 in the treatment of erectile dysfunction. Int J Impotence Res. 1999;11:21–4.
22. Porst H. Transurethral Alprostadil with MUSE™ (medicated urethral system for erection) vs intracavernous Alprostadil- a comparative study in 103 patients with erectile dysfunction. Int J Imptence Res. 1997;9:187–92.
23. Junemann KP, Alken P. Pharmacotherapy of erectile dysfunction: a review. Int J Impotence Res. 1989;1:71–93.
24. Belew D, Klassen Z, Lewis RW. Intracavernosal injection for the diagnosis, evaluation, and treatment of erectile dysfunction: a review. Sex Med Rev. 2015;3:11–23.
25. Lewis R, Puyau, Kerstein MD, Kaack MB. Corpus cavernosa outflow as defined by dynamic cavernosography. In: Ronald Virag, Helene Virag-Lappas, editors. Proceedings of the first world meeting on impotence. Paris: Les Editions du CERI; 1986. p. 138–42.
26. Lewis RW. Venous ligation surgery for venous leakage. Int J Impotence Res. 1990;2:1–19.
27. Rhee AC. Lewis RW. Vacuum systems for erectile dysfunction. In: Carson CC, Kirby RS, Goldstein I, Wyllie MG, editors. Textbook of erectile dysfunction. New York, NY: Informa Healthcare; 2009. p. 291–7.
28. Carrion R, Bochinski D, Rahman N, Lue TF. Physiology and pharmacology of erectile dysfunction. In: Broderick GA, editor. Oral pharmacotherapy for male sexual dysfunction. Totowa, NJ: Humana Press; 2003. p. 1–24.
29. deGroat WC, Steers WD. Neuroanatomy and neurophysiology of penile erection. In: Tanagho EA, Lue TF, McClure RD, editors. Contemporary management of impotence and infertility. Baltimore, MD: Williams and Wilkins; 1988. p. 3–27.
30. Carson CC, Kirby RS, Goldstein I, Wyllie MG. Textbook of erectile dysfunction. New York, NY: Informa Healthcare; 2009. p. 25–119.
31. Lewis RW, Fugl-Meyer KS, Corona G, et al. Definitions/epidemiology/risk factors for sexual dysfunction. J Sex Med. 2010;7:1598–607.
32. McCabe MP, Sharlip ID, Atalla E, et al. Definitions of sexual dysfunction in women and men: a consensus statement from the fourth international consultation on sexual medicine 2015. J Sex Med. 2016;13:135–43.
33. McCabe MP, Sharlip ID, Lewis R, et al. Incidence and prevalence of sexual dysfunction in women and men: a consensus statement from the fourth international consultation on sexual medicine 2015. J Sex Med. 2016;13:144–52.
34. McCabe MP, Sharlip ID, Lewis R, et al. Risk factors for sexual dysfunction among women and men: a consensus statement from the fourth international consultation on sexual medicine 2015. J Sex Med. 2016;13:153–67.
35. Lewis RW, Fugl-Meyer KS, Bosch R, Fugl-Meyer AR, Laumann EO, LIzza F, Martin A. Definitions, classification, and epidemiology of sexual dysfunction. In: Lue TF, Basson R, Rosen R, Giuliano F,

and Khoury S, Montorsi F, editors. Sexual medicine: sexual dysfunction in men and women. Paris Health Publications; 2004. p. 39–72.
36. Lewis RW, Parulkar BG, Johnson CM, Miller WE. Radiology of impotence. In: Lytton B, Catalona WJ, Lipshultz LI, McGuire EJ, editors. Advances in urology, vol III. Chicago: Mosby Year Book, Inc.; 1990. p. 132–53.
37. Karacan I. Clinical value of nocturnal erection in the prognosis and diagnosis of impotence. Med Asp Hum Sex. 1970;4:27–34.
38. Bradley WE, Timm GW, Gallagher JM, Johnson BK. New method for continuous measurement of nocturnal penile tumescence and rigidity. Urology. 1985;26:4–9.
39. Slob AK, Blom JHM, Van Der Werft Ten Bosch J. Erectile problems in medical practice: differential diagnosis with relatively simple method. J Urol. 1990;143:46–50.
40. Rowland DL, Den Ouden AH, Slob AK. The use of vibrotactile stimulation for determining sexual potency in the laboratory in men with erectile problems: methodological considerations. Int J Impotence Res. 1994:153–61.
41. Goldstein I. Vasculogenic impotence: its diagnosis and treatment. In: deVere White R, editor. Problems in urology. Philadelphia: Lippincott; 1987. p. 547–63.
42. Lue TF, Hrick H, Marich KW, Tanagho EA. Vasculogenic impotence evaluated by high-resolution ultrasonography and pulsed Doppler spectrum analysis. Radiology. 1985;155:777–81.
43. Quam JP, King BF, James EM, Lewis RW, Brakke DM, Ilstrup DM, Parulkar BG, Hattery RR. Duplex and color Doppler sonographic evaluation of vasculogenic impotence. Am J Roentgenol. 1989;153:1141–7.
44. Hattery RR, King BF, Lewis RW, McKusick M. Vasculogenic impotence: duplex and color Doppler imaging. Radiol Clin North Am. 1991;29(3):629–35.
45. King BF, Hattery RR, James FM, Lewis RW. Duplex sonography in the evaluation of impotence: current techniques. Semin Int Radiol. 1990;7(3–4):215–21.
46. Sikka SC, Hellstrom WJ, Brock G, Morales AM. Standardization of vascular assessment of erectile dysfunction: standard operating procedures for duplex ultrasound. J Sex Med. 2013;10:120–9.
47. Rosen RC, Riley A, Wagner G, et al. The international index of erectile function (IIEF): a multidimensional scale for assessment of erectile dysfunction. Urology. 1997;49:822–30.
48. Rosen RC, Brown C, Heiman J, et al. The female sexual function index (FSFI): a multidimensional self-report instrument for the assessment of female sexual dysfunction. J Sex Marital Ther. 2000;26:191–208.
49. Barrisford GW, O'Leary MP. Design, development, and use of questionnaires in the evaluation and management of erectile dysfunction. In: Carson CC, Kirby RS, Goldstein I, Wyllie MG, editors. Textbook of erectile dysfunction. New York, NY: Informa Healthcare; 2009. p. 347–52.
50. Padma-Nathan H. Sildenafil citrate, the classic PDE-5 inhibitor. In: Broderick GA, editor. Oral pharmacotherapy for male sexual dysfunction—a guide to clinical management, Totowa, NJ: Humana Press; 2003. p. 65–83.
51. Levine LA, Lenting EL. A surgical algorithm for the treatment of Peyronie's disease. J Urol. 1997;158:2149–52.
52. Ralph D, Gonzalez-Cadavid N, Mirone V, et al. The management of Peyronie's disease: evidence-based 2010 guidelines. J Sex Med. 2010;7:2359–74.
53. Yafi FA, April D, Powers MK, et al. Penile priapism, clitoral priapism, and persistent genital arousal disorder: a contemporary review. Sex Med Rev. 2015;3:145–59.
54. McMahon CG. Current and emerging treatments for premature ejaculation. Sex Med Rev. 2015;3:183–202.
55. Sadowski MD, Butcher J, Kohler TS. A review of pathophysiology and management options for delayed ejaculation. Sex Med Rev. 2016;4:167–76.
56. Mills TM, Lewis RW. The role of androgens in the maintenance of the erectile response: a 1999 perspective. Molecular Urology. 1999;3:75–80.
57. Maggi M, Corona G, Forti G. Endocrinolgy of male sexual function. In: Carson CC, Kirby RS, Goldstein I, Wyllie MG, editors. Textbook of erectile dysfunction. New York, NY: Informa Healthcare; 2009. p. 61–71.
58. Dean JD, McMahon CG, Guay AT, et al. The international society for sexual medicine's process of care for the assessment and management of testosterone deficiency. J Sex Med. 2015;12: 1660–86.
59. Corona G, Isidori AM, Aversa A, et al. Endocrinologic control of men's sexual desire and arousal/erection. J Sex Med. 2016;13:317–37.
60. Marson L, Giamberardino MA, Constantini R, et al. Animal models for the study of female sexual dysfunction. Sex Med Rev. 2013;1:108–22.
61. Khera M. Testosterone therapy of female sexual dysfunction. Sex Med Rev. 2015;3:137–44.
62. Parish SJ, Hahn R. Hypoactive sexual desire disorder: a review of epidemiology, biopsychology, diagnosis, and treatment. Sex Med Rev. 2016;4:103–20.
63. Davis SR, Worsley R, Miller KK, et al. Androgens and female sexual dysfunction-findings from the fourth international consultation of sexual medicine. J Sex Med. 2016;13:168–78.
64. Worsley R, Santoro N, Miller KK, et al. Hormones and female sexual dysfunction: beyond estrogens and androgens—findings from the fourth international consultation on sexual medicine. J Sex Med. 2016;13:283–90.
65. Pukall CF, Goldstein AT, Bergeron S, et al. Vulvodynia: definition, prevalence, impact, and pathophysiological factors. J Sex Med. 2016;13:291–304.
66. Santoro N, Worsley R, Miller K, et al. Role of estrogens and estrogen-like compounds in female sexual dysfunction. J Sex Med. 2016;13:305–16.
67. Levin RJ, Both S, Georgiadis J, et al. The physiology of female sexual function and pathophysiology of female sexual dysfunction. J Sex Med. 2016;13:733–59.
68. Jayne C, Simon JA, Taylor LV, et al. Open-label extension study of Flipanserin in women with hypoactive sexual desire disorder. J Sex Med. 2012;9:3180–8.
69. Gao Z, Yang D, Yu L, Cui Y. Efficacy and safety of Flibanserin in women with hypoactive sexual disorder: a systematic review and meta-analysis. J Sex Med. 2015;12:2095–104.

3
Surveys of Sexual Behavior and Sexual Disorders

Gabriel Tobia, Khushminder Chahal, and Waguih William IsHak

Introduction

Few topics elicit as much passionate discussion, debate, and controversy as that of sex. As a result, a frank public health-oriented conversation free from taboo and prejudice remains difficult, even in the early twenty-first century, as evidenced by the recent controversy regarding the administration of the quadrivalent human papillomavirus (HPV) vaccine in teenagers [1]. The ensuing moral panic echoed that which followed the publication of the *Kinsey Reports* in the 1950s and that surrounding the issue of public funding of the *National Health and Social Life Survey* (NHSLS) in the late 1980s. The polemic recurs with every public discussion about sexual health, leading former Surgeon General of the United States M. Jocelyn Elders, M.D., to write, "We have a sexually dysfunctional society because of our limited views of sexuality and our lack of knowledge and understanding concerning the complexities and joys of humanity. We must revolutionize our conversation from sex only as prevention of pregnancy and disease to a discussion of pleasure [2]. This discussion cannot occur in the absence of accurate and dispassionate data.

Furthermore, in 2002, the World Health Organization (WHO) updated its definition of sexual health which it now defines as "a state of physical, emotional, mental and social well-being related to sexuality; it is not merely the absence of disease, dysfunction or infirmity. Sexual health requires a positive and respectful approach to sexuality and sexual responses, as well as the possibility of having pleasurable and safe sexual experiences, free of coercion, discrimination and violence" [3]. In the era of HIV/AIDS, the very private sexual act may have major public health repercussions.

In order to promote better sexual health, as defined by the WHO, it is essential to gather accurate data regarding the sexual behaviors and sexual health of the population. From Kinsey to the present day, numerous surveys about sexual habits have been published (Table 3-1); some of them were rigorous and scientifically valid, others less so. All sought to satisfy the public's curiosity for this most unique topic. The following chapter aims at reviewing the major surveys of sexual behaviors and sexual disorders and to present their main findings, focusing mainly and whenever possible on surveys pertaining to the US population.

A Brief History of Sex Surveys

The first known sex surveys in the United States were the *Kinsey Reports*, published in 1948 and 1953. Alfred Kinsey was an evolutionary biologist and a professor of zoology from Indiana University who had never studied human behavior. The main focus of his early research was in fact the mating practices of gall wasps [4]. In 1938, he was asked to teach the sexuality section of a course on marriage. As he was looking up literature in preparation for his lectures, he realized that scarcely anything had been published on the topic. He then decided to conduct his own study, using taxonomic methods transposed from entomology with which he was familiar. He started by handing out questionnaires to his class students, soon switching to face-to-face interviews. Along with his three colleagues, he ended up interviewing close to 18,000 subjects. He used samples of convenience starting with his own students, later expanding to other college students, prison inmates, mental hospital patients, a group of homosexuals, and hitchhikers. His findings were published in two books, *Sexual Behavior in the Human Male* in 1948 [5], followed 5 years later by *Sexual Behavior in the Human Female* [6]. These two works were later collectively dubbed the *Kinsey Reports*. They challenged preconceived notions about sex, a topic which was previously deemed taboo. Notably, Kinsey's data was presented free of any social, cultural, or political taboos [7]. The controversial nature of the topic naturally invited a backlash. Many critics, including religious and political figures, feared that Kinsey's candid discussion of sexual practices would disrupt

W.W. IsHak (ed.), *The Textbook of Clinical Sexual Medicine*, DOI 10.1007/978-3-319-52539-6_3

Table 3-1. Comparison of the major sex surveys

	Sample size	Type of sample	Information gathering	Major findings	Major limitations
Kinsey *1930s–1950s published 1948 and 1953*	5300/8000	Convenience sample	Face-to-face interviews	10% of men had had sex exclusively with other 46% of the male subjects "reacted" sexually to persons of both sexes	Sampling bias
Masters and Johnsons *published 1966 and 1970*	694	Convenience sample	Direct observation	Four-stage model of the sexual response	Sampling bias
Sex and Morality in the U.S. *1970–1972, published 1989*	3018	Nationally representative sample	Face-to-Face interviews	48% disapproved of masturbation 29% approved of outlawing premarital sex 59% favored laws against homosexuality	Chaotic inception Unpublished for 17 years
National Health and Social Life Survey (NHSLS) *1992*	3432	Multistage area probability sample	Face-to-face surveys	Americans tend to engage in sexual intercourse with demographically similar people Most STIs are contracted by young adults 6.9% reported an STI at some point Increased number of sexual partners correlated to STI risk Increased condom use in at-risk populations	Excluded adolescents and elderly subjects Focused solely on genital sexual acts
Sexual Well Being Global Survey (SWGS) *2009*	26,032	Unknown	Online, face-to-face (Nigeria)	3/5 respondents globally said that sex was important to them 69% enjoyed sex 44% were "very or extremely satisfied" with their sexual life	Possible sampling bias
National Survey of Sexual Health and Behavior (NSSHB) *2010*	5865	Population-based cross-sectional study, randomized using random digit dialing and address-based sampling	Online survey	High condom use rates in teenagers Active sex lives in elderly, but limited condom use	Self-selection Subjects sampled were only those accessible in the community

the moral order of the nation. Nevertheless, the *Reports* soon reached the top of bestseller lists, turning their author into a celebrity.

Some of Kinsey's most famous and controversial findings concerned homosexuality. He reported that 37% of men had at least one sexual encounter with another man at some point in their life and that 46% of men "reacted" sexually to persons of both sexes. Ten percent of men had had sex exclusively with other men for at least 3 years [5]. This figure may be the basis of the oft-repeated assertion that "10% of Americans are homosexual." Kinsey himself however avoided the categories "homosexual" and "heterosexual," instead using a seven-point scale—later dubbed "Kinsey scale"—to describe a person's sexual orientation, ranging from 0, or "exclusively heterosexual," to 6 or "exclusively homosexual" [5]. Regarding women, Kinsey reported that 7% of single females aged 20–35, as well as 4% of previously married women from that same age group, had equal heterosexual and homosexual experiences or responses (a rating of 3 on the Kinsley scale). One to three percent of single females of that age group were reported to be exclusively homosexual [6].

Kinsey estimated that the average frequency of marital sex among women in their late teens was almost three times a week, and it decreased to a little over two times a week at age 30 and once a week by age 50 [6]. On the topic of masturbation, he reported that 62% of female responders partook of it, 45% of which indicated that they could achieve orgasm in less than 3 min [6]. The rate of masturbation in males was markedly higher, at 92% [5].

Kinsey reported that around 50% of all married males had had an extramarital affair at some point during their married life, as did 26% of females under 40. He estimated that between 1 in 6 males and 1 in 10 females aged 26–50 had engaged in extramarital sex. Eighty-six percent of men reported that they had engaged in premarital sex, as did half of the women who married after World War I.

Additionally, Kinsey reported that 50% of males and 55% of females endorsed having responded erotically to being bitten. Furthermore, 22% of males and 12% of females reported an erotic response to a sadomasochistic story [5, 6].

Although his reports are still regarded as foundational works in sex surveys and the study of sex in general, Kinsey's methodology was heavily criticized, especially his use of convenience samples. His rationale for not using a random sample was that he could not persuade a random sample of Americans to answer deeply personal questions about sexual behavior. The result is a sample which, despite being considerable in size, may not be representative of the general population, as is generally the case with convenience samples [8]. Some groups were overrepresented in the sample. For instance, 25% of respondents were or had been prison inmates, and 5% were male prostitutes. One vocal critic even asserted that "a random selection of three people would have been better than a group of 300 chosen by Mr. Kinsey" [9]. Additionally, many of Kinsey's respondents volunteered to be in the study. Subsequent investigations showed that individuals who volunteer for surveys are often not representative of the entire population [10]. Nevertheless, Kinsey's work has been described as "monumental" [11] and has been named as one of the factors that changed the general public's perception and eventually led to the sexual revolution of the 1960s. It also led the way for the next generation of sex researchers. Indiana University's Institute for Sex Research (later renamed Kinsey Institute) has strived to expand and update the trove of information left behind by its founder. Subsequent studies were conducted, most notably in 1970 and in 2009. They are presented below. Researchers in other countries also emulated Kinsey. A notable example is the survey conducted in the United Kingdom in 1949 by the social research organization Mass-Observation. It was dubbed "Little Kinsey" although, unlike its model, it was conducted using random sampling [12].

In the late 1950s and early 1960s, Washington University gynecologist William Masters and his research associate and eventual wife Virginia Johnson studied sexual behavior using a medical model. They described the anatomy and physiology of human sexual response by observing 382 women and 312 men engaging in "10,000 complete cycles of sexual response." Their findings were published in *Human Sexual Response* (1966) [13] and *Human Sexual Inadequacy* (1970) [14].

The next major study was funded by the NIMH and was conducted by Indiana University's Institute for Sex Research, under the direction of Albert D. Klassen, subsequently joined by Eugene E. Levitt and carried out by the National Opinion Research Center (NORC) at the University of Chicago. It was originally conceived as a survey of the public's perception of homosexuality but was later expanded to cover a wide variety of sexual behaviors and attitudes. A fairly large sample of Americans (3018 respondents) were surveyed from 1970 to 1972. The data gathering process was slower and more expensive than anticipated, and the data analysis and writing processes were mired in controversy and personal disputes. As a result, the manuscript, which was finished as early as 1979, was not published. It was not until 1988 that the text re-emerged [15]. What *Science* had dubbed "The Long, Lost Survey on Sex" [16] was eventually published in 1989 as *Sex and Morality in the U.S.* [15], with additional data published in *Science* [17]. The main interest of the study lies in the fact that it dealt primarily with perceptions of sexual practices rather than the prevalence of the practices themselves. The researchers reported that 48% of respondents disapproved of masturbation, and a vast majority disapproved of extramarital coitus and homosexual relations without affection (87 and 88%, respectively). Even homosexual relations with affection had a disapproval rating of 79%. Similarly, a majority (65–82%) disapproved of premarital sex in teenagers, whether boys or girls, with or without romantic love. Adult age and the presence of love were predictors of a lower disapproval rate. Still, 29% of responder approved of outlawing premarital sex, 59% favored laws against homosexuality, and 14% believed a person convicted of homosexuality should be sentenced to at least a year in prison [15].

In subsequent years, there were other smaller studies, targeting certain specific population groups, such as young women [18–20] or college students [21]. These studies tended to focus more on social issues, such as contraception and teenage pregnancy, rather than actual sexual practices [22].

In the absence of rigorous scientific studies of sexual practices, a number popular nonscientific or pseudoscientific reports attempted to assuage the public's curiosity about the topic. More often than not, these studies used convenience samples. For instance, a number of these studies were funded by and published in magazines, and they drew their samples from the readership of said magazines. These include *Psychology Today* [23], *Redbook* [24], and *Playboy* [25].

The samples used in the studies may be large—20,000 in the case of *Psychology Today*, more than five times more for the *Redbook* study. However, these samples are drawn from the readers of the publications, and it has been argued that these are an already preselected population not necessarily representative of the general population, especially in terms of liberalism and education [15]. An additional issue is that of response rate. In the case if the *Redbook* survey, a survey was sent out to 4,700,000 *Redbook* readers, and only 2% of them responded. Such a response rate casts doubts as to the representative abilities of the findings, a shortcoming that will plague many other such surveys, such as that conducted by American-born German sex educator Shere Hite. Hite sent out surveys to women whose names she obtained from women's organizations and subscriber lists of women's magazines. In total, she distributed 100,000 questionnaires and received 3000 of them back, a 3% response rate [26].

The *Janus Report* (1993), by Samuel S. Janus and Cynthia L. Janus, was distributed to 4550 subjects with 2795 returned and were "satisfactorily completed" [27]. These included volunteers who came to the offices of sex therapists. It presents itself as an updated snapshot of American sexual practices in the context of the AIDS epidemic that had started a decade earlier. The report claimed to be going against preconceived notions about the sexual habits of senior citizens. It reported that over 70% of Americans ages 65 and older have sex once a week. The rate reported is almost as high in men over 65 (69%) as in men aged 18–26 (72%). It even went on to claim that a similar proportion of men over 65 have sex every day (14%) as men aged 18–26 (15%). The Januses' conclusions contradicted previous—and subsequent—studies that found a gradual decline in sexual activity beginning in the fifties. The *Janus Report* was heavily criticized for its skewed sampling, which resulted in overestimating the rates of sexual behaviors. For instance, Arthur Greeley [28] systematically compared the results obtained by the Januses to results drawn from the *General Social Survey* (GSS), which was based on a national household-based probability sample conducted by the National Opinion Research Center over two decades. He found that the *Janus Report* estimates were often 2–10 times higher than those of the GSS. For instance, as mentioned above, the *Janus Report* estimates that 69% of men aged 65 and above have sex at least once a week, as do 72% of men aged 18–26. By comparison, GSS rates for these age groups are 17 and 57%, respectively. The fact that the Januses' findings were never replicated elsewhere seems to give credence to their detractors.

In 2004, ABC News Primetime Live published its own *American Sex Survey*. The researchers interviewed 630 American adults by telephone, out of a random national sample of 1501. The survey lavishly describes "eye-popping sexual activities, fantasies and attitudes in this country." Among the results is 42% of Americans call themselves "sexually adventurous," 30% of single men aged 30 and older have "paid for sex," and that half of women acknowledge having "faked an orgasm" [29].

The scarcity of serious up-to-date studies and the urgent necessity of accurate information about sexual behaviors as a matter of public health, especially in the era the HIV epidemic, were the drivers behind the *National Health and Social Life Survey* (NHSLS) in 1990 [30]. The NHSLS, sometimes dubbed the *Chicago Study* or *Chicago Survey*, sought to remedy what its authors saw as methodological flaws in all previous sex surveys, from Kinsey on. The purpose of the NHSLS, according to one of its authors, was to "collect and analyze data on the social organization of sexual behavior, particularly the social structuring of sexual action, and the ways in which that structuring influences behaviors that increase the incidence and prevalence of a variety of health-related problems" [22]. The inception of the NHSLS was not without controversy. The study of people's private sexual behaviors has long been contentious, as evidenced by the vivid reactions to the *Kinsey Reports*. The government was reluctant to fund a project which would "provide a mandate of excessive sexual expression" [31], and although the study was originally requested by the National Institute of Child Health and Human Development (NICHD), its funding was soon terminated. The researchers were thus forced to turn to private donors to fund the study, including the Robert Wood Johnson Foundation, the Rockefeller Foundation, and the American Foundation for AIDS Research. The NHSLS was headed by Edward O. Laumann, Research Associate at NORC; John H. Gagnon, Professor of Sociology and Psychology at the State University of New York at Stony Brook; Robert T. Michael, NORC founding director; and James Coleman, NORC Research Associate [8].

The NHSLS used a novel approach in sampling. It involved a multistage area probability sample designed to give each household an equal probability of inclusion. The sampling returned 4369 eligible respondents. These subjects were administered a face-to-face 90-min survey, 3432 of which responded and were thus included in the study, resulting in a response rate of 78.6%. The subjects were aged 18–59, including 75% Whites, 12% African Americans, and 8% Hispanic Americans.

NHSLS researchers reported on a wide array of topics, such as sexual fantasies, masturbation, orgasm, and emotional satisfaction. Some of the findings from this survey are highlighted later in this chapter. The results of the study were published in *Sex in America: A Definitive Survey* [8] and *The Social Organization of Sexuality* [22]. Among the NHSLS findings was the fact that Americans tend to engage in sexual intercourse with peers who are similar to themselves in age, education, and ethnicity. It also revealed that, at the time, most sexually transmitted infections were contracted by young adults. 16.9% of respondents reported that they had at some point been diagnosed with at least one sexually transmitted infection. The survey also reported a correlation between the number of both lifetime and simultaneous sexual parwtners and the likelihood of contracting a sexually transmitted infection. Those with more than 10 lifetime sexual partners were 20 times more likely to have contracted such an infection as those with only one. Interestingly, the NHSLS found that the populations at highest risk of contracting sexually transmitted infections were starting to change their sexual practices accordingly, for instance, with increased condom use.

Overall, according to Cooks and Baur, the NHSLS "stands alone as the most representative U.S. sex survey and as one that reliably reflects the practices of the general U.S. adult population in the 1990s" [31]. Nevertheless, the study had some important shortcomings. As the NHSLS was conceived in the wake of the AIDS epidemic, it was in part designed to understand sexual behaviors associated with the transmission of the disease, so the researchers focused mainly on sexual practices that may lead to infection, omitting many significant non-genital sexual acts such as hugging, kissing, and body stroking, as well as the events surrounding the act such as courtship. Another major limitation has been the exclusion of adolescents and older adults, as the NHSLS researchers have chosen to focus solely on adults aged 18–59. It was in order to remedy to these limitations that some more cohort-specific surveys have appeared in recent years. The *Youth Risk Behavior Survey* (YRBS), conducted by the *Center for Disease Control and Prevention* (CDC) has strived since 1991 to gain data in the adolescent population, studying health risk and health protective factors in 9th to 12th graders, including sexual behavior [32–34]. The *National Social Life, Health and Aging Project* (NSHAP), on the other hand, researches the elderly population [35].

An all-encompassing survey to cover all age groups remained absent until two decades later, with the *National Survey of Sexual Health and Behavior* (NSSHB) conducted by the Kinsey Institute and Indiana University. The NSSHB not only provided an expanded age group but also allowed insight into changing trends and developments in sexuality over the past 20 years [36]. The NSSHB studied nearly 6000 subjects aged 14–94 and provided the scientific community with the first batch of thorough data on human sexuality and sexual behaviors in the past two decades. The NSSHB also took into consideration new developments in society which could influence sexuality. Such changes include the use of medications to treat erectile dysfunction (sildenafil, marketed as Viagra®, was released in 1998) which had extended the sexual lives of many and increased sexual behaviors in older ages. Also, in contrast to the 1970 Kinsey survey, same-sex relationships were now viewed differently, as same-sex marriage had become legal in some states and there had been increased recognition of same-sex partnerships and lifestyles. Another major development was the possible influence of the Internet on sexual perceptions and practices. The ability of the NSSHB to consider this influence on sexuality provides data, which researchers hoped would be more representative of the national population [37].

The NSSHB set out with the expressed aim to be the most nationally representative sexual survey conducted to date. It enrolled a total of 5865 participants (2936 males and 2929 females) through a population-based cross-sectional study conducted in the spring of 2009, randomized using random digit dialing and address-based sampling. This allowed the sampling frame to cover approximately 98% of all US households. Ages included ranged from 14 to 94, with adolescents requiring consent from their parent or guardian. Sample adjustments made included gender, age, race (Black, Hispanic, White, or other), geographic region (Midwest, North, South, West), sexual orientation (heterosexual, homosexual, bisexual, asexual, or other), household income, level of education, and relationship or marital status. Participants were asked to report whether or not they had engaged in certain solo or partnered sexual behaviors and, if so, how recently (never, within the past month, within the past year, or more than a year ago). These reports were obtained via the Internet, as opposed to face-to-face interviews in past surveys. Findings were presented as 95% confidence intervals sorted by age cohorts. Sexual behaviors included masturbation (solo and partnered), vaginal intercourse, anal intercourse, and same-sex behaviors. Condom use during vaginal intercourse was also assessed [37].

The NSSHB claimed to be a more modern sexual survey in comparison to previous studies, arguing that its design and items of investigation allow for a better insight into the sexual health of the US population. Investigation of earlier ages (younger than 18) provided insights into young teens, who have been considered a higher-risk demographic. Investigation of older ages (over 60) has allowed a better understanding of sexuality in an age group which has seen an extended sexual life due to the pharmacological advancements, an expanded range of sexual enhancement products (vibrators, lubricants), and consumer marketing messages that shape expectations for sex and relationships at an advanced age. Another particularity of the NSSHB lies in its methodology for data acquisition; the researchers claimed that, since answers were sent via the Internet, they were likely to be more honest than face-to-face answers such as those of the NHSLS, the latter being thought as more anxiety provoking and not allowing for the same degree of honesty. Nevertheless, the study did have its own major limitations. In particular, in a recurrent problem common to many sex surveys, the sample may have been subject to self-selection, as those who chose to participate may represent different sexual personalities than those who chose not to participate. Also, subjects sampled were only those accessible in the community and not those in group homes, hospitals, or long-term care facilities. Such factors are important and should be taken into consideration when designing future sexual surveys.

Although this chapter focuses primarily on surveys of sexual behaviors conducted in the United States, there were many more carried out in various parts of the world. Listing them all would be far outside the purview of this volume, but one notable study is the *Sexual Well Being Global*

Survey, or SWGS, conducted by Kevan Wylie, M.D., of the United Kingdom in 2006 and published in 2009. The researchers surveyed 26,032 participants across 26 countries, including the United States, the United Kingdom, China, Brazil, and Nigeria. The study was conducted online except for Nigeria where the respondents were interviewed face-to-face. The listed objective of the study was to "identify the variety of sexual behaviors undertaken by adults across the world." The researchers found that three out of five respondents globally said that sex was important to them, with comparable findings in men and women. Sixty-nine percent of those surveyed enjoyed sex. Forty-four percent of participants were "very or extremely satisfied" with their sexual life [38].

Prevalence of Sexual Behaviors

The following data regarding the prevalence of sexual behaviors are mainly derived from the most recent nationally representative sexual surveys, the NSSHB [8, 22] and NHSLS [36–41] (Figures 3-1 and 3-2).

Sexual Fantasies

The NHSLS survey found that 54% of men think about sex at least every day, 43% of them a few times a week or a month, and 4% less than once a month or never. In contrast, 19% of women think about sex at least every day, 67% of them a few times a week or a month, and 14% less than once a month or never. The survey also reported that 84% of married couples fantasized during intercourse. The most common fantasies, in decreasing order, are sex with the partner, sex with a stranger, sex with more than one person at a time, and engaging in sexual behaviors one would not usually engage in in reality [22].

Masturbation

According to the data gathered by the NSSHB, solo masturbation was reported by more than 20% of women in all age groups during the past month and by more than 40% within the past year, with the exception of those aged 70 years and more [37]. More than half of women aged 18–49 had masturbated in the past 90 days, including more than 60% of women aged 25–29. Being in a relationship and perceived health status are not significant factors in solo masturbation practices, except for women aged 60–69 who were less likely to masturbate if in a relationship. Forty-eight percent of women aged 18–39 reported masturbation "a few times each month or more" [39].

The NSSHB also found that the majority of men in all age groups reported masturbation in the past year with the exception of those aged 14–15 and 70 and more. Solo masturbation was more commonly reported than the majority of partnered sexual behaviors for men aged 14–24 and men aged 50 years or older [37]. It also reported that about half of men aged 18–69 masturbated in the past 90 days. Men aged 25–39 were the ones who engaged most frequently in solo masturbation, including 95.5% of men who describe themselves as single and dating, and more than 80% of all unmarried men from that age group. Married men over 70, in contrast, had the lowest rate (27%). Partnered men were less likely to report masturbation than non-partnered men. Health status was not a factor, except for men over 70 for whom poor to fair health was associated with lower rates of masturbation (18%) than those with good to excellent health (40%). More than 30% of men aged 18–49 reported masturbation alone on average more than twice a week during the past year [42].

NSSHB reported that women aged 25–29 were most likely to have engaged in partnered masturbation in the past 90 days (35%), as were men aged 30–39 (33%). Women who

FIGURE 3-1. Women's rates of sexual acts by age (Based on data from Ref. [39]).

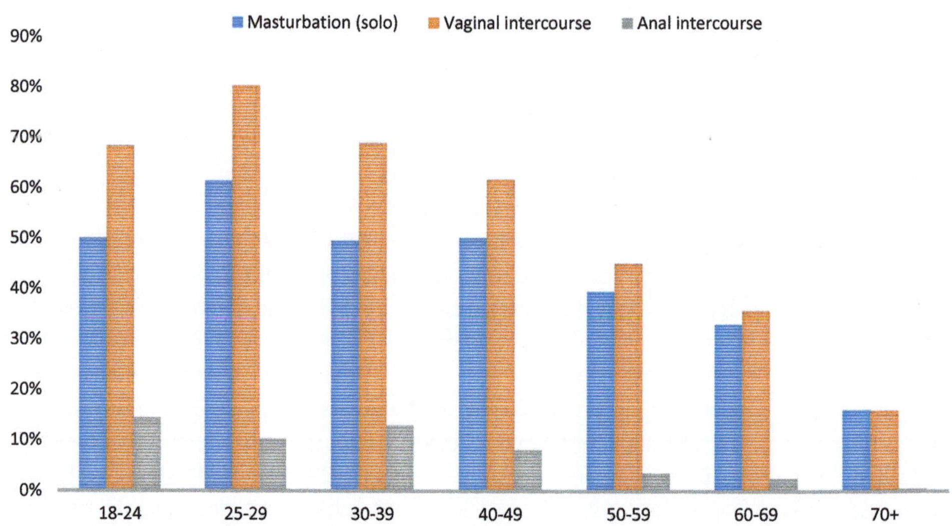

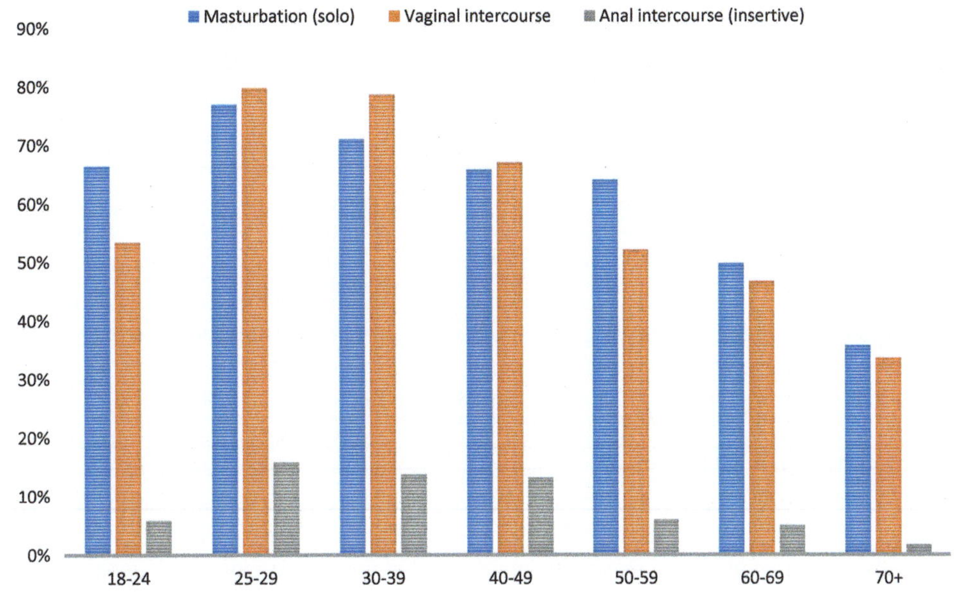

FIGURE 3-2. Men's rates of sexual acts by age (Based on data from Ref. [42]).

were in a relationship were more likely to engage in the practice than women who were not and perceived health status was not a significant factor. Men in a relationship were also more likely to engage in the practice. In women aged 25–39, the practice was most frequent in those who identified as single and dating (more than 60% engaged in it in the past 90 days). The highest rate in men when factoring all variables was among 25–29-year-olds in a relationship but not living together (44%) [37].

Two decades earlier, the NHSLS found that 63% of men and 42% of women masturbated at least once a year; 29% of men and 9% of women masturbated once a week. Eighty-one percent of men and 61% of women achieved orgasm during masturbation; 54% of men and 47% of women felt guilty afterwards. Individuals with a master's or advanced degree tended to masturbate at a higher rate (81% of men and 59% of women) than those without a high school degree (68% of men and 48% of women). Overall, the NHSLS finds that the higher the education level, the more likely the individual is to report that he or she masturbates. The NHSLS also reported that Whites masturbated more (66% of men, 44% of women) than Blacks (40% of men, 32% of women). In married individuals, the proportions of those who masturbated at least once a year is 57% in men and 37% in women, compared to 70 and 47%, respectively, in men and women who are divorced, separated or widowed, and not in a relationship. When asked for the reasons for masturbation, 40% of men and 42% of women said they sought physical pleasure; 26 and 32%, respectively, said it was to relax; 73 and 63% said they did it to relieve sexual tension; 32 and 32% cited the absence of a partner; and finally 11 and 5% said they did it out of boredom [22].

Partnered Sexual Intercourse

The NHSLS in 1992 looked at the frequency of all sexual contacts, whether vaginal, oral, anal, or others. According to the data reported, about a third of respondents (37% of men and 33% of women) engaged in sexual intercourse with a partner at least twice a week, another third (35% of men and 37% of women) engaged in intercourse a few times a month, and the rest engaged in intercourse a few times a year or not at all. Ten percent of men and 14% of women had not had sex at all in the past year. The youngest and the oldest respondents in the NHSLS survey were the least active sexually. People in their twenties were the most active, with 48% of men and 33% of women in that cohort engaging in intercourse twice a week or more. For both men and women, married and cohabiting couples engaged in sexual intercourse more frequently than non-cohabitating individuals. Contrary to perceived stereotypes, the survey did not find any significant variation in frequency of sexual activity across different racial groups, religions, or levels of education. Data from surveys showed that 40% of married people and half of people who were living together engaged in intercourse twice a week or more. Fewer than 25% of single or dating men and women engaged in intercourse twice a week. Twenty-five percent of single people not living together reported to engage in intercourse "just a few times," compared to 10% of married individuals. The length of the last sexual event of 11% of men and 15% of women was shorter than 15 min, and longer than an hour for 20% of men and 15% of women. Younger respondents appeared to have longer sexual encounters than older ones, with 31% of men and

23% of women aged 24 and less reporting that their last encounter lasted an hour or more, compared to 4% of men and 3% of women aged 55–59 [22].

Oral Sex

The NSSHB found that more than half of women aged 18–39 reported giving or receiving oral sex in the past 90 days, including 57% of women aged 25–29. Across all age cohorts, women who were in a relationship were more likely to report giving or receiving oral sex than those who were not. The highest rates were in women aged 25–29 who were living with a partner but not married, as 80% reported having received oral sex and 88% having given it in the past 90 days. Women in their thirties were most likely to receive (64%) and give (68%) oral sex among women who were single and dating. For most age cohorts, perceived health status was significantly associated with increased likelihood of oral sex in the past 90 days. Women aged 18–24 were the most likely to have reported oral sex with another woman in the past 90 days, with 3% reporting having received it and 4% having given it [39].

As for men, the NSSHB found that 64% of those aged 25–39 received oral sex from a female partner in past 90 days, and about 60% of them gave oral sex to a female partner. The men who were most likely to receive oral sex in this age cohort were in a non-cohabitating relationship (81%). In contrast, men over 70 had lower rates of receiving oral sex (15% in past 90 days). Being in a relationship was predictive of having received and having performed oral sex in the past 90 days for all men through age 69. Seven percent of men in their fifties reported having received oral sex from another man in past 90 days, and 7% reported having given it. This rate is higher than any other age cohort [42].

Interestingly, the data reported by the NSSHB is very similar to that of the NHSLS in the 1990s. At the time, the Chicago Study found that roughly three quarters of women reported cunnilingus having been performed on them by men and about the same proportion of men who reported fellatio performed on them by women. Around a quarter of respondents reported having performed oral sex on their partner during the last encounter, and about the same proportion reported receiving it. There was a sharp increase in the prevalence of these practices between those born between the 1930s and 1940s and those born afterwards, which coincided with coming of age sexually in the late 1960s and early 1970s, or the height of the so-called sexual revolution. Those respondents who reported no religious affiliation were more likely to have had experience with oral sex than Catholics or mainstream Protestants. Religiously conservative Protestants were the least likely to engage in the practice [22].

Vaginal Intercourse

The NSSHB reported that the majority of women aged 18–49 endorsed vaginal intercourse in the past 90 days (62–80%). In adult women, vaginal intercourse was the most frequently reported sexual behavior. After their thirties, more and more women reported having had no vaginal intercourse during the previous year: this was the case of about a quarter of women in their thirties, a third of women in their forties, half of women in their fifties, and finally four fifths of women over 70 [37]. Women aged 25–29 were most likely to report vaginal intercourse in the past 90 days (80%). Women in a relationship were more likely to report recent vaginal intercourse than women who were not; this difference increases with age, as 87% of women in their thirties who were in a relationship reported intercourse in the past 90 days, compared to 21% of non-partnered women. Among single women who were dating, the frequency was highest, perhaps surprisingly, in the 60–69 age cohort (81% in past 90 days). Higher perceived health status was associated with higher likelihood of vaginal intercourse in the past 90 days. The highest frequency of intercourse in women was in the 18–24 and 25–29 age groups. Women in a relationship reported more frequent intercourse, and frequency decreased with age [39].

As for men, those aged 25–30 and 30–39 were most likely to have had vaginal intercourse in the past 90 days (80 and 79%, respectively). Married men were more likely to have had intercourse than men in any other relationship status, and men in a relationship more than men who were not. The highest rates were in married men aged 18–24 and 25–29 (both 96%). Among single men who were dating, the frequency was highest among men in their thirties (76%). Health status was not a factor, except for men over 60 years as those with an excellent to good health status reported vaginal intercourse in the past 90 days at rates twice or more those with fair to poor health status [42].

Anal Intercourse

According to the NSSHB data, 10–14% of women aged 18–39 reported anal sexual intercourse in the past 90 days. The rate was highest in younger women with 14% of women aged 18–24 reporting anal intercourse in the past 90 days. Among women aged 18–24, a quarter of those who were cohabitating and a fifth of those who were married reported anal intercourse in the past 90 days. Women in a relationship were significantly more likely to report anal intercourse in the past 90 days. Among single women who were dating, those in their thirties were most likely to report such intercourse (14%). More than a quarter of married women aged 18–24 and women in a relationship aged 30–39 reported anal intercourse "once a month" to "a few times per year" [39]. As for men, insertive anal intercourse was more frequently reported in men aged 25–29 (16% in past 90 days), and men in a relationship were more likely to have practiced it if they were aged 18–24. Men aged 25–59 and in a relationship but not married were more likely to have had insertive anal intercourse than married or single men [42]. Anal intercourse among adolescents was rare (<5%) [43]. Within the past year, 13% of adult women and 3.6% of adult men reported having received anal sex. Sixteen percent of men reported insertive anal intercourse [37].

In comparison, the NHSLS had reported that 20% of women and 26% of men endorsed having had anal intercourse at some point in their lives. Of the respondents who have been active with a partner of the opposite sex in the previous year, around 9% reported anal intercourse in the previous year. There was a steady increase in rate between the cohorts born in the 1930s and 1950s, with a decrease in younger men and women, which the authors attributed to the HIV epidemic and resulting fear of transmission [22].

Homosexuality

Despite the fact that homosexuality has been documented since antiquity, its acceptance by modern Western societies as nonpathological is a fairly recent phenomenon. Alfred Kinsey asserted in *Sexual Behavior in the Human Male* (1948) that such behaviors were more common than previously thought. He also eschewed the categories "homosexual" and "heterosexual," devising instead a seven-point scale [5], suggesting that homosexuality may be part of a spectrum of sexual behaviors instead of an isolated phenomenon. Nevertheless, change in attitudes was slow to come in the psychiatric field. Kinsey's research was met mostly with indifference, if not hostility, by the specialty [44]. Homosexuality was still classified as a "sociopathic personality disturbance" in the first edition of the *Diagnostic and Statistical Manual* (DSM) in 1952 [45] and a "sexual deviation" in the second edition in 1968 [46]. A combination of a generational change in the field of psychiatry and relentless activism by members of the gay community led to an evolution in psychiatrists' approach to homosexuality [47]. Judd Marmor, M.D., in particular, was key in bringing about the "depathologization" of homosexuals. As a psychoanalyst, he challenged the prevailing psychoanalytic views regarding homosexuality. His two books *Sexual Inversion: The Multiple Roots of Homosexuality* (1965) [48] and *Homosexual Behavior: A Modern Reappraisal* (1980) [49] were highly influential. Finally, in 1973, homosexuality was eliminated as a diagnostic category by the American Psychiatric Association (APA), and in 1980, the next edition of the DSM did not contain the diagnosis [50].

Societal views on homosexuality were also slow to evolve. A 1972 survey by the University of Indiana found that a vast majority of Americans still disapproved of homosexuality. Eighty-eight percent of respondents disapproved of homosexual relations without affection, and 79% disapproved of homosexual relations with affection. Fifty-nine percent were in favor of laws against homosexuality, and 14% asserted that a person convicted of homosexuality should be sentenced to at least a year in prison [15].

The demographic of homosexuality have long been a subject of contention. Kinsey's reported that 37% of men had at least one sexual encounter with another man at some point in their life and that 46% of men "reacted" sexually to persons of both sexes [5]. His famous assertion that 10% of men had had sex exclusively with other men may be the basis of popular view that "10% of Americans are homosexual." Kinsey also reported that about 13% of women have had at least one homosexual experience and that 1–3% of single females aged 20–35 were exclusively homosexual [6]. In 1993, the NHSLS reported that 1.4% of women and about 2.8% of men were identified as homosexuals. It also found that 6% of men reported sexual attraction to other men, and 2% of the men endorsed a sexual encounter with another man in the past year. Five percent of men had a sexual encounter with another man at least once since the age of 18. The survey also found that about 5.5% of the women reported that the thought of having sex with another woman was appealing or very appealing. Fewer than 2% of the women in the study had a sexual encounter with another woman in the past year, about 4% had a sexual encounter with another woman after the age of 18, and 4% of women had a sexual encounter with a woman at some point in their lifetime. The NHSLS found that people who identified as gay or lesbian tended to reside in urban areas and tended to be more highly educated. The survey found that 9% of men in the largest 12 cities in the United States identified themselves as gay, compared to 3–4% of men living in suburbs and 1% of men in rural areas. Three percent of college-educated men identified themselves as homosexual, compared to 1.5% of men with a high school degree. Women with college educations were eight times more likely to identify as gay than women with just high school educations (4 and 0.5%, respectively) [22]. More recently, a 2012 Gallup poll (Figure 3-3) reported that 3.4% of adults in the United States identify as lesbian, gay, bisexual, or transgender (LGBT). It also reported that 6.4% of adults aged 18–29 identified as LGBT, twice as many as those aged 30–49 (3.2%) and three times as many as those 65 or older (1.9%). The difference between genders was only significant in the younger demographics (aged 18–29), where women were reported to be twice as likely to identify as LGBT as men [51].

FIGURE 3-3. Percentage of people self-identifying as lesbian, gay, bisexual, or transgender (LGBT) by age group (Based on data from Ref. [51]).

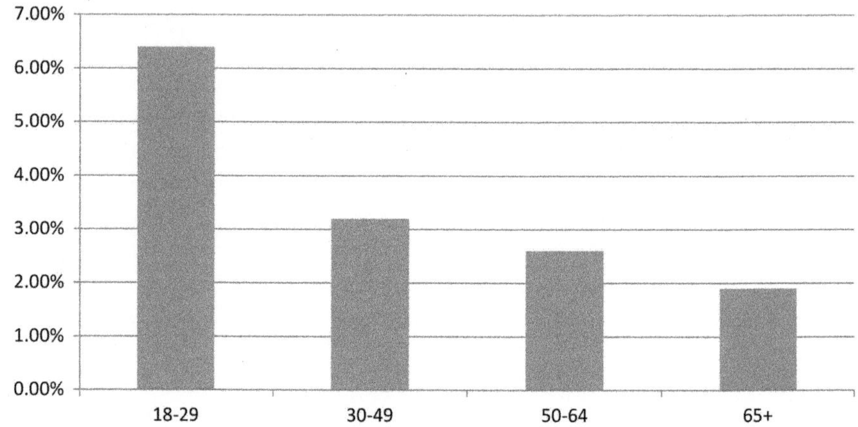

Sexually Transmitted Infections (STIs) and AIDS

The transmission of infectious diseases remains a major risk associated with sexual relations, producing public health repercussions to an otherwise private act. The CDC estimates that 20 million new cases of STIs are diagnosed every year in the United States, half of which affect those aged 15–24 [52]. The entailing direct and indirect costs are estimated at almost 16 billion dollars [53]. Yet, the exact figures remain difficult to obtain. Not all physicians report STIs, and when they are reported, it is often as individual cases, not as patients. A patient who presents repeatedly with the same infection is reported every time as a new case. Nevertheless, the NHSLS reported that more women (18%) than men (16%) have had an STI at least once in their life. Individuals with multiple sexual partners and those who rarely use condoms are ten times more likely to suffer from an STI than those with fewer or only one partner [8].

When it comes to HIV and AIDS, the highest risk groups traditionally have included men who had sex with men, intravenous drug abusers, their partners and children, and patients who had received contaminated blood products such as hemophiliacs. With drastic measures pertaining to the handling of the blood supply, the risk associated with the last group has decreased significantly. In 1993, the NHSLS reported that 27% of people who were at risk said that they had been tested. Those who were tested tended to be younger, more educated, and living in larger cities. According to NHSLS, 30% of people who were at risk of contamination admitted to have modified their sexual behaviors. Those tended to include younger individuals and those living in larger cities. African Americans and Hispanics were more likely to have been tested and to have changed their sexual behaviors than Whites. Twenty-three percent of married respondents reported being tested and only 12% of them changed their behaviors [22].

Two decades later, looking at the use of condoms during the past ten sexual encounters, NSSHB researchers found that the rate of use was higher in men (22%) than women (18%). Adolescent men (79%) and adolescent women (58%) had a particularly high rate. Condom use was highest among singles (47% of past 10 events), followed by single people in a relationship (24%), with married adults trailing behind (11%). On average, among all non-married adults, condoms were used 33.3% of past 10 events. When broken down by racial group, the rate of condom use was found to be higher among Black (31%) and Hispanic (25%) individuals than Whites (17%). Twenty-five percent of adult men and 22% of adult women reported using a condom during their most recent vaginal intercourse, compared to 80% of adolescent boys and 70% of adolescent girls. Condoms were used more often with casual sexual partners than with relationship partners across all ages and both sexes [41]. Condoms were on average used 26% of the past 10 anal intercourse events (both receptive and insertive) by men and 13% by women [37]. When asked about their most recent sexual encounter, 38% of heterosexual men who reported anal intercourse with a female partner used condoms, lower than 62% of homosexual men [40]. In adult men, those with a higher education used condoms more consistently, single men used them more consistently than married men, and Hispanics used them more consistently than other ethnic groups. In adult women, higher education, single status, and African American race were predictors of more frequent condom use. Men and women who reported a lower number of previous intercourse experiences with the partner and were not using other forms of contraception tended to use condoms more frequently. When it comes to anal intercourse, homosexual and bisexual men used condoms more consistently than heterosexual men [40]. Twenty-six percent of men and 22% of women used condoms during their most recent vaginal intercourse. More than half reported their most recent sexual partner was a relationship partner. Condom use was associated with fewer number of previous intercourse experiences with the partner and not using other forms of contraception for both men and women. Interestingly, condom use was not a significant predictor of pleasure, arousal, erection or lubrication, pain, or eventual orgasm for the participant or his or her partner [41].

A particularly noteworthy finding by the NSSHB was that the rate of condom use among adolescents was on the rise. In 2001, the *Youth Risk Behavior Survey* (YRBS) data revealed that 65% of male adolescents and 51% for females reported condom use during their last intercourse [54]. In comparison, the NSSHB figures, published in 2010, were 79 and 58%, respectively [43]. In 1988, 53% of 17-year-olds used a condom during their last vaginal intercourse [55]. The figure rises to 65% of 12th graders in 2009 [56]. In the NSSHB, 80% of males that age reported condom use during their last vaginal intercourse [43]. The authors concluded that this may have been due to public health efforts to encourage condom use [43]. However, rates of condom use are lower in young adults, suggesting that more effort should take place at educating those transitioning from adolescence to adulthood regarding maintenance of condom use, given that this may be due to entering short- and long-term relationships at this age [41].

The NSSHB reported that condom use with casual partners was lowest among men and women over the age of 50 [41]. Two thirds of men over 50 reported that they did not use a condom during their last sexual encounter. About 20% of men and 24% of women reported condom use during the last sexual encounter. This figure fluctuated depending on partner type, as men used condoms most frequently with a sex worker and women with a friend. These findings, the authors conclude, speak to the need to promote its use in this cohort, given that sexual lives are now being extended thanks to pharmacology and that the risk of sexually transmitted illnesses remains [41]. It is nowadays common for older adults to have new sexual partners, given that their old partners could be lost to divorce, death, or serious illness. Even though pregnancy may not be a concern in this age group, the risk of infection still is. The authors of the study conclude that providers should be attentive to the sexual behaviors of older patients, especially with regard to sexually transmitted infections, and that this age cohort should increasingly be the target for sexual health education (Figure 3-4).

Prevalence of Sexual Disorders

Sexual disorders are disturbances in the psychophysiological changes related to the sexual response cycle in men and women [57]. They have a relatively high prevalence in the US population [58], as suggested by the ubiquity of the advertising for pharmacological remedies such as erectile dysfunction. However, the scarcity of large-scale epidemiological data has led researchers to rely on integrating the data from smaller studies [59]. The most important recent set of data on the topic derives from the NHSLS [60] and is cited extensively in the *Diagnostic and Statistical Manual*, 5th edition (DSM-5) [57] as well as in this section.

Male Sexual Dysfunction

The exact prevalence of erectile disorder is unknown. There is a clear correlation between advancing age and increase in prevalence and incidence of erectile dysfunction [61]. Thirteen to twenty-one percent of men aged 40–80 report occasional issues with erections. Two percent of men younger than 40 report frequent issues with erections, compared to 40–50% of men older 70 who have significant erectile disorder [62]. Interestingly, on their first sexual experience, 20% of men feared problems with erection, but only 8% actually experienced an erectile issue that hindered penetration [57]. The prevalence of delayed ejaculation is also unclear, since the syndrome lacks a precise definition [57]. Seventy-five percent of men report that they always ejaculate during sex [60]; however, less than 1% of them report trouble lasting 6 months or more with achieving ejaculation [63].

One Swedish study reported that 6% of men aged 18–24 and 41% of men aged 66–74 report a decreased sexual desire [64]; however, the prevalence of male hypoactive sexual desire disorder varies with both the method of assessment and the country of origin.

Concern with premature ejaculation is reported by more than 20% of men aged 18–70 [65]. However, the actual prevalence of the disorder drops to about 1–3% if the narrow DSM-5 definition is followed (ejaculation occurring within approximately 1 min of vaginal penetration) [57]. Interestingly, men with liberal attitudes about sex were reported to be 134 times more likely to experience premature ejaculation [60].

Female Sexual Dysfunction

The epidemiology for male sexual dysfunction is scarce at best, but the data is even more lacking when it comes to female sexual dysfunction [60]. The prevalence of female orgasmic disorders has been reported as 10–42%, depending on the age, culture, duration, severity, and the method symptom assessment [57, 66]. However, only a fraction of them report distress related to the disorder [67]. Laumann estimates that about 10% of women do not experience orgasm throughout their lifetime [22].

Female sexual interest/arousal disorder is a new entry in the DSM 5, so its prevalence as such is unknown [57]. The prevalence of low sexual desire and of problems with sexual arousal, which was the disorder present in the previous edition, also varies with age, culture, and duration [68, 66].

FIGURE 3-4. Percent of past ten vaginal intercourse events in which condoms were used by age group (Based on data from Refs. [41, 43]).

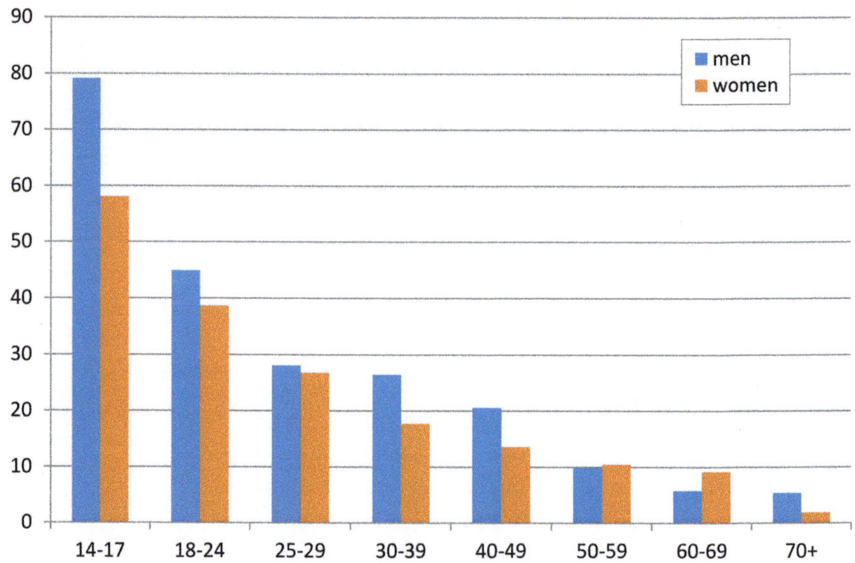

Again, only a fraction of women with the disorder report distress related to it [69, 70], and although sexual desire may decrease with age, older women often reported less distress related to the lack of sexual desire than younger women [69]. Fifteen percent of North American women report recurrent painful intercourse [60].

Conclusion

The topic of sexual behavior is a complex one, surrounded by a web of cultural and social norms, as well as ancient taboos. Although the sexual act remains one of the most private events, it continues to have major public health repercussions. Given the ever-changing nature sexual practices and the public perception thereof, the gathering of accurate data regarding sexual behaviors remains of utmost importance in order to adequately allocate resources and properly target at-risk populations. Despite the myth to the contrary, recent surveys have shown that "under the proper circumstances, adults in the United States will cooperate in a scientific survey about their sexual behavior" [30].

References

1. Ohri L. HPV vaccine: immersed in controversy. Ann Pharmacother. 2007;41(11):1899–902.
2. Elders MJ. Sex for health and pleasure throughout a lifetime. J Sex Med. 2010;7(Suppl 5):248–9.
3. World Health Organization. Defining sexual health: report of a technical consultation on sexual health. Geneva; 2006.
4. Christenson CV. Kinsey: a biography. Bloomington/London: Indiana University; 1971.
5. Kinsey AC, Mart CE. Sexual behavior in the human male. Bloomington/London: Indiana University Press; 1948.
6. Kinsey A, Pomeroy W, Martin C, Gebhard P. Sexual behavior in the human female. Philadelphia: Saunders; 1953.
7. Goldstein I. Looking at sexual behavior 60 years after kinsey. J Sex Med. 2010;7(Suppl 5):246–7.
8. Michael RT, Gagnon JH, Laumann EO, Kolat G. Sex in America: a definitive survey. Boston: Little, Brown; 1994.
9. Kinsey AC, Hyman R, Sheatsley PB, Hobbs A, Lambert R, Pastore N, Goldstein J, Terman LM, Wallin P, Wallis WA, Cochran WG, Mosteller F, Tukey JW. The Cochran-Mosteller-Tukey report on the kinsey study: a symposium. J Am Stat Assoc. 1955;50(271): 811–29.
10. Bradburn NM, Sudman S. Polls and surveys: understanding what they tell us. San Francisco: Jossey-Bass Publishers; 1988.
11. Duberman M. Jones: Alfred C. Kinsey. The Nation, p. 40–43, 1997.
12. England L. Little kinsey: an outline of sex attitudes in Britain. Public Opin Q. 1949;13(4):587–600.
13. Masters WH, Johnson VE. Human sexual response. Toronto, NY: Bantam Books; 1966.
14. Masters WH, Johnson VE. Human sexual inadequacy. Toronto, NY: Bantam Books; 1970.
15. Klassen AD. Sex and morality in the U.S.: an empirical enquiry under the auspices of the Kinsey Institute. Wesleyan: Middletown; 1989.
16. Booth W. The long, lost survey on sex. Science. 1988;239(4844):1084–5.
17. Fay RE, Turner CF, Klassen AD, Gagnon JH. Prevalence and patterns of same-gender sexual contact among men. Science. 1989;243(4889):338–48.
18. Zelnik M, Kantner JF. Sexuality, contraception and pregnancy among young unwed females in the U.S. In: Demographic and social aspects of popultion growth. Washington, DC: U.S. Government Printing Office; 1972.
19. Zelnik M, Kantner JF, Ford K. Sex and pregnancy in adolescence. New York: Sage; 1981.
20. Mosher WD, McNally JW. Contraceptive use at first premarital intercourse: United States 1965-1988. Fam Plann Perspect. 1991;23(3):108–16.
21. Gagnon JH, Simon W. Sexual conduct: the social sources of human sexuality. Chicago: Aldine; 1973.
22. Laumann EO, Gagnon JH, Michael RT, Michaels S. The social organization of sexuality: sexual practices in the United States. Chicago: The University of Chicago Press; 1994.
23. Athanasiou R, Shaver P, Tavris C. Sex. Psychol Today. 1970;37–52.
24. Tavris C, Sadd S. The redbook report on female sexuality. New York: Random House Publishing Group; 1978.
25. Louis Harris & Associates. The playboy report on American men: a survey and analysis of the views of American men in their prime years, regarding family life, love and sex, marriage and children,

the "outer" man and "inner" man, drug use, money, work, politics and leisure. Playboy. 1979.
26. Hite S. The Hite report: a national study of female sexuality. New York: Dell; 1976.
27. Janus SS, Janus C. The Janus report on sexual behavior. New York: Wiley; 1993.
28. Greeley AM. Janus report. Contemp Sociol. 1994;23:221–3.
29. ABC News. The American Sex survey: a peek beneath the sheets. 2004.
30. Michael RT. The National Health and Social Life Survey: public health findings and their implications. In: To improve health and health care. San Francisco: Jossey-Bass; 1997.
31. Cooks R, Bauer K. Our sexuality. Belmont: Thomson Wadsworth; 2010.
32. Warren C, Santelli J, Everett S, et al. Sexual behavior among US high school students. Fam Plann Perspect. 1998;30(4):170–172, 200.
33. Santelli J, Warren C, Lowry R, Sogolow E, Collins J, Kann L, Kaufmann R, Celentano D. The use of condoms with other contraceptive methods among young men and women. Fam Plann Perspect. 1997;29(6):261–7.
34. Santelli J, Lowry R, Brener N, Robin L. The association of sexual behaviors with socioeconomic status, family structure, and race/ethnicity among US adolescents. Am J Public Health. 2000;90(10):1582–8.
35. Suzman R. The National Social Life, Health, and Aging Project: an introduction. J Gerontol B Psychol Sci Soc Sci. 2009;64B(Suppl 1):i5–i11.
36. Reece M, Herbenick D, Schick V, Sanders SA, Dodge B, Fortenberry JD. Background and considerations on the National Survey of Sexual Health and Behavior (NSSHB) from the investigators. J Sex Med. 2010;7(Suppl 5):243–5.
37. Herbenick D, Reece M, Schick V, Sanders SA, Dodge B, Fortenberry JD. Sexual behavior in the United States: results from a national probability sample of men and women ages 14–94. J Sex Med. 2010;7(Suppl 5):255–65.
38. Wylie K. A global survey of sexual behaviours. J Fam Plann Reprod Health Care. 2009;3(2):39–49.
39. Herbenick D, Reece M, Schick V. Sexual behaviors, relationships, and perceived health status among adult women in the United States: results from a national probability sample. J Sex Med. 2010;7(suppl 5):277–90.
40. Reece M, Herbenick D, Schick V, Sanders SA, Dodge B, Fortenberry JD. Condom use rates in a national probability sample of males and females ages 14 to 94 in the United States. J Sex Med. 2010;7(suppl 5):266–76.
41. Sanders SA, Reece M, Herbenick D, Schick V, Dodge B, Fortenberry JD. Condom use during most recent vaginal intercourse event among a probability sample of adults in the United States. J Sex Med. 2010;7(suppl 5):362–73.
42. Reece M, Herbenick D, Schick V. Sexual behaviors, relationships, and perceived health among adult men in the United States: results from a national probability sample. J Sex Med. 2010;7(suppl. 5):291–304.
43. Fortenberry JD, Schick V, Herbenick D. Sexual behaviors and condom use at last vaginal intercourse: a national sample of adolescents ages 14 to 17 years. J Sex Med. 2010;7(Suppl 5):305–14.
44. Lewes K. The psychoanalytic theory of male homosexuality. New York: Simon and Schuster; 1988.
45. American Psychiatric Association. Diagnostic and statistical manual of mental disorders. Washington, DC: American Psychiatric Association; 1952.
46. American Psychiatric Association. Diagnostic and statistical manual of mental disorders. 2nd ed. Washington, DC: American Psychiatric Press; 1968.
47. Drescher J. Out of DSM: depathologizing homosexuality. Behav Sci. 2015;5(4):565–75.
48. Marmor J. Sexual inversion: the multiple roots of homosexuality. New York: Basic Books; 1965.
49. Marmor J. Homosexual behavior: a modern reappraisal. New York: Basic Books; 1980.
50. American Psychiatric Association. Diagnostic and statistical manual of mental disorders. 3rd ed. Washington, DC: American Psychiatric Press; 1980.
51. Gates GJ, Newport F. Special report: 3.4% of U.S. adults identify as LGBT. 18 Oct 2012. [Online]. http://www.gallup.com/poll/158066/special-report-adults-identify-lgbt.aspx. Accessed 18 Sept 2016
52. Centers for Disease Control and Prevention. Sexually transmitted disease surveillance, 2014. Atlanta, GA: U.S. Department of Health and Human Services; 2015.
53. Chesson H, Blandford J, Gift T, Tao G, Irwin K. The estimated direct medical cost of sexually transmitted diseases among American youth, 2000. Perspect Sex Reprod Health. 2004;41:217.
54. Anderson J, Santelli J, Morrow B. Trends in adolescent contraceptive use, unprotected and poorly protected sex, 1991-2003. J Adolesc Health. 2006;38(6):734–9.
55. Pleck JH, Sonenstein FL, Ku L. Changes in adolescent males' use of and attitudes toward condoms, 1988-1991. Fam Plann Perspect. 1993;25(3):106–10.
56. Centers for Disease Control and Prevention. Youth risk behavior surveillance—United States, 2009. MMWR 2010;59:1–142
57. American Psychiatric Association. Diagnostic and statistical manual of mental disorders. 5th ed. Arlington, VA: American Psychiatric Publishing; 2013.
58. Spector IP, Carey MP. Incidence and prevalence of the sexual dysfunctions: a critical review of the empirical literature. Arch Sex Behav. 1990;19(4):389–408.
59. Simons J, Carey MP. Prevalence of sexual dysfunctions: results from a decade of research. Arch Sex Behav. 2001;30(2):177–219.
60. Laumann EO, Paik A, Rosen RC. Sexual dysfunction in the United States: prevalence and predictors. JAMA. 1999;281(6):537–44.
61. Lewis R. Epidemiology of erectile dysfunction. Urol Clin North Am. 2001;28(2):209–16.
62. Prins J, Blanker M, Bohnen A, et al. Prevalence of erectile dysfunction: a systematic review of population-based studies. Int J Impot Res. 2002;14(6):422–32.
63. Mercer C, Fenton K, Johnson A, et al. Sexual function problems and help seeking behaviour in Britain: national probability sample survey. BMJ. 2003;327(7412):426–7.
64. Fugl-Meyer A, Sjögren Fugl-Meyer K. Sexual disabilities, problems and satisfaction in 18-74 year old Swedes. Scand J Sexol. 1999;2:79–105.
65. Laumann EO, Nicolosi A, et al. Sexual problems among women and men aged 40–80 y: prevalence and correlates identified in the Global Study of Sexual Attitudes and Behavior. Int J Impot Res. 2005;17(1):39–57.
66. Graham C. The DSM diagnostic criteria for female orgasmic disorder. Arch Sex Behav. 2010;39(2):256–70.
67. Oberg K, Fugl-Meyer A, Fugl-Meyer K. On categorization and quantification of women's sexual dysfunctions: an epidemiological approach. Int J Impot Res. 2004;16(3):261–9.
68. Brotto L. The DSM diagnostic criteria for hypoactive sexual desire disorder in women. Arch Sex Behav. 2010;39(2):221–39.
69. Bancroft J, Loftus J, Long J. Distress about sex: a national survey of women in heterosexual relationships. Arch Sex Behav. 2003;32(3):193–208.
70. Dennerstein L, Koochaki P, Barton I, Graziottin A. Hypoactive sexual desire disorder in menopausal women: a survey of Western European women. J Sex Med. 2006;3(2):212–22.

4
The Human Sexual Response Cycle

Roy J. Levin

Abbreviations

EPOR model	Excitation, plateau, orgasm, resolution
DEOR model	Desire, excitation, orgasm, resolution
STP model	Sexual tipping point
PERT	Post-ejaculation refractory time
SIS	Sexual inhibition scale
SES	Sexual excitation scale
DSM	Diagnostic and statistical manual of mental disorders

Introduction

The Modelling Concept in Relation to Human Sexual Responses

Early detailed accounts of human sexual responses had to be obtained from lay erotic writings and pornography, but the validity of the descriptions was always suspected. It could be argued that the history of the scientific study of human sexual arousal began in the "sexual hygiene literature" with the attempts to characterise the various stages of the arousal process; in modern parlance, we call this "modelling the system". Modelling biological processes and mechanisms have become an essential and inseparable part of scientific activity. Two important questions should be asked in relation to models, the first is "what kind of models can be used to describe sexual arousal responses?", while the second is "what properties should a good model possess?" The answers to the first question are shown in Table 4-1. This lists five categories of models that can be applied to characterise sexual arousal responses. The most familiar and popular are the descriptive ones using words and the graphic either of a line graph or a flow chart. A number of examples of these will be described later. Mathematical models, while being ordered and elegant, are extremely rare [1–3] although computational models have been used to investigate penile erectile processes [4]. Artificial or simulated sexual models have been used occasionally to examine a particular aspect of the sexual response, for example, the axial strength of the rigidity of the penis during erection or how the shape of the glans and its coronal ridge could be involved in removing another man's ejaculate from the vagina during coitus [5]. Finally, animal models are used to investigate aspects of the sexual response that would be unethical to undertake in humans or to allow an in-depth analysis of possible physiological factors involved [6, 7].

What Properties Should a Good Model Possess?

A number of the important properties that a good model should possess are listed in Table 4-2. What do, and what should, such models try to accomplish? The listing in Table 4-2 describes eight suggested functions that any model should possess; these are ideals, and most current models do not tick all the "yes" boxes. Moreover, in relation to the discipline practised by the user, some of the functions will be more important than others. For example, a clinician dealing with sexual dysfunctions would clearly be more interested in a model that ticks "yes" to number 4 than say to number 3, while a scientist involved in laboratory studies would be more interested in "yes" ticks to 1, 2 and 3. Those teaching about human sexual responses would clearly prioritise 6 and 7.

The Development of the Sexual Response Model

Early Models

Our present models of the human sexual response have been developed and refined from earlier proposals. The first four-phased word/text model for the human sexual response was that of Moll [8] as shown in Figure 4-1. His four

W.W. IsHak (ed.), *The Textbook of Clinical Sexual Medicine*, DOI 10.1007/978-3-319-52539-6_4

TABLE 4-1. The type of models used to describe/characterise the sexual cycle response

1. *Text*—descriptive—words used alone
2. *Diagrammatic*—graphic
   - Flow charts
   - Descriptive
   - Analytic pathways
3. *Mathematical*—use of equations—catastrophe theory
   - Computational models
4. *Physical*—artificial models penis/vagina
5. *Animal*—variety of animals used (rat, rabbit, dog, cat) to study penile/vaginal haemodynamics, muscular activity, brain activity

TABLE 4-2. A checklist to assess the possible usefulness of a model

Does it	Yes	No
1. Have a predictive power function?		
2. Add to our understanding of sexual arousal?		
3. Help researchers to design better studies?		
4. Contribute to clinical practice?		
5. Store information in a convenient format?		
6. Create a useful summary?		
7. Aid in teaching?		
8. Reduce uncertainty?		
9. Allow modifications in the light of new discoveries?		

How many boxes have to be ticked "yes" before we accept it as a significant advance on "previous models?".

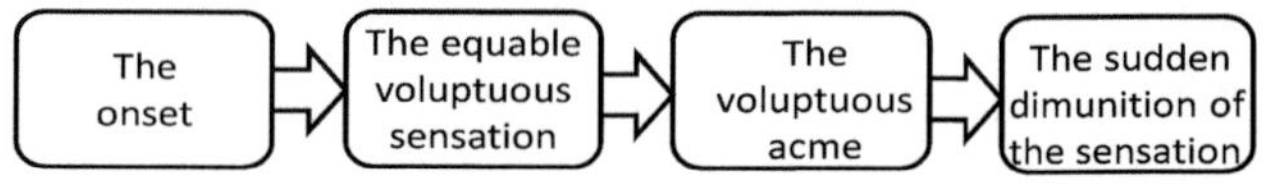

FIGURE 4-1. The four-phase human sexual response model of Moll [8] (Based on data from Ref. [8]).

descriptive phases were non-specific in terms of the various genital structures involved thus were applicable to both females and males. Havelock Ellis [9] oversimplified the model into just two phases, namely, "tumescence" (the swelling of genital tissues) and "detumescence" (their resolution to baseline), a model that had poor explanation of the facts, viz., little consilience. Van de Velde [10], in his popular book *Ideal Marriage*, published diagrams that used a continuous graphic line to represent the sexual arousal (accumulated tension) of the female (and male) from their basal state ascending to a peak at which orgasm occurred and then rapidly falling away back to the basal state. He acknowledged, in a footnote, that earlier authors had also published such curves. The weakness of his line graphs was that they did not identify the nature of the two graphic axes although they could be surmised to be the degree of sexual arousal (vertical or ordinate *y*-axis) and its duration (horizontal or abscissa *x*-axis). Reich [11], a pupil of Freud and a controversial sexologist, published a graphic line, unisexual model showing a slow ascent to an apex (orgasm) followed by a rapid descent that described "the orgastically satisfying sexual act pertaining only to the course of a few, typical naturalistic phase and modes of behaviour" that lasted for 5–20 min. After the "forepleasure" (now renamed as foreplay), he divided up his line graph into five distinct naturalistic phases (penile penetration, phase of voluntary control of excitation, phase of involuntary control of muscle contractions, sudden and steep ascent to climax, orgasm). Dickenson [12] modelled the human sexual response as various types of coital scenarios plotting the line graphs of male and female "sensations" graphically against time in minutes. He acknowledged, like van de Velde [10], that similar graphs of coitus had been published by a number of other authors but without the actual timings (see Dickenson [12] for references). Whether the "sensations" were central or peripheral or a combination was not described. In some respects, the early models adopted an elementary "nomothetic" approach, that is, establishing the common generalisations of the sexual arousal. Much later was the development of "idiographic" models (see biopsychosocial models of Basson, the Sexual Tipping Point and the Sexual Man models below) where the underlying "zeitgeist" was to characterise what makes sexual arousal individually unique. The methodologies used by the two approaches differ in that the nomothetic uses surveys, experimentation with measurements, statistical evaluations and analysis, psychometric testing and quantitative methodology, while the idiographic uses interviews, case studies, "focus" groups and qualitative methodology (e.g. Grounded Theory, observation, open-ended questions, iterative study design).

Triphasic Model of Wenger, Jones and Jones

Wenger, Jones and Jones [13] published their simple, triphasic model of the human sexual response in their book *Physiological Psychology* in 1956 (Figure 4-2). Its three phases were suggested to be mediated by first the parasympathetic nervous system and then the sympathetic returning to the parasympathetic for resolution. The model was never seriously endorsed probably because:

1. It was published only in a book.
2. The difficulty in assigning the specific neural mediations to the three phases.

The EPOR Model of Masters and Johnson (1966)

Masters and Johnson [14] were aware of the publications of all four authors and incorporated their concepts into their own descriptive unisex model that had both graphic and text modes of presentation. The major difference was that they used their empirical findings from their laboratory physiological and observational studies to create and establish their model unlike previous authors' mental conceptualisations. In their concise, sequential, text model of sexual arousal based on their laboratory observations, they arbitrarily categorised

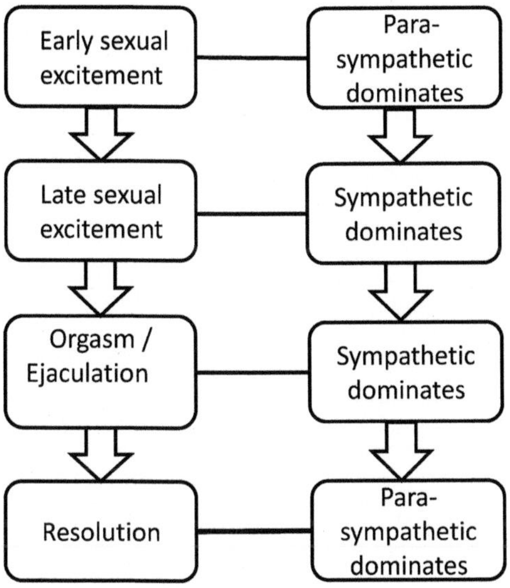

FIGURE 4-2. The triphasic sexual response model of Wenger, Jones and Jones [13]. See text for details (Based on data from Ref. [13]).

four phases described as excitation (E), plateau (P), orgasm (O) and resolution (R) often referred to by its acronym as the *EPOR* model (Figure 4-3). While the concepts of the excitation, orgasm and resolution phases are practically self-explanatory, that of the plateau phase is not. According to the descriptive accounts of Masters and Johnson [14], in the female plateau phase, mottling occurs on the breast skin, the colour of the engorged minor labia changes to a pink or bright red, the clitoral shaft and glans retract beneath the clitoral hood (retraction reaction), the outer third of the vagina becomes distended with venous blood that reduces the size of the entrance to the vaginal cavity (the orgasmic platform) and the full elevation of the uterus (vaginal tenting) is accomplished. In the male, a number of features occur, namely, a pre-ejaculation of secretion from Cowper's (bulbourethral) gland, a small increase in the size of the penile coronal glans, maximum testicular elevation to the perineum and enlargement of the testes by vasocongestion.

The model, while conceptually useful, has not been without criticism [15, 16] although it is often overlooked that Masters and Johnson themselves stated "in apologia" that:

1. The division of the male and female sexual cycles into the specific phases "is inadequate for evaluation of fine psychogenic aspects of elevated sexual tensions".
2. Only one pattern was diagrammed for the male despite the fact that there were variations in male sexual reactions but most were of duration rather than intensity.
3. While three different sexual responses were characterised for the female sexual response cycle, it was emphasised that "these patterns are simplifications of those most frequently observed and are only representative of the infinite variety in the female sexual response".
4. The models of the sexual responses although presented as a contribution to understanding the human sexual response patterns "the prejudiced source of this information must always be borne in mind. Until a representative cross section of the general population can be available to research interests, even admittedly prejudiced information is of inordinate value in the study of human behaviour" (a "prejudiced source" would today be referred as a "sample of convenience"). It should be noted that no published laboratory study has yet accomplished a "cross section of the general population representation" (what is now called a representative statistical sample of the population), and it is highly unlikely that one ever will as undertaking observed and recorded sexual arousal for scientific examination in a laboratory is far from everyone's passion despite the ubiquity of free porn on television!

Robinson [17] argued convincingly that the plateau phase was misnamed as the sexual excitement did not actually plateau but was still rising towards the orgasmic climax and that all the changes described occurred simply in the late part of the excitement phase. There appeared to be no reason to create a different phase allowing its abandonment. The newer version of the model thus became the *EOR* model. Despite this, authors who apparently are not familiar with the various developments still include the plateau phase in the model. Another peculiarity is that the original EPOR model when described against the "circular" Basson model (see section below) has been named as the "linear model" as it is the assumption that each EPOR phase occurs linearly from the previous phase. Yet Masters and Johnson [14], in the heading of the first chapter of their book, called their model "the sexual response cycle", and their Figures 1.1 and 1.2 have legends the "male sexual cycle" and the "female sexual cycle" presumably because after the orgasm the resolution phase could return the individual's status to basal. An important feature of the Master and Johnson's model was that the females were able to have multiple, sequential orgasms unlike the males (see Figure 4-5).

The DEOR Model of Kaplan [18, 19]

Major weaknesses of the *EPOR* model were its overly strong genital focus and a lack of a phase of being aware of a desire for sexual activity. Two sexual therapists, Helen Kaplan [18, 19] and Harold Lief [20], reported that some of their female patients had an absence of a desire to undertake sexual activity even with their loved ones. She surmised that there must a period before the so-called excitation phase when the individual felt a need to undertake sexual activity and named this phase the "desire phase". The model (Figure 4-3) then became the *DEOR* model, viz., desire (D), excitation (E), orgasm (O) and resolution (R). It should be noted

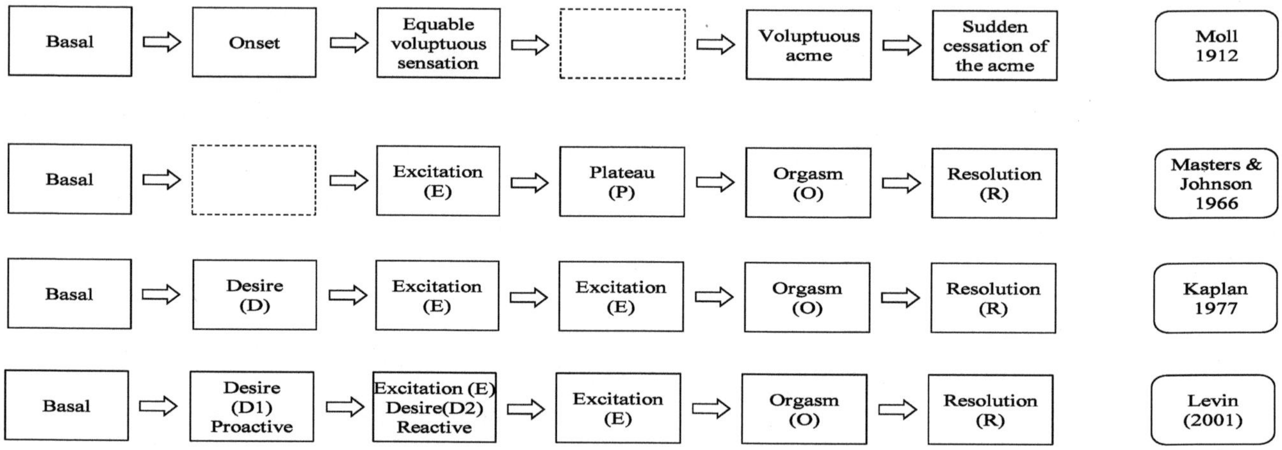

FIGURE 4-3. Development of the "text/word model" of the human sexual response. Note that the blank dotted line boxes have been added only for visual alignment and all the models obviously start from a basal beginning. Kaplan [18] added the desire phase and deleted the plateau phase. The suggestion of the two desire phases was discussed by Levin [23] and others. The open arrows indicate the apparent linearity of the progression of the phases of the models, but see text for further discussion (Based on data from Refs. [18, 23]).

that Kaplan created this phase simply from her work with patients and never surveyed "normal" subjects to ascertain whether they actually experienced such a "desire phase" before partaking of sexual arousal activity. She was the first to identify disorders of sexual desire as a distinct entity. When Garde and Lunde [21] surveyed normal Danish women who were orgasmic, they reported that some 32% had never experienced "spontaneous" desire. In a later random sample survey of American women, Michael, Gagnon, Laumann and Kolata [22] found that some 33% of women (one out of three) answered "yes" to the question "During the last 12 months has there ever been a period of months or more when you lacked interests in sex?" Levin [23] suggested that these surveys indicated that some 33% of orgasmic women did not appear to have a desire phase preceding their excitation phase. Laqueur [24] summarised the earlier literature that questioned "the very existence of a female sexual desire". No scientific epidemiological information about the incidence of female sexual desire was available in the nineteenth century. Kaplan and others automatically placed the desire phase before the excitation phase because at the time it was conceived that only one presentation of sexual desire was activated. While the "spontaneous" or endogenous desire has to be placed before the excitation phase, Levin [23] questioned the position of the desire phase in the model and suggested that a second desire phase could well be positioned during the excitation phase (Figure 4-3). This concept which is now called a "reactive desire" phase (D2) activated by sexual arousal per se compared to the "proactive desire phase" (D1) (Figure 4-1) has been accepted by many as a significant advance on the previous *DEOR* model (Basson, 16). Its shortened, acronymic form is the *D1D2EOR* model.

Other authors produced criticisms of the Masters and Johnson [14] model. Hoon [25] voiced his dissatisfaction in relation to its definitional and sequential reliability as there was no interobserver agreement about the changes observed, while Guttman scaling was not applied. Tiefer [15] questioned many aspects of the study from a clinical and feminist point of view as she argued that it was based on biased subject selection, experimenter bias and biases in methods. Basson [16], in her analysis, tabled a number of the major flaws in its conceptualisation and offered a new model of female sexual arousal (see below). Morrow [26] criticised it from a sociological perspective, while Levin [27] highlighted some unexamined mechanisms and some incorrect features involved in the sexual arousal processes and proposed specific modifications and corrections. It should be remembered, however, that despite all the criticisms the basic model, albeit with some modifications, has survived for more than 50 years, and many of the descriptions of what happens during human sexual arousal are still those of Masters and Johnson.

The Circular Model of Whipple and Brash-McGreer [28]

Whipple and Brash- McGreer proposed a circular model of the female sexual response composed of the four stages of Reed's (1998) Erotic Stimulus Pathway, namely, seduction (desire, attraction), sensations (excitation and plateau), surrender (orgasm) and reflection (resolution) [29]. The phases in brackets represent the phases of the EPOR model in juxtaposition to

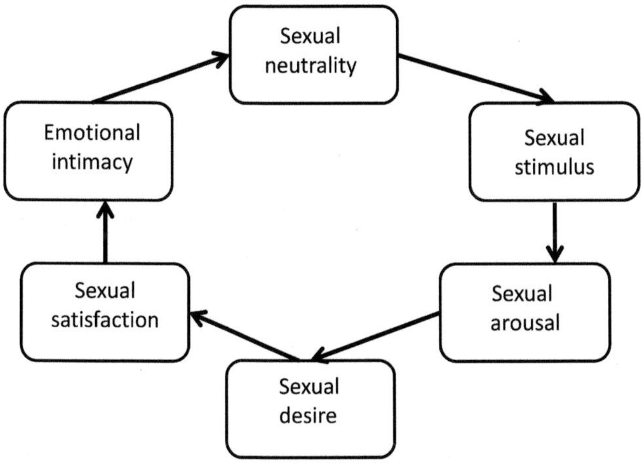

FIGURE 4-4. Brief schema for the Basson model [30] (Based on data from Ref. [30]).

the four new phases. The authors suggested that if the sexual experience was agreeable and satisfying, it would have a positive feedback to undertake a further "seduction" experience. Apart from the circularity, the four new phases made little or no impact to the development of the arousal literature.

The Biopsychosocial Female Models of Basson [30]

The next significant development in modelling the female sexual response was that of Rosemary Basson [16, 30], a medical sex therapist working in Canada. Based on her clinical experiences treating women with sexual difficulties, she conceptualised a qualitative biopsychosocial model that has become known as the "circular model" of the female sexual response. While she accepted that women in new sexual relationships usually followed the DEOR model of sexual responses, she argued that women, especially those in long-term relationships, are not always activated to undertake sexual activity prefaced by a desire phase (Figure 4-4). She proposed that many started from a position that she called "neutrality" (i.e. basal) and that subsequent sexual stimulation then activated their sexual desire. Moreover, they did not necessarily undertake the sexual activity to obtain sexual release but more for other rewards or gains such as intimacy needs and feelings for the partner. The model has become very popular as an alternative to the *DEOR*, but its general applicability to all groups of women has been questioned (see section on empirical testing below).

Empirical Testing of the Female Models

With the publication of different models of female sexual arousal, the problem of evaluating their validity becomes critical. One obvious way of empirically testing their validity is to ask women which model best fits their own sexual behaviour/activity. The study of Sand and Fisher [31] was the first to empirically test the endorsement of the *EPOR*, *DEOR* and the biopsychosocial models in a community sample of women (registered nurses, $n = 133$) with and without sexual dysfunction as to what model best fitted their sexual experience. Their possible dysfunctional aspects were assessed using the validated Female Sexual Function Index (FSFI; Wiegel, Meston and Rosen [32]). They found that equal proportions endorsed the *EPOR*, *DEOR* and biopsychosocial model, but those with the lowest FSFI score, indicating possible sexual difficulties, chose the latter model. They argued that this showed heterogeneity of women's sexual response and that the biopsychosocial model best reflected women with sexual concerns.

Since the Sand and Fisher [31] study, a number of other investigations on how women with and without sexual dysfunction endorse the various sexual response models have been published, and there is now significant controversy over which groups of women endorse the different models. Giles and McCabe [33] used an anonymous online survey that was completed by 404 women. They concluded, like Sand and Fisher, that the linear model more accurately represented the sexual responses of women without sexual dysfunction, while a modified circular model of Basson best fitted that of women with female sexual dysfunction. Hayes [34] undertook a systematic review of papers that compared the linear and circular models published since 1990. Of the 898 studies identified of which 13 met the inclusion criteria, only two compared the linear and circular models with limited evidence that most women identified with the linear model although some aspects of the female response fitted the circular model. Basson's [35] recent, but delayed, response to such studies was "that the FSFI questionnaire used to assess sexual concerns although validated reflected a non-evidence based conceptualization of the sexual response simplified as a linear entity of discrete sequential phases, beginning with the desire at the outset of sexual activity, arousal that is focussed on genital events rather than the subjective excitement". Other reviews of female sexual response models can be found in Wylie and Mimoun [36] and Perelman [37].

More recently, Giraldi, Kristensen and Sand [38], using an online study, investigated further which sexual response model represents a large cross-sectional sample of sexually active Danish men and women endorsed. In the case of the women, 34% chose the *EOR* model (Kaplan), 28% the linear *EPOR* model (Masters and Johnson 14), 25.6% the circular Basson model and 12.5% none of the models presented. Those women that showed sexual dysfunction (assessed by the FSFI) and most importantly also suffering distress significantly related to the circular Basson model. They concluded that women with no sexual dysfunction who were satisfied with

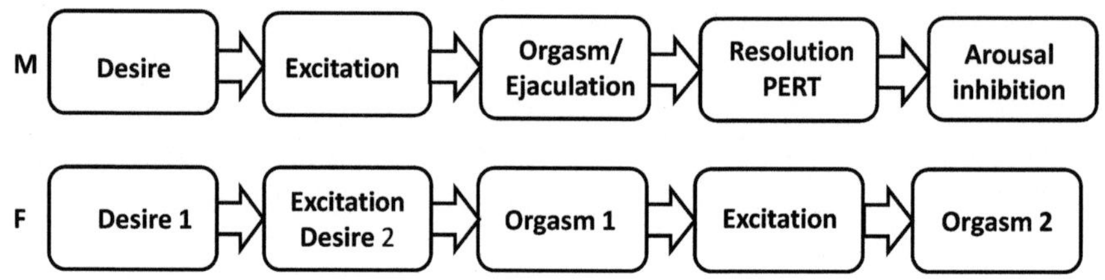

FIGURE 4-5. Comparison of the male (M) and female (F) sexual response models based on the modified DEOR model of Masters and Johnson [14]. Note that in the male, after orgasm and ejaculation, there is a resolution phase involving post-refractory ejaculation time (PERT) when no further arousal can occur (arousal inhibition) for a variable time dependent on age. This does not occur in the female (F) model when multiple orgasms can be induced before the cessation of resolution, just two are shown in the diagram. See text for details (Based on data from Ref. [14]).

their sexual life endorsed the linear EPOR model. This study was criticised by Basson, Correia, Driscoll, Laan, Toates and Tiefer [39] on a number of aspects. First, questioning why the authors only chose to ask about one type of sexual experience, and secondly the descriptions of the models used was questioned and whether the women understood the important aspects of the model, and it was suggested that the women could have been confused by the descriptions and chose the simplest formulation. It was argued that the "way in which the items tapping into sexual desire are worded, use of the FSFI and IEF (Index of Erectile Function) biases against participants who rarely acknowledge non-triggered desire". Those more likely to endorse non-sexual desire will score higher on the desire domains of these two questionnaires. Given that there are no questions that tap into responsive desire persons with more of the latter will of course score in the "dysfunctional range". The rebuttal by Giraldi, Kristensen and Sand [40] discounted the second criticism as they claimed they employed the wording used by Basson herself to describe the models. Their counter against criticism of the use of the FSFI and the IEF was that while they were not perfect they were the best validated questionnaires to use. Furthermore, they also assessed sexual distress and satisfaction with sexual life, and the women with a low FSFI score and high distress endorsed the Basson model. This result was in line with other quoted epidemiological studies. The dispute remains unsettled.

The Sexual Tipping Point Model

This unisexual, biopsychosocial behavioural and cultural model developed by Perelman [41] embraces both mental and physical aspects of sex. It is based on the concept that both mental and physical (MAP) factors can either "activate" or "inhibit" sexual arousal and in this respect has similarities to the dual control model. The obvious difference is that the Sexual Tipping Point (STP) model is usually portrayed using a graphic model of a classic two-pan weighing balance. One pan is weighted by inhibiting or negative factors of sexual arousal while the other pan by excitatory or positive factors. Whichever weighting is the heaviest upsets the balance to the negative or positive side of sexual arousal. The model was trademarked in 2013 and assigned to the MAP Education and Research Fund to allow it to freely distribute Sexual Tripping Point resources (explanatory video and related animations, publications and presentations) worldwide. A detailed history of the STP model development can be accessed on the Internet at www.maped.org/history/ [42].

Male Sexual Response Models

The early models for human sexual responses were unisexual covering the same phases for both sexes. Thus the previously described models for the female, viz., Moll [8], van de Velde [10], Reich [11] and Dickenson [12], equally apply for the male sexual response. The obvious difference that Masters and Johnson [14] detailed in their graphic model was the fact that unlike the female, with males there was a phase after the ejaculation/orgasm of a post-ejaculation refractory period (PERT) when they could not have a further erection or ejaculation/orgasm (see Figure 4-5) until after a significant duration has passed which becomes longer with ageing. Interestingly, this occurrence was not included in any of the earlier models. Even today, the neural mechanism(s) for this feature of male sexual physiology is poorly understood (see Levin [43], Bancroft [44] for reviews) and without an obvious explanation, apart from the fact that the males have an ejaculatory mechanism and women, normally, do not. However, in those women that have a urethral emission of fluid at orgasm, it has been suggested that they also have a post emission refractory state and do not have the ability to have further sequential orgasms (Levin [43]).

Unlike that of the female, the male sexual response has always been represented as relatively simple and straightforward and presumed to be initiatory and spontaneous (Perelman [37]) so there has been little controversy over the male EPOR model of Masters and Johnson although some specific aspects needed revision and change (Levin [27, 43]).

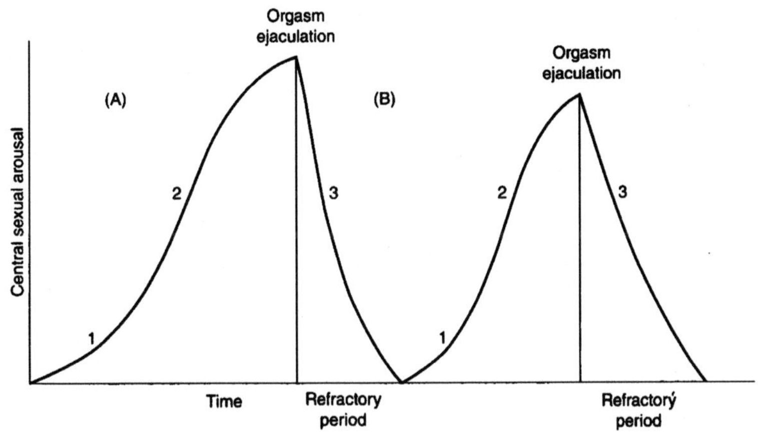

FIGURE 4-6. A graphic "cusp" representation of two serial male sexual response cycles. Orgasm is an example of a "cusp catastrophe". In the first response, (**A**) a desire phase (1) precedes the excitation phase (2) which increases the central sexual arousal until a cusp is reached that trips over to activate an orgasm and ejaculation. The subsequent resolution phase (3) returning to the basal level initiates a post-ejaculation refractory time (PERT) inhibiting a further orgasm/ejaculation until the PERT has ended. A second sexual response (**B**) can then occur with the same sequence as the first but usually with less intensity shown by the lower central arousal. See text for details (from Levin RJ. Anatomy and Physiology in the male. In Wylie K. ed. ABC of Sexual Health, 3rd edition. Oxford; Wiley & Sons, Wiley Blackwell; 2014:7–11. With permission of John Wiley & sons, Wiley Blackwell).

Some authors, however, have claimed that not all males follow the model (Zilbergeld [45]), but this has had little follow-up although one study, published only as an abstract, indicated that men used different sexual response models during their lifespan [46].

The original graphic *EPOR* model possessed a number of obvious weaknesses. These have been discussed in Levin [43]. In brief:

1. The designations of the two axis were not explicit, the vertical simply being the labelled with the phases "excitement, plateau, orgasm" presumably indicating the excitement levels at each phase but unclear as to whether it is that of the central or peripheral or combined nervous systems, while the unlabelled horizontal axis is "time", but no units were supplied.
2. The refractory period was incorrectly labelled.
3. The timescale of the orgasm duration was completely out of proportion to the other phases. Corrections for these features were made in the "cusp" model described below (Levin [43]).

The Four Es Model

A four-phase model or schema for the male sexual arousal that represents the named physiological mechanisms involved is the "Four Es" model; its designation comes from the acronym of the four phases, namely:

1. *Excitation*—sexual arousal that is activated by sight, sound, touch, taste, smell and fantasy
2. *Erection*—rigidity of the penis that cannot be bent, if it can then it is just tumescent (swollen)
3. *Emission*—genital fluids and spermatozoa moved into the prostatic urethra
4. *Ejaculation*—forceful ejection of the semen along the urethra mediated initially by urethral smooth muscle peristalsis and then 5–30 expulsive contractions of the striated bulbocavernosus muscle which is normally accompanied with orgasm

Each of these phases, together with orgasm, has its own independent mechanism (Levin [47]). Although this "physiological" phase model is the only one that actually describes the explicit mechanisms of the male sexual response, it is hardly ever used in the literature on its own but normally as an explanatory adjunct to the male *EOR/DEOR* model detailing the mechanisms involved in the phases [47].

Simple and Complex Models

The Cusp Catastrophe Model

The sexual response is usually one of a smooth, continuous slow change usually culminating in a discontinuous rapid change, the point of the transition is known as a "cusp". Orgasm is an example of a "cusp catastrophe" as the sexual excitation increases up to a "cusp" and then the system tips over into a completely different behaviour and orgasm occurs for both males and females with added ejaculation in the former (Figures 4-6 and 4-7). Such cusp diagrams of the male

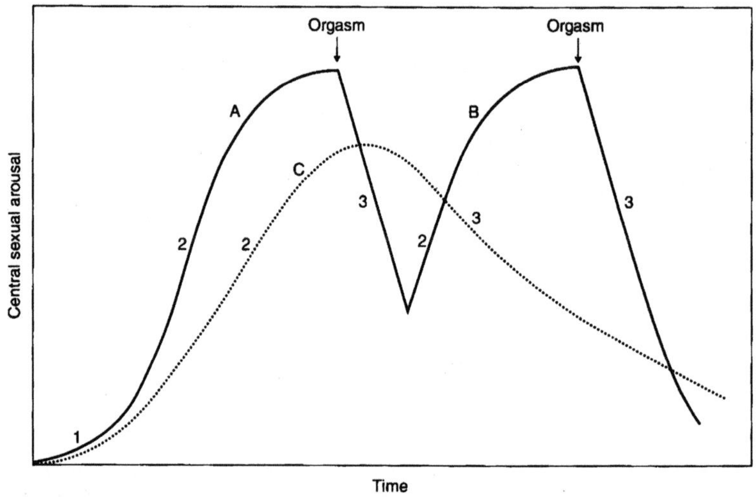

FIGURE 4-7. A graphic "cusp" representation of two serial female sexual response cycles. Orgasm is an example of a "cusp catastrophe". In the first response (A, *solid line*) a desire phase (1) precedes the excitation phase (2) which increases the central sexual arousal until a cusp is reached that trips over to initiate an orgasm. A partial resolution phase (3) then occurs until a second bout of sexual stimulation (B) creates another excitation phase leading to a second orgasmic cusp and a final resolution phase (3). The second scenario (C, *dotted line*) again has an initial desire phase (1) preceding the excitation phase (2), but as the central sexual arousal does not reach the level required to activate the orgasm cusp, orgasm does not occur, and the resolution phase (3) takes much longer to resolve back to the basal state (from Levin RJ. Anatomy and Physiology in the female. In: Wylie K. ed. ABC of Sexual Health, 3rd edition. Oxford: Wile & Sons, Wiley Blackwell; 2014:12–5. Reprinted with the permission of John Wiley & sons, Wiley Blackwell).

and the female sexual response were first shown by Levin [43, 48, 49]. This combination is characterised by the branch of mathematics described as Catastrophe Theory (see also section below on Unusual models). The Cusp line models (Levin [43, 48, 49]) are based on the EPOR model but now corrects a number of the weak features of the original EPOR model and is a more accurate graphic display model of the sexual response for the various phases.

The Dual Control Model

The dual control model is a unisexual model, superficially of relative simplicity (Figure 4-8). The theoretical basis of the model is the balance between central excitation and inhibition. Individuals vary in their abilities for the excitation and inhibition of their sexual responses. It began with Helen Kaplan's [50] concept of a "psychosomatic" dual control of sexual motivation emphasising "inhibition and excitation" as processes derived from the Kupferman [51] ideas of inhibitory and excitatory control in physiology. The concept was developed theoretically for the male sexual response (Bancroft and Janssen [52]) which was then formulated into a dual control model by Bancroft and co-workers at the Kinsey Institute (Bancroft, Graham, Janssen, Sanders [53]). Initially, two psychometric scale questionnaires were created to assess the degree of sexual inhibition and excitation in men, an inhibitory scale (SIS) and an excitatory scale (SES).

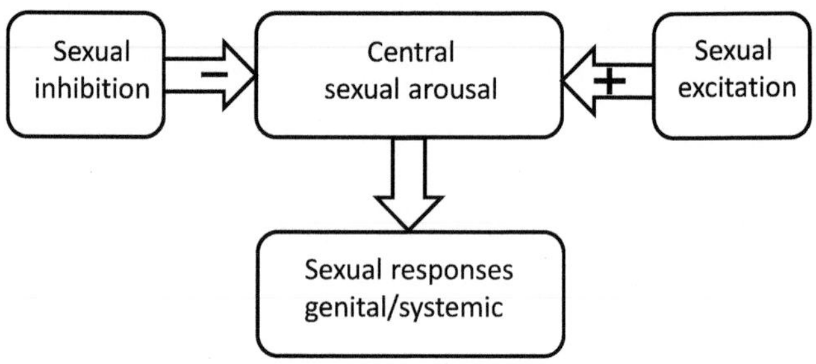

FIGURE 4-8. The essence of the dual control model [52, 53, 55] (Based on data from Refs. [52, 53, 55]).

Two inhibition factors were found, one thought to be associated with fear of performance failure (SIS1) while the other (SIS2) to external threats (e.g. unwanted pregnancy, being seen or heard having sex) within the relationship. Subsequently similar scales (SESII-W) were developed for women [54] and later a combined scale (SESII-W/M) for both men and women [55]. Kurpisz, Mak, Lew-Starowicz, Nowosielski and Samochowiec [56] have recently reviewed the practical issues involved with the model.

The "Sexual Man" Model

In an attempt to categorise the complexity of human sexual responses, the highly complex flow chart model of "Sexual Man" (Figure 4-9) was created (Levin [57]). This model

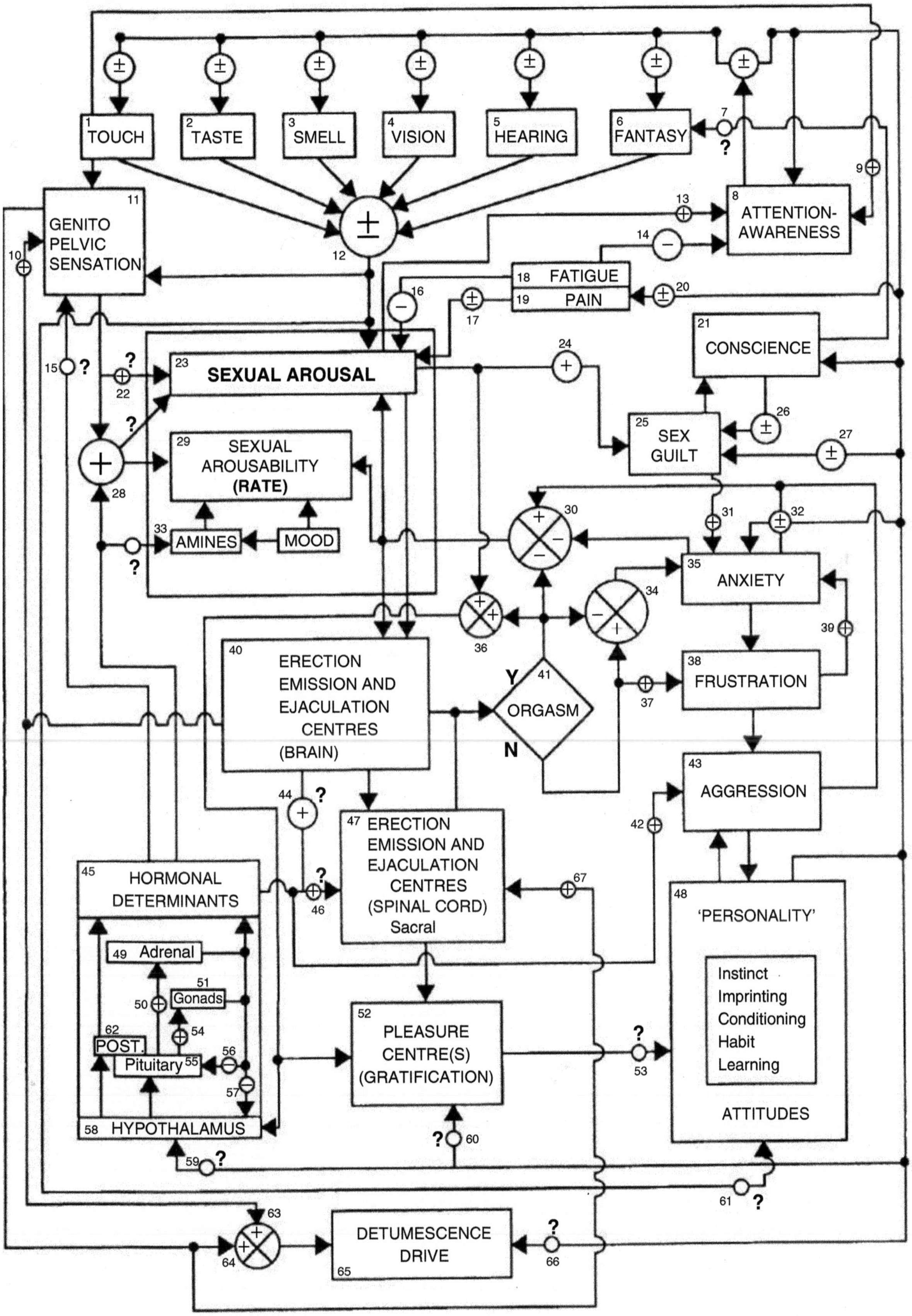

FIGURE 4-9. The sexual man model [57]. This is a flow chart model where the various paths are designated by numbers so that they can easily be followed. The positive signs indicate enhancement, while the negative signs indicate inhibition or reduction and the pathways are delineated in the text in round brackets. The question marks indicate pathways that had not yet been identified as positive or negative (or both). Central to the model is "sexual arousal", the state, while "Sexual arousability" is the rate of its attainment. Orgasm (41) can either occur (=Y path) or not (=N path) with resultant pathway effects (From Levin RJ. Human male sexuality: appetite and arousal, desire and drive. In: Legg CR, Booth DA. eds. Appetite- neural and behavioural basis. Oxford: Oxford University Press: 1994: 127–64. Reprinted with the Permission from Oxford University Press).

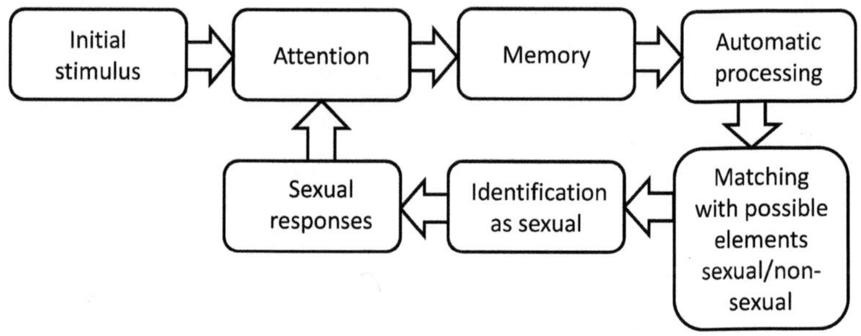

FIGURE 4-10. A brief schema for the information processing model [60] (Based on data from Ref. [60]).

incorporated and integrated not only the physiological and hormonal aspects involved in sexual arousal but also the psychological. These interacting aspects were characterised by numbers, allowing the simple designation of specific pathways by a linked chain of numbers. The model characterises sexual man as a "positive feedback-negative feedback relaxation oscillator". The relaxation oscillation occurs because there is a build-up of sexual arousal (23) which finally discharges through the emission and ejaculation (40, 47). When this happens, it inhibits (23–41) sexual arousal and arousability for a finite time (post-ejaculation refractory time, PERT). After a variable period, the PERT wears off and the circuit can be reset ready for a further arousal and its orgasmic discharge.

While the model obviously incorporated many features that previous models avoided, such as indicating that a single pathway does not exist for sexual functions or dysfunctions, e.g. sexual motivation has two dimensions, sexual arousal (23) and sexual arousability (29). The latter is influenced by the sensory modalities of touch (1), taste (2), smell (3), vision (4), hearing (5) and hormones (45). The model's complexity and just book publication undoubtedly limited its diffusion to a larger audience. The model was created over 20 years ago when little was published about brain imaging, actions of central transmitters and neuromodulators and reward centre circuitry. Updates on these aspects can be found in Pfaus [58] and Kingsberg, Clayton and Pfaus [59].

Unusual Models of Sexual Response

There are a few atypical and unusual models of the human sexual response. The cusp catastrophe model of sexual arousal previously described for both sexes has a mathematical equation to model the behaviour of a slow change reaching a cusp that suddenly creates a different behaviour. This equation was developed by Huby [1] for the male sexual response but not for the female because the latter was too complicated. Unsurprisingly, the equation has generally been ignored and has not made any impact in the field. Janssen, Everaerd, Spiering and Janssen [60] tentatively proposed a theoretical "information processing" model of sexual arousal, elaborated from the sexual dysfunction model of Barlow [61], based on the concept that such arousal involved physiological, psychological (cognitive and affective) and behavioural components. A rudimentary schema for this model is shown in Figure 4-10. In brief, stimuli activate attention and are then encoded automatically and compared with those in memory. If a match is found, it can be appraised as a sexual stimulus, and it then activates genital/systemic responses which focus the attention towards the stimulus creating a positive feedback loop. Further developments of the model have been made by Spiering, Everaerd and Laan [62]. In an effort to study the effect of the appraisal of sexual stimuli on sexual arousal in sexually functional women (controls) and those with superficial dyspareunia, Brauer et al. [63] undertook an experimental study. They found that those with dyspareunia reported marginally significantly more negative affect than the controls when fed sexual pain instructions compared to sexual enjoyment instructions. Their interpretation was that this provided preliminary evidence of the modulatory effects of the appraisal of sexual stimuli on subsequent genital response in women.

A rather unusual model, developed by Chiang and Chiang [64], was that of an "ideal cognitive model of sexual desire" using textual analysis of 27 languages and based on conceptual metaphors, metonymies (figures of speech) and related concepts. Comparing, on a linguistic perspective, their ideal cognitive model with related emotions, they proposed that "sexual desire" was an emotion closely related to those of love and happiness as all consist of physiological, cognitive, psychological and expressive components, but they also have specific components of their own. However, defining what sexual desire is has troubled many workers, and no single definition has been accomplished [23, 65–68].

The Contribution of Sexual Response Models to Clinical Practice

One important suggested function (Table 4-2) that a model should try to accomplish was "does it contribute to clinical practice?" The relevance of the sexual response models to clinical practice might at first be questioned especially as they do not reveal details of the physiological and possible pathophysiological process involved in the mechanisms of arousal (Levin, Both, Georgiadis, Kukkonen, Park and Yang [69]). Undeniably, however, the original female *EPOR* model of Masters and Johnson [14] was extensively utilised to support numerous aspects of the Diagnostic and Statistical Manual of Mental Disorders (DSM IV, American Psychiatric Association [70]), a key resource for many clinicians treating sexual problems. While being extremely useful in helping characterise various features of male sexual function and dysfunction, criticisms were levelled, however, as an approach to categorising female dysfunctions (Basson, Leiblum, Brotto et al. [71, 72]). The most recent revision of the DSM, DSM V, has an increased disregard of the unisexual *EPOR* model of sexual arousal (Ishak, Tobia [73]) and now prefers the "circular model" for female sexual function and dysfunction and identifies differences between male and female sexual dysfunctions. A similar preference was advocated by Rosen and Barsky [74].

A number of authors have promoted their models as possible useful contributions to clinical practice. Janssen, Everaerd, Spiering and Janssen [60] suggested that their information processing model was relevant to understanding the inhibition of sexual response in people with sexual arousal disorder. However, it has not gained much clinical popularity and seems to have been superseded by the "dual control model" [53]. While these authors discussed the relevance of their model to the clinical management of sexual problems, they stated that the evidence of its utility is very limited and restricted to men and that the focus is on sexual arousal rather than orgasm. Sanders, Graham and Milhausen [75] suggested that the scores obtained on the SESII-W could well have a predicted utility in identifying women likely to experience sexual difficulties and that the scales might be used as prognostic for possible treatments. Basson [35] claimed that her "circular model of overlapping phases of variable order reflects the well-documented typical co-morbidity of dysfunction in women", such co-morbidity was described by Lewis, Fugl-Meyer and Corona et al. [76]. In her opinion, "therapy begins by explaining the sexual response cycle, clarifying the points of interruption in the patient's own cycle so as to guide treatment". Perelman [41, 77] suggested, in regard to his Sexual Tipping Point® model, that "the greatest advantage of the STP model is the ease with which it provides clinicians as well as their patients (and their partners) with a common sense explanation of sexual problems and potential solutions". He has recently promoted the model as an integrated approach to the aetiology, diagnosis and treatment of men with delayed ejaculation [77]. Another claimed feature is that when appropriate drug medication is created for the specific dysfunction, the model can support such medication. Rellini [78] produced a highly specific theoretical model to facilitate understanding the sexual problems of women who had a history of child sexual abuse. She claimed that the model had advantages over others because it included the ability to guide the selection of cognitive and behavioural interventions for patients presenting for treatment.

Some Final Thoughts on Human Sex Response Models

The history of the modelling of the human male and female sexual response reveals the various facets that have gone into its productions from initially non-evidence-based conceptualisation later bolstered by physiology, psychology, neurology and sociology, and, like science, it is work in progress [79]. Most models are simplifications of reality, no one model is perfect, and no one model ticks all the boxes in Table 4-2, but significant developments can easily be seen over the 100 plus years between the model of Moll [8] and the contemporary ones. However, according to Perelman [37], the "differences in the conceptualizations of the female sexual response have not, surprisingly, led to a lack of diagnostic consensus and created contentious debates in sexual medicine circles". Should we expect models to conform to the Popperian standard of being scientific [80]—that is, to be able to be falsified? As Bancroft [44] has pointed out, this is not always possible as such rigour needs experimentation and the control of the circumstances which cannot take place in the real world. But there is little doubt that with further research and findings, models will become more comprehensive and more inclusive, making them more complex, less facile and perhaps less popular. One final comment, it is interesting to note that none of the sexual response models relate to how the changes induced by sexual arousal in the male, but especially in the female, are involved in the mechanisms of reproduction; these have been reviewed by Levin [81, 82].

References

1. Huby HM. Catastrophe theory and the human sexual response. 3rd international symposium on systems research, informatics and cybernetics. Baden Baden, Germany, 1991.
2. Gillon G, Barnea O. Erection mechanisms of the penis: a model based analysis. J Urol. 2002;168:2711–5.
3. Blanchard R, Kuban ME, Blak T, Klassen PE, Dickey R, Cantor JM. Sexual attraction to others: a comparison of two models of alloerotic responding in men. Arch Sex Med. 2012;41:13–29.
4. Gefen A, Chen J, Elad D. Computational tools in rehabilitation of erectile dysfunction. Med Eng Phys. 2001;23:69–82.
5. Gallup GG, Burch RL, Zappieri ML, Parvez R, Stockwell M, Davis JA. The human penis as a semen displacement device. Evol Human Behav. 2003;24:277–89.
6. Pfaus JG, Kippin TE, Coria-Avila G. What can animal models tell us about human sexual response? Annu Rev Sex Res. 2003;14: 1–63.

7. Ventura-Aquino E, Paredes RG. Animal models in sexual medicine: the need and importance of studying sexual motivation. Sex Med Rev. 2016; 1–15. http://dx.doi.org/10.1016/j.sxmr.2016.07.003.
8. Moll A. The sexual life of the child. New York, NY: Macmillan Co; 1912.
9. Ellis H. Studies in psychology of sex. Vol 2. New York: Random House; 1936.
10. Van de Velde TH. Ideal marriage. Its physiology and technique. Great Britain: William Heineman Medical Books Ltd; 1940. p. 181–91.
11. Reich W. The function of the orgasm. New York: Farrar, Straus & Giroux: 1973. p. 103.
12. Dickenson RL. Human sex anatomy. 2nd ed. Baltimore: The Williams & Wilkins Company; 1949.
13. Wenger MA, Jones FN, Jones MH. Physiological psychology. New York, NY: Holt, Rinehart & Winstone Inc.; 1956.
14. Masters WH, Johnson V. Human sexual response. 1st ed. Boston: Little, Brown & Company; 1966.
15. Tiefer L. Historical, scientific, clinical and feminist criticisms of the "human sexual response cycle" model. Annu Rev Sex Res. 1991;2: 1–23.
16. Basson R. Female sexual dysfunctions—the new model. Br J Diabetes Vasc Dis. 2002;2:267–70.
17. Robinson P. The modernisation of sex. London: Paul Elek; 1976.
18. Kaplan HS. Hypoactive sexual desire. J Sex Mar Ther. 1977;3: 3–9.
19. Kaplan HS. Disorders of sexual desire. New York: Simon & Schuster; 1979.
20. Lief HI. What's new in sex research? Inhibited sexual desire. Med Aspects Hum Sex. 1977;7:94–5.
21. Garde K, Lunde I. Female sexual behaviour. A study in a random sample of 40-year-old women. Maturitas. 1980;2:225–40.
22. Michael RT, Gagnon JH, Lauman EO, Kolata G. Sex in America: a definitive survey. London: Little Brown & Co; 1994.
23. Levin RJ. Sexual desire and the deconstruction and reconstruction of the human female sexual response model of Masters & Johnson. In: Everaerd W, Laan E, Both S, editors. Sexual appetite, desire and motivation: energetics of the sexual system. Amsterdam Royal Netherlands Academy of Arts and Science; 2001. p. 63–93.
24. Laqueur T. Making sex: body and gender from the Greeks to Freud. Cambridge MA: Harvard University Press; 1990.
25. Hoon PW. The assessment of sexual arousal in women. Prog Behav Modif. 1979;7:1–61.
26. Morrow B. Sex research and sex therapy: a sociological analysis of Masters and Johnson. New York: Routledge Taylor and Francis Group; 2008.
27. Levin RJ. Critically revisiting aspects of the human sexual response cycle of Masters & Johnson: correcting errors and suggesting modifications. Sex Relat Ther. 2008;23:393–9.
28. Whipple B, Brash-McGreer KB. Management of female sexual dysfunction. In: Sipski ML, Alexander CJ, editors. Sexual function in people with disability and chronic illness. A health professional's guide. Gaithersburg, MD: Aspen Publishers, Inc.; 1997. p. 509–34.
29. Greenberg JS, Bruess CE, Haffner DW. Exploring the dimensions of human sexuality. Burlington, MA: Jones & Bartlett Publishers; 2004.
30. Basson R. The female response: a different model. J Sex Marital Ther. 2000;26:51–65.
31. Sand M, Fisher WA. Women's endorsement of models of female sexual response: the nurses' sexuality study. J Sex Med. 2007;4: 708–19.
32. Wiegel M, Meston C, Rosen R. The female sexual function index (FSFI): cross validation and the development of clinical cut-off scores. J Sex Marital Ther. 2005;31:1–24.
33. Giles KR, McCabe MP. Conceptualizing women's sexual function: linear vs. circular models of sexual response. J Sex Med. 2009; 6:2761–71.
34. Hayes RD. Circular and linear modelling of female sexual desire and arousal. J Sex Res. 2011;48:130–41.
35. Basson R. Human sexual response. Chapter 2. In: Vodušek DB, Boller F, editors. Handbook of clinical neurology. Vol 180. 3rd series, Neurology of sexual and bladder disorders. 2015. p. 11–8.
36. Wylie K, Mimoun S. Sexual response models in women. Maturitas. 2009;63:112–5.
37. Perelman MA. History of sexual medicine. In: Diamond L, Tolman D, editors. APA handbook of sexuality and psychology handbook. Washington, DC: American Psychological Association; 2013. p. 138–79.
38. Giraldi A, Kristensen E, Sand M. Endorsement of models describing sexual response of men and women with a sexual partner: an online survey in a population sample of Danish adults 20-65 years. J Sex Med. 2015;12:116–28.
39. Basson R, Correia S, Driscoll M, Laan E, Toates F, Tiefer L. Problematic endorsement of models describing sexual response of men and women with a sexual partner. J Sex Med. 2015;12: 1948–850.
40. Giraldi A, Kristensen E, Sand M. Response and rebuttal of "endorsement of models describing sexual response of men and women with a sexual partner: an online survey in a population sample of Danish adults ages 25-65". J Sex Med. 2015;12:1848–50.
41. Perelman MA. Why the sexual tipping Point® model? Cur Sex Health Rep. 2016;8:39–46.
42. History of the sexual tipping point model at Www.Mapedf.Org/History. Accessed 21 Sept 2016.
43. Levin RJ. Revisiting post ejaculation refractory time—what we know and what we don't know in males and females. J Sex Med. 2009;6:2376–89.
44. Bancroft J. Human sexuality and its problems. 3rd ed. Edinburgh: Churchill Livingstone; 2012.
45. Zilbergeld B. Men and sex—a guide to sexual fulfilment. London: Souvenir Press; 1979. p. 105.
46. Nakopoulou E, Macaskill A, Wylie K, Hatzichristou D. Men use different response models during their lifespan: the role of erectile dysfunction and sexual motives. J Sex Med. 2010;7(Suppl 6):S377.
47. Levin RJ. The physiology of male and female sexual arousal. Chapter 26. In: Payne-James J, Busuttil A, Smock W, editors. Forensic medicine-clinical and pathological aspects. London: Greenwich Medical Media Limited; 2003. p. 379–98.
48. Levin RJ. Anatomy and physiology in the male. Chapter 3. In: Wylie K, editor. ABC of sexual health, 3rd ed. Oxford: Wiley; 2014. p. 7–11.
49. Levin RJ. Anatomy and physiology in the female. Chapter 4. In: Wylie K, editor. ABC of sexual health, 3rd ed. Oxford: Wiley; 2014. p. 12–5.
50. Kaplan HS. The sexual desire disorders: dysfunctional regulation of sexual motivation. New York, NY; Brunner/Mazel Inc.; 1995.
51. Kupferman I. Hypothalamus and limbic system motivation. In: Kandel ER, Schwartz JH, Jessel TM, editors. Principle of neural science. 3rd ed. New York: Elsevier; 1991. p. 751–5.
52. Bancroft J, Janssen E. The dual control model of male sexual response: theoretical approach to centrally mediated erectile dysfunction. Neurosci Biobehav Rev. 2000;24:571–9.
53. Bancroft J, Graham CA, Janssen E, Sanders SA. The dual control model: current status and future directions. J Sex Res. 2009;46: 121–42.
54. Graham CA, Sanders SA, Milhausen RR. The sexual excitation/sexual inhibition inventory for women: psychometric properties. Arch Sex Behav. 2006;35:397–409.

55. Milhausen RR, Graham C, Sanders SA, Yarber WL, Maitland SB. Validation of the sexual excitation/ inhibition inventory for men and women. Arch Sex Behav. 2010;39:1091–104.
56. Kurpisz J, Mak M, Lew-Starowicz M, Nowosielski K, Samochowiec J. The dual control model of sexual response by J. Bancroft and E. Janssen. Theoretical basis, research and practical issues. Postępy Psychiatrii I Neurologia. 2015;24:156–64.
57. Levin RJ. Human male sexuality: appetite and arousal, desire and drive. In: Legg CR, Booth DA, editors. Appetite-neural and behavioural basis. Oxford: Oxford University Press; 1994. p. 127–64.
58. Pfaus JG. Pathways of sexual desire. J Sex Med. 2009;6:1506–33.
59. Kingsberg SA, Clayton AH, Pfaus JG. The female sexual response: current models, neurobiological underpinnings and agents currently approved or under investigation for the treatment of hypoactive sexual; desire disorder. CNS Drugs. 2015;29:915–33.
60. Janssen E, Everaerd W, Spiering M, Janssen J. Automatic processes and the appraisal of sexual stimuli: toward an information processing model of sexual arousal. J Sex Res. 2000;37:8–23.
61. Barlow DH. Causes of sexual dysfunction: The role of anxiety and cognitive difference. J Consult Clin Psychol. 1986;54:140–8.
62. Spiering M, Everaerd W, Laan E. Conscious processing of sexual information: mechanisms of appraisal. Arch Sex Behav. 2004;33:369–80.
63. Brauer M, ter Kuile MM, Laan E. Effects of appraisal of sexual stimuli on sexual arousal in women with and without superficial dyspareunia. Arch Sex Behav. 2009;38:476–85.
64. Chiang AY, Chiang W-Y. Behold, I am coming soon! A study on the conceptualization of sexual orgasm in 27 languages. Metaphor Symb. 2016;31:131–47.
65. Everaerd W, Laan E. Sexual motivation and desire. In: Everaerd W, Laan E, Both S, editors. Sexual appetite, desire and motivation: energetics of the sexual system. Amsterdam, The Netherlands: Royal Netherlands Academy of Arts and Sciences; 2001. p. 96–110.
66. Heiman JR. Sexual desire in human relationships. In: Everaerd W, Laan E, Both S, editors. Sexual appetite, desire and motivation: energetics of the sexual system. Amsterdam, The Netherlands: Royal Netherlands Academy of Arts and Sciences; 2001. p. 117–34.
67. Buss DM. The evolution of desire: Strategies of human mating New York. New York: Basic Books; 1994.
68. Toates F. How sexual desire works. The enigmatic urge. Cambridge; Cambridge University Press; 2014.
69. Levin RJ, Both S, Georgiadis J, Kukkonen T, Park K, Yang CC. The physiology of sexual function and the pathophysiology of sexual dysfunction (Committee 13A). J Sex Med. 2016;13:733–59.
70. American Psychiatric Association. Diagnostic and statistical manual of mental disorders. 4th ed. Washington DC: American Psychiatric Association; 1994.
71. Basson R, Leiblum S, Brotto L, et al. Definitions of women's sexual dysfunction reconsidered: advocating expansion and revision. J Psychosom Obstet Gynecol. 2003;24:221–9.
72. Basson R, Leiblum S, Brotto L, et al. Revised definitions of women's sexual dysfunction. J Sex Med. 2004;1:40–8.
73. Ishak WW, Tobia G. DSM-5 changes in diagnostic criteria of sexual dysfunctions. Reprod Syst Sex Disord. 2013;2.2: http://dz.doi.org/10.4172/2162-038X.1000122.
74. Rosen RR, Barsky JL. Normal sexual response in women. Obstet Gynecol Clin North Am. 2006;33:515–26.
75. Sanders SA, Graham C, Milhausen RR. Predicting sexual problems in women: the relevance of sexual excitation and sexual inhibition. Arch Sex Behav. 2008;37:241–51.
76. Lewis RW, Fugl-Meyer KS, Corona G, et al. Definitions/epidemiology/risk factors for sexual dysfunction. J Sex Med. 2010;7:1598–607.
77. Perelman M. Psychosexual therapy for delayed ejaculation based on the sexual tipping point model. Transl Androl Urol. 2016;5:563–75.
78. Rellini A. Review of the empirical evidence for a theoretical model to understand the sexual problems of women with a history of CSA. J Sex Med. 2008;5:31–46.
79. Rutherford A. A brief history of everyone who ever lived: the stories in our genes. Weidenfield & Nicolson; 2016.
80. Popper K. The logic of scientific discovery. London: Routledge Classics; 2002.
81. Levin RJ. Sexual arousal—its physiological roles in human reproduction. Annu Rev Sex Res. 2005;16:154–89.
82. Levin RJ. Recreation and procreation: a critical view of sex in the human female. Clin Anat. 2015;28:339–54.

5 Facilitators and Barriers in Sexual History Taking

Ana Virgolino, Luis Roxo, and Violeta Alarcão

"It is pointless to ask: Why then is sex so secret? What is this force that so long reduced it to silence and has only recently relaxed its hold somewhat, allowing us to question it perhaps, but always in the context of and through its repression?"

——Michel Foucault, The History of Sexuality: An Introduction: 1.

Abbreviations

AIDS	Acquired immune deficiency syndrome
FSD	Female sexual dysfunction
FSW	Female sex workers
GP	General practitioner
HIV	Human immunodeficiency virus
HSDD	Hypoactive sexual desire disorder
IV	Intravenous
LGBT	Lesbian, gay, bisexual, transgender
LGBTQ	Lesbian, gay, bisexual, transgender, queer or questioning
MESH	Medical subject headings
MSM	Men who have sex with men
OB/GYN	Obstetrician/gynaecologist
PCP	Primary care physicians
SD	Sexual dysfunction
STD	Sexual transmitted diseases
STI	Sexual transmitted infections

Introduction

In a contemporary pluralistic society, sex is envisaged as an adult recreation, a saleable commodity, the personal orientation of desire and the usual method for procreation [1]. Throughout history, civilizations have attempted to repress sexual expression in an effort to define what is considered normal sexuality. More recently, however, within a context of sexual revolution and new movements, the topic of sex has moved from the confines of private discussions to an accepted presence in most of public domains [1, 2]. Modern Western culture is now impregnated with colourful and sometimes explicit images of sexuality and intimacy to advertise and market products using all media and communication technology available [3].

Over the years, on the vanguard of this fever, clinical practice has witnessed a similar reverse. Sex and sexuality once considered taboo subjects started being approached from a more inclusive perspective [4]. Health professionals come to agree on the importance of integrating sex-related questions into a general health history [2], and some residency programmes and medical schools have endeavoured to gradually adjust their curricula to incorporate these topics [4, 5]. Furthermore, the advent of HIV/AIDS and child sexual abuse has markedly changed attitudes towards talking about sexual issues in health settings [6].

Yet, sexual history taking is not readily and easily incorporated into patient assessments [7]. Several barriers still impede the discussion of intimacy and sexual functioning. Sex continues to be embedded in misconceptions and stereotypes, and for most health-care providers, talking about specific issues of sexuality creates a degree of discomfort and embarrassment as sexual issues are regarded as very "private" and "personal" matters [8, 9].

Sexual history taking is vital for diagnostic, therapeutic and preventive reasons, being one of the best ways to lessen the potential impact of medical conditions and improve quality of life [7, 10]. Omitting it may have negative consequences for care. For example, not inquiring about sexual difficulties might lead patients to believe them unimportant, insignificant or not amenable to treatment which might buffer the initiation of or delay of proper treatment or referrals [9, 11, 12].

W.W. IsHak (ed.), *The Textbook of Clinical Sexual Medicine*, DOI 10.1007/978-3-319-52539-6_5

The purpose of this chapter is to undertake a review on the barriers and facilitators health professionals[1] encounter when taking a sexual history. The map of the circumstances under which sexual histories are obtained will help in identifying important areas for further research and tailored interventions.

In a period of changing assumptions, perceptions and attitudes towards sex and sexuality, given the unique position they hold, the consideration of the viewpoint of health professionals is a structural element in the evaluation procedure of the quality of the provided sexual health-care services. Within the intersection with patients' opinions, the look at providers' perspectives will allow an in-depth understanding of the ongoing improvement processes which ultimately have an impact on the functioning of health systems.

This chapter is organized into five parts. On the first part, we describe the fundamental theoretical concepts that are on the basis of the current work. The second part presents the study itself, including the main objectives and the operational framework adopted. The followed methodology for data collection and analysis is described on the third part. The fourth and fifth parts are dedicated to the description, discussion and interpretation of the results, with the identification of barriers and facilitators to sexual history taking.

Taking a Sexual History

Sexuality is a central part of human life and general wellbeing, encompassing feelings that are experienced and expressed in language, thoughts, beliefs, attitudes, values, behaviours, practices and relationships [13, 14]. As awareness on issues of sexuality has been increasing, sexual health history is ever more thought of as an indispensable part of the general health assessment [9, 15].

The main purpose of taking a sexual history is to assess a patient's sexual background and current functioning [16]. It provides a firm basis for gaining a good understanding of sexual health and sexual problems as well as setting the agenda for issues regarding specific risks to be further explored [17, 18]. A detailed sexual history should allow:

1. A careful assessment of symptoms which will guide the examination and testing
2. An exposure history to identify which sites need to be sampled and the sexual transmitted diseases (STDs) to which the patient may be at risk
3. An assessment of contraception use and risk of pregnancy
4. An assessment of other sexual health issues (including a discussion of psychosexual problems)
5. An assessment of HIV, hepatitis B and C risk for both testing and prevention
6. An assessment of risk behaviours, which will then facilitate sexual health promotion activities [19, 20]

[1]Sexual history taking is relevant in different clinical specialties. The terms "health-care professional", "health-care provider", "provider" and "clinician" are interchangeably used throughout the chapter since there are other professional areas (e.g. nursing, psychology, among others) that are also in advantageous positions to address these topics by the reason that their work in clinical practice also involves the need to build a therapeutic relationship with the patient.

General Guidelines for Sexual History Taking

Taking a sexual history should begin in the initial stage of care [16, 21]. From the very first moment, the health professional needs to take into consideration how to put the patient at ease, find out what the real problem is, discover his/her background and clinical history and then work out a management plan [22]. To that end, several communication strategies and skills can enhance the efficiency and effectiveness of this process (Box 5-1) [2, 20, 23, 24].

Box 5-1. Key Aspects of Taking a Sexual History

- *The first contact with the patient*
- *The use of appropriate body language*
- *The initiation of the consultation with open-ended questions (including the assurance of privacy and confidentiality) followed by an exploration of previous concerns and the use of more closed questions as the interview continues (emotionally charged questions and areas should be approached gradually and may be deferred for a second or subsequent interview)*
- *The adoption of a direct, sensitive, non-judgmental approach with inquiry*
- *The explanation of the rationale for some of the questions asked*
- *The use of clear, geared to the lay person–language and with which both clinician and patient feel comfortable (sexually explicit terminology may serve to desensitize to any embarrassment or hesitation but should be used after a very careful judgement in deciding if it would be appropriate)*
- *The quest for details that must be balanced by sensitivity to the patient's concerns and feelings as the information is collected and the interview proceeds*
- The *awareness of the signs of distress and anxiety from the patient*
- *The observation of non-verbal cues from the patient (body language and facial expressions)*

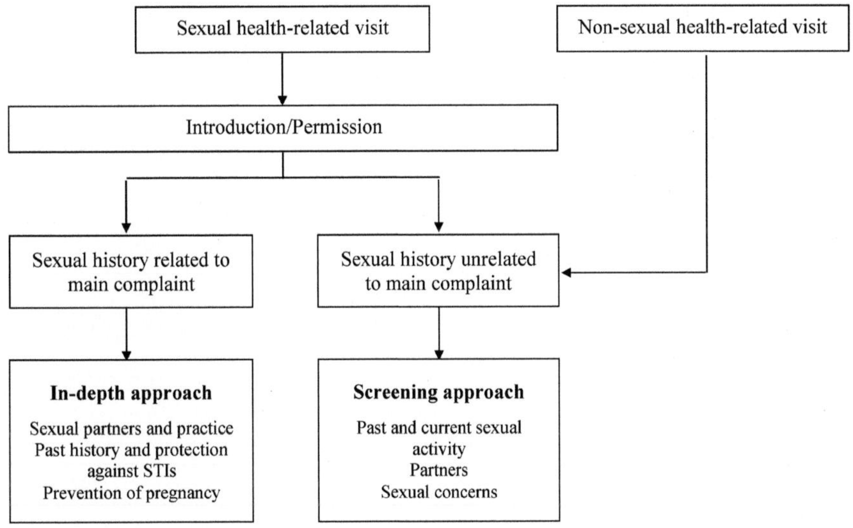

FIGURE 5-1. Screening and in-depth sexual health history.

A key to facilitate taking a sexual history is communication [9] which might be an important element in improving health outcomes [20, 25]. Establishing rapport and putting patients at ease are important first steps and help patients feeling comfortable when reporting their sexual concerns [2].

The health professional sets the tone for the conversation. Talking about "sex" is what begins this process and is the key to the search for understanding sexual thoughts, sexual feelings and sexual actions—ultimately it is the key to helping patients [6]. Though experience and skills in taking a sexual history are pivotal foundations, so patients can be sympathetically encouraged to reveal the intimate details of their private life [2, 17].

A Comprehensive Approach: Screening or In-Depth Sexual Health History

Numerous health-related conditions, life events and developmental milestones can be associated with the development of sexual problems. The best occasion to undertake a sexual history or initiate a discussion of sexual concerns varies depending on the nature of the visit [2]. The clinician needs to adjust the scope of the history and physical examination to the situation at hand [26].

The transition to the sexual health history can be done throughout the introduction of a routine way to elicit the patient's sexual history by linking the sexual history to the patient's medical history or current health problem which will make it easier to gather the needed data [27].

There are two ways to approach the interview in sexual history taking: the screening and the in-depth approach (Figure 5-1). An abbreviated basic assessment with a minimal number of specific screening questions will be sufficient if the sexual history appears unrelated to the main complaint brought by the patient. These questions which focus past and current sexual activity, partners and sexual concerns will guide the determination of possible sexual health needs of the patient [2, 27].

If the patient's sexual history seems directly related to the main complaint, a complete history is indicated for a thorough sexual assessment [27]. Relevant information ought to include[2] sexual and reproductive history and current status (sexual partners and practice, past history and protection against STIs and prevention of pregnancy) in addition to past medical history and current health status (viz., endocrine system, neurologic diseases, cardiovascular disease, psychiatric illness and current use of prescription and over-the-counter medicines). A physical examination or laboratory testing could be used complementary to determine the physiologic factors involved in a sexual complaint [2].

Screening and In-Depth Sexual Health History

In obtaining a detailed sexual history alongside the assessment of each domain of function as to its individual or combined impact [2], the biopsychosocial model [28] provides a comprehensive holistic framework for it takes into account medical, psychological, intrapsychic, interpersonal, social, cultural and ethnic variables that may affect sexual health and function [7, 18] (Figure 5-2). Since sexual health encompasses many facets of a person's life, the clinician needs to guard against simplistic thinking about the cause and treat-

[2]More detailed examples of screening and in-depth sexual history approaches are available elsewhere [6, 27].

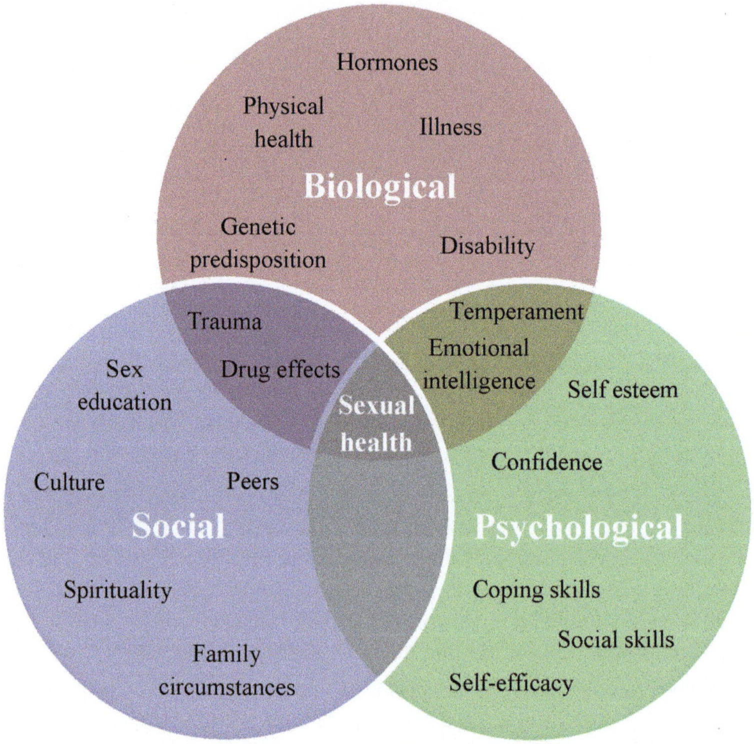

Figure 5-2. Biopsychosocial model of sexual health. [Adapted from Wylie KR. ABC of Sexual Health. John Wiley & Sons; 2015. With permission from Wiley].

ment of sexual problems and take time to perform a comprehensive biopsychosocial assessment. This is essential to identify the predisposing, precipitating, maintaining and contextual factors[3] responsible for the problem [10, 29].

Only by bearing this structure in mind while taking a sexual history, clinicians can offer more efficacious, efficient and better tolerated treatments by patients and their partners [18].

Barriers to Effective Sexual History Taking

Sexual health is important throughout the entire lifespan. Individuals of all ages and backgrounds are at risk and should have access to the knowledge and services necessary for optimal sexual health. Given the public health impact that these risks have, health professionals are instrumental in promoting sexual health. Nonetheless, issues around sexuality can be difficult to discuss because they are intimate and because there is great diversity in how they are perceived and approached [30].

Patients are becoming more demanding and clamour for explicit information and clear guidance in dealing with sexual problems and complaints. Most expect their health-care provider to be an expert in all aspects of sexual health [6]. Nonetheless, several obstacles impede the communication about sexual topics. The obstacles can be categorized as patient based and health-care provider based.

General barriers pointed out by patients are the lack of opportunity to discuss the subject, a sense of discomfort, embarrassment or shame when there is openness to approach it during consultation [23, 31]. Feelings of uncertainty whether sexual problems/concerns are part of health care and if the provider is the suitable specialist to treat sexual problems/concerns often undermine a transparent dialogue [23, 32]. Taboos held by society against the open discussion of sexuality can also constitute an impediment to seek professional help [33, 34].

The most commonplace health-care provider-based obstacle is the inadequate or insufficient training in sexual health [35] (Table 5-1). Despite much progress in the past years, medical schools often lack trained sexuality educators [36] and still have inadequate sex education curricula which fail to emphasize the importance of sexual functioning [5, 37]. This gap becomes even more pronounced attending to the fact that health providers are interested and recognize the

[3]Predisposing factors are defined as the long-term experiences that might influence sexual thoughts, feelings and behaviours (e.g. restricted family views of sex, early life experiences of sex and intimacy, chronic conditions, child sexual abuse or attachment difficulties). Precipitating factors are those which might be understood as "triggers" and are likely to have occurred just before the onset of the problem (e.g. a recent medical diagnosis, change in medication, job loss or family transitions). Maintaining factors are the patterns of interaction and/or behaviour that influence the problem and "keep it going" and may be displayed as communication difficulties in couples, sexual boredom, depression in one partner or cognitive interference [7, 18].

Table 5-1. Health-care providers' barriers to effective sexual history taking

Inadequate/insufficient education or training in sexual health
Time constraints
Reimbursement concerns
Personal conservative sexual beliefs
Deficits in communication skills
Growing knowledge gap between developments in sexual medicine and the clinical skills of the clinician
Generational obstacles
Cultural differences of the practitioner and the patient

importance in attaining expertise in sexual history taking but ended up showing marked deficit communication skills when in a consultation [35].

Limited time and concerns about insurance reimbursement can also hinder clinician's capacity to take an open discussion about sexual issues, especially as sexual topics are often raised by patients towards the end of a consultation. Many providers are unaware that a simple query about sexual concerns and one or two follow-up questions only add 2 to 3 min to an appointment. If a more complete sexual history or assessment is warranted, a follow-up visit can be scheduled (and billed appropriately with ICD-9 codes), or a referral to a specialist in treating sexual dysfunctions can be made [2, 35].

When working with specific populations, conflicting attitudes and perceptions may emerge, and providers may have difficulties disconnecting from their own personal belief system. Also, they often rationalize not talking to clients about sexual issues by saying that clients do not raise the issue [36].

Moreover, the growing knowledge gap between developments in sexual medicine and the clinical skills of the clinician is also a reason elicited by providers for not taking a sexual history. This might be a consequence of lack of formal education and training which often leads to a lack of confidence in knowledge and mastery in this area [2, 32].

Finally, the age and gender of either the patient or the provider as well as cultural differences between both may also play a role in how information is exchanged [37]. Within a multicultural society, where cultural and religious differences are inevitable, these discrepancies are worrisome. The concern is that, because of these barriers, health professionals may shy away from taking sexual histories from patients and, thus, be unable to identify patients' health needs [32].

So what are the remedies for this situation? How can the clinician become proficient in taking a sexual history? One way in which the clinician will gain comfort and ease in obtaining a sex history and performing a general examination is by practice [34]. If clinicians take the step of including sexual history more routinely into their daily practice, much ground can be gained. Increasing the frequency of sexual health inquiries will substantially improve sexual health care through earlier identification of sexual problems and intervention. Routine assessment of sexual health also provides opportunities for preventive care, such as immunization against hepatitis B and counselling on sexual risk taking [27, 37].

Barriers to sexual health care can also be removed by assuring medical education that teaches sexual health care as integral to health care in general [27]. For clinicians who remain uncomfortable with taking a detailed history, written sexual history inventories are also effective. Similarly, referral to clinicians with special interest in sexual function is always an appropriate alternative [37].

The Study

The main objective of this work was to explore, integrate and summarize current knowledge on the perceived obstacles and facilitators for taking a sexual history encountered by health professionals in their clinical practice. The exploration of providers' perspectives is justified by the fact that health-care providers hold clinical and institutional knowledge nurtured with relevant information about the practices surrounding sexual history taking when examining patients.

The adopted posture was one of the eliciting emergent redundancies or disparities in terms of optimal care provision in specific settings and intervention areas, namely, sexual health education/promotion; STDs; sexuality and disease; sexual dysfunction; lesbian, gay, bisexual, transgender, queer or questioning (LGBTQ); and sexual violence. This way, we aim to uncover key areas which require further research and tailored interventions in the context of sexual health promotion.

For this purpose, we employed a narrative review approach, preceded by a scoping analysis [38, 39], to determine the adequate and most cited terms in scientific search databases. This combined strategy seems well suited for first identifying the appropriate parameters of a review and its potential scope.

The Collected Information

Search Strategy and Selection Criteria

A narrative review of literature was conducted through a search of published studies contained in the PubMed and Web of Science electronic databases. Publication date (from January 1, 1995, to December 31, 2015) and language of the documents (English) were used as restriction filters. The search was undertaken on April 27, 2016, using both free-text and "medical subject headings" (MeSH) terms combined as

TABLE 5-2. The search strategy

Search terms and sequence	#2 "sexual history" AND "facilitators"
#1 "sexual history" AND "barriers"	#4 "sexual history" AND "sexual dysfunction"
#3 "sexual history" AND "attitude of health personnel"	#6 "sexual history" AND "patient-centered care"
#5 "sexual history" AND "sexual disorder"	#8 "sexual evaluation" AND "barriers"
#7 "sexual history" AND "biopsychosocial model"	#10 "sexual evaluation" AND "attitude of health personnel"
#9 "sexual evaluation" AND "facilitators"	#12 "sexual evaluation" AND "sexual disorder"
#11 "sexual evaluation" AND "sexual dysfunction"	#14 "sexual evaluation" AND "biopsychosocial model"
#13 "sexual evaluation" AND "patient-centered care"	#16 "sexual assessment" AND "facilitators"
#15 "sexual assessment" AND "barriers"	#17 "sexual assessment" AND "sexual dysfunction"
#17 "sexual assessment" AND "attitude of health personnel"	#20 "sexual assessment" AND "patient-centered care"
#19 "sexual history" AND "sexual disorder"	#22 "sexual interview" AND "barriers"
#21 "sexual history" AND "biopsychosocial model"	#24 "sexual interview " AND "attitude of health personnel"
#23 "sexual interview" AND "facilitators"	#26 "sexual interview " AND "sexual disorder"
#25 "sexual interview " AND "sexual dysfunction"	#28 "sexual interview " AND "biopsychosocial model"
#27 "sexual interview " AND "patient-centered care"	

alternatives: "sexual history", "sexual evaluation", "sexual assessment", "sexual interview", "barriers", "facilitators", "attitude of health personnel", "sexual dysfunction", "sexual disorder", "patient-centred care" and "biopsychosocial model". Details of the search terms are given in Table 5-2. Screening of the lists of references in the identified articles was used as additional strategy to identify otherwise unfound published articles.

Screening Process

All citations identified by the above searches were downloaded and duplicates removed. Titles and abstracts of the identified papers were independently screened by at least two authors for consensus on eligibility and content. In case of disagreement, the third author made a decision on whether to maintain or exclude the paper from the review. Potentially relevant papers were assessed according to the following inclusion criteria: (1) empirical and self-contained research documents, (2) articles in which the population under study was consisted of health professionals, (3) papers that explore the views of health professionals with regard to facilitators and barriers in taking a sexual history and (4) full texts which are in English. Studies published before 1995 and after 2015, without a focus on the sexual history taking and on professionals' knowledge, attitudes or perceptions on that process, were excluded. Opinion articles and conceptual papers were also discarded from the review.

The screening covered an initial 10% of the articles to determinate the necessity to perform alterations in inclusion and exclusion criteria, being made redefinitions at this stage. Subsequently, all article titles and abstracts were appraised taking the reformulated inclusion/exclusion criteria into consideration.

Data Extraction and Quality Assessment

Data was extracted into a standardized matrix that included the area of the article (sexual health education/promotion, STDs, sexuality and disease, sexual dysfunction, LGBTQ, and sexual violence), authors, year of publication, sample characteristics, variables/measures, study design, major findings (including facilitators and barriers) and comments.

The authors independently appraised the quality of the evidence produced by studies, attending to the purposes of this review of enlightening the barriers and the facilitators for sexual history taking and identifying important areas for further research and tailored interventions.[4]

The papers were categorized by study design using the following categories: cross-sectional survey, literature review, qualitative study and intervention study.

Results

The study selection process is shown in Figure 5-3. A total of 56 (60%) articles from an initial list of 94 citations were considered eligible for this review. These articles were published between 1995 and 2015, the majority (n = 39; 70%) within the last 10 years. Not only the last decade was more prolific, but also new areas of research emerge, such as LGBTQ and sexuality and disease. In fact, six different research areas and one miscellaneous (with more than one area) were identified among the eligible studies, as it is shown in Figure 5-4.

Four major study methodologies were identified, as it can be seen in Figure 5-5 and Table 5-3. The majority of the analysed articles were cross-sectional surveys (n = 36; 64%), but also qualitative studies (n = 11; 20%), interventions studies (n = 6; 11%) and literature reviews (n = 3; 5%) were included.

For a more detailed outline of each of these 56 articles, please see our supplemental table (Table 5-4).

Health professionals perceived barriers and facilitators for taking sexual history derived from the selected articles

[4]This review does not deeply evaluate the methodological quality of all available studies.

FIGURE 5-3. Fluxogram for article selection.

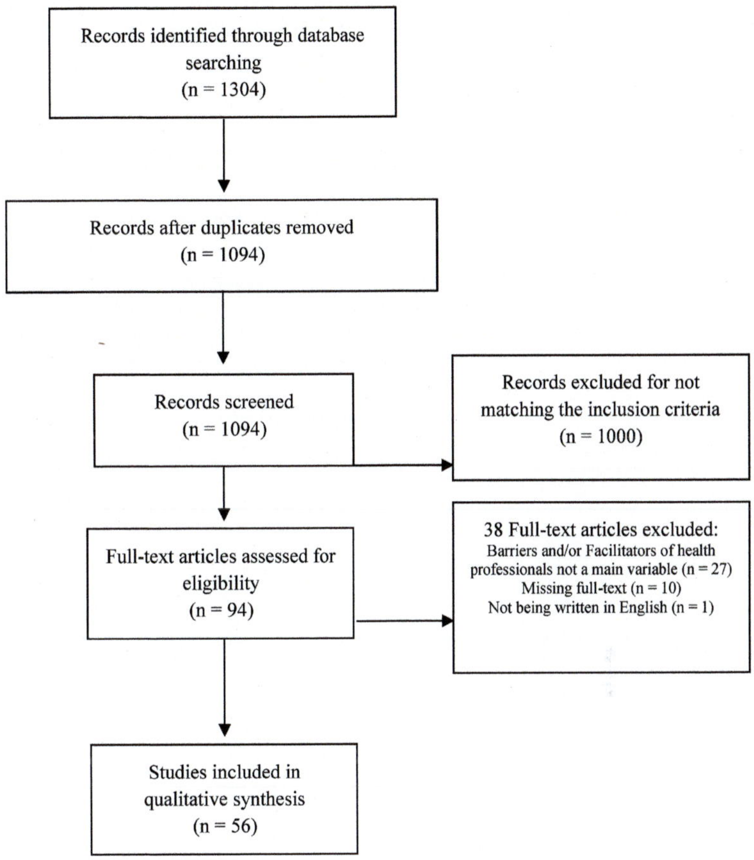

FIGURE 5-4. Studies' research areas.

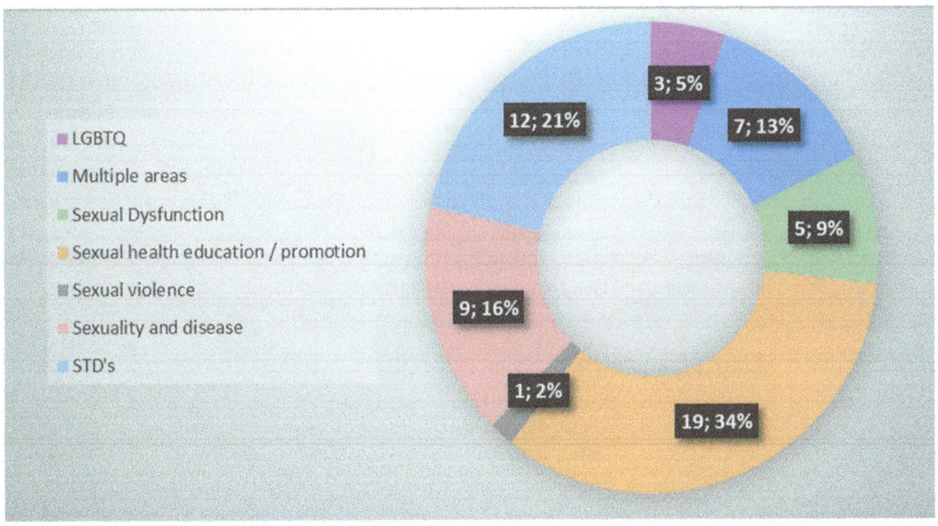

Figure 5-5. Studies' methods.

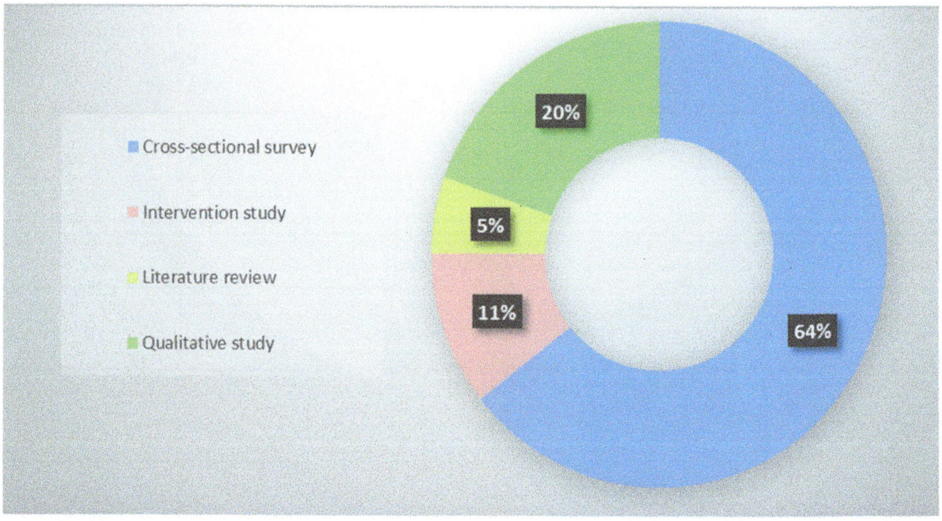

Table 5-3. 1995–2015 Peer-reviewed studies and methodologies and areas

Methodology	Areas	Studies
Cross-sectional survey ($n = 36$; 64%)	Sexual health education/ promotion ($n = 14$; 39%)	(Ariffin et al. 2015) (Bouman and Arcelus 2001) (Bull et al. 1999) (Burd et al. 2006) (Dadich and Hosseinzadeh 2013) (Jolley 2002) (Morand et al. 2009) (Sobecki et al. 2012) (Stokes and Mears 2000) (Temple-Smith et al. 1999) (Tsai and Hsiung 2003) (Tsai 2004) (Tsimtsiou et al. 2006) (Vieira et al. 2015)
	STDs ($n = 8$; 22%)	(Do et al. 2015) (Khan et al. 2007) (Khan et al. 2008) (Maheux et al. 1995) (McGrath et al. 2011) (Tucker et al. 2012) (Verhoeven et al. 2003) (Webber et al. 2009)
	Sexual dysfunction ($n - 5$; 14%)	(Abdolrasulnia et al. 2010) (Goldstein et al. 2009) (Humphery and Nazareth 2001) (Platano et al. 2008) (Ribeiro et al. 2014)
	Sexuality and disease ($n = 4$; 11%)	(Byrne et al. 2013) (Cort et al. 2001) (Doherty et al. 2011) (Oskay et al. 2014)
	LGBTQ ($n = 3$; 8%)	(Hayes et al. 2015) (Kitts 2010) (Sanchez et al. 2006)
	Multiple areas ($n = 2$; 6%)	(Barber et al. 2011) (Wiggins et al. 2007)
Qualitative study ($n = 11$; 20%)	Multiple areas ($n = 5$; 46%)	(Carter et al. 2014) (Collins 2006) (Hinchliff et al. 2005) (Stead et al. 2003) (Wendt et al. 2011)
	Sexuality and disease ($n = 2$; 18%)	(Hordern and Street 2007) (Mellor et al. 2013)
	Sexual health education/ promotion ($n = 2$; 18%)	(Gott et al. 2004) (Schweizer et al. 2013)
	Sexual violence ($n = 1$; 9%)	(Leder et al. 1999)
	STDs ($n = 1$; 9%)	(Woodbridge et al. 2015)
Intervention study ($n = 6$; 11%)	Sexual health education/ promotion ($n = 2$; 33%)	(Cushing et al. 2005) (Leeper et al. 2007)
	STDs ($n = 2$; 33%)	(Lanier et al. 2014) (Patel et al. 2009)
	Sexuality and disease ($n = 2$; 33%)	(Quinn and Happell 2013) (Quinn et al. 2013)
Literature review ($n = 3$; 5%)	Sexuality and disease ($n = 1$; 33%)	(Quinn and Happell 2013)
	Sexual health education/ promotion ($n = 1$; 33%)	(Kingsberg 2006)
	STDs ($n = 1$; 33%)	(Emmanuel and Martinez 2011)

(continued)

N.A.: Articles miscellaneous were classified as multiple areas.

TABLE 5-4. 1995–2015 Peer-reviewed studies and methodologies related to health professionals' facilitators and barriers in sexual history taking

Areas[a]	Author, year	Sample	Measures	Study design	Facilitators and barriers	Comments and commonalities
Sexual health education/ promotion ($n = 19$)	(Ariffin et al. 2015)	$N = 379$, final-year medical students	Attitudes and perceptions regarding training on taking sexual histories	Cross-sectional survey	*Barriers* (1) feeling uncomfortable in taking sexual histories from patients, (2) cultural and religious differences between the doctor and the patient, (3) having received training not adequate to prepare doctors to take sexual histories	Participants reported high interest in sexual health and felt it was important for doctors to know how to take a sexual history. The delivery of sexual health education programme should incorporate confidence building and to make students feel comfortable to take sexual histories from patients
	(Bouman and Arcelus 2001)	N[20;24], general consultant psychiatrists	Perceptions on taking a sexual history and management of sexual dysfunction	Cross-sectional survey	*Barriers* (1) conflicting attitudes and perceptions of the patients who rarely volunteer their symptoms, (2) difficulties of the psychiatrists in disconnecting from their own personal belief system regarding aged sexuality, (3) lack of awareness of physiological, pharmacological and psychosocial bases of sexual problems, (4) referral of middle-aged patient with sexual dysfunction to sexual therapy and elderly patients to community psychiatric nurses, (5) sexual therapy not included in the training schemes of community psychiatric nurses	Sexual history is often omitted in the psychiatric assessment of elderly men; elderly men with sexual dysfunction do not receive appropriate referral and treatment
	(Bull et al. 1999)	$N = 121$ clinic sites, 208 service providers (physician extenders, nurses, nonclinical administrators, nursing or medical assistants or clerical staff)	Sexual history	Cross-sectional survey	*Facilitators* (1) good communication skills, (2) training and experience, (3) provider comfort *Barriers* (1) client emotional response to sexual transmitted diseases (STDs), (2) lack of time, (3) client reluctance to talk about STDs, (4) client reluctance to change behaviour, (5) client resistance to discuss STDs	Practice patterns for the elicitation of sexual history were inconsistent. Sexual history taking was described as routine in 57% of sites
	(Burd et al. 2006)	$N = 78$, physicians (obstetrician/ gynaecologist—ob/gyns, family practitioners, internists, paediatricians and surgeons)	Discomfort during interviews	Cross-sectional survey	*Barriers* (*Characteristics causing discomfort*) (1) patient's age <18 and >65, (2) patient's academic achievement below college level, (3) patient's marital status (divorced or single), (4) interviewing opposite gender patients	88% reported taking sexual histories; 13% reported asking about sexual dysfunction in every patient interview
	(Cushing et al. 2005)	$N = 192$, medical students attending a workshop	Attitudes, behavioural intentions, behaviour (pre- and postworkshop evaluations)	Intervention study	*Facilitators* (*By the end of the workshop*) (1) students more likely to think they would initiate discussion of patients' sexual problems and to think that patients want doctors to make such enquiries; (2) students more likely to think that sexual problems could be an issue for patients with serious illnesses such as gynaecological cancers, (3) students more likely to ask patients' questions about sex in situations when it could be relevant	Attendance at the sexual health workshops or any one particular teaching session on sexual health was not a predictor of whether students asked patients about sexual health in subsequent clinical settings, but those students who had attended an additional teaching session were more likely to have done so. Predominantly it was in obstetrics and gynaecology or infectious disease clinical settings where students asked questions. A minority had asked such questions in general practice settings

(continued)

TABLE 5-4. (continued)

Areas[a]	Author, year	Sample	Measures	Study design	Facilitators and barriers	Comments and commonalities
	(Dadich and Hosseinzadeh 2013)	$N = 431$ clinicians (214generalpractitioners—GP—and 217 practice nurses)	Awareness, use and perceived impact of six resources to promote sexual health care: a placard that guides sexual health consultations, an interactive course, a face-to-face programme of active learning, an independent learning programme booklet, a practice nurse postcard to help practice nurses undertake a preventative women's health check, an online interactive training course	Cross-sectional survey	*Facilitators* (1) six different resources were reported to improve the delivery of sexual health care, (2) the reorganization of the primary care sector, (3) the removal of particular medical benefits scheme items *Barriers* (1) limited time, (2) limited perceived need, (3) limited access to and familiarity with the resources	The results highlight (1) the translation of evidence-based practices into patient care is viable despite reform, (2) the potential value of a multimodal approach; (3) the dissemination of relatively inexpensive resources might influence clinical practices, (4) reforms to governance and/or funding arrangements may widen the void between evidence-based practices and patient care
	(Gott et al. 2004)	$N = 22$, GP working in demographically diverse primary care practices	Sex and sexual health in primary care: effect of patient age upon GPs' management of sexual health issues	Qualitative study	*Barriers* (1) sexual health priorities within primary care not perceived as relevant to older people, (2) communication and training issues, (3) sex as "private" for older people and the risk of causing offence, (4) understandings of sexuality and old age	GPs do not address sexual health proactively with older people; sexual health is equated with younger people and not seen as a "legitimate" topic for discussion with this age group; beliefs are based on stereotyped views of ageing and sexuality, rather than personal experience of individual patients
	(Jolley 2002)	Gynaecology nurses	Frequency of sexual history and barriers for taking sexual history	Cross-sectional survey	*Facilitators* (1) guidance on taking a sexual history	The results of the survey suggest that gynaecology nurses need clear guidelines and policies for sexual history taking, supported by education and training
	(Kingsberg 2006)	Clinicians	Barriers for taking sexual history and assess current sexual function in women	Literature review	*Barriers* (1) insufficient medical education or training, (2) lack of confidence, (3) underestimation of sexual dysfunction prevalence, (4) time pressure, (5) few perceived treatment option, (6) patient discomfort	The importance of sexual health to a woman's quality of life is often understated. The most effective treatment is to ask
	(Leeper et al. 2007)	$N = 92$, medical students	Satisfaction with the course, content learned (sexual history taking skills)	Intervention study	*Facilitators* (1) knowledge on how to effectively apply different questions for different patient age groups and situations, (2) practice of exercises and feedback in the course, (3) role playing the discussion of difficult topics such as human immunodeficiency virus (HIV) with patients *Barriers* (1) Deficiency in sexual history-taking education	The need of more information on legal aspects of reporting and minor confidentiality, sexual assault, information about taking a sexual history from children, the elderly and intravenous (IV) drug users was identified
	(Morand et al. 2009)	$N = 56$, medical students and residents in a paediatric emergency department	Barriers to taking a sexual history	Cross-sectional survey	*Barriers* (1) young age of the patient (adolescent girls presenting to the emergency department with abdominal pain), (2) presence of the patient's parents during the consultation, (3) unsubstantiated beliefs that the patient was chaste, (4) lack of training	The barriers to taking a sexual history in adolescent girls are multifaceted. Further training is needed to expose learners' preconceived notions of sexuality as barriers to taking a sexual history, to provide practical methods for overcoming those barriers and to further instil in learners the importance of doing so

(Schweizer et al. 2013)	$N = 30$, gynaecologists	Approaching sexuality during gynaecological consultations, the place of sexuality during consultations and training in sexology	Qualitative study	*Facilitators* (1) keeping the discussion open, by offering, from the gynaecologist's perspective, the opportunity for the patient to address sexuality; (2) training in sexology *Barriers* (1) lack of tools, (2) a sense of modesty, (3) eroticization of the relationship	The decision to integrate questions relating to sexuality seems to depend on non-medical factors such as the personal experience, interest or gender of the doctor The majority of interviewed gynaecologists claimed that they asked their patients if they had "pain during intercourse" or if they had "any concerns in that area". Male gynaecologists asked questions relating to methods of contraception. Female gynaecologists asked questions relating to the patient's relationships. Only gynaecologists trained in sexology widened the field of enquiry by asking if the patient felt pleasure during intercourse, or if the patient's partner is a man or a woman
(Sobecki et al. 2012)	$N = 1.154$, practising ob/gyns	Practices of communication with patients about sex	Cross-sectional survey	*Facilitators* (1) Practising predominately gynaecology *Barriers* (1) communication	63% reported routinely assessing patients' sexual activities; 40% routinely asked about sexual problems. 28.5% asked about sexual satisfaction, 27.7% about sexual orientation/identity, 13.8% about pleasure with sexual activity (13.8%). A quarter of ob/gyns had expressed disapproval of patients' sexual practices. There are areas for improvement in ob/gyn practices with respect to communication with patients about the comprehensive range of sexual matters that relate to women's health. Ob/gyns' comfort and willingness to discuss sexual identity and orientation with patients remains an important area for further research; improved care for women of sexual minority groups may require interventions tailored to the age and/or gender of the ob/gyn physician
(Stokes and Mears 2000)	$N = 234$, practice nurses	Reported practice and training in sexual health, attitudes towards sexual health, barriers to discussing sexual health with patients and training needs	Cross-sectional survey	*Facilitators* (1) Having received training *Barriers* (1) lack of time (2) lack of training, (3) concern about not being able to cope with the issues raised	93% of practice nurses would attend a local training course in sexual health. Nurses were more comfortable discussing sexual health issues with female patients and teenagers than with male patients and those of different sexual orientations
(Temple-Smith et al. 1999)	$N = 520$, high activity GPs, under 65 years old	Clinical features of STDs, investigations, treatment, public health issues, epidemiology and demographic information	Cross-sectional survey	*Facilitators* (1) GPs' feelings of confidence about taking a sexual history where the need to do so is obvious to the patient, (2) finding of an acceptable way of making the patient aware of the need for sexual history taking, (3) display of posters advertising the importance of sexual behaviour to the patient's overall health and GPs asking the patient about this during the consultation *Barriers* (1) patient's embarrassment in discussing sexuality, (2) length of the standard first consultation which allows insufficient time to take a sexual history (sexual topics are often raised by patients towards the end of a consultation), (3) lack of training, (4) infrequent STD consultations, (5) GPs' lack of confidence in discussing this issues	The importance of educating both patients and GPs about sexual history taking is discussed

(continued)

Table 5-4. (continued)

Areas[a]	Author, year	Sample	Measures	Study design	Facilitators and barriers	Comments and commonalities
	(Tsai 2004)	*N* = 391, nurses	Perceived facilitators and barriers nurses encounter when taking a sexual history	Cross-sectional survey	*Facilitators* (1) nurse's desire to know whether or not a patient's sexual history was related to his/her illness, (2) patient specifically mentioned a sexual problem, (3) having a bachelor of science or master's degree in nursing, (4) having experience in taking a sexual history lead to higher perceived facilitators and lower perceived barriers *Barriers* (1) patients' feeling of embarrassment about the issues of sexuality, (2) sexuality unrelated to the treatment, (2) lack of professionals for referral of patients for further consultations	88.2% of the nurses had not attended any formal course about human sexuality. Half of the participants reported having taken a sexual history
	(Tsai and Hsiung 2003)	*N* = 206, aboriginal nurses	Facilitators and barriers to sexual history taking	Cross-sectional survey	*Facilitators* (1) have attended a communication training course, (2) have experienced a needle stick accident (they want to prevent themselves or colleagues from becoming infected) *Barriers* (1) patients' feelings of embarrassed and not knowing how to answer the questions, (2) purposely concealing of information on the part of patients	Decreasing barriers and reinforcing facilitators about taking a sexual history are an important task for nursing education, and nurses can play an important role in promoting aborigines' sexual health and decreasing the prevalence of STDs in this population
	(Tsimtsiou et al. 2006)	*N* = 316, physicians participating in educational courses on erectile dysfunction	Involvement in taking sexual histories, patient–practitioner orientation scale (beliefs about the doctor–patient relationship), Physician Belief Scale (psychosocial aspects of patient care), Derogatis Sexual Functioning Inventory (sexual attitudes)	Cross-sectional survey	*Facilitators* (1) previous training in communication skills, (2) medical specialty (possibly reflecting level of education in sexual medicine), (3) having liberal sexual attitudes, (4) physicians in private practice, (5) physicians addressing patients' psychosocial concerns *Barriers* (1) female physicians and GPs reported more difficulty in dealing with sexual problems	Physicians' training in communication skills seems to be fundamental for sexual history taking and the management of sexual problems, as it improves their level of comfort in dealing with sexual issues; exposure to sexual medicine courses and psychosocial orientation, as well as physicians' personal sexual attitudes, are also important factors affecting their involvement in sexual medicine
	(Vieira et al. 2015)	*N* = 197, obstetrician and gynaecologist residents enrolling in an online sexology course	Training in sexuality during medical school and residency and attitudes and practice on sexual issues during pregnancy	Cross-sectional survey	*Barriers* (1) lack/few hours of training about sexuality in medical school, (2) lack/few hours of formal training about sexuality during residency up to that moment, (3) feeling of incompetence and lack of confidence to answer pregnant patients' questions about sexuality, (4) lack of specific knowledge on the topic	Almost two-thirds of the participants stated that they did not receive any training at all about sexuality in medical school

STDs ($n = 12$)	(Do et al. 2015)	$N = 371$, physicians	Frequency of sexual history and barriers for taking sexual history among female sex workers (FSW)	Cross-sectional survey	*Facilitators Factors associated with always taking a sexual history* (1) being doctor, (2) training in STIs, (3) working at provincial level facilities. *Factors inversely associated with physician's discomfort* (1) Training on communication with patients, (2) seeing 15 or fewer patients a week, (3) working at provincial level facilities *Barriers* (1) physicians' and patients' discomfort (2) time constraints	27% respondents always obtained and 19% respondents never obtained a sexual history from FSW patients. Improvements in sexual history taking in general practice require strategies to improve physicians' knowledge, skills and attitude towards sexual history taking from FSW and other at risk groups. Tools that allow physicians to quickly and comprehensively obtain patients' sexual history and empower FSW to be more proactive about their sexual health are also needed
	(Emmanuel and Martinez 2011)	Physicians (mainly paediatricians)	Epidemiological data about routine HIV screening	Literature review	*Barriers (to routine HIV testing)* (1) physicians' lack of knowledge with local laws (concerning consent and confidentiality for HIV care and treatment that vary among states), (2) reimbursement and disclosure to parents via insurance billing, (3) lack of knowledge with regard to available resources for referral in communities	Paediatricians can play a key role in preventing and controlling HIV infection by promoting risk-reduction counselling and offering routine HIV testing to adolescent and young adult patients
	(Khan et al. 2007)	$N = 409$, GPs	Sexual risk assessment and barriers in eliciting sexual histories from patients	Cross-sectional survey	*Facilitators* (1) further training in sexual history taking *Barriers* (1) lack of time, (2) a concern that patients might feel uncomfortable if a sexual history was taken, (3) the presence of another person in the consultation room, (4) physician's embarrassment	Although nearly 70% of GP regularly elicited a sexual history from commercial sex workers whose presenting complaint was not an STI, this history taking was much lower (<10%) among GPs for patients who were young or heterosexual. About 23% never took a sexual history from indigenous patients and 19% never elicited this history from lesbian patients. Inconsistent involvement by GP in taking sexual histories was identified, which can result in missed opportunities for early detection of many STIs. Sexual history taking needs to be extended beyond symptomatic and "high-risk group" patients and history taking more routinely is needed
	(Khan et al. 2008)	$N = 409$, GPs	GPs' self-reported comfort in dealing with STI patients with different sexual orientations	Cross-sectional survey	*Facilitators Practitioners who were comfortable* (1) offer sexual risk assessment, (2) offer safe-sex counselling and (3) are less likely to report limited ability to influence patients' risk behaviours *Practitioners who were more proactive in sexual history taking from patients with different sexual orientations* (1) are older, (2) practising in rural areas, (3) have a postgraduate training in STI *Barriers Practitioners who were uncomfortable* (1) constraints in sexual history taking, (2) little capacity to influence patients' risk behaviour perceived, (3) patient's embarrassment, (4) lack of training on sexual health	Although over two-thirds of GPs were comfortable in managing STI in heterosexual or young patients, fewer than half felt comfortable caring for patients who were sex workers, indigenous, people who inject drugs, gay or lesbian. Practitioners' comfort was positively associated with offering information on preventive measures against STI, mode of transmission and the importance of partner treatment. Having STI leaflets for patients was more common among GPs who were comfortable Practitioners' care and support for patients with STI are influenced by their inexperience, lack of skills and/or attitudes

(continued)

TABLE 5-4. (continued)

Areas[a]	Author, year	Sample	Measures	Study design	Facilitators and barriers	Comments and commonalities
	(Lanier et al. 2014)	$N = 26$, physicians serving high-risk group for HIV infection	Practice characteristics	Intervention study	*Facilitators* (1) widespread implementation of a brief, routine sexual history tool, (2) training of medical personnel to take sexual histories routinely during clinical visits, (3) creation of clinical performance indicators to track routine sexual history taking and HIV/STD measures, (4) sexual history training and conduction of brief sexual histories can be strengthened as part of medical and nursing school training *Barriers (Individual-level barriers)* (1) stigma, (2) physician and patient's comfort with discussions of same-sex behaviours	Providers were willing to utilize a sexual history tool in clinical practice in support of HIV/STD prevention efforts
	(Maheux et al. 1995)	$N = 148$, family physicians	Frequency of sexual history and barriers for taking sexual history	Cross-sectional survey	*Barriers* (1) patients' discomfort, (2) uneasy discussion of sexual matters, (3) inadequate training in sexual history taking	The physicians reported taking a sexual history less frequently than a drug use history when seeing patients for a general medical examination or a first pregnancy visit. Although infections from STDs and the HIV are important causes of morbidity and mortality, family physicians are still not actively involved in their prevention. When taken, the sexual history was often too superficial to detect risk behaviours. Consequently, safe-sex counselling was infrequent. Medical education may be deficient in this area and more training in human sexuality should be provided for family physicians
	(McGrath et al. 2011)	$N = 128$, licenced paediatricians, obstetrician/gynaecologists and family practitioners	Chlamydia screening practices and beliefs	Cross-sectional survey	*Barriers* (1) cost-related concerns, (2) provider discomfort with discussing sexuality or STD screening, (3) lack of knowledge of urine-based and self-collected vaginal swabbed specimens (providers do not know that screening can be done without a pelvic examination)	There is a need to address these issues through targeted provider educational interventions
	(Patel et al. 2009)	$N = 19$, HIV care providers of the programme	Prevention needs of providers of HIV-infected patients, their attitudes towards prevention and their experiences in providing prevention counselling to HIV-infected patients	Intervention study	*Barriers For discussing prevention with patients* (1) time, (2) competing medical priorities	The Positive Steps Programme (a provider-delivered HIV transmission risk-reduction intervention for HIV-infected patients) was successfully integrated in an infectious disease clinic and was received well by patients
	(Tucker et al. 2012)	$N = 62$, STI care providers	Reasons for not offering HIV testing routinely: physical examination, sexual history taking practices, frequency of HIV test offer	Cross-sectional survey	*Barriers* (1) low perceived prevalence of disease; (2) not recommended by current guidelines; (3) HIV stigma	There was substantial variability across providers in the frequency of offering testing, ranging from 3 to 100%. 76% reported asking about same-sex behaviours rarely or never

	(Verhoeven et al. 2003)	$N = 122$, primary care physicians	Problems and difficulties in sexual counselling	Cross-sectional survey	*Barriers* (1) language and comprehension problems, (2) ethnic differences, (3) insufficient training, (4) lack of time, (5) presence of the patient's partner or mother, (6) first contact with a patient, (7) fear of embarrassing the patient, (8) patient without genital complaints	Only 44.3% of the participants provide some form of counselling (asking about sexual history, informing about safe sex or about STIs) regularly, at least once a week
	(Webber et al. 2009)	$N = 358$, health-care providers	HIV knowledge and attitudes and predictors of intentions to take a sexual history	Cross-sectional survey	*Facilitators* (1) future training of skills in sexual history taking	Attitudes about taking a sexual history did not contribute to intention; attitudes were often not positive towards people living with HIV
	(Woodbridge et al. 2015)	$N = 17$, GP	Risk assessment and perceptions of risk, pre- and post-testing conduct and the operation and functions of the practice, during the previous 5 years	Qualitative study	*Facilitators* (1) nature of the doctor's interaction with men influences the quality of sexual health services utilization, (2) optimal sexual health consultations require sufficient time and recognition of the "delicacy" of the consultation content for both patient and health practitioner *Barriers* (1) inadequate consultation time, (2) male utilization of GP consultations challenges in discussing sexual health topics within the consultation, (3) doctor's gender, (4) sexual health with low priority if other demands were present	Sexual health consultations by men in general practice are usually initiated by the patient. GPs appear to have a consistent rationale for their risk assessments in terms of STI testing
Sexuality and disease ($n = 9$)	(Byrne, Doherty et al. 2013)	$N = 121$, hospital cardiac rehabilitation staff and GPs	Background and training characteristics and views concerning sexual problems in general practice	Cross-sectional survey	*Barriers For GPs* (1) lack of time, (2) patient's lack of readiness, (3) lack of training, (4) concerns about increasing patients' anxiety and discomfort, (5) patients perceived as too ill to address sexual issues *For cardiac rehabilitation staff* (1) lack of training, (2) patient's lack of readiness, (3) lack of knowledge, (4) issues relating to culture and religion, (5) issues relating to language and ethnicity	Patients reported that sex was rarely discussed, yet nearly half of patients said they would have liked this opportunity. A gap exists: patients, who generally want sexual issues to be addressed, perceive fewer barriers to communication than health-care providers, who fear causing anxiety and discomfort by raising sexual issues with their patients
	(Cort et al. 2001)	$N = 122$, community mental health nurses	Sexual ideology scale	Cross-sectional survey	*Facilitators* (1) clinician taking responsibility (and feeling comfortable with that) for initiating discussion of sexual matters, (2) talking with a professional of the same or different gender *Barriers* (1) reticence of the clinician to take a history—acceptability of discussing sexuality with clients, (2) lack of training concerning specific topics encountered in clinical practice (e.g. client's being sexually aroused when administering depot medication), (3) need of specific sexual health programme which includes training and support for nurses, (4) low knowledge in relation to the sexual side effects of psychotropic medication	Though clients may be expected to have sexual difficulties, only 52.4% respondents agreed that a sexual history should be routinely included in the assessment. This reticence to take a history may relate to concerns about the acceptability of discussing sexuality with clients in general or within the community setting

(continued)

TABLE 5-4. (continued)

Areas[a]	Author, year	Sample	Measures	Study design	Facilitators and barriers	Comments and commonalities
	(Doherty et al. 2011)	$N = 60$, cardiac rehabilitation staff members (coordinators, nurses, physiotherapists and psychologists)	Sexual health management: current practice, staff attitudes, beliefs and perceived barriers to discussing sexual problems	Cross-sectional survey	*Barriers* (1) lack of assessment and counselling protocols for addressing sexual health problems, (2) lack of confidence of the staff (perception that the patient is not ready to discuss sexual health issues), (3) lack of knowledge of sexual health issues, (4) lack of training, (5) cultural issues, (6) language problems	Staff reported a lack of assessment and counselling protocols for addressing sexual health problems, with little or no onward referral system available
	(Hordern and Street 2007)	$N = 82$, health professionals from hospitals	Constructions of intimacy and sexuality in cancer and palliative care: communication process between patients and health professionals	Qualitative study	*Barriers* (1) structural constraints, (2) lack of education (which prevents health professionals from communicating with patients about sexual and intimate changes after cancer), (3) gender and culture of the patients	Feelings of personal vulnerability and uncertainty drove the majority of health professionals away from the topic, even when they were aware that patients had these concerns
	(Mellor et al. 2013)	$N = 30$, health-care professionals (nurses, doctors, therapists, support coordinator, health-care assistant)	Experiences of discussing sexual wellbeing with patients who have had a stroke and resources available to assist them	Qualitative study	*Facilitators* (*Strategies*) (1) To information patients when leaving the hospital that they are free to raise what they liked (including sexual wellbeing) with the acknowledgement that the health-care professional would deal with what they could and direct them to relevant services, (2) trying to create an environment that was conducive to such conversations (changes to home life, relationship, etc.), (3) "sex after stroke" information leaflet *Barriers* (1) structural care pathway level (sexual wellbeing not an area of concern in the hospital, lack of specialist service, time limitations on visits), (2) health-care professionals level (perception that sexual wellbeing was not within their role, and someone else was better suited to deal with it, lack of training, fear of being unable to deal with the magnitude of the issues, embarrassment, lack of formal support), (3) patient level (sexual wellbeing not a priority for patients or the staff, particularly during the acute phase, problems perceived to be mechanical and purely medical, fear of harming the patient with psychological effects), (4) health-care professionals—patient interface (fear of harming the relationship, potential to embarrass or offend the patient or fear that the patient would think badly of the health-care professionals, patients may not want partners present for discussions, fear of making false assumptions about patients, sexual wellbeing not worth raising)	Sexual wellbeing is a topic that participants do not raise with patients and is infrequently raised by patients

	(Oskay et al. 2014)	*N* = 87, nurses from oncology departments	Views and attitudes regarding sexual counselling	Cross-sectional survey	*Barriers* (1) absence of routine regarding sexual counselling in oncology departments, (2) belief that the patient may become ashamed, (3) self-evaluation of insufficient skills and education to counsel in this subject	Most nurses do not evaluate or provide counselling to patients regarding their sexual problems and many difficulties prevent them from focusing on sexual health
	(Quinn and Browne 2009)	N/A	Attitudes and practices of mental health nurses regarding sexual history taking in people with mental illness	Literature review	*Barriers* (1) lack of sexual knowledge, (2) possible de-emphasis in nurse education, (3) insufficient time, (4) not part of the role to discuss sexual issues, (5) illness of consumers that prevent the discussion of sex, (6) discussing sexuality causes the consumers'/nurses' anxiety, (7) burden associated with the discussion of sex, (8) discomfort asking for peer help	Nurses recognize the importance of sexual health; however, it has not as yet been integrated into their practice. Consumers perceive nurses as more approachable and as a safe person to discuss sexual problems that they experience There is a need for research to explore models to support mental health nurses to include sexuality in their assessments to ensure practice standards are met and to provide holistic care
	(Quinn and Happell 2013)	*N* = 14, mental health nurses	Perceptions of how consumers of mental health services have responded to mental health nurses discussing sexuality with them	Intervention study	*Facilitators* (1) the *better* model is a simple and effective intervention that can assist mental health nurses to include sexuality as part of nursing care	Given the reluctance of nurses to address these concerns, educational programmes are needed to assist nurses to develop both comfort and confidence in talking about issues of sexuality with consumers
	(Quinn et al. 2013)	*N* = 14, mental health nurses	Inclusion of sexual issues as a topic in their assessments and interactions with consumers	Qualitative study	*Facilitators* (1) Provision of education and opportunities to nurses to improve their self-awareness *Barriers* (1) Time constraints, (2) increased workloads (create a situation where it is difficult for nurses to be released from patient care to attend training)	Nurses tend to avoid discussing sexual issues in their practice. Given that the skills and knowledge can be easily taught; this type of education needs to become a priority in mental health nursing preparation and professional development
Sexual dysfunction (*n* = 5)	(Abdolrasulnia et al. 2010)	*N* = 505, primary care physicians (PCPs) and ob/gyn	Practice patterns and confidence in managing FSD: diagnostic tests ordered, treatment recommendation, confidence in treating hypoactive sexual desire disorder (HSDD), barriers to initiating a dialogue about sexual health with female patients and sexual history taking	Cross-sectional survey	*Barriers* (1) time constraints, (2) perceived lack of effective therapies, (3) perceptions regarding patient–physician gender discordance, (3) years in practice, (4) number of patients seen per week, (5) perceptions regarding continuing medical education and practice experience	21% of ob/gyns and 38% of PCPs stated that they were not at all confident in treating HSDD
	(Goldstein et al. 2009)	*N* = 137, clinicians involved in the treatment of female sexual dysfunction (FSD)	Language used by clinicians	Cross-sectional survey	*Barriers* (1) FSD as a difficult subject to discuss, (2) frustration by the lack of effective treatment options for HSDD (which contributed to reluctance in discussing sexual health with patients), (3) fear of opening "Pandora's box" about a problem for which they felt there were few, if any, viable treatment options	More carefully constructed definitions, based on understanding the common language between clinicians and patients, would improve doctor–patient communications and set common expectations for treatment of HSDD. Defining HSDD in simpler, nonpsychiatric terms such as "decreased sexual desire" illustrates how HSDD can be translated into more patient-friendly language

(continued)

TABLE 5-4. (continued)

Areas[a]	Author, year	Sample	Measures	Study design	Facilitators and barriers	Comments and commonalities
	(Humphery and Nazareth 2001)	$N = 133$, GPs	Views on the clinical importance of sexual dysfunction, barriers to the management of sexual dysfunction, suggestions for tackling these barriers	Cross-sectional survey	*Barriers* (1) contextual/structural barriers (lack of time, lack of treatments, lack of freedom to prescribe, stigma about sex), (2) doctor barriers (lack of training, embarrassment, lack of experience, fear of opening floodgates), (3) patient barriers (patients' reluctance, difficult area, lack of knowledge, awareness, indirect presentation), (4) doctor–patient interaction (different genders, sensitive subject, different cultures, embarrassment)	6% GPs had a special interest in sexual health. Postgraduate training received: 33% in taking a sexual history, 33% in diagnosis of a sexual problem, 36% in management of sexual dysfunction, 29% in psychosexual counselling
	(Platano et al. 2008)	$N = 50$, GPs and urologists	Male sexual dysfunction in SHT, active initiation of discussion about male sexual dysfunction by patients, self-reported sense of competence in discussing and treating male sexual dysfunction	Cross-sectional survey	*Barriers* (1) Discussion of sexual dysfunction with certain patient groups (e.g. "immigrants", "macho men")	Urologists reported a significantly higher frequency of actively asking male patients about sexual dysfunction. GPs reported a significantly lower percentage of male patients who spontaneously address sexual problems. Both physician groups emphasized erectile dysfunction in SHT. Urologists reported having significantly greater competence in discussing and treating sexual dysfunction than the GPs. Competence in discussing correlated positively with competence in treating sexual dysfunction for GPs and urologists. The majority of GPs and urologists reported a need for continuing education in sexual issues
	(Ribeiro et al. 2014)	$N = 50$, GPs working in primary health-care units	GPs' consultation of guidelines, active exploration of sexual dysfunction (SD) in male and female patients and focus on sexual history taking	Cross-sectional survey	*Facilitators* (1) guidelines' consultation *Barriers* (1) lack of time, (2) low accessibility to health care	15.5% actively ask their patients about SD. 14.0% of the GPs reported being asked by patients about sexual problems (SP). Routine sexual history taking appears as one of the least mentioned motives
Lesbian, gay, bisexual, transgender, queer or questioning (LGBTQ) ($n = 3$)	(Hayes et al. 2015)	$N = 159$, medical students and resident/fellows	Knowledge, comfort and training related to sexual history taking with attention to LGBTQ care	Cross-sectional survey	*Facilitators* (1) specific training for taking sexual histories with general population and with LGBTQ patients (format: interviewing standardized patients, lectures, videotaped examples, patient panel discussions, and on-line modules), (2) institutional culture, (3) curricular material focused on LGBTQ-related health and health disparities, (4) having faculty who were willing to teach LGBTQ-related content, (5) increased clinical exposure to LGBTQ patients *Barriers* (1) feeling uncomfortable in taking sexual histories and discussing safe sexual practices from LGBTQ patients (when compared with other patients)	Medical students and resident/fellows reported a significantly lower level of comfort with sexual history taking and management of sexual issues in the LGBTQ population

	(Kitts 2010)	$N = 184$, physicians in paediatrics, internal medicine, obstetrics gynaecology, psychiatry, emergency medicine and family practice	Practice, knowledge and attitude pertaining to LGBTQ adolescents	Cross-sectional survey	*Barriers* (1) practice: physicians leave the door closed or barely open for adolescents to discuss their sexuality or potentially related issues, (2) knowledge: lack of knowledge for understanding LGBTQ adolescents and the multiple psychosocial stressors and issues that they may face, (3) attitude (non-judgemental) between physicians and LGBTQ adolescents	Barriers in providing optimal care for LGBTQ adolescents can be found with regard to practice, knowledge and attitude regardless of medical field and other demographics collected
	(Sanchez et al. 2006)	$N = 248$, third- and fourth-year medical students	Ability to care for LGBT patients (attitudes, knowledge and clinical skills pertaining to the health care of LGBT patients)	Cross-sectional survey	*Facilitators* (1) Being a medical student with greater clinical exposure to LGBT (had more positive attitude scores and possessed higher knowledge scores than students with little or no clinical exposure)	High desire and willingness to provide health care to LGBT patients. Less than half of respondents reported screening for same-sex activity "always" or "often" when taking a sexual history. Gaps in the current curriculum's history-taking instruction (screening for same-sex intimate partners, screening for household dependents) and LGBT health instruction (cancer risk, mental health, nutrition)
Sexual violence ($n = 1$)	(Leder et al. 1999)	$N = 65$, paediatric primary care providers and child psychiatrists and psychologists	Approach to management, terminology used in discussions with families, barriers to inquiry	Qualitative study	*Barriers* (1) to give anticipatory guidance about sexual abuse inconsistently, (2) lack of training to recognize red flags for sexual abuse, (3) lack of a consistent approach to cases of suspected abuse, (4) feeling uncomfortable discussing sexual issues, (5) lack of time, (6) fear/uncertainty, (7) lack of appropriate referral services, (8) belief that child protective services are inadequate/counterproductive, (9) concern regarding false accusations	Paediatric practitioners reported that they are not trained to recognize sexual abuse and that they do not have a consistent approach to cases of suspected abuse. Additionally, they reported that they are not comfortable discussing sexual issues and that they miss cases of sexual abuse primarily because of lack of training
Multiple areas ($n = 7$) STDs and LGBTQ ($n = 2$) Sexual health education and LGBTQ ($n = 1$) Sexual health education and sexuality and disease ($n = 2$) Sexual health education and sexual violence ($n = 1$) Sexual dysfunction and sexuality and disease ($n = 1$)	(Barber et al. 2011)	$N = 354$, GPs	Attitudes and practices regarding sexual history taking and screening for HIV in men who have sex with men (MSM)	Cross-sectional survey	*Barriers (to HIV screening)* (1) being unlikely to take a sexual history, (2) fear of patient embarrassment *Barriers to sexual history taking* (1) time constraints, (2) feeling inadequately trained, (3) discomfort discussing sex, (4) fear of patient embarrassment, (5) being male, (6) moral or religious views	63% GP reported they would offer HIV screening 3–6 monthly for MSM with casual partners; 16% would offer screening only on request. GP often fails to take a sexual history from MSM, limiting opportunities to offer HIV screening. Strategies are required to increase GPs' awareness of sexual health as a priority for MSM

(continued)

Table 5-4. (continued)

Areas[a]	Author, year	Sample	Measures	Study design	Facilitators and barriers	Comments and commonalities
	(Carter et al. 2014)	$N = 40$, health-care providers (physicians, midlevel providers, nurses and health educators) of HIV-infected MSM	STD screening practices and barriers to conducting sexual risk assessments	Qualitative study	*Barriers Obstacles that prevented routine chlamydia and gonorrhoea screening* (1) time constraints, (2) difficulty obtaining a sexual history, (3) language and cultural barriers, (4) patient confidentiality concerns	Most health-care providers reported routine syphilis screening, screening for chlamydia and gonorrhoea at exposed anatomical sites was less frequent. Interventions are needed to help to mitigate barriers to STD screening, such as structural and patient-directed health services models that might facilitate increased testing coverage of these important preventive services
	(Collins 2006)	$N = 46$, mental health-care providers (of clinical, rehabilitation or administrative services)	HIV vulnerability and prevention, perceptions of patients' attitudes towards sexuality	Qualitative study	*Barriers* (1) providers' views of psychiatric illness, (2) transitions occurring in the mental health-care system, (3) shifting of social attitudes towards sexuality	Barriers operate at the individual level, institutional level and societal level. At the individual level, providers' perceptions of psychiatric symptoms shape their outlook on intervention with psychiatric patients. At the institutional level, disruptive transitions in service delivery relegate HIV services to lesser importance. At the societal level, personal beliefs about sexuality and mental illness have remained slow to change despite major political changes
	(Hinchliff et al. 2005)	$N = 22$, GPs	Difficulties GPs face when discussing sexual health issues with lesbian and gay patients in primary care consultations	Qualitative study	*Facilitators Suggestions* Improving communication about sexual health with lesbian and gay patients (training at undergraduate and postgraduate levels, taking a proactive role during consultations, not making assumptions about patients' sexual orientation and having a non-discriminatory policy for their practice) *Barriers* (1) feeling shy, uncomfortable and not wanting to be intrusive, (2) ignorance of lesbian and gay lifestyles and sexual practices, (3) concerns about the appropriate language to use, (4) assumptions about the nature of gay men's relationships, (5) homophobic attitudes	(non-hetero)sexual orientation could form a barrier to talking about sexual health matters for almost half of this GP sample

(Stead et al. 2003)	$N = 43$, doctors and nurses treating women with ovarian cancer	Knowledge of the frequency and types of sexual problems/ concerns in ovarian cancer, attitudes and behaviours towards discussing sexual issues, knowledge of written information currently available for women about sexual issues	Qualitative study	*Facilitators* (1) age of the patients (younger age), (2) confidence in talking to patients, (3) comfort about sex (seen as a bodily function like all others that are discussed) *Barriers* (1) health professional' unaccountability, (2) consideration that that it is not appropriate to talk to patients, (3) embarrassment, (4) lack of knowledge and experience, (5) lack of resources to provide support if needed, (6) lack of time or privacy, (7) age of the patients (old age), (8) low priority at diagnosis and during treatment, (9) inadequate timing (should wait until the patient asked about sex), (10) taboo subject, (11) lack of role model to follow, (12) fear of the consequences, (13) patients may be taken aback if they were asked about sex, (14) consideration that people do not talk about those sort of things, (15) it is medical tradition not to ask	98% health-care professionals thought that the majority of women with ovarian cancer would experience a sexual problem. Only a quarter of doctors and a fifth of nurses discussed sexual issues with the women Suggestions: written information
(Wendt et al. 2011)	$N = 26$, midwives, gynaecologists, GPs	Sexuality and sexual abuse (including bi- and homosexual women)	Qualitative study	*Facilitators* (1) support from the organization and the use of personal skills and assets, (2) creation of a respectful encounter (being sensitive and open, displaying a respectful attitude, focusing on the individual, inviting woman to participate, offering a calm and undisturbed environment), (3) strengthening women (promoting knowledge, encouraging positive sexuality, relieving pressure), (4) organizational support (education and knowledge, appropriate tools, supervision, guidelines), (5) the use of personal skills and assets (experience, positive attitude, reflecting on actions and behaviour) *Barriers* (1) Lack of organizational support (lack of knowledge, lack of guidelines, lack of time, lack continuity, expectation of exclusively medical focus), (2) communication skills (leaving to the woman to ask, superficial communication, being influenced by own mood), (3) difficult emotions (feeling stunned, feeling frustrated)	The participants described the respectful encounter that can be created when young women meet midwives and clinicians in the context of a gynaecological consultation. In this situation, there was a potential to strengthen women while attempting to improve their sexual health. Increased knowledge, support and opportunities for reflection concerning dialogue regarding sexual issues might evoke the interest and intent of health professionals to approach these issues
(Wiggins et al. 2007)	$N = 35$, specialists in gynaecologic oncology	Barriers for taking sexual history	Cross-sectional survey	*Barriers* (1) no sufficient time to devote to exploring sexual issues, little time for sensitive discussions on sexuality, fertility and intimacy issues, (2) perceived lack of support once a problem has been identified	Although the majority of gynaecologic oncologists were comfortable discussing issues related to sexuality in their cancer patients, less than half performed a sexual history and only 20% did so. Aspects of sexual dysfunction in women with gynaecologic cancer may be neglected by gynaecologic oncology providers. There is a need for cancer programmes to develop formal resources for women with questions regarding sexuality following a diagnosis of cancer

[a]Areas appear in descending order per number of citations, with those most commonly cited appearing first. Articles assessing multiple areas ($n = 7$) appear at the end of the table. Areas: LGBTQ, sexuality and disease, sexual dysfunction, sexual health education/promotion, sexual violence, STDs.

Table 5-5. Recommendations for future research, education actions and intervention programmes derived from the selected articles

Research	1.	Conduct research to develop and test the effectiveness of guidelines for taking a sexual history
	2.	Further exploration of the reasons for health professionals discomfort in managing STI patients is needed as does its impact on patient care
	3.	Investigation of the comfort and willingness to discuss gender identity and sexual orientation with patients remains an important area for further research
Education/training	4.	Educational programmes should expand their curriculum on human sexuality, by specifically addressing why taking a sexual history is so important and offering practicums in how and when to do patient teaching
	5.	More comprehensive continuing education, so that sexual aspects of diseases and treatments and gender and sexual orientation issues are routinely considered
Intervention	6.	Interventions should focus on increasing physician self-efficacy for assessing sexual health in gender discordant and race/ethnicity concordant patient interactions
	7.	Interventions for older adults should increase education about sexual health and sexual risk behaviours as well as empower individuals to seek information from their health-care providers

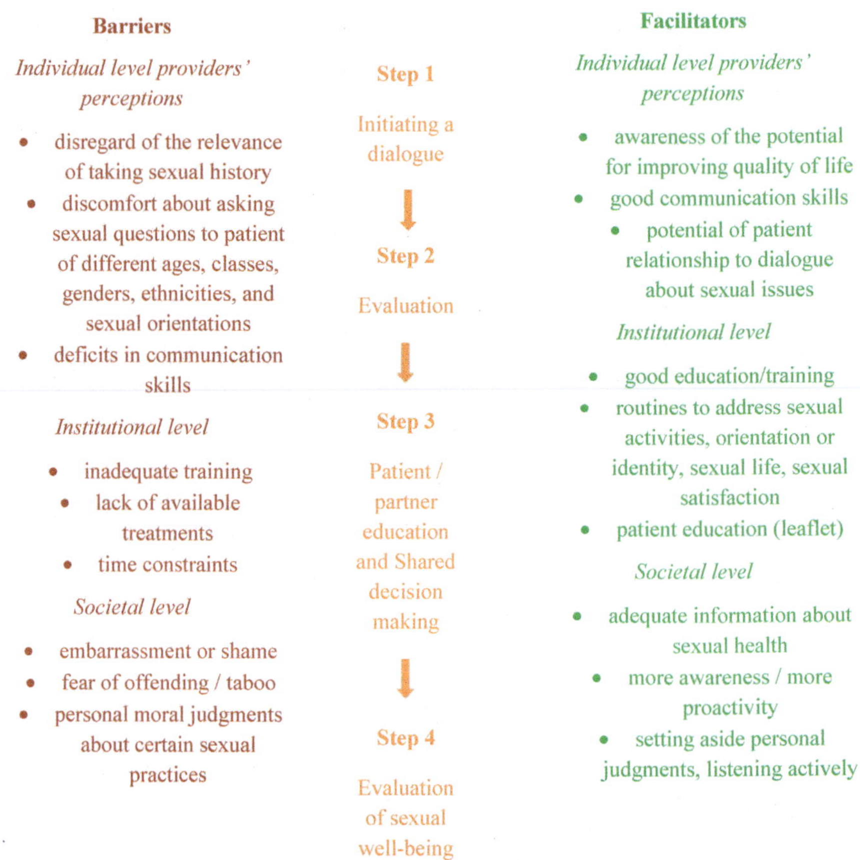
Barriers
Individual level providers' perceptions
disregard of the relevance of taking sexual history
discomfort about asking sexual questions to patient of different ages, classes, genders, ethnicities, and sexual orientations
deficits in communication skills
Institutional level
inadequate training
lack of available treatments
time constraints
Societal level
embarrassment or shame
fear of offending / taboo
personal moral judgments about certain sexual practices
Step 1
Initiating a dialogue
Step 2
Evaluation
Step 3
Patient / partner education and Shared decision making
Step 4
Evaluation of sexual well-being
Facilitators
Individual level providers' perceptions
awareness of the potential for improving quality of life
good communication skills
potential of patient relationship to dialogue about sexual issues
Institutional level
good education/training
routines to address sexual activities, orientation or identity, sexual life, sexual satisfaction
patient education (leaflet)
Societal level
adequate information about sexual health
more awareness / more proactivity
setting aside personal judgments, listening actively

Figure 5-6. Health professionals perceived barriers and facilitators for taking sexual history derived from the selected articles.

are synthetized in Figure 5-6. Barriers and facilitators operate at the individual, institutional and societal levels. At the individual level, providers' perceptions of sexuality influence their attitudes on sexual health history taking; at the institutional level, organizational factors are major determinants; and at the societal level, personal beliefs about sexuality shape their outlook.

Cross-Cutting Themes Related to the Barriers and Facilitators Perceived by the Health Professionals

The first major barrier that crossed the generality of the studies was the *deficiency in sexual history taking education and training*. Secondly, a reticence to take a history related to concerns about *the acceptability of discussing sexuality with the patient* was commonly testified. Finally, *stigma and society's attitudes to sex* appeared as an important barrier to talking about sexual health matters.

Discussion of Sexual Health Issues with the Patients' Interaction with the Patient

- *Health professionals have interest in sexual health and feel it is important to know how to take a sexual history* (Ariffin et al. 2015; Tsai and Hsiung 2003).
- *Health professionals are more willing to adhere to sexual history taking where the need to do so is obvious to the patient* (Temple-Smith et al. 1999), *with disregard to sexual wellbeing* (Mellor et al. 2013) *or sexual identity and orientation* (Sobecki et al. 2012).
- *Health professionals feel greater discomfort in taking a sexual history with opposite gender patients* (Abdolrasulnia et al. 2010; Burd et al. 2006), *with cultural or religious differences* (Ariffin et al. 2015; Humphery and Nazareth 2001; Verhoeven et al. 2003), *LGBTQ population* (Hayes et al. 2015; Platano et al. 2008), *sex workers, drug users and risk groups* (Carter et al. 2014; Do et al. 2015; Khan et al. 2007, 2008).
- *The decision to integrate questions relating to sexuality seems to depend more on non-medical factors such as the personal experience or interest* (Schweizer et al. 2013).

Health professionals need the appropriate skills to ask sensitive questions that are non-judgemental and empathetic. These skills must include comfort in addressing these topics for patients of different ages, classes, genders, ethnicities and sexual orientations.

Stigma/Society's Attitudes Towards Sex

- *Health professionals do not address sexual health proactively with older people, being sexual health equated with younger people and not seen as a "legitimate" topic for discussion with this age group. Beliefs are based on stereotyped views of ageing and sexuality, rather than personal experience of individual patients* (Gott et al. 2004).
- *Personal beliefs about sexuality and mental illness are a barrier to address sexual health issues with psychiatric patients* (Collins 2006; Quinn and Browne 2009; Quinn and Happell 2013; Quinn et al. 2013).
- *Feelings of personal vulnerability and uncertainty drive the majority of health professionals away from discussing sexuality and intimacy with cancer patients* (Hordern and Street 2007; Oskay et al. 2014; Stead et al. 2003; Wiggins et al. 2007).
- *Health professionals' knowledge and attitudes towards LGBTQ population is a barrier in providing optimal care* (Barber et al. 2011; Hayes et al. 2015; Hinchliff et al. 2005; Kitts 2010; Sanchez et al. 2006).

Ignorance, incorrect assumptions and discriminatory attitudes form a barrier to talking about sexual health matters.

Final Considerations

In pursuing the aim of uncovering the barriers and facilitators health professionals encounter when taking a sexual history, we undertook a review of literature on scientific evidence in this area.

Overall, clinical practice in the field of sexuality is still embedded in preconceived ideas that hamper an adequate sexual history taking. Due to lack of training, time pressure and (sometimes inappropriate) personal beliefs, health professionals often worry about how, where and when to ask the questions, of whom to ask and what to do with the collected information [2, 18]. Thereby, not surprisingly, sexual history taking remains slow to learn in terms of how to help patients with problems and complaints, and many health professionals simply avoid the topic entirely since they often feel unprepared to tackle the topic of sexual health in the detail and with the sensitivity it deserves [6]. As Warner and colleagues [10] stressed out, "every human being has a sexual dimension. We can learn to talk most effectively with our patients about sexuality by setting aside personal judgments, listening actively, and becoming adequately informed about sexual health".

The concept of sexual health emphasises the need to promote health by education and information. It encourages a further step in the public and medical acceptance that sexual activity is and should be a healthy and fulfilling behaviour. In that sense, sexual inquiry holds the key to the practice of sexual health and provides the basis for treatment, prevention, education and comprehensive sexual health care and promotion [40].

Still, there are deficits at different levels in this area that must be addressed (Table 5-5). Research, education/training and intervention actions are a few examples of neglected topics in the literature that has been published with regard to sexual health and assess.

Acknowledgements. We want to thank André Silva for his valuable and tireless help in the identification and access to some of the articles included in the review.

References

1. Goodwach R. Fundamentals of theory and practice revisited. Sex therapy: historical evolution, current practice. Part I. Aust New Zeal J Fam Ther. 2005;26(3):155–64.
2. Kingsberg SA. Taking a sexual history. Obstet Gynecol Clin North Am. 2006;33(4):535–47.
3. Hordern AJ, Street AF. Constructions of sexuality and intimacy after cancer: patient and health professional perspectives. Soc Sci Med. 2007;64(8):1704–18.
4. Burd ID, Nevadunsky N, Bachmann G. Impact of physician gender on sexual history taking in a multispecialty practice. J Sex Med. 2006;3(2):194–200.
5. Leeper H, Chang E, Cotter G, MacIntosh P, Scott F, Apantaku L, et al. A student-designed and student-led sexual-history-taking module for second-year medical students. Teach Learn Med. 2007;19(3):293–301.
6. Maurice WL. Sexual medicine in primary care. London: Mosby; 1999.
7. Cohen MAA, Alfonso CA. A comprehensive approach to sexual history-taking using the biopsychosocial model. Int J Ment Health. 1997;26(1):3–14.
8. Verhoeven V, Bovijn K, Helder A, Peremans L, Hermann I, Van RP, et al. Discussing STIs: doctors are from Mars, patients from Venus. Fam Pract. 2003;20(1):11–5.
9. Andrews WC. Approaches to taking a sexual history. J Womens Health Gend Based Med. 2000;9(Suppl 1):21–4.
10. Warner PH, Rowe T, Whipple B. Shedding light on the sexual history. Am J Nurs. 1999;99(6):34–40.
11. Peck SA. The importance of the sexual health history in the primary care setting. J Obstet Gynecol Neonatal Nurs. 2001;30(3):269–74.
12. Van Sickle M, Rosenstock H. Taking a sexual history: which questions to ask. Female Patient (Parsippany). 1999;24(7):43.
13. Bernhard LA. Sexuality and sexual health care for women. Clin Obstet Gynecol. 2002;45(4):1089–98.
14. World Health Organization. Defining sexual health, report of a technical consultation on sexual health, 28–31 January 2002, Geneva. 2006.
15. Tsimtsiou Z, Hatzimouratidis K, Nakopoulou E, Kyrana E, Salpigidis G, Hatzichristou D. Predictors of physicians' involvement in addressing sexual health issues. J Sex Med. 2011;3(4):583–8.
16. Tsai Y-F. Nurses' facilitators and barriers for taking a sexual history in Taiwan. Appl Nurs Res. 2004;17(4):257–64.
17. Jones R, Barton S. Introduction to history taking and principles of sexual health. Postgrad Med J. 2004;80(946):444–6.
18. Wylie KR. ABC of sexual health. New York: Wiley; 2015.
19. Wimberly YH, Hogben M, Moore-Ruffin J, Moore SE, Fry-Johnson Y. Sexual history-taking among primary care physicians. J Natl Med Assoc. 2006;98(12):1924–9.
20. Brook G, Bacon L, Evans C, McClean H, Roberts C, Tipple C, et al. 2013 UK national guideline for consultations requiring sexual history taking. Clinical Effectiveness Group British Association for Sexual Health and HIV. Int J STD AIDS. 2014;25(6):391–404.
21. Fogel CI. Sexual health promotion. In: Lauver D, editor. Saunders; 1990.
22. Tomlinson J. ABC of sexual health: taking a sexual history. Br Med J. 1998;317(7172):1573.
23. Althof SE, Rosen RC, Perelman MA, Rubio-Aurioles E. Standard operating procedures for taking a sexual history. J Sex Med. 2013;10(1):26–35.
24. Tomlinson J, Milgrom EC. Taking a sexual history. West J Med. 1999;170(5):284–6.
25. Griffin SJ, Kinmonth A-L, Veltman MWM, Gillard S, Grant J, Stewart M. Effect on health-related outcomes of interventions to alter the interaction between patients and practitioners: a systematic review of trials. Ann Fam Med. 2004;2(6):595–608.
26. Bickley L, Szilagyi PG. In: Wilkins LW, editor. Bates' guide to physical examination and history-taking. 2012.
27. Nusbaum MRH, Hamilton CD. The proactive sexual health history. Am Fam Physician. 2002;66(9):1705–12.
28. Engel GL. The need for a new medical model: a challenge for biomedicine. Science. 1977;196(4286):129–36.
29. McCabe M, Althof SE, Assalian P, Chevret-Measson M, Leiblum SR, Simonelli C, et al. Psychological and interpersonal dimensions of sexual function and dysfunction. J Sex Med. 2010;7(1):327–36.
30. Nusbaum M, Rosenfeld JA. Sexual health across the lifecycle: a practical guide for clinicians. Cambridge University Press; 2004. 198 p.
31. Temple-Smith M, Hammond J, Pyett P, Presswell N. Barriers to sexual history taking in general practice. Aust Fam Physician. 1996;25(9 Suppl 2):S71–4.
32. Ariffin F, Chin KL, Ng C, Miskan M, Lee VK, Isa MR. Are medical students confident in taking a sexual history? An assessment on attitude and skills from an upper middle income country. BMC Res Notes. 2015;8(1):248.
33. Kingsberg SA, Malemud CJ, Novak T, Cole-Kelly K, Wile MZ, Spanos P, et al. A comprehensive approach to enhancing sexual health education in the Case Western Reserve University School of Medicine. Int J Impot Res. 2003;15(5):S51.
34. Nadelson C. Treatment interventions in human sexuality. New York: Springer; 2012.
35. Dadich A, Hosseinzadeh H, Starfield B, Shi L, Macinko J, Skinner C, et al. Healthcare reform: implications for knowledge translation in primary care. BMC Health Serv Res. 2013;13(1):490.
36. Risen CB. A guide to taking a sexual history. Psychiatr Clin North Am. 1995;18(1):39–53.
37. Kuritzky L. Taking a male sexual history. Curr Sex Health Rep. 2006;3(2):61–6.
38. Arksey H, O'Malley L. Scoping studies: towards a methodological framework. Int J Soc Res Methodol. 2005;8(1):19–32.
39. Armstrong R, Hall BJ, Doyle J, Waters E. Cochrane Update. "Scoping the scope" of a cochrane review. J Public Health (Oxf). 2011;33.
40. Jones R, Barton S. Introduction to history taking and principles of sexual health. Postgrad Med J. 2004;80(946):444–6.

Selected Articles

Abdolrasulnia M, Shewchuk RM, Roepke N, Granstaff US, Dean J, Foster JA, Goldstein AT, Casebeer L. Management of female sexual problems: perceived barriers, practice patterns, and confidence among primary care physicians and gynecologists. J Sex Med. 2010;7(7):2499–508.

Ariffin F, Chin KL, Ng C, Miskan M, Lee VK, Isa MR. Are medical students confident in taking a sexual history? An assessment on attitude and skills from an upper middle income country. BMC Res Notes. 2015;8:248.

Barber B, Hellard M, Jenkinson R, Spelman T, Stoove M. Sexual history taking and sexually transmissible infection screening practices among men who have sex with men: a survey of Victorian general practitioners. Sex Health. 2011;8(3):349–54.

Bouman WP, Arcelus J. Are psychiatrists guilty of "ageism" when it comes to taking a sexual history? Int J Geriatr Psychiatry. 2001;16(1):27–31.

Bull SS, Rietmeijer C, Fortenberry JD, Stoner B, Malotte K, VanDevanter N, Middlestadt SE, Hook III EW. Practice patterns for the elicitation of sexual history, education, and counseling among providers of STD services: results from the gonorrhea community action project (GCAP). Sex Transm Dis. 1999;26(10):584–9.

Burd ID, Nevadunsky N, Bachmann G. Impact of physician gender on sexual history taking in a multispecialty practice. J Sex Med. 2006;3(2):194–200.

Byrne M, Doherty S, Murphy AW, McGee HM, Jaarsma T. Communicating about sexual concerns within cardiac health services: do service providers and service users agree? Patient Educ Couns. 2013;92(3):398–403.

Carter Jr JW, Hart-Cooper GD, Butler MO, Workowski KA, Hoover KW. Provider barriers prevent recommended sexually transmitted disease screening of HIV-infected men who have sex with men. Sex Transm Dis. 2014;41(2):137–42.

Collins PY. Challenges to HIV prevention in psychiatric settings: perceptions of South African mental health care providers. Soc Sci Med. 2006;63(4):979–90.

Cort EM, Attenborough J, Watson JP. An initial exploration of community mental health nurses' attitudes to and experience of sexuality-related issues in their work with people experiencing mental health problems. J Psychiatr Ment Health Nurs. 2001;8(6): 489–99.

Cushing A, Evans D, Hall A. Medical students' attitudes and behaviour towards sexual health interviewing: short- and long-term evaluation of designated workshops. Med Teach. 2005;27(5):422–8.

Dadich A, Hosseinzadeh H. Healthcare reform: implications for knowledge translation in primary care. BMC Health Serv Res. 2013;13:490.

Do K, Minichiello V, Hussain R, Khan A. Sexual history taking in general practice: managing sexually transmitted infections for female sex workers by doctors and assistant doctors in Vietnam. Int J STD AIDS. 2015;26(1):55–64.

Doherty S, Byrne M, Murphy AW, McGee HM. Cardiac rehabilitation staff views about discussing sexual issues with coronary heart disease patients: a national survey in Ireland. Eur J Cardiovasc Nurs. 2011;10(2):101–7.

Emmanuel PJ, Martinez J. Adolescents and HIV infection: the pediatrician's role in promoting routine testing. Pediatrics. 2011;128(5): 1023–9.

Goldstein I, Lines C, Pyke R, Scheld JS. National differences in patient-clinician communication regarding hypoactive sexual desire disorder. J Sex Med. 2009;6(5):1349–57.

Gott M, Hinchliff S, Galena E. General practitioner attitudes to discussing sexual health issues with older people. Soc Sci Med. 2004;58:2093–103.

Hayes V, Blondeau W, Bing-You RG. Assessment of medical student and resident/fellow knowledge, comfort, and training with sexual history taking in LGBTQ patients. Fam Med. 2015;47(5):383–7.

Hinchliff S, Gott M, Galena E. "I daresay I might find it embarrassing": general practitioners' perspectives on discussing sexual health issues with lesbian and gay patients. Health Soc Care Community. 2005;13(4):345–53.

Hordern AJ, Street AF. Constructions of sexuality and intimacy after cancer: patient and health professional perspectives. Soc Sci Med. 2007;64(8):1704–18.

Humphery S, Nazareth I. GPs' views on their management of sexual dysfunction. Fam Pract. 2001;18(5):516–8.

Jolley S. Taking a sexual history: the role of the nurse. Nurs Times. 2002;98(18):39–41.

Khan A, Plummer D, Hussain R, Minichiello V. Sexual risk assessment in general practice: evidence from a New South Wales survey. Sex Health. 2007;4(1):1–8.

Khan A, Plummer D, Hussain R, Minichiello V. Does physician bias affect the quality of care they deliver? Evidence in the care of sexually transmitted infections. Sex Transm Infect. 2008;84(2): 150–1.

Kingsberg SA. Taking a sexual history. Obstet Gynecol Clin North Am. 2006;33(4):535–47.

Kitts RL. Barriers to optimal care between physicians and lesbian, gay, bisexual, transgender, and questioning adolescent patients. J Homosex. 2010;57(6):730–47.

Lanier Y, Castellanos T, Barrow RY, Jordan WC, Caine V, Sutton MY. Brief sexual histories and routine HIV/STD testing by medical providers. AIDS Patient Care STDS. 2014;28(3):113–20.

Leder MR, Emans SJ, Hafler JP, Rappaport LA. Addressing sexual abuse in the primary care setting. Pediatrics. 1999;104(2 Pt 1):270–5.

Leeper H, Chang E, Cotter G, MacIntosh P, Scott F, Apantaku L, Lazarus C. A student-designed and student-led sexual-history-taking module for second-year medical students. Teach Learn Med. 2007;19(3):293–301.

Maheux B, Haley N, Rivard M, Gervais A. STD risk assessment and risk-reduction counseling by recently trained family physicians. Acad Med. 1995;70(8):726–8.

McGrath CM, Katz AR, Lee MV, Rochat RW. Chlamydia screening of adolescent females: a survey of providers in Hawaii. J Community Health. 2011;36(2):274–80.

Mellor RM, Greenfield SM, Dowswell G, Sheppard JP, Quinn T, McManus RJ. Health care professionals' views on discussing sexual wellbeing with patients who have had a stroke: a qualitative study. PLoS One. 2013;8(10):e78802.

Morand A, McLeod S, Lim R. Barriers to sexual history taking in adolescent girls with abdominal pain in the pediatric emergency department. Pediatr Emerg Care. 2009;25(10):629–32.

Oskay U, Can G, Basgol S. Discussing sexuality with cancer patients: oncology nurses attitudes and views. Asian Pac J Cancer Prev. 2014;15(17):7321–6.

Patel SN, Golin CE, Marks G, Grodensky CA, Earp JA, Zeveloff A, O'Daniels C, Gardner L, Boland MS, Davis R, Quinlivan EB. Delivery of an HIV prevention counseling program in an infectious diseases clinic: implementation process and lessons learned. AIDS Patient Care STDS. 2009;23(6):433–41.

Platano G, Margraf J, Alder J, Bitzer J. Frequency and focus of sexual history taking in male patients—a pilot study conducted among Swiss general practitioners and urologists. J Sex Med. 2008;5:47–59.

Quinn C, Browne G. Sexuality of people living with a mental illness: a collaborative challenge for mental health nurses. Int J Ment Health Nurs. 2009;18(3):195–203.

Quinn C, Happell B. Talking about sexuality with consumers of mental health services. Perspect Psychiatr Care. 2013;49(1):13–20.

Quinn C, Happell B, Welch A. Talking about sex as part of our role: making and sustaining practice change. Int J Ment Health Nurs. 2013;22(3):231–40.

Ribeiro S, Alarcao V, Simoes R, Miranda FL, Carreira M, Galvao-Teles A. General practitioners' procedures for sexual history taking and treating sexual dysfunction in primary care. J Sex Med. 2014;11(2):386–93.

Sanchez NF, Rabatin J, Sanchez JP, Hubbard S, Kalet A. Medical students' ability to care for lesbian, gay, bisexual, and transgendered patients. Fam Med. 2006;38(1):21–7.

Schweizer A, Bruchez C, Santiago-Delefosse M. Integrating sexuality into gynaecological consultations: gynaecologists' perspectives. Cult Health Sex. 2013;15(2):175–90.

Sobecki JN, Curlin FA, Rasinski KA, Lindau ST. What we don't talk about when we don't talk about sex: results of a national survey of U.S. obstetrician/gynecologists. J Sex Med. 2012;9(5):1285–94.

Stead ML, Brown JM, Fallowfield L, Selby P. Lack of communication between healthcare professionals and women with ovarian cancer about sexual issues. Br J Cancer. 2003;88(5):666–71.

Stokes T, Mears J. Sexual health and the practice nurse: a survey of reported practice and attitudes. Br J Fam Plann. 2000;26(2):89–92.

Temple-Smith MJ, Mulvey G, Keogh L. Attitudes to taking a sexual history in general practice in Victoria, Australia. Sex Transm Infect. 1999;75(1):41–4.

Tsai YF. Nurses' facilitators and barriers for taking a sexual history in Taiwan. Appl Nurs Res. 2004;17(4):257–64.

Tsai YF, Hsiung PC. Aboriginal nurses' perception of facilitators and barriers for taking a sexual history in Taiwan. Public Health Nurs. 2003;20(4):281–6.

Tsimtsiou Z, Hatzimouratidis K, Nakopoulou E, Kyrana E, Salpigidis G, Hatzichristou D. Predictors of physicians' involvement in addressing sexual health issues. J Sex Med. 2006;3(4): 583–8.

Tucker JD, Walensky RP, Yang LG, Yang B, Bangsberg DR, Chen XS, Cohen MS. Expanding provider-initiated HIV testing at STI clinics in China. AIDS Care. 2012;24(10):1316–9.

Verhoeven V, Bovijn K, Helder A, Peremans L, Hermann I, Van Royen P, Avonts D. Discussing STIs: doctors are from Mars, patients from Venus. Fam Pract. 2003;20(1):11–5.

Vieira TC, de Souza E, da Silva I, Torloni MR, Ribeiro MC, Nakamura MU. Dealing with female sexuality: training, attitude, and practice of obstetrics and gynecology residents from a developing country. J Sex Med. 2015;12(5):1154–7.

Webber G, Edwards N, Graham ID, Amaratunga C, Gaboury I, Keane V, Ros S, McDowell I. A survey of Cambodian health-care providers' HIV knowledge, attitudes and intentions to take a sexual history. Int J STD AIDS. 2009;20(5):346–50.

Wendt EK, Marklund BR, Lidell EA, Hildingh CI, Westerstahl AK. Possibilities for dialogue on sexuality and sexual abuse—midwives' and clinicians' experiences. Midwifery. 2011;27(4):539–46.

Wiggins DL, Wood R, Granai CO, Dizon DS. Sex, intimacy, and the gynecologic oncologists: survey results of the New England Association of Gynecologic Oncologists (NEAGO). J Psychosoc Oncol. 2007;25(4):61–70.

Woodbridge MR, Dowell AC, Gray L. "He said he had been out doing the traffic": general practitioner perceptions of sexually transmitted infection and HIV testing strategies for men. J Prim Health Care. 2015;7(1):50–6.

6
Biopsychosocial Evaluation of Sexual Dysfunctions

Prem K. Pahwa and Sallie M. Foley

Introduction

Sexuality is defined by the World Health Organization (WHO) as "a biopsychosocial phenomenon comprised of physiologic functioning, psychological factors specific for each person, and sociologic/interpersonal/cultural environment contributors to personal sexual health and well-being" [1]. The DSM-5 in its diagnostic criteria for sexual dysfunction issues looks at not only the relevant medical factors associated with the presenting issue, but also what are the psychological and social factors. Sexual function can be impacted by a range of factors that need to be understood, not just in isolation as discrete issues, but as part of a larger complex system where each part of the system impacts one another. Approximately 43% of women and 31% of men in the USA are impacted by some form of sexual dysfunction, making it very common for the general population to have sexual function concerns at some point in their life [2]. Women are most impacted by decrease in desire, whereas the most common issues for men are erectile dysfunction (ED) and premature ejaculation (PE) [2, 3].

Integrative practice, which combines medical and psychosocial interventions, has become an increasing focus for healthcare professionals working within a range of specialties. The often low levels of attention to psychosocial variables among medical practitioners may reflect both discomfort in addressing sexual issues and a low level of core competency in the treatment of psychosexual problems [4].

This overview of sexual assessment comes from the perspective of psychotherapeutic assessment and certified sex therapy. It looks at subjective experience of person and partner focusing on the intrapersonal and interpersonal, while also considering the patient's distress and the partner's distress. Sexual health is considered as part of peoples' overall quality of life. The biopsychosocial approach to assessment is followed here.

Biopsychosocial

Psychiatrist, George Engel, developed the biopsychosocial (BPS) model in 1977. This model moved away from the biomedical model of understanding illness to a formulation that looked at a person's overall being to understand disease and illness, as well as health and wellness. According to the BPS model, neither illness nor health is the result of physiology alone, but rather is the result of how three distinct areas of a person's life intersect: the biological or physiological components, the mental health or psychological components, and the social and cultural components. When looking at disease or ill health, the BPS model believes that it is the social/cultural environment and the psychological state that helps or worsens the condition [5–7].

Engel offered a holistic alternative to the dominant biomedical model at a time when science overall was changing from a simplistic and exclusively analytic approach to a more interdisciplinary approach based in context. He posited that clinicians would yield better outcomes if they provided empathy to patients and addressed the biological, psychological, and sociocultural components of their illness [5–7].

The approach of the biopsychosocial model is to consider the potential impact of any parts of the overall systems on the sexual health of the individual patient. George Engel formulated the biopsychosocial model as a dynamic, interactional, but dualistic view of human experience in which there is mutual influence of mind and body [8].

The biopsychosocial model is also known as the "mind–body" connection in dominant culture, and is an important way to understand and treat health issues, and specifically sexual health issues. There has been significant evidence for the role of the mind in disease and healing, leading to a greater acceptance of "mind–body" medicine. In the past 40 years, research into the link between overall health and psychological, social, and cultural factors has moved the mind-body connection from the fringe of biomedical science into the mainstream [9].

W.W. IsHak (ed.), *The Textbook of Clinical Sexual Medicine*, DOI 10.1007/978-3-319-52539-6_6

When evaluating patients, the BPS model tries to take both a macro and micro perspective in understanding the patient's experience. This includes the individual picture of what is going on for the patient from a biological perspective, as well as the bigger picture of how the patient's psychological sense of well-being and the impact that their culture or environment is having on their particular experience. The model empowers patients to view their relationship with the provider as a partnership in which each take an active role. The individual and his or her support community play a vital part in the psychological and social recovery through enhancing mental health and adapting healthy lifestyle habits. The clinician is responsible for any physiological treatment. Patients can also use this model, or the skills they have learned through it, in a preventative manner surrounding sexual health issues.

The biopsychosocial model can be viewed as a framework for providing clinical understanding, as well as a practical guide for evaluation. It is a way for clinicians to understand how health and illness are impacted through many levels of organization, from the macro societal level to the micro molecular one. BPS is a way of understanding and accounting for the patient's subjective experience as a vital part of formulating a correct evaluation of the patient's health and treatment issues [10].

The three biopsychosocial factors impacting health, wellness, and disease:

The biological part of the biopsychosocial model has to do with awareness of the physiological causes of a disease or dysfunction. The physiological causes, however, are often accompanied by the other parts of the model, which will increase the complexity of the illness or dysfunction. Many sexual dysfunctions do have biological factors at their root; a few are hypertension, diabetes, hormones, and physical trauma.

The psychological part of the BPS model evaluates what may be some underlying mental health issues that can contribute to the manifestation of a sexual dysfunction. The clinician wants to identify any psychological issues that may be impacting the patient's physical or sexual health directly or indirectly, such as depression, anxiety, addiction, body image issues, negative thinking, etc.

The social part of the BPS model refers to the sociocultural environment that surrounds the patient. This part evaluates the dysfunction from a sociological point of view, and examines what external factors may have influenced the onset and maintenance of the sexual dysfunction. These external sociocultural factors could be anything from religion, to economic background, primary relationships, cultural environment, peer group, etc. For example, media messages suggesting that only thin women are "attractive" or "sexually desirable" may influence a young woman's development of body image issues.

Engel, in an article he authored in the American Journal of Psychiatry (1980), firmly brings the biopsychosocial model into overall patient care. It discusses how any presenting patient concern can be seen narrowly from a solely biological perspective or more broadly as a concern that may have psychological and social components, which will inform a patient's understanding of his or her condition and will impact how it develops. Engel believed that the biomedical model, which was predominantly used at the time, had significant limitations, which are outlined out below [5–7].

Engel's Critique of Biomedicine

1. A biochemical alteration does not translate directly into an illness. The appearance of illness results from the interaction of diverse causal factors, including those at the molecular, individual, and social levels. And the converse, psychological alterations may, under certain circumstances, manifest as illnesses or forms of suffering that constitute health problems, including, at times, biochemical correlates.
2. The presence of a biological derangement does not shed light on the meaning of the symptoms to the patient, nor does it necessarily infer the attitudes and skills that the clinician must have to gather information and process it well.
3. Psychosocial variables are more important determinants of susceptibility, severity, and course of illness than had been previously appreciated by those who maintain a biomedical view of illness.
4. Adopting a sick role is not necessarily associated with the presence of a biological derangement.
5. The success of the most biological of treatments is influenced by psychosocial factors, for example, the so-called placebo effect.
6. The patient–clinician relationship influences medical outcomes, even if only because of its influence on adherence to a chosen treatment.
7. Unlike inanimate subjects of scientific scrutiny, patients are profoundly influenced by the way in which they are studied, and the scientists engaged in the study are influenced by their subject.

Medical and psychological therapies for sexual dysfunctions should evaluate the multidirectional systems and biopsychosocial influences of the patient, the partner, and the couple where relevant. The biopsychosocial model provides a compelling reason to doubt that any single cause will be enough to explain the experience of sexual dysfunction for most patients. For effective evaluation and treatment of sexual dysfunction, it is useful to have cross-disciplinary collaboration amongst providers. Frequently, both psychotherapy and medical treatment are needed to help patients achieve a lasting resolution to their sexual problems. Evaluation of male, female, or couples' sexual dysfunction issues should include an investigation of factors that may have caused the dysfunction, are involved in its maintenance, and are contextual factors for its treatment. Sexual dysfunction issues that are chronic in nature need to be understood as different from those that are acquired more recently.

According to Berry, "contextual assessment models continue to place a great deal of emphasis on the use of a predisposing, precipitating, and maintaining factor model of assessment. This model allows biological, psychological, and social-cultural-relational factors to be organized in terms of vulnerability factors, immediate causes, and ongoing issues that might be reversed in order to functioning. Evidence-based process of care guidelines prescribe the use of a patient-centered approach as a core principle of clinical assessment. Patient-centered care aims to allow the treating clinician to adopt the patient's perspective and account for his subjective biopsychosocial experience in assessing sexual dysfunction" [4].

Assessment of Sexual Problems: A Proposed Model

Sallie Foley has proposed a model for Sex Therapy and Evaluation that is detailed in the section below. She lays out specific questions for clinicians to ask their patients. The DOUPE Model, an approach for understanding and evaluating patients presenting symptoms, developed by Foley, is also explained in this section.

Many adults have a need for sexual health information that can address concerns and educate about treatment. Medical and mental health care providers can open the conversation by including questions about sexual health in the general review of systems (ROS) or early in the interview: [1]

Ask: "We've been talking about your general health and your sexual health is part of your general health. Do you have any questions about your sexual health?"

"We've been talking about your general concerns and often sexual concerns are part of general concerns. Do you have any sexual concerns or need for more information?" [1]

Some individuals may answer "No," but others will welcome this opportunity. Many will say "No" and bring up their questions later. They may have difficulty describing their concern [1].

Some professionals do not ask about sex for fear of looking stupid when they do not know the answer. Research indicates that older adults don't expect professionals to know everything; rather, they value the discourse. Providers can model collaboration: "That's a good question. I don't know the answer, but will check and get back to you" [1].

Ask: "Do you have a spouse or partner?" Rather than asking, "Do you have a wife?" Use of inclusive questioning shows respect for all patients/partner relationships. Pronoun sensitivity empowers the patient to more comfortably disclose the nature of his/her sexual orientation and relationship status, providing more accurate information about sexual activity. Sadly, because providers so commonly use assumptive pronouns, LGBT people, regardless of age, are faced with constantly coming out every time they see a new provider [1].

DOUPE—an Assessment. Algorithm. A standard interview assessment called DOUPE was developed by the coauthor, Sallie Foley, to allow professionals to gain information quickly and concisely. Useful in any assessment, it is especially helpful when weaving sexual health assessment into a more general interview. It follows the lines of routine medical history-taking such as the OPQRST (onset, provocation, quality, radiation, severity, time).

Description— "What is the concern?" or "What is a typical situation when this happens?"

Onset—Lifelong or more recent? Paired with any other change? Every time or just in one situation or with one person.

Understanding—"What's your understanding of why this is happening?" allows HCP to understand level of distress and the person's reasoning. "God is punishing me." is a different interview than "I think it happens a lot to older women."

Past—"What's your experience trying to fix the problem?" Almost everyone has thought of or tried something. This also elucidates the "why now" of seeking help.

Expectations—How motivated and how realistic is the person? [1].

Once DOUPE is established, further questions usually "deepen the conversation" and include discussion of pain or discomfort, changes in amount of stimulation needed for arousal, and other challenges. "How satisfied overall are you with your sex life?" sheds light on presence or absence of satisfaction and pleasure in spite of functionality challenges. Use real language rather than euphemisms (i.e., "intercourse" or "masturbation/manual stimulation" rather than vague references to "having relations" and "taking care of yourself") [11]. Finally, model an affirmative outlook on sexuality by taking a permission-giving stance [1, 12].

An informed health care professional (HCP) can treat many sexual problems within a clinical practice. Treatment often begins with the recognition and treatment of underlying medical problems, encouraging the inclusion of the partner, and comfort with addressing both partners' concerns. The professional listens carefully, encourages couples to openly discuss concerns and enhance their skills in communication. Interventions frequently useful in addressing sexual problems include asking permission to proceed with discussion, explaining the causes and physiology of the problem, regularly checking in with the individual or couple to make sure they are "following" the discussion, recommending patients read sexual problem specific self-help books, addressing co-occurring problems like anxiety or sleep apnea, and integrating medical (including pharmacologic) and physical therapy as needed. If problems persist, if individuals have a history of trauma affecting their sexual lives, if the couple is unable to work collaboratively, or if mental health or substance abuse problems predominate, it is best to refer to a sex therapist. Sex therapists have extensive training in treatment of complex sexual problems as well as couples therapy. Couples and individuals may need the HCP's assurance that trying out new things with curiosity and non-judgment is good. Use of ubiquity ("Many individuals think about use of a vibrator but wonder if it's okay to try something like that. Lots of people of all ages and sexes explore new options for sexual pleasure. Focusing in and trying new things may take some work, but it is a good work to do.") is affirming [1, 12–19].

Assessment

In assessment it is important to measure sexual function before and after any medication, treatment, health/mental health condition. This allows us to get a better picture of any changes in an individual's or couple's sexual health. Sexual norms, behavior, and function vary greatly from person/couple to person/couple that getting a sense of an individual's norm will serve us better in our assessment process [20] (Figure 6-1).

Biological

Physical Health

Aging

Sexual problems are common in older adults, but physical health and aging tend to impact male sexual health more than female sexual health. Challenges with lubrication are a common challenge for older adult women, where for men it can include decreased libido, erectile dysfunction, and ability to achieve orgasm [21].

For older adults, emphasis on what does not work sexually must be balanced with a curiosity about "what does"—the resiliencies and capabilities of the individual and couple in a broader context than that based solely on "sexual performance" [1].

There is no common agreement about when older age actually begins. In this chapter, 65 years—the onset in the USA for Medicare health coverage—is used to demarcate the socially defined beginning of older age. Older adults are the fastest growing segment of the population in the USA. In 2000, one in ten persons was over 65, and in 2030, one in five will be over 65. Currently, 14.1% of the US population is 65 or older [1].

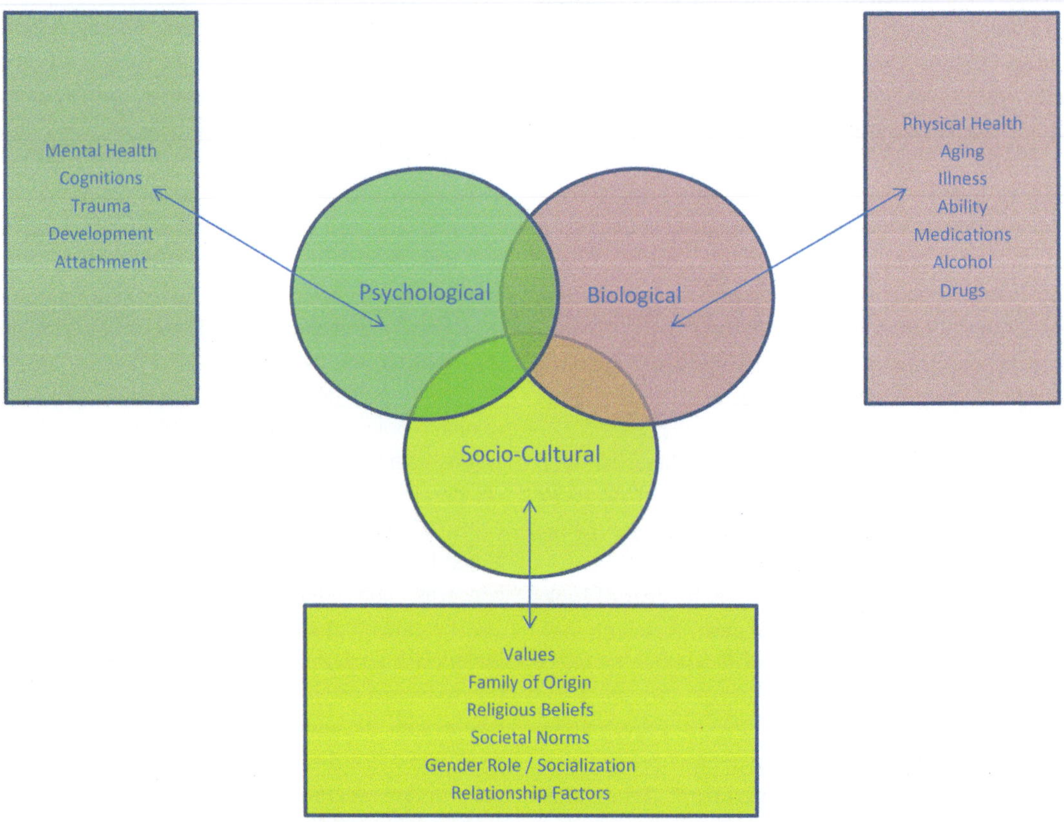

FIGURE 6-1. Biospychosocial model of sexual dysfunction.

Rosemary Basson and colleagues have introduced a nonlinear model of the female sexual response cycle that includes physical and emotional satisfaction and sexual pleasure. The Basson model is well researched and represents an accurate understanding of sexual arousal and responsivity for many women. The model emphasizes willingness, motivation, intentionality, and individual sexual satisfaction rather than a performance model. Although the triphasic model continues to be endorsed by some, the Basson model calls into question the need for "desire" to exist as a separate distinct category prior to arousal. By indicating that interest/desire and arousal are neither distinctly separate nor exactly the same for all, Basson's model supports individual variances in sexual response and also endorses the biopsychosocial nature of sexual response. In assessment of older adult females, it is vital to assess desire through the lens of the Basson model, as opposed to a linear model with desire as the starting point [1, 22–24].

AARP conducts semi-decennial research on "Sex, Romance, and Relationships: AARP Survey of Midlife and Older Adults." The 2009 survey employs a representative sample of the US population aged 45 and older. Thirty percent of men report that they "never" or "just sometimes" are able to maintain erections sufficient for penetrative sex, indicating a high correlation with illness and medication related problems [25]. Despite promising integrative treatments for erectile dysfunction (ED), older men will continue to have treatment resistant ED due to confounding factors [4]. Interestingly, many men in the AARP study continue to report sexual satisfaction even if they are not able to have penetrative sex [25]. The more "performance" or "erection focused" male models simply do not reflect all older men's experiences of continued sexual satisfaction even if erection does not occur [26–28]. Wittmann describes a model for survivors of prostate cancer and their partners, a model with more emphasis on pleasure and satisfaction that could well be adapted. It is important for clinicians in their assessment of sexual functioning to be aware of the differing models, as well as clinician bias, as we work to understand, assess, and help our patients [1].

As men age, they often experience a decrease in their testosterone levels, and often an increase in their Body Mass Index (BMI). Weight gain and muscle loss are factors in sexual dysfunction. Older adult men experience lower libido/sexual desire due to both low testosterone and to higher BMI. Low testosterone however is not a contributing factor to erectile dysfunction issues for most men. Benign enlarged prostate, diabetes, hypertension are also all factors that can negatively impact male sexual function. All of these are common factors impacting men's health as they age.

At menopause, some women experience a decrease in arousal when masturbating or engaging in partnered sex. Many remark that the pleasant sense of "fullness, tingling, and swelling" in and around the vulva is only vaguely represented [29]. Several valuable studies reflect the growing interest in understanding and treating postmenopausal changes for older women, especially those associated with vaginal atrophy (VA) and vulvar vaginal atrophy (VVA) [30–33]. REVIVE (REal Women's VIews of Treatment Options for Menopausal Vaginal ChangEs) survey [31] found VVA symptoms negatively affected sexual enjoyment (59%), including problems with spontaneity, intimacy, and partner relationship. Loss of sexual intimacy was of "concern" for 47% of women with a partner, with 85% stating "some problems" related to loss of intimacy due to VVA. Most common concerns were dryness (55%), dyspareunia (44%), and irritation (33%). This study and others confirm that vulvovaginal changes—and, for some, decreased sensitivity and increased dryness and thinning of vaginal walls—are associated with vaginal pain, negatively affecting sexual activity, with decreases in desire, arousal, and pleasure [31].

Sexual function for older women includes the passage through menopause and, for most, changes in sensation and some decreased sensitivity as well as vulvovaginal changes with increased dryness and thinning of vaginal walls. There may be increases in vaginal pain associated with drying thinning tissues. The associated discomfort often results in increased avoidance of sexual thought or activity—both penetration and vulvar stimulation—since it is no longer pleasurable and pain free [1].

Illness

Cancer in Women

Sexual issues related to women in all stages of cancer are very common. The cancer diagnosis and resulting treatment can bring about many sexuality related social/emotional issues in addition to the physical side effects that treatment can have on self-esteem, desire, and sexual function. The sexual issues associated with cancer (such as dyspareunia, poor body image, and relationship distress) can be on-going and can get worse over time if not addressed. Sexuality is an integral part of what makes up quality of life for most female cancer survivors. However, these concerns for women dealing with cancer related sexual issues are rarely asked about or addressed. Providers can ask simple questions, such as: "Do you have any questions/concerns about: fertility, menopause, or sexual health?" Or questions that are a little more specific, such as: "Are you experiencing any vaginal dryness, pain, or sexual issues?" [34–42]

Breast Cancer

Breast cancer, and the treatments for it, cause many women to have significant changes in their relationship to their body and their body image. This holds true for both women who have had breast reconstruction and those that have not. These changes can impact sexual self-esteem, body image, and self-efficacy, from a mental health stand point. Physical effects come from chemotherapy and hormone therapy causing vulvovaginal atrophy, loss of libido, and dyspareunia. Prescribed medications also contribute to vulvar and vaginal atrophic change, especially when used long term [43].

Prostate Cancer

Post recovery from prostate cancer surgery, 90% of men will experience issues with erectile dysfunction. What that exactly looks like depends on a variety of factors, the key ones being: the age and overall health of the individual, their preoperative erectile functioning, and the skill/expertise of the surgeon. Even with an experienced surgeon, using a nerve sparing procedure, patients will likely experience erectile function issues post-surgery. Erectile function is treatable in a variety of ways when aggressively approached from a biopsychosocial perspective, as all areas can be impacted. Many men and their partners, however, are often unprepared for and unaware of the post-surgical impacts to sexual health, and the approaches to recovery, leaving 75% of prostate cancer survivors with unresolved sexual problems 5 years post-surgery [44–46].

It is important for providers to understand the sexual hopes of the individual and their partner, when appropriate, around the importance of sexual connection to the individuals and within the relationship. According to Daniela Wittmann, "There are many psychological and relationship strengths that people can employ to get back or retain their sex lives." Satisfaction with sex life and not erectile function is the focus in sexual dysfunction interventions with this population. Feelings of grief and loss are a normative part of this process and if not dealt with can leave patients more susceptible to depression and anxiety, which in turns can negatively impact sexual desire [44, 47–49].

According to Dr. Wittmann, "After PCa treatment, all aspects of sexual health are affected, including the man's erectile function, self-image, mental health, and relationship with his partner; therefore, it affects not only his quality of life but also that of his partner. Furthermore, most PCa survivors' partners are postmenopausal women whose sexual function also requires assistance. The challenge is to help men and partners restore sexual health in the context of significant functional loss. For men and partners to recover sexual health in survivorship, all components of sexuality and sexual health must be addressed because known psychological barriers, such as overly optimistic expectations about erectile function outcomes, unresolved grief about functional loss, poor sexual communication, and difficulty accepting sexual aids, may lead survivors and their partners to reject the idea of a sexual relationship that does not rely on a natural erection" [47, 50].

Benign Prostatic Hyperplasia/Lower Urinary Tract

Approximately 50% of men in their 50s and 90% of men in their 80s are impacted by an enlarged prostate of benign prostatic hyperplasia (BPH). Often men who experience BPH also are impacted by lower urinary tract symptoms (LUTS). Sexual dysfunction is a known symptom of lower urinary tract symptoms in men. The sexual dysfunction primarily shows up as erectile dysfunction or ejaculatory dysfunction falling in the range of 50–70% of the male population affected. Additionally, some of the treatments for both BPH and LUTS also are known to have significant sexual side effects as well, including erectile dysfunction, ejaculatory dysfunction, and hypoactive sexual desire, which can make the sexual dysfunction issues more complex [51].

Two 5-a reductase inhibitors can be used to treat BPH, with two of them also being used to treat male pattern hair loss (MPHL). Finasteride is one that is used for treatment of both issues, and in multiple randomized studies significant sexual dysfunction was found to be associated with its use. According to Irwig and Korokula, "A subset of otherwise healthy men taking finasteride for MPHL developed persistent sexual side effects in temporal association with the medication. Most men developed sexual dysfunction in multiple domains with 94% experiencing low libido, 92% experiencing erectile dysfunction, 92% experiencing decreased arousal, and 69% experiencing problems with orgasm. The mean duration of the persistent sexual side effects was at least 40 months, with 20% of subjects reporting durations of over 6 years. The mean number of sexual episodes per month dropped from 25.8 before finasteride to 8.8 after finasteride" [52].

Diabetes

Diabetes is a chronic disease that has become increasingly common, impacting more than 371 million people around the world in 2012. It is associated with sexual dysfunction in both women and men. Diabetes is a known risk factor for sexual dysfunction in men, with a threefold increased risk of erectile dysfunction over nondiabetic men. Evidence showing an association between diabetes and sexual dysfunction in women is less conclusive. Female sexual function is more connected to social and psychological components than to the physical impacts of diabetes, but most studies do report a higher prevalence of female sexual dysfunction in diabetic women [53]. Sexual disorders reported in women with diabetes include decreased libido, difficulties with lubrication and arousal, dyspareunia, and for some anorgasmia [53–55].

Heart Disease

Sexual dysfunction and a decrease in sexual activity are common in people living with cardiovascular disease. Often times there is significant psychological stress connected to being sexual and fear that sexual activity will worsen the heart health or possibly even cause death. This anxiety can be experienced by patient or partner, but leads to decreased sexual activity and satisfaction. It can be the decline in sexual satisfaction that may bring about other issues, such as strain in romantic or marital relationships. Depression and anxiety are not uncommon and often are a significant factor, when coupled with age and other health issues, leading to erectile dysfunction in men, and of a variety of sexual function issues in women, including dyspareunia, decreased desire, and difficulty with arousal and orgasm [56–63].

People with cardiovascular disease are able to engage in sexual activity, but it is often suggested for them to have a complete physical beforehand to ensure their symptoms are controlled and stable, and if not they should be treated and stabilized first. Medications for heart disease are often a cause of ED in men, but can be countered with PDE5 inhibitors. PDE5 inhibitors should never be used in conjunction with nitrates [56, 57].

Other Health Issues

Sexual issues commonly associated with Parkinson's disease in women include difficulty with desire, arousal, and orgasm. Men living with Parkinson's disease can experience erectile dysfunction and premature ejaculation, in addition to overall sexual dissatisfaction. Some of the other physical issues associated with Parkinson's disease, such as challenges with speech and posture can also make sexual behavior more challenging. As with other health issues, many people also experience depression with Parkinson's disease, which further exacerbates sexual difficulties, as do many antidepressants [64].

People living with Multiple Sclerosis often experience symptoms including pain, numbness, fatigue, coordination, and body image. All of which have a significant impact on sexual functioning both physically, as well as emotionally [65].

On the other hand, achieving orgasm through sexual activity can alleviate pain for some people. A European study of 63 women living with fibromyalgia found that sexual intercourse actually gave relief from continuous pain [66].

Ability Issues

When working with people with disabilities (PWD) around sexual issues, it is important for the provider to be cognizant of their biases toward these populations. Society has created negative or dismissive narratives around the sexuality of PWD, which can be infantilizing, stigmatizing, or both, and many providers have unconsciously internalized those same societal biases [67].

Dr. Mitchell Tepper, in his work on sexuality and disability, encourages providers to recognize that the discourse surrounding sexuality and disability focuses on deviance and inappropriate behavior, abuse and victimization, as well as reproductive issues in women and men. He notes that there seems to be missing a discourse around pleasure. Pleasure is an important part of sexual health for all people, including people who are living with a range of ability issues, and it is an important factor for which to assess in an evaluation [68].

Physical

A spinal cord injury's (SCI) impact upon sexual function depends on where the injury takes place in the spine and the level of severity [69, 70]. Men and women who have experienced an SCI frequently report both lower libido and a decreased frequency of sexual behavior [71]. Dealing with both the psychological elements (e.g., body image, self-esteem) and sociocultural elements (gender, age, and religion) all impact the conceptualization of the sexual self of the person with an SCI [72]. Problems with both orgasm and arousal due to struggles with coordination and self-image also significantly impact people with SCIs [73, 74].

Men who experience spinal cord injuries can also have sexual dysfunction issues, with erectile function being a significant impact factor upon quality of life. Studies have shown success for men in this area with penile injections, sildenafil, and for more challenging cases penile implants. All have shown success in helping men as one part of rehabilitation.

Many aspects of physical sexual functioning can be impacted for women following an SCI. A few of the important areas for clinicians to assess include: sexual arousal and vaginal lubrication, orgasm, urinary incontinence, bowel incontinence, and spasticity—particularly with regard to stiffness and pain [75].

Intellectual

Sexual health knowledge and attitudes in people living with intellectual disabilities (ID) is poor, but they express sexual health needs and desires comparable to the general population. There is less sexual activity among people with moderate to severe intellectual disabilities, but they remain very vulnerable to sexual abuse [76].

According to Eastgate, "People with intellectual disability experience the same range of sexual needs and desires as other people. With appropriate education and good social support, people with intellectual disability are capable of safe, constructive sexual expression and healthy relationships. Providing such support is an essential part of supporting people with an intellectual disability" [77].

The sexuality of people living with intellectual disabilities can be a challenge for the people that work with them [78]. For the individual with the disability, they may find barriers to their sexual expression from an institutionalized living system that does not afford them access to privacy or even information about healthy sexuality and healthy sexual expression, and in many scenarios they are given misinformation about their sexuality [79]. Some care providers maintain the idea of people with intellectual disabilities as eternal children and thus restrict their social and relational opportunities, thus denying them the right to self-fulfillment [80, 81].

People with intellectual disabilities will have normative desires and feelings around sex as they develop. It is normal for them to want to masturbate and can be a healthy form of expression. Masturbation can be used as a way of self-soothing or having pleasure when bored. It may also seem to happen sometimes in inappropriate places. All of this can be dealt with through attention to the overall well-being and healthy education of the person with the intellectual ability. They will also benefit by understanding self-care for the body, good sexual expression, and what constitutes inappropriate behavior or abuse [78, 81–83].

Although a lot of the current discourse for people with ID focuses on sexual rights, in evaluating the sexual needs of this population there is also a strong need for reproductive health information to help with unplanned pregnancy, as well as information around safer sex to help prevent STIs including HIV. Sexual hygiene, gynecological care, and sexual abuse are other areas that consistently need to be addressed for overall sexual health [76].

Medications

Sexual dysfunction issues that are already common in the general population are often increased for people being treated for mental health issues. Many people being treated for mental health issues are prescribed psychotropic medications. Psychotropic medications, which are often helpful to deal with a patient's mental health, frequently have a negative effect on a person's sexual health or sexual functioning. Looking at a sexual history from a biopsychosocial perspective can help to separate out what sexual function issues are connected to mood, what is related to antidepressant medication, and what might be related to other medical or social factors [84].

Antidepressants

Antidepressants can affect the same areas of sexual functioning that depressive disorder does, mainly desire, arousal, and orgasm. There is some evidence to suggest that delayed orgasm is the most significant side effect. Selective serotonin reuptake inhibitors (SSRIs) are a group of antidepressant medications that increase the availability of serotonin in the synapse by inhibiting the serotonin transporters. Increased synaptic serotonin has an inhibitory effect on sexual functioning. Individual SSRIs vary in their exact pharmacological impact, with a range of impact on the serotonin transporter, and some impacting other receptors [84].

Antipsychotics

Similarly to antidepressants and depression, antipsychotic medication and schizophrenia both will have significant impact on a person's sexual functioning. Antipsychotics, although impacting libido, arousal, and orgasm, seem to have the most significant impact upon sexual desire. The first generation of antipsychotic medications has greater impact upon sexual functioning than the second generation, but both have significant impact [84].

Mood Stabilizers

Studies looking at the impact of lithium upon people living with bipolar disorder found that there is sexual dysfunction reported, but the frequency is low and the severity of the impact upon sexual functioning is mild [84].

Blood Pressure Medications

Sexual dysfunction is a common issue that arises for patients living with hypertension. The available data suggests that sexual function issues are more common for patients that have been treated for the condition than in those patients that remain untreated. This would indicate that antihypertensive therapy is correlated with sexual dysfunction issues. Several studies indicate differences on the impact of sexual function for various antihypertensive drugs. The older antihypertensive drugs (diuretics, beta blockers) have more of a negative impact upon erectile function whereas the newer drugs (nebivolol, angiotensin receptor blockers) have little or in some cases beneficial effects upon sexual function [85].

Alcohol and Other Drugs

The initial connection between drugs and sex was one that attempted to enhance sexual functioning. Some drugs can indeed enhance sexual response in the early stages of their use, particularly with people who have had previous sexual function issues. Most significantly, males with early ejaculation often report increased satisfaction with the delayed orgasm caused by many drugs. For women, alcohol and drugs can cause an initial heightened sense of relaxation or pain management. Chronic use of substances tends to negatively impact sexual function in every stage (desire, arousal, orgasm) of sexual function over time for both male and female users [86].

Tobacco

Cigarette smoking has a negative impact on erectile function. It can have an immediate effect on a man's ability to get and maintain a good erection. Male smokers have a 1.5 greater probability of developing erectile dysfunction then nonsmokers. The physical components of the arousal phase require blood to flow to the genital areas for both males and females, but Nicotine is a potent vasoconstrictor and reduces blood circulation in these areas. The more a person smokes, the longer they have been smoking, and increased age all are significant risk factors for sexual dysfunction [86].

Alcohol

Alcohol is often used as a precursor to sexual activity, because it can be a dis-inhibitor and make people more open to sexual activity. However, alcohol used in large quantities can bring about significant sexual function issues. It can cause erectile dysfunction and inhibit orgasm in men (even in young men). Women who use alcohol heavily may have difficulty with vaginal lubrication, inhibited orgasm, menstrual irregularities, and dyspareunia. More chronic users may experience inhibited desire, arousal and orgasm [86].

Cannabis

There are pros and cons to the use of marijuana when it comes to sexual function. Marijuana is reported by many users, both male and female, to increase sexual desire and arousal. THC, for some users, can help them to feel more relaxed, and stimulate sexual fantasy. There are mixed results in terms of sexual dysfunction with some studies showing that ongoing use can cause erectile dysfunction, and daily use can lead to trouble achieving orgasm for some men, while other studies show no significant negative impact on sexual function [86].

Cocaine

As with marijuana usage, cocaine usage can have differing impacts on sexuality based upon how it is used. People who use this drug infrequently may feel an enhanced sense of sexual desire, arousal, and sensuality, but may also experience their ability to achieve orgasm as delayed. Some male users who have concerns about PE may like this side effect, while other male users and most female users find delayed orgasm distressing. For more chronic users, their cardiovascular system may be negatively impacted, which speaks to the increased reports of erectile dysfunction in men, along with an ultimate decrease in sexual desire for many long-term users, and further delays in achieving orgasm [86].

Methamphetamine

Most users of methamphetamine strongly connect it to sexual experiences. The drug itself does not impact the sexual response cycle, but it is rather an overall nervous system stimulator bringing about increased senses of confidence, energy, and reducing inhibitions. The general sense of well-being and excitement provided can enhance a user's sense of sexual pleasure. This drug is highly addictive, and for many users turns quickly to more habitual usage. The chronic stage of methamphetamine use is correlated with more sexual dysfunction. As more of the drug is consumed, users are more likely to not be able to achieve orgasm, and ultimately see their overall interest in sexual behavior decline significantly [86].

Opiates

Many users report that heroin can bring about intense feelings of pleasure, similar to those experienced through orgasm. Women who experience vaginismus or dyspareunia may feel greater levels of relaxation and reduced pain as a result of the analgesic qualities of this drug. And men with rapid ejaculation may also see initial benefit with orgasm delayed. There are also many sexual dysfunctions caused by the ongoing usage of heroin. In one study of regular users, decreased libido was reported in 68% of women and 75% of men. Sixty percent of women and 71% of men felt that their sexual arousal was negatively impacted by heroin use over time. Also, 60% of female and male users reported difficulty achieving orgasm with prolonged use of opiates. A second study found erectile dysfunction in over 50% of regular opiate users. Both heroin and methadone usage cause a decrease in testosterone levels which can quickly rebound once use of the drugs are stopped [86].

Psychological

Mental Health

People living with mental health issues have higher rates of sexual dysfunction issues than those people without them. This is particularly true for the people whose mental health issues are being treated with psychotropic medications. Sexual dysfunction negatively impacts between 30 and 60% of people living with schizophrenia who are treated with antipsychotic medications, up to 78% of those living with depression and being treated with antidepressants, and up to 80% of people who are living with anxiety disorders. Working with the challenges and complexities of mental health and sexual function, it is important for the clinician to identify the specific sexual dysfunctions and how it is impacted by the individual's mental health condition, current medications, and their interpersonal relationships [2].

As discussed, many patients living with mood disorders have sexual difficulties. An estimated half of all people with mood disorders will experience some form of sexual dysfunction [84]. Loss of sexual interest is the most common form of sexual dysfunction. Often this will have a substantial negative effect upon interpersonal romantic relationships, as withdrawal from partners is common, thus demonstrating the multidirectional impact of various factors involved in sexual dysfunction [84]. Depression can also impact a patient's level of arousal, as well as their ability to achieve orgasm. All of which can lead to subsequent sexual performance anxiety [84].

Depression

It's estimated that about 10% of the population suffers from depression at a level strong enough to impact overall life functioning and quality of life. One significant side effect that often accompanies major depression is a decrease in or loss of sexual desire. Casper et al. [87], reported that the majority of participants in their study of moderate to severe patients hospitalized for depression, who were not on any form of drug, reported significant loss of libido. For patients with depression alone it was 72%, and for patients with bipolar disorder 77% reported loss of libido. The more severe the depression or anxiety the greater the negative impact on sexual desire. People experiencing depression also can experience difficulty maintaining sexual arousal or achieving orgasm. All of which can lead to subsequent sexual performance anxiety [4]. Men living with severe depression can experience rates of erectile dysfunction as high as 90% [2, 88].

The understanding of both depression and sexual functioning is important for all clinicians as both mood disorders and sexual function issues are very common, are believed to be comorbid, and may even share a common origin [89, 90]. Waldinger reports "that the relationship between depressive mood and sexual dysfunction is bidirectional and further complicated by the sexual side-effects of antidepressant" [91, 92].

The empirical evidence confirms a prominent role of depression in sexual dysfunction. While the exact direction of causality is difficult to ascertain, the data not only indicate a close correlational relationship between depression and sexual disorders but also support a functional significance of mood disorders in causing and maintaining sexual dysfunction. Compared with functional controls, sexually dysfunctional men and women exhibit both higher levels of acute depressive symptoms and a markedly higher lifetime prevalence of affective disorders [92].

Anxiety

The DSM-5 recognizes numerous anxiety disorders and it is believed that about 15% of the population is impacted to varying degrees. People who are impacted by more severe anxiety issues are also shown in research studies to have higher rates of sexual dysfunction [2]. Anxiety and sexual function issues can be bidirectional, meaning that anxiety can cause sexual dysfunction, but sexual dysfunction can also cause people to develop anxiety issues. Anxiety is a frequent player in the development of sexual dysfunctions, and it is a common way that many biological, psychological, social, and religious factors interact to impair human sexual response. Anxiety can also negatively impact both arousal and orgasm, as well as decrease overall libido. Corretti and Baldi state that "the complex relationship between anxiety disorders and desire disorders is rarely clarified in the medical literature. Kaplan underlines a strong prevalence of panic disorder (25%) in patients affected by sexual aversion disorder. Anxiety is also relevant in sexual arousal. Induced by different stressors, anxiety can distract from erotic stimuli and impair sexual arousal, principally through an increased sympathetic tone [93, 94]. This may result in poor erection in males and a reduction in lubrication and clitoral tumescence in females" [95].

Performance anxiety is one type of anxiety that often shows up in men who are worried about achieving erection and, subsequently, the quality and duration of the erection. The worry itself often creates a vicious cycle where the anxiety causes the erectile dysfunction [2, 95]. Post-traumatic stress disorder (PTSD) can also have a significant impact on sexual function. A study of combat veterans with PTSD showed 69% struggling with erectile dysfunction. These veterans also reported problems with orgasm, and overall a poor level of sexual satisfaction. In addition to desire and arousal, orgasm may also be impaired by anxiety. Anxious thoughts and feelings can have a negative impact on female orgasm. Women who experience dyspareunia have also been found to have high levels of anxiety. Sexual satisfaction and pleasure, for people with social phobias, is often a diminished experience. Women with social phobias are more likely to also have sexual desire disorders (46%), experience pain during sex (42%), and have less frequent sexual thoughts, as well as sexual intercourse. Women with obsessive compulsive disorder have high rates of sexual dysfunction, with about 39% reporting some negative impact, and 73% experiencing lower levels of sexual pleasure and expressing a strong dissatisfaction with their overall sexual health as well [95].

Cognitions

Studies have shown that the best predictors of sexual desire in men are associated with cognitive factors, including their general beliefs and values around sexual health, as well as the automatic thoughts they have during sexual activity. The specific negative beliefs or restrictive attitudes toward sexuality, worries about erection, and lack of erotic thoughts in sexual context, all have the effect of significantly reducing sexual desire. However, positive cognitions can also be factors that help to reduce problems with health issues and age, and sexual desire [96].

Sexual desire is more often significantly impacted by the lack of erotic thoughts during sexual activity then it is by other factors. Lack of overall erotic focus when coupled with erection concerns during sexual activity is a process that brings about the decline in sexual response. Cognitive distractions during sexual intercourse (specifically related to poor sexual performance) pay a significant role in sexual dysfunction [96–100].

Cognitive factors related to sociocultural and religious values can engender beliefs leading to sexual dysfunction. A similar process around automatic thoughts can be distracting during sexual interactions, also leading to dysfunction. Research has indicated the need to include an understanding of cognitive dimensions in the evaluation of sexual desire issues. They can be viewed as either vulnerabilities or resiliencies in sexual desire. These cognitions can be even more significant than many biological factors in the overall impact upon sexual health [96].

Sociocultural

Sociocultural factors play a vital role when evaluating clients presenting issues. Not all of the sexual symptoms that will present will be recognized as sexual dysfunction in dominant western culture, but it is important that clinicians evaluate through the lens of the client's intersecting cultural frameworks. In many clinical settings, the sociocultural parts in assessment of sexual dysfunction are overlooked or minimized. However, these factors are vital, as culture is the lens through which people interpret and communicate their experiences, and informs what our clients do and don't talk about. According to Atallah et al., "political correctness, lack of knowledge of various cultural mores, or a micro rather than macro view of sexual dysfunction often prevent adequate investigation of the possible role of culture, religion, and social norms that may influence sexual behavior and functioning" [101].

Sue and Sue, et al., stress the awareness of both patient and clinician beliefs, the attainment of background knowledge about the patient (including his or her worldview), and the development of culturally competent skills [102]. As with all clinical interactions the clinician should demonstrate strong empathy, but even more so when working cross-culturally. To develop an accurate cultural understanding of a client, the clinician needs to start by gaining awareness of the client's cultural identities, how those identities and experiences impact the client's understanding of self and how they experience the world, the other systems that interact upon the client, including support systems, family, community, and religion. Additionally, clinicians should inquire as to the client's perspective of what is going on, what they believe is causing it, and what else was happening at the time of onset. All of this is taken into account when evaluating the client's sexual presenting issues or dysfunction [103].

The biopsychosocial model is enhanced by paying attention to culture when evaluating diverse clients. This keeps a focus on the way in which culture impacts the experience, understanding, and expression of sexual dysfunction, distress, or even illness. The way in which a client presents can be very much influenced by their religious, cultural, and social beliefs. It is also vital that clinicians are aware of their own cultural understandings and lenses, as this impacts how we understand health, normative behavior, and illness [103].

Guidelines for Clinicians Carrying Out a Culturally Sensitive Assessment of Individuals and Couples Presenting With Sexual Concerns by Cardernil and Battle [101, 104]

- Suspend preconceptions about clients' race/ethnicity/gender/sexuality and that of their family members.
- Recognize that clients may be quite different from other members of their racial/ethnic/gender/sexual group.
- Consider how racial/ethnic/sexual and other differences in background and experience between therapist and client might affect therapy.
- Acknowledge that power, privilege, racism, and sexual prejudice might affect interactions with clients.
- When in doubt about the importance of race, ethnicity, gender, and sexuality in treatment, err on the side of discussion; be willing to take risks with clients.

Cultural Sensitivity in Sex Therapy, according to Atallah et al. takes into account the following factors [101]:

1. Assess personal values and attitudes—we don't always need to agree with our client's values, but we do need to show respect and acceptance without judgment.
2. Ask about culture—evaluation needs to include how culture impacts the presenting issue.
3. Acknowledge and address culturally based challenges in discussing sex—recognize language barriers, effective language styles, and the culture-bound challenges that may be present when discussing sexual issues.
4. Clarify the triangle of love—Sternberg's Triangle of Love includes intimacy, passion and commitment. It can be helpful to understand the client's experience in this context.
5. Assess Sexual Knowledge and Preparation—a client's lack of sexual knowledge can lead to dysfunction, as they are not prepared to be sexual.
6. Be mindful of religious conflicts—religion plays a strong role in developing our client's sexual values and informing how clients engage sexually.
7. Sociological considerations in practice—our client's sexual function is also influenced by their social worlds.

Cultural Values

Culture is a very powerful influence upon people's feelings, thoughts, and understanding of self. It is what everyone in a particular group knows that everyone else within that group knows. It can include values, patterns of behavior, the way in which thoughts are constructed, and the ways in which people make meaning. Culture can be passed generation to generation, while still being active and evolving.

In some cultures young people, particularly young women, are taught that sexual activity is not something that one engages in for pleasure, but rather for procreative purposes only. If there is pleasure to be experienced it is about the male partner's sexual pleasure, and the female experience is often subjugated to that of the male. The level of religiosity and the literalness of religious teachings can cause client distress when they detour from the strict instruction, often causing or exacerbating sexual dysfunction. Understanding the level of sexual education, the values from the family of origin as well as sub community, and religious teachings around sexual health can help to uncover what is often underneath the presenting sexual dysfunction [103].

How one makes sense of their personal self or identity varies from culture to culture. In the West there is a strong emphasis on the individual and autonomy, in many Eastern cultures there is a much greater emphasis on the collective experience and understanding oneself in the context of a group identity. Eastern cultures also focus on a mind and body integration, with emotions impacting physical health. In general Western culture separates out the mind and the body as two discrete parts [101].

In cultures where people become relationally committed prior to the experiences of intimacy and passion (Sternberg's Triangular Theory of Love), the challenge to function in a sexually intimate way can be daunting for new couples. Going from relative sexual abstinence to sexual intimacy with someone one does not know well can bring up sexual function issues for both males and females [101].

Family of Origin

Norms surrounding how couples live or how people have access to privacy can impact sexual health significantly. Couples living in extended family situations, or sometimes even with their own children, may have struggles with privacy, particularly lower income families. Pressure from parents or in-laws for new couples to have children can cause sexual dysfunction issues in both men and women. Limited sexual opportunities or private time can lead to the development of premature ejaculation in men. Men can train themselves through masturbation to reach orgasm quickly when they have limited time [101].

Religious Beliefs

Religious beliefs and values around sexuality are important to evaluate, as they are common contributors to sexual dysfunction issues in both men and women. Guilt and anxiety are two common feelings that come up for clients when integrating their religious beliefs with their sexuality. Asking questions of our clients to understand their unique practices, rituals, meanings, and traditions around sexuality will help to understand their level of sexual health knowledge and understanding, as well as giving information as to potential causes of sexual distress. Some conservative religions may restrict access to information and may also have a narrow perspective on the role of human sexuality. Understanding meanings, values, and traditions, including any restrictions—such as when and where a male may ejaculate—can inform how we evaluate a client's sexual functioning [101, 105].

Societal Norms

Lack of education or knowledge about sexual health issues is what is most often connected to sexual dysfunction. People from all cultural backgrounds can have challenges with obtaining accurate sexual education. Sometimes the conflicting messages that young people get from dominant culture and subcultures can lead to confusion about sexuality often leading to sexual dysfunction. Lack of comprehensive, scientifically accurate sexual health education in schools leave young people with limited access to information about what is healthy sexuality. This is also a common situation for people who have immigrated from developing countries [102, 106].

What motivates sexual behavior varies in cultures. Some cultures view sexual behavior as a way of connecting with one's partner, experiencing pleasure and intimacy, and expressing feelings of love. Others view its function as part of marital responsibility or duty, as well as for procreation. Depending upon the meaning of sexual behavior in a relationship and culture, sexual dysfunction can represent anything from a challenge to relational satisfaction to not living up to one's duty within a marriage [101].

Gender Roles/Socialization

Societal messages about what the appropriate way for males and females to understand and display their sexuality is very connected to the concept of patriarchy. This can have negative impacts for both men and women, and ultimately be an underlying cause of sexual dysfunction. Clinicians need to gather an understanding of what the client has learned about what it means to be a sexual person and how that gendered sexuality is to be performed. There can be conflicting messages, particularly for females, between dominant culture and messages and those from the culture of origin. In some cultures the role of a female is to be submissive to her partner and to put his needs ahead of hers [101].

The role expectations of men and women can also have significant impact upon sexual dysfunction. In a traditional role example, women who may be exhausted from working, childcare, and household duties may find lack of sexual desire. Men who are experiencing work, financial, or family stress may feel added pressures around sexual function causing erectile difficulties. Men are taught that they should always want to engage sexually and women are taught that it is not appropriate to be seen as having sexual needs outside of a committed relationship. Both of these narratives can lead to sexual dysfunction and even shame.

Shame can bring about a sense of severe disconnection from others. Diagnosis of sexual dysfunction can also bring about shame for people. It can be a strong emotion that, left unaddressed, can have a negative circular impact on a person's sense of well-being and healthy sexuality [1, 59, 107].

Generally taken for granted and invisible, but yet woven into social fabric, is gender inequality. This has been transformed by popular media into stereotypes about men's and women's sexuality and natures. Sexual health challenges for men and women are fairly equal in numbers of complaints and there can be a resulting assumption that their concerns are equally represented. However, women's legacy of subordination is reflected in incomplete health care; greater social pressure to marry, and trading of sex for socioeconomic advantages; Women also carry greater responsibilities in homecare, child care, and eldercare, all of which limit energy for sex, as well as other activities to care and nurture the self [108, 109].

Women's sexual health issues arise from a few different areas. (1) Medical and physical issues. (2) Mental Health challenges or psychological conflicts. (3) Partner or relationship issues. (4) Social and cultural issues. Issues falling into categories (1–3) can benefit from professional intervention. The issues falling into category (4) can benefit from being named and addressed on both individual, as well as systemic level in order to create broader change [108, 110].

Relationship Factors

It can be challenging to assess if sexual issues in a relationship are caused by or the result of problems or discord within a relationship. Sexual function and relationship function are connected and the impact needs to be understood as a whole. Consider—did the low sexual desire or performance anxiety cause one partner to avoid being sexual and lead to a non-physically intimate relationship? Or did disconnection in the romantic relationship lead to sexual avoidance? [2] Unhappiness within a relationship, unresolved anger or resentment can lead to a sexual distancing between couples.

Many couples with sexual function issues have never talked to each other about the problems that they are having, let alone with anyone else. Couples often misread their partner's experiences, with one study finding discrepancies between the male and female partner's narratives of their experiences 78% of the time for the study participants [108, 111]. An overfocus on genital function, erection, orgasm, and goal-oriented sexual behavior adds to sexual pressure and dysfunction in many couples [108]. Communication patterns between couples and an understanding of how couples discuss their sexual relationship can help to evaluate what is connected to lack of communication, as opposed to a differing etiology [108, 111]. Fear of intimacy and not having an understanding of what healthy sexual behavior is are two additional issues that lead to sexual dysfunction in couples.

Conclusion

Patients who present with sexual dysfunction may be dealing with a simple sex therapy situation or a complex sex therapy situation. A simple sex therapy case is one in which the presenting issue and symptomology is easily dealt with through one direct intervention. More complex cases are ones that are impacted by several factors and need to have interventions on multiple levels, often concurrently. The biopsychosocial model for evaluating sexual dysfunction allows the provider to gain an understanding of all the potential factors that may be causing or contributing to problems, be it a simple issue or a more complex one, and to formulate an effective treatment plan. Without a comprehensive approach in more complex cases, the patient may find himself or herself struggling to experience any sense of symptom relief despite having what appears to be an appropriate medical intervention. Through tending to all aspects of the BPS model, the multi-pronged understanding of factors contributing to dysfunction will be identified and the patient will be more likely to receive comprehensive and effective treatment.

Historically, the biomedical approach has been the dominant model for evaluating sexual dysfunction issues, particularly in the medical field. However, an increasing awareness of the psychological impact, and sociocultural and religious influence on a person's overall sense of wellness highlighted the need for a more comprehensive model in health and wellness, and particularly in the field of sexual health. It was important to maintain the strengths of evaluating disease from a biomedical approach, while enhancing that approach to include other factors that have a significant effect on sexual functioning to gain a more complete picture. The biopsychosocial model takes that more comprehensive approach to understanding all the varying factors that can impact a person's sense of overall sexual wellness, paying attention to the physiological components, the mental health components, and the broader social context and messages that impact all people. This approach for evaluating and understanding a person's experience has allowed for more consistently effective interventions and treatments.

References

1. Foley SM. Biopsychosocial assessment and treatment of sexual problems in older age. Curr Sex Health Rep. 2015;7:80–8. doi:10.1007/s11930-015-0047-9.
2. Balon R, editor. Sexual dysfunction. The brain body connection. Adv Psychsom Med. Vol 29. Basel: Karger; 2008, p. 89–106.
3. Laumann EO, Paik A, Rosen RC. Sexual dysfunction in the United States prevalence and predictors. JAMA. 1999;281:537–44.
4. Berry MD, Berry PD. Integrative approaches to the treatment of erectile dysfunction. Curr Sex Health Rep. 2014;6:114–23.
5. Engel GL. The need for a new medical model: a challenge for biomedicine. Science. 1977;196:129–36.
6. Engel GL. The clinical application of the biopsychosocial model. Am J Psychiatry. 1980;137:535–44.
7. Engel GL. From biomedical to biopsychosocial: being scientific in the human domain. Psychosomatics. 1997;38:521–8.
8. Borrell-Carrió FF. The biopsychosocial model 25 years later: principles, practice, and scientific inquiry. Ann Fam Med. 2004;2(6): 576–82.
9. Brower V. Mind–body research moves towards the mainstream. EMBO Rep. 2006;7(4):358–61.
10. Borrell-Carrió F, Suchman AL, Epstein RM. The biopsychosocial model 25 years later: principles, practice, and scientific inquiry. Ann Fam Med. 2004;2(6):576–82.
11. Laumann EO, et al. Sexual problems among women and men aged 40–80 years: prevalence and correlates identified in the global study of sexual attitudes and behaviors. Int J Impot Res. 2005;17(1):39–57.
12. Maurice WL. Sexual medicine in primary care. St. Louis: Mosby; 1999.
13. Gottman JM, Silver N. The seven principles for making marriage work: a practical guide from the country's foremost relationship expert. New York: Random House; 2000.
14. Gottman JM. Principia amoris: the new science of love. New York: Routledge; 2014.
15. McCarthy BW, Metz ME. Coping with premature ejaculation: how to overcome PE, please your partner and have great sex. New York: New Harbinger; 2004.
16. McCarthy BW, Metz ME. Coping with erectile dysfunction: how to regain confidence and enjoy great sex. Oakland, CA: New Harbinger; 2004.
17. Levine S, Risen CB, Althof SE. Handbook of clinical sexuality for mental health professionals. 2nd ed. NY: Routledge; 2010.
18. Binik YM, Hall KSK. Principles and practice of sex therapy. 5th ed. New York: Guilford; 2014.
19. Kleinplatz P. New directions in sex therapy: innovations and alternatives. 2nd ed. New York: Routledge; 2012.
20. Jean CY, Syrjala KL. Sexuality after hematopoietic stem cell transplantation. Cancer J. 2009;15(1):57.
21. Laumann EO. Sexual problems among women and men aged 40–80y: prevalence and correlates identified in the global study of sexual attitudes and behaviors. Int J Impot Res. 2005;17(1):39.
22. Basson R. The female sexual response: a different model. J Sex Marital Ther. 2000;26(1):51–65.
23. Basson R. A model of women's sexual arousal. J Sex Marital Ther. 2002;28(1):1–10.
24. Basson R. Women's sexual dysfunction: revised and expanded definitions. CMAJ. 2005;172(10):1327–33.
25. Fisher L. Sex, romance, and relationships: AARP survey of midlife and older adults. AARP. 2010. http://assets.aarp.org/rgcenter/general/srr_09.pdf. Accessed 22 Aug 2016.
26. DeLamater J. Sexual expression in later life: a review and synthesis. J Sex Res. 2012;49(2–3):125–41.
27. Chao J-K, et al. Relationship among sexual desire, sexual satisfaction, and quality of life in middle-aged and older adults. J Sex Marital Ther. 2011;37(5):386–403.
28. Corona G, et al. Frequency of sexual activity and cardiovascular risk in subjects with erectile dysfunction: cross-sectional and longitudinal analyses. Andrology. 2013;1:864–71.
29. Foley S, Kope S, Sugrue D. Sex matters for women: a complete guide to taking care of your sexual self. 2nd ed. New York: Guilford; 2012.
30. Nappi RE, et al. The CLOSER (clarifying vaginal atrophy's impact on sex and relationships) survey: implications of vaginal discomfort in postmenopausal women and in male partners. J Sex Med. 2013;10(9):2232–41.
31. Kingsberg S, et al. Vulvar and vaginal atrophy in postmenopausal women: findings from the revive (real women's views of treatment options for menopausal vaginal changes) survey. J Sex Med. 2013;10:1790–9.
32. Parish S, et al. Impact of vulvovaginal health on postmenopausal women: a review of surveys on symptoms of vulvovaginal atrophy. Int J Women's Health. 2013;13(5):437–47.
33. Reiter S. Barriers to effective treatment of vaginal atrophy with local estrogen therapy. Int J Gen Med. 2013;6:153–8.
34. Wang LY, Pierdomenico A, Lefkowitz A, Brandt R. Female sexual health training for oncology providers: new applications. Sex Med. 2015;3(3):189–97.
35. Ganz PA, Desmond KA, Leedham B, Rowland JH, Meyerowitz BE, Belin TR. Quality of life in long-term, disease-free survivors of breast cancer: a follow-up study. J Natl Cancer Inst. 2002;94:39–49.
36. Kedde H, Van de Wiel HBM, Schultz WW, Wijsen C. Sexual dysfunction in young women with breast cancer. Support Care Cancer. 2013;21:271–80.
37. Zebrack BJ, Foley S, Wittmann D, Leonard M. Sexual functioning in young adult survivors of childhood cancer. Psychooncology. 2010;19:814–22.
38. Davis SR, Panjari M, Robinson PJ, Fradkin P, Bell RJ. Menopausal symptoms in breast cancer survivors nearly 6 years after diagnosis. Menopause. 2014;21:1075–81.
39. Schover LR, Baum GP, Fuson LA, Brewster A, MelhemBertrandt A. Sexual problems during the first 2 years of adjuvant treatment with aromatase inhibitors. J Sex Med. 2014;11:3102–11.
40. Ussher JM, Perz J, Gilbert E. Information needs associated with changes to sexual well-being after breast cancer. J Adv Nurs. 2013;69:327–37.
41. Hill EK, Sandbo S, Abramsohn E, Makelarski J, Wroblewski K, Wenrich ER, McCoy S, Temkin SM, Yamada SD, Lindau ST. Assessing gynecologic and breast cancer survivors' sexual health care needs. Cancer. 2011;117:2643–51.
42. Scanlon M, Blaes A, Geller M, Majhail NS, Lindgren B, Haddad T. Patient satisfaction with physician discussions of treatment impact on fertility, menopause and sexual health among premenopausal women with cancer. J Cancer. 2012;3:217–25.
43. Krychman ML, Katz A. Breast cancer and sexuality: multi-modal treatment options (CME). J Sex Med. 2012;9(1):5–13.
44. Maximizing Sexual Health After Prostate Cancer. Medscape. Nov 13, 2015.
45. Darwish-Yasine M, Berenji M, Wing D, et al. Evaluating long-term patient centered outcomes following prostate cancer treatment: findings from the Michigan Cancer Survivor study. J Cancer Surviv. 2014;8:121–30.
46. Sherer BA, Levine LA. Current management of erectile dysfunction in prostate cancer survivors. Curr Opin Urol. 2014;24:401–6.
47. Wittmann D, Skolarus TA, Montie JE. Are we targeting the right outcome for sexual health after prostate cancer treatment? Eur Urol. 2015;68:550–1.
48. Wittmann D. Coping with losses, grief, and mourning in prostate cancer. Adv Psychosom Med. 2015;34:109–22.
49. Wittmann D, Foley S, Balon R. A bisopsyhcosocial approach to sexual recovery after prostate cancer surgery: the role of grief and mourning. J Sex Marital Ther. 2011;37:130–44.

50. Wittmann D, Northouse L, Crossley H, et al. A pilot study of potential pre-operative barriers to couples' sexual recovery after radical prostatectomy for prostate cancer. J Sex Marital Ther. 2015;41:155–68.
51. Seftel A, Rosen R, Kuritzky L. Physician perceptions of sexual dysfunction related to benign prostatic hyperplasia (BPH) symptoms and sexual side effects related to BPH medications. Int J Impot Res. 2007;19(4):386–92.
52. Irwig MS, Kolukula S. Persistent sexual side effects of finasteride for male pattern hair loss. J Sex Med. 2011;8(6):1747–53.
53. Maiorino M, Bellastella G, Esposito K. Diabetes and sexual dysfunction: current perspectives. Diabetes, Metabolic Syndrome and Obesity: Targets and Therapy. March 2014.
54. Tyrer G, Steel JM, Ewing DJ, Bancroft J, Warner P, Clarke BF. Sexual responsiveness in diabetic women. Diabetologia. 1983;24(3):166–71.
55. Enzlin P, Mathieu C, Vanderschueren D, Demyttenaere K. Diabetes mellitus and female sexuality: a review of 25 years' research. Diabet Med. 1998;15(10):809–15.
56. Gandaglia G. A systematic review of the association between erectile dysfunction and cardiovascular disease. Eur Urol. 2014;65(5):968.
57. Levine GN. Sexual activity and cardiovascular disease: a scientific statement from the American Heart Association. Circulation. 2012;125(8):1058.
58. Moser DK, Dracup K, Evangelista LS, Zambroski CH, et al. Comparison of prevalence of symptoms of depression, anxiety, and hostility in elderly patients with heart failure, myocardial infarction, and a coronary artery bypass graft. Heart Lung. 2010;39:378–85.
59. Roose SP, Seidman SN. Sexual activity and cardiac risk: is depression a contributing factor? Am J Cardiol. 2000;86(2):38–40.
60. Mosack V, Steinke EE. Trends in sexual concerns after myocardial infarction. J Cardiovasc Nurs. 2009;24:162–70.
61. Lai YH, Hsieh SR, Ho WC, Chiou AF. Factors associated with sexual quality of life in patients before and after coronary artery bypass grafting surgery. J Cardiovasc Nurs. 2011;26:487–96.
62. Phan A, Ishak WW, Shen BJ, Fuess J, et al. Persistent sexual dysfunction impairs quality of life after cardiac transplantation. J Sex Med. 2010;7:2765–73.
63. Kazemi-Saleh D, Pishgou B, Assari S, Tavallaii SA. Fear of sexual intercourse in patients with coronary artery disease: a pilot study of associated morbidity. J Sex Med. 2007;4:1619–25.
64. Wiwanitkit V. Sexuality in Parkinsonism. Sex Disabil. 2008;26:105–8.
65. Esmail S, Munro B, Gibson N. Couple's experience with multiple sclerosis in the context of their sexual relationship. Sex Disabil. 2007;25:163–77.
66. Kool MB, et al. Low relationship satisfaction and high partner involvement predict sexual problems of women with fibromyalgia. Sex Marital Ther. 2006;32(5):409–23.
67. Binik Y, Hall KS, editors. Principles and practice of sex therapy. 5th ed. New York: Guilford Press; 2014. p. 462.
68. Tepper M. Sexuality and disability: the missing discourse of pleasure. sexuality and disability. 2000;18(4).
69. Sipski ML, Alexander CJ, Rosen R. Sexual arousal and orgasm in women: effects of spinal cord injury. Ann Neurol. 2001;49:35–44.
70. Biering-Sorensen F, Sonksen J. Sexual function in spinal cord lesioned men. Spinal Cord. 2001;39:455–70.
71. Alexander CJ, Sipski ML, Findley TW. Sexual activities, desire, and satisfaction in males pre- and post-spinal cord injury. Arch Sex Behav. 1993;22:217–28.
72. Sipski ML, Alexander CJ. Sexual activities, response and satisfaction in women pre- and post-spinal cord injury. Arch Phys Med Rehabil. 1993;74:1025–9.
73. Taylor Gomez M. The S words: sexuality, sensuality, sexual expression and people with intellectual disability. Sex Disabil. 2012;30(2):237.
74. Alexander MS, Alexander CJ. Recommendations for discussing sexuality after spinal cord injury/dysfunction in children, adolescents and adults. J Spinal Cord Med. 2007;30:S65–70.
75. Forsythe E, Horsewell JE. Sexual rehabilitation of women with a spinal cord injury. Spinal Cord. 2006;44:234–41.
76. Servais L. Sexual health care in persons with intellectual disabilities. Ment Retard Dev Disabil Res Rev. 2006;12:48–56.
77. Eastgate G. Sexual health for people with intellectual disability. Salud Publica Mex. 2008;50(Suppl 2):S255–9.
78. Tarnai B. Review of effective interventions for socially inappropriate masturbation in persons with cognitive disabilities. Sex. Disabil. 2006;24:151–68.
79. Cuskelly M, Gilmore L. Attitudes to sexuality questionnaire (individuals with an intellectual disability): scale development and community norms. J Intellect Dev Disabil. 2007;32(3): 214–21.
80. McVilly KR, et al. Self-advocates have the last say on friendship. Disabil Soc. 2006;21(7):693–708.
81. Swango-Wilson A. Caregiver perceptions and implications for sex education for individuals with intellectual and developmental disabilities. Sex. Disabil. 2008;26(2):75–81.
82. Elders MJ. Sex for health and pleasure throughout a lifetime. J Sex Med. 2010;7(Suppl 5):248–9.
83. Noonan A, Taylor Gomez M. Who's missing? awareness of lesbian, gay, bisexual and transgender people with intellectual disability. Sex. Disabil. 2010;29(2):175–80.
84. Balon R, editor. Sexual dysfunction. The brain body connection. Adv Psychsom Med. Vol 29. Basel: Karger; 2008. p. 107–30.
85. Manolis A. Antihypertensive treatment and sexual dysfunction. Curr Hypertens Rep. 2012;14(4):285.
86. Balon R, editor. Sexual dysfunction. The brain body connection. Adv Psychsom Med. Vol 29. Basel: Karger; 2008. p. 131–49.
87. Casper RC, Redmond DE, Katz MM, Schaffer CB, Davis JM, Koslow SH. Somatic symptoms in primary affective disorder. Arch Gen Psychiatry. 1985;42:1098–104.
88. Feldman HA, Goldstein I, Hatzichristou DG, Krane RJ, McKinlay JB. Impotence and its medical and psychosocial correlates: results of the Massachusetts Male Aging Study. J Urol. 1994;151: 54–61.
89. Waldinger MD. Lifelong premature ejaculation: from authority-based to evidence-based medicine. BJU Int. 2004;93:201.
90. McMahon CG, Abdo C, Incrocci L, Perelman M, Rowland D, Waldinger M, Xin ZC. Disorders of orgasm and ejaculation in men. J Sex Med. 2004;1(1):58–65.
91. Waldinger MD. The neurobiological approach to premature ejaculation. J Urol. 2002;168:2359.
92. Althof SE. Original research—psychology: psychological and interpersonal dimensions of sexual function and dysfunction. J Sex Med. 2005;2(6):793.
93. Maggi M, Filippi S, Ledda F, et al. Erectile dysfunction: from biochemical pharmacology to advances in medical therapy. Eur J Endocrinol. 2000;143:143–54.
94. Filippi S, Marini M, Vannelli GB, et al. Effects of hypoxia on endothelin-1 sensitivity in the corpus cavernosum. Mol Hum Reprod. 2003;9:765–74.
95. Corretti G, Baldi I. The relationship between anxiety disorders and sexual dysfunction. Psychiatr Times. 2007;24(9):16–21.
96. Carvalho J. Biopsychosocial determinants of men's sexual desire: testing an integrative model. J Sex Med. 2011;8(3):754.
97. Beck JG, Barlow DH, Sakheim DK, Abrahamson DJ. Shock threat and sexual arousal: the role of selective attention, thought content and affective states. Psychophysiology. 1987;24: 165–72.
98. Geer JH, Fuhr R. Cognitive factors in sexual arousal: the role of distraction. J Consult Clin Psychol. 1976;44:238–43.
99. Dove NL, Wiederman MW. Cognitive distraction and women's sexual functioning. J Sex Marital Ther. 2000;26:67–78.

100. Elliot AN, O'Donohue WT. The effects of anxiety and distraction on sexual arousal in a non-clinical sample of heterosexual women. Arch Sex Behav. 1997;26:607–24.
101. Attalah S, Johnson-Agbakwu C, Rosenbaum T, et al. Ethical and sociocultural aspects of sexual function and dysfunction in both sexes. J Sex Med. 2016;13:591e606.
102. Sue D, Arredondo P, RJ MD. Multicultural counseling competencies and standards: a call to the profession. J Couns Dev. 1992;70(4):477–86.
103. Lu FG, Lim RF, Mezzich JE. Issues in the assessment and diagnosis of culturally diverse individuals. Am Psychiatr Press Rev Psychiatr. 1995.
104. Cardemil E, Battle C. Guess who's coming to therapy? Getting comfortable with conversations about race and ethnicity in psychotherapy. Prof Psychol Res Pract. 2003;34: 278–86.
105. Kellogg SS, Rosenbaum TY, Dweck A, Millheiser L, PillaiFriedman S, Krychman M, et al. Sexual health and religion: a primer for the sexual health clinician. J Sex Med. 2014;11:1606–19.
106. Atallah S, Johnson-Agbakwu C, Rosenbaum T, et al. Ethical and sociocultural aspects of sexual function and dysfunction in both sexes. J Sex Med. 2016;13(4):591–606.
107. Herman J. Trauma and recovery: the aftermath of violence–from domestic abuse to political terror. New York: Basic Books; 1997.
108. Tiefer L. A new view of women's sexual problems: why new? why now? J Sex Res. 2001;38(2):89.
109. Kramarae C, Spender D (Eds). The knowledge explosion: generations of feminist scholarship. New York: Columbia University Teachers College Press; 1992.
110. Cole E, Rothblum ED (Eds). Women and sex therapy. New York: Haworth Press; 1988.
111. Tiefer L, Melman A. Interview of wives: a necessary adjunct in the evaluation of impotence. Sex Disabil. 1983;6:167–75.

7
Biopsychosocial Treatment of Sexual Dysfunctions

Klaus M. Beier and Kurt K. Loewit

Abbreviations

BEDIT Berlin dissexuality therapy
DSM Diagnostic and statistical manual of mental disorders
ICD International statistical classification of diseases
SST Syndyastic sexual therapy

Introduction

Sexual medicine occupies a special position among medical disciplines because it can neither be considered a specialty of its own regarding theory and practice nor can it directly be associated with one specific specialty. On the contrary, in striving to meet the complexity of its subject—human sexuality—clinical sexual medicine must work across disciplines by definition in order to offer help to its target group, i.e., men and women, or couples, suffering from sexual disorders. General practitioners, internists, gynecologists, urologists, surgeons, pediatricians, psychiatrists, or psychotherapists could uncover the roots of many diseases within their specialties and activate salutogenic potentials by inquiring about the degree of satisfied psychosocial needs within the partnership and sexuality—without thereby appropriating sexual medicine as part of their own disciplines.

A holistic or comprehensive medicine perspective rather calls for a conception of the individual in its entirety, taking into account all relevant aspects of life. Whereas practitioners do not need to be fully trained in sexual medicine, they should at least have a basic knowledge of the field in order not to fearfully avoid the subject of sexuality. A holistic approach also demands not to perceive the individual as composed of separate fictional parts. Initially expressed through the concept of psychosomatics, the holistic perspective was refined into the biopsychosocial approach by George Engel in 1977 [1], who declared it a "challenge for biomedicine." While the biopsychosocial approach in fact applies to all disciplines concerned with the human, its unique potential is revealed in particular in the treatment of sexual disorders. By means of thorough anamnesis, a dualistic either/or perspective (e.g., somatic or psychic) usually proves to be non-exhaustive, as in fact both aspects contribute to an individual's functions or dysfunctions. Even the so-called "biomedicine" is ultimately concerned with the result of an organic process marked by a simultaneous interaction between physiological, psychological, and relationship-related factors. We can neither assume purely physical functions or dysfunctions, nor purely psychological disorders. Hence, concepts such as somatic or psychosocial are misleading in that they invoke a purely biological body, an independent psyche and a social surrounding operating by and for itself—an artificial construct obscuring the real, inseparable entity at hand.

In theory, these facts are known and undisputed. However, in medical practice, a holistic approach and attitude towards patients is far from established. In addition, patients themselves have adopted this kind of either/or thinking: "Are you really saying my problem is psychological? There is nothing wrong with my mind." Hence, patients slowly need to be reacquainted with a holistic approach and the ideas of equivalence, simultaneity, and biopsychosocial interaction. Because human sexuality is, at least de facto, a social phenomenon, sexual medicine is not concerned with the diseased individual as a "symptom carrier," as it is mostly the case in medical disciplines. Quite the contrary, sexual medicine is the only discipline to focus on the couple and the relationship above all else. Whatever happens in a relationship concerns both partners, i.e., every sexual disorder causes a relationship disorder and, most likely, vice versa. Using the example of an erectile disorder, Figure 7-1 illustrates how an interaction of overlapping vicious circles in the couple can lead to disadvantages for both partners and their relationship on the functional as well as on the partnership level.

Comparing sexual medicine with reproductive medicine, which equally deals with couples and sexuality, the differences in approach become evident: Even when the couple is

W.W. IsHak (ed.), *The Textbook of Clinical Sexual Medicine*, DOI 10.1007/978-3-319-52539-6_7

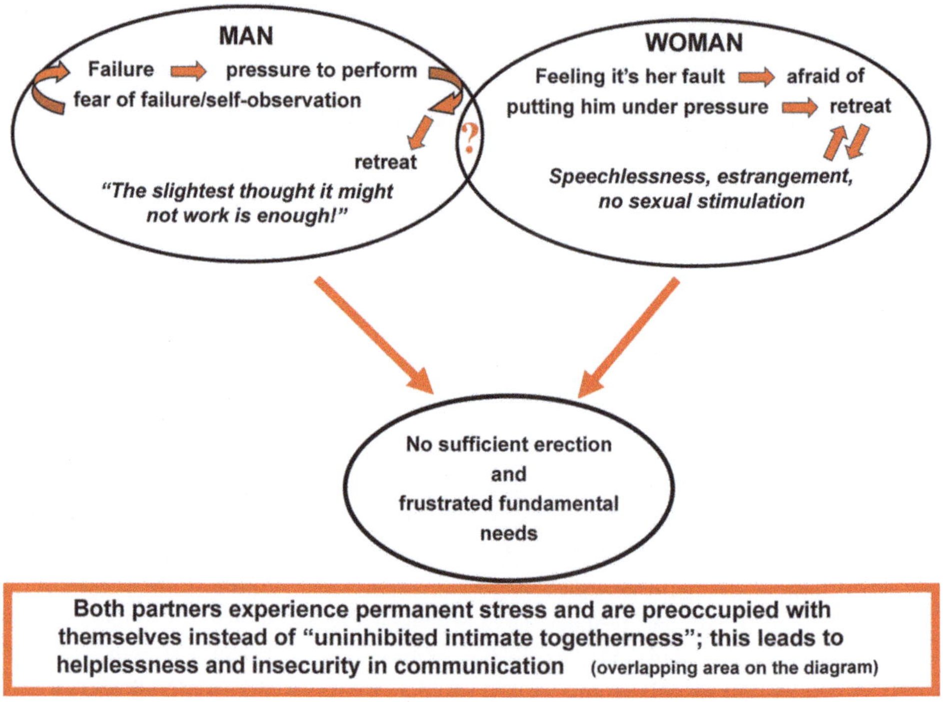

FIGURE 7-1. Overlapping vicious circles in erectile dysfunction and consequences for the partnership.

invited for an assessment interview (to invite both partners is not imperative), the focus of reproductive medicine is placed on the child to be conceived and on the technological aspects necessary to achieve pregnancy rather than the relationship quality, effectiveness of parenting, motivation, and sexual functioning. In so doing, sexuality is reduced to only one dimension, the dimension of reproduction, which constitutes a too narrow focus on sexuality as a whole.

The Three Dimensions of Sexuality

From a holistic medicine perspective, a multifunctional understanding of sexuality is deployed, comprising three dimensions which interact with one another: the dimensions of desire, attachment, and reproduction.

- The *dimension of desire* encompasses sexuality in all conceivable ways of experiencing and increasing desire by sexual stimulation. It provides sexuality with the unique sensual experience of sexual arousal and orgasm, which distinguishes it from other human experience. It establishes the motivational quality of sexuality and simultaneously provides the impulse and reward of sexual behavior. The dimension of desire can predominate in subjective experience in auto-eroticism and in experienced erotic interactions, passion, and ecstasy. It can be an isolated experience, without any connection to the reproductive dimension and the attachment dimension of sexuality. It is, however, difficult to view this dimension completely on its own, because it is so closely connected to the other dimensions and is obviously influenced by various factors outside and within the realm of sexuality.
- The *dimension of attachment* emphasizes the importance of sexuality for the fulfillment of biopsychosocial fundamental needs for acceptance, closeness, warmth, and security by sexual communication in partnership [2, 3]. In the animal kingdom, sexuality has been attributed to social significance, to enhancing pair and group bonding in the sense of a change in meaning and function [4, 5]. In human beings—distinguishing themselves from their primate relatives mainly by the capability of speech and creating culture—the attachment dimension of sexuality specifically becomes one with a communication function: Attachment develops by communication, so communication and attachment are interchangeable terms. With reference to the fact that "you cannot not communicate" [6], "you cannot not interact" in relationships, and therefore, the function of social attachment in sexuality is an obligatory and lifelong relevant function. At the same time, this social function illustrates the specific human elements of sexuality.
- The *dimension of reproduction* stands for the significance of sexuality in reproduction. Of the three dimensions, the reproductive dimension of sexuality is the phylogenetically oldest in higher animals. While at the stage of single-celled organisms multiplication is performed asexually, the more sophisticated multicellular organisms combined genetic recombination and multiplication to operate reproduction as we know it. Taking into account the gender difference, the significance of the dimension of reproduction varies, and is limited for women to the time

span of reproductive capability extending from puberty to menopause. Furthermore, it is dependent on biographical decisions, making it optional. The availability of reliable contraceptive methods on the one hand, and the progress of reproductive medicine on the other, has made it possible to separate the dimension of reproduction from the other two dimensions of desire and attachment.

From a sexual medicine perspective, all three dimensions of sexuality contribute to sexual functions or dysfunctions. Furthermore, the biopsychosocial treatment of sexual disorders is not confined to the restoration of disturbed functions, but places, along with the couple itself, the quality of the relationship at the center of attention [7]. Since the human being is a relational being with a "social brain," i.e., phylogenetically programmed to lead a life in pairs (Aristotle: syndyastikós), the relationship quality has a lifetime salutogenic and/or pathogenic importance, as has been revealed long ago by attachment research. The quality of relationship is even an indicator for the human's morbidity and mortality risk, as can be seen in the extreme case of death from a "broken heart" (Tako-Tsubo cardiomyopathy).

When it comes to prevention and therapy, medicine—and not only sexual medicine—should attend more to the quality of essential relationships, especially love relationships. Therefore, when assessing sexual desire, arousal or orgasm dysfunctions, aspects of the sexual relationship need to be taken into account, as well [8]. This involves the question of whether or to which degree fundamental needs as, for example, the need to be accepted and respected the way one is have been frustrated or violated (see above).

However, on the part of the therapist or counselor it does not suffice to assess mere facts during anamnesis, but to understand their individual meaning for each person seeking help [9]. In spite of the universal validity of fundamental needs, their emotional significance, i.e., their subjectively felt meaning and urgency, can only be understood from personal history. The fulfillment or frustration of fundamental needs is achieved in everyday life through nonsexual couple interactions, but also—in a very intensive and intimate way—through the "language of sexuality" [10]. Given the attachment dimension of sexuality, sexuality itself can become a means of communication expressing, for example, acceptance, belonging, openness, closeness, and warmth through body language in genital union. As such, it is not a symbolic, but rather physical and at the same time psychosocial, sensual reality.

The Communication Aspect

Taking into account the communication aspect of sexuality also contributes to a more complex understanding of sexual desire. The aspect of genital desire as being exclusively and one-dimensionally aimed at sexual arousal and orgasm is thereby complemented by the aspect of *relationship reward*, the stimulating joy of being chosen and accepted, of being released from loneliness into the new commonness of the couple-relationship. The more both genital desire and relationship reward are experienced consciously, the more they can reinforce each other. Although this perspective might appear unfamiliar to most couples and needs to be acquired first, it quickly leads to evidence-based experience: "Somehow this had always been inside of me, I have just never been consciously aware of it."

What might at first appear to be a merely theoretical construct is put into effective clinical practice by *Syndyastic Sexual Therapy* (SST). The SST is distinguished by a variety of features among other treatment methods of sexual disorders: First, while consequently assuming the treatment of the couple as a general rule, the SST does not focus on sexual dysfunctions or the intensification of genital desire in the first place, but on improving the relationship quality in general. It is concerned with the role of the couple-relationship as the condition of a primary or secondary deeper cause for dysfunctions. The fulfillment or frustration of the biopsychosocial fundamental needs serves as the crucial measurement criterion (syndyastic focus), because the degree of fulfillment of those needs forms the basis of relationship quality and couple (dis-)satisfaction. Hence, the SST combines the (re-)fulfillment of biopsychosocial needs and desires with the aspect of sexuality, or, more precisely, with sexuality as a way of communicating through body language. From kiss to coitus sexuality can be experienced as the embodiment of acceptance, belonging, openness, closeness, etc., being naked can signify a liberating, authentic revelation of oneself instead of mere exposure, and so forth.

Perceived in this way, the to date often isolated and orgasm-centered perspective on "sex" is changed to describe a means of communicating through body language vital desires and values central to—and often searched for in—(love) relationships. Table 7-1 demonstrates the difference between typical statements made by patients expressing an isolated view on sexuality compared to statements by patients after treatment. The aim of an integrated approach to sexuality is to overcome the pathogenic opposition between sex and love, so that a new meaning can be discovered to unfold its salutogenic potentials.

However, this should not result in a neglect of the dark sides of sexuality. Especially in light of the apparent predominance of compulsive sexual violence, abuse, exploitation, humiliation, or the global dispersion of commercialized, completely non-syndyastic pornographic sexuality (without any relationship aspect), the intent to emphasize, make aware of, and therapeutically utilize the joyful side of sexual communication might as well seem utopian, idealistic, or even cynical. What remains as a fact is that fundamental human needs are present in every individual seeking help, which—in case of prompt evidence-based experience and successful

TABLE 7-1. Patients' quotations on isolated and integrated sexuality

Isolated sexuality (not perceived on a communicational level)	Integrated sexuality (consciously applied as a way of communication)
I could do without sex without missing anything	On this level, sex is a way of reaching me
Always the same procedure: direct foreplay . . . sleeping away afterwards	It's deeper than just sex—not only him reducing his arousal. I respond differently to his ejaculation—it was something like pleasure
Sex was physical sports—nothing more	Now it's more like *us* sleeping together
Sex does nothing for me. When sex begins, I retreat	For the first time my thoughts were involved—I didn't think about anything else, that was liberating
Sex was a one-way street to orgasm	You were different, you connected more to me
I could live without sex, but not without love, tenderness and warmth	Romance is revived, it is like being married for not more than 6 months
Sex drive—I don't know what that is. I need you to be there, hugging me and caressing me, without *it* being there	Now, for the first time I have experienced sexual intercourse and cuddling not as two different things
There are more important aspects to a partnership than sex	I have never looked at it that way—I was not aware of it, but it had been inside of me all the time
Sex just belongs to a partnership	For us that is a completely revolutionary insight

(re-)fulfillment of these needs—is likely to mobilize salutogenic energies to an unexpected extent. Therefore, SST, despite conceptually being a short-term therapy, can lead to long-lasting and sustainable results.

Meaning as a Salutogenic or Pathogenic Element

Because in sexual therapy, as in other fields, the decisive factor is the question of meaning, we will now expand on the already mentioned concept of *Syndyastic Sexual Therapy* in order to enable a more conscious access to the subjectively felt meaning of sexuality. This is necessary and helpful, given that the individual attribution of meaning can be an essential pathogenic element.

As already mentioned, sexuality is commonly perceived as a purely genital act, i.e., aimed at sexual arousal and orgasm. This genital sexuality is then again lived and experienced as isolated and separate from attachment and affection. However, a lack of subjectively felt meaning cannot be replaced by (arousal-increasing) "techniques"; on the contrary, those techniques themselves in fact presuppose meaning.

In a 2007 interview-study on "building blocks toward optimal sexuality" [11] among men and women involved in long-term partnerships, the interviewees did not refer to strong sexual desire, easy sexual arousability, optimal erectile or orgasmic functions, etc. as important elements of sexuality, but to focused attention for each other, authenticity, intense emotional connection, erotic intimacy, communication, and transcendence (understood as supra-individual experiences in the common sexual intimacy). Consequently, optimal sexual functions do not guarantee optimal sex, whereas optimal sexuality is possible even if function disorders exist, as long as the relationship as a whole conforms to the "building blocks" described above.

Principles of Biopsychosocial Assessment: As a Part of Treatment

In sexual medicine, diagnostics and therapy are interrelated more closely than in other medical fields: From the very beginning, we are dealing with a diagnostic-therapeutic process, because the diagnostic assessment is already indicative of the therapist's perspective on sexuality and its disorders.

The Spectrum of Sexual Disorders

The suggested categories of the clinical classification systems ICD-10 [12] and DSM-5 [13] are purely descriptive concepts which fail to do justice to the complexity of human sexuality. Already by taking into account the sexologically required differentiation of the three dimensions of sexuality, the inadequacy of such categorization is unmasked. Thus, sexual disorders cannot only influence the dimension of desire, but very likely the dimension of attachment as well and hence not only the disturbed sexual function, but, moreover, the disturbance of partnership comfort turns out to be the actual reason for suffering.

According to present knowledge, chronic lack of feelings of security conveyed by body communication (frustration of psychosocial fundamental needs) increases the probability of developing psychological and physical disorders. Furthermore, it hinders overcoming prevailing illnesses [14]. The symptoms presented by patients seen in clinical practice are usually described as "psychosomatic disorders," "depressive state of mood," "anxiety and/or nervous restlessness," i.e., "nervous anxiety, tension and restlessness" or, additionally, as "emotionally caused state of restlessness." Therefore, it can be assumed that in many areas of medicine male and female patients with varying disorders or dysfunctions consult a practitioner because of a lack of availability of a

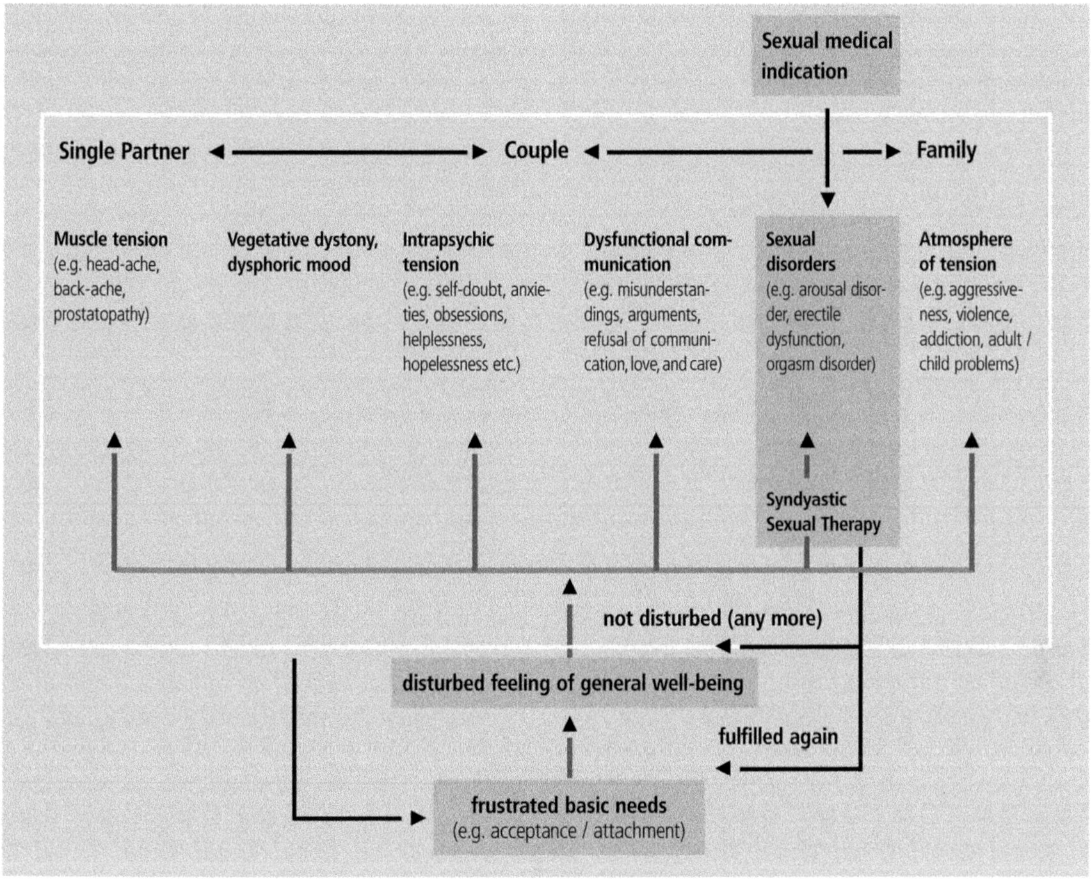

FIGURE 7-2. Connection between psychological fundamental needs and various symptoms.

functioning and therefore emotionally stabilizing intimate attachment. Also included are chronically ill or older persons suffering from psychosocial destabilization due to reduced opportunities for social contacts.

This explains why very different symptoms can dominate the clinical impression and, as a result, various medical disciplines may come into contact with the patients concerned: orthopedics for muscle tension; gynecology and urology for pelvic floor tensions, disturbances of micturition, etc.; general practice for symptoms of the autonomic nervous system; psychiatry for intrapsychic tension or states of depression; or andrology concerning involuntary childlessness. Also, sexual dysfunction may perhaps be only one of the many possible symptoms (apart from, of course, sexual disorders caused by illness, e.g., condition after paraplegia). The special quality of sexological therapy options (see section "Principles of Biopsychosocial Treatment of Sexual Disorders") lies in the fact that it deals explicitly with the actual roots (the frustrated fundamental needs) of possible causes at a level not reached elsewhere, while it aims at restoring the feeling of complete attachment by physical acceptance through intimacy with the partner, which also has curative effects on symptoms and positive consequences in other areas of life (Figure 7-2).

Notwithstanding these limited and only partially useful systematic categorizations, clinically significant sexual disorders are compactly characterized as follows:

1. Disorders of sexual function.
2. Disorders of sexual development.
   (a) Disorder of sexual maturity.
   (b) Disorder of sexual orientation.
   (c) Disorder of sexual identity.
   (d) Disorder of sexual relationship.
3. Disorders of gender identity/gender dysphoria.
4. Disorders of sexual preference/paraphilic disorders.
5. Disorders of sexual behavior/dissexuality.
6. Disorders of sexual reproduction.

Each sexual disorder is itself capable of causing other disorders which are encoded (e.g., chronic prostatitis, fluor genitalis, etc.), but they can also occur overlapping with one another: Disorders of sexual function are very often closely linked to disorders of sexual relationship. For those disorders of sexual preference which are not integrated into self-concept this is regularly the case (see section "Treatment of Sexual Preference Disorders"), often additionally involving disorders of sexual function (e.g., erectile disorder). This, again, underlines the serious impact of unfulfilled psychosocial fundamental needs, which play, in the end, a key role in all sexologically relevant disorders.

Assessment of the Sexual Disorder

In order to tackle the problem of a disturbed partnership and/or sexual life, it is essential to address the issue adequately and to explore sexual disorders, the level of syndyastic function (i.e., the extent of fulfillment of psychosocial fundamental needs for acceptance and appreciation within the relationship), as well as to evaluate physical findings and laboratory parameters in a qualified way.

At this point, the previous strict approach "first diagnosis, then therapy" should be changed into a dynamic, process orientated "diagnostic therapeutic circle" [15]: Every interview for assessment, empathically carried out, has a therapeutic effect in itself and every further therapeutic step produces new diagnostic material for the duration of the relationship between therapist and patient(s).

This calls for attentiveness on the part of the therapist on three information levels simultaneously: (1) on the level of given facts, (2) on the level of the significance these facts have for the patient(s), (3) on the level of partnership dynamics by observation of couple interaction. This demands complete awareness, never to be confused with not maintaining a professional distance to the involved couple.

At the same time the therapist offers a role model by speaking openly about sexuality as a basic element of human life. This is one of the most important foundations of sexological skills and definitely shows therapeutic effects. It has been long proven that patients actually wait for certain signals from the therapist concerning mentioning the issue of sexuality [16–19]. For instance, on prescribing a new medication, the therapist can provide a signal in terms of a question like: "Should the illness or its treatment lead to problems or changes in your sexual life, then we can talk about that and look for solutions." It is essential, however, that the therapist should never retreat into the role of the "expert." He/she will always be confronted by subjective interpretations—the patient's as well as his/her own—making personal compassion inevitable.

Successfully carrying out treatment with decisiveness is based on extensive information on the specific sexual experience and behavior of a patient/couple. In the case of partnership involvement, the information has to provide the investigator with insight into the level of sexual functions and the sexual preference structure of *both* partners; otherwise therapeutic steps remain ineffective or can even cause harm (e.g., if a preference disorder remains undetected as a reason for a dysfunction). When couples are concerned, it must be decided whether the sexual assessment should be taken on with each partner alone or immediately with both partners together from the beginning.

Single anamnesis has the advantage that the partner may be more uninhibited and speak more openly than in the presence of the other, particularly on subjects like masturbation fantasies or topics like paraphilic inclinations and past relationships. The advantage of *couple-interviews*, on the other hand, is that all information issues are gathered together and processed from the beginning, which can demonstrate and increase the extent of openness and trust among the partners involved.

It is crucial to know which kind of disorder (e.g., direct or indirect disorder of sexual function; disorder of sexual partnership) is being dealt with and under which circumstances or conditions it arises (e.g., lifelong or acquired type; generalized or situational type). What is the partner's opinion on this disorder? What attitude does each partner have toward sexuality, irrespective of the disorder in question? What kind of sex education are opinions based on? Does each partner know the opinions of the other and can they talk about them? Such generalized questions are imperative in order to put specific questions into the greater context of the partnership and to be able to judge their significance for each partner, e.g.: Who takes the initiative in sexual contact? Are there differences and where and how are they expressed? Which preferences or aversions are there and how are they dealt with?

This inevitably leads to the analysis of possibly existing peculiarities of the sexual preference structure, which should and can be systematically explored (see overview).

Overview Sexual Preference Structure: Exploration Tools

Three Axes

The human sexual preference structure is generally configured on three axes, i.e.,

- *Gender* (of the desirable partner): the other or the same gender (or both);
- *Age* (of the desirable partner): children, adolescents, adults, or the elderly; and
- *Way* (of the desirable partner or object or of an interaction): type, object, mode, procedure, etc., all intermingling with one another and of which all (from non-conform to paraphilic) should be explored.

Three Levels

Sexual experience and behavior should be investigated into on three different levels, i.e.,

- The *sexual self-concept*
- The *sexual fantasies*; and
- The concrete *sexual behavior*,

all intermingling with one another and of which all should be explored.

Three Forms

The concrete sexual behavior should again be explored within three forms:

- *Masturbation:* self-stimulation and self-satisfaction;
- *Extragenital sexual interaction:* e.g., stroking, cuddling, kissing; and
- *Genital stimulation:* manual, oral, or other stimulation, e.g., petting incl. sexual intercourse, penis or penis surrogate penetrating vagina or anus, and these should also all be explored.

The extent of naturalness conveyed by the therapist during exploration has direct influence on the information flow. It obtains diagnostic-therapeutic relevance and underlines the necessity of acquiring a professional repertoire of knowledge and skills, which can be learned in the context of sexological advanced training (see section "The Dual Role of the Therapist as an Expert and an Attendant").

Conducting partner interviews, which are an essential part of sexological practice, the following questions are of particular diagnostic interest: What is communication like within the partnership in general and in sexual matters in particular? Can personal feelings, needs and wishes be communicated and does this happen? Are boundaries respected? Are there self-strengthening mechanisms, "vicious circles" or self-fulfilling prophecies, and how do these affect partnership communication? Might problems result from misunderstandings due to misinterpretations of partner-behavior?

Exploration of the Three Dimensions of Sexuality

The assessment of the attribution of meaning regarding the three dimensions of sexuality (reproduction, desire, attachment) by each patient/couple is of essential—diagnostic and therapeutic—importance. Inquiring about the meaning of sexuality ("What does it mean for you to have sex?"), many patients/couples begin to realize that some things are not as obvious as previously assumed ("This is something I/we have not considered so far.").

Dimension of attachment: Which needs or values are indispensable for a relationship? To what degree are those human fundamental needs realized within the couple relationship? How far is sexuality perceived as a form of communication through body language by which fundamental needs are communicated and simultaneously realized as "bodily expression and gestures" of the relationship? Is there an awareness of the communicative aspect of sexuality, is it lived implicitly, or does it lack any—"real-life" or mental—significance?

Dimension of reproduction: What role do the ability of reproduction and children play in the relationship? Is there a difference in attitude between the partners? Are there any problems affecting an unfulfilled desire to have children?

Dimension of desire: What is the importance attributed to genital desire within the three dimensions of sexuality? (How) did this change over the course of the relationship? Is there an awareness regarding the complexity of experiencing sexual desire?

Interaction of the three dimensions on the individual and relationship level: Are there any imbalances possibly related to the sexual disorder, e.g., potential discrepancies between fantasized and lived sexuality, a predominance of one dimension at the expense of the other two, or a strongly diverging distribution of the dimensions between both partners?

History of Diseases and Somatic Findings

All significant diseases treated medically at the present time or previously should be taken into account, but particularly those, which might be connected with the sexual disorder. This includes all urological, gynecological, or psychosomatic illnesses and surgery; any medication and/or substance abuse or addiction; and/or information concerning pregnancies (abortions and miscarriages) and childbirth.

In addition, any therapy relevant to sexual disorders and previous psychotherapeutic treatment need to be looked into. Biopsychosocial anamnesis needs to include diagnostics for somatic findings. This concerns *sexual functions* as well as *general physical functions*. An overview of the necessary physical diagnostics concerning sexual dysfunctions in males is shown in Table 7-2 [20].

Principles of Biopsychosocial Treatment of Sexual Disorders

Generally, similar to every medical branch, sexual medicine can be interpreted and practiced in two ways: focusing on disease or focusing on the patient. In sexual medicine, the ideal is: focusing on the couple and their partnership.

The first-mentioned approach deals primarily with "disorders" of sexual function, of gender identity, of sexual

TABLE 7-2. Organ diagnostics in sexual disorders in men

Physical diagnostics	Diagnostic method	For exclusion	Indication
Clinical examination	Inspection, palpation, pulse, exercise tolerance test	Urogenital, neurological, and cardiovascular diseases	General examination in connection with risk factors (e.g., age, overweight)
Laboratory	BS, lipids, testosterone, prolactin	Diabetes mellitus, dyslipidosis, hypogonadism, prolactinoma	General examination General examination If necessary in arousal disorder or erectile dysfunction (ED), depending on further hypogonadism symptoms
Imaging	Duplex sonography with intracavernous pharmaco testing Neurophysiology (e.g., corpus-cavernosum-*EMG*) Penile angiography	Cavernous insufficiency Neurogenic deficit (e.g., following an accident) Pelvic vascular occlusion	if necessary in ED in the case of no response to oral medication and wish for *SKAT* If necessary in ED when expertise or scientific issues are concerned Only in planned revascularisation surgery

ED erectile disorder.

[Reprinted from Rösing D, Klebingat KJ, Berberich HJ, Bosinski HAG, Loewit KK, Beier KM. MEDIZIN Übersichtsarbeit-Sexualstörungen des Mannes Diagnostik und Therapie aus sexualmedizinisch-interdisziplinärer Sicht. Dtsch Arztebl. 2009;106(50):821–8. With permission from Deutsches Ärzteblatt].

preferences and of sexual behavior. The pathogenesis is in the center of scientific interest. Anatomy, physiology, neuroendocrinology, etc. are favored subjects. Diagnostics are made according to common classifications by assessment of facts, clinical examinations, laboratory results including hormone analysis and function tests, and are recorded in a "case history." The therapy is aimed at fast and efficient elimination of the disorder, i.e., at the reestablishment of normal function. Until the end of the sessions with the therapist, pharmacological, surgical, and technical methods are available and most times applied to the one single person with such symptoms. Examples for this are, for instance concerning the most frequent indications, the disorders of sexual function, the reflex-like prescription of PDE5-inhibitors in erectile disorder without carrying out any differentiated assessment, not to speak of talks to the couple involved; or the treatment of vaginism with dilating measures, without ever having spoken to the male partner; or the administration of hormones, e.g., testosterones for hypoactive sexual desire disorder as first choice therapy, and so forth.

The Dual Role of the Therapist as an Expert and an Attendant

In contrast to a solely disease-centered approach, a biopsychosocial, couple- and relationship-centered sexual therapy focuses on the disease *and* the patient. This means a challenge concerning *two* emphases or roles of the physician/therapist: the medical (or psychotherapeutic) expert and the empathic assistant with their respective identity.

During standard undergraduate medical training a certain image of a physician may still be conveyed, which depicts him/her as a caring helper and healer but at the same time as a person thinking in terms of natural science, occasionally as a distanced expert-observer. He/she is the responsible problem-solver and solution-finder, the success of therapy depending on his/her skills and knowledge. He/she knows, what is best for his/her patients, clarifies, educates, teaches, gives authoritative orders and advice to be followed in trust by his/her patients.

The second—also aspired—image of the doctor aims at exactly that patient-focused conduct as an empathic companion, a good patient-listener who "reads between the lines," who tries to assess the patient—in this case the couple—in their overall situation. To achieve this he/she applies his/her own reflected feelings, impressions, experiences at each ongoing doctor–patient relationship as a diagnostic instrument, as has been previously worked out, particularly by Balint [21, 22]. Within the "Balint groups," named after him, these abilities can be learned and practiced [23], which is done more and more in regular medical training, while in psychology and psychotherapy it is general state of the art. Sexual medicine, however, is no "psycho subject" and sexual therapy is not a specialized form of psychotherapy, which is why specialists like urologists, andrologists, gynecologists, dermatologists, GPs and psychiatrists, who want to gain additional qualification in sexual medicine, definitely need to learn and train role security in this new identity as a companion, catalyst, mirror, midwife, and aide to problem-solving with the patient or the couple.

Beyond the necessity for every physician and therapist to develop his/her "second identity," this comes especially true for the couple-centered approach in diagnosis and treatment in sexual medicine. In this—for many—unfamiliar or unsettling situation there is no means of reassurance according to customs and this may lead to wanting to return to the well-rehearsed role security of the expert and knowledgeable scientist. Fact is, however, that concerning the particular couple in question, one is actually the "not knowledgeable one," having to rely on inquiries and observations, leaving the solving of the couple's problems to the couple itself.

The couple heals itself, the therapist offers the necessary "sheltered workshop" and supplies the continuity of the process. He/she would be out of his/her depth with the role of the expert as far as the couple relationship goes.

Thus, it is crucial for him/her to be conscious of both his/her roles, the one of the expert and the one of the assistant, to have both roles available, feel comfortable in both, and to be able to apply any one of both wherever needed, particularly in a couple setting. This is a skill which needs to be taught and practiced. It represents an indispensable demand to every training program in sexual therapy.

Taking as an example the treatment of post-prostatectomy erectile disorder caused by prostatic cancer, a German study showed that in long-term exclusive use of medication or mechanical treatment options, the patients were clearly less satisfied than their treating urologists would have imagined (see [24]). Even concerning selection of therapy options the patients' comments were clearly discrepant to the judgment of their treating physicians. Questions concerning the importance of partnership, of non-genital sexuality (the exchange of affectionate words and gestures) and genital sexuality (intercourse) put to prostate cancer patients and their partners *before and after radical prostatectomy* showed that only the importance of genital sexuality decreased and not the non-genital kind. Partnership in general and the meaning of physical attachment maintained an unchanged high value [25]. The high rating of satisfaction of psychosocial intimacy, closeness, and security in comparison to aiming at sexual erotic satisfaction has also been validated by other studies [26].

Sexological interventions, therefore, are imperatively based on consideration of biopsychosocial aspects of sexuality and on systematic involvement of partnership issues and communication (e.g., the couple is the patient). Such modifications of conventional patient concepts also lead to a different understanding of therapy.

The familiar concept of the "therapist–patient relationship" is extended—especially in the case of sexual disorders—to a new "therapist–couple relationship." Advocacy for the patient turns into plural advocacy for the couple and their partnership, as long as this is the mandate given to the therapist. Furthermore, the dimension of attachment is taken into account beyond any function disorders and is considered as being an essential resource for sexual contentedness. In many cases, this turns out to be a helpful approach for the patients because an idea for behavioral change is given—within quite a short time (usually not more than two to three sessions) —and this is often enough to get things going. If this proves not to be sufficient, supportive sexual therapeutic interventions can be supplied systematically to achieve the aspired modification of attitude and behavior over a longer period of time.

Sexological Counseling

It is obvious that sexological counseling concerned with more than functional disorders is a very high-quality job, demanding not only vast knowledge, but also much empathic capability and self-restraint. Again and again it is a challenge, because it is about finding a new and individual path for each individual patient/couple. Here, again, it is true that diagnosis and therapy in sexological practice are knitted together creating a mutual and complementing whole: integral diagnostic assessment is already a part of therapy and each therapeutic step leads to further diagnostic insights. So it can be said that sexological counseling may have a "therapeutic" impact, if it were qualified, and on the other hand cause consequential damage, if not.

Here, too, the foremost principle is to make patients/couples aware of the attachment dimension of sexuality and to apply this therapeutic aspect (see section "The Dual Role of the Therapist as an Expert and an Attendant"). Many patients/couples do not realize that genital/coital sexuality is only one of many ways of satisfying wishes within a partnership concerning needs for authenticity, appreciation, satisfaction, closeness, security, etc. Accordingly, sexological counseling will be adapted to the specific needs of the patient/couple, in which the following priorities, alone or combined, may be of significance:

Passing on knowledge (where deficits are obvious) concerning anatomical, physiological or psychological processes of sexual reaction, and, if necessary, correcting false ideas in the sense of sexual myths (e.g., masturbation causes harm), which one or both of the partners may believe in. It would be quite appropriate to refer to the issue of "typical" gender differences in sexual/partnership feelings and behavior in males and females (i.e., in this particular partner, male or female), meaning to aim at understanding and realizing differences instead of finding fault in such differences.

Assessment of mutual hopes and expectations concerning sexuality and partnership.

Teaching communicative strategies, if general communication difficulties are a reason for the development or continuation of the disorder concerned.

When primary illnesses are involved, specific information must be obtained (1) about the length of elapsed time between surgery and resumption of sexual contact (usually after approx. 6 weeks); (2) about the use of lubrication gel, if, for instance, the vaginal epithelium is altered by radiological or chemotherapy or due to menopause; (3) in some cases concerning the use of auxiliaries (tools such as an erection ring, a vacuum pump, any oral or invasive medication options). However, the first step should be to deal with discrepancies in the relationship between the partners concerning the significance of the different dimensions of sexuality.

The Syndyastic Focus: A Case History on Partnership Counseling

The following is a case example of sexological counseling, starting out with two individual face-to-face sessions and a concluding couple session. The example demonstrates the importance, and at the same time great difficulty, to focus on the (re-)fulfillment of psychosocial fundamental needs ("syndyastic focus") and to keep this perspective all the way through sexological counseling.

Case Report 1

First session with the husband

The 63-year-old man is a retired civil servant, married for 31 years, his wife is 4 years younger. He describes briefly, what leads him to the outpatient clinic: He is "impotent" and wants to know, whether, at his age, there is anything "to be done" here, considering that he has an enlarged prostate gland and has been taking "medication against high blood pressure" since his heart attack 6 years ago. Possibly it might all be connected with the medication? On the other hand, he feels it might just as well be caused by his high masturbation frequency, which—next to coital intimate contact—has been a fixed component of his sexuality throughout his whole marriage.

More detailed assessment revealed that the patient had been treated for 5 years with a beta receptor antagonist (propanolole) due to a moderate hypertonia. Exactly since 5 years he has been in early retirement and at about this time he first experienced erectile dysfunctions. These were not at all always prominent, particularly not during masturbation, which took place approx. Once a week, in former times 2 to 3 times a week. Since 2 years there had been no sexual contacts with his wife. It becomes obvious that the patient had withdrawn more and more, because he was sure that he was "a burden for his wife" alone for the existence of the erectile disorder. In fact, during intimate contact he would always be worried about the erection receding or he was dissatisfied, if it were "not sufficient." He could hardly imagine his wife still being interested in him, however, both were suffering from this complete standstill of mutual sexuality. The assessment of this patient gave insight on many influencing factors, all with a tendency of unfavorably effecting sexual experience and behavior: firstly, the current condition following the heart attack with the consequence of early retirement and high blood pressure needing treatment including possible side-effects through medication; secondly, his personal image of "impotency," for him already a fact, just because he was not in all circumstances—by own arousal or wishes from his partner—capable of an erection, even though principally sexual function was still given (such as during masturbation and morning erection); finally, the comprehensible psychological dimension of his conduct (anxious self-observation of his own sexual reaction; fear of failure toward his wife). Furthermore, there was a certain worry that he may have "used up" his sexual potency by masturbating too frequently in the past, claiming two to three times per week to be excessive, perhaps linked with feelings of guilt toward his wife.

This patient was suffering from a condition of frustrated needs for acceptance, closeness, etc. concerning the relationship to his wife and—most important!—during the initial interview this became quite obvious to himself. Because he loved his wife and wished for (re-)accomplishment of the syndyastic dimension of their sexuality, it seemed reasonable to him that this might be achieved by including the wife in the assessment and the counseling, particularly as there had never been any conversation between the couple on this subject.

First session with the wife

The wife is 59 years old and until 3 years ago had worked as a clerk in a housing management company. She is of slender stature, seems fragile and lowers her eyes during conversation. She very well knows that her husband is always worrying about his "erection problems," it is depressing for her as well that there had been no intimate contact whatsoever now since 4 years (not 2 years, like the husband said). In other ways they were such a good match, had always gotten on well together and have mutually raised three fine children. Her own sexual experience is restricted to intimate contacts to her husband, she had always liked having sex. She is quite capable of orgasm and sometimes, perhaps once a month, she reaches climax by masturbation. All the more she regrets that some time ago her husband had withdrawn altogether following several coitus attempts which had failed due to his erectile disorder. She had accepted this and let him be, even

(continued)

though she herself would still have liked some sexual activity and actually does not really want to do without it altogether. After all, he had had a heart attack and suffers from high blood pressure, presumably his poor health has led to physical demands he could not cope with. Even so, their mutual sexuality was never really as pleasurable as she might have wished for—her husband had always had a very early orgasm, which he resented, too (this disorder of sexual function—a premature orgasm—was not mentioned by the husband). She, on the other hand, was still very appreciative for endearments and interested in an extended foreplay. She believes he is putting himself under extreme pressure, although she does not put pressure on him because she does not expect such performance. She would be very pleased about a revival of their sexual intimacy, even if this would not lead to intercourse. She loves her husband and would very much like to be intimately and physically close to him.

Here, only by involving the wife, the different views of both partners on their mutual sexuality became clear, but also on both sides the frustrated psychosocial needs while at the same time strong wishes existed in both for syndyastic fulfillment with and by each other. All this information now makes it possible to discuss with the couple, how to reactivate the partnership sexuality they both long for.

Often, the syndyastic focus can be limited to few sessions whenever the involvement of the partner is possible and the couple is ready for a change in their relationship. This can be achieved by helping the couple to realize:

- that it is possible to talk about a sexual problem;
- that their difficulties are in good hands and that there is no need to be ashamed of anything;
- that the new information might help to readjust their view on the world of sexuality;
- that they can help themselves by broadening their sexual behavior repertoire, attaining new alternatives for themselves to fulfill their (mutual) needs for closeness, caring and acceptance;
- that by this fulfillment, no matter how difficult the barriers or restrictions might be, self-confidence arises; and
- that coping strategies are now available for cases of possible adverse reactions from the partner, e.g., after surgical interventions with physical impairments like in the case of implementing a stoma or an artificial bladder.

Concluding Couple Session

During the couple session it became obvious that the patient's sexual difficulties were experienced quite differently by his wife. Misunderstandings were cleared impressively. In fact, the wife described how she had always thought, throughout the whole marriage, that she could never satisfy him sexually, because she knew about his frequent masturbation practice; he, on the other hand, had always assumed that she took him for an insufficient lover because of his premature climaxes. She used this opportunity to explain, how important for her non-genital practice as part of sexuality was. This again, was quite relieving for him, because he, too, loved to just lie close to her and to "feel her closeness." So both declared that they had been taking wrong attitudes of the partner for granted and that improved sexual communication is to be acquired by mutual syndyastic fulfillment. They resolved for the future to talk about their sexual wishes, to create opportunities of enjoying these and to do this quite pragmatically, e.g., if they felt like it, to make use of a morning erection.

A further session after 3 months showed that these resolutions were kept. Both appeared quite changed, fresh and alive as a couple. They had revived their mutual sexuality and were very relaxed about enjoying their intimate contact. They had had sexual intercourse several times, in which no erectile disorder had arisen and the man did not experience his early orgasm as premature at all, even though he did not have the feeling of being able to control the arousal progression. Most important was: He was now completely sure that his wife did not mind this. She, herself, was extremely happy about the expansion of the non-coital sex (i.e., changed view on significance of sexual arousal and desire). This way, both experienced appreciation and acceptance in physical closeness, i.e., fulfillment of fundamental needs, and had, thus, found access for themselves to the syndyastic dimension of sexuality.

Shortly after this session the wife wrote a grateful letter to the therapist, expressing her happiness about the revived marital sexuality ("It's a great feeling, to be man and woman again") and she also expressed her surprise about the fact that "a third party could play such an important role in partnership togetherness."

Conclusions

This case report shows clearly that the worrying erectile disorder of the man was only to be understood and successfully treatable under the aspect of a biopsychosocial viewpoint on sexuality as well as under consideration of the attachment aspect of sexual disorders which means the syndyastic dimension of sexuality. In this case there was no need for any deep understanding of the life history and the sexual experiences, but most of all awareness to what was troubling both partners and to pick up their need for physical communication—extra-genital and genital. Only by involving the partner, this neediness became evident and the syndyastic fulfillment was made attainable for both.

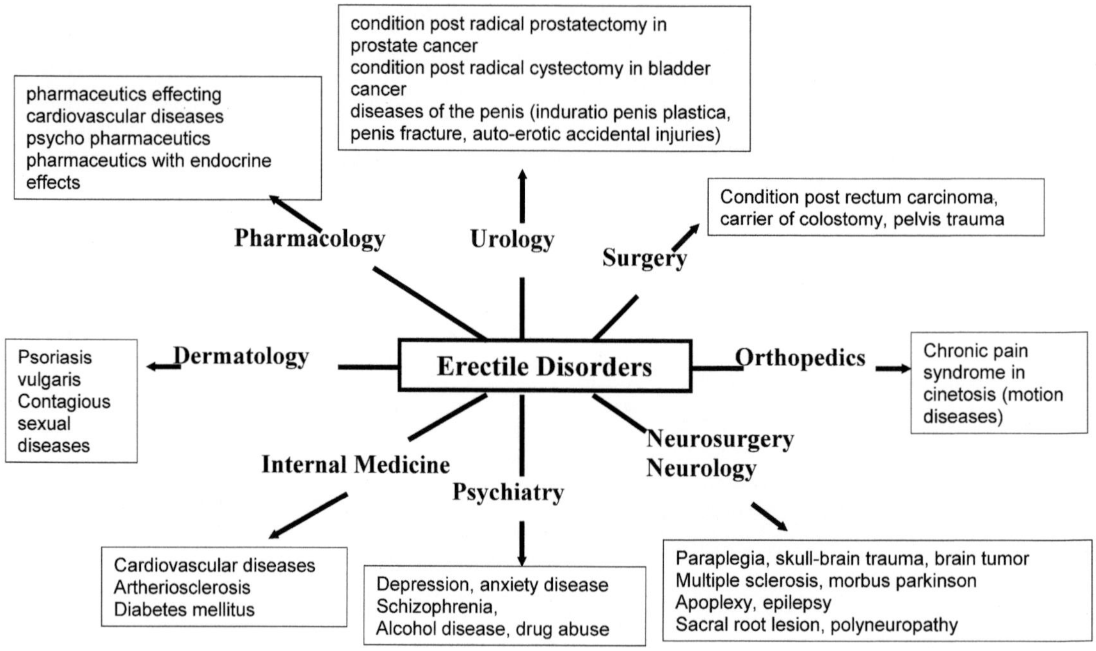

FIGURE 7-3. Erectile disorders caused by illnesses and/or their treatment.

It must be said, however, that this case was dealing with an ideal course of sexological counseling with a syndyastic focus—in every-day practice this not always proceeds so smoothly. Often, for example, the involvement of the partner is not a simple matter. And even if the partner does come along, the conversation with the couple might find one or both of the couple unable to cope with the idea of the "reorganisation" of the sexual relationship, especially when different inhibiting factors exist at the same time, e.g., an erectile disorder due to a radical prostatectomy and impairment of physical mobility with pain in certain positions. But also in such cases it should always be attempted to improve the requirements for the fulfillment of psychosocial needs in both partners by applying the syndyastic focus. Very often, talks about male myths and anxiety caused by a bad conscience (masturbation is sometimes seen as betrayal of the partner, sometimes even as immoral) are just as helpful as a survey concerning wishes of closeness and how to make them happen.

During sexological counseling there are often a great number of influencing factors on the biological, psychosocial and sexual level, which are all important to take note of, but on the other hand must not concentrate the attention of the therapist in such a way as to neglect the syndyastic focus. Such factors are:

- possible effects of a primary disease (e.g., hypertonia, condition after heart attack) and connected anxieties;
- possible effects of medication (e.g., beta receptor antagonists, often suspected of causing disorders of sexual function and this is often given as an explanation by patients;
- physical changes due to aging;
- change of social status (e.g., retirement)
- dynamics of sexual myths ("a man has to be ready at all times")
- wrong ideas about the needs and expectations of the (female) partner combined with feelings of guilt, not to be able to live up to them;
- similar wrong ideas in the (female) partner, also combined with feelings of guilt and insufficiency (not to be good enough as a woman etc.);
- lacking opportunities of mutual correction concerning misjudgements due to communication barriers;
- chronification with increasing psychological stress and development of self-reinforcement mechanisms such as failure anxieties and performance pressure—these could lead to maintaining the symptoms.

The multitude of possible reasons for the development of erectile disorders caused by illness or treatment is shown in Figure 7-3.

Syndyastic Sexual Therapy

As mentioned previously, the general aim of sexual therapy is to enable both partners to satisfy each others' fundamental needs—based on full acceptance—through their sexual behavior, i.e., their positive sexual communication in partnership. Negative sexual experiences create and sustain sexual disorders which are bound to put strain on a partnership.

The priority is not to restore sexual *function in the first place*, the therapeutic aim is to broaden the *understanding* of sexuality (particularly to appreciate the dimension of attachment), thereby gathering new experiences of (sexual) body communication and improving (sexual) partnership satisfaction on the whole. The option of effective medication or other aids is no contradiction and can be a helpful supplement at times.

Thus, within the course of therapy, new, mutually agreed upon, intimate experiences for the couple emerge, allocating a new significance of sexuality in a much broader sense. These are no "prescriptions," because it is not possible to "prescribe" anything in a relationship; they are genuine, holistic and consciously lived partnership experiences.

It is important to note that the syndyastic focus involves the activation of basically already existing potentials. Something is retrieved and nothing is "added," but brought into consciousness. In rare cases of total syndyastic deprivation (e.g., from infant development on), syndyastic therapy would be stretched to its limits and individual psychotherapy be required.

Finally, it must be stressed that the SST method is not restricted to certain specialized fields or schools. It merely relies on a basic biopsychosocial understanding and the willingness not to project oneself into the role of the objective expert, but to actually concentrate on the syndyastic focus—trusting in the knowledge that improvement of the fulfillment of psychosocial fundamental needs can lastingly effect all other areas of life, health and well-being. In what follows, the different aspects and phases of an SST-process are outlined.

Initial Phase: Motivation for Therapy

In the (quite common) case of a patient/couple being fixated on purely somatic causes it will be crucial not to fall into the "*organic or psychological*" *trap.* It would be best to flatly avoid using the often negatively understood term "psychological causes" altogether, e.g.: *You are here as a whole person with a body, a mind and feelings, living human relationships. All these things exist simultaneously and influence each other. Perhaps you are not used to doctors taking all these aspects into account instead of concentrating on the body alone.*

This course will be kept up by asking about "partnerships" instead of only asking about sexuality, usually (mis-)understood as genital sexuality—e.g.:. . *everyone needs a place to feel accepted, where somebody cares for you, where you can speak openly, be yourself and feel safe, etc.—where is such a place in your life? What is your partnership like? What part does sexuality play within this relationship?*

So if during a one-to-one conversation the impression is that relationship, partnership, and/or sexuality play a significant part in genesis and continuation of a particular disorder, it will be necessary to motivate the patient to involve the partner and to accept the offer of couple counseling. For example: *...whatever happens within a partnership concerns both partners and only both together can work on a solution. Both are suffering from this problem and most probably both could use some help. Without your partner it would be like doing things half right from the beginning. What do you think and do you think your partner would agree to come?* If the answer is: *"I'm not quite sure"* or *"my husband/my wife/my friend will definitely not come"* it will be necessary to go into the anxiety behind this and also to react to the "invitation," such as: *That would really surprise me. In my experience it is extremely seldom that a partner would refuse this offer—and this in itself would be significant—but how would you put the matter to him/her?* Under some circumstances a dialog involving role play might be encouraging and lead to an acceptable manner of announcement, not allowing for misunderstandings such as sounding like *"a legal summons to a trial."* In any case, success very much depends on the convincing manner and resoluteness of the therapist. Possibly, the patient and the therapist unconsciously do not want a third party to join their relationship; in that case, the invited partner would most likely refuse participation. At this stage of discussion the question could arise, whether an upcoming therapy should be carried out personally or if the case should (or needs to) be passed on to a specialist? Very often, this question remains academic, because the patient/the couple have already inspired confidence: *"If we/I do decide to do it, then only with you."*

No matter whether in individual sessions or sessions together with the couple, from the beginning the conversation should be run like the most natural thing in the world. If things like inhibitions or shame, uncertainty, feelings of guilt or embarrassment are in the air, this should directly be addressed, e.g.: *From my experience I know quite well that it can be a huge effort to talk to a third party about personal and intimate issues. Many people believe that only they themselves have such problems, in reality, these are quite common, but not many try to solve them professionally. Therefore, making the effort of asking for help is a sign of caring and looking out for a continuation of the partnership.*

If it is a couple session from the start, it begins before the first words are spoken with the perception of the partners' interaction, their performance, e.g., *How do both enter the room (overall impression, body language, facial expression, etc.)? Who leads the way, opens the door, assists at taking off the coat, looks for a seat, is seated first? What is the sitting position like: next to one another, opposite each other or across the corner?* A reply to the question *"Where should we be seated?"* could be like *"wherever you like,"* noting that the therapist takes his seat after the couple. A table with four chairs or several freely placed chairs is more appropriate than a small sofa, on which the couple would be forced to sit next to each other. (No need to say that the therapist should not hide behind his desk, nor computerize data simultaneously!). Which one of them begins the conversation, do the individuals look at each other or do both just look at the therapist, do they interrupt each others' speech? etc.

If a patient has been able to motivate his/her partner to take part in a session, quite a lot of movement has come into the partnership, even if it might seem as if someone "uninvolved" has just come along to support his/her partner. Generally, men are more inhibited when it comes to discussing relationship issues, therefore the positive decision to come along deserves recognition such as: *good of you to come—I expect it wasn't so easy?*

After an open invitation to the couple to start with whatever seems to them to be most important, the therapist should choose the right moment to define his own role, e.g.: *Maybe I should say something about my role in our talks, so that from the beginning you do not misinterpret it or get the wrong idea. I am neither judge nor referee, who makes decisions about which one of you is in the right. This is not about judgments or guilt, it is about causes and the understanding of how things are connected. It is also not my job to solve your problems, you need to do that yourselves and I can try to help you do so. I am not the expert on your relationship, so you won't be getting any advice from me, only suggestions/ideas. It will be crucial to put the ideas we develop here and whatever you "prescribe" to yourself to work in the outside world. I will not take sides with either one of you, but will step in for both of you and your partnership, as long as it is in your intention. Should one of you still have a feeling of partiality on my part or coalition being built up, please don't hesitate to refer to it.*

Usually—depending on the gender of the therapist—one male and two females or one female and two males will sit opposite one another and—again—it is important to ask, if there is any suspicion of coalitions or worries of any kind.

On the other hand, usurpation efforts on the part of the patient/couple have to be immediately opposed. Statements like: "Doctor, see for yourself…., what do you say to that?, you have to confess, I'm right… tell my partner, he doesn't believe me…," etc. could be retorted by saying: *Are you looking for an ally?* Or: *You want to make me a referee, which I am not! Or: What would it mean to you if I were to say you were right, or you were wrong?* Or *I can't take that off your shoulders, but this would be a great opportunity to tell your partner personally what is really bothering you. Do try to make him/her understand and perhaps we can find out, what it is all about.*

In such situations it is important not to directly answer the questions reflex-like with regard to content, like one would in organic medicine, but to keep out of the content level and to stay on the meta or interpretation level, in order to be able to continue work with both parties.

Often, right at the beginning there is the situation of having to directly refer to anxieties and to disperse these, for instance the fear of being given the death sentence for the relationship or the inevitability of a separation. The anxious question: *"According to your experience, do we still have a chance?"* is often put forward already in the first session. It has to be taken up on, but must not be dealt with in a direct way, for example: *"You're asking me?—You know yourself and your relationship much better than I know you, how much chance do you yourself think you have?* Or: *Whether or not you do have a chance depends on, whether or not you give yourself one and you would probably not be here if you didn't, right?* Or, for example in particular function disorders: "*I can generally say, that in the case of these disorders there are statistically very good chances of success, but statistics say nothing about an individual case. So I can't say whether you belong to the 80% success rate or to the other 20%—this you decide yourself.*

Before therapy begins, however, it is inevitable to negotiate the practical procedure in detail and to clarify the essential parameters, because it is crucial for success of therapy to comply to these. In accordance, for the whole duration of therapy, both partners need to be able to concentrate on each other and the new common experiences. Therefore, maintained external sexual relationships are incompatible with these requirements and any desire for having children should not be a key issue. Generally, this is easily conveyed, because the time period of a therapy is seldom more than 3 to 6 months. Furthermore, there would be no point in beginning with a *Syndyastic Sexual Therapy*, if the couple has not enough opportunity to gather intimate experiences with one another. This needs to be seen as a specific obligation prior to therapy by both partners.

In same-gender partnerships, there are modifications to consider insofar as the typical gender differences of sexual behavior (see [3]) in the partners very probably do not occur complementarily. Therefore it could, perhaps, be expected in a male couple that both partners show a higher willingness for occasional sexual contacts and for them the general significance of infidelity may allow for a relaxed reaction, thus not questioning the syndyastic fulfillment within the partnership. But exactly this is the determining point: The partnership is in danger only if the biopsychosocial elementary needs—existent in both genders, independent of their sexual orientation—are frustrated. The syndyastic dimension of partnership can, however, be strengthened in many ways, namely always by giving the partner the feeling that he/she is appreciated, taken seriously and accepted and when they feel mutually secure in each others' company. If an external sexual contact does authentically not mean destabilization (which is practically never the case in two-gendered couples), then the syndyastic experience is not threatened.

Nevertheless, sexual communication is a particularly intensive opportunity of finding syndyastic fulfillment and this also applies to one-gendered couples, in which trust in mutual intimacy usually reaches a deeper experience level than one found in occasional external sexual contacts.

New Experiences with Intimacy: The Practical Approach

The principles of *Syndyastic Sexual Therapy*—the central role of the fulfillment of fundamental needs, the communicative dimension of sexuality—can only be achieved through plausible self-evident experiences by the patient(s)/the couple, enabling them to change their former "view on the world of sexuality." It is inevitable that the couple needs to *organize* these new experiences to *make them happen*. It is all about *practicing improved biopsychosocial communication* (sensual body language) at certain previously appointed times, which will lead to a new experience. This obviously implies that communication on the partnership level itself has to be improved. Which means, the first experiences will often touch on the partnership communication as such. This automatically points out the significance of the time between the therapy sessions in which the patient(s)/couples themselves do the main work concerning the intended change of their situation. They put into effect their own previously made resolutions for meaningful new experiences from one session to the next.

In this respect, it can be called a "self-devised experience" or a mutually conceived resolution. Here, the difference to previous well-known popular terminology becomes obvious—no more "home work," "exercises," "sensuality training" or "prescribed experiences." During the *syndyastic focus*, it is exactly *not the therapist* who organizes the experiences for the couple and virtually imposes these upon them; rather, the couple finds an own way of creating opportunities for the fulfillment of fundamental needs and finally their connection to sexual arousal and pleasure. The therapist accompanies the couple along this path. Consequently, a further significant difference to classic sexual therapy emerges as it provides for achieving a final goal (namely the restoration of sexual function(s)) in stages. Those various preliminary steps are only a means to an end, whilst, according to the SST, the therapy goals are to be fully reached at any stage: With each new experience, the couple may reach the therapy goal completely—it is the task and the responsibility of the therapist to convey this adequately.

Because the "new experiences" are organized by the couples themselves, Masters and Johnson's [27] established "Sensate Focus"-steps can at most (and not least for the therapists) serve as reference points in the background. In most cases, their internal logic—to gradually obtain closeness via nonsexual tenderness, i.e., tenderness not directed at sexual arousal and orgasm, by way of sensual exploration of one another, momentarily leaving aside the negatively burdened genital sexuality—corresponds with the aims of the couple.

However, in the beginning couples do not aim at "sexuality" in the first place, but at conversation, joint activities, more time for and with each other, etc. These activities can also result in closeness and they emphasize the essential role of body language, which almost automatically leads to the need for a more extensive physical closeness and intimacy, as, for example, in "cuddling." In this case, therapists can make further inquiries: What is this need about and how are you planning to reach your goal? What seems necessary to you, what does not? Do you have any fears or anxieties, and if yes, which ones? How could those be avoided?

First, the planned steps need to be understood and internalized as body language communication, so that from the beginning, they are more than a training program for all sensory functions. They are, as a matter of fact, personal body language communication and encounter, and thus receive a new allocation of significance. Before this is not fully understood, the planned steps should not be started with by the couple.

This is also important given that many couples are already familiar with the "Sensate Focus Exercises" from the internet or state that "we already know about this, we have already tried it, but it did not help"—precisely because the new significance has not been understood. In this sense, the six steps in Masters and Johnson [27] shall be recalled briefly, bearing in mind that the respective practical applications are as variable as the couples and their needs. Instead of a fixed program to be "executed," the six steps constitute possibilities, guideposts for the couples to plan their future experience.

First Step: Mutual Body Discovery, Omitting Breast and Genitals

The agreement to omit the erogenous zones of breast and genitals from the body language communication as well as to abstain from the (often problematic) intercourse (the so-called ban on intercourse by Masters and Johnson) usually arises and makes sense during the discussion of the concrete situation and is often suggested by the couple themselves. For instance, it gives a woman suffering from hypoactive desire disorder or sexual aversion the necessary security that out of a tender display of affection "nothing more" will arise, but the fulfillment of fundamental needs and that it will not "end in sex." A man with problems of erection or orgasm obtains the security that "he can't go wrong" and doesn't have to worry that again "it won't work." As a rule—apart from rare exceptions—the strict abstaining from sexual intercourse is the precondition to make really new experiences on the communicative level which have their value in their own right and should not be degraded to "a step on the ladder up to the real thing."

Second Step: Involvement of the Female Breast

Again, in the next move the female breast can become involved in the exploring and caressing in a pleasurable tentative way not aimed at sexual arousal. In communicative meaning, the attention to this particular zone of femininity can express, e.g., appreciation, attractivity, invitation, pleasure, being welcome—once again mutual acceptance, not reduced to sex appeal.

Third Step: Involvement of the Genitals

In this step, too, the coitus still remains banned, but now the genitals can be included into the playful caressing. By now, for the couple, there should be an understood difference between "purposeful" sexual arousal (with one thing in mind) and "random playfulness" on the level of body language communication, so that exhilarating experiences can be made without erection and/or orgasm. It is extremely important that both partners take joint responsibility for mutually satisfying intimacy (and therefore for example direct the partner's hand to the place they like to be caressed). This promotes the most important goal of the therapy: internalization of the syndyastic dimension of sexuality.

Fourth Step: Teasing and Arousal

If the couple focuses on the topic of desire (which may be present from the beginning), lust is also connected to the dimension of attachment, because it arises on the basis of mutual acceptance. This way it is easy to explain to the patients that they can experience a syndyastic enhancement of their passion respectively a sensual–orgastic enhancement of their partnership. From a therapeutic point of view it is all about connecting the dimension of desire with the syndyastic dimension, meaning a changed view on and significance of sexual arousal and desire.

Fifth Step: Non-demanding Coitus

The next step could add sexual intercourse, but still with the intention of getting to know one's own reaction better and to make new experiences with the partner, in order to, for instance, consciously experience the body language messages during the intercourse like in "slow motion," stripping off anxieties, gaining security, etc. They have mutually agreed to relax after penetration. So this non-demanding intromission (sometimes termed "quiet vagina") is not about spontaneous complete coitus. This step can also be applied in the treatment of orgasm praecox.

Sixth Step: Spontaneous, Whole Coitus

Here, the connection between the syndyastic system and the system of desire should be so stable that it remains internalized, even when not thinking about it all the time. Sexual desire should now be consciously experienced in the context of fulfilled fundamental needs and be therefore more intensive and more intimate as a whole. Sex and love should no longer be in any way separated in the partner, but be molded into one. Only in this entity, desire can really develop freely, as long as the communication is experienced as authentic.

As in classical sexual therapy, special techniques such as "stop-start" or "squeeze" can be integrated into *Syndyastic Sexual Therapy*, but need to be understood and utilized on the basis of the treatment's focal point, the attachment dimension of sexuality. The woman might stimulate the penis to near climax but would need the response from the partner, in order to interrupt at the right moment; this only works, if, on the basis of their relationship understanding, she really feels involved and not just as being used like a random physiotherapist.

Detailed Exploration

During this kind of work with the couple it is important right from the start (as by the way also in the partnership) to pay attention to details and nuances and particularly to the significance it has for each individual of the couple. In addition to the usual (macro-)anamnesis, there has to be the micro-anamnesis, the inquiring into and asking for elaboration of the slightest details: *What exactly was that like? How did you experience it? What exactly was normal about it, good or dreadful? What did it mean to you in that situation/at that time?*

In the—not so rare—case that the couple or one partner does not adhere to the mutual agreement to abstain from full sexual intercourse (or any other agreement), a micro-anamnestic investigation is of special importance. Instead of blaming or exhorting the couple, the therapist could ask: *What were the consequences of the broken agreement? How did the partner feel? How did the evening continue? How long did it take until the atmosphere was rectified? What conclusions do you draw? Do you now understand what the agreement to abstain from any intercourse is about? etc.*

However, in some cases the "transgression" might be perfectly right, because coitus became syndyastically necessary, but was leading to feelings of guilt on the part of the couple: *"We did not behave well."* Here, the therapy goal needs to be positively emphasized: *How did this happen? What were the feelings leading to full sexual expression? What did this mean for your experiencing of intimacy? What overall effects did it have?* etc. (see section "Introduction," Figure 7-1).

Doing this, it is not primarily about working through "psychotherapeutic pathways," it is about the "syndyastic focus" on the violated (or fulfilled) elementary needs of being acknowledged, desired and respected, feeling accepted, trusting, experiencing closeness and being sheltered, etc. Which of these needs have been frustrated and what kind of significance have they obtained during the biography of this person? At the same time the partner will be asked questions like: *Is that the way you saw it too? Are you agreeing cognitively or emphatically? Were you aware of the significance for your partner?* Often, one partner (normally the man) uses facts for argument, the other partner is on a level of feelings and meanings, which results in them not really talking to each other and the whole argument escalates.

In many cases, there will be uncontrollable disputes or, e.g., long pauses where both partners are silent. These must be given room and endured for the patient's/couple's contemplation and thought tracking. There is, of course, the possibility of asking about their significance. In this case, own ideas could indicate a diagnostic direction of the patient's/couple's state of mind and could be, reflectively, offered as a question (see frame below).

Perceiving One's Own Feelings in the Context of the *Syndyastic Sexual Therapy*

- consciously reflecting one's own feelings instead of (re-)acting in an unreflected spontaneous way
- can these feelings be clearly named, are they understandable or are they contradictory, vague, not concrete?
- in what way are they "my own" feelings connected closely to my own personality/life history/present situation—and how far are they induced by the patient/the couple and what might this reveal about his/her/their situation?

After all, the consent to doing a session as a couple is in itself a therapy contract, so decision-making should be given thought, discussion, and time. After terminating a couple therapy experienced as successful, the answer to the question "what helped you most" was "the fact that you did not give up on us."

Case Reports

To explicitly integrate this communication approach into the treatment of sexual disorders means to raise awareness of a hitherto only implicit, but not sufficiently registered perspective, which therefore did not have the desired impact. Almost all patients and/or couples seeking sexual therapy in both authors' clinical practice described the couple-, relationship-, and communication-centered approach as a fundamentally new, even revolutionary way of thinking and experiencing. The approach has proven to be key to therapy success; a success driven by emotional experiencing and practice, rather than information and cognitive understanding. It has proven useful to build on the most recent behaviors experienced and interpreted as positive by the couples, i.e., to proceed from healthy and successful experience instead of being deficit-oriented: "Now you are again talking about what did not work out—where (and when) have you been successful?"

Missing Orgasm

A couple, in the beginning of their 30s, suffering from the woman's anorgasmia for 8 years, experienced the new, self-conceptualized practices and the learning and reorientation process encouraged through therapy as follows: The husband, who had hitherto insisted on daily sexual intercourse, reported to now see sexuality "in a different light" and became "as tender as possible." This helped his wife, who had strictly differentiated between love and sexuality before, to overcome her anorgasmia through new experience rather than pornographic films, as has unsuccessfully been tried before. Consequently, she stated: "Now it is more like *we* are sleeping together, while before it was just a sexual act." Because now "a new aspect was added and I am able to really understand how this also has a deeper meaning," she was able to dedicate herself emotionally, at the same time experiencing more self confidence, ("because I felt that my husband was concerned with me as a whole person"), security, and freedom, "because like this, you make less mistakes and there is less to lose." Thereby, physical receptivity was increased and the woman became capable of orgasm with her husband. This change was achieved in the course of ten appointments with the couple, where other aspects were addressed as well, and where mutual understanding and insight into the multilevel biographical specificities were initiated.

With this new perspective of sexual communication—proceeding from the concept by Masters and Johnson [27] and practiced as *Syndyastic Sexual Therapy* for more than a decade—the hitherto isolated "sex" can become a conscious, twofold sensual and personal dialogue in a sexual way and thereby gain an additional dimension of significance. At the same time, sexuality is fully integrated into the couple relationship, reversing the split between sex and love. In the positive event, the self-developed new experiences can lead to holistic personal encounters in accordance with individual needs and desires; in the negate event, they can lead to an inevitable confrontation with the reality of the relationship.

The syndyastic approach can lead to questioning fixed roles, reduces anxieties and the pressure to perform, and hence helps to restructure behaviors in the everyday partnership and sexuality. A syndyastic perspective also facilitates the reconciliation between shame and sexuality, disgust and sexuality, or religion and sexuality, thereby addressing potential pathogenic disturbances. It can also help addressing problems of sexuality in old age, which usually do not result from functional changes caused by age, but from social stigmatization of sexuality during this life stage. A syndyastic perspective could help to abandon irrational myths and preconceptions about this life stage in favor of a more adequate and human attitude and practice [28, 29].

Sexual Traumatization in Personal History

A 16-year-old middle school student, female, seems approximately 5 years older than her age, calm and considerate in appearance, but not very emotionally responsive. She had been in a relationship with a 20-year-old apprentice, whom she referred to as her "prince" and whom she wanted to "start a family" with. An increasingly serious problem was pain during sexual intercourse ("feelings of pain when his penis enters my vagina," "lack of lubrication," "nothing happens"). She had never experienced an orgasm, nor had she tried self-stimulation. She reported that her partner was worried ("You get nothing out of it"), which made her feel "uncomfortable."

When inquiring about negative sexual experiences in her biography, she reported to have been sexually abused several times by her mother's boyfriend at the age of ten (having to stimulate him manually or orally until he reached climax). He forced her to remain silent and threatened to leave her mother and to withdraw his financial support of family (the patient had two younger sisters). Shortly after, he left her mother ("because of another woman"); the mother did not only "mourn after him" but also "blocked" all intents to talk about the sexual abuses, accusing her of "only trying to make him look bad." The patient had not told her boyfriend about her experience, because she "felt embarrassed."

The traumatization had not been therapeutically processed. The first interview aimed to relieve the juvenile from her experience and to strengthen the relationship with her boyfriend as the first-time opportunity to (re-)fulfill her psychosocial fundamental needs (for acceptance, security, etc.), which had been frustrated by the abuse. It was explained how this was the precondition for a pleasurable integration of the body and the genitals into an intimate encounter with a loved person. It was therefore recommended to ensure the boyfriend's support and tell him about her experience. After doing so, the boyfriend was involved in the appointments (altogether 5), which proved to be useful. Because he felt an authentic affection for the patient ("she is perfect for me"), they were able to build up confidence in the success of the relationship, in which she would not feel used any more, but accepted and loved.

As can be seen from the case example, the development of a sexual function disorder can be closely related with experiences of sexual abuse. Therefore, it is necessary not to avoid this topic during treatment, but to address it carefully, for example by the question whether the patient ever had any sexual experiences in her life (thereby explicitly mentioning childhood, as childhood is often taken to be the "non-sexual part" of life) which she perceived as uncomfortable or embarrassing, which happened against her will, and which she was unable or unwilling to talk about so far. The communication-oriented approach to human sexuality encourages patients to include potential experiences of abuse into the couple therapy, even, and especially, if they had been kept secret from the partner. Thereby, the relationship can be used as a valuable resource to overcome the effects of distressing experience. Again, the syndyastic focus is helpful, because most people can be encouraged to open up towards addressing their fundamental needs.

The *Syndyastic Sexual Therapy* served to carry the problematic beyond the functional aspect of sexuality. A more detailed engagement with the individual life and learning history and with partnership problems is the precondition for this new "sexual world view." Potential resistance, which would usually be activated with the first practical therapy steps, can thereby be identified and tackled beforehand, whereas patients/couples should define the speed of progress themselves. However, it is important to encourage concrete changes from the very beginning of the therapy, while at the same time not losing sight of the new meaning of sexuality. From our therapeutic experience, the couple can gain considerably regarding the profundity of experiencing and salutogenic effectiveness: "Our whole life has changed!"

Treatment of Sexual Preference Disorders

According to DSM-5, a diagnosis of a sexual preference disorder (paraphilia) is only possible if the individual suffers from his/her paraphilic inclination or if this inclination has lead to impairments in important social or professional fields, or, in the case of paraphilias potentially endangering others (e.g., a pedophilic inclination), if the individual has acted according to these endangering impulses (independent of potential psychological distress). Only in these cases a paraphilic disorder is diagnosed; otherwise, it is considered only being a paraphilia which is not causing disease and needs no diagnostic classification.

The human sexual preference structure manifests on three axes (see section "Assessment of the Sexual Disorder"), is constituted during adolescence, and thereafter remains stable over lifetime in its fundamental characteristics. This also involves the unchangeability of specific sexual preferences, which equally manifest during adolescence and which can partly (non-exclusive type) or entirely (exclusive type) characterize the sexual preference structure (see [3]).

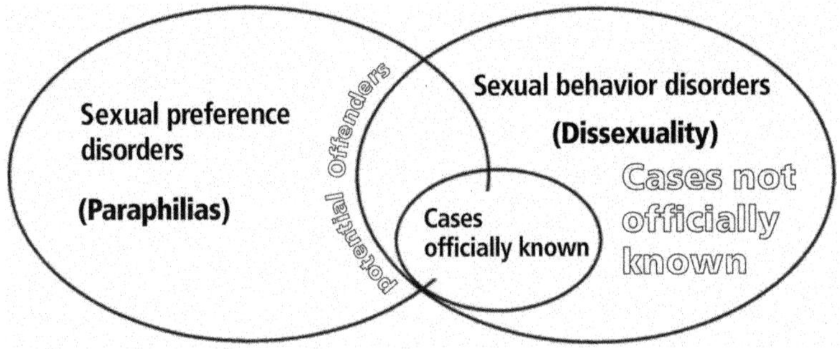

FIGURE 7-4. Spectrum of sexual preference and sexual behavior disorders.

TABLE 7-3. Disorders of sexual preference/paraphilic disorders by ICD-10/DSM-5

ICD-10: disorders of sexual preference	DSM-5: paraphilic disorders
F65.0 Fetishism	302.81 Fetishistic disorder
F65.1 Transvestic fetishism	302.3 Transvestic disorder
F65.2 Exhibitionism	302.4 Exhibitionistic disorder
F65.3 Voyeurism	302.82 Voyeuristic disorder
F65.4 Pedophilia	302.2 Pedophilic disorder
F65.5 Sadomasochism	302.83 Sexual masochism disorder
	302.84 Sexual sadism disorder
	302.89 Frotteuristic disorder
F65.6 Multiple disorders of sexual preference	
F65.8 Other disorders of sexual preference	302.89 Other specified paraphilic disorder
F65.9 Sexual disorder not otherwise specified	302.9 Unspecified paraphilic disorder

Table 7-3 gives an overview of the most important disorders of sexual preference/paraphilic disorders according to ICD-10 [12]/DSM-5 [13].

Sexual preference disorders need to be differentiated from sexual behavior disorders. The latter involve intended or carried out sexual acts in front of or passively or actively involving children [the so-called "pedo-sexual acts"; in criminal law: "child sexual abuse (CSA)"], prepubescent or pubescent minors, or other persons unable to consent to these sexual acts. If these acts can be attributed to acting out certain paraphilias, they are considered *acts of inclination*; if they are related to a different primary problem, they can be understood as *substitute acts,* compensating the actually desired sexual interaction with an adult and consenting partner, which is not obtainable in a socially acceptable manner. For sexological diagnosis this implies that disorders of sexual preference and sexual behavior have to be well differentiated and not confused, or even equated.

Figure 7-4 shows that within the whole spectrum of paraphilias, the dominant part is *not* related to sexually abusive behavior (dissexuality). Conversely, dissexuality usually *does not* date from a sexual preference disorder. In simple terms: The majority of men with a sexual preference disorder are not dissexual, and the majority of men with a sexual behavior disorder are not paraphilic. In addition, only a small part of dissexual behavior is committed in the "Hellfeld" (i.e., cases that are legally registered), whereas most cases remain undetected by legal authorities in the "Dunkelfeld" (literally "dark field"), yet playing an important role in everyday clinical practice.

The treatment of sexual disorders that can immediately involve the endangerment of others, e.g., pedophilia or sexual sadism, entails specific therapeutic responsibilities. It is assumed that a person is not responsible for his/her sexual preference, but the resulting sexual behavior. Hence, the presence of a pedophilic preference demands a life-time sexual self-regulation and behavioral control, whereas the development of appropriate coping strategies is often complicated by the fear of social stigmatization (see [30]). During the last 10 years, primary prevention therapy programs have been developed to address these issues. These programs aim at adults (see [31, 32]), and, more recently, also at juveniles (see [33]), and have proven successful.

Based on a multidimensional understanding of sexuality (dimensions of desire, reproduction and attachment; see section "The Three Dimensions of Sexuality"), it needs to be taken into account that individuals with a pedophilic preference pursue fulfillment in the dimension of attachment with a child as a partner. It is therefore necessary to support the fulfillment of these emotionally stabilizing factors by establishing alternative relationships. For that purpose, the *Berlin Dissexuality Therapy* [34] was developed as a treatment program aiming to increase self-efficacy and behavioral control (including sexual fantasies and interests); to substitute emotion- and avoidance-oriented sexualized coping strategies by more adequate behaviors; to strengthen social functioning (by focusing on the dimension of attachment); to decrease offense-supportive attitudes and behaviors; and to increase empathy with children involved in CSA to prevent further child sexual abuse and the use of child abuse images (see [35]).

A biopsychosocial approach also includes pharmacological therapy options. In clinical practice, three groups of medications are important, which differ in pharmacological mechanism [36]:

Selective Serotonin-Reuptake-Inhibitors (SSRI)

Applied for the treatment of sexual impulsivity, SSRI was found to decrease sexual impulses [37, 38]. The medical effect of a decrease in sexual appetence, usually an undesirable adverse drug reaction in other indications, might contribute to the effectiveness of SSRI. The influence of SSRI on sexual experiencing and behavior is well documented [39] and it is applied regularly (see [40]).

Antiandrogenic Medications (CPA and GnRH-Analog)

The antiandrogen cyproterone acetate (CPA) blocks receptors for testosterone in the organs, leading to a strong reduction of sexual fantasies and behavior [41]. The administration of gonadotropin-releasing hormone analog (GnRH-Analog) reduces the endogenous production of testosterone in the testicles via the brain areas in control of hormone production, resulting in a significant decrease in sexual urges and behavior.

Opioid Antagonists

In promising case reports [42–44] it was shown that Naltrexon improved the controllability of sexual urges. Hypothetically, this is indirectly related to the influencing of the dopaminergic reward system. So far, the medication is only applied as an individual curative trial, yet with a favorable side-effect profile.

The medication described above can help to reduce sexual impulses and fantasies and can complement psychotherapeutic interventions [36, 45, 46]. The overall aim is for patients to accept their sexual preferences ("accepting what is") and to assume responsibility for their sexual behavior. By now, the prevention network "Do not become an offender!" has opened 11 project offices all over Germany, offering preventive therapy to individuals with a pedophilic disorder according to defined quality standards, which includes specialized competence in diagnostics and therapy of sexual disorders (see [35]).

Excursus: *Syndyastic Sexual Therapy* with Patients Suffering from Disorders of Sexual Preference and Without Potential Harm for Others

Clinical experience shows that disorders of sexual preference can often lead to disorders of sexual relationship. In the end, it depends on the question of whether or not the partner would be able to accept these and be able to cope, if fantasy contents were made known to him/her—even, if their execution were not intended. Such uncertainties have the power of destabilizing the syndyastic system so severely that relationships are very difficult to enter into or they put existing ones at great risk (see section "Treatment of Sexual Preference Disorders"). If, however, a partnership does exist and both partners have an authentic interest in a mutual perspective, the *Syndyastic Sexual Therapy* can be effectual in improving partnership contentment. The following 4 factors are crucial:

1. The proportion of the paraphilic pattern in relation to the sexual preference structure.
   It makes a big difference whether the paraphilic experience affects the whole sexual preference structure, or whether there might be other, non-paraphilic parts, which can be acted out with the partner. For example, in the case of an exclusive masochistic inclination, in which a (gynephilically orientated) man, in order to get sexually aroused, exclusively fantasizes scenes in which he is mutilated by his (female) partner, then there is no way for him to build up a comparable sexually arousing situation any other way with his partner. This, again, would very likely lead to disorders of sexual function and would burden the partnership severely, if the partner were kept in the dark and she were not able to understand why there were such difficulties in sexual communication.
2. Sexual function disorders emerging additionally.
   Just as every disorder of sexual function can be a symptom of another disease (e.g., a disorder of orgasm in multiple sclerosis), there is always the possibility that it might be caused by a paraphilia—precisely because the individual involved does not want to further burden the partnership with his paraphilic stimulus, making him insecure in intimate contact because he fears that the emergence of paraphilic fantasy images would keep him away from his partner, while all he wants is to be close. On the other hand, a functional disorder (e.g., an erectile disorder) is a visually obvious symptom for the partner and generally both partners communicate a wish to change this situation, so that here would be a starting point regarding the therapeutic work, keeping in mind that the explanation about the connection with the feelings of paraphilic experience in itself is an important step within the therapy context.
3. The significance of the paraphilic stimulus within self-experience.
   The fact that an attachment to the paraphilic stimulus can exist (as, e.g., in the case of a fetishistic inclination), affecting the syndyastic experience in such a way that in contact with the stimulus, not only sexually arousing but also psycho-emotionally stabilizing feelings (comparable to those in attachment to another person) are experienced, makes a clear statement concerning the limits of therapeutic intervention. This applies when the attachment to the paraphilic stimulus (e.g., a fetish) has the same or greater significance for the individual as the attachment to

a real partner. An especially extreme example for this is the so-called "Cannibal from Rothenburg" whose feelings of attachment were constricted in such a way that he could only experience real "love" toward another person, when this other person was inside of him, whereas other forms of sexual fulfillment were not available, at least not in regard to the desired attachment experience. Diagnostically this meant a special form of fetishistic orientation (namely toward male flesh; DSM-5: 302.81; ICD-10: 65.0) without any further psychopathological disorders (see [47, 48]). However, clinical experience has shown that particularly in fetishistic preference patterns (e.g., diaper fetishism) the attachment toward the fetish is so strong that a real partner has little chance to reach this level of significance, so that, from the beginning, there certainly are limits concerning couple-centered intervention.

4. Ability of self-retraction.
The significance of the paraphilic pattern in self-experience is not the only therapeutically limiting factor (see above), but also—however, in no way coincident—the ability of self-retraction with regard to the partnership is an issue: In the case of an exclusively paraphilic pattern (e.g., sadism with exclusive and not acceptable stimulus-enhancing content, involving injury or mutilation of the partner) it may be of importance for the individual involved, to aim at improvement of the attachment contentedness, because for him it may be a resource of life quality which he wants to make use of within a functioning partnership. From a clinical point of view it is striking that this criterion is often found in women with an exclusive type of paraphilia (e.g., a sexual masochism), who much more often emphasize the syndyastic function level in comparison to the dimension of desire. Without doubt there are also women with paraphilias, in whom this is not so, but this is more seldom the case than in men. Additionally, an important motivational factor in this context—for men as well—is a feeling of responsibility for existing (or planned) mutual children (see [49]).

Treatment of Gender Identity Disorders/Gender Dysphoria

This field of indication involves insecurities, irritations, and paresthesia regarding the individual gender identity, subsumed under the category "gender dysphoria" in the current *Diagnostic and Statistical Manual of Mental Disorders* by the American Psychiatric Association (DSM-5; see [13]), or, respectively, under "Gender Identity Disorders" in the current International Classification System of the World Health Organization (ICD-10; see [12]).

Of clinical relevance is an individual's subjective feeling not to belong to the gender they were assigned at birth, the feeling to have to live in the "wrong" body (resulting in the wish to change this condition), and a feeling of unease with the assigned gender. The diagnostic category comprises different grades and manifestations, which can have different backgrounds, requiring different treatments. This does not apply to a temporary unease with the birth gender, discontent and insecurity concerning the individual gender role, cosmetic or other needs for body-altering measures.

Individuals with gender identity disorders usually receive a specialized psychotherapeutic treatment. The therapy goal is not to "combat" or "reverse" the wish to change one's gender, but solely to offer these persons a strategy for tackling their own gender identity insecurity over a long period of time and with an open outcome. At the same time, therapeutic guidance allows the patient to test real-life conditions in the desired gender in all social fields (the so-called "real-life test"—however, this does not mean the "testing" of the person, but the person "tests" him- or herself in everyday life, gaining experience in the desired gender role; see [50]). With skilled counseling and advice the patient is able to understand and process the developing impressions, experiences, and feelings. The central and difficult task for further diagnoses is to adequately estimate the given unease with the birth gender and perceived belonging to the other gender in the context of the individual development for each singular case. In this regard, it is of interest how the concerned person has implemented his/her wish to belong to the other gender in real life to the present point, which difficulties were encountered, and how they were processed.

In many cases, concerned persons have very concrete ideas and aims regarding future proceedings, therefore quickly feeling impeded by the health system. When the self-attributed diagnosis of "transsexuality" is perceived as absolutely central, it can result in the tendency to avoid dealing with individual developmental aspects. However, it is indispensable for the diagnostic-therapeutic process to come to terms with the physical gender development, as it is necessary to reconstruct the development of the gender identity—always against the background of the general personality development (see [51]).

The strongest and irreversible form of gender identity disorder is described as *transsexuality*. These cases involve a lifelong persisting, irreversible disintegration of one's own gendered body feeling, which is usually treated with cross-gender hormone medication and in some cases with sex-reassignment surgery, along with the necessary psychotherapeutic support. This procedure is internationally recognized within sexual medicine (see [52, 53]).

In non-transsexual manifestations of gender dysphoria, body-altering measures (hormones, surgery) are usually not indicated; the priority is on psychotherapy accompanying attainment of a suitable identity. In biological adult men, transvestic fetishism is one of the most important and frequent differential diagnoses; in biological women it is a not integrated (ego-dystonic) homosexual orientation. Moreover, personality disorders are of particular clinical relevance. Complicating the assessment process, they may explain the problems of gender identity (e.g., a borderline personality disorder), but can also be found additionally.

Sexuality and Partnership in the Elderly

Particularly in older age with its various burdens, general changes and losses, not least the imminence of life's end, signals of love and caring, esteem, concern, closeness and security—also in the nonverbal language of sexuality—are more than ever vital and directly responsible for feelings of self-respect and self-esteem, attitude to meaning of life and happiness. Accordingly, the grounds for relationships in older men and women can be the desire of not wanting to be alone, living love and companionship, caring and being cared for, with or without sexuality, living apart or together, having a long-term partnership or marriage, or affairs with different partners—all kinds of relationship modes are possible and practiced in reality [54]. Limitations are set, most of all, by the unequal ratio of women to men. Biopsychosocially based sexual medicine wants to feature the salutogenic potential of a communicative sexuality and to keep it available for a lifetime, making it necessary to also work on questions concerning sexuality during older age.

This is even more important, seeing that the subject of sexual life in the elderly undergoes stronger taboos than the demographic development and sexological facts might imply: People do not only grow older, but they are fit and healthy far longer, keeping their sexual interests and fantasies awake (but old prejudices and educational encumbrances may also remain active). Sexual functions generally age slower than other physical functions.

Basically it can be said that there is no such thing as old-age sexuality. Every individual remains a sexual being and grows old with his or her lifelong mode of sexuality, regardless of his or her sexual orientation: A person who has been living a fulfilled sexual life will want to keep it that way, for others, age could be a welcome excuse to put an end to this chapter in life as soon as possible.

Wherever possible and desired, sexual activity (within a partnership and/or autoerotic) remains a part of life into old age (empirically, at any age, coitus and masturbation are more frequent in men). There are, however, "normal" age-related changes as well as effects in the case of comorbidity: In men, sexual reaction usually gradually becomes slower and weaker.

The amount of seminal fluid and the intensity of sexual feeling decreases. Erections may be less strong and not as long lasting, the nightly and morning spontaneous erections may decrease, refractory time may be prolonged. This would make stronger and more direct stimulation necessary. Despite the gradual hormonal conversion (in contrast to women), sexual functions in men are more inclined to disturbances than in the aging women and their self-confidence is (too) closely linked to their "potency." In both genders, sexual activity has a positive influence on the functions: "Use it or lose it" was a key phrase by Masters and Johnson [27] regarding sexuality in older age.

Women experience a drastic hormonal conversion during their menopause and the end of fertility with consequences on body image (relocation of fat distribution) and questioning their self-esteem (still attractive and loved?). It may come to problems such as decrease of vaginal elasticity (perhaps irritable bladder and correlated problems during coitus), atrophy of the vaginal tissue, lack of lubrication fluid, less orgastic contractions as well as changes in skin and general sensitivity in the breast and an altogether slowing down of the sexual reaction, making a longer duration of coitus necessary. Such changes may result in hypoactive sexual desire disorders, disorders of sexual arousal, dyspareunia, and disorders of sexual orgasm. Desire, arousal and orgastic capability are influenced more by psychosocial partnership factors than by hormonal conditions. At the same time, disorders may take place in the older person of the partnership, so that sexual activity in the couple is reduced. In any case, talks with both partners and within the couple or, in the case of a single person, with this individual, to avoid misinterpretations of situations are extremely important [women tend to blame themselves, men believe not to be a good lover without full erectile function, both retreat from the partner(-ship)].

Reaching a certain age does, however, also offer new chances for an active sexual life, e.g., larger amount of freedom in life organization and a greater amount of intimacy through long years of closeness, more spontaneity due to lack of contraception or fear of pregnancy, longer coitus duration before orgasm, vitalization of the cardiovascular system, activation of the "syndyastic system" (hormone/neurotransmitter release), prevention of atrophic processes, strengthening of the immune system, general biosocial harmonization and "well-being" as a lifestyle reality.

It is more of academic interest, whether or not these statements can be objectified. According to the Masters and Johnson sentence "use it or lose it" there is some credibility

Case Report 2
A Brief Sexological Counseling with a Couple Aged 70 and 72

A vital, fit-looking couple with silver hair visits the urological outpatient department in order to have the vacuum pump explained to them. The man speaks about the loss of his potency (meaning, in fact, erection capability) 2 years before, probably in connection with his heart disease. According to the surgeon the corporacavernosa of the penis "were damaged."

Some months later, he has heart transplantation surgery and is released to go home 4 weeks later. Erection capability does not return within the following 2 years, he does, however, now and again perceive slight erections during the night time and in the mornings. Sometimes, with manual help by his wife, these would enable coitus lying on the side. Implantation of a penis prosthesis does not come into consideration due to the ongoing immune suppressive therapy.

The couple has a very positive attitude towards sexuality, is keen on a mutual sexual life, the wife as much as the husband, and both claim not to have any other problems within the partnership. They consider sexuality as a passionate form of communication, both radiating optimism and happiness. Issues concerning sexuality after heart transplantation surgery are discussed, the significance of sexual communication emphasized and on this basis the vacuum pump and its working mechanisms and capabilities are explained and demonstrated.

It is known from literature that long-term use of the device (in approx. 25 %) may have positive effects on returning erection capability and actually, a certain training effect could take place. Both partners can come to terms with the idea of utilizing the device, the wife would help "hands on," they would purchase it and report their experience by telephone.

After 8 weeks the husband calls to say that he has been using the device for 5 weeks, 15–20 min daily for training purposes and that he is quite satisfied with it. He wants to "train my penis" without involving the penis ring and explains cheerfully that the nightly and morning erections are completely restored to their previous state. During spontaneous sexuality they find the device interfering, so his wife stimulates him manually and intercourse takes place in the described manner (lying on the side) and he already has a feeling of steady improvement. His report sounds very enthusiastic and motivated, the couple is satisfied with this solution.

in that and the psychosocial effect of daily "penile training sessions" in favor of the own as well as the mutual sexuality is definitely not to be underestimated.

Integration of Somatic Therapy Options

The integration of somatic options within sexual therapy complies with the biopsychosocial character of sexual dysfunctions [55, 56]. It often makes less invasive somatic interventions necessary, but could shorten the time period of sexual therapy and improve the compliance and the prognosis of all treatment approaches. It is hardly, however, ever conducted in practice [57]. As in all therapy methods, a combined approach can come up with problems as well as chances. Involvement of somatic options may produce the following problems:

- the patient/the couple might mistake the use of a medication as an uncomplicated "rapid repair" method, which would
- paralyze the self-healing qualities of the couple and could
- reduce the motivation to tackle personal or partnership problems.

On the positive side, a combined approach

- improves effectiveness and prognosis of the treatment in many patients;
- conveys to the patient that the therapist takes his worries, often fixated on somatic causes, seriously;
- enables establishment of an initial working bond and
- in the sense of taking the patient seriously meeting him "from where he is standing" and by this means opening up an approach also to the psychosocial side of things.

Particularly in male patients, practical clinical work in sexual medicine often means having to lead the patient—who usually takes it for granted that his problem is related to physical causes—to understand the psychological burden and partnership-relevant angles and to convince him of the biopsychosocial concept of sexuality [58].

This can only succeed (or succeed much better) if the therapist is well-informed about the advantages and disadvantages of medical treatment options (which are—in the sense of the method proclaimed here—an acclaimed part of sexual therapy), discusses them with the patient signalizing readiness to try certain methods, if the examination findings suggest this and the patient agrees to go along with this approach. If the therapist succeeds in conveying to the patient that it is not about "withholding" certain somatic options such as self-injection or oral medication, but that he is trying to find out their possibilities and their limits, particularly

TABLE 7-4. Medication as a possible option in sexological treatment

Substance	Application	Mechanism of action	Symptoms which may make further medication necessary
Yohimbine	Oral	Central alpha-2 antagonist, enforces erection benefit	Erection disorder (no effect in ED with somatic correlation)
Sildenafil, vardenafil, tadalafil	Oral	Selective PDE-5-inhibitor, relaxes smooth cavernous muscle tissue by inhibiting the c-GMP-reduction	Erection disorder
	Intracavernous injection therapy (SKAT), transurethral (MUSE)	Prostanoid, leads to relaxation of smooth muscle tissue	Erection disorder
Lidocaine, Prilocaine	Local (glans penis)	Locally anesthetizing, diminishes arousal of the penis	Premature orgasm
Fluoxetine, sertraline, paroxetine, dapoxetine	Oral	Serotonine re-uptake inhibitor, stimulation of sexually attenuating central serotonine receptors	Premature orgasm
Testosterone	Oral, transcutaneous, intramuscular	Central, stimulates the T-synthesis, release and storage of proerectile neurotransmitters (oxytocin, dopamine, NO), testosterone deprivation leads to apoptosis of the smooth cavernous muscle tissue	Substantiated hypogonadism with effects on appetence and erection

SKAT intracavernous injection therapy, *MUSE* medicated urethral system for erection, *NO* nitric oxide, *T* testosterone, *ED* erectile disorder.
[Reprinted from Rösing D, Klebingat KJ, Berberich HJ, Bosinski HAG, Loewit KK, Beier KM. MEDIZIN Übersichtsarbeit-Sexualstörungen des Mannes Diagnostik und Therapie aus sexualmedizinisch-interdisziplinärer Sicht. Dtsch Arztebl. 2009;106(50):821–8. With permission from Deutsches Ärzteblatt].

with reference to the couple relationship. This way an acceptable working bond can be developed, allowing work on the psychological effects as well as the partnership problems (Table 7-4).

Outlook for the Future of (Intimate) Relationships

As far as the future of intimate relationships is concerned, we may definitely, in possession of our knowledge on the evolution of the "socially organized mammal," take for granted that the longing for attachment and relationship will be, as in the past, much stronger and more durable than the varying tides of time. Intimate relationship does, however, need caring for and, if necessary, a helping hand, because the gulf between the longing for a functioning partnership and making it work is widening, following the process of individualization having been promoted by the so-called "post-modern times" of our day and age. Alone the high geographical flexibility taken for granted concerning the place of work may put tight limitations on the taking up, cultivation and continuation of intimate partnerships.

This is where sexual medicine has its preventive task in supporting sexual health and its specific therapeutic task where it is necessary to regain sexual health. In this context, the *Syndyastic Sexual Therapy* conducts a methodical focus, which is quite different from all other sex therapy approaches: For example, Schnarch [59, 60] and also Clement [61] concentrate on the dimension of sexual desire, most likely meeting the (still undifferentiated) expectations of most patients. All this may be an appealing prospect (and promotional at that), but cannot reach the fundamental variable for the development of desire: the attachment dimension of sexuality.

Indeed, particularly Schnarch, emphasizes its particular significance, but only to—in the long run—regard it as a vehicle to enhance desire. In *Syndyastic Sexual Therapy* it is exactly the other way around: The dimension of attachment is therapeutically focused on in the first place, then differentiates the conditions and issues concerning intimacy, as does Schnarch, as well, thus creating a common basis for mutual sexually arousing experiences. This construction is all the more necessary, because for many partners desire and relationship are (at least to begin with) two different realms of experience, connecting gradually during therapy progress and—at its best—evolving into an encompassing experience of lust, when "orgastic" and "attachment" desire blend together. The widespread dualism or opposition of "sex" and "love" is radically (literally from the roots) revoked by the *Syndyastic Sexual Therapy*, thus restoring the longed for unity of "desire and attachment."

References

1. Engel GL. The need for a new medical model: a challenge for biomedicine. Science. 1977;196:129–36.
2. Beier KM, Loewit KK. Lust in Beziehung. Einführung in die Syndyastische Sexualtherapie. Heidelberg: Springer; 2004.
3. Beier KM, Bosinski HAG, Loewit KK. Sexualmedizin. 2. Aufl ed. Elsevier Urban & Fischer: München; 2005.
4. Wickler W. Sind wir Sünder? Naturgesetze der Ehe. München: Droemer; 1969.
5. Wickler W, Seibt U. Männlich, Weiblich. Der große Unterschied und seine Folgen. München: Piper; 1984.
6. Watzlawick P, Beavin JH, Jackson DD. Menschliche Kommunikation. Bern: Huber; 1969.
7. McCabe M, Althof SE, Assalian P, Chevret-Measson M, Leiblum SR, Simonelli C, et al. Psychological and interpersonal dimensions of sexual function and dysfunction. J Sex Med. 2010;7(1 pt 2):327–36.
8. Althof SE, Leiblum SR, Chevret-Measson M, Hartmann U, Levine SB, McCabe M, et al. Original research—psychology: psychological and interpersonal dimensions of sexual function and dysfunction. J Sex Med. 2005;2(6):793–800.
9. Carvalho J, Nobre P. Biopsychosocial determinants of men's sexual desire: testing an integrative model. J Sex Med. 2011;8(3):754–63.
10. Loewit KK. Die Sprache der Sexualität. Frankfurt: Fischer; 1992.
11. Kleinplatz PJ, Ménard AD. Building blocks toward optimal sexuality: constructing a conceptual model. Fam J. 2007;15:72–8.
12. World Health Organization. ICD-10: international statistical classification of diseases and health related problems. 10th Revision (ICD-10). Volume III Alphabetical Index; 1993.
13. American Psychiatric Association. Diagnostic and statistical manual of mental disorders. 5th ed. (DSM-5). Washington, DC: APA-Press; 2013.
14. Egle UT, Hoffmann SO, Steffens M. Psychosoziale Risiko- und Schutzfaktoren in Kindheit und Jugend als Prädisposition für psychische Störungen im Erwachsenenalter. Nervenarzt. 1997;68: 683–95.
15. Wesiack W. Psychosomatische Medizin in der ärztlichen Praxis. München: Urban & Schwarzenberg; 1984.
16. Vincent CE. Human sexuality in medical education and practice. Springfield: Thomas; 1964.
17. Buddeberg C. Sexualberatung. Eine Einführung für Ärzte, Psychotherapeuten und Familienberater. 3rd ed. Stuttgart: Enke; 1996.
18. Zettl S, Hartlapp J. Sexualstörungen durch Krankheit und Therapie. Ein Kompendium für die ärztliche Praxis. Berlin: Springer; 1997.
19. Fröhlich G. Psychosomatik männlicher Sexualität. Sexuologie. 1998;5(4):203–11.
20. Rösing D, Klebingat KJ, Berberich HJ, Bosinski HAG, Loewit KK, Beier KM. Sexualstörungen des Mannes Diagnostik und Therapie aus sexualmedizinisch-interdisziplinärer Sicht. Dtsch Arztebl. 2009;106(50):821–8.
21. Balint, M. Der Arzt, sein Patient und die Krankheit. Stuttgart: Klett; 1957.
22. Balint M. Forschung in der Psychotherapie. Fünf Minuten pro Patient. Suhrkamp: Frankfurt; 1975.
23. Loewit KK. Sexualmedizin und Balintarbeit. Sexuologie. 2005;12:67–70.
24. Herkommer K, Niespodziany S, Zorn C, Gschwend JE, Volkmer BG. Versorgung der erektilen Dysfunktion nach radikaler Prostatektomie in Deutschland. Urologe. 2006;45(3):336–42.
25. Rösing D, Berberich HJ. Krankheits-und behandlungsbedingte Sexualstörungen nach radikaler Prostatektomie. Der Urologe A. 2004;43(3):291–5.
26. Deneke FW. Psychische Struktur und Gehirn. Die Gestaltung subjektiver Wirklichkeiten. Stuttgart/New York: Schattauer; 1999.
27. Masters WH, Johnson VE. Human sexual response. Boston: Little, Brown & Co.; 1966.
28. Scheingold LD, Seiz-Hauser A, Wagner NN. Herz,Alter, Sexualität; medizinische Aspekte der zweiten Lebenshälfte. Wiesbaden: Verlag Medical Tribune; 1976.
29. Giesen RM, Schuhmann G. An der Front des Patriarchats. Bensheim: Päd-Extra; 1980.
30. Jahnke S, Imhoff R, Hoyer J. Stigmatization of people with pedophilia: two comparative surveys. Arch Sex Behav. 2015;44(1):21–34.
31. Beier KM, Ahlers CJ, Goecker D, Neutze J, Mundt IA, Hupp E, et al. Can pedophiles be reached for primary prevention of child sexual abuse? First results of the Berlin Prevention Project Dunkelfeld (PPD). J Forens Psychiatry Psychol. 2009;20(6):851–67.
32. Beier KM, Grundmann D, Kuhle LF, Scherner G, Konrad A, Amelung T. The German Dunkelfeld Project: a pilot study to prevent child sexual abuse and the use of child abusive images. J Sex Med. 2015;12(2):529–42.
33. Beier KM, Oezdemir UC, Schlinzig E, Groll A, Hupp E, Hellenschmidt T. Just dreaming of them: the Berlin project of primary prevention of child abuse by Juveniles (PPJ). Child Abuse Negl. 2016;52:1–10.
34. Berliner Institut für Sexualwissenschaft und Sexualmedizin. BEDIT—the Berlin dissexuality therapy program. Weimar: Gutenberg; 2013.
35. Scherner G, Konrad A, Grundmann D. Diagnostik im Präventionsprojekt Dunkelfeld. Sexuologie. 2015;22(3–4):165–74.
36. Hill A, Briken P, Kraus C, Strohm K, Berner W. Differential pharmacological treatment of paraphilias and sex offenders. Int J Offender Ther Comp Criminol. 2003;47(4):407–21.
37. Greenberg DM, Bradford JM, Curry S, O'Rourke A. A comparison of treatment of paraphilias with three serotonin reuptake inhibitors: a retrospective study. J Am Acad Psychiatry Law. 1996;24(4): 525–32.
38. Greenberg DM, Bradford JM. Treatment of the paraphilic disorders: a review of the role of the selective serotonin reuptake inhibitors. Sex Abuse. 1997;9(4):349–60.
39. Guay DR. Drug treatment of paraphilic and nonparaphilic sexual disorders. Clin Ther. 2009;31(1):1–31.
40. Thibaut F, Barra FDL, Gordon H, Cosyns P, Bradford JM. The World Federation of Societies of Biological Psychiatry (WFSBP) guidelines for the biological treatment of paraphilias. World J Biol Psychiatry. 2010;11(4):604–55.
41. Bradford JM, Pawlak A. Effects of cyproterone acetate on sexual arousal patterns of pedophiles. Arch Sex Behav. 1993;22(6): 629–41.
42. Raymond NC, Grant JE, Kim SW, Coleman E. Treatment of compulsive sexual behaviour with naltrexone and serotonin reuptake inhibitors: two case studies. Int Clin Psychopharmacol. 2002;17(4):201–5.
43. Raymond NC, Grant JE, Coleman E. Augmentation with naltrexone to treat compulsive sexual behavior: a case series. Ann Clin Psychiatry. 2010;22(1):55–62.
44. Ryback RS. Naltrexone in the treatment of adolescent sexual offenders. J Clin Psychiatry. 2004;65(7):982–6.
45. Berner W (Ed). Sexualstraftäter behandeln: mit Psychotherapie und Medikamenten. Berlin: Deutscher Ärzteverlag; 2007.
46. Beier KM, Amelung T, Pauls A. Antiandrogen therapy as part of the prevention of child sexual abuse in the "Dunkelfeld". Forens Psychiatr Psychol Kriminol. 2010;4(1):49.

47. Beier KM. Sexueller Kannibalismus. München, Jena: Elsevier, Urban & Fischer; 2007.
48. Beier KM. Comment on Pfäfflin's (2008) "good enough to eat". Arch Sex Behav. 2009;38(2):164–5.
49. Beier KM. Sexuelle Präferenzstörungen und Bindungsprobleme. Sexuologie. 2010;17(1–2):24–31.
50. Becker S, Bosinski HA, Clement U, Eicher W, Goerlich TM, Hartmann U, et al. Standards der Behandlung und Begutachtung von Transsexuellen. Sexuologie. 1997;4:130–8.
51. Becker S. Transsexualität—Geschlechtsidentitätsstörungen—Geschlechtsdysphorie. Diagnostik, Psychotherapie und Indikation zur somatischen Behandlung. HIV&More. 2012;2:26–35.
52. Coleman E, Bockting W, Botzer M, Cohen-Kettenis P, DeCuypere G, Feldman J, et al. Standards of care for the health of transsexual, transgender, and gender-nonconforming people. Version 7. Int J Transgend. 2012;13(4):165–232.
53. Zucker KJ, Lawrence AA, Kreukels BPC. Gender dysphoria in adults. Annu Rev Clin Psychol. 2016;12:217–47.
54. Zank S. Sexualität im Alter. Sexuologie. 1999;6(2):65–87.
55. Althof SE. What's new in sex therapy (CME). J Sex Med. 2010;7 (1 pt 1):5–13.
56. Meana M, Jones S. Developments and trends in sex therapy. In: Balon R, editor. Sexual dysfunction: beyond the brain-body connection. Vol 31. Basel: Adv Psychosom Med Karger; 2011, p. 57–71.
57. Berry MD, Berry PD. Contemporary treatment of sexual dysfunction: reexamining the biopsychosocial model. J Sex Med. 2013; 10(11):2627–43.
58. McCarthy BW, Fucito LM. Integrating medication, realistic expectations, and therapeutic interventions in the treatment of male sexual dysfunction. J Sex Marital Ther. 2005;31(4):319–28.
59. Schnarch DM. Constructing the sexual crucible: an integration of sexual and marital therapy. New York: WW Norton & Company; 1991.
60. Schnarch DM. Passionate marriage: love, sex, and intimacy in emotionally committed relationships. WW Norton & Company: New York; 1997.
61. Clement U. Systemische Sexualtherapie. Stuttgart: Klett-Cotta; 2004.

Part II
Sexual Dysfunctions

8 Evaluation of Male Hypoactive Sexual Desire Disorder

Demetria Pizano and Waguih William IsHak

Introduction

For as long as mankind has existed, sex has provided our species the means for our continuation. This chapter focuses on the lack of desire, the core driver of sexual activity. Hypoactive sexual desire disorder (HSDD) is the decrease, deficiency, or absence of sexual thoughts, fantasies, and desire for sexual activity; these symptoms, if severe enough, are known to cause personal distress [1]. At what point did we, as humans, stop having automatic sexual urges? How did this sexual disorder evolve? Most importantly, how could the causes be identified and addressed? Throughout this chapter, we explore the aforementioned questions to understand a relatively under-researched sexual disorder affecting men.

What Is Sexual Desire?

Sexuality is often described as the interplay of multiple factors including anatomical, physiological, psychological, development, cultural, and relational factors [2]. Sexuality is comprised of several components: gender identity, orientation, intention, desire, arousal, orgasm, and emotional satisfaction. Therefore, it is pertinent to observe and understand a person's sexual response cycle, which consists of five components: desire, arousal, plateau, orgasm, and resolution. Sexual desire is the "psychobiological energy that precedes and accompanies arousal and tends to produce sexual behavior" [3]. We will continue to explore, sexuality and how it is also connected to partner's sexuality, drive, and experiences.

Sexual desire is comprised of three components [3]: sexual drive, sexual motivation, and sexual wish. (1) Sexual drive (biological) includes the anatomical and neuroendocrinal, and other biological mechanisms. (2) Sexual motivation (psychological) includes one's mood, sexual identity, self and partner regulation, quality of relationship, and transference from past attachment. Specifically, motivation played a key role in the controversy that iniated the change of terms that once describe the disorder. The terminology change from inhibited sexual desire to hypoactive sexual desire raised questions whether patients had low levels of motivation or were truly inhibited [4]. (3) Sexual wish (cultural) includes factors external to the individual, such as societal rules of sexual expression.

The biopsychosocial influences on sexual function are balanced between sexual excitation and inhibition around a Sexual Tipping Point® hypothesized by Perelman [5] throughout the phases of the sexual response cycle including sexual desire as seen in Figure 8-1.

What Got Us Here? The History of Male HSDD

Masters and Johnson's research remains to be the most prominent and representative for patients who suffer from HSDD [6]. Prior to Masters and Johnson, Harold Leif was the first to formalize the term for low sexual desire or inhibited sexual desire (ISD) [7]. In 1980, the American Psychiatric Association (APA) included ISD in the Diagnostic and Statistical Manual of Mental Disorders (DSM) 3rd edition (DSM-III) [8]. In the 1987 DSM-III-R, ISD was replaced by two disorders: Hypoactive sexual desire disorder (HSDD) and sexual aversion disorder [9]. In 1994, in the DSM-IV, the diagnostic criteria required marked distress or interpersonal difficulty in order to make the diagnosis [10]. The DSM-IV-TR [11] published in the year 2000 did not include any changes for sexual desire disorders. However, in 2013, the DSM-5 separated male and female sexual desire disorders into male hypoactive sexual desire disorder, merged female desire and arousal disorders into female sexual interest/arousal disorder, and deleted sexual aversion disorder [12].

Epidemiology

How Common Is Male HSDD?

In 1970, researchers identified that there was an estimated 16% of males that were struggling with low sexual desire.

W.W. IsHak (ed.), *The Textbook of Clinical Sexual Medicine*, DOI 10.1007/978-3-319-52539-6_8

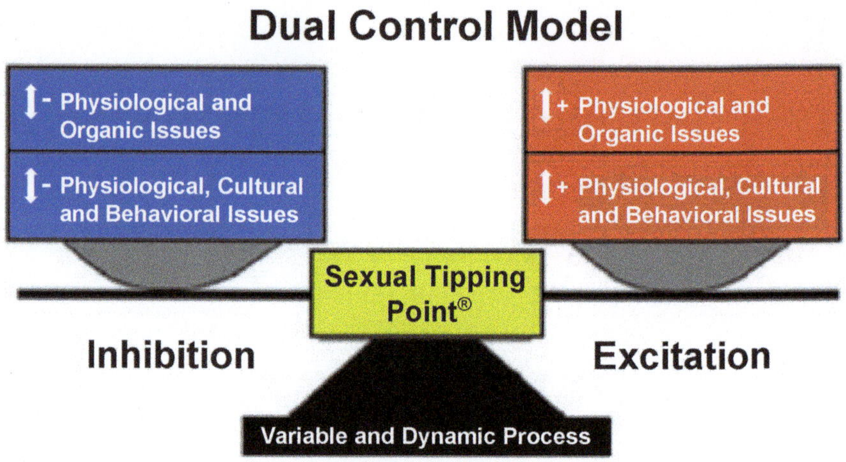

FIGURE 8-1. Perelman's sexual tipping point and the balance between sexual excitation and inhibition [Reprinted from Pfaus JG. Pathways of sexual desire. J Sex Med. 2009;6(6): 1506–33.with permission from Elsevier].

In 1980 this statistic changed slightly when the American Psychiatric Association (APA), stated that roughly 20% of the population struggled with lack of or lowered sexual desire, which included women. The National Health and Social Life Survey revealed that 15% of men experience a lack of sexual interest or desire [13]. Research shows that 1 in 4 men over the age of 70 have lower levels of bioavailable testosterone compared to their younger counterparts [14]. According to Araujo and colleagues [15] each decade after a males' 40s they will experience a successive decrease in desire. That is why ageing is the most significant risk factor [6]. In fact, age-based surveys showed that 6% of men 18–24 years as opposed to 41% of men 66–74 years experienced sexual desire problems [16]. However, Beutel, Stobel-Ritcher and Brahler [17] report that only 11% of males that have identified a loss or lack of sexual desire will contact their physician regarding this issue. HSDD's prevalence is still debated by many researchers as being an under-diagnosed disorder [2, 3, 17, 18].

Etiology

When identifying the etiology of any disease or disorder, it is essential to look at all biopsychosocial predisposing, precipitating, and perpetuating factors in order to understand the 'whole picture.' Male HSDD is caused by a number of factors that affect individuals and couples, which could be divided into biological and psychosocial factors (Figure 8-2). Medical conditions including hormonal deficiencies, relationship difficulties, and negative impact of medications, are a few examples [2]. Weeks and Gambescia [19] proposed systemic etiological model in HSDD: (1) Individual: including both biological and psychological factors, (2) Interactional: "the relationship" including couple/dyadic factors, and (3) Intergenerational: the internalized message we inherit from the families of origin [19].

Biological Factors

Biological influences include genetic, age-related, hormonal, neurological, and vascular systems, and not only general medical conditions but also their associated treatments [20]. By the ages of 40–70, males' sexual desire and frequency of fantasies decrease with age [21]; an effect that is made worse with associated medical conditions and their associated treatment. Overall, men's health is correlated with high blood pressure, enlarged prostate, anticoagulants, and medications for hypertension. Hormone levels decrease at a steady rate each year age, in addition to a decline in androgen receptors [20].

Genetic

Genetic factors are under-explored in male sexual desire. However, the dopamine D4 receptor gene (DRD4) was shown to contribute to individual differences in human sexual desire in a group of 148 nonclinical university students [22]. More studies are needed to explore the role of genetics in Male HSDD.

Ageing

Age is one of the most significant factors associated with male HSDD [6, 23]. Approximately each year there approximately a loss of 0.12 pg/ml, and total decline of testosterone concentration decreased at a steady rate of 18.5 pg/ml every year [6]. It is important to remember that the research found a strong relationship between age and bioavailable testosterone, and not concentrated testosterone. Explaining the findings that Beck [24] gained when exploring HSDD male patients and control group, unraveling that levels of testosterone were lower. However, according to a study conducted by Kimura [25] there are significant fluctuations of testosterone in men [26]. Although many researchers support the correlation between testosterone and low desire, researchers such as Feldhaus-Dahir [27] state cautiously that the correlation may

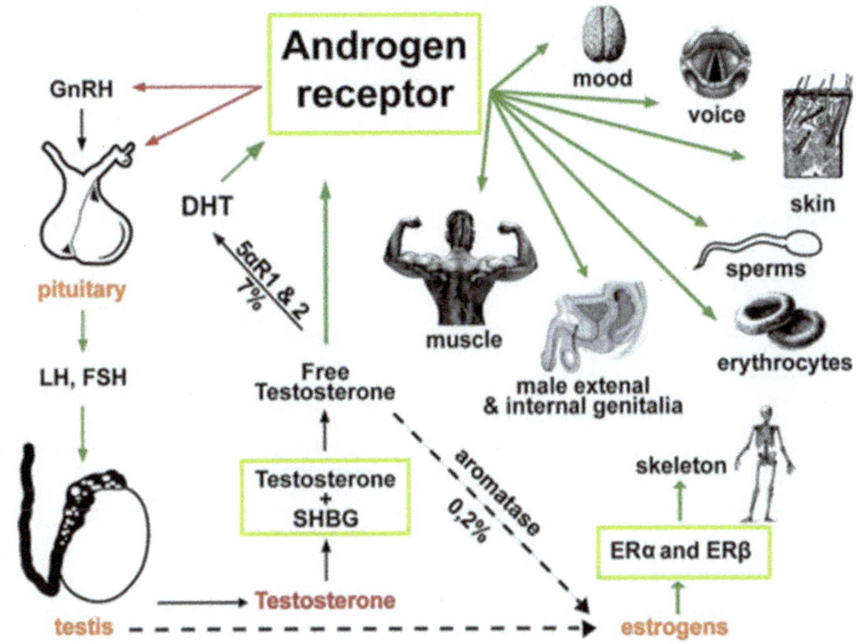

FIGURE 8-2. Conceptual model of male HSDD [Reprinted from DeRogatis L, Rose RC, Goldstein I, Werneburg B, Kempthorne-Rawson J, Sand M. Characterization of hypoactive sexual desire disorder (HSDD) in men. J Sex Med 2012; 9(3): 812–920with permission from Elsevier].

play a role, but the criticial levels beyond which clinically significant impairments of desire, are yet to be established.

Andropause is a term coined to describe the decrease of produced testosterone [28]. According to Laumann and fellow researchers [13], they found that lack of sexual interest is associated with the belief that age reduces sexual desire. Stahl [29, 30] suggested that HSDD may be a result of hyperfunction inhibition of the reward pathways, prompting exploration of treatments that block inhibitory paths, potentially disinhibiting sexual rewards, and providing a potential for improved sexual function.

Medical Conditions

Medical conditions could have a significantly negative impact on sexual desire [6]. The following are some of the common disorders associated with low desire: Anemia, cardiovascular diseases, endocrine diseases, hypertension, diabetes, mellitus, thyroid, muscular sclerosis, lupus, PCOS, HIV, traumatic brain injury potentially due to stroke, changes in sex hormones [13, 31–38]. Moreover, cardiovascular disorders constitute a major factor behind loss of sexual drive. Prostate cancer is still known to be widely associated with lowered sexual desire. Being the second most prevalent cancer in aging men, nerve-sparing operations are not efficient enough to prevent psychological side effects. Thirty-nine percent of patients with hepatitis C experience low desire, with an increase to 58% after several weeks of treatment [34]. Impairment in sexual desire function and satisfaction was present throughout treatment. Older participants had a greater decline in desire than younger participants according to a study conducted by Dove and colleagues [34].

Other researchers noted that additional symptoms or aliments that affecting sexual desire. For example, physical debilitation, bowel and bladder incontinence, and both hyperthyroid and hypothyroid functioning, are encountered more frequently than expected [39].

Sex Hormones

Sex hormones or sex steroids are secreted to the circulation at a very low concentration with specific specialized receptors concentrated heavily in the brain and the reproductive system. Sex steroids include testosterone and estrogen, and their levels constitute an important biological factor influencing sexual desire [2].

Levels of testosterone, luteinizing hormone, and prolactin should be tested as part of the clinical evaluation of male HSDD. Hypogonadism with impaired testosterone secretion is the product of testicular failure, malfunction of pituitary, or hypothalamic level [19, 28, 40]. (Figure 8-3)

Hyperprolactinemia, or the increased production of prolactin, is well known to negatively affect sexual desire [41]. Corona and colleagues [28] found that patients with moderate or severe low desire had significantly high levels of prolactin. Dopamine, in contrast, tends to promote sexual desire [2, 18, 42]. Other biological responses include responses to sexual cues that activate the hypothalamic, limbic norepinephrine, and oxytocin—leading to heightened sexual desire [43].

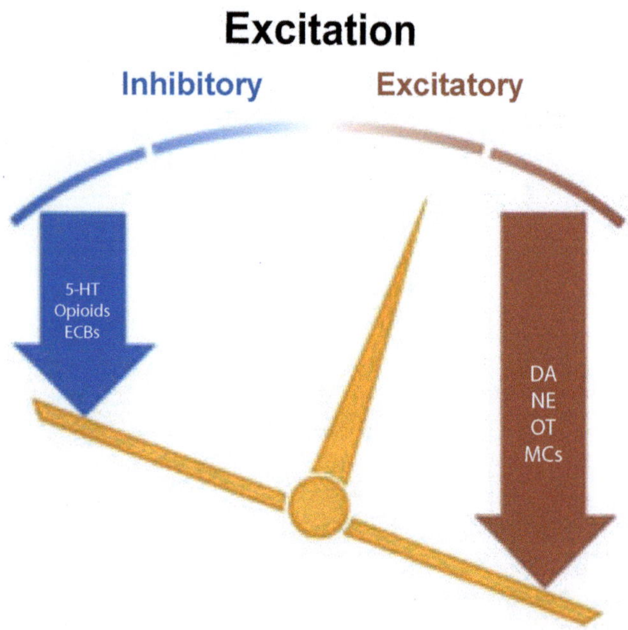

FIGURE 8-3. Testosterone formation and activity in the male. Green arrows represent stimulatory pathways, red arrows represent inhibitory ones. In target tissues, T cab be reducted to dihydrotestosterone (DHT), through two distinct 5 α reductase (5αR) isoforms, 5αR type 1 (5αR1) which is androgen-independent, and a more tightly androgen-controlled one, 5αR type 2 (5αR2). In addition, T and its precursor, delta-4 androstenedione, can be actively transformed through P450 aromatase to estrogens, which activate estrogen receptors (ERs) [Reprinted from Buvat J, Maggi M, Guay A, Torres LO. Testosterone deficiency in men: systematic review and standard operating procedures for diagnosis and treatment. J Sex Med. 2013; 10(1):245–84. with permission from Elsevier].

Medications and Substances

Selective serotonin reuptake inhibitors, SSRI, are recognized as the most commonly prescribed medications that could cause low or lack of sexual desire. Multiple medications could contribute to low desire in men as well, but more commonly are: beta-blockers, anti-androgens, and substances of abuse like alcohol, methadone [44, 45]. For example, drugs with hypotensive effects are likely to affect drive; these include adrenergic and diuretics agents. Prescriptions used for seizures, chemotherapy, heart failure, glaucoma, and excessive appetite—are all types of medications that will hinder the sexual drive as a common side effect. After depression, the most frequently affected are patients with schizophrenia, especially those on neuroleptic medication. Although not a medication, one of the most common side effects of methadone use is lack of sexual desire in many males on methadone maintenance. Researchers suggest potentially adjusting opioid maintenance to buprenorphine to normalize sexual drive. Alcohol and recreational drugs may lead to low sexual response by affecting vascular and neural functioning. Narcotics especially heroin and prescription opiates have been shown to significantly decrease sexual desire [19]. Ecstasy users experienced lower sexual desire compared to controls whereas cannabis showed no difference [46]. However, the data remains mixed about cannabis; interestingly, a 1981 review pointed that small amounts of cannabis are reported to improve sexual pleasure, whereas higher doses are linked to decreased sexual desire [47].

Psychological Factors in Male HSDD

While biological factors may take a toll on sexual desire, it is important to remember the impact that psychological components can also have. Psychological factors include not only information about sex, attitudes towards sexual expression, and previous sexual experiences, but also psychiatric disorders such as depression/treatment for depression, body image, and stressors [20].

Depression and Anxiety

Low desire is associated with depression, and their comorbid relationship remains bidirectional [15] where it is considered both a symptom and a product of depression, as also seen in other sexual dysfunctions. Seventy percent of patients with depression experience a loss of libido or sexual drive [19]. Similarly, 88% males in a clinical study were found to have depressive episodes preceding HSDD [38]. HSDD patients were found to have the highest and most significant scores on the Beck Depression Inventory in comparison to a control group and asexual subject pool [48, 49]. The more significant the depression, the lower the sexual desire [38]. Therefore, the treatment of depression is necessary for the treatment for HSDD [50]. In contrast, a study by Fabre, Clayton, Smith, Goldstein, and Derogatis [51], which showed that sexual desire was preserved and that orgasm was the most impaired sexual function in males diagnosed with major depressive disorder, and atypical depression. It should be noted, most studies since 1986, had shown the strong association of depression and low sexual desire [6, 28, 52]. Moreover, an analysis of the STAR*D study, IsHak and colleagues [53] showed that impaired sexual satisfaction was present in 64.3% of MDD patients at pretreatment, but that percentage declined to 47.1% at post-treatment with citalopram ($P < 0.0001$). More importantly, 61.3% of patients who did not achieve remission status still experienced impaired sexual satisfaction versus only 21.2% in remitters [$P < 10(-8)$].

Although depression and substance use tend to be the most highly associated psychological comorbid disorders with HSDD, there still are several others that can have a negative impact on sexual desire. Studies showed that OCD is associated with mild HSD whereas anxiety is correlated with mild to severe HSD [28, 52].

Body Image

A patient with a body image issue struggle to find themselves attractive, and therefore they find it particularly difficult to understand why anyone else would find them attractive. This feeling could contribute to low sexual desire, feeling disappointed, hopeless, and ashamed, due to their perception of their body [50]. Becoming highly self-conscious interferes with the pleasurable components of sex.

Eating disorder are associated with lack of or low sexual desire due to anxiety and performance anxiety surrounding body image and how they perceive their body appearance to their partner [6, 19]. Patients with Eating disorders tend to underrate their physical appearance, and have difficulties with feeling comfortable with their genitals and sexual activity.

Self-inflicted negative thoughts such as penis size, body size/weight, and/or a partner's negative attention may worsen self-consciousness [54, 55]. Ferrini and Barrett-Connor [33] noted the importance of a patient's age, obesity level, and nutrition on circulation levels of bioavailable sex steroids. This research revealed a statistically significant negative correlation between testosterone levels and weight, body mass index, and waist-to-hip ratio. A positive correlation has been identified between bioavailable estradiol and weight, and BMI [56].

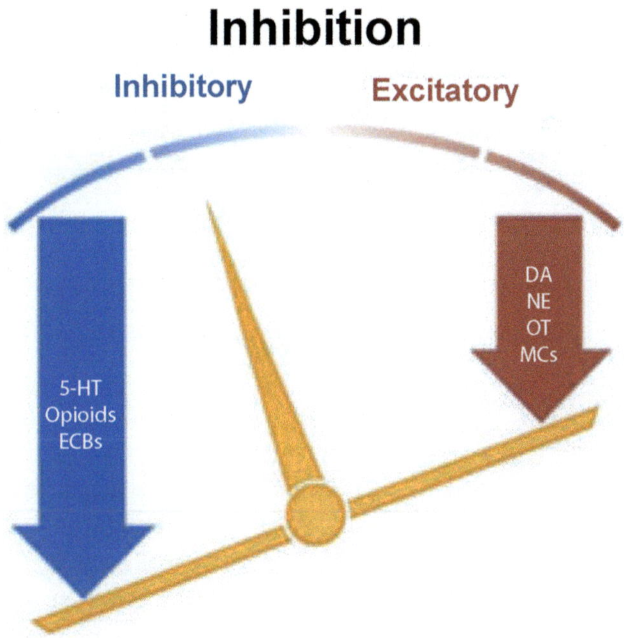

FIGURE 8-4. Excitatory mechanisms. *5-HT* serotonin, *ECB* endocannabinoid, *DA* dopamine *NE* noradrenaline, *OT* oxytocin, *MC* melanocortin, *ECBs* endocannabinoid, *MCs* melanocortins [Reprinted from Pfaus JG. Pathways of sexual desire. J Sex Med. 2009;6(6):1506–33.with permission from Elsevier].

Other Psychological Factors

Everyday stressors include work stress, relationships and marriage, financial issues, perception of poor health, and emotional problems, and they correlate with lower levels of sexual desire [12, 24, 26, 48]. Individuals in long-term partnered relationships are more likely to develop HSDD than divorced or never married [48]. This finding is supported by other studies by identifying to their older age, and long-term relationships are being associated with low sexual desire [12, 57]. Male's sexuality is influenced by cultural environment especially with negative attitudes from the patient's family of origin, e.g., strict religious household and negative stigma associated with sexual activity [20].

Pathophysiology

It was believed that the natural state of the libido is controlled and functions the same way our hunger, thirst, and sleepiness cues work [54, 55, 58], implying that sexual desire is an effortless and an unconscious act. The urge or desire for sex is all balanced by excitatory and inhibitory mechanisms (Figures 8-4 and 8-5).

As highlighted by Pfaus [59, 60], sexual excitatory mechanisms involves the activation of noradrenaline (NE) and oxytocin (OT), which stimulate dopamine (DA) and melanocortins (MCs), leading to stimulation of attention and desire, within regions of the hypothalamus and limbic system, in response to sexual cues. Brain opioid, endocannabinoid, and serotonin systems released in the cortex, limbic system, hypothalamus, and midbrain during an orgasm, dampen excitatory mechanisms at the end of the sexual response cycle and the refractory period or "sexual satiety." Stress, hypogonadism, and medications such as SSRIs or tranquilizers, could contribute to the blunting of excitatory neurochemical systems. Steroid hormones, sexual incentives, and drugs such as stimulants could contribute to the activation of excitatory mechanisms [59, 60].

Although Kaplan, like many others, after her, believed that a human's sexual drive was controlled similarly to other drives such as the urge for food, drink, and sleep—her research was the first to discuss brain neurotransmitters as mediators of the process [54]. As the field progressed, the role of the hypothalamic–pituitary–adrenal axis have on sexual desire, was delineated [24]. The role that the limbic system, preoptic area, and hypothalamus, play in having an active or lowered drive, has also been highlighted especially with signal pathways from the prefrontal cortex and serotonin or dopamine response [42]. Patients with symmetric brain damage to the amygdala or cortical, commonly seen in stroke patients tend to have hypoactive sexual behaviors. On the contrary, some stroke patients will present hyperactive desire behaviors [6]

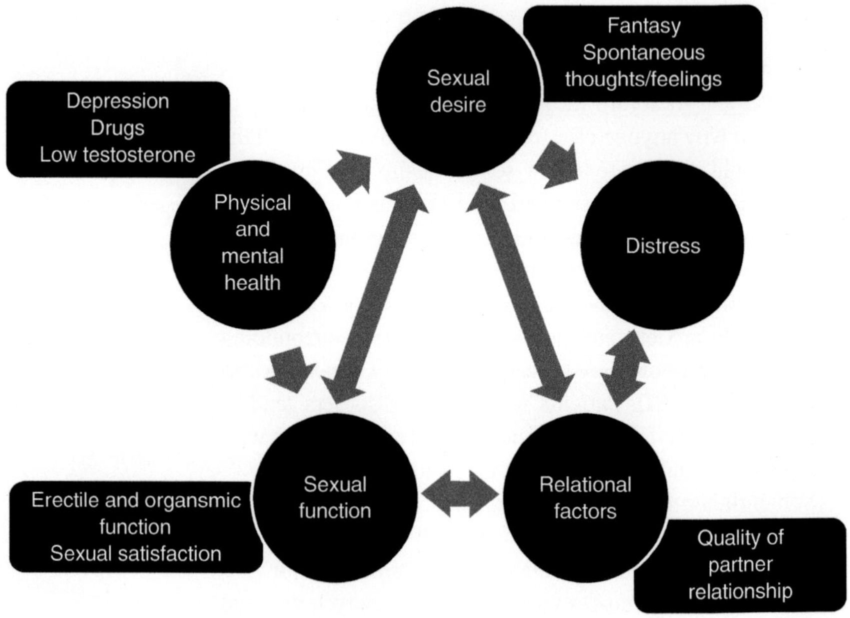

FIGURE 8-5. Inhibitory mechanisms [Reprinted from Pfaus JG. Pathways of sexual desire. J Sex Med. 2009;6(6):1506–33.with permission from Elsevier].

TABLE 8-1. DSM-5 Diagnostic Criteria for Male Hypoactive Sexual Desire Disorder 302.71 (F52.0)

A. Persistently or recurrently deficient (or absent) sexual/erotic thoughts or fantasies and desire for sexual activity. The judgment of deficiency is made by the clinician, taking into account factors that affect sexual functioning, such as age and general and sociocultural contexts of the individual's life
B. The symptoms in Criterion A have persisted for a minimum duration of approximately 6 months
C. The symptoms in Criterion A cause clinically significant distress in the individual
D. The sexual dysfunction is not better explained by a nonsexual mental disorder or as a consequence of severe relationship distress or other significant stressors and is not attributable to the effects of a substance/medication or another medical condition
Specify whether:
Lifelong: The disturbance has been present since the individual became sexually active
Acquired: The disturbance began after a period of relatively normal sexual function
Specify whether:
Generalized: Not limited to certain types of stimulation, situations, or partners
Situational: Only occurs with certain types of stimulation, situations, or partners
Specify current severity:
Mild: Evidence of mild distress over the symptoms in Criterion A
Moderate: Evidence of moderate distress over the symptoms in Criterion A
Severe: Evidence of severe or extreme distress over the symptoms in Criterion A

[Reprinted with permission from the Diagnostic and Statistical Manual of Mental Disorders, Fifth Edition, (Copyright 2013). American Psychiatric Association].

Diagnosis and DSM-5 Criteria

The Diagnostic and Statistical Manual of Mental Disorders—fifth edition (DSM-5), has described the criteria for Male HSDD as "persistently and/or recurrently deficient (or absent) sexual/erotic thoughts or fantasies and desire for sexual activity" as judged by the clinician accounting for factors that affect sexual functioning, such as age and general and sociocultural contexts. Criteria B Symptoms in Criteria A have persisted for. Some of the new additions never previously seen in the past DSM revisions include minimum duration of approximately 6 months, the presence of clinically significant distress, and that the dysfunction is not better explained by a nonsexual mental disorder or the consequence of severe relationship distress, or other significant stressors and is not attributable to these effects of substance and/or medication or another medical condition (Figure 8-4). The DSM-5 has three specifications under these new criteria: lifelong or acquired, generalized or situational, and severity (mild, moderate, severe) [12]. Lifelong is used to describe the disturbance that has been present since the individual became sexually active, whereas acquired is used to describe the disturbance that began after a period of relatively normal sexual function. Another specification is identifying if the dysfunction is generalized or situational. Generalized is defined as pervasive across the board, whereas situational is only occurring when there are certain types of stimulations, situations, or partners. Lastly, the new addition to the criteria is the specification of mild, moderate or severe/extreme distress in the individual. The DSM-IV specifier of dysfunction due to psychological or combined factors was removed from the DSM-5 [12] (see Table 8-1).

Best Practice in Evaluation of HSDD: What's the First Step?

"Sexual well-being is not a luxury but a right" [61]. Nevertheless, many patients may find the topic uncomfortable or "awkward" to bring up with their physician. Thus it our job, as physician and clinicians, to create an environment that is not only comfortable but allows our patients to feel safe about explaining their symptoms, especially low sexual desire, which is sometimes perceived as less grave than erectile dysfunction or ejaculatory problems. Maurice [32] suggests the following steps to creating a safe environment: (1) Use simple terms when speaking to the patient, and be matter of fact, in order to minimize confusion and embarrassment. (2) Start with the easier subjects, as this would allow patients to gradually open up and not feel so exposed. (3) Ask pointed questions and request clarification that will result in sufficiently specific data about the patient's symptoms. This would help avoid misinterpretations of information and potential misdiagnosis. (4) Be sensitive to the optimal time to ask more emotionally charged questions, i.e., be sensitive not to interrupt and be mindful of the appropriate times to speak. (5) Look for and respond to nonverbal cues that may signal discomfort or concern. Being aware of the patient's body language may allow to further facilitating the conversation despite discomfort. (6) Be sensitive to the impact of emotionally charged words. Some patient with HSDD may have had exposure to rape, abortions, or other sexual or emotionally abusive situations. (7) If you are not sure of the patient's sexual orientation, use gender-neutral language in referring to his or her partner in order to avoid the perception of being judgmental which could further inhibit the process. (8) Explain and justify your questions and procedures. (9) Similarly, teach and reassure as you examine. (10) Lastly, intervene to the extent that you are qualified and comfortable, this means referring patients to qualified medical or mental health specialist as necessary.

The PLISSIT model is easy and readily applicable in the evaluation of HSDD [61, 62]. It is an acronym for Permission, Limited Information, Specific Suggestion, and Intensive Therapy. Permission is about creating a judgment-free atmosphere about sex. The next step, limited information is about sexual development, and male to female gender differences in terms of genital anatomy, and the potential of sexual pleasure enhancement or functioning. Specific suggestions include simple things like techniques, activities, and being more supportive. Lastly, intensive therapy, this stage includes bringing in a skilled professional to improve sexual dysfunction.

Another important step of intervention is the referral process, i.e., could this patient with male HSDD be treated in a primary care setting, or is specialized care needed. Even if needed, some patients may be reluctant to visit a specialist or a sex therapist, even more so if they have never been to any type of mental health professional. A 'help' checklist that physicians should ask themselves prior to giving any referral, the list includes: (1) Does the patient wish for or accept referral? (2) Does patient have a treatable sexual dysfunction? (3) Has the patient been educated about their dysfunction to your fullest capabilities? (4) Has the patient tried a first-line medication or therapy, if indicated, and failed or had a negative experience? (5) Are there relationship issues involved that should be addressed? (6) Does the partner of the patient have a sexual problem that may be independent, preexisting, or secondary to the sexual problem by the primary patient? (7) Is there any diagnostic information obtained so far, including specific concerns and/or symptoms as described by the patients that can be passed forward? (8) What are the time frames of the intervention(s)? (9) Is there any result of the intervention to report, or pass forward to the specialist? (10) Are there any current medical conditions that may be considered problematic? (11) What is the list of current medications the patient is receiving? (12) Are there any important individual psychological issues that have been identified? (13) What are any relevant pieces of information obtained about the patient's relationship or problems with their partner? (14) Lastly, make sure to refer to the appropriate specialist for the sexual disorder.

It is essential to explore all evidence based approaches prior to any diagnosis, several types of tests that can be requested to reassure appropriate diagnosis is through administering surveys or hosting a semi-structured interview, a physical examination, or running blood work. If an interview if preferred, Gagnon [63] recommends having two interviews, one with the patient, and one with the partner if they have one. This allows both the patient and their partner to include information about any issues that may be occurring within the relationship. This often may lead to the patient or partner feeling as though they need to report discomforts within the relationship, which is may be beneficial in terms of assessment.

Conducting a physical examination and getting full information about medical history to identify general medical problems, is of vital importan. Potential medication side effects and medical problems might be the reasons for the onset of lower desire. Running lab test will allow a physician to examine Testosterone and DHEA-5 levels, and specifically measure the level of bioavailable testosterone that is free [64]. Examine whether testosterone levels are within the range of 300–1100 ng/dl, seeing that this is the normal critical level and can significantly impact sexually functioning [2, 6]. Important lab test to order includes: sex hormone binding globulin (SHBG), estrogen, prolactin, ferritin, follicle stimulating hormone (FSH), luteinizing hormone (LH), and thyroid stimulating hormone (TSH).

After ruling out medical and medication-related causes, it is wise to run a psychiatric evaluation to rule out any other potential disorder. Controversially, Jacobson and Gurman [50] believed that there were three reoccurring problems that would resurface in formal assessments and interviews, namely individual, interpersonal, and sociocultural patterns [38]. Individual ones include current and historical illness, surgeries, medication, alteration in psychological function, change in gender identity or sexual orientation. While interpersonal patterns look at current and historical relationships, family patterns, and sexual relationships. It's also important to look at potential intimacy, or trust problem, including conflicts over power and control and loss of physical attraction to partner [35]. Lastly, sociocultural patterns include the examination of current and historical beliefs about sex, gender, sexual orientation, and the importance of religion.

Instruments

There are several measures used by clinicians and researchers to identify and quantify HSDD. The most commonly used instruments created specifically to measure sexual desire are displayed in Table 8-2.

Translating Evaluation of HSDD to Treatment Selection

The first steps in treatment would be seeking out ways to engage the patient's willingness to partake in sexual activity and actively removing the biological and psychosocial barriers to sexual desire. Receiving hormone treatment, dietary changes, and additional rest, might be further steps towards addressing HSDD [52]. Figure 8-1 show all the elements that could be identified for the clinician to tailor a personalized plan for the patient.

In order to counter act and begin to enhance the diminished state of desire, several forms of treatment were utilized [67] who believed that individual therapy was unlikely to work due to the critical need of the couple's interaction in a treatment that addresses both partners. Most research will discuss the importance of couple and sex therapy, however, Crowe, Gillon, and Golombok is one of the few to discuss the important of relaxation training, and the positive effects it can have as an alternative treatment [24].

It is important to for therapist to understand and communicate effectively the treatment goals and how they align with the patient. It may seem obvious that there is only one goal, and that would be to increase overall desire and drive. Jacobson and

Table 8-2. Measures and instrument to measure sexual desire and sexual desire disorders

Name	Description
1. Sexual desire inventory [6] created by Spector, Carey, and Steinberg	A 14-item scale that has a total score range from 0 to 109. It can be broken down into two subscales dyadic and solitary [42]
2. Index of sexual desire by Hulbert [6]	A 25-item questionnaire focusing solely on sexual desire
3. Sexual experience scale by Frenken and Vennix	A 29-item scale where participants rate statements about own sexual behavior as true or false
4. International Index of Erectile Function [6]	IIEF contains a sub-scale for sexual desire. The IIEF was administered in more than 50 clinical trials
5. Golombok Rust's inventory of sexual satisfaction [6]	A scale that examines the level of satisfaction in a heterosexual couple. As well as looking at each partner's individual sexual function in the relationship, all examined with 11 questions
6. The sexual desire relationship distress scale	A 17-item scale that measures the distress caused by the decreased sexual desire [42]
7. Sexual history form (SHF) of the multiaxial diagnostic system for sexual dysfunction by Schover, Freidmen, Weiler, Heiman, and LoPiccolo	A 28-item questionnaire with six items most predictive of sexual desire disorders [24]
8. Male desire scale	A 35-item instrument that assesses sexual desire, sexual pleasure/satisfaction, desire distress, partner relationship, and social relationships [42]. All measured on a 5-point likert-type scale
9. Derogatis' sexual functioning inventory [65]	Measures the successfulness of individual sexual behavior, their drive, and satisfaction. Similar to establishing treatment, many of these questionnaires and scales were not produced until after 1970. In fact, it is approximately 90% that were created after this timeline [65]
10. NIH PROMIS interest in sexual activity scale [66]	A 4-item scale to measure the sexual desire subdomain, specifically measuring the "conscious awareness of wanting to engage in sexual activity". The measures which used cutting edge methodology using item-response theory were validated in a significant effort by the NIH [66] to be interpreted using a T-score where 50 is considered "normal" and SD=10 above or below the normal values

Gurman [50] offer two helpful questions that would guide the therapist or clinician in building treatment goals, those being: (1) Can sexual desire become integrated into an individual's experience and identity of himself? (2) Can sexual desire become integrated into each spouse or partner's experience of the relationship? Through the continuation of therapy, if there is ever a no to either of these questions it becomes more evident that further individual and relationship exploration must take place. To effectively treat HSDD, the clinician must evaluate if the patient has experienced significant pacification of loss of sexual desire, and their levels of distress [68]. A multiple-dynamics approach highlighted by McCabe [52], is necessary to treat includes the use and exploration of sexual fantasies, and assignments used to increase sensual awareness and sexual communication, and sensate focus exercises. The use of cognitive restructuring in CBT, and behavioral intervention are used to combat the negative feelings, and increase the sensation of sexuality, placing a particular emphasis on the quality and satisfaction of the sexual relationship and not the goal of just having sex.

References

1. Wierchx K, Elaut E, Van Hoorde B, Heylens G, De Cuypere G, Monstrey S, Weyers S, Hoebeke P, T'Sjoen G. Sexual desire in trans persons: associations with sex reassignment treatment. J Sex Med. 2014;11(1):107–18.
2. Montgomery KA. Sexual desire disorders. Psychiatry (Edgemont). 2008;5(6):50–5.
3. Levine SB. Hypoactive sexual desire disorder in men: basic types, causes, and treatment. Psychiatric Times. 2010;1:40–5.
4. Stoleru S, Redoute J, Costes N, Lavenne F, Le Bars D, Dechaud H, Forest MG, Pugeat M, Cinotti L, Pujol JF. Brain processing of visual sexual stimuli in men with hypoactive sexual desire disorder. Psychiatry Research: Neuroimaging. 2003;124(2):67–86.
5. Perelman MA. A new combination treatment for premature ejaculation: a sex therapist's perspective. J Sex Med. 2006;3:1004–12.
6. Meuleman EJH, Van Lankveld JJDM. Hypoactive sexual desire disorder: an underestimated condition in men. BJU International. 2004;95:291–6.
7. Irvine JM. Disorders of desire: sexuality and gender in modern American sexology. Philadelphia, PA: Temple University Press; 2005.
8. American Psychiatric Association. Diagnostic and statistical manual of mental disorders. 3rd ed. Arlington, VA: American Psychiatric Publishing; 1980.
9. American Psychiatric Association. Diagnostic and statistical manual of mental disorders. 3rd ed. Arlington, VA: American Psychiatric Publishing; 1987.
10. American Psychiatric Association. Diagnostic and statistical manual of mental disorders. 4th ed. Arlington, VA: American Psychiatric Publishing; 1994.
11. American Psychiatric Association. Diagnostic and statistical manual of mental disorders. 4th ed. Arlington, VA: American Psychiatric Publishing; 2000.
12. American Psychiatric Association. Diagnostic and statistical manual of mental disorders. 5th ed. Arlington, VA: American Psychiatric Publishing; 2013.
13. Laumann EO, Nicolosi A, Glasser DB, Paik A, Gingell G, Moreira E, Wang T. Sexual problems among women and men aged 40-80 y: prevalence and correlates identified in the global study of sexual attitudes and behaviors. International Journal of Impotence Research. 2004;17(1):39–57.
14. Panser LA, Rhodes T, Girman CJ, Guess HA, Chute CG, Oesterling JE, Lieber MM, Jacobsen SJ. Sexual function of men ages 40 to 79 years: the olmsted county study of urinary symptoms and health status among men. Journal of the American Geriatrics Society. 1995;43:1107–11.
15. Araujo AB, Beth MA, Mohr A, McKinlay JB. Changes in sexual function in middle-aged and older men: longitudinal data from the Massachusetts male aging study. J Am Geriatr Soc. 2002;52(9):1502–9.
16. Fugl-Meyer AR, Sjögren Fugl-Meyer K. Sexual disabilities, problems and satisfaction in 18-74 year old Swedes. Scandinavian Journal of Sexology. 1999;2:79–105.
17. Beutel ME, Stobel-Ritcher Y, Brahler E. Sexual desire and sexual activity of men and women across their lifespans: results from a representative German community survey. Journal Compilation BJU International. 2007;101:78–82.
18. Giagiari TD, Mahaffey AL, Craighead WE, Hutchinson KE. Appetitive response to sexual stimuli are attenuated in individuals with low levels of sexual desire. Archives of Sexual Behavior. 2005;34(5):547–56.
19. Weeks GR, Gambescia N. Hypoactive sexual desire: integrating sex and couple therapy. New York, NY: W.W. Norton & Company, Inc.; 2002.
20. DeLamater JG, Sill M. Sexual desire in later life. Journal of Sex Research. 2005;42(2):138–49.
21. McKinlay JB, Feldman HA. Age-related variation in sexual activity and interest in normal men: results from the Massachusetts male aging study. In: Rossi AS, editor. Sexuality across the lifecourse: proceedings of the Macarthur foundation research network on successful mid-life development, 1992. New York, NY: University of Chicago Press; 1994. p. 261–85.
22. Ben Zion IZ, Tessler R, Cohen L, Lerer E, Raz Y, Bachner-Melman R, Gritsenko I, Nemanov L, Zohar AH, Belmaker RH, Benjamin J, Ebstein RP. Polymorphisms in the dopamine D4 receptor gene (DRD4) contribute to individual differences in human sexual behavior: desire, arousal and sexual function. Mol Psychiatry. 2006 Aug;11(8):782–6.
23. Bacon CG, Mittleman MA, Kawachi I, Giovannucci E, Glasser DB, Rimm EB. Sexual function in men older than 50 years of age: Results from the health professionals follow-up study. Annals of Internal Medicine. 2003;139(3):161–8.
24. Beck JG. Hypoactive sexual desire disorder: an overview. Journal of Consulting and Clinical Psychology. 1995;63(6):919–27.
25. Kimura D. Sex, sexual orientation and sex hormones influence human cognitive function. Curr Opin Neurobiol. 1996;6(2):259–63.
26. Van Anders SM. Testosterone and sexual desire in healthy women and men. Arch Sex Behav. 2012;41(6):1471–84.
27. Feldhaus-Dahir M. The causes and prevalence of hypoactive sexual desire disorder: part I. Urologic Nursing. 2009;29(4):259.
28. Corona G, Mannucci E, Petrone L, Giommi R, Mansami R, Fei L, Forti G, Maggi M. Psycho-biological correlated of hypoactive sexual desire in patients with erectile dysfunction. International Journal of Impotence Research. 2003;16(3):275–81.
29. Stahl SM. Targeting circuits of sexual desire as a treatment strategy for hypoactive sexual desire disorder. J Clin Psychiatry. 2010;71(7):821–2.
30. Stahl SM. Circuits of sexual desire in hypoactive sexual desire disorder. J Clin Psychiatry. 2010;71(5):518–9.
31. IsHak WW. The guidebook of sexual medicine. Beverly Hills, CA: A&W Publishing Group; 2008.

32. Maurice WL. Sexual medicine in primary care. St Louis, MO: Mosby, Inc.; 1999.
33. Ferrini RL, Barrett-Connor E. Sex hormones and age: a cross-sectional study of testosterone and estradiol and their bioavailable fractions in community dwelling men. American Journal of Epidemiology. 1997;*147*(8):750–4.
34. Dove LM, Rosen RC, Ramcharran D, Wahed AS, Belle SH, Brown RS, Hoopnagle JH. Decline in male sexual desire, function, and satisfaction during and after therapy for chronic hepatitis c. Gastroenterology. 2009;137(3):873–84.
35. Rosen RC. Prevalence and risk factors of sexual dysfunction in men and women. Curr Psychiatry Rep. 2000;2(3):189–95.
36. Carvalho J, Nobre P. Biopsychosocial determinants of men's sexual desire: Testing an integrative model. J Sex Med. 2011;8(3):754–63.
37. Carvalho J, Nobre P. Gender differences in sexual desire: how do emotional and relationship factors determine sexual desire according to gender. Sexologies. 2011;20:207–11.
38. Carvalho J, Nobre P. Gender issues and sexual desire: the role of emotional and relationship variables. J Sex Med. 2010;7(7): 2469–78.
39. Carani A, Isidori AM, Granata A, Carosa E, Maggi M, Lenzi A, Jannini EA. Multicenter study on the prevalence of sexual symptoms in male hypo-and hyperthyroid patients. J Clin Endocrinol Metab. 2006;90(12):6472–9.
40. Zitmann M, Nieschlag E. Hormone substitution in male hypogonadism. Mol Cell Endocrinol. 2000;161(1–2):73–88.
41. Melmed S, Casanueva FF, Hoffman AR, Kleinberg DL, Montori VM, Schlechte JA, Wass JA. Diagnosis and treatment of hyperprolactinemia: an endocrine society clinical practice guideline. J Clin Endocrinol Metab. 2011;96(2):273–88.
42. DeRogatis L, Rose RC, Goldstein I, Werneburg B, Kempthorne-Rawson J, Sand M. Characterization of hypoactive sexual desire disorder (HSDD) in men. J Sex Med. 2012;9(3):812–920.
43. Clayton AH, Kim DH. Hypoactive sexual desire disorder: separating fact from fiction. CNS Spectrums. 2016;21(1):9–11.
44. Yee A, Loh HS, Hisham Hashim HM, Ng CG. The prevalence of sexual dysfunction among male patients on methadone and buprenorphine treatments: a meta-analysis study. J Sex Med. 2013;11(1):22–32.
45. Mintz LB, Balzer AM, Zhao X, Bush HE. Bibliotherapy for low sexual desire: evidence for effectiveness. Journal of Counseling Psychology. 2012;59(3):471–8.
46. Kumsar NA, Kumsar Ş, Dilbaz N. Sexual dysfunction in men diagnosed as substance use disorder. Andrologia. 2016. doi: 10.1111/and.12566.
47. Abel EL. Marihuana and sex: a critical survey. Drug Alcohol Depend. 1981 Aug;8(1):1–22.
48. Brotto LA, Yule MA, Gorzalka BB. Asexuality: an extreme variant of sexual desire disorder. J Sex Med. 2015;12(3):646–60.
49. Brotto LA. The DSM diagnostic criteria for hypoactive sexual desire disorder in men. J Sex Med. 2015;7(6):2015–30.
50. Jacobson NS, Gurman AS. Clinical handbook of couple therapy. New York, NY: The Guilford Press; 1995.
51. Fabre LF, Clyaton AH, Smith LC, Goldstein IM, Derogatis LR. Association of major depression with sexual dysfunction in men. J Neuropsychiatry Clin Neurosci. 2013;25(4):308–18.
52. McCabe MP. A program for the treatment of inhibited sexual desire in males. Psychotherapy. 1992;29(2):288–96.
53. IsHak WW, James DM, Mirocha J, Youssef H, Tobia G, Pi S, et al. Patient-reported functioning in major depressive disorder. Therapeutic Advances in Chronic Disease. 2016;7(3):160–9 .http://doi.org/10.1177/2040622316639769
54. Kaplan HS. Disorders of sexual desire and other new concepts and techniques in sex therapy. New York, NY: Brunner/ Mazel Publication; 1979.
55. Kaplan HS. The new sex therapy: active treatment of sexual dysfunctions. New York, NY: Brunner/Mazel Publication; 1974.
56. Bonthuis PJ, Cox KH, Rissman EF. X-chromosome dosage affects male sexual behavior. Hormones and Behavior. 2012;61(4): 565–72.
57. Regan PC, Berscheid E. Gender differences in beliefs about the causes of male and female sexual desire. Personal Relationships. 1995;2:345–58.
58. Stein E. The Mismeasure of desire: the science, theory, and ethics of sexual orientation. New York, NY: Oxford University Press; 2001.
59. Pfaus JG. Treatment of hypoactive sexual desire. Cell. 2015; 163:533.
60. Pfaus JG. Pathways of sexual desire. J Sex Med. 2009 Jun;6(6): 1506–33.
61. Plaut SM, Graziottin A, Heaton JPW. Sexual dysfunction (fast facts). UK: Health Press; 2004.
62. Annon JS. The PLISSIT model: a proposed conceptual scheme for the behavioral treatment of sexual problems. J Sex Educ Ther. 1976;2:1–15.
63. Gagnon JH. An interpretation of desire: essays in the study of sexuality. Chicago, IL: The University of Chicago Press; 2004.
64. Hoboken GB. SMIP—sexual medicine in practice: hormonal therapy for male sexual dysfunction (1). Wiley-Blackwell; 2011.
65. American Psychiatric Association. Measure of psychiatric tools. Arlington, VA: American Psychiatric Publishing; 2000.
66. Weinfurt KP, Lin L, Bruner DW, Cyranowski JM, Dombeck CB, Hahn EA, Jeffery DD, Luecht RM, Magasi S, Porter LS, Reese JB, Reeve BB, Shelby RA, Smith AW, Willse JT, Flynn KE. Development and initial validation of the PROMIS(®) sexual function and satisfaction measures version 2.0. J Sex Med. 2015 Sep;12(9):1961–74.
67. Kolody RC, Masters WH, Johnson VE. Textbook of sexual medicine. Boston, MA: Little, Brown and Company; 1979.
68. Pyke RE, Clayton AH. Psychological treatment trials for hypoactive sexual desire disorder: a sexual medicine critique and perspective. J Sex Med. 2015;12(12):2451–8.

9 Treatment of Male Hypoactive Sexual Desire Disorder

Barry McCarthy and Danielle M. Cohn

Introduction

The new mantra in sex therapy is desire/pleasure/eroticism/satisfaction [1]. Desire is the core dimension, especially for couple sexual vitality and satisfaction. When clinicians addressed desire problems, the traditional focus had been on female desire problems, namely female sexual interest/arousal disorder (FSIAD). However, a little known fact is that when couples stop being sexual, especially after age 50, it is usually the man who makes the decision. He usually does so unilaterally and conveys it nonverbally. The primary cause of male secondary hypoactive sexual desire disorder (HSDD) is loss of confidence with erection, intercourse, and orgasm. He falls into the negative cycle of anticipatory anxiety, performance-oriented intercourse, frustration, embarrassment, and ultimately avoidance. The sexual avoidance cycle becomes self-perpetuating, becoming stronger and more controlling over time. This leads to a nonsexual relationship.

The message of the media and pharmacological advertising is to turn to a biomedical intervention (e.g., Viagra, Cialis, testosterone, penile injections) as a stand-alone approach to restore male confidence. Although pro-erection medications can and do improve sexual function, they are not a "magic pill" as touted by the advertisements. The problem is that men expect a return to easy, totally predictable erections they experienced in their teens and twenties. When this is not the outcome, they feel like "Viagra failures."

The great majority of men learn sexual response as autonomous; they experience erection, intercourse, and orgasm needing nothing from their partner. Entirely predictable sex function is viewed as the measure of a man and the model for "real male sex" [2]. This model is not appropriate for males as they and their relationship age. Yet peers and the media demand perfect sex performance from men.

Over 90% of male HSDD is secondary, caused by sexual dysfunction, especially erectile dysfunction (ED) and, to a lesser extent, delayed ejaculation (DE). It is important to note that 8–10% of males experience primary HSDD [3]. Typically, the man denies primary HSDD, saying, "How can I have a desire problem when I have three children?" At the core of primary HSDD is the fact that man does not value intimate, interactive couple sexuality. That does not mean he cannot perform intercourse or have reproductive sex. The typical cause of primary HSDD is a sexual secret. Contrary to the myth that male sexual problems are caused by sexual orientation issues, the most common sexual secrets involve: (1) a variant (atypical) arousal pattern, such as fetishes, cross-dressing, BDSM scenarios; (2) he is confident with masturbatory sex (with or without porn), but is an anxious performer during couple sex; and (3) a history of sexual trauma which has not been disclosed and processed.

The male model of sex is: "A real man is ready and able to have sex with any woman, any time, in any situation." This oppressive model focuses on individual sex performance, rather than sexuality as an intimate couple experience. The core issue in treatment planning and change goals for HSDD is whether the focus is on totally predictable male individual sex performance or the goal is restoring comfort and confidence with sexuality as a couple process of giving and receiving pleasure-oriented touching using the criterion of Good Enough Sex (GES) [4]. The traditional treatment focus has been an individual, biomedical, performance-oriented approach. This chapter will advocate for a comprehensive, couple biopsychosocial model of assessment, treatment, and relapse prevention of HSDD, with a focus on the couple GES approach rather than on perfect individual sex performance. Regaining and maintaining comfort and confidence with desire, pleasure, eroticism, and satisfaction is the core strategy. As this book is primarily for a medical audience, this chapter utilizes a biopsychosocial framework. However, as psychologists we prefer the strategies and interventions embodied in the psychobiosocial model [5]. What is clear is that successful treatment involves addressing biological/

W.W. IsHak (ed.), *The Textbook of Clinical Sexual Medicine*, DOI 10.1007/978-3-319-52539-6_9

medical, psychological, and social/relational factors. A major mistake made both in the media and by clinicians is the simplistic belief in the efficacy of a stand-alone medication or medical intervention. The reality of male and couple sexuality, especially desire, is that by its nature it is variable and flexible rather than totally predictable [6]. Media advertisements and physician expectations are that the medication will return the man to totally predictable, autonomous sexual function. The message is that when the man takes a pro-erection medication he will experience a 100% predictable erection like he did in his teens. The data, which is not empirically validated, is that successful intercourse occurs in 65–85% of encounters [7]. This is a positive and realistic outcome, but it is not what the man expects. The dropout rate for pro-erection medications and other medical interventions (i.e., testosterone enhancement, penile injections, external penile pumps) is quite high, an estimate of 70% after 2 years [8]. The man is disappointed and frustrated, feels stigmatized, and avoids partner sex. Many clinicians believe that Viagra has caused more nonsexual relationships since 1998 than anything else in history [6]. This is not the drug's fault as much as it is that no one tells the man (or couple) how to integrate the medical intervention into their couple style of intimacy, pleasuring, and eroticism. In addition, the physician or clinician does not help enable the man or couple to establish positive, realistic expectations for erections and intercourse. Based on media expectations of 100% predictable erection, almost all men are "Viagra failures."

The reason that psychological and relational factors are so important in treatment of HSDD is they establish a genuine sense of male sexual self-efficacy based on GES expectations rather than on perfect performance. The relational dimension emphasizes that the essence of couple sexuality is giving and receiving pleasure-oriented touch rather than sex as an individual pass–fail test. Couple sex therapy emphasizes an anti-perfectionistic approach. Women accept GES more easily because it is compatible with female sexual socialization and her lived sexual experiences. Few women experience autonomous sexual response and do not feel pressure to be a perfect sex performer. The oppressive performance myth for men is strongly reinforced in porn videos, where the man always has a firm erection and needs nothing from the woman.

GES is much more likely to be accepted in the context of couple therapy than among male peers, with whom the man is unwilling to share sexual questions or anxieties. Male peers judge GES as "wimpy" and "not man enough," and fear that GES feminizes male sexuality. Clinically, the intervention is to say to the man and couple that "traditional men stop being sexual in their 50s or 60s, whereas 'wise men' can be sexual in their 60s, 70s, and 80s" [9]. Wise men turn toward their partner, embrace variable, flexible couple sexuality, accept GES, and value sensual, playful, and erotic sexuality in addition to intercourse. These concepts are congruent with psychological and social/relational perspectives, but stand in stark contrast with traditional male beliefs and the biomedical model of male sex performance. The comprehensive couple biopsychosocial model promotes change and guards against relapse. A key component is to affirm the mantra of desire/pleasure/eroticism/satisfaction, with an emphasis on the core role of desire. This requires the man (and couple) to give up the traditional model of male sex as totally predictable erection, intercourse, and orgasm. Autonomous sex function is the way most males learn sex response and is mistakenly believed to be "natural." Although this approach might be functional for young adult men, after age 40 and certainly for men in their 50s and 60s this self-defeating approach must be replaced by a positive, realistic model of male sexuality.

Female–male sexual equity promotes emotional and sexual relationships. Hyde [10] found that there are more similarities than differences intellectually, emotionally, behaviorally, and sexually between men and women. The traditional gender split underlies the double standard that it is the man's role to initiate sex and that sex must involve intercourse. Intercourse frequency and eroticism is the man's domain. In this gender split, women are to value intimacy, touching, and relational security. The "pop psych" approach to gender differences was illustrated by Gray's [11] best-selling book, *Men are from Mars, Women are from Venus*. Although this perspective is clearly described, it is fundamentally lacking in scientific validation. The data is clear that intellectually, emotionally, behaviorally, and sexually, there are many more sexual similarities than differences between adult men and women. This is especially true for adults over 40 and those in married and partnered relationships. Couples who adopt the female–male sexual equity model have a valuable sexual resource [12].

It is crucial to address the conceptual and clinical factors of the biopsychosocial model when trying to assess, treat, and prevent relapse of HSDD. Since secondary HSDD is so much more common than primary HSDD, this chapter addresses secondary HSDD through the use of a case study format.

Best Practice/Evidence-Based Approach to Treatment

There is a great need for empirical and clinical research to establish the best treatment approach for HSDD. However, present data and clinical guidelines suggest that a couple biopsychosocial approach is most likely to be efficacious for the man and couple. HSDD is multicausal, multidimensional, and complex; thus, "Sexually, one model never fits all."

The couple sex therapy approach is likely to be most efficacious because it addresses the core issues underlying

HSDD. Secondary HSDD, which is far more common, is typically caused by sex dysfunction, including ED as well as secondary delayed ejaculation (ejaculatory inhibition). The man has lost confidence with erection, intercourse, and orgasm and has fallen into a cycle of anticipatory anxiety, performance-oriented intercourse, frustration, embarrassment, and avoidance. The more he avoids and the more shame he feels, the more chronic and severe the HSDD.

The comprehensive couple biopsychosocial approach to HSDD enables the man and woman to explore and address the causes of the HSDD as well as to utilize all needed biomedical, psychological, and relational resources to rebuild sexual comfort and confidence. Although the man wants an easy answer and a quick sexual fix, his partner is usually aware of the complexity and variability of couple sexuality and encourages him to view intimacy and sexuality as a couple issue. The typical male learning history about desire, spontaneous erections, and totally predictable sex performance interferes with successful treatment of HSDD. The partner's active role as his intimate and erotic friend who accepts Good Enough Sex (GES) expectations is a crucial factor in successful treatment.

The couple biopsychosocial approach is just as relevant to the treatment of primary HSDD. The combination of high secrecy, high eroticism, and high shame poisons desire for couple sexuality. Usually, the woman is less judgmental of the man's sexual secret life than he is. Together, they discuss and determine whether acceptance, compartmentalization, or necessary loss is the best strategy to rekindle desire in the relationship.

The clinician (whether medical or mental health) is ideally pro-sexual and pro-relationship, but not anti-divorce. Sometimes HSDD is indicative of a fatally flawed relationship or of the lack of value the man has for couple sexuality. Ideally, the clinician would be empathic and respectful of both traditional couples and sexually nontraditional individuals and couples. Ideally, the clinician would be competent in the assessment of biomedical, psychological, and relational factors and comfortable either treating all necessary dimensions or making referrals to specialists.

The following detailed case study illustrates the couple biopsychosocial approach to assessment, treatment, and relapse prevention of HSDD.

Brian and Claudia

Fifty-four-year-old Brian and 53-year-old Claudia were referred to a couples therapist, with a subspecialty in sex therapy, by their primary care physician. Two years prior to that, Brian had complained about increasing frequency of erectile dysfunction (ED). The internist conducted an assessment of Brian's cardiovascular function and checked for diabetes and testosterone status before prescribing Viagra. He scheduled a 6-month follow-up appointment. At the follow-up, Brian reported he was very disappointed in the results of Viagra, and had stopped taking it after 2 months. He reported ED was worsening and causing marital distress. The internist made a referral to a urologist for a more extensive assessment, including an evaluation of whether penile injection therapy was appropriate. Brian attended two appointments, was given a testosterone gel to be used daily and taught to do penile self-injection of a vascular agent in the urologist's office. Brian did not speak to Claudia about penile injections. He tried this injection three times. The first two attempts resulted in intercourse, but it was not successful the third time. Brian felt quite awkward with the injection procedure and stopped using it without saying anything to Claudia. He continued to use the testosterone gel for 2 more months, but he did not tolerate the side effects of increased irritability (including Claudia's complaint about his bad temper) and sleep disturbance. Again, Brian discontinued use without speaking to Claudia or his physician.

At the next 6-month appointment, Brian was reluctant to discuss ED with the internist. Instead he expressed concern about Claudia's unhappiness with him and wondered if, at 54, it was time to put sex behind them. Claudia was also a patient of the internist. Thus, the physician was not surprised when she scheduled an appointment. The internist considered Brian and Claudia healthy people with a stable marriage and family, and not prone to mental health problems. He was reluctant to make a referral for couple therapy. However, he was convinced by Claudia's evident distress about Brian's avoidance not only of intercourse but also of any intimate touching. She worried that he no longer loved her and thought that he might be having an affair or keeping some other sexual secret. Claudia wanted to be sure the couple therapist was properly credentialed and that the therapist was pro-marriage rather than someone who promoted opening the marriage to other sex partners. The internist promised to do research on mental health referrals, which he turned over to his secretary. She researched websites for the American Association of Marriage and Family Therapy (www.therapist locator.net) and the American Association of Sex Educators, Counselors, and Therapists (www.assect.org). She found three therapists listed on both sites.

Typically, it is the woman who calls for the initial appointment. The couple therapist utilizes the four-session assessment model, whether the problem is sexual or involves general couple concerns. The four-session assessment model involves scheduling the first session as a couple, followed by sessions 2 and 3 which are individual psychological/relational/sexual histories, and the fourth session is a 90-min couple feedback session which bridges the assessment and treatment phases [13].

By conducting the first session as a couple, they receive a powerful message that intimacy and sexuality are best approached as a couple issue. Often, therapy begins with the woman alone and the man is invited to join the sessions after 6 weeks or even 6 months. In such instances, he enters therapy in the "one down" position, feeling blamed and stigmatized. Most therapy in the USA is conducted as individual therapy rather than couple therapy. The data indicate that couple therapy has a better outcome, especially much lower relapse rates [14]. One of the best predictors of divorce is a woman in individual therapy for marital problems [15]. In the four session assessment model, the man is invited as an equal partner from the beginning. The therapist does not assume that the male is the "bad guy."

Sexual problems often degenerate into a pattern of blame and counter-blame. This is especially true of desire problems and sexual avoidance. In the initial couple session, the therapist takes the stance that the "desire problem is the joint enemy." Brian felt the therapist was respectful and empathic, rather than blaming or demonizing him. Claudia also felt listened to and that the therapist was trying to help her as well as the relationship. This approach calmed Claudia's feelings of panic and distrust. The therapist asked both Brian and Claudia to sign release of information forms so he could consult with the internist. Brian signed a form so the therapist could consult with the urologist. Rather than waiting for a written report, the therapist wrote on the form that he would call next week. Clinicians (e.g., physicians, individual therapists, couple therapists, psychiatrists, ministers) are more likely to be honest and forthcoming during a phone call. Ideally, the therapist discusses the clinician's assessment and treatment summary as well as future recommendations. If possible, the therapist works in a synergistic manner with other clinicians, but at a minimum avoids an adversarial approach. The internist wanted to be able to share information. The internist indicated a willingness to prescribe medication the therapist recommended. The urologist was clearly irritated that Brian stopped penile injections and suggested he might be a candidate for a penile prosthesis.

An important question to ask in the initial couple session is whether sexuality ever had a positive role in their relationship. Brian and Claudia agreed they had begun, as do most couples, as a romantic love/passionate sex/idealized couple (i.e., limerance phase) that had lasted a little over a year [16]. Both had positive memories of the limerance phase, especially in terms of desire and frequent, satisfying sex. Brian felt that sex had been a positive factor in the relationship until the past 3–4 years. Claudia agreed that sex had been positive, but better for Brian than for her. Claudia had not resented that difference. Her female peers would joke about their husbands wanting more sex and about touching always ending in intercourse. Claudia noted that there was never just sexual play.

Claudia believed that their sexual relationship changed 7–8 years ago, at which point she felt that Brian began been rushing to intercourse as soon as he obtained an erection. Often, she was not subjectively aroused enough to enjoy intercourse. Traditionally, Claudia was orgasmic during 50% of sexual encounters, either before or during intercourse. However, that had decreased to less than 20% in the last few years. Brian had attributed that to menopause and her decreased libido, but Claudia wondered aloud for the first time whether it was caused by Brian's rush to intercourse. Brian became defensive, saying he wanted to be sure they had intercourse so that Claudia could have an orgasm. This quickly degenerated into an attack-counterattack pattern, which gave the therapist an opportunity to describe the negative impact of couple power struggles. The issue in a power struggle is not winning, but rather not losing and being labeled the "bad" partner. Sex problems bring out the worst in a couple. The therapist contrasted the good feelings that came from discussing the limerance phase with the bad feelings of whose fault it was when intercourse was not successful. These observations, particularly the fact that Claudia said that neither sex nor talking about sex had been fun in the past few years, caught Brian's attention. Instead of counterattacking, Brian agreed.

In the first session, it is crucial to explore how each spouse understands the sexual problem and what they have tried to do to address it. The therapist does not want to repeat the same mistakes. Claudia's objection was that she was not included in any discussion nor was she aware that Brian had used Viagra, injections, or testosterone. Her assumption had been that he denied problems and stonewalled. Her fear was that there was a major sexual secret, namely an affair or worse. Brian was initially offended. He had tried medical means to solve the sex problem and felt like a failure. Brian was demoralized and Claudia was confused.

Claudia was optimistic that they could renew couple intimacy, which Brian heard as a "sexual put-down." He felt she did not view him as man enough to have "real sex." Often when couples use the terms "intimacy" and "sex," they are speaking different languages. The therapist reflected that they were speaking like Democrats and Republicans, using adversarial language and misunderstanding each other. He encouraged them to talk normally to each other, instructing them to "speak English to each other about intimacy and sexuality." These are not adversarial terms or concepts. Intimacy refers to emotional and sexual experiences of warmth, closeness, attachment, affection, sensual touch, security, and predictability. Sexuality includes intercourse and orgasm, but is much more than that. Sexuality involves sensual, playful, and erotic touch in addition to intercourse. Eroticism involves unpredictable sexual scenarios and techniques, intense emotions and sensations, mystery and creativity, and uninhibited sexuality. Intimacy and eroticism are crucial parts of sexuality for the man, woman and the couple. Both the man and woman can value intimacy and sexuality. They do not need to fall into the traditional gender split in which men value eroticism and women value intimacy. A core issue throughout therapy is integrating intimacy and eroticism to develop a couple sexual style which reinforces strong, resilient sexual desire [17]. Ideally, Brian and Claudia would accept the female–male sexual equity model to replace Brian's traditional approach to intercourse.

An important question to ask in the initial couple session is: "Are each of you committed to a satisfying, secure, and sexual marriage?" It's important to directly assess this rather than assume it is true. This was a particularly sensitive issue for Brian and Claudia. Although both wanted these elements in their marriage, Claudia was quite concerned with satisfaction and sexuality. Brian was sexually demoralized and felt ready to give up on the sexual relationship; however, he also wanted marital stability and family and was concerned with pleasing Claudia, wanting her to feel loved and satisfied. The answers to that open-ended question were surprising to each spouse. Brian learned that the core issue for Claudia was not intercourse and orgasm, but rather touching as well as reassurance that he did not have a secret sexual life. Claudia was pleased to learn that Brian still loved her and valued their marriage, but was shocked at how sexually demoralized he was. Speaking the same language about intimacy and sexuality was enlightening for both, but especially Claudia. She was motivated to address issues as a couple. Brian was feeling pessimistic sexually, but better about having Claudia as his intimate ally.

A helpful therapeutic intervention was their reading material between sessions. The therapist never sells clients a book nor asks them to read a whole book, but rather assigns a short reading. In this case, the therapist gave them Chap. 2, "Whose Problem is It? His, Hers or Ours?" from *Rekindling Desire* [17]. Reading the chapter separately, marking up personally relevant sections, and then discussing it at home and in therapy were surprisingly valuable, especially for Brian. It clarified Claudia's role as an emotional supporter and erotic ally in addressing HSDD and ED. Brian learned that he had to be responsible for his sexuality. He liked the concept that he deserved sexual pleasure. It also introduced Brian to the value of sexual knowledge, especially regarding ED. In Brian's individual history session, the therapist told him that no man reacts as positively to Viagra as in television advertisements. Based on the media criterion, all men were "Viagra failures." This awareness was invaluable in destigmatizing ED and set the stage for Brian and Claudia to read a section of an ED book during therapy [18]. Reading does not cure ED or HSDD; however, it does normalize the problem and creates positive, realistic expectations for change.

The first individual psychological/relational/sexual history was scheduled with Brian. The therapist began by saying, "I want to understand your psychological, relational, and sexual strengths and vulnerabilities both before you met Claudia and since she has been in your life. I want you to be as honest and forthcoming as possible. At the end, I will ask you to identify anything you do not want shared with her. I will not share it without your permission, but I would like to know everything I can in order to help you resolve these problems."

Typically, the history is conducted using a chronological format, moving from less anxiety-provoking topics to more challenging ones. Open-ended questions are superior to yes-no questions, as the latter make it easy to deny and just say no. Open-ended questions give the therapist the opportunity to explore positives and problems.

It is imperative to find out about educational background generally, and sex education specifically. Following this, open-ended questions about religious background, and specifically religious sex education, are useful. The question about family background and his parents as a marital and sexual model was particularly revealing for Brian. He loved and appreciated them as parents and grandparents, but never thought of them as a marital or sexual model. Brian, like many men, had low expectations of marriage and marital sex. He enjoyed being married to Claudia and having sex, but he had emphasized intercourse frequency rather than satisfying couple sexuality. In later sessions, the issue of parenting was discussed. Brian had been a dutiful father to their son (now 26), but not been emotionally attentive in his parenting. Brian felt badly that the son was much closer to Claudia than he.

In reviewing his psychological and sexual development, Brian labeled it "normal" and gave it little thought. However, with gentle probing, Brian identified the fear that his penis was smaller than average (a fear shared by the majority of males). He also recognized his hatred of being bullied, and believed he had received the message that he was deficit as a male. Brian left home at age 18 for college. When asked what his best psychological, relational, or sexual learning had been before leaving home, Brian answered with no hesitation that being accepted at a prestigious college had reinforced his self-esteem. The therapist then asked, "What was the most confusing, guilt-inducing, negative, or traumatic experience before leaving home?" Brian was very hesitant and embarrassed before admitting to his belief that he was a compulsive masturbator who had a strange pattern of rubbing his genitals against the bed rather than use direct penile stimulation. Brian worried that this might be a cause of his ED. It was clear that Brian, like most men, was not sexually well educated. He was reluctant to ask questions or to read scientifically validated books or articles about sexuality.

In college, Brian did well academically and was sexually active, but not in the context of increased comfort and confidence. Almost all of his sexual encounters involved alcohol. Like most young males, he began as a premature ejaculator, but with experience gained ejaculatory control. Brian had a difficult time identifying his best sexual experiences during college. Without giving it much thought, Brian assumed he would eventually marry and have a family.

At age 24, Brian met Claudia, and they married 2 years later. Claudia was a college graduate and he found her an attractive, engaging partner. Brian was glad he had married Claudia, and felt they were a loving couple. He viewed intimacy and family planning as her domain. Their peer group was getting engaged and beginning to marry, and Brian was swept up in the momentum.

Although he joked about it, he was very concerned about his bachelor party experience. His friends hired two strippers, who took him into a private room and took turns fellating him. In previous experiences with girlfriends and with Claudia, Brian had always functioned autonomously; he had a spontaneous erection, intercourse with his first erection, and was easily orgasmic. Brian had not been sexually self-conscious. However, this stag party experience ended his autonomous sexual function. Brian had a difficult time maintaining his erection, although he did ejaculate easily. Afterwards, he bragged to his friends how good he had been sexually and that the women offered to pay him. However, he felt embarrassed by his performance anxieties and the autonomous sexual function pattern was broken.

Brian felt best about sex with Claudia before marriage. The romantic love/passionate sex/idealization experience (limerance phase) was the sexual highlight of his life. They were sexual almost every time they were together, and every sexual experience flowed to intercourse and orgasm. Although he recalled the sex as loving and passionate, his focus was on intercourse frequency. Both remembered the limerance phase with positive feelings.

As Brian and Claudia settled into married life with two jobs and household tasks, sex frequency decreased; however, sex function, especially for Brian, was still predictable. Their son was planned and wanted, but the pregnancy signaled a dramatic change sexually. There was almost no sex during the last trimester and for 8 weeks after the birth. Since Brian defined sex as intercourse, other than affectionate touch there was no sexuality. For both Brian and Claudia, the return to intercourse after their son was born was awkward. Claudia was sleep-deprived and much less sexually responsive. Brian was irritated and pushed for more frequent intercourse. They no longer felt they were on the same sexual team.

For the next 20 years, their sexual relationship was functional, especially for Brian. However, it was not special or energizing. They fell into the traditional male–female power struggle of "intercourse or nothing." Claudia built resentment about Brian's focus on intercourse frequency. Brian felt Claudia was no longer his sexual friend, but rather that she had power as the sexual gatekeeper.

Brian first experienced intermittent ED in his mid-40s. Like most males, rather than accept variable sexuality as normal and not become anxious, Brian overreacted. This made the ED worse by rushing to intercourse as soon as he became erect. That common self-defeating reaction had two negative impacts. First, it reinforced the cycle of anticipatory anxiety, performance-oriented intercourse, and frustration and embarrassment. Second, it subverted Claudia's sexual desire and response. She was neither subjectively nor objectively aroused; as a result, intercourse was less pleasurable, and her desire decreased over time. Claudia's orgasmic response decreased from 80% during the limerance phase, to 40% during the adult years, and then to less than 15% during the erectile anxiety phase. Claudia felt that Brian was a less involved partner and negated her role as his sexual friend. Brian was largely unaware of this pattern, and complained about Claudia's lack of sexual desire and enthusiasm.

The most difficult section of the history was the exploration of Brian's attempts to use medical interventions to resolve the ED. Brian thought of ED as an individual performance problem and did not mention sexual desire until the therapist asked him directly. Brian attributed his low desire and sexual avoidance to ED. He stated, "How can I enjoy sex when I fail most of the time?" When asked how often he was orgasmic each month, Brian looked very embarrassed. He initially said less than once a month; however, when the therapist defined being orgasmic as involving any means (i.e., masturbation, intercourse, manual or oral stimulation, with another partner, with the use of Internet material), Brian admitted he was orgasmic 8–10 times a month. It was not true that Brian lacked sexual desire or was incapable of an orgasm; rather, he had desire and valued orgasm, but avoided couple sexuality because he feared intercourse failure. The crucial question when assessing for the presence of HSDD is whether it is generalized or specific to couple sex. Rather than feeling bad or embarrassed, the therapist assured Brian that masturbating to orgasm was normal and a good prognostic indicator.

Like the majority of men, Brian had masturbated throughout their marriage. For the last few years, Brian had been much more confident with masturbation than with couple sex. When asked about his self-efficacy with erections during masturbation, Brian reported firm erections the great majority of time. Neither the internist nor urologist had asked whether he experienced erections and in what context. Equally important was to explore his use of erotic fantasies and materials during masturbation. Like many males, Brian regularly used online porn while masturbating. The key dimensions when assessing porn use are: is it narrow and controlling, or diverse and a facilitator of erotic flow. Although many women label use of porn during masturbation as "porn addiction," this is usually a misnomer to punish and shame the man. Of men who use porn, 85% utilize porn in a manner that is not harmful to him or his relationship [19]. This was the case with Brian. His masturbation and porn use illustrated his confidence with masturbation and eroticism as well as his lack of confidence with erection and intercourse during couple sex.

Brian had not shared his concerns about erection with Claudia, nor had he spoken with her about his need for manual and oral stimulation to increase his subjective and objective arousal. For Brian, the only criterion was objective arousal (i.e., an erection sufficient for intercourse). Brian was unaware of the concept of subjective arousal, and was therefore surprised when the therapist focused on the importance of increasing subjective arousal as a key resource in rebuilding comfort and confidence with erections. Brian sensed becoming "turned-on" when he masturbated, but in couple sex, his sole focus was on whether he was erect enough to attempt intromission.

When the internist prescribed Viagra, Brian was very optimistic that this would resolve his ED. Brian had told neither Claudia nor the internist that he had purchased a cheap Viagra brand from the Internet; when it did not provide dramatic results, he quickly stopped using it. Brian was confident that the prescription Viagra would provide the dramatic results shown on the TV ads, and was therefore bitterly disappointed when that did not occur. He did not contact the internist; rather, he just gave up and stopped taking it. All of this was unknown to Claudia.

The referral to the urologist was more problematic. Brian did not trust medical specialists and did not feel at ease with the urologist, whom Brian described as detached and uninterested. The urologist used the analogy of male "plumbing" and stated that he treated ED as a plumbing problem. Brian did not understand the reason for penile injections. Brian did not experience any technical problems with the injection and did experience a firm erection. There was no guidance from the urologist about how to integrate the injections into their couple sexuality.

Brian was more comfortable using the testosterone gel. The idea of being "more of a man" appealed to him. Again, Brian was not encouraged to discuss testosterone enhancement with Claudia. In fact, Brian had no desire to share anything sexually with Claudia.

Brian utilized the injection in the bathroom, and he moved to intercourse immediately upon meeting Claudia in the bedroom. Brian was pleased because intercourse was very easy with the injection-induced firmness; however, Claudia was not lubricated and seemed uncomfortable. Brian did not understand why it was difficult for him to reach orgasm, although he eventually succeeded. What caused him to feel awkward and self-conscious is that his erection did not dissipate after orgasm. Although he could sense that Claudia was puzzled, he chose to say nothing and turned away. He had no answers and wanted no questions. The third time he used the penile injection, he was unable to reach orgasm even though he tried as hard as he knew how. His frustration was evident to Claudia, especially since his erection did not decrease even when he felt turned-off. This time Claudia asked Brian what was wrong, and he left the bedroom out of desperation. This was a thoroughly negative experience for both of them.

Brian continued to use the testosterone gel even after he gave up on penile injections. He wondered if testosterone alone would enhance erectile response. Although he felt better with the testosterone, his irritability and sexual frustration increased. It was Claudia's complaints about his irritability and anger that caused him to stop using testosterone gel. Internally, Brian blamed Claudia for the testosterone failure.

The therapist asked, "What do you make of the lack of success with Viagra, testosterone, and penile injections?" Brian was quite agitated and responded, "I'm a sexual failure and there's nothing that can help me." He asked the therapist, "Will Claudia still love me even though we don't have sex?" The therapist said he needed to hear Claudia's psychological/relational/sexual history, but wanted to know whether it was in Brian's perceived best interest to focus on masturbatory sex and ignore intimacy, touching, and sexuality with Claudia. It was clear that Brain had not thought of his approach to Claudia and sexuality in that way. Brian was sensitive to feeling blamed; thus, the therapist was empathic and respectful while challenging Brian's secrecy and narrow approach to sex. Brian needed to share information and perspectives with Claudia and explore healthy alternatives for him, her, and their relationship. Brian felt sexually at fault and stigmatized rather than positively motivated.

Even though the history is done in a chronological, comprehensive manner, asking open-ended wrap-up questions is strongly recommended. Typically, the therapist attempts to complete the history in one 55-min session. Some clinicians recommend a 90-min history session. Some clients require three sessions and others are finished in 30 min.

The first wrap-up question is either, "What else should I know about you psychologically, relationally, or sexually?" or "What do you not want me to know that I should know?" Often, the client discloses an important sensitive issue in response to one of these questions. Brian said he wanted the therapist to understand how much he loved Claudia and that he did not want a separation or divorce. A second question is, "As you think about your entire life, what was the most confusing, negative, guilt-inducing, or traumatic thing that has ever happened to you?" Contrary to clinical lore, the majority of clients with a history of child sex abuse, incest, or rape report the most negative thing as what is happening at the present. This was true of Brian, who had always thought of himself as pro-sexual; however, sex was now a source of stigma and depressive feelings of failure. A third question is, "Is there anything you have told me that you do not want shared with your spouse?" Brian had a number of sensitive/secret issues: (1) his belief that he had a small penis; (2) his frequency of masturbation and use of porn to masturbate; (3)

his use of Viagra, testosterone, and penile injections; (4) his fear that Claudia would leave him: (5) his avoidance of couple sex because of ED. Approximately 80% of clients with sexual problems have sensitive/secret material. The therapist then asks, "What is the positive reason for keeping this secret?" Almost never is there a positive motivation. Secrecy is driven by guilt, embarrassment, or fear of the partner's reaction. The therapist encourages the client to disclose sensitive/secret material in over 90% of cases and is given permission to do so in over 85% of cases. Unless there is an issue of potential suicide, homicide, or sexual abuse, the therapist does not disclose information without permission. In the great majority of cases, the sensitive/secret material is an integral component of the client's psychological/relational/sexual narrative. Brian was reluctant to give permission, but the therapist made two cogent points. First, too much of Brian's approach to sexuality was controlled by secrecy and shame. Second, these materials were integral to his genuine sexual narrative. Brian realized the therapist did not have an agenda to blame or shame him, and gave permission to share all five secrets.

The final wrap-up question is: "I've been asking you questions for 55 min; is there anything you want to ask me?" The most common question is, "Are we the worst couple you have ever seen?" Reassurance that this is not true is helpful. Brian asked, "If there is no way you can help us, will you tell us that?" The therapist's answer was well received by Brian: "I need to speak with Claudia and the two physicians you have consulted, but if I am not able to help, I will tell you that at the couple feedback session. I do not want to take your time and money if it is not helpful to you."

Brian left the session feeling that it had been worthwhile. He processed more information about himself and sexuality than ever in his 54 years. Brian felt understood and respected. The therapist had given him a number of things to think about, especially regarding sexual desire and erections during masturbation.

The psychological/relational/sexual history with Claudia followed the same format. The most striking issue was how different Claudia's narrative was in regard to both her sexual desire and her understanding of ED. Claudia wanted to stay married, but was very confused about what was happening sexually and was very suspicious about Brian's sexual agenda. She agreed with Brian that their best sex was during the limerance phase. She enjoyed intercourse, but felt Brian did not support her arousal and orgasm pattern even before the ED. Ever since his erectile anxiety began, he ignored her sexual feelings entirely. She always viewed him as very sexually interested, and thought it strange that he now avoided sex. When asked, "In a typical month, how often will you be orgasmic?" Claudia was embarrassed to report that she masturbated 1–3 times a month. She did not use porn, but she did enjoy erotic fantasies that consisted of other men, group sex, and a man from work on whom she had a "crush," though she did not intend to act upon it. When asked whether she thought that Brian masturbated, Claudia responded that she hoped so. Claudia very much wanted to resume touching and sexuality with Brian. It was she who raised the issue of erotic, non-intercourse sexuality. In the past, she had manually and orally stimulated Brian. He had done traditional "foreplay" with manual stimulation to get her ready for intercourse. She enjoyed being touched, but not the focused genital stimulation and did not agree with Brian's belief that intercourse was the only real type of sex. When asked whether she was always passive during foreplay, Claudia responded, "That's the way Brian likes it." When asked, "What would be your requests to improve couple sexuality?" Claudia felt overwhelmed. It was easier for her to say what she did not want than what she wanted. She did want Brian to stop avoiding touching, she wanted to be reassured he did not have a secret sex life or affair, and she wanted to stop feeling old and sexless. The therapist affirmed she had a right to get the "poisons" out of their relationship, but continued to gently prod her about what she positively wanted. Claudia had truly lost her "sexual voice." She spoke vaguely about wanting more intimacy.

In terms of sensitive/secret material, Claudia wanted to "red flag" the following: (1) her masturbation, (2) her erotic fantasies, (3) her "crush," and (4) the fact that she had been successfully treated for Chlamydia prior to meeting Brian. Her guilt and embarrassment were unnecessary. She was urged to process these issues with Brian at the couple feedback session. Claudia reluctantly agreed to share these issues in the next session.

The 90-min couple feedback session is a crucial component of this couple sex therapy model. The session bridges the assessment and treatment phases. There are three components: (1) create a new and genuine narrative for each spouse with psychological/relational/sexual strengths and vulnerabilities, (2) devise a therapeutic agreement around sexual goals as well as a therapeutic contract, and (3) assign the first psychosexual skill exercise to be done at home, ideally 2–4 times between therapy sessions.

The individual narrative typically takes 20–25 min per person and begins with the less motivated spouse. In this case, we began with Claudia because of the message to Brian that she would have a positive, integral role in the change process so that he would not feel as though all the pressure was on him. This was quite motivating for Claudia, who wanted an active therapeutic role.

The therapist moved his chair so that he was looking directly at Claudia while Brian attentively listened to the new narrative. With most clients, about a third of the narrative is new; with Brian it was over 60%. We began by describing Claudia's genuine strengths, including her intentionality. She wanted a satisfying, secure, and sexual marriage with Brian.

Another strength was that she valued sexuality, as demonstrated by her masturbation and erotic fantasies. She respected and loved Brian and had special memories of the limerance phase. She had enjoyed their sexual relationship before the ED. Claudia was motivated to understand the ED and avoidance, and wanted to be Brian's intimate and erotic ally. In addition, Claudia had genuine vulnerabilities. Her major vulnerability was confusion about the sexual avoidance. She had the mistaken fear that Brian had a hidden sexual life, which made her distrustful and vigilant. Like Brian, Claudia had a very difficult time discussing sexual issues and was ashamed of masturbation, erotic fantasies, and her history of an STI. She had difficulty seeing ways in which these illustrated her courage and resilience; rather, they had served as a source of shame. Claudia had not focused on the challenge of regaining her sexual voice, which would be good for her and their relationship. Another vulnerability was that Claudia had allowed Brian's definition of sex as intercourse to control their sexual relationship. She did not understand his ED; rather, she viewed it as a rejection of her. Finally, neither Claudia nor Brian focused on desire, which was their core issue (as it is for most middle-years couples).

The therapist checked in with Claudia to determine whether this was her narrative. Claudia said that she had not previously thought of herself in this comprehensive manner with strengths and vulnerabilities. She felt that the therapist understood her and her approach to sexuality better than she had. The narrative was not just new to Brian, but also to Claudia. She now felt more optimistic that she could become Brian's ally in building a new couple sexual style.

The therapist turned to Brian and said, "Much of this is new to you. What facts and perceptions do you need to clarify?" This is much superior to the traditional, "How do you feel about this?" The therapist emphasized moderate emotion and processing of the new material. Although clinicians fear a major emotional drama (i.e., a "Jerry Springer" reaction), the greater danger is that the spouse will deny or minimize the new information. It is important that the couple "speak English" to each other about psychological, relational, and sexual strengths and vulnerabilities. Secrecy and avoidance had been very costly for both Claudia and Brian.

Brian's individual narrative acknowledged his very real strengths as a person, spouse, and sexual man, especially his commitment to Claudia and their marriage. The therapist noted Brian's courage to seek help and acknowledged that he had a right to be disappointed in the bio-medical approach that had previously been used, which stood in contrast to the present couple comprehensive biopsychosocial approach to assessment and treatment. Brian needed to feel understood and validated rather than blamed. His masturbation with erections was an excellent prognostic sign. This demonstrated that he felt genuine sexual desire. The therapist said, "You have a right to choose to be non-sexual, but it is not a wise decision for either you or Claudia. What is your positive motivation for being non-sexual?" Brian's motivation was negative; specifically, it was to avoid feeling like a failure as a man and lover. His emotions were frustration, embarrassment, and shame. Brian's dilemma was now clear to Claudia. She did not want him to feel badly about himself sexually, nor did she want to be his "caretaker" and pretend that she did not want to feel desire and desirable. Talking about sexual issues was challenging for Brian and Claudia. The therapist congratulated them on trying to understand and reach out to each other. He reinforced the concept of needing to take personal responsibility for sex, and that the essence of sexuality is ultimately that it is a team activity. This was particularly helpful for Claudia, who needed to redefine sexual touching for herself and to share these new understandings and experiences with Brian.

In terms of a therapeutic contract, the therapist recommended a 6-month "good faith" effort to build a healthy marriage with vital marital sexuality. In his clinical experience, three of four couples like Brian and Claudia were able to reach these goals. It would take a great deal of work on Brian's part, Claudia's part, and the therapist's part; however, he was optimistic that they could develop a satisfying couple sexuality. This would be reevaluated after 6 months; they agreed to remain focused on this goal during the 6 months. If Brian decided to be nonsexual, he could make that decision later. However, for this 6-months period, he committed to trying a new approach to desire, pleasure, eroticism, and satisfaction.

The third component in the couple feedback session was the assignment of the first psychosexual skill exercise. When clinicians consider sex therapy, they assume it centers on the sensate focus exercise with a prohibition on intercourse. Sensate focus is a very valuable strategy for anxious and poorly skilled couples. However, it is not the optimal strategy for desire problems. The desire psychosexual skill exercises of comfort, attraction, trust, and create your preferred scenario is the optimal strategy [9]. Rather than focus on ED, Brian and Claudia focused on rebuilding touch and sexual desire. The therapeutic narrative was that avoidance was the joint enemy and that touch was the optimal way to rekindle desire.

They began with the comfort exercise. Claudia was asked to take the first initiative by setting up a sexual date involving comfort with pleasure-oriented touching. In this psychosexual skill exercise, they explored mutual touching versus taking turns; touching nude versus clothed; touching in the bedroom versus touching in other rooms; being silent versus talking while touching; and experimenting with sensual and playful touch. Although intercourse was not expected, there was not a prohibition on intercourse. Desire exercises involve an anti-avoidance approach to touching and sexuality. Rather than depending on spontaneous desire with a focus on intercourse and orgasm, the focus is on non-demand pleasuring. Desire is responsive to touch and emotional connection. The essence of couple sexuality is giving and receiving pleasure-oriented touch.

Each spouse has a chance to initiate. Initiation can be compared to a ping-pong game in which each person gets a "ping." The hope is that they will have at least two pleasuring experiences a week; ideally, they will have four (daily exercises is too much pressure). Not surprisingly, Claudia was more enthusiastic than Brian. She looked forward to reestablishing an intimate touching relationship. Brian was unsure of what to do and what was expected of him. The therapist asked Brian if he would be more comfortable with a prohibition on intercourse to reduce performance anxiety. To the therapist's surprise, Brian said no. Claudia said she was looking forward to enjoying comfortable sensual and sexual touch without intercourse.

At the end of the couple feedback session, the therapist commented that they must feel a bit overwhelmed with these new personal narratives and sexual suggestions. He appreciated their willingness to engage with the exploration and change process. He encouraged them to call if questions or concerns arose during the week, rather than wait for the next therapy session. The therapist expected a call from one or both and was surprised that this did not occur.

The next couple session began with the therapist asking what the most positive experience had been during that week. Claudia said it was their most intimate week in years. She felt closer to Brian emotionally and physically. She noted he was more turned-on and erect, but she was also glad they had not tried to have intercourse. Brian's reaction was more muted, but when asked his most positive experience, he said it was receiving a chest massage from Claudia. Her touch felt good, and he did not feel awkward. They had discussed subjective arousal as being rated on a ten-point scale. Brian said for him it was a 3–4, which pleased Claudia. She had initiated twice and Brian once. The therapist asked Brain whether Brian was more comfortable initiating or having Claudia initiate. Brian said it was much better for him if she initiated. That surprised her, but she agreed that for the rest of the month she would do the "ping" for their sexual dates. This gave Brian the clarity he needed.

The focus of the next psychosexual skill exercise was to find the trust position that allowed them to feel secure and connected. Half of the therapy occurs in the privacy of their home. The trust position exercise was a major breakthrough for Brian's sexual self-esteem. Claudia initiated a trust position in which her back was to Brian's chest and she laid her head on his shoulder. He could caress her legs and thighs as well as enjoy kissing. Claudia was very receptive and responsive to Brian's touch, feeling both safe and turned-on. She guided his hand to her vulva and he was thoroughly involved in pleasuring her to orgasm with manual stimulation. This was her first orgasmic response with Brian in 2 years. What she learned through masturbation was transferable to couple sexuality. For Brian, seeing Claudia reach orgasm with non-intercourse erotic stimulation was a life-changing experience. Rather than fear sex and have it be a source of frustration and embarrassment, Brian felt like a sexual partner who could pleasure Claudia for the first time in years. They lay together in the trust position for 10 min, feeling like an intimate sexual team.

Two days later, they explored a trust position in which Brian lay on his back and Claudia sat beside him so her hands were free to caress his body. For the first time in his life, Brian was able to accept pleasure without rushing to intercourse. As he opened himself to her gentle, rhythmic touch and kisses on his body, Claudia was aware of his growing erection. Rather than focusing on his penis, she continued playful non-demand pleasuring and enjoyed his emotional and sexual response. As she continued kissing and caressing him, she was surprised when he began touching his penis, and he reached orgasm 2 min later. This had never happened before; Brian had never been orgasmic with erotic sexuality. Both Brian and Claudia celebrated this breakthrough. Brian in particular was pleased by the strength of his erection in response to her touch. Claudia's sexual enthusiasm continued to grow. She felt they deserved to share sexual pleasure. Brian was less optimistic about the long-term role of erection, intercourse, and orgasm, but was clearly enjoying this new intimacy, pleasure, and eroticism.

At the next couple therapy session, Claudia asked whether the therapist could give them reading about ED. The therapist turned to Brian and asked if he thought this was the right opportunity to read about EDs. Brian was not interested in reading at this time; he wanted to continue to explore the desire exercises. He suggested that the reading might be of value to Claudia, and the therapist agreed to assign readings as long as she did not pressure Brian to read with her.

Brian was particularly interested in the attraction exercise. The focus on building a new pattern of sexual desire was important for Brian. He was especially intrigued by what would increase Claudia's attraction to him. As with other psychosexual skill exercises, touching is a crucial component. Claudia took the first ping. She began by telling Brian all the psychological, physical, relational, emotional, and sexual things she found attractive about him. Brian was genuinely surprised by her list of 24 attractive factors, which included the way he combed his hair, his reliability as a life partner, his willingness to give erotic touch from their trust position, and more. He was even more surprised by her requests that would increase her attraction to him. Her three requests were: (1) genuinely enjoy helping her be orgasmic during erotic stimulation; (2) stay connected to her even if he did not have an erection and even if they did not have intercourse, and (3) to say at least once a week that he loved and valued her. These requests were very emotional for Brian, and he had no hesitation in agreeing to all three. He felt welcome, rather than forced or coerced. The concept of sexuality as sharing pleasure was becoming more real and concrete. Brian told Claudia he was committed to being a sexual couple, although he still worried about ED and intercourse. Brian asked to delay his part of the attraction exercise until the next week because he needed time to prepare. Brian asked Claudia to initiate the trust position again in which she lay against him. He held and stroked her and again this transitioned to her being orgasmic with his stimulation. Afterward, Brian requested that Claudia pleasure him and this time he was orgasmic with her manual stimulation. Brian particularly enjoyed Claudia kissing him as he built erotic flow to orgasm. Her use of manual stimulation was more erotic than self-stimulation had been. There were new feelings and sensations for Brian as well as growing confidence in erections with non-intercourse eroticism.

The process of sexual change is usually "two steps forward and one step back." The day before the next therapy session, they had their first negative sexual encounter. After engaging in mutual genital pleasuring, Brian felt highly aroused and tried to initiate intercourse from the male on top position. As he approached intromission, his erection weakened. He tried unsuccessfully to insert his penis three times. Brian was visibly upset and turned away from Claudia, feeling embarrassed and disgusted with himself. Claudia pulled him close and requested he follow through on his commitment to not abandon her. They transitioned to the trust position. When Brian began to stimulate her, she said, "No just hold me, I want touch and connection." This brought tears to Brian's eyes. He now had a better understanding of Claudia's emotional and sexual needs. More importantly, it helped Brian make an emotional transition to valuing touch and sexuality as a couple rather that narrowly defining sex as intercourse (an individual pass–fail performance test).

The therapist had not yet spoken about the Good Enough Sex (GES) model. However, Claudia was already reading about GES in *Men's Sexual Health* [20], and was sure it would be valuable for Brian and her. Although the therapist agreed, his sense of Brian was that experiential learning was more impactful than cognitive and reading strategies. In terms of experiential learning, the therapist congratulated Claudia for implementing the touch strategies and encouraged Brian to follow her model.

After five weekly couple therapy sessions, the clinician recommended switching to scheduling sessions every other week rather than weekly, with which Brian enthusiastically agreed. The therapist urged them to keep the reserved scheduled time for themselves. They could engage in a psychosexual skill exercise, have an enjoyable walk, talk about an important nonsexual issue, shower together, take a nap, or share a concern from the past. The theme was to value and utilize their couple time and learn that they did not need a therapy appointment or the therapist to be able to engage with each other. This set the foundation for their relapse prevention program. A major contribution of couple therapy is to reinforce the importance of couple time.

The focus of therapy and the psychosexual skill exercises continued to be on intimacy, non-demand pleasuring, eroticism, and sexual desire in particular. The next set of psychosexual skill exercises was called, "Bridges to desire." At Brian's request, Claudia continued to be the initiator of the planned and semi-planned dates. The difference is that Brian was now considerably more open, receptive, and responsive. Whether the date was sensual, playful, or erotic, Brian was a full partner, both giving and receiving touch. Claudia relished the opportunity to be creative in the execution of the sexual date, and Brian responded to her enthusiasm.

Brian followed through on his part of the attraction exercise. The list of positive factors was powerfully validating for Claudia. He made two requests of Claudia to enhance his attraction to her: to renew their marital vows on their next anniversary, and plan a weekend getaway to a sex-themed hotel in the mountains. Claudia was very positive about the first request and asked that they invite their son and a small group of extended family and friends to witness and lend support for their renewed commitment.

Claudia offered an alternative to the second request, as she was turned-off by the gaudiness of the sex hotel. She proposed a couple weekend at a historic inn in a small town, where there was a claw foot tub in which to bathe and play sexually. Brian was fine with that alternative, and put the event on their calendar.

While processing sexual dates, the therapist raised the issue of synchronous and asynchronous sexual experiences. Like most couples, Brian and Claudia endorsed synchronous couple sexuality: both partners experience equal desire, pleasure, eroticism, and satisfaction. Brian, Claudia, and the therapist agreed that this was optimal couple sexuality. The therapist noted that for most couples, the sexual experience was positive, but not synchronous. This means the sex was better for one partner than the other. In fact, that had been their sexual pattern before ED. Sex, especially intercourse, had been better for Brian than for Claudia. This is a common pattern, especially for couples under age 40. This insight was more compelling for Claudia than for Brian. He agreed with the observation, but feared being labeled a "selfish lover." The therapist was clear that was not the intention; rather, he wanted to get them to speak about present sexual experiences and expectations for the future, and to consider whether they could affirm synchronous couple sexuality and still enjoy asynchronous sexuality [7]. Claudia observed that this was what they had experienced in the last few weeks; sexuality was best when mutual and synchronous, but asynchronous sexuality was worthwhile and fun. For the first time, sexuality was better for Claudia than Brian. Asynchronous experiences were more than okay; in fact, they were good. The therapist observed that one of the strategies of middle-years and aging couples was to embrace asynchronous sexuality. He also explained that asynchronous sex could be better for the woman and might increase in frequency over time. The concept of variable, flexible individual and couple sexuality is particularly relevant for middle-years and aging couples. Brian was more hesitant and ambivalent about this new approach, but agreed that he enjoyed Claudia's intense sexual responsiveness. The therapist affirmed the value of both synchronous and asynchronous sexuality as long as it was not at the expense of the partner or the relationship. This was congruent with what Claudia was valuing. She assured Brian that she would never want sexuality to be at Brian's expense or the expense of the marriage.

In the next 2 weeks, Brian and Claudia focused on the psychosexual skill exercises involving "Bridges to Desire." Claudia asked Brian if he was interested in taking "pings." He said their system was working so well that he wanted to stay with it. Although she would have preferred he initiate, she was willing to initiate sexual activity 2–4 times a week. Claudia especially enjoyed the exercise, "Overcoming differences in sexual desire." Claudia was sold on the strategy of touch as the core for her desire and that variable, flexible, responsive couple sexuality would ensure they stayed sexual in their 60s, 70s, and 80s [21].

The "Discrepancies" psychosexual skill exercise allowed Claudia to be sexually playful and creative. She was eager to take full advantage of the new sexuality definition, which valued sensual, playful, and erotic touch in addition to intercourse. Brian continued to prioritize intercourse. She prioritized playful and erotic touch. Since it was her "ping," Claudia introduced scenarios that focused on sharing erotic sexuality to orgasm for both her and Brian.

Claudia was especially influenced by the concept that, "If couples had to wait until both partners were equally desirous, frequency of sex would dramatically decrease." Claudia emphasized "responsive sexual desire." For Claudia, playful sexuality, rather than sensual touch, was her key for desire. In initiating playful touch scenarios, she felt freedom from the traditional female sexual role of being the "gatekeeper" and overemphasizing intimate touch. She valued the structure of the exercise, which enabled them both to become comfortable saying "no" so they had the freedom to say "yes" to playful and erotic sexuality. When the partner said no, it was his responsibility to introduce an alternative sensual or sexual scenario; avoidance was not acceptable. Claudia's favorite erotic alternative was pleasuring Brian to orgasm. Claudia enjoyed feelings of power to elicit erotic responsiveness. Brian would reliably become erect and she enjoyed his erotic flow to orgasm. At first, Brian felt "sexually selfish," but he clearly relished the erotic scenario. Claudia was clear that this was not an inviting scenario for her in the receiving role. It brought back bad memories of being passive in traditional "foreplay." Instead, Claudia's favorite erotic scenario was mutual, interactive, playful, and erotic touch. Being active in the pleasuring/eroticism process was a key for her sexual desire. Another key was her accepting while getting Brian to also accept that variable, flexible sexuality—both the process and outcome—was integral to Claudia's sexual voice. The preference for partner interaction arousal and variable response, as opposed to Brian's preference for self-entrancement, predictable arousal and orgasm, illustrated that they were not clones of each other. This insight was motivating and empowering and added spice to couple sexuality.

In exploring playful and erotic scenarios, Claudia discovered that when her subjective arousal was at a 5 or 6, mutual stimulation facilitated her sexual responsiveness. This involved giving as well as receiving stimulation. Brian's receptivity and responsiveness added to hers. In the recent past, Brian's fears of erectile failure and rush to intercourse had reduced Claudia's sexual response. Tentativeness, anxiety, and self-consciousness had subverted her and their sexuality. Now, Brian and Claudia valued the "give to get" pleasuring guideline and "piggy-backing" each partner's arousal on the other's.

The third exercise from the "Bridges to desire" series was the breakthrough in treatment. The "Sources of erotic desire" exercise was the impetus for Brian's enhanced desire. Brian finally adopted the insights that he did not need erection and intercourse in order to feel desire, and that Claudia need not be the source of all of his sexual desire. Brian could enjoy playful and erotic sexuality, including orgasm, without a firm erection. He now felt free to use erotic fantasies about others and nonsocially acceptable fantasies to promote desire. Fantasies, movies, TV, the Internet, people on the street, and more could serve as a bridge to desire. A prime bridge for desire for Brian was erotic fantasies. For most people, sexual fantasies serve to increase desire, involvement, eroticism, and orgasm.

Brian was enthusiastic about Claudia's playful and erotic scenarios. He was able to "piggyback" his arousal on hers. He had confidence that even if Claudia was not feeling erotic at that time, she was still enthusiastic about pleasuring him to orgasm.

At the next therapy session, it was Brian who suggested it was time to focus on increasing self-efficacy with arousal and erection. Claudia was enthusiastic about incorporating the "Arousal and erection" psychosexual skill exercises as long as Brian agreed he would not turn away from their progress if intercourse did not occur. Claudia affirmed the value of intercourse for her personally and them as a couple, but she did not allow it to control their sexual relationship. Brian agreed and asked the therapist whether he should again utilize a medical intervention. The therapist called the internist, and they jointly agreed that Brian would be prescribed a daily low dose of Cialis for 3 months. The therapist was clear in speaking to Brian and Claudia not to consider this a "magic pill," but rather an additional medical resource to enhance confidence in erectile function. There were three factors in rebuilding erectile confidence: (1) Brian's sexual voice, which emphasized desire and sexual pleasure; (2) turning toward Claudia as his intimate and erotic ally who valued sensual, playful, and erotic touch in addition to intercourse; and (3) Cialis to improve vascular function. When Brian felt subjectively aroused, Cialis made his vascular system more functional and promoted maintaining his erection. The therapist was clear with Brian that expecting 100% predictable erection and intercourse would set him up for failure. The therapist said what he says to almost all men, which was, "Whether it happens once a month, once every ten times, or once a year, it is normal to not have an erection sufficient for intercourse. I know you are cured of ED when you don't panic or apologize if sex does not flow to intercourse."

The Good Enough Sex (GES) model sets the expectation that in approximately 85% of sexual encounters, the experience will flow from desire, to pleasure, to eroticism, to intercourse, and then to orgasm. Rather than trying to force it when sex does not flow, the couple transitions to an erotic scenario (synchronous or asynchronous) to orgasm, or to a sensual, cuddly scenario, which ensures that the encounter ends in a positive manner. Another alternative is to say, "This isn't going to be an intercourse night. Let's take a rain check and be sexual during the next few days when we're aware, awake, and responsive." The key for GES is to affirm that couple sexuality is about sharing pleasure-oriented touch and that it is not an individual pass–fail intercourse test. Increasing erectile self-efficacy is a healthy strategy, whereas demanding perfect erectile function and intercourse performance is self-defeating and reinforces the ED. The biopsychosocial approach featuring positive, realistic expectations stands in sharp contrast to the biomedical approach to ED.

As most women do, Claudia affirmed GES for erection and couple sexuality. GES is congruent with the lived female sexual experience. Almost all women experience sexuality as variable, flexible, and interactive, rather than autonomous and perfectly predictable. GES was much more challenging for Brian, as it is for most men. The fact that physicians, advertisements, and male peers expect perfect erectile function serves as a major barrier to acceptance of GES. A strategy to convince the man is for the therapist to say, "Traditional men typically stop being sexual in their 50s and 60s; wise men are sexual in their 60s, 70s, and 80s. Wise men turn toward their partner and embrace GES."

The major factors that enabled Brian to accept GES included Claudia's support and encouragement as well as his experiences with erotic, non-intercourse sexuality. As they began to explore the "Arousal and erection" psychosexual skill exercises, the therapist urged them to retain their focus on the primacy of sexual desire and reminded them that "pleasure is the measure" [22].

The psychosexual skill exercise of "Waxing and Waning of Erections" is crucial. Brain was not expected to enjoy the exercise, but to experientially learn that it is physiologically normal for erections to wane. If he does not panic or try to force an erection, the erection will wax (i.e., grow) again with relaxation and sexual playful touch. Like almost all men, Brian expected and wanted to proceed to intercourse and orgasm on his first erection. This is a healthy preference, but becomes self-defeating when it is a mandate. In the exercise, Brian is the receiving partner with self-entrancement arousal. When he becomes erect, Claudia stops stimulation, so the erection will naturally wane. If Brian remains physically and psychologically relaxed, mindful, and open to sensual and playful touch his erection will wax again. Then, for a second time, allow it to wane and then wax. When practicing this skill, Claudia pleasured Brian to orgasm with his third erection. Brian understood the purpose of the exercise, which was to make him aware that he need not panic when his erection waned. The key to regaining an erection was not to work at or rush it, but rather to remain mindful of touch. This lesson was clearer to Claudia, and she found it intriguing. Like almost all men, Brian found it a difficult exercise and had no desire to repeat it; however, he now accepted the "wax and wane of erection" process.

Brian did enjoy the second exercise, "Playing With Your Penis Around Her Vagina." Brian was open to Claudia's playful and erotic manual and oral penile stimulation. Both understood that unless Brian's subjective arousal was at least a 5, penile stimulation was counter-productive, thereby increasing self-consciousness and reducing arousal. The next two exercises involved integrating intercourse into the pleasuring/eroticism process. Claudia decided when to move to intromission and guided Brian's penis inside her vagina. Brian was actively involved in giving and receiving erotic touch, which dramatically reduced "spectatoring." Rather than fearing intercourse as an individual pass–fail performance test, intercourse was a couple process and a natural extension of the pleasuring/eroticism process. At the next therapy session, Brian affirmed Claudia's point that if sex did not flow to intercourse, he would turn toward her to share an erotic scenario. His challenge was to stay emotionally and physically involved, rather than panic or apologize.

At this point, Brian and Claudia had integrated concepts of desire, pleasure, eroticism, and satisfaction. When sex was not positive for one or both, they could still appreciate broad-based sexuality. Variable, flexible GES was the foundation for their continued growth as a sexual couple.

The last set of psychosexual skill exercises was "Maintaining resilient couple sexuality." Relapse prevention is an integral component of comprehensive sex therapy. Relapse prevention strategies and techniques are ignored in most therapy programs, much to the detriment of individuals and couples. The most demoralized couples are those who are successfully treated and then relapse. They ask themselves, "Should I blame myself, my partner, our relationship, or the therapist?" Usually it is the therapist who failed to help them develop an individualized relapse prevention plan.

In the next-to-last formal therapy session, Brian and Claudia were given the handout, "Relapse Prevention Strategies and Guidelines" [6]. Their homework assignment was to choose 2–4 guidelines as the basis of their individualized relapse prevention program. At the last therapy session, Brian and Claudia made an emotional commitment to maintain strong, resilient couple sexuality that focused on desire. The most common relapse prevention strategy is how to prevent a sexual lapse from becoming a relapse. This was particularly important to Claudia. She knew, both from reading and experience, that it is normal for 5–15% of sexual encounters to be dissatisfying or dysfunctional. She wanted to be sure that Brian could accept that and not use it as a cue to avoid. Brian had a proposal: Claudia would commit to initiating a sexual date within 72 h of a negative experience to ensure that avoidance did not have a chance to grow. She enthusiastically agreed.

Brian and Claudia agreed that they would schedule 6-month check-in sessions with the therapist over the next 2 years. The check-in session would have two areas of focus: to be sure gains were maintained, and to set a new couple sexual goal for the next 6 months. The goal could be any one of a number of things, including trying a new pleasuring lotion, taking a couple weekend trip, developing a new afterplay scenario, trying a multiple stimulation technique during intercourse, or trying a role enactment scenario. The message is not to treat couple sexuality with benign neglect. Vital, satisfying sexuality requires new energy, inputs, creativity, and unpredictability. Of course, if there were a problem, they were encouraged to schedule a "booster session." Claudia committed to call for a booster session if a month went by without a sexual encounter. Brian and Claudia had come too far to allow a relapse. They were committed to desire, pleasure, eroticism, and satisfaction.

Biological Treatments

The major biomedical treatment for HSDD is testosterone enhancement therapy. Ideally, this would be under the care of an endocrinologist who specializes in the assessment and treatment of hormonal function and sexuality. Testosterone is often prescribed by an internist, psychiatrist, urologist, or sexual medicine specialist.

Assessing for free testosterone is a challenging task that is ideally carried out by a specialty lab. Testosterone levels are difficult to measure and can vary widely. Also, many men are overly influenced by the barrage of "low T" advertisements. When there is no available testosterone or extremely low levels, it is appropriate to prescribe testosterone enhancement therapy, most often in a gel form. What is not appropriate is expecting testosterone to be a stand-alone medication to cure HSDD. The integration of testosterone into the couple sexual style of intimacy, pleasuring, and eroticism is crucial. Ideally, the prescribing physician would have at least one consultation with the man and his partner to discuss how to successfully integrate testosterone and to establish positive, realistic expectations.

When ED causes HSDD, the use of Viagra, Cialis or penile injections can promote sexual desire by reducing anticipatory and performance anxiety. However, this does not automatically cure HSDD. Discussing with the man (ideally the couple) the concepts of responsive male sexual desire and Good Enough Sex (GES) is critically important in rebuilding resilient sexual desire.

Another important biomedical intervention is the promotion of good health, especially behavioral health habits. Anything that is good for the man's physical body is good for his sexual body. Understanding that no illness and no disability stops sexual desire is empowering. The major biomedical cause of HSDD is side effects of medications. The client (ideally the couple) schedules a consultation with the internist or specialist to address how to be an involved, active patient while reducing the negative impact that the disease or disability has on sexuality. In addition, the man is urged to improve behavioral health habits such as: refraining from smoking, engaging in moderate or no drinking, adopting healthy sleep patterns, participating in regular exercise, and maintaining healthier eating patterns. He wants sexuality to maintain a positive 15–20% role in his life and relationship.

Psychosocial Treatments

The biopsychosocial model views psychological and relational interventions as integral to treatment of HSDD. The treatment of choice for men in a married or partnered relationship is couple sex therapy. However, individual sex therapy or counseling can be of great value.

A crucial strategy is the use of psychosexual skill exercises to build sexual comfort and confidence. A series of psychosexual skill exercises includes building sexual desire, arousal and erection, and enhanced erotic flow and orgasm. These are most effective when practiced as a couple, but they can also be rehearsed using masturbation or guided imagery.

Cognitive restructuring involves addressing the traditional male sex socialization to confront the myth that "sex=intercourse" and that autonomous sex performance is the norm. This is replaced with a model in which sexuality is focused on the couple sharing pleasure rather than on erection and intercourse as an individual pass–fail sex test. Again, this is more effective in the context of the woman being his intimate and erotic ally.

Teaching physical and psychological relaxation skills (including mindfulness) is a critical area of learning for the man. The foundation for sexual response is relaxation, the understanding of which most males are not aware.

Another crucial psychosocial intervention is to change the definition of sexual satisfaction. Although arousal, intercourse, and orgasm are highly valued, satisfaction is more than orgasm. Satisfaction involves feeling good about himself as a sexual man and energized as a sexual couple. Perhaps the most important change is to accept the Good Enough Sex (GES) model and let go of the individual perfect sex performance model. In the traditional approach, the man is always one negative sexual experience from feeling like a "sexual failure." GES frees him from the oppressive model of individual sex performance. This increases self-acceptance and sexual self-esteem.

Complexity of HSDD

Although this chapter follows the dichotomous diagnostic categories of primary versus secondary HSDD and generalized versus specific contexts, the reality is that HSDD is complex in both assessment and treatment. The biopsychosocial model provides a framework for understanding HSDD as multicausal and multidimensional with large individual, couple, cultural, and value differences. Sexual secrecy and couple dynamics frequently play a crucial but underappreciated role in subverting sexual desire. The traditional male model consisting of spontaneous erection, totally predictable sex performance, and an unconditional desire for sex is not motivating or empowering for the adult man, particularly one who is in a serious relationship and over age 40. In fact, it is oppressive and destructive. In many ways, male HSDD has the same variability and complexity as FSIAD does for women. Desire is strongly influenced by expectations about arousal and erection, especially with ED. Some researchers believe that the rate of HSDD is 15–25% [23].

Although testosterone enhancement has been promoted as the cure for "low T," careful assessment of testosterone levels is not common, and the level of free testosterone is quite variable. Males (and females) who lack testosterone or whose levels are abnormally low can benefit from testosterone enhancement. However, testosterone is not an effective stand-alone intervention [24].

Anxiety and depression, as well as the side effects of the medications used to treat these problems, are common biomedical factors in HSDD. Social/relational factors have to be carefully assessed and addressed as possible causes, especially of primary HSDD. Common causes of primary HSDD include having a secret sexual life; a variant (atypical) arousal pattern; a preference for masturbation; or a history of sexual trauma that is not shared with the spouse (partner). The man treats these issues as "shameful secrets" and often blames his partner for the sexual problem. The secret sexual pattern can go on for years. When the partner discovers the secret, her reaction is similar to that of a PTSD response; she feels shocked and betrayed. Often, it is not discovered until the assessment process, and it is then disclosed in the couple feedback session. The therapist faces the challenge of simultaneously supporting the man in the session so that he does not feel shamed while supporting the woman in her sense of confusion, hurt, and anger. The therapist emphasizes how important it is for the couple to process HSDD issues. They now have the information and resources to address these hidden desire problems. The therapist emphasizes that the past cannot be changed; rather, the power of change is in the present and future. They can process and learn from the themes of the past, but they do not have the opportunity for a "do-over."

In dealing with primary HSDD, the personal responsibility/intimate team model is crucial. The core question is: what is thc man's motivation and intentions regarding change? The therapist helps him deal with ambivalence and confront sexual shame. The clinician needs to be sure that the man's motivation is genuine and that he is not simply giving the "socially desirable" response. The woman's motivation and needs are as important as the man's are. The therapist must make sure that the woman is open to being the man's intimate and erotic ally in developing a new couple sexual style, and that she is not intent on punishing/shaming him. They must address whether she can overcome her sense of betrayal and be an active partner in building a new couple sexual style.

In working with couples facing HSDD, there are five clients in the room: (1) the man; (2) the woman; (3) their general relationship; (4) their sexual relationship; and (5) the most difficult client: their history as an emotional and sexual couple. It is imperative to conduct a comprehensive biopsychosocial assessment with both the man and woman. Issues pertaining to desire, especially primary HSDD, are extremely challenging clinical problems.

Variant Arousal as the Cause of HSDD

The most common sexual secret causing primary HSDD is a variant (atypical or kinky) arousal pattern. This includes fetishes, cross-dressing, BDSM scenarios, and more. Traditionally, the man never disclosed the variant arousal pattern to his partner. Approximately 4% of men experience variant arousal [25]. This pattern is established in childhood or adolescence; it seldom develops during adulthood. Commonly, the pattern is controlled by high secrecy, high eroticism, and high shame. This controls the man's sexuality. Although he is usually able to function sexually, especially early in the relationship, his ability to do so decreases over time because his sexual desire is controlled by the variant arousal rather than by the desire for intimate, interactive couple sexuality. It is not that he cannot perform intercourse or succeed at reproductive sex; rather, he does not value couple sexuality. He uses masturbatory sex with fetish fantasies, and sparingly uses couple sex as a way to service his partner so that she does not complain. Over time, he resents sex with the woman and falls into a negative sexual cycle in which she pursues sex and he avoids it. When they are sexual, it is often dysfunctional for him or dissatisfying for her. Over time, sex is marked by anticipatory anxiety, tense performance-oriented intercourse, frustration, embarrassment, and eventually avoidance. The contrast between masturbating to the fetish and couple sex becomes even starker.

This negative pattern can last for years. In essence, the man and woman are speaking different languages about intimacy and sexuality, often trading charges and put-downs. A common occurrence is that the man's secret sexual life is ultimately discovered with a great deal of ensuing drama.

There are three basic treatment strategies: acceptance, compartmentalization, and necessary loss. At this time, there is little clinical or empirical data to support one strategy over the others. Typically, the man is hoping for acceptance and the woman is hoping he will give up the variant arousal and accept necessary loss. In assessing the man, woman, relationship, and their intimacy and sexuality pattern, the clinician carefully assesses cognitive, behavioral, and emotional factors, as well as each partner's motivation. Specifically, it is important to identify how the man views the spouse and the relationship: does he value it, marginalize the woman, or endure the marriage for the sake of the children or social acceptance? It is imperative to identify whether the woman values him and their bond, or whether the variant arousal and history of betrayal gives her freedom to terminate the relationship. It is crucial for the clinician to provide first class treatment with a curious, nonjudgmental stance, rather than assume the presence of psychopathology.

"Kink-friendly" therapists advocate for acceptance, which is much better than assuming pathology. The primary issue is whether the affirming therapist considers the whole picture, including the needs and motivations of the woman. Both partners have a right to feel that the therapist is addressing the problem in a respectful, empathic manner.

The acceptance strategy requires emotional acceptance, not just of the variant arousal but also of the ability of both partners to incorporate this into couple sexuality. This can be a challenge for both the man and woman. For the man, his variant arousal (whether a fetish, cross-dressing, or being submissive in a BDSM scenario) has always been in the context of a secret arousal. Some men find that acting out the variant scenario in an intimate relationship strips away the erotic charge. Some women emotionally accept that the variant arousal is integral to his authentic sexuality, but experience activities such as putting on fetish material, being sexual when he is cross-dressed, or taking the dominant sexual role as anti-erotic. Couples who adopt the acceptance strategy usually experience the new sexual scenario as better for him than her. Asynchronous sex is common and healthy, but not all their sexual experiences are based on the variant arousal. An important question is whether they can develop mutual, synchronous scenarios or value asynchronous scenarios that are better for her than for him. The key to the successful therapeutic implementation of the acceptance strategy is for the couple to take pride in "beating the odds" and creating a new sexual style that integrates the variant arousal into their desire/pleasure/eroticism/satisfaction pattern. It is important that the therapist focus the couple on the present and future, without allowing the couple to get stuck in the "what if" questions or feelings of betrayal about past sexual secrecy. Clients can learn from the past and process and honor new learning, but they cannot change the past. The power of change is in the present and future.

With greater cultural awareness and acceptance of variant (kinky) sexual scenarios, a new guideline is that the man discloses his sexual patterns in the first 6 months of a new relationship so that the woman can decide whether she can accept it. This problem is prevented when the couple meets through a "kink-friendly" website. The couple celebrates kinky sex while rejecting "vanilla sex."

The "necessary loss" strategy is the other extreme. This occurs when it is not possible or acceptable to incorporate the variant arousal pattern into couple sexuality. The man has to accept that his special erotic charge will not work in this relationship. He is not being shamed or coerced. She is being honest in saying that the variant arousal is anti-erotic for her. The challenge is to develop a new couple sexual style that affirms desire/pleasure/eroticism/satisfaction. The man has to be honest with himself and his partner about the fact that the erotic charge is not as intense as it is with the variant arousal, but that their new couple sexual style is a better fit, with eroticism integrated into couple sexuality. Rather than compare intensity of erotic sensations/feelings, he accepts the integrated eroticism and learns to "piggyback" his arousal on hers.

Some men find even if the partner were willing to play out his variant erotic scenario, it is not erotically satisfying for him. Sharing the variant erotic scenario results in a lessened erotic charge and in some cases, it is an erotic "dud."

The third strategy, compartmentalization, is the traditional secret strategy. The man acts out the variant arousal with other partners or uses Internet stimuli for masturbation. He utilizes variant arousal fantasies during couple sex in order to function sexually. When disclosed, most couples will choose either the acceptance or necessary loss strategies. However, some couples purposefully choose the compartmentalization strategy. For example, a woman might say that she could accept that her husband valued being sexual when cross-dressed, but that sexual activity with him wearing her slip or in make-up is an erotic turn-off for her. They agree that he can utilize cross-dressing fantasies while engaged in couple sex, but not verbalize them. When she was out of town, he is free to cross-dress and go to clubs where he can be sexual, as long as he practices safe sex.

The core therapeutic issue is to find an acceptable emotional/sexual agreement that works for the man, woman, and couple so that sex does not have a destructive role, but rather a 15–20% positive role.

Deviant Sexual Arousal

Less than 1% of men have a deviant arousal pattern. Deviant sexuality refers to illegal sexual behavior that is harmful to others. The most common deviant behaviors are exhibitionism, voyeurism, frotteurism, pedophilia, and obscene phone calls [26]. Therapeutically, the goal is to stop acting out deviant behavior entirely, although there is wide disagreement about therapeutic strategies and techniques. There is agreement that shaming the man is counter-therapeutic, reducing his self-esteem and reinforcing a secret sexual life. A multi-dimensional biopsychosocial treatment approach involving his partner is likely to increase success, with a much lower relapse rate. There is a need for empirical and clinical research on which strategies are most efficacious in stopping deviant sexual behavior.

Men Who Prefer Masturbation to Couple Sex

There has been a misplaced emphasis on the concept of "porn addiction" in both the media and professional literature. In the sex therapy field, there is little support for the sex addiction model, which tends to shame men and overemphasizes the negative impact of pornography for all men. The "out of control male sexual behavior" model [27] is an empirically validated sexual health approach to problematic sexual behavior.

In primary HSDD, the man is comfortable and confident with masturbation, but he is an anxious performer in couple sex. Diagnostically, the question to ask the man is: "In a typical month, how often are you orgasmic by any means?" Men who identify (or are labeled by their partners) as low sex interest disclose that in masturbatory sex, they are orgasmic 20–30 times per month. Follow-up questions pertain to what erotic fantasies or materials are used. Sometimes, the core issue is a variant arousal pattern. However, often the issue is his sexual preference for masturbation. The analogy is: " I am an A+ masturbator, but a D- at couple sex."

This pattern reflects the poisonous combination of high secrecy, high eroticism, and high shame. Almost invariably, the partner is kept in the dark, although she is suspicious that something is going on sexually. Often, the man blames the woman for the no-sex relationship, which is both unfair and unkind. In the extreme case, the man chooses to marry (or partner) with this woman for anti-erotic reasons (i.e., specifically because he did not want to be sexual with her and could thus blame her for the sexual problem).

When the secret sexual life is revealed, whether by accident at home or in the couple feedback session, the woman's reaction is similar to a PTSD response whereas the man's reaction is one of guilt or shame. The therapist's role is to be empathic and respectful of each partner while challenging them to process the new sexual information in a non-destructive manner. The man has to accept responsibility for the secret sexual life, rather than minimize it or wallow in guilt, shame, or cognitions that he is a bad man and that sex is bad. He is responsible for his own sexuality and needs to be honest with himself (and his partner) about his genuine motivation and intention to utilize change strategies. It is important to identify whether he is proposing acceptance, compartmentalization, or necessary loss. Too often, the therapist is faced with the woman blaming or demonizing the man, and the man being silent and shameful. He agrees to something he is not committed to in order to placate her. Rather than change based on positive motivation, it is driven by guilt or by the need to pretend. As with other examples of negative motivation, this almost never results in positive change. The man is driven by shame and embarrassment, rather than by wanting to be intimate and sexual. For this type of HSDD, intimacy and eroticism are totally separate.

In an empathic manner, the therapist confronts the destructive power struggle that has been driven by shaming the man and his sexuality. He has a right to say what strategy is healthy for him, rather than be driven by the partner's agenda. The core issue in working with desire problems caused by a secret sexual life is to create a new genuine couple sexuality that meets each partner's preferences and feelings. Ideally, the clinician is pro-sexual and pro-relationship but also able to help couples divorce in a non-destructive manner. Divorce is usually the woman's decision because she feels there is not a genuine intimate sexual relationship. Typically, a man who prefers masturbation to couple sex, whether there is a variant arousal or not, does value the relationship, but is too anxious to enjoy couple sexuality. The therapeutic strategy is to build a new couple sexual style that integrates desire/pleasure/eroticism/satisfaction. The man accepts that sexuality will not be as predictable and erotically charged as the masturbation pattern and learns that sexuality becomes better integrated into his and their sexual relationship. In healthy relationships, sexuality is not the most important factor. Sexuality has a positive, motivating role to promote feelings of desire and desirability and bond the couple. Primary HSDD has the opposite role, in that it demoralizes the couple.

History of Sexual Trauma as a Cause of Primary HSDD

The third major sexual secret causing HSDD is a history of sexual trauma or emotional neglect. Sexual trauma is less common for males, but it is a pervasive shameful secret that controls his sexual self-esteem. Most males do not disclose the trauma history to anyone, especially not their spouse/partner. Public awareness and professional literature emphasize female trauma. The mistaken assumption is that male children and adolescents do not experience trauma. As the great majority of perpetrators are males, there is the additional stigma of same sex interactions. To compound the stigma, a common form of male sexual abuse is being fellated to orgasm. This leads the client to question how can it be abuse if he responded sexually. The essence of child sexual abuse is that the older male's sexual wants are met at the expense of the child or adolescent's emotional needs. The majority of sexual abuse incidents occur with someone the boy knows, do not involve anal intercourse, and are not physically violent, which is the opposite of the stereotype. Sadly, this makes it harder to disclose and process the sexual trauma in a healing manner. Instead, it serves as a "shameful secret." The man has a contingent sexual self-esteem, believing if his partner knew the abuse history, she would not respect or love him.

In many ways, neglect has a greater degree of negative impact on emotional and interpersonal development than trauma does. Neglecting the young boy's physical, psychological, and emotional needs sends a message that he has no value. He is not even important enough to abuse.

When addressing a history of trauma or neglect with the adult man, the clinician is mindful of being empathic, rather than sympathetic, as well as respectful of the client's feelings. It is especially important not to blame or shame the man, but rather to convey the message that processing his psychological, relational, and sexual history is crucial to the healing process. He needs to verbalize and honor the trauma history without giving it control over his life and sexuality. Typically, the partner is more accepting and supportive of him than he is of himself. Common misperceptions that the man harbors include: (1) he was responsible for the abuse; (2) he was chosen for abuse because he was a weak male; (3) if he responded sexually, he must be gay; (4) if his partner or male friends were to find out, they would blame him or deem him to be "damaged goods"; and (5) the abuse history has destroyed his sexual self-esteem.

Cognitive restructuring is a core therapeutic strategy. In honoring the themes of the trauma history, the goal is to shift his sexual self-esteem from that of a shameful or angry victim to that of a proud survivor. He can learn from the past, but he cannot change the past. The power of change is in the present and future. The treatment of choice where there is a history of trauma is couple sex therapy [28]. When he feels deserving of sexual pleasure and is able to experience desire/pleasure/eroticism/satisfaction in the milieu of an intimate sexual relationship, he has taken back control of his body and sexuality; he is no longer controlled by the trauma history.

A crucial therapeutic strategy is to give him the power to veto a sexual scenario or technique. He has confidence that his partner will honor the veto, which is the opposite of what happened in the trauma. However, he does not have the right to avoid sexual activity. When he avoids, this builds sexual anxiety. If he becomes anxious or has a flashback, a useful strategy is to switch to their "trust position" and regain a sense of mindful control. Trauma-informed couple sex therapy is a sophisticated approach that honors the sensitivities of the trauma history without giving it power in the present sexual relationship [29]. The woman takes the role of "a partner in healing" and supports the belief that as an adult, he deserves sexual pleasure. Sexuality now has a positive 15–20% role in his life and relationship. They develop a new couple sexual style that affirms desire/pleasure/eroticism /satisfaction. The core dimension is strong, resilient sexual desire.

Secrets Regarding Sexual Orientation

When males report sexual problems, the most common reaction from male peers, partner, physician, and mental health professionals is to ask, "Are you gay?" This is a major cause of prejudice that straight men have against gay men. Although the clinician does need to assess for sexual orientation issues, it is imperative not to assume that is the problem; most of the time, that is not the issue. As the culture becomes more accepting of gay men and gay marriage, there is less need to be secretive, and certainly less shame regarding sexual orientation. For most men, sexual orientation is "hard-wired" rather than a choice behavior. For the 3–4% of men whose sexual orientation is gay, the challenge is to live their lives psychologically, relationally, and sexually as first class people. In the great majority of cases, reparative and change therapies are not only unsuccessful; they are harmful. Typically, sexual desire is a strength for gay men.

The scientific community has now accepted that sexual orientation is much more complex than the old model depicted, which centered on the gender of those that the man fantasies about and with whom he has sex. A better understanding of sexual orientation involves with whom the man feels emotionally attached to and shares genuine intimacy. The second factor is with whom he experiences a genuine erotic charge [30].

There are at least four sexual orientations: (1) homosexual, (2) heterosexual, (3) pan-sexual, and (4) asexual. Pan-sexual (which includes bi-sexual) is a genuine orientation. The clinical challenge is to help the client develop a sexuality that affirms a 15–20% role in the man's life and relationship. His sexual self-acceptance and ability to negotiate expectations and behavioral boundaries with partners is crucial. Most pansexual men adopt a nontraditional approach to relational fidelity and consensual non-monogamy [31].

Asexuality

Over the past 5–10 years, the scientific study of asexuality has grown [32]. Approximately 0.5% of men are asexual, which means they lack sexual desire for a physical relationship with another person. However, many asexual men are able to procreate and desire marriage and family. To evaluate the complexity of asexuality, the clinician needs to conduct a careful biopsychosocial assessment. Asexual men deserve first class mental health services with a clinician who does not assume that asexuality is psychopathological or caused by a lack of testosterone. It is important to assess testosterone levels as well as to identify whether trauma, a sexual secret, shame, fear of intimacy, or a self-misdiagnosis is present. However, it is a mistake to assume that any of these factors are the cause of asexuality.

Prognosis

Male HSDD has been understudied both empirically and clinically. In general, the traditional treatment approaches, whether biomedical or psychodynamic, have been pessimistic about change. Meana 3 identified the core issues in HSDD: psychological, relational, and sexual secrets. The couple biopsychosocial model is much more likely to promote a genuine understanding and successful resolution of HSDD because it explores a range of causes and dimensions and directly confronts the man's secrets.

The stand-alone medication approach to ED has been unsuccessful for two core reasons. First, it reinforces the individual perfect sex performance model, which sets the man up to feel like a "Viagra failure" and subsequently avoid couple sex. Second, the woman is someone for whom he is supposed to perform, rather than someone he can turn to as his intimate and erotic ally when sex does not flow to intercourse. Unless the man's core assumptions about healthy male sexuality are confronted and changed, the prognosis for HSDD is poor. However, when the man (and couple) adopt a variable, flexible approach to couple sexuality that both values sharing pleasure more than individual sex performance as well as accepts that sensual, playful, and erotic sexuality are valid in addition to intercourse, this new model promotes strong, resilient sexual desire. This is an anti-perfectionistic approach to male sexual function and desire. The partner uses a positive influence process, which enables the man to value variable, flexible couple sexuality. The focus is on sharing pleasure and embracing GES.

A clinical intervention that dramatically increases prognosis is urging the man to take pride in "beating the odds" and being a "wise man" rather than a traditional man. A key for positive prognosis is to accept that this approach to male and couple sexuality is superior to the traditional, rigid, individual predictable performance model. The concept of "male responsive sexual desire" is the foundation of this new model of desire. Rather than be driven by spontaneous erection, eroticism, and orgasm, responsive male desire emanates from the giving and receiving of pleasure-oriented touching and mindfulncss of his cmotions and those of his partner.

Recognition that couple sexuality can have a number of roles, meanings, and outcomes allows a range of bridges to desire. The man and couple's openness to the use of all resources—including biomedical, psychological, and relational—to facilitate desire is an empowering strategy that promotes a positive outcome.

A crucial element in successful treatment is the development of an individualized relapse prevention plan. The sign of resilient desire is the ability to ensure that a lapse (i.e., a negative sexual experience) does not become a relapse (i.e., a pattern of anticipatory anxiety and performance-oriented intercourse that leads to avoidance). Creating a couple sexual style that integrates intimacy and eroticism and allows the man to have his sexual voice and turn toward his partner sexually in both good and bad times ensures strong, resilient sexual desire.

Relapse Prevention of HSDD

Comprehensive assessment and treatment using all biopsychosocial resources is crucial in the successful treatment of HSDD. The most ignored issue is relapse prevention [6]. The most demoralized men and couples are those who regained desire and then relapsed into HSDD and sexual avoidance. The client wonders whether he should blame himself or his partner, or whether this is a fatally flawed relationship. However, it is usually the fault of the clinician, who did not help the man and couple develop an individualized relapse prevention plan. Whether the HSDD was treated using a couple therapy format or individually using a biomedical model, a relapse prevention plan is part of comprehensive treatment.

Two sessions before termination in the couple sex therapy approach, the couple receives a ten-item set of relapse prevention guidelines. The couple is asked to choose 2–4 guidelines that provide the basis for their individualized relapse prevention plan. During the last formal therapy session, they discuss their plan in detail. The most common guideline chosen is how to ensure a lapse (i.e., a negative sexual experience) does not become a relapse (i.e., reversion to the pattern of anticipatory anxiety, tense performance-oriented intercourse, frustration, embarrassment, and avoidance). Other commonly utilized guidelines include reinforcing the concept that sensual, playful, and erotic touch are sexual; scheduling a non-demand pleasuring date every 4–8 weeks; and setting aside quality couple time without children. Clinically, the most important guideline is to schedule a check-in session at 6-month intervals for 2 years. This sends a powerful message that the therapist cares about the man and couple and wants them to maintain gains. Sexuality cannot be treated with benign neglect. There are two areas of focus in the 6-month session: (1) ensure gains are maintained; and (2) set a new growth goal for the next 6 months. The message is to continue to nurture and grow their intimate sexual relationship. Examples of goals include: try a different intercourse position, type of thrusting, or afterplay scenario; use a new body lotion for pleasuring; plan a couple weekend without children; participate in a role enactment scenario; or process an incident from the past so that it no longer causes psychological pain. Affirming their couple sexual style and the value of desire/pleasure/eroticism/satisfaction is at the core of relapse prevention.

Summary

Male HSDD is a crucial issue that has been understudied both empirically and clinically. This chapter focuses on a comprehensive couple biopsychosocial approach to the treatment of primary and secondary HSDD. There is a range of approaches, from stand-alone medications such as testosterone enhancement to long-term individual psychodynamic therapy. In dealing with secondary HSDD caused by ED, Viagra or Cialis can be a valuable therapeutic resource. However, for most men, ED medications have limited success as a stand-alone intervention because the man has unrealistic expectations of a return to the autonomous, totally predictable erections he experienced as a young adult. After a sensitizing experience of ED, men do not return to totally predictable erectile function. This is why psychological and relational approaches are so valuable when integrated with medical interventions. A key to rebuilding erectile comfort and confidence is adopting positive, realistic expectations promoted by the Good Enough Sex (GES) model [4]. Regaining erectile self-efficacy is key to rebuilding male sexual desire. Positive anticipation, sense of deserving pleasure, and freedom and choice with sensual and erotic scenarios in addition to intercourse facilitate strong, resilient sexual desire. Rather than be pressured to perform for the woman with intercourse as an individual pass–fail sex test, he embraces variable, flexible couple sexuality, which includes, but is not limited to, intercourse. This approach to sexual desire and function has received support from the sex therapy community and from female mental health clinicians, but not from drug companies, physicians, male peers, or the media. Ideally, medical clinicians and mental health clinicians would work in a synergistic manner to promote male sexual health with a special focus on resilient sexual desire.

The more invasive the medical procedure is, the more it promotes erectile function, but not necessarily desire. For example, penile injections are more effective for erectile function than pro-erection medications are; however, unless it is integrated into the couple sexual style of intimacy, pleasuring, and eroticism, it will be discontinued. Predictable erections do not guarantee enhanced desire if the man or couple does not experience comfort while utilizing the injections. An even better example is penile prosthesis, which does guarantee functional erections. The unkind joke is "even if you build it, no one will come." The prosthesis does not invite desire for either partner.

The hope for the future is that medications and medical devices will become more user-friendly and efficacious. However, psychological, relational, psychosexual, and social factors will need to be assessed and treated. It is especially crucial to adopt a new approach to male sexuality that accepts individual differences, a pleasure-orientation, and the female–male equity model. The traditional male model of autonomous, totally predictable sex performance is oppressive for men and ultimately undermines the man and woman as intimate and erotic allies. Male sexual desire cannot be defined as "the man is willing and able to have sex with any woman, any time, and in any circumstance." This is a crazy-making model for the man, woman, couple, and the culture. With men over 50, the model of "responsive male sexual desire" is motivating and empowering. The new model of male desire involves a biopsychosocial approach, which accepts sexual desire that is integrated. The man values intimacy, non-demand pleasuring, and eroticism, and accepts the woman as an equitable sexual partner who is his intimate and erotic friend. This model of male and couple sexuality promotes strong, resilient sexual desire.

References

1. Foley S, Kope SA, Sugrue D. Sex matters for women: a complete guide to taking care of your sexual self. 2nd ed. New York, NY: Guilford; 2012.
2. Zilbergeld B. The new male sexuality. New York, NY: Bantam; 1999.
3. Meana M, Steiner E. Hidden disorder/hidden desire: presentations of low sexual desire in men. In: Binik I, Hall K, editors. Principles and practice of sex therapy. 5th ed. New York, NY: Guilford; 2014. p. 42–60.
4. Metz M, McCarthy B. The good enough sex (GES) model. In: Kleinplatz P, editor. New directions in sex therapy. 2nd ed. New York, NY: Routledge; 2012. p. 213–30.
5. McCarthy B, Wald L. The psychobiosocial model of couple sex therapy. In: Peterson Z, editor. Wiley-Blackwell handbook of sex therapy. New York, NY: Wiley-Blackwell; 2017.
6. McCarthy B. Sex made simple. Eau Clair, WI: PESI Publishing; 2015.
7. Berry M. Historical revolutions in sex therapy. J Sex Marital Ther. 2013;39:21–39.
8. Althof S, Leiblum S, Chevret-Measson M, Hartman U, Levine S, McCabe M. Psychological and interpersonal dimensions of sexual function and dysfunction. J Sex Med. 2005;2:793–818.
9. McCarthy B, McCarthy E. Rekindling desire. 2nd ed. New York, NY: Routledge; 2014.
10. Hyde J. The gender similarities hypothesis. Am Psychol. 2005;60: 581–92.
11. Gray J. Men are from mars, women are from venus. New York, NY: Harper-Collins; 1988.
12. Kelly S, Shelton J. African-American couples and sex. In Hall K, Graham C, editors. The cultural context of sexual pleasure and problems. New York, NY: Routledge; 2012. p. 48–83.
13. McCarthy B, Thestrup M. Men, intimacy, and eroticism. J Sex Med. 2009;6:588–94.
14. Whisman M, Snyder D, Beach S. Screening for marital and relationship discord. J Fam Psychol. 2009;22:247–54.
15. Snyder D, Whisman M. Treating difficult couples. New York, NY: Guilford; 2003.
16. Tennov D. Love and limerance. New York, NY: Scarborough; 1988.
17. Perel E. Mating in captivity. New York, NY: Harper-Collins; 2006.
18. Metz M, McCarthy B. Coping with erectile dysfunction. Oakland, CA: New Harbinger; 2004.
19. Bancroft J, Vukadinovic Z. Sexual addiction, sexual compulsivity, or what? J Sex Res. 2004;41:225–34.
20. McCarthy B, Metz M. Men's sexual health. New York, NY: Routledge; 2008.
21. Lindau S, Schumm L, Laumann E, Levinson W, O'Muircheartaigh C, Waite L. A study of sexuality and health among older adults in the United States. N Engl J Med. 2007;357:762–74.
22. Nagoski E. Come as you are. New York, NY: Simon and Schuster; 2015.
23. Brooks G, Elder W. Sex therapy for men. In: Kleinpatz P, editor. New directions in sex therapy. 2nd ed. New York, NY: Routledge; 2012. p. 37–50.
24. Toates F. An integrative theoretical framework for understanding sexual motivation, arousal, and behavior. J Sex Res. 2009;46:168–93.
25. Kafka M. Nonparaphilic hypersexuality disorders. In: Binik I, Hall K, editors. Principles and practice of sex therapy. 5th ed. New York, NY: Guilford; 2014. p. 280–304.
26. Abel G, Becker J, Cunningham-Rathner J, Mittleman M, Rouleau J. Multiple paraphilic diagnoses among sex offenders. Bull Am Acad Psychiatry Law. 1988;16:153–68.
27. Braun-Harvey D, Vigorito M. Treating out of control sexual behavior. New York, NY: Springer; 2015.
28. Maltz W. The sexual healing journey. 3rd ed. New York, NY: William Morrow; 2012.
29. Zoldbrod A. Sexual issues in treating trauma survivors. Curr Sex Health Rep. 2015;7:3–11.
30. Herek G, Garnets L. Sexual orientation and mental health. Annu Rev Clin Psychol. 2007;3:353–75.
31. Nichols M. Therapy with LGBTQ clients. In: Binik I, Hall K, editors. Principles and practice of sex therapy. 5th ed. New York, NY: Guilford; 2014. p. 309–33.
32. Brotto L, Kudson G, Inskip J, Rhodes K, Erskine Y. Asexuality. Arch Sex Behav. 2010;39:599–618.

10
Evaluation of Female Sexual Interest/Arousal Disorder

Cindy M. Meston and Amelia M. Stanton

Female sexual interest/arousal disorder (FSIAD) is the result of merging female hypoactive sexual desire disorder (HSDD) and female arousal disorder (FSAD) in the *DSM-5* (APA, 2013).

Epidemiology (Incidence/Prevalence)

As FSIAD is a new diagnosis, prevalence studies have yet to be published. However, previous work has examined the prevalence of low sexual interest (HSDD) and low sexual arousal (FSAD) in women. Desire concerns are the most frequently reported sexual complaint among women. One of the most frequently cited prevalence studies reported low sexual interest in 22% of women in the general US population [1]. A survey of women from 29 countries yielded rates of self-reported low sexual interest ranging from 26 to 43% [2]. For a clinical diagnosis of HSDD, which requires the presence of significant levels of distress, rates range from 7.3 [3] to 23% [4], depending on a woman's age, cultural background, and reproductive status. In the National Health and Social Life Survey, the first large-scale assessment of the prevalence of sexual problems in the USA, low sexual desire was more common in African-American women compared to Caucasian women [1]. In this survey, low sexual desire was also more common in women with a history of sexually transmitted diseases and in women of low socioeconomic status.

Prevalence studies of sexual arousal problems in women have focused primarily on self-reported lack of vaginal lubrication. These studies have found that 8–15% of all women and 21–31% of sexually active women report experiencing such difficulties (for review, see [5]). Similarly, Bancroft and colleagues [3] found that 31.2% of heterosexual women in the USA reported lubrication problems over the past month. Within the UK, the prevalence of persistent lubrication problems, lasting three months or more, ranged from 2.6 [6] to 28% [7]. The incidence of lubrication problems is higher among peri- and postmenopausal women, with one study reporting that 44% of postmenopausal women experience persistent or recurrent lubrication problems [8]. These studies have not always included all the information necessary to diagnose FSAD, as many did not inquire about distress or level of stimulation. However, research that did assess distress indicated that lubrication problems do not lead to significant distress in many women [3, 9].

Etiology/Pathophysiology

Factors Associated with Female Sexual Interest/Arousal Disorder

Factors associated with FSIAD have not yet been examined. However, past research has elucidated a number of causes of and contributors to HSDD and FSAD in women. These elements are broken down into biological factors, which include medical health, hormones, and medications, and psychological factors, such as stress, relationships, comorbid mental illness, and history of sexual abuse.

Biological Factors Associated with Low Desire

Endocrine levels are the most commonly discussed biological factor that is associated with low sexual interest in women. Decreased ovarian function during menopause, which results in lower estrogen production, has been related to lack of sexual desire. Surgically induced menopause (such as by oophorectomy) causes a sharp drop in estradiol and testosterone, as opposed to the more gradual decline that is characteristic of natural menopause. Epidemiological studies point to this drastic hormonal change as a more prominent risk factor for HSDD than natural menopause, particularly among younger cohorts [10, 11]. Increased sexual desire has been found in women near the time of ovulation [12, 13], and research has shown that decreased sexual desire occurs after chemical suppression of ovarian hormones [14].

W.W. IsHak (ed.), *The Textbook of Clinical Sexual Medicine*, DOI 10.1007/978-3-319-52539-6_10

Sex hormones, specifically androgens, estrogens, and progestins, are also thought to affect female sexual interest and function, but there is still some uncertainty as to which hormones are most important. Estrogens and androgens govern the structure and function of the cervix, vagina, labia, and clitoris. Androgens, which represent the immediate precursor to estrogen synthesis, may be most influential with respect to sexual interest, mood, and energy. There is some controversy surrounding the notion of androgen insufficiency as a potential cause of low sexual desire in women. Researchers originally believed that androgen depletion occurred as an organic result of natural menopause, due to age-related decline in adrenal and ovarian androgen production; now, the field recognizes that the decline in androgen production begins in the early 20s [15]. Though low androgen levels may contribute to low sexual desire in women, the lack of reference ranges for androgens in women has made it difficult to determine when clinical insufficiency is present.

Testosterone levels have been correlated with solitary desire, which is thought to be a "true" measure of desire. In contrast to dyadic desire, or the desire to be sexual with another person, solitary desire is less influenced by social context and more responsive to endogenous physiology. Several studies have indicated that higher levels of testosterone are associated with increased solitary desire [16, 17]. In these same studies, dyadic desire showed no or negative correlation with testosterone. Masturbation, which is considered to be a behavioral index of solitary desire, has been linked to testosterone, such that masturbation frequency was more strongly related to solitary desire when testosterone was low [18]. In other words, women with low testosterone and high masturbation reported higher solitary desire than women with low testosterone and low masturbation.

There has also been recent interest in whether the hormonal changes caused by oral contraception use can lead to low sexual interest in women. Oral contraceptives involve a combination of estrogens and progesterone in varying amounts. The combination of these two hormones may produce substantial increases in the sex hormone-binding globulin, which can lower testosterone levels. It is possible that this decrease in testosterone could contribute to the low sexual desire that is reported by some women who take oral contraceptives. Research on the relationship between oral contraceptives and sexual desire has produced mixed results with studies reporting that oral contraceptives increase, decrease, or do not change women's sexual desire.

Despite the fact that oral contraceptives have been shown to decrease androgen levels, they have not been consistently associated with decreases in sexual desire. When McCall and Meston [19] assessed cues for sexual desire, they determined that contraceptive use did not influence sexual desire in women with or without HSDD. Other studies have shown that oral contraceptives do have a negative impact on libido. For instance, a recent study revealed that women taking oral contraceptives reported significantly lower levels of sexual thoughts and sexual interest compared to nonusers [20]. Similarly, a study of over 1000 German medical students showed that oral contraceptive users had significantly lower scores on the desire subscale of the FSFI than did nonusers [21]; however, the direction of causality could not be determined. It is important to note that, for some women, the benefits derived from the use of oral contraception, such as freedom from the fear of pregnancy and a reduction in menstrual symptoms, may serve to enhance, rather than inhibit, sexual desire.

Certain brain regions and neurotransmitters have been associated with sexual desire. Specifically, research has pointed to the involvement of the prefrontal cortex, locus coeruleus, nucleus accumbens, paraventricular nucleus, and the reward-processing center of the ventral tegmental area. Excitation of these areas involves the action of several neurotransmitters, including dopamine, oxytocin, norepinephrine, and vasopressin, and inhibition of these areas is facilitated by the serotonin, opioid, and endocannabinoid systems. Disruption in any of these processes may result in clinically relevant decreases in sexual desire. Changes in brain structure and chemistry may be additionally reinforced by individual experience, which has been referred to as experience-based neuroplasticity. This construct is not unique to HSDD, as it has been discussed in the context of other conditions [22, 23].

It is well known that many psychoactive medications affect sexual desire. Stahl [24] and Pfaus [25] suggest that drugs may inhibit sexual interest via three distinct pathways: a decrease in dopamine levels, an increase in serotonin at specific serotonin receptors, and an increase in opioids at mu receptors. Among all psychoactive medications, antidepressants are most often associated with low sexual desire. With respect to effects on sexual desire, there are both intra-class and interclass variations among antidepressants. These variations are largely dependent on neurotransmitter receptor profiles and genetics [26]. Selective serotonin reuptake inhibitors (SSRIs), which are most commonly used for the treatment of depression and anxiety, increase serotonin levels and produce a variety of negative sexual side effects in both men and women, including decreased desire. Sexual dysfunction secondary to SSRI use is believed to result, in part, from activation of the serotonin$_2$ receptor. Newer generations of antidepressants that act as antagonists (blockers) at the serotonin$_2$ receptor (e.g., agomelatine (Valdoxan), bupropion (Wellbutrin), moclobemide (Amira), and reboxetine (Edronax)) are associated with fewer sexual side effects [27]. Clayton and colleagues [26] suggest that future research should seek to validate genetic factors associated with antidepressant medications. Doing so would enable personal genotyping and the development of individualized treatment approaches.

General health status can also influence sexual desire. Fatigue, pain, and mood disturbance caused by chronic illness can all contribute to decreased sexual desire. In a large population-based study of postmenopausal women, participants with low sexual desire reported poorer health on several domains of the widely used SF-36 health status measure than did women with no sexual concerns [11]. Physical activity also appears to play a role in sexual desire and overall sexual function, such that greater physical activity may be linked to better sexual function [28, 29].

Biological Factors Associated with Low Arousal

Research has shown that hormones play a unique role in female sexual arousal. Specifically, estrogens influence the physiologic function of tissues, including the lower genital tissues. Estrogens have vasodilatory and vasoprotective effects that regulate blood flow into and out of the vagina and clitoris. Reductions in estradiol during menopause and lactation have been associated with reduced vaginal blood flow, which results in reduced vaginal lubrication. One of the major biological changes that occurs during menopause is a decrease in circulating estrogen, which helps account for decreased genital lubrication and arousal. However, the lack of a precise estrogen "cut off" that indicates whether one's estrogen levels are adequate for sexual arousal makes it is hard to determine if estrogen deficiency can be deemed a specific cause of sexual arousal problems.

Both the sympathetic and the parasympathetic nervous systems (SNS and PNS) play a role in genital arousal in women. Norepinephrine (NE) is the primary neurotransmitter involved in SNS communication, and when measured after exposure to a sexually arousing film, blood levels of NE are higher than pre-film levels [30]. The spinal cord literature provides strong support for the role of the SNS in female sexual arousal. Women with spinal cord injuries between areas T11 and L2 in the spinal cord show a lack of lubrication during psychological sexual arousal [31]. According to Sipski and colleagues [32], this region is associated with sympathetically mediated genital vasocongestion. That is, this is the area of the spinal cord where sympathetic nerves project to the genital region.

Laboratory studies have also provided evidence for the role of the SNS in women's sexual arousal. Meston and colleagues reported that moderate activation of the SNS using either exercise [33–35] or ephedrine [36] increased genital sexual arousal, and suppression of the SNS using clonidine inhibited genital arousal [37]. A recent study proposed that there is an optimal level of SNS activation for women's physiological sexual arousal [38]. Specifically, Lorenz and colleagues [38] found that a moderate increase in SNS activation was associated with greater physiological sexual arousal, while both very low and very high SNS activation were associated with lesser physiological sexual arousal. Similarly, low resting state heart rate variability has been associated with a risk for sexual arousal problems [39]. Heart rate variability is a noninvasive index of autonomic imbalance [40] and has been used to examine the relative role of SNS activity during arousal in women [38]. Mechanisms that interfere with normal SNS activity, such as stress, can lead to sexual arousal concerns.

Various vascular and neurological problems may also negatively impact a woman's ability to become sexually aroused. Researchers have shown reduced sexual arousal in patients with multiple sclerosis [41, 42], pelvic vascular disorder [43], and diabetes [44]. Antidepressants (namely, SSRIs and SNRIs) and other prescription drugs may also decrease sexual arousal and vaginal lubrication in women [45, 46]. Some six forms of hormonal contraceptives have also been shown to reduce arousal [47].

Psychological Factors

Low sexual interest and/or arousal has also been linked with a number of psychosocial factors in both men and women. Murray and Milhausen [48] found that, after controlling for age, relationship satisfaction, and sexual satisfaction, relationship duration significantly predicted variance in sexual desire. Specifically, women's sexual desire decreased as relationship duration increased. Among married women, feelings of overfamiliarity and institutionalization of the relationship are thought to lead to decreased desire. Daily hassles such as worrying about children and paying the bills and high-stress jobs are offenders for suppressing sexual desire, as are a multitude of relationship or partner-related issues. In regard to the latter, couples reporting sexual difficulties have been characterized by sex therapists as being less satisfied with their relationships compared to couples without sexual problems. According to sex therapists, couples with sexual difficulties have an increased number of disagreements, more difficulties with communication and conflict resolution, and more sexual communication problems, including discomfort discussing sexual activities. Warmth, caring, and affection within the relationship are undoubtedly linked to feelings of sexual desire. Beliefs and attitudes about sexuality acquired over the course of sexual development can influence sexual desire and sexual response across the life span. Internalizing passive gender roles or negative attitudes toward sexuality may put women at greater risk of experiencing sexual problems [49, 50].

Societal factors, which differ greatly by region and by culture, may also contribute to low sexual interest and arousal. When women are socialized to believe that being interested in sex is shameful, they may experience guilt and shame both of which have been associated with low levels of sexual desire and arousal [51]. Moreover, women who have negative attitudes toward sexuality and sexual behavior may have difficulty forming healthy sexual relationships. Feminist perspectives on low sexual desire among women in heterosexual relationships place the couple in a larger sociocultural context wherein men's desires are valued and women's either minimized or denied [52]. Wanting to be the object of men's sexual attraction and desire is culturally reinforced, and deviations from such sexual scripts are often socially rejected. In this context, the very notion of discrepant desire between partners becomes suspect. Among lesbian and bisexual women, internalized homophobia may be a source of shame and inhibition toward same-sex sexual activity.

McCall and Meston [19] reported four distinct factors that describe triggers or cues for sexual desire in women. These include emotional bonding cues (e.g., "Feeling a sense of love with your partner," "Feeling a sense of commitment from your partner"), erotic/explicit cues (e.g., "Watching an erotic movie," "Asking for or anticipating sexual activity"), visual/proximity cues (e.g., "Seeing/talking with someone famous," "Seeing a well-toned body"), and romantic/implicit cues (e.g., "Having a romantic dinner with your partner," "Laughing with a romantic partner"). Not surprisingly, when compared to sexually healthy women, women diagnosed with HSDD reported significantly fewer cues in each of these domains.

It is not surprising that sexuality becomes less of a priority when an individual experiences substantial distress in other areas of her life. Psychological conditions such as generalized anxiety disorder, social phobia, obsessive-compulsive disorder, panic disorder, and mood disorders (depression in particular) are all commonly associated with a lack of sexual interest. Anxiety specific to sexual concerns plays a unique role in the development of sexual arousal problems. Barlow [53] proposed that the cognitive distraction of performance anxiety directs attention from sexual to nonsexual cues, which then interferes with arousal. In men, performance anxiety typically relates to attaining and maintaining an erection; in women, "performance" concerns are broader and may be directed at body image or perceived sexual attractiveness. Studies of women indicate that self-consciousness about body image and sexual desirability predicts sexual esteem, sexual assertiveness, and sexual function [54, 55]. Low sexual desire is also comorbid with depression. Rumination about negative events, a common cognitive aspect of depression, likely contributes to this decrease in desire, as women may be focusing exclusively on aspects of sexuality that are unpleasant. Individuals who are experiencing a major depressive episode are more likely to attribute negative events to stable and global causes. This cognitive style could negatively affect one's perception of sexuality.

A history of unwanted sexual experiences can also negatively affect sexual desire. Many, but not all, women with a history of childhood sexual abuse fear sexual intimacy during adulthood. Women with such histories are likely to avoid sexual interactions and are often less receptive to sexual approaches from their partners [56]. Sexual self-schemas, which are defined as cognitive generalizations about sexual aspects of the self that guide sexual behavior and influence the processing of sexually relevant information [57], have been shown to differ between women with and without a history of childhood sexual abuse [58, 59]. A high proportion of women with a history of childhood sexual abuse engage in risky sexual behaviors, such as sexual intercourse with strangers while intoxicated [60]. It is unknown whether this behavior is reflective of high levels of sexual desire, emotional avoidance, an inability to maintain or enforce physical boundaries, or some combination of these reasons. Other studies have found that prior sexual abuse is associated with low sexual interest [61].

Although individual factors may contribute to low sexual desire and decreased sexual arousal, it is valuable to conceptualize these difficulties in the context of the greater relationship with the partner. It is possible that a woman's lack of enthusiasm for sex is a perfectly normal reaction to problems within the relationship, such as a lack of sexual activities that are stimulating and pleasurable to the woman, a highly restricted sexual repertoire, or poor sexual knowledge or skill on the part of her partner. It is not uncommon for a woman's sexual problems to develop concomitantly with sexual problems in her partner. Although previous research has identified partner sexual dysfunction as a frequent reason that women avoid sexual activity, the influence of the partner's sexual problems on sexual interest and arousal has received relatively little study until recently. Women involved with men who have premature ejaculation or erectile dysfunction are at increased risk for sexual desire and arousal problems. Goldstein and colleagues [62] reported that pharmacologic treatment of male erectile dysfunction was associated with improved sexual desire, arousal, and satisfaction among their female partners.

Many of the factors affecting women's sexual desire also affect women's sexual arousal. According to the dual control model proposed by Bancroft and colleagues [63], sexual arousal is the combination of both excitatory and inhibitory forces. Five main themes have been described as potential inhibitors or enhancers of sexual arousal for women ages 18–84 years: feelings about one's body, negative consequences of sexual activity (e.g., bad reputation, pregnancy), feeling desired and accepted by a sexual partner, feeling used by a sexual partner, and negative mood [64].

Definition/Phenomenology/Diagnostic Criteria

In the *DSM-5*, female sexual interest/arousal disorder (FSIAD) is defined as a complete lack of, or significant reduction in, sexual interest or arousal. A woman must have three of the following six symptoms in order to receive the diagnosis: absent or reduced interest in sexual activity, absent or reduced sexual thoughts or fantasies, no or reduced initiation of sexual activity and typically unreceptive to a partner's attempts to initiate, absent or reduced sexual excitement or pleasure in almost all or all sexual encounters, absent or reduced sexual interest/arousal in response to any internal or external sexual cues, and absent or reduced genital or nongenital sensations during sexual activity in all or almost all sexual encounters. These symptoms must have persisted for a minimum of six months and result in clinically significant distress. There must be no indication of a physical, biological, or substance-induced cause for the distressing lack of interest or arousal. The disorder is specified by severity level (mild, moderate, and severe) and subtyped into lifelong versus acquired, generalized versus situational (see Table 10-1).

TABLE 10-1. DSM-5 Diagnostic Criteria for Female Sexual Interest/Arousal Disorder. 302.72 (F52.22)

A. Lack of, or significantly reduced, sexual interest/arousal, as manifested by at least three of the following:
   1. Absent/reduced interest in sexual activity
   2. Absent/reduced sexual/erotic thoughts or fantasies
   3. No/reduced initiation of sexual activity and typically unreceptive to a partner's attempts to initiate
   4. Absent/reduced sexual excitement/pleasure during sexual activity in almost all or all (approximately 75–100%) sexual encounters (in identified situational contexts or, if generalized, in all contexts)
   5. Absent/reduced sexual interest/arousal in response to any internal or external sexual/erotic cues (e.g., written, verbal, visual)
   6. Absent/reduced genital or nongenital sensations during sexual activity in almost all or all (approximately 75–100%) sexual encounters (in identified situational contexts or, if generalized, in all contexts)

B. The symptoms in Criterion A have persisted for a minimum duration of approximately 6 months

C. The symptoms in Criterion A cause clinically significant distress in the individual

D. The sexual dysfunction is not better explained by a nonsexual mental disorder or as a consequence of severe relationship distress (e.g., partner violence) or other significant stressors and is not attributable to the effects of a substance/medication or another medical condition

Specify whether:

Lifelong: The disturbance has been present since the individual became sexually active

Acquired: The disturbance began after a period of relatively normal sexual function

Specify whether:

Generalized: Not limited to certain types of stimulation, situations, or partners

Situational: Only occurs with certain types of stimulation, situations, or partners

Specify current severity:

Mild: Evidence of mild distress over the symptoms in Criterion A

Moderate: Evidence of moderate distress over the symptoms in Criterion A

Severe: Evidence of severe or extreme distress over the symptoms in Criterion A

In past editions of the DSM, sexual interest and sexual arousal have been conceptualized as separate, though related, constructs. Most recently, the *DSM-IV-TR* had separate diagnoses for low or absent interest and arousal, hypoactive sexual desire disorder (HSDD), and female sexual arousal disorder (FSAD), respectively. HSDD was characterized by persistently or recurrently deficient (or absent) sexual desire and fantasies, while FSAD was characterized by continuous or recurrent inability to achieve or maintain sufficient physiological arousal, such as vaginal lubrication or swelling.

During the formulation of the *DSM-5*, the Sexual Dysfunction Subworkgroup referenced various forms of evidence to suggest that desire and arousal cannot be reliably distinguished in women. Sarin and colleagues [65] reported that differentiating desire and arousal in women has been complicated by four specific types of evidence. First, quantitative data has indicated that there is a high degree of comorbidity of desire and arousal disorders [66]. Second, qualitative data has suggested that women may have trouble discriminating between desire and arousal [64, 67, 68]. Third, researchers have found that women's sexual response is nonlinear, as desire may precede or follow arousal within any given sexual encounter [64, 69]. Finally, Sarin and colleagues [65] noted that psychophysiological data (such as vaginal pulse amplitude) does not differentiate sexually healthy women from women who report difficulties becoming genitally aroused [70]. It was also suggested that FSAD as a distinct disorder was problematic in that it focused exclusively on the impairment of genital response and did not incorporate women's subjective perceptions of arousal [71].

The merging of HSDD and FSAD into one diagnosis has led to substantial controversy in the field, as some experts disagree with this new conceptualization [72]. Balon and Clayton [73] reviewed the evidence against the establishment of the new disorder, namely, the lack of field trial testing, and the lack of attention paid to problems with lubrication and other genital sensations that have long been associated with absent or impaired genital sexual arousal. Other evidence cited by Balon and Clayton [73] included unclear symptom distinction (i.e., based on the established six symptoms, a diagnosis of FSIAD can be made without any impairment of physiological arousal) and no proposed underlying pathology. Additionally, recent findings suggest that there is significant genetic sharing between arousal, lubrication, and orgasm, which is independent of desire [74]. Balon and Clayton [73] conclude that the establishment of the new diagnosis risks harm to women who meet *DSM-IV-TR* diagnostic criteria for FSAD or HSDD, but not for FSIAD, as their insurance companies may not cover treatment for their sexual problems. This controversy has led to a number of debates among experts in the field. Ultimately, some organizations, such as the International Society for the Study of Women's Sexual Health (ISSWSH) and the US Food and Drug Administration (FDA), chose to maintain the *DSM-IV* diagnostic criteria for HSDD and FSAD and to preserve the conceptualization of desire and arousal as distinct constructs.

Assessment of Female Sexual Interest/Arousal Disorder

Given that FSIAD is new to *DSM-5*, there are no assessment tools based on the new diagnostic criteria. Therefore, this section draws on the HSDD and FSAD literature.

Assessment

Comprehensive assessment of women's sexual dysfunction includes a detailed clinical interview to gather information on the presenting problem, the woman's sexual and relationship history, her psychosocial history, and her medical history. A gynecological exam may also be warranted.

The assessment of sexual interest in women is difficult due to the subjective and complex nature of sexual desire. Basson's [69] model of the female sexual response introduced the concept of receptive desire. She explained that many women respond sexually when approached by their partner despite not seeking out sexual activity. Therefore, it may be important to gauge a woman's level of responsiveness to sexual stimuli for a thorough assessment of her sexual desire.

When assessing for low sexual desire, clinicians may inquire about sexual thoughts, fantasies, and daydreams; examine the degree to which patients seek out sexually suggestive material; question how often patients have the urge to masturbate or engage in sensual self-touching; and determine level of motivation for partnered sexual activity. Clinicians should also focus on identifying situations or cues that may have stimulated the woman's interest in sex in the past.

If a woman endorses certain "turn-ons," it is useful to determine whether these cues or fantasies are currently absent from her life, fail to interest her any longer, or have been deemed unacceptable to her for some reason. A candid discussion of the woman's attraction to and feelings toward her partner is useful as well. The desire for sex is only one of a multitude of factors informing the choice to be sexual; therefore, frequency of sexual activity should not be considered indicative of a sexual desire problem (or lack thereof). Women engage in sexual activity for a variety of reasons unrelated to sexual desire, including fear, duty, and revenge [75]. Overall, assessment of sexual desire needs to be carefully considered within the context of the dyadic relationship (when relevant) and must take into consideration factors known to affect sexual functioning such as the person's age, religion, culture, the length of the relationship, the partner's sexual function, and the context of the person's life.

Given the close relationship between androgens and sexual desire, laboratory testing may be appropriate. To rule out hormonal causes, clinicians should consider performing assays for prolactin, total testosterone, free testosterone, sex hormone binding globulin (SHBG), dehydroepiandrosterone (DHEA), estrogens, and cortisol. Although diagnostic laboratories routinely provide reference values for these hormones, there is some disagreement as to what differentiates "normal" from "low" and "deficient" hormonal states [76]. Hormone deficiencies are therefore defined primarily by symptoms rather than quantitative cutoff points [77].

Assessment of arousal problems should focus on both the mental and genital aspects of the woman's sexual response. Specifically, the clinician should ascertain the degree of mental excitement the woman experiences in various sexual situations (e.g., when reading erotica alone, when stimulating herself, when her partner stimulates her), the degree and type of genital sensations that are common during her sexual encounters (e.g., pulsing, swelling, tingling, warmth), and the level of genital wetness or lubrication that occurs during sexual activity. Levels of physiological sexual arousal can also be assessed indirectly using a vaginal photoplethysmograph to assess vaginal blood flow, as well as by sonograms (pictures of internal organs derived by sound waves bouncing off organs and other tissues), thermograms (images of radiation in the long-infrared range of the electromagnetic spectrum), and fMRI (imaging techniques that track changes in blood concentration in inner organs) to assess blood engorgement in the genitals. However, these techniques are more commonly used for research purposes than as clinical diagnostic tools.

If it is suspected that vulvovaginal atrophy or compromised pelvic floor muscle function may be contributing to a patient's sexual interest and/or arousal concerns, patients should receive a gynecological examination. A gynecologist can evaluate a woman's level of voluntary control of the pelvic floor muscles, her pelvic floor muscle tone, as well as the presence of vaginal tissue atrophy or infection. It is important to rule out these potential contributors to low sexual desire/arousal before commencing treatment.

Diagnostic Tests, Instruments, or Rating Scales

In addition to the clinical interview, there are a number of validated measures that may help elucidate the degree of sexual dysfunction the woman is experiencing and may also be useful for monitoring treatment-related changes. These include the Brief Index of Sexual Functioning for Women [78], the Changes in Sexual Functioning Questionnaire [79], the Derogatis Interview for Sexual Functioning [80], the Female Sexual Function Index [81], and the Sexual Satisfaction Scale [82] (for review of validated measures, see [83]). Questionnaires that specifically address relationship issues include the Dyadic Adjustment Scale [84], the Relationship Beliefs Scale [85], and the Locke-Wallace Marital Adjustment Test [86]. Scales for measuring female sexual desire are currently in development.

In an effort to create a set of high-quality, self-report assessment tools to measure physical, mental, and social health, the US National Institutes of Health established the Patient-Reported Outcomes Measurement Information System (PROMIS) network (http://nihpromis.org). The first PROMIS Sexual Function and Satisfaction measure (SexFs; [87]) was constructed to assess sexual function and satisfaction in both male and female cancer patients. The second version of the SexFs [88], which was published in 2015, improved upon the original scale by expanding its validity beyond patients with cancer, centering scores around norms for sexually active US adults, and establishing new content domains. The domains that are most relevant to FSIAD include interest in sexual activity and vaginal lubrication for sexual activity. This measure offers researchers and clinicians a flexible and reliable tool for assessing self-reported sexual function and satisfaction.

In general, assessment of both sexual desire and sexual arousal should comprise a complete sexual, medical, and psychosocial history, which can be obtained through standardized interviews and validated self-administered questionnaires mentioned above [89]. The clinician should explore the onset of the sexual problem, taking into account the dates of pregnancies (if applicable), surgeries, medication changes, and diagnoses of medical conditions. In addition to ruling out or identifying various medical factors, the exam serves to educate women about their anatomy and what is normal or problematic. It is also important to assess the context of the problem, especially situations or cues that have stimulated sexual desire and arousal in the past. It should be determined if previous cues for sexual desire or specific instances in which she previously felt aroused are now absent from her life or no longer of interest. The clinician may also explore the woman's feelings about her current sexual partner to look for relationship factors that could be contributing to the sexual difficulties.

Conclusion

Female sexual interest/arousal disorder is associated with a number of biological and psychological factors. The disorder is diagnosed when women are distressed by a persistent absence or notable reduction of mental interest in sexual activity and/or physiological responsiveness to sexual cues for at least six months. Given that the disorder encompasses both sexual desire and sexual arousal concerns, women with FSIAD may have variable symptom profiles. Therefore, a thorough assessment of women who report low sexual desire and/or low sexual arousal is warranted.

References

1. Laumann EO, Paik A, Rosen RC, Page P. Sexual dysfunction in the United States. JAMA. 1999;282(13):1229.
2. Laumann EO, Nicolosi A, Glasser DB, Paik A, Gingell C, Moreira E, et al. Sexual problems among women and men aged 40–80 y: prevalence and correlates identified in the global study of sexual attitudes and behaviors. Int J Impot Res. 2005;17(1):39–57.
3. Bancroft J, Loftus J, Long JS. Distress about sex: a national survey of women in heterosexual relationships. Arch Sex Behav. 2003;32(3):193–208.
4. Witting K, Santtila P, Varjonen M, Jern P, Johansson A, Von Der Pahlen B, et al. Female sexual dysfunction, sexual distress, and compatibility with partner. J Sex Med. 2008;5:2587–99.
5. Lewis RW, Fugl-Meyer KS, Bosch R, Fugl-Meyer AR, Laumann EO, Lizza E, et al. Epidemiology/risk factors of sexual dysfunction. J Sex Med. 2004;1(1):35–9.
6. Mercer CH, Fenton KA, Johnson AM, Wellings K, Macdowall W, McManus S, et al. Sexual function problems and help seeking behaviour in Britain: national probability sample survey. BMJ. 2003;327(7412):426–7.
7. Dunn KM, Croft PR, Hackett GI. Sexual problems: a study of the prevalence and need for health care in the general population. Fam Pract. 1998;15:519–24.
8. Rosen R, Taylor JF, Leiblum SR, Bachmann GA. Prevalence of sexual dysfunction in women: results of a survey study of 329 women in an outpatient gynecological clinic. J Sex Marital Ther. 1993;19(3):171–88.
9. Shifren JL, Monz BU, Russo PA, Segreti A. Sexual problems and distress in United States women. Obstet Gynecol. 2008;112(5):970–8.
10. Dennerstein L, Koochaki P, Barton I, Graziottin A. Hypoactive sexual desire disorder in menopausal women: a survey of Western European women. J Sex Med. 2006;3:212–22.
11. Leiblum SR, Koochaki PE, Rodenberg CA, Barton IP, Rosen RC. Hypoactive sexual desire disorder in postmenopausal women: US results from the Women's International Study of Health and Sexuality (WISHeS). Menopause. 2006;13(1):46–56.
12. Diamond LM, Wallen K. Sexual minority women's sexual motivation around the time of ovulation. Arch Sex Behav. 2011;40(2):237–46.
13. Pillsworth EG, Haselton MG, Buss DM. Ovulatory shifts in female sexual desire. J Sex Res. 2004;41(1):55–65.
14. Schmidt PJ, Rubinow DR. Sex hormones and mood in the perimenopause. Ann N Y Acad Sci. 2009;1179:70–85.
15. Sandhu KS, Melman A, Mikhail MS. Impact of hormones on female sexual function and dysfunction. Female Pelvic Med Reconstr Surg. 2011;17(1):8–16.
16. Van Anders SM, Brotto LA, Farrell J, Yule M. Associations among physiological and subjective sexual response, sexual desire, and salivary steriod hormones in healthy premenopausal women. J Sex Med. 2009;6:739–51.
17. Van Anders SM, Gray PB. Hormones and human partnering. Annu Rev Sex Res. 2007;18:60–93.
18. Van Anders SM. Testosterone and sexual desire in healthy women and men. Arch Sex Behav. 2012;41(6):1471–84.
19. McCall KM, Meston CM. Cues resulting in desire for sexual activity in women. J Sex Med. 2006;3(5):838–52.
20. Davison SL, Bell RJ, LaChina M, Holden SL, Davis SR. Sexual function in well women: stratification by sexual satisfaction, hormone use, and menopause status. J Sex Med. 2008;5:1214–22.

21. Wallwiener CW, Wallwiener LM, Seeger H, Muck AO, Bitzer J, Wallwiener M. Prevalence of sexual dysfunction and impact of contraception in female German medical students. J Sex Med. 2010;7:2139–48.
22. Wexler BE. Review article neuroplasticity , cultural evolution and cultural difference. World Cult Psychiatry Res Rev. 2010;Summer: 11–22.
23. Wittenberg GF. Experience, cortical remapping, and recovery in brain disease. Neurobiol Dis. 2010;37(2):252–8 .Elsevier B.V
24. Stahl SM. Targeting circuits of sexual desire as a treatment strategy for hypoactive sexual desire disorder. J Clin Psychiatry. 2010;71(7):821–2.
25. Pfaus JG. Pathways of sexual desire. J Sex Med. 2009;6(6):1506–33.
26. Clayton AH, El Haddad S, Iluonakhamhe J-P, Ponce Martinez C, Schuck AE. Sexual dysfunction associated with major depressive disorder and antidepressant treatment. Expert Opin Drug Saf. 2014;13(10):1361–74.
27. Keks NA, Hope J, Culhane C. Management of antidepressant-induced sexual dysfunction. Australas Psychiatry. 2014;22(6):525–8.
28. Dennerstein L, Lehert P. Women's sexual functioning, lifestyle, mid-age, and menopause in 12 European countries. Menopause. 2004;11(6 Pt 2):778–85.
29. Gerber JR, Johnson JV, Bunn JY, O'Brien SL. A longitudinal study of the effects of free testosterone and other psychosocial variables on sexual function during the natural traverse of menopause. Fertil Steril. 2005;83(3):643–8.
30. Exton NG, Chau Truong T, Exton MS, Wingenfeld SA, Leygraf N, Saller B, et al. Neuroendocrine response to film-induced sexual arousal in men and women. Psychoneuroendocrinology. 2000;25: 187–99.
31. Sipski ML, Alexander CJ, Rosen RC. Physiological parameters associated with sexual arousal in women with incomplete spinal cord injury. Arch Phys Med Rehabil. 1997;78:305–13.
32. Sipski ML, Alexander CJ, Rosen R. Sexual arousal and orgasm in women: Effects of spinal cord injury. Ann Neurol. 2001;49(1): 35–44.
33. Meston CM, Gorzalka BB. Differential effects of sympathetic activation on sexual arousal in sexually dysfunctional and functional women. J Abnorm Psychol. 1996 Nov;105(4):582–91.
34. Meston CM, Gorzalka BB. The effects of immediate, delayed, and residual sympathetic activation on sexual arousal in women. Behav Res Ther. 1996;34(2):143–8.
35. Meston CM, Gorzalka BB. The effects of sympathetic activation on physiological and subjective sexual arousal in women. Behav Res Ther. 1995;33(6):651–64.
36. Meston CM, Heiman JR. Ephedrine-activated physiological sexual arousal in women. Arch Gen Psychiatry. 1998;55(7):652–6.
37. Meston CM, Gorzalka BB, Wright JM. Inhibition of subjective and physiological sexual arousal in women by clonidine. Psychosom Med. 1997;59:339–407.
38. Lorenz TA, Harte CB, Hamilton LD, Meston CM. Evidence for a curvilinear relationship between sympathetic nervous system activation and women's physiological sexual arousal. Psychophysiology. 2012;49(1):111–7.
39. Stanton AM, Lorenz TA, Pulverman CS, Meston CM. Heart rate variability: a risk factor for female sexual dysfunction. Appl Psychophysiol Biofeedback. 2015;40(3):229–37.
40. Xhyheri B, Manfrini O, Mazzolini M, Pizzi C, Bugiardini R. Heart rate variability today. Prog Cardiovasc Dis. 2012;55(3):321–31.
41. Hulter, B. (1999). Sexual function in women with neurological disorders (Doctoral dissertation, Acta Universitatis Upsaliensis).
42. Lew-Starowicz M, Rola R. Prevalence of sexual dysfunctions among women with multiple sclerosis. Sex Disabil. 2013;31(2):141–53.
43. Schover LR, Jensen SB. Sexual problems and chronic disease: a comprehensive approach. New York, NY: Guilford Press; 1988.
44. Spector IP, Leiblum SR, Carey MP, Rosen RC. Diabetes and female sexual function: a critical review. Ann Behav Med. 1993;15(4):257–64.
45. Frohlich PF, Meston CM. Evidence that serotonin affects female sexual functioning via peripheral mechanisms. Physiol Behav. 2000;71(3–4):383–93.
46. Kennedy SH, Rizvi S. Sexual dysfunction, depression, and the impact of antidepressants. J Clin Psychopharmacol. 2009;29(2):157–64.
47. Smith NK, Jozkowski KN, Sanders SA. Hormonal contraception and female pain, orgasm, and sexual pleasure. J Sex Med. 2014;11(2):462–70.
48. Murray SH, Milhausen RR. Sexual desire and relationship duration in young men and women. J Sex Marital Ther. 2012;38(1):28–40.
49. Nobre PJ, Pinto-Gouveia J. Dysfunctional sexual beliefs as vulnerability factors to sexual dysfunction. J Sex Res. 2006;43(1):68–75.
50. Nobre PJ, Pinto-Gouveia J. Differences in automatic thoughts presented during sexual activity between sexually functional and dysfunctional men and women. Cognit Ther Res. 2008;32(1): 37–49.
51. Woo JST, Brotto L. a, Gorzalka BB. The relationship between sex guilt and sexual desire in a community sample of Chinese and Euro-Canadian women. J Sex Res. 2012;49(2–3):290–8.
52. Richgels PB. Hypoactive sexual desire in heterosexual women: a feminist analysis. Women Ther. 1992;12(1–2):123–35.
53. Barlow DH. Causes of sexual dysfunction: The role of anxiety and cognitive interference. J Consult Clin Psychol. 1986;54(2):140–8.
54. Dove NL, Wiederman MW. Cognitive distraction and women's sexual functioning. J Sex Marital Ther. 2000;26(1):67–78.
55. Wiederman MW. Women's body image self-consciousness during physical intimacy with a partner. J Sex Res. 2000;37(1):60–8.
56. Rellini A. Review of the empirical evidence for a theoretical model to understand the sexual problems of women with a history of CSA. J Sex Med. 2008;5(1):31–46.
57. Andersen BL, Cyranowski JM. Women's sexual self-schema. J Pers Soc Psychol. 1994;67(6):1079–100.
58. Meston CM, Rellini AH, Heiman JR. Women's history of sexual abuse, their sexuality, and sexual self-schemas. J Consult Clin Psychol. 2006;74(2):229–36.
59. Stanton AM, Boyd RL, Pulverman CS, Meston CM. Determining women's sexual self-schemas through advanced computerized text analysis. Child Abuse Negl. 2015;46:78–88.
60. Bensley LS, Van Eenwyk J, Simmons KW. Self-reported childhood sexual and physical abuse and adult HIV-risk behaviors and heavy drinking. Am J Prev Med. 2000;18(2):151–8.
61. Leonard LM, Follette VM. Sexual functioning in women reporting a history of child sexual abuse: review of the empirical literature and clinical implications. Annu Rev Sex Res. 2002;13(1): 346–88.
62. Goldstein I, Fisher WA, Sand M, Rosen RC, Mollen M, Brock G, et al. Women's sexual function improves when partners are administered vardenafil for erectile dysfunction: a prospective, randomized, double-blind, placebo-controlled trial. J Sex Med. 2005;2(6):819–32.
63. Bancroft J, Janssen E. The dual control model of male sexual response: a theoretical approach to centrally mediated erectile dysfunction. Neurosci Biobehav Rev. 2000;24(5):571–9.
64. Graham CA, Sanders SA, Milhausen RR, Mcbride KR. Turning on and turning off: a focus group study of the factors that affect women's sexual arousal. Arch Sex Behav. 2004;33(6):527–38.
65. Sarin S, Amsel R, Binik YM. A streetcar named "Derousal"? A psychophysiological examination of the desire–arousal distinction in sexually functional and dysfunctional women. J Sex Res. 2015;53(6):711–29.

66. Basson R, Leiblum SR, Brotto LA, Derogatis LR, Fourcroy JL, Fugl-Meyer KS, et al. Definitions of women's sexual dysfunction reconsidered: advocating expansion and revision. J Psychosom Obstet Gynecol. 2003;24:221–9.
67. Brotto LA, Heiman JR, Tolman DL. Narratives of desire in mid-age women with and Without arousal difficulties. J Sex Res. 2009;46(5):387–98.
68. Mitchell KR, Wellings KA, Graham C. How do men and women define sexual desire and sexual arousal? J Sex Marital Ther. 2014;40(1):17–32.
69. Basson R. The female sexual response: a different model. J Sex Marital Ther. 2000;26(1):51–65.
70. Laan E, Van Driel EM, Van Rik H.W. Van Lunsen. Genital responsiveness in healthy women with and without sexual arousal disorder. J Sex Med. 2008;5(6):1424–35.
71. Graham CA. The DSM diagnostic criteria for female sexual arousal disorder. Arch Sex Behav. 2010;39(2):240–55.
72. Clayton AH, Derogatis LR, Rosen RC, Pyke R. Intended or unintended consequences? The likely implications of raising the bar for sexual dysfunction diagnosis in the proposed DSM-V revisions: 2. For women WITH loss of subjective sexual arousal. J Sex Med. 2012;9(8):2040–6.
73. Balon R, Clayton AH. Female sexual interest/arousal disorder: a diagnosis out of thin air. Arch Sex Behav. 2014;43(7):1227–9.
74. Burri A, Greven C, Leupin M, Spector T, Rahman Q. A multivariate twin study of female sexual dysfunction. J Sex Med. 2012;9(10):2671–81.
75. Meston CM, Buss DM. Why women have sex. New York: St. Martin's Press; 2009.
76. Guay AT, Spark R. Pathophysiology of sex steroids in women. In: Goldstein I, Meston CM, Davis SR, Traish AM, editors. Women's sexual function and dysfunction: study, diagnosis, and treatment. New York: Taylor & Francis Group; 2006. p. 218–27.
77. Bachmann G, Braunstein G, Burger H, Dennerstein L, Leiblum S. Female androgen insufficiency: the Princeton consensus statement on definition, classification, and assessment. Fertil Steril. 2002;77(4):661–5.
78. Taylor JF, Rosen RC, Leiblum SR. Self-report assessment of female sexual function: psychometric evaluation of the brief index of sexual function for women. Arch Sex Behav. 1994;23:627–43.
79. Clayton AH, McGarvey EL, Clavet GJ. The Changes in Sexual Functioning Questionnaire (CSFQ): development, reliability, and validity. Psychopharmacol Bull. 1997;33:371–45.
80. Derogatis L. The Derogatis interview for sexual functioning (DISF/DISF-SR): an introductory report. J Sex Marital Ther. 1979;23:291–04.
81. Rosen R, Brown C, Heiman J, Leiblum S, Meston C, Shabsigh R, et al. The Female Sexual Function Index (FSFI): a multidimensional self-report instrument for the assessment of female sexual function. J Sex Marital Ther. 2000;26(2):191–208.
82. Meston C, Trapnell P. Development and validation of a five-factor sexual satisfaction and distress scale for women: the SEXUAL Satisfaction Scale for Women (SSS-W). J Sex Med. 2005;2(1):66–81.
83. Meston CM, Derogatis LR. Validated instruments for assessing female sexual function. J Sex Marital Ther. 2002;28:155–64.
84. Spanier GB. Measuring dyadic adjustment: new scales for assessing the quality of marriage and similar dyads. J Marriage Fam. 1976;38:15–28.
85. Fletcher G, Kininmonth L. Measuring relationship beliefs: an individual differences scale. J Res Pers. 1992;26:371–97.
86. Locke H, Wallace K. Short marital adjustment and prediction tests: their reliability and validity. J Marriage Fam Living. 1959;2:251–5.
87. Flynn KE, Lin L, Cyranowski JM, Reeve BB, Reese JB, Jeffery DD, et al. Development of the NIH PROMIS® sexual function and satisfaction measures in patients with cancer. J Sex Med. 2013;10(01):43–52.
88. Weinfurt KP, Lin L, Bruner DW, Cyranowski JM, Dombeck CB, Hahn EA, et al. Development and initial validation of the PROMIS® sexual function and satisfaction measures version 2.0. J Sex Med. 2015;12(9):1961–74.
89. Stewart E. Physical examination and female sexual dysfunction. In: Goldstein I, Meston CM, Davis S, Traish A, editors. Women's sexual function and dysfunction: study, diagnosis, and treatment. Boca Raton: Taylor & Francis Group; 2005. p. 347–55.

11
Treatment of Female Sexual Interest/Arousal Disorder

Cindy M. Meston and Amelia M. Stanton

Introduction

Female sexual interest/arousal disorder (FSIAD) is a new diagnosis in *DSM-5* for which there are currently no published treatment studies. Therefore, this chapter is based on the treatment research literature for hypoactive sexual desire disorder (HSDD) and female sexual arousal disorder (FSAD), which were included in *DSM-IV-TR*.

Biological Treatments

Androgens

For peri- and postmenopausal women experiencing low sexual desire as a result of biologically compromised natural levels of androgens, testosterone replacement therapy can sometimes be an effective treatment option. There are currently no testosterone products for the treatment of low sexual desire in women that have been approved by the FDA, due in part to lack of long-term safety studies assessing the potential risk for cardiovascular disease and breast cancer. However, many clinicians prescribe "off-label" testosterone, in the form of patches or pills, to women who are distressed by low sexual desire [1]. One estimate suggests that 4.1 million prescriptions for off-label testosterone are made annually in the United States [2]. The use of transdermal testosterone for low sexual desire in women with surgically induced menopause was approved by the European Medicines Agency in 2010 but has yet to be approved by the FDA or Health Canada. In addition, Androfeme, a 1% daily testosterone cream that is only available in Australia, has been shown to increase sexual motivation in women [3].

Estrogen/Tibolone

Estrogen treatment and tibolone therapy are other hormonal therapies for low sexual desire. Estrogen treatment is particularly efficacious for desire problems that stem from vulvovaginal atrophy. Given the established relationship between low levels of estrogen and atrophy, estrogen therapy is the first-line treatment for this particular condition [4]. Tibolone is a 19-nortestosterone derivative and a selective tissue estrogenic activity regulator with estrogenic, progestogenic, and androgenic properties [5]. Available in 90 countries (but not in the United States), tibolone is typically used for the treatment of endometriosis and as hormone therapy for postmenopausal women. It has also been shown to increase sexual desire and lubrication. Nijland and colleagues [6] demonstrated an overall improvement in sexual function in women receiving tibolone. There are some concerns, however, that tibolone may increase the risk of breast cancer recurrence [7] and stroke [8] in older women.

Flibanserin

Flibanserin (Addyi) was approved by the FDA in 2015 for the treatment of HSDD in premenopausal women after studies showed that the drug increased self-reports of sexually satisfying events and led to significant increases in desire, as measured by the FSFI [9]. Flibanserin (Addyi), a multifunctional serotonin agonist and antagonist (MSAA), acts on different neurotransmitters in the brain. The drug increases levels of norepinephrine and dopamine while reducing levels of serotonin in the prefrontal cortex, nucleus accumbens, and medial preoptic area, all three of which are brain regions that regulate sexual desire in women.

A recent systematic review and meta-analysis of the effects of flibanserin (Addyi) on sexual desire in women revealed that, on average, treatment with the drug resulted in one-half additional sexually satisfying events per month, and women's mean global impression of improvement scores indicated minimal improvement to no change [10]. The authors of the review suggested that the overall quality of the current evidence supporting the use of the drug in clinical practice was low.

W.W. IsHak (ed.), *The Textbook of Clinical Sexual Medicine*, DOI 10.1007/978-3-319-52539-6_11

Nonhormonal Centrally Acting Agents

There is some research on other nonhormonal, centrally acting medications for low desire and arousal problems in women. Bupropion (Wellbutrin) is a norepinephrine-dopamine reuptake inhibitor (NDRI) that has been approved by the FDA as an antidepressant and as a smoking cessation aid (branded as Zyban). When used to treat hypoactive sexual desire among nondepressed premenopausal women, bupropion (Wellbutrin) led to modest improvements in sexual interest and arousal [11]. Buspirone (BuSpar), a serotonin 5-HT1A partial agonist, is typically prescribed for the treatment of generalized anxiety disorder or for relief from acute anxiety symptoms. When administered to counteract the sexual side effects of an SSRI, buspirone (BuSpar) led to a significant increase in sexual function compared to placebo [12]. There is preliminary evidence to suggest that intranasal bremelanotide may also be beneficial for treating low sexual desire in women [5].

Vasodilator Drugs/PDE-5 Inhibitors

Since the success of using PDE-5 inhibitors (e.g., sildenafil (Viagra), tadalafil (Cialis), vardenafil hydrochloride (Levitra)) to treat erectile dysfunction, researchers have attempted to find a comparable drug for women with sexual desire or arousal concerns.

Evidence from limited placebo-controlled studies indicates that sildenafil (Viagra) increases genital engorgement in healthy, premenopausal women [13] and in postmenopausal women with severe levels of genital arousal concerns [14]. Despite reports of increased physiological sexual arousal, studies in general have not found that these drugs positively impact a woman's psychological experience of sexual arousal. This suggests that, for women, psychological factors such as relationship satisfaction, mood state, and sexual scenarios may play a more important role in facilitating increased sexual arousal than do physiological genital cues. If this is the case, drugs that target increasing vasocongestion are likely to be most effective in women whose primary complaint is decreased genital responding, experienced as decreases in lubrication and/or feelings of vaginal fullness or engorgement. Patients with this primary complaint would most likely be women who are postmenopausal, women who have undergone oophorectomy, or women who suffer from arterial vascular problems. For some women, if a drug increases vaginal engorgement to the extent that the sensations are detected and labeled as *sexual feelings*, vasodilator drugs may also enhance general, psychological arousal.

Studies on vasodilator drugs for women have revealed a notable placebo effect on women's sexual arousal. Up to 40% of women in the placebo groups of randomized clinical trials for sildenafil (Viagra) and other pharmacological agents report significant improvements in sexual arousal [15]. It appears that nonspecific factors such as treatment expectancies, having contact with a sexuality professional, and monitoring sexual response can exert a powerful influence on women's sexual arousal and satisfaction at large.

Combination Drugs

Lybrido and Lybridos are combination drugs that are currently in development for the treatment of FSIAD. Lybrido is the combination of sublingual testosterone and a PDE-5 inhibitor [16]. Designed for women who have a low sensitivity to sexual cues, Lybrido has been associated with statistically significant increases in sexual satisfaction compared to placebo [17, 18]. Lybridos is the combination of sublingual testosterone and buspirone, a 5-HT_{1A} receptor agonist [16]. Buspirone is believed to counter the sexual inhibition mechanism, so Lybridos was developed specifically for women who experience sexual inhibition during sexual stimulation or partnered sexual activity. Compared to placebo, the combination of testosterone and buspirone increased sexual satisfaction in sexually dysfunctional women [19].

Topical Lubricants

Though some studies have tested the effects of pharmacological agents on genital arousal, decreased physiological sexual arousal is most commonly treated with topical lubricants. Topical lubricants help mask impairments in vaginal lubrication but do not, however, enhance genital/clitoral blood flow or increase other genital sensations, such as warmth, fullness, and tingling.

EROS Clitoral Therapy Device

Though there are no FDA-approved pharmacological treatments for sexual arousal problems in women, the EROS clitoral therapy device (Urometrics, St. Paul, Minnesota) has been approved by the FDA to address arousal concerns. This small handheld device increases vasocongestion in the clitoral and labial region via a suction mechanism and has been reported to increase vaginal lubrication and sensation [20].

Herbal Supplements

Several herbal supplements, including gingko biloba, ginseng, and maca, have been examined in relation to female sexual arousal and desire. Gingko biloba, a living fossil tree that is typically grown in China, contains glycosides and terpenoids, which have been used in traditional Chinese medicine to stimulate blood flow and improve memory. Despite some initial case studies highlighting of the facilitatory effect of gingko biloba on sexual function, several randomized placebo-controlled trials have found that gingko biloba neither significantly increases sexual arousal or desire in women (e.g., [21]) nor improves antidepressant-induced sexual dysfunction [22, 23]. Ginseng, a slow-growing perennial plant with fleshy roots, is common ingredient in many contemporary Asian medicines. Anecdotal reports suggest that ginseng may increase sexual interest, particularly in women with antidepressant-induced sexual dysfunction. Specifically, ginseng's phytoestrogen activity may increase libido, but research has yet to verify this hypothesis [24]. Maca is a Peruvian plant that is characterized by its hypocotyl, which can be eaten as a root vegetable or employed as a medicinal herb. Native Andean populations have used dried hypocotyls to enhance sexual function and fertility [25]. The results of one small, placebo-controlled trial suggested that maca decreases symptoms of sexual dysfunction in healthy postmenopausal women [26]. In general, researchers have concluded that, though some herbal supplements may hold promise as treatments for female sexual dysfunction, there is no plant that currently has a strong enough level of evidence to be considered efficacious [27].

Psychosocial Treatments

Psychological treatments for low desire include education about factors that affect sexual desire, relationship-building exercises (e.g., scheduling times for physical and emotional intimacy), communication training (e.g., opening up about sexual needs and concerns), cognitive restructuring of problematic beliefs (e.g., a good sexual experience does not always end with an orgasm), sexual fantasy training (e.g., training people to develop and explore mental imagery), and sensate focus. Sensate focus, introduced by Masters and Johnson in the 1970s, is a behavioral technique that emphasizes increased focus on pleasurable sensations brought about through touch and decreased attention on goal-directed sex (e.g., achieving orgasm). In the beginning stages of sensate focus, couples are asked to touch each other's bodies and assess for sexual sensations but to refrain from touching breasts or genitals and engaging in intercourse. Over time, couples touch more and more areas in order to build organic desire, in preparation for intercourse. When desire has been fully heightened, couples are encouraged to have intercourse. Cognitive-behavioral techniques may be useful when traditional sex therapy and education alone are not effective or appropriate. These therapies are distinguished in large part by techniques used to challenge beliefs that undermine sexual desire and arousal, such as unrealistic expectations of performance, self-consciousness, and the notion that one is innately dysfunctional.

Mindfulness-based approaches, which cultivate active awareness of the body and its sensations in a present-centered, nonjudgmental manner, have recently been implicated as potentially beneficial for women with FSIAD [5, 28]. Mindfulness may affect sexual function through improved interoceptive awareness [29] and increased attention to sexually relevant physiological cues [30]. By focusing on the physical sensations of sexual activity instead of being preoccupied with sexual performance or with current level of desire or arousal, couples can learn to be present and respond to their partner during the sexual situation.

Psychosocial treatment for problems with sexual desire and arousal may also include identifying distracting or negative thoughts, and encouraging women to let go of these thoughts during sexual activity. Leiblum and Wiegel [31] described four such types of distracting thoughts in women: negative emotions, body image concerns (e.g., focusing on unattractive aspects of one's body), performance anxiety, and myths and misconceptions (e.g., "Women are not supposed to enjoy sex"). Behavioral techniques designed to help men and women explore their sexual likes and dislikes, alone or with their partners, can help create associations between sexual behaviors and positive experiences or affect. For individuals who are distracted by feelings of shame or embarrassment about their bodies, cognitive restructuring might involve helping them to identify their fears (e.g., a fear of rejection) and maladaptive beliefs (e.g., "My partner thinks my body is not sexy") and then test the accuracy of these beliefs through a series of behavioral experiments. For example, a woman who keeps her clothing on during sex because she feels that her partner would reject her if he saw her naked would be encouraged to incrementally remove pieces of clothing and test the reaction of her partner. These experiments aim to reduce avoidance behavior and provide corrective experiences to counteract maladaptive beliefs.

Conclusion

Women who present with symptoms of FSIAD require individualized treatment strategies that may include some combination of biological, pharmacologic, and behavioral approaches. Most primary care providers will refer patients with symptoms of FSIAD to qualified sexual medicine specialists, who will guide women through the treatment process. Women with FSIAD may have more than one sexual complaint; therefore, careful treatment planning is essential to ensure that all problems are addressed. Researchers and clinicians agree that there is a need to continue to develop safe and effective treatments for sexual desire and arousal concerns. Future research may also explore novel ways to disseminate FSIAD interventions into both primary care and general gynecology in order to reach the greatest number of women who are in need of services.

References

1. Kingsberg SA, Knudson G. Female sexual disorders: assessment, diagnosis, and treatment. CNS Spectr. 2011;16(2):49–62.
2. Davis SR, Braunstein GD. Efficacy and safety of testosterone in the management of hypoactive sexual desire disorder in postmenopausal women. J Sex Med. 2012;9(4):1134–48.
3. El-Hage G, Eden JA, Manga RZ. A double-blind, randomized, placebo-controlled trial of the effect of testosterone cream on the sexual motivation of menopausal hysterectomized women with hypoactive sexual desire disorder. Climacteric. 2007;10(4):335–43.
4. Tan O, Bradshaw K, Carr BR. Management of vulvovaginal atrophy-related sexual dysfunction in postmenopausal women: An up-to-date review. Menopause. 2012;19(1):109–17.
5. Brotto L, Luria M. Sexual interest/arousal disorder in women. In: Binik YM, Hall KSK, editors. Principles and practice of sex therapy. 5th ed. New York: Gilford Press; 2014. P. 17–41.
6. Nijland EA, Weijmar SW, Nathorst-Boos J, Helmond FA, Van Lunsen RH, Palacios S, et al. Tibolone and transdermal E2/NETA for the treatment of female sexual dysfunction in naturally menopausal women: results of a randomized active-controlled trial. J Sex Med. 2008;5(3):646–56.
7. Kenemans P, Bundred NJ, Foidart JM, Kubista E, von Schoultz B, Sismondi P, et al. Safety and efficacy of tibolone in breast-cancer patients with vasomotor symptoms: a double-blind, randomized, non-inferiority trial. Lancet Oncol. 2009;10(2):135–46.
8. Cummings SR, Ettinger B, Delmas PD, Kenemans P, Stathopoulos V, Verweij P, et al. The effects of tibolone in older postmenopausal women. N Engl J Med. 2008;359(7):697–708.
9. Rosen R, Brown C, Heiman J, Leiblum S, Meston C, Shabsigh R, et al. The female sexual function index (FSFI): a multidimensional self-report instrument for the assessment of female sexual function. J Sex Marital Ther. 2000;26(2):191–208.
10. Jaspers L, Feys F, Bramer WM, Franco OH, Leusink P, Laan ETM. Efficacy and safety of flibanserin for the treatment of hypoactive sexual desire disorder in women: a systematic review and meta-analysis. JAMA Intern Med. 2016;176(4):453–62.
11. Segraves RT, Clayton A, Croft H, Wolf A, Warnock J. Bupropion sustained release (SR) for the treatment of hypoactive sexual desire disorder (HSDD) in nondepressed women. J Sex Marital Ther. 2004;27(3):303–16.
12. Landen M, Eriksson E, Agren H, Fahlen T. Effect of buspirone on sexual dysfunction in depressed patients treated with selective serotonin reuptake inhibitors. J Clin Psychopharmacol. 1999;19(3):268–71.
13. Laan E, Smith MD, Boolell M, Quirk F. Development of a sexual function questionnaire for clinical trials of female sexual dysfunction. J Womens Health Gend Based Med. 2002;11(3):277–89.
14. Basson R, Brotto LA. Sexual psychophysiology and effects of sildenafil citrate in oestrogenised women with acquired genital arousal disorder and impaired orgasm: a randomised controlled trial. BJOG. 2003;110(11):1014–24.
15. Basson R, McInnes R, Smith MD, Hodgson G, Koppiker N. Efficacy and safety of sildenafil citrate in women with sexual dysfunction associated with female sexual arousal disorder. J Womens Health Gender Based Med. 2002;11(4):367–77.
16. Van Rooij K, De Leede L, Frijlink HW, Bloemers J, Poels S, Koppeschaar H, et al. Pharmacokinetics of a prototype formulation of sublingual testosterone and a buspirone tablet, versus an advanced combination tablet of testosterone and buspirone in healthy premenopausal women. Drugs R D. 2014;14(2):125–32.
17. Poels S, Bloemers J, van Rooij K, Goldstein I, Gerritsen J, van Ham D, et al. Toward personalized sexual medicine (part 2): testosterone combined with a PDE5 inhibitor increases sexual satisfaction in women with HSDD and FSAD, and a low sensitive system for sexual cues. J Sex Med. 2013;10(3):810–23.
18. Van Der Made F, Bloemers J, Yassem WE, Kleiverda G, Everaerd W, Van Ham D, et al. The influence of testosterone combined with a PDE5-inhibitor on cognitive, affective, and physiological sexual functioning in women suffering from sexual dysfunction. J Sex Med. 2009;6(3):777–90.
19. van Rooij K, Poels S, Bloemers J, Goldstein I, Gerritsen J, van Ham D, et al. Toward personalized sexual medicine (part 3): testosterone combined with a serotonin1A receptor agonist increases sexual satisfaction in women with HSDD and FSAD, and dysfunctional activation of sexual inhibitory mechanisms. J Sex Med. 2013; 10(3):824–37.
20. Billups KL, Berman L, Berman J, Metz ME, Glennon ME, Goldstein I. A new non-pharmacological vacuum therapy for female sexual dysfunction. J Sex Marital Ther. 2001;27(5):435–41.
21. Meston CM, Rellini AH, Telch MJ. Short- and long-term effects of *Ginkgo biloba* extract on sexual dysfunction in women. Arch Sex Behav. 2008;37(4):530–47.
22. Kang B-J, Lee S-J, Kim M-D, Cho M-J. A placebo-controlled, double-blind trial of *Ginkgo biloba* for antidepressant-induced sexual dysfunction. Hum Psychopharmacol. 2002;17(6):279–84.
23. Wheatley D. Triple-blind, placebo-controlled trial of *Ginkgo biloba* in sexual dysfunction due to antidepressant drugs. Hum Psychopharmacol. 2004;19(8):545–8.
24. Rowland DL, Tai W. A review of plant-derived and herbal approaches to the treatment of sexual dysfunctions a review of plant-derived and herbal dysfunctions. J Sex Marital Ther. 2003;29(3):185–205.
25. Gonzales GF. Ethnobiology and ethnopharmacology of *Lepidium meyenii* (Maca), a plant from the peruvian highlands. Evid Based Complement Altern Med. 2012;2012:193496.
26. Brooks NA, Wilcox G, Walker KZ, Ashton JF, Cox MB, Stojanovska L. Beneficial effects of *Lepidium meyenii* (Maca) on psychological symptoms and measures of sexual dysfunction in postmenopausal women are not related to estrogen or androgen content. Menopause. 2008;15(6):1157–62.
27. Mazaro-Costa R, Andersen ML, Hachul H, Tufik S. Medicinal plants as alternative treatments for female sexual dysfunction: utopian vision or possible treatment for climacteric women? J Sex Med. 2010;7(11):3695–714.
28. Brotto LA, Basson R. Group mindfulness-based therapy significantly improves sexual desire in women. Behav Res Ther. 2014; 57:43–54.
29. Silverstein RG, Brown AC, Roth HD, Britton WB. Effects of mindfulness training on body awareness to sexual stimuli: implications for female sexual dysfunction. Psychosom Med. 2011;73(9):817–25.
30. de Jong D. The role of attention in sexual arousal: Implications for treatment of sexual dysfunction. J Sex Res. 2009;46(2–3):237–48.
31. Leiblum SR, Wiegel M. Psychotherapeutic interventions for treating female sexual dysfunction. World J Urol. 2002;20(2):127–36.

12 Evaluation of Erectile Disorder

Ahmed I. El-Sakka

Introduction

Erectile dysfunction (ED) has been defined clinically as the inability to attain and/or maintain penile erection sufficient for satisfactory sexual performance [1]. Our modern understanding of erectile physiology and pathophysiology began relatively recently in the seventies of the last century and has led to the discovery of numerous organic etiologies [2]. In recent years research has been focused on not only developing better treatments, but also at enhancing the diagnosis that are constantly being evaluated and refined to yield optimal and cost effective results.

The eventual ambition of treating a man with ED is to convert the sexually crippled patient and his disappointed partner to a satisfied, sexually active couple. The therapeutic strategy is either to interfere with the underlying cause of ED or to bypass the etiology and offer a nonspecific, personally and socially accepted treatment. Nevertheless, important considerations such as patient age, general health, as well as patient and partner desires and expectations should not be neglected. Nowadays, a variety of treatment options are available. A tailored diagnostic approach for each treatment option is strongly recommended. Whereas an extensive investigation was previously reported to diagnose ED, recent treatment guidelines promote a more minimalist, goal-oriented approach. For a satisfactory and cost-effective treatment, the evaluation methods should address these issues: (1) the etiology of ED whether organic or psychogenic; (2) the severity and possible reversibility of ED; (3) the patient and partner's goals and expectations.

Hence, a thorough workup should be applied for any patient complaining of sexual dysfunction. In most of the cases treatment plan can be created after a thorough history, focused physical exam and basic lab work. In more complex cases sophisticated testing can be employed. The major etiologies can be subdivided into psychological and organic that includes vascular, neurologic, endocrine, and cavernosal smooth muscles causes. The preliminary clinical evaluation should direct the specific testing to approach etiology diagnosis. These tests vary in degree of invasiveness, precision, and worthiness to reach final diagnosis or guiding therapy. In this chapter, we review the epidemiology (incidence/prevalence), etiology, pathophysiology, phenomenology/DSM-5 diagnostic criteria, best practice or evidence-based approach to diagnosis including diagnostic tests and rating scales.

Epidemiology (Incidence/Prevalence)

Erectile dysfunction is a highly prevalent health problem that affects about 30 million men in the USA. It is a common worldwide clinical problem, with thousands of new cases per year. Worldwide, the affected population is predicted to increase from 152 million in 1995 to 322 million in 2025. The range in ED prevalence varies widely, depending on patient population and defining criteria. Due to the increasing life span and the high incidence of ED in this ageing population, a further increase in patients with ED can be expected [3, 4]. The Massachusetts Male Aging Study surveyed 1709 men aged 40–70 years in the greater Boston area between 1987 and 1989 and reported a prevalence of ED of 52%, with 9.6% of respondents reporting complete ED [5]. In 2000 the overall prevalence of erectile dysfunction in this study population was reestimated to be 44%.

The prevalence of ED is fourfold higher for men in their 70s compared to their 20s. Approximately 52% of men between the ages of 40 and 70 have some degree of sexual dysfunction [3]. A survey of 3009 men aged 18–70 years from all regions of Canada revealed a similar high prevalence of ED [6]. In cross-sectional office-based studies of >1500 male patients, El-Sakka showed that ED was very prevalent in the Middle East region and ED risk factors were also very common in this community. In all patients presented with sexual disorders, 92.6% had ED, 50.8% had premature ejaculation, and 7.6% had low sexual desire. Furthermore, 20% of the patients had psychogenic while 80% had organic causes of ED. Of the patients, 10% had mild, 40% had moderate, and 50% had severe ED [7, 8].

W.W. IsHak (ed.), *The Textbook of Clinical Sexual Medicine*, DOI 10.1007/978-3-319-52539-6_12

In a cross-sectional community-based random sample of Egyptian men, Seyam et al. reported on the prevalence of ED and its correlates in Egypt [9]. Shaeer et al. reported on the prevalence of ED and its correlates among men attending primary-care clinics in Pakistan, Egypt and Nigeria. They found that the age-adjusted prevalence rates of ED were 57.4% in Nigeria, 63.6% in Egypt, and 80.8% in Pakistan [10]. Until seventies of the last century ED in young men was thought to be psychogenic. However, several studies have identified organic causes in 15–72% of this population [11].

The Global Online Sexuality Survey (GOSS) is a worldwide epidemiological study using an online survey to evaluate the prevalence and perceptions of sexuality and sexual disorders in different communities. It is conducted online using validated questionnaires, of the 804 male respondents in the Middle East GOSS report, there was a collective ED prevalence rate of 47%, with a higher prevalence in patients with infertility and concerns over genital size, among other associated factors such as hypertension, diabetes, depression, subjective reports of severe penile deviation, interpersonal distress, PE, and low libido [12]. In their report on the USA-based GOSS, Shaeer et al. studied the responses from 1133 English-speaking men. The GOSS findings from both regions identified concerns over genital size as a novel risk factor (35.4% in the USA and 30% in the Middle East) which might be a reversible cause of ED that can be addressed during medical consultation. In the Middle East, infertility was a more significant social stigma that was closely associated with ED [13].

Erection Physiology and Pathophysiology of ED

Physiology of Penile Erection

Integration of neural and vascular functions is the cornerstone in the process of erection. Relaxation of trabecular smooth muscle results in increased distension of the sinusoids that host inflow of blood to the corpora cavernosa and allows erection. This expansion causes mechanical compression of the emissary veins running through the tunica albuginea, which impedes their ability to drain blood and thereby results in penile rigidity. The autonomic nervous system provides parasympathetic (S2–S4) and sympathetic (T12–L2) input to the pelvic plexus, including the cavernous nerves. These nerves are responsible for the delivery of nitric oxide which results in relaxation of the trabecular smooth muscle [14, 15]. Nitric oxide activates guanylate cyclase to produce cyclic guanosine monophosphate (cGMP); the biochemical cascade results in decrease in cytosolic calcium concentration and ultimately causes trabecular smooth muscle relaxation and increased regional blood flow [16, 17]. Phosphodiesterase enzymes (PDEs) type 5 can reverse this pathway by inactivating cGMP, which results in elevated cytosolic calcium concentrations and smooth-muscle contraction [18].

The somatic motor nerve supply arises from the sacral spinal cord, whose fibers join the pudendal nerve innervating the bulbocavernosus and ischiocavernosus muscles. Adrenergic stimulation causes cavernous smooth-muscle contraction and detumescence while cholinergic stimulation may contribute to the erectile process through adrenergic inhibition as well as release of nitric oxide from the endothelium [19].

Different types of erection were documented: psychogenic, reflexogenic, and centrally originated (nocturnal erections). Psychogenic erections occur through stimulatory pathways such as sound, smell, sight, and touch that travel from the spinal erection centers and induce a dopaminergic initiation of erection from the medial pre-optic area [20]. Reflexogenic erections, induced by direct genital stimulation, send ascending pulses to the central erection centers and direct messages to the autonomic nuclei, which explains preservation of erection in patients with upper spinal cord injuries. Nocturnal erections, initiated in the pontine reticular formation and amygdalae and are believed to be caused by a relative decrease in sympathetic inhibition with augmentation of the pro-erectile centers. Furthermore, androgens play a principally modulating role by their effect on libido and sexual behavior. Testosterone acts on different aspects of sexual function including enhances of sexual interest and the frequency of sexual acts; increases the frequency of nocturnal erections however does not effect reflexogenic or psychogenic erections [21].

Pathophysiology of Erectile Dysfunction

Erectile dysfunction is thought to be a result of psychologically based factor especially in young population however nowadays it is well known that the most common causes of ED is organic-based such as neurological, hormonal, pharmacological, and end-organ (penile) factors, especially in older patients [22]. Either central or peripheral neurological causes, may lead to ED. Among cerebral diseases as well as spinal cord injury, 95% of those who have upper motor neuron lesions are capable of reflexogenic erections, 25% of patients who have lower motor neuron lesions are capable of psychogenic erections, and more than 90% of patients who have incomplete lesions of either kind retain their erectile function [23]. Injury to the neurovascular bundle supply may occur during therapy for prostate cancer whether by surgery or external beam radiation therapy and consequently ensure ED [24]. Most of antihypertensive medications have been implicated in ED [25].

The mechanisms vary from central-acting sympatholytics, depression of libido as well as higher blood pressure requirement to achieve erection in atherosclerotic patients taking diuretics and vasodilators. More recently sexual dysfunctions associated with thiazide-class diuretics, β-blockers, and centrally acting sympathoplegics were addressed by half of the recent guidelines with one-third of the guidelines are vague about individual β-blockers and diuretics, and there is no statement on third-generation β-blockers and thiazide-like diuretics that can improve erectile function [26]. While there is evidence to suggest that older antihypertensive drugs (diuretics, beta-blockers, centrally acting agents) have a negative impact on erectile function, newer agents seem to have either neutral (ACE inhibitors, calcium antagonists) or beneficial effects (i.e., angiotensin receptor blockers, nebivolol) [27].

The role of smoking in causing ED remains a source of controversy. Smoking seems to amplify other risk factors, such as hypertension and coronary artery disease [28]. Recent experimental studies demonstrated that exposure to chronic smoking increases apoptosis and oxidative stress and decreases nNOS, endothelial and smooth muscle contents, and ICP in a dose dependent fashion [29].

Male androgen deficiency is a global health issue [30]. Testosterone (T) deficiency or hypogonadism has been recently associated with cardio vascular morbidity and mortality [31]. Low T is the most common hormonal cause of ED. El-Sakka et al. reported a possible association between sexual dysfunction, e.g., (ED, premature ejaculation (PE) and low desire) and hypogonadism. The most frequent endocrine changes were a low testosterone level [32] Hyperprolactinemia leads to sexual dysfunction, due to low testosterone concentrations. Increased prolactin concentration leads to the inhibition of gonadotropin-releasing hormones, which, in turn, decreases the secretion of luteinizing hormone, which is responsible for testosterone secretion [33]. In addition to vasodilatory actions of T it is critical to the health of the vascular beds, stimulating endothelial cell proliferation via an androgen receptor/vascular endothelial growth factor-mediated mechanism (AR/VEGF), and promoting angiogenesis, Furthermore, because T deprivation is known to decrease the availability of nitric oxide (NO) and because NO is a key marker of endothelial function, it can be inferred that testosterone may have a direct effect on endothelial function and development and the differentiation, maturation, migration, and homing of circulating endothelial progenitor cells (EPCs) [34].

Sexual complaints represent the most specific symptoms associated with late onset hypogonadism, while central obesity is the most specific sign. In addition, although hypogonadism can exacerbate obesity-associated ED, recent data suggest that a direct contribution of fat-derived factors could be hypothesized. In particular, fat accumulation induces several hepatic pro-inflammatory genes closely linked to corpora cavernosa endothelial dysfunction. Lifestyle modifications and weight loss are the first steps in the treatment of ED patients with obesity or metabolic diseases. In symptomatic hypogonadal men with metabolic impairment and obesity, combining the effect of testosterone substitution with lifestyle modifications could result in better outcomes [35].

Etiology, Risk Factors, and Medical Comorbidities

Age

Recent studies highlighted that even in young men the organic etiology of ED should not be neglected. The authors determined that 14.8% of men under the age of 40 had organic ED. The etiology was further subdivided into arteriogenic (32.1%), venogenic (16.7%), neurogenic (12.8%), endocrinologic (2.6%), drug-induced (7.7%), mixed (11.5%), and unknown (16.6%) [11, 36]. The main risk factors were determined to be current smoking (41.4%), diabetes mellitus (27.1%), hypertension (17.3%), hyperlipidemia (18.5%), perineal trauma (5.1%), spinal cord injury (4.5%), and drug consumption (4.5%). Another study done at the University of California San Francisco reviewed 100 men under the age of 40, who had ED, and determined that only 13% had exclusively psychogenic ED [37]. These findings have raised the issue that young men with sexual dysfunction should not be dismissed without proper evaluation.

Medical Comorbidities

Comorbidities such as hypertension, diabetes mellitus, dyslipidemia, coronary artery disease (CAD), and depression have been described as primary risk factors for the development of ED [38]. Several studies in the Middle East showed that the prevalence of ED was >40% in Arab men, which is higher than in other parts of the world. At least five Arab countries are included in the top 10 countries worldwide with a high prevalence of diabetes mellitus [39].

Cardiovascular Events "CAD, Hypertension, and Stroke"

The independent association between ED and cardiovascular (CV) events like angina, myocardial infarction, and stroke had been well established in earlier epidemiological studies [40]. However, the relationship between ED and CV deaths as a result of the CV events remains unclear. In the Massachusetts Male Aging Study, where a prospective population-based cohort of 1709 men was followed up, ED was associated with all-cause mortality. Although there was no formal significance detected between ED and CV deaths in this study, the trend suggested that CV deaths were a significant part of the all-cause mortality [41]. In a prospective population-based Australian study called 'The 45 and Up Study', Men with severe ED had double the risk of death during the follow-up than men with no ED. That study reinforced ED as a risk marker in men with and with no known CV disease [42]. A meta-analysis to assess the overall risk of CV events in patients with ED and diabetes was reported by Yamada et al. [43]. The relative risk of CV disease in men with diabetes and ED was 1.74, which was higher than the combined relative risk of about 1.5 from two previous meta-analyses which were not limited to diabetic patients [41, 44]. ED should be recognized as an independent risk factor for CV disease and screening for CAD in patients with severe vasculogenic or diabetes-associated ED might enhance the therapeutic outcome.

El-Sakka et al. evaluated risk factors for CAD in patients with ED. They found that reduced PSV of the cavernous artery is associated with IHD and of these patients, 26.9% had different degrees of ischemic heart disease (IHD), of whom 84.8% were aged >50 years. Overall, 92.1% of the patients with ED had one or more coronary artery risk factors [45, 46]. Jackson et al. evaluated the link between ED and CAD. They stated that ED can arise before CAD becomes symptomatic, with a time window of 3–5 years. ED and CAD share the same risk factors, and endothelial dysfunction is the common denominator [47, 48]. Treating ED in cardiac patients is safe, provided that their risks are properly evaluated. El-Sakka et al. further assessed the association between the severity of ED and left ventricular diastolic dysfunction (LVDD) in patients with no overt cardiac complaint. There were significant associations between an increased severity of ED and the following categorical echo variables; grade 1 and 2 of E/A ratio, deceleration time, IVRT, and grades 1, 2, and 3 of the E/Em ratio ($P < 0.05$ for each). They concluded that LVDD is prevalent among patients with ED-associated medical comorbidities but no overt cardiac complaint [49].

Diabetes Mellitus

The association between diabetes and ED is very well established. The prevalence has been reported as high as 75% in certain populations. In a prospective study, the incidence of ED in diabetic patients was 68 cases per 1000 patients per year compared to 25.9 cases per 1000 patients per year in the general populous. In addition, ED was reported as an independent risk factor for poor quality of life in diabetic patients [50].

El-Sakka and Tayeb reported that, of all patients with type 2 DM, 86.1% had various degrees of ED, including mild in 7.7%, moderate in 29.4%, and severe in 49.1%. The prevalence of ED was 25% in patients aged <50 years, which increased to 75% in those aged >50 years. Of those without ED, 70% were aged <50 years and 30% were >50 years ($P < 0.001$). Patients with a history of DM for >10 years were three times more likely to report ED than those with a history of <5 years. Men with poor metabolic control were 12.2 times more likely to report ED than those with good metabolic control. Of diabetic patients with ED, 53% had one or more diabetic-related complications compared with 20.5% with no ED [51].

El-Sakka reported a study on the association between DM and changes in penile Doppler ultrasonography and axial penile rigidity variables in patients with ED. There was a statistically significant association between the presence of DM and a poor response to intracorporeal injection and decreasing PSV values and Rigidometer values [52]. In another study assessing the relation between DM and other sexual problems, El-Sakka and Tayeb evaluated the prevalence of Peyronie's disease (PD) in patients with type 2 DM who were screened for ED. Of a total of 1133 male diabetic patients, 8.1% were diagnosed as having PD. There were also significant associations between PD and age, obesity, smoking, duration and number of cigarettes smoked per day. Dyslipidemia, psychological disorders, and the presence of at least one risk factor were significantly associated with PD [53]. In another study they also assessed the impact of type 2 DM and PD, solely and together, on impairment of the vascular status of erection in patients with ED. They found that the means of the Erectile Function (EF) domain of the International Index of Erectile Function, and Questions 3 and 4, were significantly lower in patients with both DM and PD than in patients with either of the conditions alone. They concluded that type 2 DM and PD solely and together negatively affect the vascular status of erection [54].

In other related factors for the relation between DM and androgen alteration, El-Sakka et al. assessed the prevalence and impact of the control of DM on the androgen pattern in men with type 2 DM-associated ED. Of all patients, 25.8%, 6.3%, and 30.2% had low total testosterone, low dehydroepiandrosterone sulfate, and hyperinsulinemia, respectively, at the baseline visit. There were significant associations between a good control of DM or decreased fasting blood sugar and normal levels of total testosterone at the 3- and 6-month visits [55, 56].

Other Risk Factors and Medical Comorbidities

A long list of additional risk factors was reported in different studies, which included liver disease, arthritis, peptic ulcer, prostate disease, LUTS, history of pelvic surgery, chronic renal failure, lead exposure, lower household income, physical inactivity, caffeine consumption, use of recreational drugs, alcoholism, and drug addiction [57].

Vasculogenic Erectile Dysfunction

Common vascular disorders that lead to ED include atherosclerosis, endothelial dysfunction, and PD. Vasculogenic ED could be arteriogenic (cavernosal artery insufficiency), venogenic (dysfunction of penile venous system), or mixed arteriogenic and venogenic ED. Arteriogenic ED can be due to atherosclerotic or traumatic arterial occlusive disease [58]. Arterial insufficiency causes an upregulation of connective tissue synthesis and inhibits vascular smooth muscle growth. This mechanism disrupts functional penile compliance, ultimately leading to ED [59].

Endothelial dysfunction may also predispose men to ED [60]. The pivotal role in the occurrence of ED is loss of the functional integrity of endothelium and subsequent endothelial dysfunction. ED, aging, hypogonadism and endothelial dysfunction are closely related to each other. The vascular endothelium plays a critical role in the vasculature [61]. Endothelial monolayer regulates relevant biological events, such as the maintenance of balanced vascular pressure, patency and perfusion, inhibition of thrombosis, induction of fibrinolysis, regulation of inflammation and platelet aggregation, and the behavior of the underlying vascular smooth muscles [62].

Endothelial cells lining the internal surface of penile arteries and sinusoids of the cavernosal tissue exert this action through the release of relaxing factors such as (NO, prostanglandin-E2, and C-type natriuretic peptide) and vasoconstrictor agents such as (endothelin-1 and angiotensin-II) [63]. The small diameter of the cavernosal arteries and the high content of endothelium (compared with other organs) suggest that the penile vasculature may be a sensitive indicator of systemic vascular disease [64]. In fact, it has been described that men with penile vascular dysfunction have also endothelial dysfunction in other vascular beds. In vasculogenic ED, the regulatory role of the endothelium is hindered, resulting in decreased bioavailability and/or responsiveness to vasodilatory mediators; this may also be combined with increased levels of and/or sensitivity to vasoconstricting agents [65].

Although some patients may not have overt cardiovascular disease, they may still possess subclinical risk factors that predispose them to ED. Peyronie's disease is also strongly associated with sexual dysfunction. Larger plaque size, veno-occlusive dysfunction, and impaired cavernosal arterial inflow may all contribute to ED in these men [66]. There is also a significant degree of physical and psychological burden in PD, which contributes to a multifactorial etiology [67]. In a qualitative study of men with PD, four core domains were found to have an impact on sexual and psychosocial health in these patients: self-image, sexual function, pain and discomfort, and social isolation [68]. These findings are suggestive of a mixed picture with psychogenic and organic contributors.

Neurogenic Erectile Dysfunction

The neurologic system is intimately involved in proper erectile function. Peripheral, spinal, supraspinal, as well as somatic and autonomic pathways, are integrated with erectile physiology. Iatrogenic causes such as cavernous nerve injury during radical prostatectomy (RP) were reported as a common cause of neurogenic ED [69]. In patients with spinal cord or cauda equina lesions, autonomic failure (including multiple system atrophy (MSA)) and normotensive hydrocephalus, ED is part of the clinical picture. In focal brain lesions, there are locations particularly related to ED (temporal). In multiple sclerosis (MS), Parkinson's disease and polyneuropathies, ED typically appears with progression of the disease. Spinal and peripheral lesions may similarly affect both functions, but not brain disease; such as epilepsy [70]. Sexual disorder commonly appears as loss of function, but "hyperfunction" may also occur; this is most typically manifested as an increase in desire, as for instance in the context of dopaminergic treatment in Parkinson's disease [71]. In men under 40, common neurologic etiologies of ED include multiple sclerosis, epilepsy, intramedullary nailing of femoral fractures, and lumbar spine procedures [11].

Endocrinogenic Erectile Dysfunction

Hypogonadism, hyperprolactinemia, hyperthyroidism, and hypothyroidism, are frequent endocrinopathies that can potentially affect erectile function. El-Sakka et al. reported that androgen deficiency has been observed in as low as 2% and as high as 33% of all men with ED. The most frequent endocrinal changes in ED patients were low testosterone level (15%), hyperprolactinemia (13.7%), and hypothyroidism (3.1%) [72].

The diagnosis of endocrinopathies is basically a laboratory evaluation of serum hormonal levels. However, several screening questionnaires and scales have been proposed particularly for evaluation of hypogonadism. Yet they still have a limited clinical utility due to lack of sensitivity and specificity. Two main forms of hypogonadism are documented. Primary i.e., gonadal dysfunction, in addition to Kleinfelter's syndrome and cryptorchidism fall into the primary category. Secondary (i.e., central dysfunction), in addition to head trauma, prolactinoma, pituitary surgery, alcohol or illicit drug abuse, and certain infiltrating disorders such as hemochromatosis fall into the secondary category [73]. Both hypothyroidism or hyperthyroidism have negative impact on erectile function [74].

In one study, 63% of men with hypothyroidism and 70% with hyperthyroidism had ED, compared to 34% in the control group [75]. Although endothelial dysfunction has been suggested, the mechanism of ED in thyroid dysfunction remains unknown.

Phenomenology/DSM-5 Diagnostic Criteria

The Diagnostic and Statistical Manual of Mental Disorders, Fifth Edition (*DSM-5*) is the 2013 update to the American Psychiatric Association's (APA) classification and diagnostic tool.

The DSM-5 was published on May 18, 2013, superseding the DSM-IV-TR, which was published in 2000. Notable changes include a revised treatment and naming of *gender identity disorder* to *gender dysphoria.* The DSM-5 field trials included test–retest reliability which involved different clinicians doing independent evaluations of the same patient—a common approach to the study of diagnostic reliability [76].

DSM-5 has sex-specific sexual dysfunctions. For females, sexual desire and arousal disorders are combined into female sexual interest/arousal disorder. Sexual dysfunctions (except substance–/medication induced sexual dysfunction) now require a duration of approximately 6 months and more exact severity criteria. A new diagnosis is genito-pelvic pain/penetration disorder which combines vaginismus and dyspareunia from DSM-IV [77]. Sexual aversion disorder was deleted. Subtypes for all disorders include only "lifelong versus acquired" and "generalized versus situational" (one subtype was deleted from DSM-IV). Two subtypes were deleted: "sexual dysfunction due to a general medical condition" and "due to psychological versus combined factors" [77].

According to the DSM-5 the diagnosis of erectile disorder requires marked difficulty in obtaining, maintaining, or decrease in erectile rigidity, experienced on almost all or all sexual activity, for a minimum duration of 6 months, causing significant distress, and cannot be explained nonsexual mental disorder, severe relationship distress or other stressors, or due to substance/medication or another medical condition (Table 12-1).

Best Practice and Evidence-Based Approach to Diagnosis

Background of ED Diagnosis

Numerous consensus meetings have attempted to formulate best-practice guidelines to diagnose and treat ED patients. The International Consultations on Sexual Medicine was one such series of meetings, first convened in 1999 with subsequent conferences in 2004, 2009 and 2015. This eventually reflects the interest of clinicians to achieve the optimal diagnostic and therapeutic tools to mange patients with ED. The goal-directed approach was combined with evidence-based practice to create diagnostic and therapeutic algorithms and establish standard-of-care practices [2, 78]. A two-level diagnostic approach is a logical guide for treating patients with ED. Currently, a tailored diagnostic pathway with full consideration of the patient's goals is recommended. Lue [2] proposed the "goal-directed approach to diagnose and treat ED" more than 20 years ago, and this approach is still valid. In general, a detailed medical and psychosexual history that includes standardized questionnaires such as the International Index of Erectile Function (IIEF) is useful for assessing the severity of ED [79]. A thorough physical examination, although does not usually reveal the cause of ED its use is recommended to identify information of value such as Peyronie's plaques, atrophic testes in hypogonadism, uncontrolled hypertension and neurological disorders [50]. Appro-

Table 12-1. DSM-5 Diagnostic criteria of Erectile Disorder

302.72 (F52.21)
A. At least one of the three following symptoms must be experienced on almost all or all (approximately 75–100%) occasions of sexual activity (in identified situational contexts or, if generalized, in all contexts):
1. Marked difficulty in obtaining an erection during sexual activity
2. Marked difficulty in maintaining an erection until the completion of sexual activity
3. Marked decrease in erectile rigidity
B. The symptoms in Criterion A have persisted for a minimum duration of approximately 6 months
C. The symptoms in Criterion A cause clinically significant distress in the individual
D. The sexual dysfunction is not better explained by a nonsexual mental disorder or as a consequence of severe relationship distress or other significant stressors and is not attributable to the effects of a substance/medication or another medical condition
Specify whether:
Lifelong: The disturbance has been present since the individual became sexually active
Acquired: The disturbance began after a period of relatively normal sexual function
Specify whether:
Generalized: Not limited to certain types of stimulation, situations, or partners
Situational: Only occurs with certain types of stimulation, situations, or partners
Specify current severity:
Mild: Evidence of mild distress over the symptoms in Criterion A
Moderate: Evidence of moderate distress over the symptoms in Criterion A
Severe: Evidence of severe or extreme distress over the symptoms in Criterion A

Reprinted with permission from the diagnostic and statistical manual of mental disorders, Fifth Edition, (Copyright 2013). American Psychiatric Association.

priate laboratory investigations are useful for uncovering potentially serious comorbidities. Complete blood count, fasting blood glucose, lipid profile, kidney function, and others if indicated should be obtained [80, 81]. Additional tests such as serum testosterone, prolactin, and thyroid function tests can be included at the physician's discretion, based on the clinical scenario [82]. For an appropriate treatment the evaluation methods should address these inquiries, whether the cause of ED is organic or psychogenic; the severity and possible reversibility of ED; and the patient's and probably the partner's ambition and expectations. The tailored diagnosis of ED not only allows the physician to avoid further costly evaluation, but also saves the patient from invasive diagnostic techniques. Dynamic color Doppler ultrasonography of the penis is not necessary for all patients with ED. However, penile hemodynamics assessment is useful in evaluating thePDE5-Is nonresponders, young men with primary or secondary ED and a history of pelvic trauma or drug abuse, or before surgical interventions for treating PD, differentiating psychogenic from organic ED, undiagnosed penile pain with occult septal scarring and in medico-legal cases [83, 84]. Invasive diagnostic tools such as penile angiography and cavernosography/cavernosometry can be used in certain undiagnosed cases. The recent years has focused on neuroimaging, biomarkers of vascular health to further refine and personalize workup. There are ongoing investigations which stabilize the role of gene, stem cell, as well as tissue engineering therapies [85].

Diagnostic Tests

Medical and Psychosexual History

A multifaceted comprehensive approach is required for a full evaluation to diagnose ED. Despite the availability of innovative diagnostic tests, a detailed sexual and medical history remains the key to the diagnosis of ED. It can also differentiate between different disorders of sexual function. Psychosexual and medical history should address any unstable interpersonal relationships, or emotional stressors that can play a huge role in sexual health. Further, it should focus on the concurrent risk factors, medical comorbidities, and medications which are pivotal parts of the diagnostic evaluation. As by far the most common presenting complaint is reduction of rigidity and duration of erection rather than complete absence of erection, sexual desire and inventory of sexual partners, therefore they should also be included in history. Assessment of the onset of ED, the presence of morning erection, and any psychological conflict may help to classify psychogenic from organic ED.

Sexual history can also direct further evaluation and treatment of ED associated with other conditions especially endocrinopathy in patients who may present with a recent history of ED and low libido [80]. Early recognition of psychogenic ED not only allows the physician to avoid further costly workup, but also save the patient from unnecessary, sometime invasive diagnostic techniques. As ED is known to be associated with many risk factors, common medical comorbidities and medications, thorough inquiring may yield insights regarding peripheral vascular or coronary artery disease, diabetes, psychological, neurologic, chronic debilitating disease, or tobacco and alcohol consumption. These risk factors may direct further evaluation. Clinically, patients with multiple risk factors and medical comorbidities such as old age, long history of diabetes, and vascular disease are likely to have ED secondary to vascular and neuropathic disease [45].

On the other hand, young patients with psychiatric illness are more likely to have psychogenic or possibly secondary ED due to psychotropic medications. A patient's past surgical history of abdomen and pelvis such as radical prostatectomy, abdominoperineal resection, pelvic trauma, and irradiation are well known to be associated with ED [86, 87].

Distinguishing Organic from Psychogenic ED

Clues to suggest a psychogenic etiology include sudden onset, good quality spontaneous or self-stimulated erections, major life events, or previous psychological problems. Conversely, gradual onset, lack of tumescence, and normal libido are more suggestive of an organic etiology [88]. Recent study classified men with ED into those that have difficulty achieving an erection. The authors reported that patients who cannot achieve tumescence are more likely to have organic etiologies. While maintaining an erection appears to have a considerable psychologic component [89]. Supporting to that men who struggle with maintaining an erection were younger, healthier, had a lower degree of penile insufficiency and a higher prevalence of normal nocturnal erections [90].

Physical Examination

The physical examination should focus on the vascular, neurological, and endocrine systems [91, 92]. Physical examination with particular attention to sexual and genital development may reveal micropenis, penile chordee, Peyronie's plaque. Furthermore, small soft atrophic testes or gynecomastia may necessitate an endocrine evaluation. A careful neurologic examination should also be performed. Testing for genital and perineal sensation and the bulbocavernosus reflex is important in assessing possible neurogenic ED. Patients with certain genetic syndromes, such as Kleinfelter's, or Kallmann's may present with obvious physical signs of hypogonadism and a distinctive body habitus. Signs of either hyper or hypothyroidism as well as stigmata of end stage organs disorders such as liver, renal, cardiac failure should be assessed. Hypertension, arrhythmia and anemia should also be excluded. The presence of obesity noted by waist circumference, high blood pressure, or abnormal pulses may require more extensive vascular workup. In many cases, a careful history and physical examination will direct the physician to the most expedient and cost-effective approach, and eliminate the need for unnecessary diagnostic tests [93].

Laboratory Investigation

The laboratory investigation is directed to identify undetected medical illnesses that may contribute to ED, e.g., metabolic disturbances such as renal insufficiency, diabetes, and endocrine abnormalities (hypogonadism, hyperprolactinemia). Laboratory investigations should follow clinical suspicion of specific disorders. Hemoglobin A1c and serum glucose may be measured to detect occult diabetes, and a lipid screen performed to assess the presence of dyslipidemia [92, 94]. A complete laboratory evaluation includes serum chemistry, renal function, a complete blood count, urine analysis, and hormonal evaluation, i.e., generally serum testosterone and prolactin should be done in the initial evaluation.

Further Investigations when Needed

Vascular Workup

Penile Brachial Pressure Index (PBI)

The penile brachial index represents the penile systolic blood pressure divided by the brachial systolic blood pressure. A penile brachial index of 0.7 or less has been used to indicate arteriogenic ED [95]. This test gained some initial popularity because of its low cost and noninvasiveness. However this test has limited clinical utility because measurement in the flaccid state will not reveal the full functional capacity of the cavernous arteries in the erect state; also because the data are based on superficial and deep penile arterial pressure, whereas erectile function depends on the deep arteries exclusively. Therefore, a normal PBI cannot be relied upon to exclude arteriogenic ED. Since PBI is inaccurate and poorly reproducible no justification for its continued use is suggested [96].

Penile Plethysmography (Penile Pulse Volume Recording)

This test is performed by connecting a 2.5- or 3-cm cuff to an air plethysmograph. The cuff is inflated to a pressure above brachial systolic pressure, which is then decreased by 10-mmHg increments and tracings are obtained at each level. In patients with vasculogenic ED the waveform shows a slow upstroke, a low rounded peak, slow downstroke, and no dicrotic notch. Its height varies considerably; patients with vascular insufficiency usually have the lowest mean height [97]. However due to the inconsistence of results, its clinical uses is abandoned.

Combined Intracavernosal Injection and Stimulation Test (CIS)

A vascular workup aims to evaluate arterial blood inflow, subsequent engorgement, and blood retention within corporeal bodies. Combined intracavernosal injection and stimulation is a first-line easy to carry with high yielding option. Vasoactive drugs (e.g., papaverine, phentolamine, alprostadil) can be used. This pharmacologic screening test allows the clinician to bypass neurogenic and hormonal influences and to evaluate the vascular status of the penis directly and objectively.

Assessment of penile rigidity and duration of response is then conducted. Normally, a full erection is achieved within 15 min (i.e., an erection > 90° that is firm to palpation) and lasts longer than 15 min [98]. Carful interpretation of the data is required due to the occasional false-positive results due to improper response secondary to anxiety, needle phobia, or inadequate injection dosage or false-negative results particularly in men with penile arterial insufficiency with an intact veno-occlusive mechanism [99, 100].

Duplex Ultrasonography

Intracavernosal injection test is a subjective evaluation of penile rigidity by the assessor. Duplex ultrasound, on the other hand, provides a quantitative component to the evaluation of blood flow. A high-resolution ultrasonography and color-pulsed Doppler is used in this technique. In 1985, Lue and associates introduced high-resolution sonography and pulsed Doppler blood flow analysis (duplex ultrasonography) with intracavernosal injection of a vasoactive agent such as papaverine (15–30 mg) or Alprostadil (10 μg) [101, 102]. Sonographic assessment of the penis is then repeated 3–5 min after the injection. Each main cavernous and dorsal artery is individually assessed. Cavernous arterial diameter and pulsation are recorded.

Flow velocities are measured after vasodilator injections. In a normal Doppler study, the peak systolic velocities (PSV) have been used to establish normal from abnormal erectile response. The mean PSV typically ranges from 35 to 47 cm/s. If velocities are below 25 cm/s, abnormal pudendal arteriography is confirmed with 100% sensitivity, 95% specificity [103].

Hence, patients with a peak velocity of >35 cm/s are supposed to have normal cavernous arterial inflow, while those with values <25 cm/s are diagnosed with cavernous arterial insufficiency. In regards to veno-occlusive dysfunction, resistive index (RI) can be a useful tool. RI =Peak systolic flow – End diastolic velocity/Peak systolic flow

Hence, the RI calculation approaches a value of one. Patients with an RI >0.9 have normal veno-occlusive function, and those with an RI <0.75 raise suspicion for veno-occlusive dysfunction, that is, dysfunctional corporal retention. In a study that investigated the association between RI and cavernosography, in men with an RI >0.9, 90% had normal cavernosography while in those with a RI <0.75, 95.5% had corporal leakage [104]. Ultrasonography has some limitations such as anatomic arterial variants that affect the accuracy of testing and the high false-positive results especially in young men [105].

Comparison with Other Tests

Duplex sonography provided significant advantages over previous techniques especially, is noninvasive and can be performed in the office setting; allows the ultrasonographer to image the individual cavernous arteries and provides an additional advantage of easier assessment of direction of blood flow and communication among the cavernous, dorsal and spongiosal arteries, which are crucial in penile vascular and reconstructive surgeries. Attempts to correlate duplex sonography with pudendal arteriography have been achieved with varying degrees of success and showed reasonable correlation [106, 107]. Previous study compared duplex ultrasonography with NPT monitoring and reported a good correlation, except in patients with neurogenic ED [108]. A good correlation in 71% of patients between color-coded duplex sonography and penile blood gas measurements was reported [109].

Pitfalls of Ultrasonography

Ultrasonography has some limitations; it is performed in a nonsexual setting with little privacy and can increase the patient's anxiety level and cause a sympathetic response that will inhibit his response to injection [110]. The result of the sonographic study may also be influenced by the temporal response to intracavernosal injection. Arterial flow decreases significantly during the full erection phase, and ultrasonography performed during this period will yield a deceptively low peak velocity. Anatomic arterial variants that affect the accuracy of testing and the high false-positive results especially in young men [105] are also reported. Lastly, ultrasonography is operator-dependent that is influenced by the clinician experience.

Penile Angiography

Penile arteriography was introduced by the pioneering work of Michal and Pospichal [111]. Currently, selective pudendal arteriography performed with the aid of intracavernosal injection is considered by many to be the gold standard for evaluating penile arterial anatomy [107]. Penile angiography is typically reserved for nonsmoking, less than 40 years patients with post-traumatic arterial injury and as a preparation for revascularization surgery [15, 94].

In this test, the internal pudendal artery is selectively cannulated, and then radiographic contrast is injected for visualization of the internal pudendal and penile arteries. A true limitation of the utility of this modality is penile vascular anatomic variations that exists and making it difficult for the angiographer to determine congenital from acquired abnormalities. Furthermore, like all invasive radiographic tests, the study is performed under artificial conditions, which may produce a significant sympathetic response and inhibit the erectile response. Penile angiography is potentially serve as a diagnostic tool and recently limited clinical data demonstrated contemporary endovascular utility as a therapeutic option in select patients [112].

Penile Magnetic Resonance Imaging

Penile magnetic resonance imaging (MRI) has promise in detailing penile anatomy and microcirculation. Another technique of assessing penile function was reported by using sequential contrast-enhanced MRI of the penis in a flaccid state. Subjects with normal erectile function showed gradual and centrifugal enhancement of the corpora cavernosa, while those with ED showed poor enhancement with abnormal progression [113]. The use of MRI during the workup of prostate cancer has recently become more popular. Owing to the vicinity of the genital organs, penile anatomy and vasculature are often depicted on these imaging studies. In a study that investigated pelvis MRI for staging prostate cancer in patients who underwent prostatectomy. On MRI a correlation between a patient's self-reported sexual function and perfusion-related parameters was also noted [114].

Cavernosometry and Cavernosography

The current standard diagnostic study for veno-occlusive dysfunction is pharmacologic cavernosometry and cavernosography. Cavernosometry involves simultaneous saline infusion and intracorporeal pressure monitoring. Wespes et al. (1984), introduced dynamic cavernosometry and cavernosography during artificial erection produced by saline infusion [115]. Veno-occlusive dysfunction is indicated by either the inability to increase intracorporeal pressure to the level of the mean systolic blood pressure with saline infusion or a rapid drop of intracorporeal pressure after cessation of infusion [116]. Cavernosography involves the infusion of radiocontrast solution into the corpora cavernosa during an artificial erection to visualize the site of venous leakage.

It should always be performed after activation of the veno-occlusive mechanism by intracavernosal injection of a vasoactive agent, various leakage sites to the glans, corpus spongiosum, superficial and deep dorsal veins, and cavernous and crural veins can then be detected [117]. The phenomenon of incomplete trabecular smooth-muscle relaxation (in a nonsexual setting) will falsely suggest veno-occlusive dysfunction in some normal subjects [118]. The normal maintenance rate in patients with complete smooth-muscle relaxation is reported to be less than 5 ml/min with a pressure diminish from 150 mmHg of less than 45 mmHg in 30 s.

Neurologic Workup

Background of Neurologic Testing

Neurologic testing should assess peripheral, spinal, and supraspinal centers and both somatic and autonomic pathways associated with all three types of erection (nocturnal, psychogenic, and reflexogenic) and sexual arousal. However, although post radical prostatectomy cavernosal nerves injury may completely eliminate spontaneous erection, a high percentage of patients with complete upper spinal cord injury are known to have adequate erections. Therefore, it is clear that the effect of neurologic deficit on penile erection is a complicated phenomenon and, with a few exceptions, neurologic testing will rarely direct management. Moreover, there is no reliable test to assess neurotransmitter release, which reflects a real deficiency in the current assessment of overall neurologic function associated with penile erection. In the clinical assessment, the aim of neuro-urologic testing should aim to reveal reversible neurologic disease such as dorsal nerve neuropathy secondary to long-distance bicycling; assess the extent of neurologic deficit from a known neurologic disease such as diabetes mellitus or pelvic injury; and determine whether a referral to a neurologist is mandatory [80].

Somatic Nervous System

Although numerous neurologic tests had been proposed to evaluate the neurologic system as a cause of sexual dysfunction, however, they carry limited clinical utility due to limited impact on management of ED, poor reproducibility, and sensitivity.

Penile Glans Biothesiometry

This test is designed to measure the sensory perception threshold to various amplitudes of vibratory stimulation produced by a handheld electromagnetic device (biothesiometer) placed on the pulp of the index fingers, both sides of the penile shaft, and the glans penis. Questions regarding utility of this test have been raised as it does not accurately mimic the neurophysiologic function of the glans penis. In addition, there is a marked intra-individual variation in vibration sensitivity, raising the issue of reproducibility and accuracy [119].

Sacral Evoked Response—Bulbocavernosus Reflex Latency

This test is designed to evaluate the somatosensory reflexogenic mechanism of erections. Two electrodes with direct stimulator are placed on the penis, one at the corona and one approximately 3 cm proximal to the corona. Concentric needle electrodes are placed in the right and left bulbocavernous muscles to record the response. Latency period is defined as the time from the electrical impulse delivery to the muscle response. The mean response time is approximately 30 ms, and an abnormal response is defined as > 3 standard deviations from the mean. However, pudendal nerve conduction appears relatively late in various forms of neurogenic ED including diabetes, making it an unreliable diagnostic test [120].

Dorsal Nerve Conduction Velocity

Two electrodes are placed on the penis, one at the glans and another at the base. A stimulus is delivered from each electrode. Conduction velocity is then calculated by dividing the distance between the electrodes by the difference in latency times recorded at each site. Slower conduction velocity has been associated with neurogenic ED. In men with neurologic ED, the most frequently observed finding was decreased conduction of the penile dorsal nerve [121].

Genitocerebral Evoked Potential Studies

This test involves electrical stimulation of the dorsal nerve of the penis as described for the BCR latency test. Instead of recording EMG responses, this study records the evoked potential waveforms overlying the sacral spinal cord and cerebral cortex. This study might provide an objective assessment of the presence, location, and nature of afferent penile sensory dysfunction in patients with subtle abnormalities on neurologic examination [80].

Autonomic Nervous System

Heart Rate Variability and Sympathetic Skin Response
Testing the autonomic system remains less sensitive and reproducible even than the somatic system. Although autonomic neuropathy is an important cause of ED, direct testing is not available. The test of heart rate control (mainly parasympathetic) and blood pressure control (mainly sympathetic) are indirect methods of assessment. Because heart rate and blood pressure responses can be affected by many external factors, these tests must be done under standardized conditions [122]. Sympathetic skin response (SSR) measures the skin potential evoked by electric shock stimuli. SSR was absent in 11 of 30 cases but was normal in all patients with non-neurogenic ED [123]. In a more recent study Yiou et al. reported that, post-radical prostatectomy, penile sensory thresholds for warm and cold sensations increased significantly after non-nerve sparing technique only [124]. This paper supported the idea of testing penile sensation to evaluate the extent of cavernous nerve damage caused by prostatectomy.

Smooth-Muscle EMG and Single Potential Analysis of Cavernous Electrical Activity

Direct recording of cavernous electrical activity with a needle electrode during flaccidity and with visual sexual stimulation was reported [125]. The normal resting flaccid electrical activity from the corpora cavernosa was a rhythmic slow wave with an intermittent burst of activity. Patients with suspected autonomic neuropathy demonstrated a discoordination pattern with continuing electrical activity during visual sexual stimulation. In normal subjects, single potential analysis of cavernous electrical activity (SPACE) shows a regular pattern of activity [126]. In patients with disruption of the peripheral autonomic supply, asynchronous potentials with higher frequencies and an irregular shape are typical. In those with complete spinal cord lesions, abnormal as well as normal electrical activity is found.

Endocrine and Hormonal Workup

Hypogonadism

In 2010, the Endocrine Society published "Testosterone Therapy in Men with Androgen Deficiency Syndromes: An Endocrine Society Clinical Practice Guideline" which addressed important issues surrounding the diagnosis and treatment of male hypogonadism [127]. A more recent systematic analysis critically updated the endocrine society clinical practice guidelines for male hypogonadism [128]. Theoretically, the best measurement of androgenic milieu is determined by calculating bioavailable testosterone, that is, the summation of free and albumin-bound testosterone. However, for screening purposes total serum testosterone is thought to be adequate. Blood draws should occur in the morning, when serum testosterone levels peak. The normal range is large, typically quoted between 280 and 1000 ng/dl. However, if an initial testosterone level falls below normal range, a repeat confirmatory test is recommended [79].

If hypogonadism is suspected based on symptoms and serum testosterone, further workup with serum luteinizing hormone (LH) and prolactin should be applied. In primary hypogonadism (i.e., gonadal dysfunction), LH and follicle-stimulating hormone (FSH) levels are elevated in response to low androgen level. Many men will present with ED or infertility and some of them may present with the classic features of Kleinfelter's (i.e., micropenis, microorchidisism, eunuchoid body habitus). Of men with Kleinfelter's, 22.7% experienced severe ED, and 60.9% had hypoactive sexual desire [129].

In secondary hypogonadism (i.e., central dysfunction), LH and FSH levels are inappropriately normal or low. Hyperprolactinemia can ultimately lead to secondary hypogonadism through suppression of gonadotropin-releasing hormone and pulsatile secretion of LH secretion. When prolactin levels are very high (>200 ng/ml, MRI imaging of the pituitary should be considered to exclude prolactin secreting tumors. Medications, i.e., antipsychotics, tricyclic antidepressants, opiates, prolactin-secreting tumors, hypothyroidism, cirrhosis, and hypothalamic lesions are contributory factors for secondary hypogonadism [130].

Thyroid Dysfunction

During endocrine workup of ED, serum thyroid function tests should also be considered. Hyperthyroidism may increase aromatization of testosterone into estrogen, ultimately raising levels of SHBG and decreasing percent of bioavailable testosterone. Fatigue, weight loss, hyperactivity, palpitations, and heat intolerance are common symptoms that help in diagnosis of this condition. Laboratory diagnosis reveals high thyroid hormone concentrations (total or free T4) with low serum thyroid-stimulating hormone (TSH) levels [130]. In contrast, diagnosis of hypothyroidism is made when serum basal TSH is elevated, and thyroid hormone concentrations are low.

Further Investigations

Nocturnal Penile Tumescence Testing (NPT)

The NPT test was one of the earliest tools to study ED. Nocturnal penile tumescence or sleep-related erection is a recurring cycle of penile erections associated with REM sleep in potent men. The association between sleep and erections was documented as early as 1940 by Halverson, and further studies revealed the association with the REM phase [131]. In 1970, Karacan suggested that NPT could be used to evaluate ED, as its mechanism is presumed to rely on neurovascular responses similar to those of erotically induced erections. The primary goal of NPT testing is to distinguish psychogenic from organic causes of ED [132]. Morales et al. (1994) found that patients with documented erections at night also exhibited erectile episodes during napping and proposed that diurnal penile tumescence is a summary reflection of NPT episodes [133].

In 1985 the Rigiscan was introduced. This combines the sophisticated monitoring of rigidity, tumescence and number and duration of events with the convenience and economic advantage of an ambulatory monitoring system [134]. Because the Rigiscan measures radial rigidity (compressibility), the validity of this measurement has been questioned. Allen et al. (1993) reported that, when Rigiscan base and tip radial rigidity exceeded 60% of maximum, correlation with axial rigidity and observer ratings was poor [135]. Normal NPT results include at least four erections, with a mean duration of 30 min, with a maximal rigidity above 70% [85]. Many investigators have advocated the use of NPT studies to differentiate organic from psychologenic ED [108]. The shortcomings associated with various NPT tests, such as false-negative results were documented. NPT was abandoned as a routine part of the ED evaluation. However, in some patients with complex and confusing histories NPT is a useful tool in confirming the clinical diagnosis.

Rating Scales

A complete medical and sexual history is the most important component of ED diagnosis. First step is to distinguish ED from other sexual dysfunctions, such as premature ejaculation and loss of libido. Several well tested sexual questionnaires, such as the IIEF (International Index of Erectile Function) and EDITS (Erectile Dysfunction Inventory of Treatment Satisfaction), allow identification of ED severity and post treatment satisfaction. The IIEF is composed of 15 questions; an abridged 5-item version, called the sexual health inventory for men (SHIM), has been developed and validated [136].

The International Index of Erectile Function (IIEF)

The NIH Consensus Panel on ED outlined several goals for basic and clinical research on ED [1]. Creation of a staging system for the quantitative and qualitative classification of ED is an important goal. For research and management purposes, the goal is to: (1) quantifying the specific type of patient population to include in a clinical trial; (2) determining and comparing responder rates associated with different treatments; (3) improving clinical decision-making and patient care; (4) fostering educational initiatives; and (5) supporting claims for reimbursement. In particular, the EF domain of the IIEF was considered as a valid, sensitive, and specific for this purpose [137].

The ability of the EF domain to serve as a diagnostic tool to detect ED, as well as to classify the degree of severity of the disorder, was investigated [138]. The results supported the EF domain as an excellent diagnostic tool. Based upon a classification-tree analysis, the optimal cutoff score was found to be 25, with men scoring less than or equal to 25 classified as having ED and those scoring above 25 as not having ED. Subsequently, among men in a stable relationship severity of ED was classified into five diagnostic categories: no ED, EF score (26–30); mild ED, EF score (22–25); mild to moderate, EF score (17–21); moderate EF, score (11–16); and severe, EF score (6–10) [138].

The validity of this diagnostic classification was evaluated in a separate, independent study comparing severity with a single-item self-assessment of ED severity adapted from the Massachusetts Male Aging Study before and after treatment. Results showed a moderate-to-high degree of correlation between the two diagnostic measures, with a high correlation at 12 weeks of treatment [139].

Brief Screening Version

An abridged 5-item version of the IIEF, also known as the Sexual Health Inventory for Men (SHIM), was developed and validated as a brief, easily administered widely used screening tool in clinical practice. The SHIM includes four of the original 6-item EF domain, in addition to a single item on intercourse satisfaction domain (IIEF item numbers 2, 4, 5, 7, 15) [136]. Of the 15 items on the IIEF, these five items were found to discriminate most highly between men with and without ED. Validity and sensitivity of the abridged scale were evaluated and its results were similar to those found with the EF domain. A classification-tree analysis suggested an optimal cutoff score of 21 or less for diagnosis of ED. Among men in a stable relationship, classification of ED was partitioned into five severity grades: no ED (SHIM total score, (22–25), mild ED (17–21), mild to moderate (12–16), moderate (8–11), and severe ED (5–7). Like the EF domain score, the SHIM showed a moderate-to-high degree of correlation with patient self-assessment of ED severity at baseline, at end of treatment, and change from baseline. Additionally, a high sensitivity (81.8%) and moderate specificity (57.7%) for detection of ED in patients scoring below 21 was reported [140].

Limitations of the IIEF

Despite its widespread utilization and strong psychometric properties, the IIEF has potential limitations in different scenarios. Some of these limitations related to the inherent design and construction of the instrument, while others are intrinsic to the use of brief questionnaires. The IIEF focuses only on current sexual functioning particularly erection and provides superficial assessment of domains of sexual functioning [137]. The IIEF provides a limited assessment of the domains of sexual desire and orgasmic dysfunction. The instrument is not entitled to differentiate between different types of sexual desire disorders (e.g., primary vs. secondary) or to distinguish between acquired or long life premature ejaculation and other types of male orgasmic disorders. Furthermore, it does not provide any precise information about the sexual functioning of the partner or the couple relationship that might be important areas for assessment in clinical practice. For this reason, it is only recommended for use in clinical or research contexts in which assessing erectile function is the primary goal on heterosexual activity, including vaginal intercourse.

Regarding the utility of IIEF in assessment of erectile function, the instrument provides accurate and reliable information as a quantitative index of ED severity or evaluating the patient's response to treatment [137]. However, two important clinical limitations of the IIEF are its sole focus on current sexual function and inability to ascertain etiology of the disorder.

In assessing sexual function over the 4-week period prior to completing the questionnaire should not be considered as a substitute for a detailed clinical history including onset, course, and progression of the disorder, relationship to other risk factors or medical comorbidities, and overall impact on the patient's life [141, 142]. However, the validation in different settings and cultures and extensive clinical trial use with high degree of sensitivity and specificity of the instrument make the IIEF ideally suited for efficacy evaluation in clinical trials of ED. Despite the mentioned limitations, the IIEF has met or exceeded expectations as a highly reliable and valid measure of erectile function. It is undoubtedly the questionnaire instrument of choice for clinical trials of ED [143].

Single Item, Self-Assessment ED Question

Based on epidemiological perspective, it has been noted that the IIEF may be longer than necessary, thus leading to poorer compliance. Derby et al. compared responses to the EF domain (six items) with a single item, self-assessment ED question [139]. Results indicated that a higher percentage of respondents completed the single item and overall, single-item responses correlated well with the EF domain scores. Thus, while a single-item question is useful in a case-finding context, it generally provides a more limited assessment of ED severity—no information on specific components of erectile function (e.g., ability to achieve or maintain erection), and no information on other domains of sexual function, and therefore not recommended in clinical trials [139, 143].

PROMIS® (Patient-Reported Outcomes Measurement Information System)

This system is a set of person-centered measures that evaluates and monitors physical, social, and emotional health in adults and children. It can be used with the general population and with individuals living with chronic conditions. The National Institutes of Health (NIH) Patient-Reported Outcomes Measurement Information System (PROMIS) Roadmap initiative (www.nihpromis.org) is a 5-year cooperative group program of research designed to develop, validate, and standardize item banks to measure patient-reported outcomes (PROs) relevant across common medical conditions. The NIH PROMIS network derived a consensus-based framework for self-reported health, systematically reviewed available instruments and datasets that address the initial PROMIS domains. Qualitative item research led to the first wave of network testing which began in the second year [144].

The PROMIS ® Sexual Function and Satisfaction Measure (SexFS)

The PROMIS ® Sexual Function and Satisfaction measure (SexFS) version 1.0 was developed with cancer populations. The SexFS version 2.0 has several improvements and enhancements over version 1.0 and other extant measures, including expanded evidence for validity, scores centered around norms for sexually active US adults, new domains, and a final set of items applicable for both men and women and those sexually active with a partner and without. The SexFS is customizable, allowing users to select relevant domains and items for their study [145].

The PROMIS Sexual Function and Satisfaction Measures Brief Profile (PSxFBP)

This profile provides scores on seven different subdomains of sexual function: Interest in Sexual Activity, Vaginal Discomfort (women only), Lubrication (women only), Erectile Function (men only), Orgasm, and Global Satisfaction with Sex Life. The PSxFBP is intended for broad use, although almost all of the development work was with cancer populations. (Research is ongoing to expand development beyond cancer.) The PSxFBP is available for men and women and consists of the best items selected from each subdomain for general purposes. Each question asks respondents to report on their experiences over the past 30 days [145].

Conclusions

Although previously thought to be frequently psychogenic, currently, the etiology of ED is documented to be mostly organic in origin. Since ED has been shown to be an early indicator for future morbidity and mortality and overall poor health, increasing awareness, making the diagnosis, and targeting men at higher risk is of utmost importance. Specifically, ED may be the first indicator of cardiovascular disease. Therefore, patients with vasculogenic ED and multiple risk factors should be referred to a cardiologist for further evaluation of overt or subclinical cardiovascular disorders.

Urologists have a unique opportunity and responsibility to evaluate and direct patients with ED complaints who might be exposed to higher risk factors that could affect his overall health in the future. In summary, the current evaluation of ED is still far away from the ideal one. We expect to see new methods and technologies that may revolutionize diagnosis and treatment of ED especially in complex cases. The dream of ED become a curable condition may come true with advancement of the proper etiology related evaluation tools and techniques in the near future.

References

1. NIH Consensus Development Panel on Impotence. NIH consensus conference: impotence. JAMA. 1993;270:83–90.
2. Lue TF. Physiology of penile erection and pathophysiology of erectile dysfunction. In: Wein AJ, Kavoussi LR, Novick AC,

Partin AW, Peters CA, editors. Campbell—Walsh urology. 10th ed. Philadelphia: Saunders Elsevier; 2007. p. 718–49.
3. Feldman HA, Goldstein I, Hatzichristou DG, Krane RJ, Mckinlay JB. Impotence and its medical and psychosocial correlates: results of the Massachusetts male aging study. J Urol. 1994;151:54–61.
4. United States Bureau of Census 1992. Statistical abstract of the United States 112th ed. Washington, DC; 1992. p. 19.
5. Kleinman KP, Feldman HA, Johannes CB, Derby CA, McKinlay JB. A new surrogate variable for erectile dysfunction status in the Massachusetts male aging study. J Clin Epidemiol. 2000;53(1): 71–8.
6. Brock G. Erectile dysfunction update education forum summary. Can J Urol. 2000;8:1416–8.
7. El-Sakka AI. Characteristics of erectile dysfunction in Saudi patients. Int J Impot Res. 2004;16:13–20.
8. El-Sakka AI. Association of risk factors and medical comorbidities with male sexual dysfunctions. J Sex Med. 2007;4:1691–700.
9. Seyam RM, Albakry A, Ghobish A, Arif H, Dandash K, Rashwan H. Prevalence of erectile dysfunction and its correlates in Egypt: a community-based study. Int J Impot Res. 2003;15:237–45.
10. Shaeer KZ, Osegbe DN, Siddiqui SH, Razzaque A, Glasser DB, Jaguste V. Prevalence of erectile dysfunction and its correlates among men attending primary care clinics in three countries, Pakistan, Egypt, and Nigeria. Int J Impot Res. 2003;Suppl 1:S8–S14.
11. Ludwig W, Phillips M. Organic causes of erectile dysfunction in men under 40. Urol Int. 2014;92:1–6.
12. Shaeer O, Shaeer K. The global online sexuality survey (GOSS.): erectile dysfunction among Arabic-speaking internet users in the Middle East. J Sex Med. 2011;9:2152–63.
13. Shaeer O, Shaeer K. The global online sexuality survey (GOSS). The United States of America in 2011. Chapter I. Erectile dysfunction among English-speakers. J Sex Med. 2012;9:3018–27.
14. Andersson KE, Wagner G. Physiology of penile erections [review]. Physiol Rev. 1995;75:191–236.
15. Burnett AL. Nitric oxide in the penis: physiology and pathology. J Urol. 1997;157:320–4.
16. Lincoln TM. Cyclic GMP and mechanisms of vasodilation. Pharmacol Ther. 1989;41:479–502.
17. Saenz de Tejada I. Molecular mechanisms for the regulation of penile smooth muscle contractility. Int J Impot Res. 2000;12(Suppl 4):S34–8.
18. Stief CG, Uckert S, Becker AJ, Truss MC, Jonas U. The effect of the specific phosphodiesterase (PDE) inhibitors on human and rabbit cavernous tissue in vitro and in vivo. J Urol. 1998;159(4): 1390–3.
19. Saenz de Tejada I, Blanco R, Goldstein I, Azadzoi K, de las Morenas A, Krane RJ, et al. Cholinrergic neurotransmission in human corpus cavernosum. Response of isolated tissue. Am J Physiol. 1988;254(3 Pt 2):H459–67.
20. Giuliano F, Allard J. Apomorphine SL (Uprima): preclinical and clinical experiences learned from the first central nervous system-acting ED drug [review]. Int J Impot Res. 2002;14(Suppl 1): S53–6.
21. Mulligan T, Schmitt B. Testosterone for erectile failure. J Intern Med. 1993;8:517–21.
22. Fazio L, Brock G. Erectile dysfunction: management update. CMAJ. 2004;170(9):1429–37.
23. Bors E, Comar AE. Neurological urology: physiology of micturition, its neurological disorders and sequelae. Baltimore: University Park Press; 1971.
24. Siegel T, Moul JW, Spevak M, Alvord G, Costabile RA. The development of erectile dysfunction in men treated for prostate cancer. J Urol. 2001;165:430–5.
25. Brock GB, Lue TF. Drug-induced sexual dysfunction: an update. Drug Saf. 1993;8:414–26.
26. Al Khaja KA, Sequeira RP, Alkhaja AK, Damanhori AH. Antihypertensive drugs and male sexual dysfunction: a review of adult hypertension guideline recommendations. J Cardiovasc Pharmacol Ther. 2016 May;21(3):233–44.
27. La Torre A, Giupponi G, Duffy D, Conca A, Catanzariti D. Sexual dysfunction related to drugs: a critical review. Part IV: cardiovascular drugs. Pharmacopsychiatry. 2015;48(1):1–6.
28. McVary KT, Carrier S, Wessells H. Subcommittee on smoking and erectile dysfunction socioeconomic committee, sexual medicine society of North America. Smoking and erectile dysfunction: evidence based analysis. J Urol. 2001;166(5):1624–32.
29. Huang YC, Chin CC, Chen CS, Shindel AW, Ho DR, Lin CS, Shi CS. Chronic cigarette smoking impairs erectile function through increased oxidative stress and apoptosis, decreased nNOS, endothelial and smooth muscle contents in a rat model. PLoS One. 2015;10(10):e0140728.
30. Grossmann M, Wu F. Male androgen deficiency: a multisystem syndrome. Asian J Androl. 2014;16(2):159–60.
31. Corona G, Rastrelli G, Monami M, Guay A, Buvat J, Sforza A, Forti G, Mannucci E, Maggi M. Hypogonadism as a risk factor for cardiovascular mortality in men: a meta-analytic study. Eur J Endocrinol. 2011;165(5):687–701.
32. El-Sakka AI, Hassoba HM, Sayed HM, Tayeb KA. Pattern of endocrinal changes in patients with sexual dysfunction. J Sex Med. 2005;2(4):551–8.
33. Chung SD, Chen YK, Lin HC, Lin HC. Increased risk of stroke among men with erectile dysfunction: a nationwide population-based study. J Sex Med. 2011;8:240–6.
34. Kelly DM, Jones TH. Testosterone: a vascular hormone in health and disease. J Endocrinol. 2013;217(3):R47–71.
35. Corona G, Bianchini S, Sforza A, Vignozzi L, Maggi M. Hypogonadism as a possible link between metabolic diseases and erectile dysfunction in aging men. Hormones (Athens). 2015;14(4): 569–78.
36. Caskurlu T, Tasci AI, Resim S, Sahinkanat T, Ergenekon E. The etiology of erectile dysfunction and contributing factors in different age groups in Turkey. Int J Urol. 2004;11:525–9.
37. Donatucci CF, Lue TF. Erectile dysfunction in men under 40: etiology and treatment choice. Int J Impot Res. 1993;5:97–103.
38. Glina S, Sharlip ID, Hellstrom WJG. Modifying risk factors to prevent and treat erectile dysfunction. J Sex Med. 2013;10: 115–9.
39. Ahmed I, El-Sakka A. Erectile dysfunction in Arab countries. Part I prevalence and correlates. Arab J Urol. 2012;10:97–103.
40. Guo W, Liao C, Zou Y, Li F, Li T, Zhou Q, et al. Erectile dysfunction and risk of clinical cardiovascular events: a metaanalysis of seven cohort studies. J Sex Med. 2010;7:2805–16.
41. Araujo AB, Travison TG, Ganz P, Chiu GR, Kupelian V, Rosen RC, et al. Erectile dysfunction and mortality. J Sex Med. 2009;6:2445–54.
42. Banks E, Joshy G, Abhayaratna WP, Kritharides L, Macdonald RJ, Korda RJ, et al. Erectile dysfunction severity as a risk marker for cardiovascular disease hospitalisation and all-cause mortality: a prospective cohort study. PLoS Med. 2013;10:e1001372.
43. Yamada T, Hara K, Umematsu H, Suzuki R, Kadowaki T. Erectile dysfunction and cardiovascular events in diabetic men: a meta-analysis of observational studies. PLoS One. 2012;7:e43673.
44. Dong JY, Zhang YH, Qin LQ. Erectile dysfunction and risk of cardiovascular disease: meta-analysis of prospective cohort studies. J Am Coll Cardiol. 2011;58:1378–85.
45. El-Sakka AI, Morsy AM, Fagih BI, Nassar AH. Coronary artery risk factors in patients with erectile dysfunction. J Urol. 2004;172:251–4.
46. El-Sakka AI, Morsy AM. Screening for ischemic heart disease in patients with erectile dysfunction. The role of penile Doppler ultrasonography. Urology. 2004;64:346–50.

47. Jackson G, Montorsi P, Adams MA, Anis T, El-Sakka A, Miner M, et al. Cardiovascular aspects of sexual medicine. J Sex Med. 2010;7:1608–26.
48. Jackson G, Montorsi P, Adams MA, Anis T, El-Sakka A, Miner M, et al. Cardiovascular aspects of sexual medicine. In: Montorsi R, Basson R, Adaikan G, et al., editors. Sexual medicine, sexual dysfunctions in men and women. Paris, France: Health Publication Ltd; 2010. p. 351–402. [chapter VIII].
49. El-Sakka AI, Morsy AM, Fagih BI. Severity of erectile dysfunction could predict left ventricular diastolic dysfunction in patients without overt cardiac complaint. J Sex Med. 2011;8:2590–7.
50. Malavige LS, Jayaratne SD, Kathriarachchi ST, Sivayogan S, Ranasinghe P, et al. Erectile dysfunction is a strong predictor of poor quality of life in men with type 2 diabetes mellitus. Diabet Med. 2014;31:699–706.
51. El-Sakka AI, Tayeb KA. Erectile dysfunction risk factors in noninsulin dependent diabetic Saudi patients. J Urol. 2003;169: 1043–7.
52. El-Sakka AI. Penile axial rigidity and Doppler ultrasonography parameters in patients with erectile dysfunction: association with type 2 diabetes. Urology. 2003;62:525–31.
53. El-Sakka AI, Tayeb KA. Peyronie's disease in diabetic patients being screened for erectile dysfunction. J Urol. 2005;174: 1026–30.
54. El-Sakka AI, Tayeb KA. Vascular impairment of erection in patients with diabetes and Peyronie's disease: Is that accumulative? J Sex Med. 2009;6:1736–42.
55. El-Sakka AI, Sayed HM, Tayeb KA. Diabetes-associated androgen alteration in patients with erectile dysfunction. Int J Androl. 2008;31:602–8.
56. El-Sakka AI, Sayed HM, Tayeb KA. Androgen pattern in patients with type 2 diabetes associated erectile dysfunction: impact of metabolic control. Urology. 2009;74:552–60.
57. El-Sakka AI. Erectile dysfunction in Arab countries. Part I: prevalence and correlates. Arab J Urol. 2012;10(2):97–103.
58. Siroky M, Azadzoi K, Kloner M, Lue T, Shabsigh R, Burnett A, Steers W, Andersson K. Vasculogenic erectile dysfunction: newer therapeutic strategies. J Urol. 2003;170(2):S24–30.
59. Sommer F, Goldstein I, Korda JB. Bicycle riding and erectile dysfunction: a review. J Sex Med. 2010;7:2346–58.
60. Yao F, Huang Y, Zhang Y, Dong Y, Ma H, et al. Subclinical endothelial dysfunction and low-grade inflammation play roles in the development of erectile dysfunction in young men with low risk of coronary heart disease. Int J Androl. 2012;35:653–9.
61. Vercellotti GM, Moldow CF, Jacob HS. Complement, oxidants, and endothelial injury: how a bedside observation opened a door to vascular biology. J Clin Invest. 2012;122:3044–5.
62. Esper R, Nordaby R, Vilariño J, Paragano A, Cacharrón J, Machado R. Endothelial dysfunction: a comprehensive appraisal. Cardiovasc Diabetol. 2006;5:4.
63. Kun A, Kiraly I, Pataricza J, Marton Z, Krassoi I, Varro A, Simonsen U, Papp J, Pajor L. C-type natriuretic peptide hyperpolarizes and relaxes human penile resistance arteries. J Sex Med. 2008;5:1114–25.
64. Vlachopoulos C, Rokkas K, Ioakeimidis N, Stefanadis C. Inflammation, metabolic syndrome, erectile dysfunction, and coronary artery disease: common links. Eur Urol. 2007;52(6):1590–600.
65. Sáenz de T, Angulo J, Cellek S, Gonzalez-Cadavid N. Physiology of erectile function. J Sex Med. 2004;1:254–65.
66. Chung E, De Young L, Brock GB. Penile duplex ultrasonography in men with Peyronie's disease: is it veno-occlusive dysfunction or poor cavernosal arterial inflow that contributes to erectile dysfunction? J Sex Med. 2011;8:3446–51.
67. Miner MM, Seftel AD. Peyronie's disease: epidemiology, diagnosis, and management. Curr Med Res Opin. 2014;30:113–20.
68. Rosen R, Catania J, Lue T, Althof S, Henne J, et al. Impact of Peyronie's disease on sexual and psychosocial functioning: qualitative findings in patients and controls. J Sex Med. 2008;5:1977–84.
69. Mulhall JP, Bivalacqua TJ, Becher EF. Standard operating procedure for the preservation of erectile function outcomes after radical prostatectomy. J Sex Med. 2012;10:195–203.
70. Fowler CJ, Panicker JN, Emmanuel A. Pelvic organ dysfunction in neurological disease. Cambridge: Cambridge University Press; 2010. ISBN:9780521198318.
71. Vodušek DB. Lower urinary tract and sexual dysfunction in neurological patients. Eur Neurol. 2014;72(1–2):109–15.
72. El-Sakka AI, Hassoba HM, Sayed HM, Tayeb KA. Pattern of endocrinal changes in patients with sexual dysfunction. J Sex Med. 2005;2:551–8.
73. Young J. Approach to the male patient with congenital hypogonadotropic hypogonadism. J Clin Endocrinol Metab. 2012;97: 707–18.
74. Veronelli A, Masu A, Ranieri R, Rognoni C, Laneri M, et al. Prevalence of erectile dysfunction in thyroid disorders: comparison with control subjects and with obese and diabetic patients. Int J Impot Res. 2006;18:111–4.
75. Krassas GE, Tziomalos K, Papadopoulou F, Pontikides N, Perros P. Erectile dysfunction in patients with hyper and hypothyroidism: how common and should we treat? J Clin Endocrinol Metab. 2008;93:1815–9.
76. Reliability and Prevalence in the DSM-5 Field Trials, January 12, 2012 http://www.dsm5.org/Documents/ Reliability_and_Prevalence_in_DSM-5_Field_Trials_ 1-12-12.pdf
77. "Highlights of changes from DSM-IV-TR to DSM-5" (PDF). American Psychiatric Association. May 17, 2013. Archived from the original (PDF) on 26 Feb 2015.
78. Papagiannopoulos D, Khare N, Nehra A. Evaluation of young men with organic erectile dysfunction. Asian J Androl. 2015; 17(1):11–6. doi:10.4103/1008-682X.139253.. Review.
79. Morgentaler A, Khera M, Maggi M, Zitzmann M. Commentary: who is a candidate for testosterone therapy? A synthesis of international expert opinions. J Sex Med. 2014;11:1636–45.
80. El-Sakka AI, Lue TF. A rational approach to investigation of the sexually dysfunctional man. In: Morales A, editor. Erectile dysfunction: issues in current pharmacotherapy. Martin Dunitz; United Kingdom 1998. p. 49–69.
81. Lue TF, El-Sakka AI. Erectile dysfunction. In: Weiss RM, George NJR, O'Reilly PH, editors. Comprehensive urology. London, UK: Mosby Harcourt Sciences; 2001. p. 597–612.
82. Hatzichristou D, Rosen RC, Derogatis LR, Low WY, Meuleman EJH, Sadovsky R. Recommendations for the clinical evaluation of men and women with sexual dysfunction. United Kingdom J Sex Med. 2010;7: 337–48.
83. Sikka SC, Hellstrom WJG, Brock G, Morales AM. Standardization of vascular assessment of erectile dysfunction. J Sex Med. 2013; 10:120–9.
84. Bella AJ, Sener A, Foell K, Brock GB. Nonpalpable scarring of the penile septum as a cause of erectile dysfunction: an atypical form of Peyronie's disease. J Sex Med. 2007;4:226–30.
85. Burnett A. Campbell-walsh urology. Evaluation and management of erectile dysfunction. Ch. 24. Philadelphia: Elsevier Inc.; 2011.
86. Walz J, Epstein JI, Ganzer R, Graefen M, Guazzoni G, Kaouk J, Menon M, Mottrie A, Myers RP, Patel V, Tewari A, Villers A, Artibani W. A Critical Analysis of the Current Knowledge of Surgical Anatomy of the Prostate Related to Optimisation of Cancer Control and Preservation of Continence and Erection in Candidates for Radical Prostatectomy: An Update. Eur Urol. 2016 Aug;70(2):301-11
87. Weyne E, Mulhall J, Albersen M. Molecular pathophysiology of cavernous nerve injury and identification of strategies for nerve

function recovery after radical prostatectomy. Curr Drug Targets. 2015;16(5):459–73.
88. Ralph D, McNicholas T. UK management guidelines for erectile dysfunction. Br Med J. 2000;321:499–503.
89. Corona G, Petrone L, Mannucci E, Mansani R, Balercia G, et al. Difficulties in achieving vs maintaining erection: organic, psychogenic and relational determinants. Int J Impot Res. 2005; 17:252–8.
90. Bivalacqua TJ, Usta MF, Champion HC, Kadowitz PJ, Hellstrom WJ. Endothelial dysfunction in erectile dysfunction: role of the endothelium in erectile physiology and disease. J Androl. 2003; 24:S17–37.
91. Canadian Urological Association Guidelines Committee. Erectile dysfunction practice guidelines. Can J Urol. 2002;9(4):1583–7.
92. Ralph D, McNicholas T. UK management guidelines for erectile dysfunction. BMJ. 2000;321:499–503.
93. Davis-Joseph B, Tiefer L, Melman A. Accuracy of the initial history and physical examination to establish the etiology of erectile dysfunction. Urology. 1995;45:498–502.
94. Chun J, Carson III CC. Physician–patient dialogue and clinical evaluation of erectile dysfunction. Urol Clin North Am. 2001;28(2):249–58.
95. Metz P, Bengtsson J. Penile blood pressure. Scand J Urol Nephrol. 1981;15:161.
96. Aitchison M, Aitchison J, Carter R. Is the penile brachial index a reproducible and useful measurement? Br J Urol. 1990;66:202–4.
97. de Wolfe VG. Non-invasive vascular evaluation. In: Montague DK, editor. Disorders of male sexual function. Chicago: Year Book Publishers; 1988. p. 44–59.
98. Lue TF, Tanagho EA. Physiology of erection and pharmacological management of impotence. J Urol. 1987;137:829–36.
99. Pescatori ES, Hatzichristou DG, Namburi S, Goldstein I. A positive intracavernous injection test implies normal veno-occlusive but not necessarily normal arterial function: a hemodynamic study. J Urol. 1994;151:1209–16.
100. Erdogru T, Kadioglu A, Cayan S, Tellaloglu S. Does the positive intracavernous papaverine test always indicate a normal penile vascular system? Eur Urol. 1997;31:323–8.
101. Lue TF, Hricak H, Marich KW, Tanagho EA. Vasculogenic impotence evaluated by high-resolution ultrasonography and pulsed Doppler spectrum analysis. Radiology. 1985;155:777–81.
102. Mueller SC, Lue TF. Evaluation of vasculogenic impotence. Urol Clin North Am. 1988;15:65–76.
103. Quam JP, King BF, James EM, Lewis RW, Brakke DM, et al. Duplex and color Doppler sonographic evaluation of vasculogenic impotence. AJR Am J Roentgenol. 1989;153:1141–7.
104. Naroda T, Yamanaka M, Matsushita K, Kimura K, Kawanishi Y, et al. Clinical studies for venogenic impotence with color Doppler ultrasonography – evaluation of resistance index of the cavernous artery. Nihon Hinyokika Gakkai Zasshi. 1996;87:1231–5.
105. Shamloul R. Peak systolic velocities may be falsely low in young patients with erectile dysfunction. J Sex Med. 2006;3:138–43.
106. Jarow JP, Pugh VW, Routh WD, Dyer RB. Comparison of penile duplex ultrasonography to pudendal arteriography. Variant penile arterial anatomy affects interpretation of duplex ultrasonography. Invest Radiol. 1993;28:806–10.
107. Rajfer J, Canan V, Dorey EJ, Mehringer CM. Correlation between penile angiography and duplex scanning of cavernous arteries in impotent men. J Urol. 1990;143:1128–30.
108. Shabsigh R, Fishman IJ, Shotland Y, Karacan I, Dunn JK. Comparison of penile duplex ultrasonography with nocturnal penile tumescence monitoring for the evaluation of erectile impotence. J Urol. 1990;143:924–7.
109. Knispel HH, Anderson R. Evaluation of vasculogenic impotence by monitoring of cavernous oxygen tension. J Urol. 1993;149: 1276–9.
110. Donatucci F, Lue TF. The combined intracavernous injection and stimulation test: diagnostic accuracy. J Urol. 1992;148:61–2.
111. Michal V, Pospichal J. Phalloarteriography in the diagnosis of erectile impotence. World J Surg. 1978;2:239–48.
112. Philip F, Shishehbor M. Current state of endovascular treatment for vasculogenic erectile dysfunction. Curr Cardiol Rep. 2013;15(5):360. doi:10.1007/s11886-013-0360-8.. Review.
113. Kaneko K, De Mouy EH, Lee BE. Sequential contrast-enhanced MR imaging of the penis. Radiology. 1994;191:75–7.
114. Vargas HA, Donati OF, Wibmer A, Goldman DA, Mulhall JP, et al. Association between penile dynamic contrast-enhanced MRI-derived quantitative parameters and self-reported sexual function in patients with newly diagnosed prostate cancer. J Sex Med. 2014;11(10):2581–8.
115. Wespes E, Delcour C, Struyen J, Schulman CC. Cavernometry-cavernography: its role in organic impotence. Eur Urol. 1984;10: 229–32.
116. Rudnick J, Bodecker R, Weidner W. Significance of the intracavernosal pharmacological injection test, pharmacocavernosography, artificial erection and cavernosometry in the diagnosis of venous leakage. Urol Int. 1991;46:338–43.
117. Lue TF, Hricak H, Schmidt RA, Tanagho EA. Functional evaluation of penile veins by cavernosography in papaverine-induced erection. J Urol. 1986;135:479–82.
118. Montague DK, Lakin MM. False diagnoses of venous leak impotence. J Urol. 1992;148:148–9.
119. Bemelmans B, Hendrixkx L, Koldewijn E, Lemmens W. Comparision of biothesiometry and neurophysiological investigations for the clinical evaluation of patients with erectile dysfunction. J Urol. 1995;153:1483–6.
120. Kaneko S, Bradley WE. Penile electrodiagnosis. Value of bulbocavernosus reflex latency versus nerve conduction velocity of the dorsal nerve of the penis in diagnosis of diabetic impotence. J Urol. 1987;137:933–5.
121. Amarenco G, Kerdraon J. Perineal electrophysiological studies in erectile dysfunctions. Study of 423 cases. Ann Med Interne (Paris). 1993;144:383–8.
122. Abicht JH. Testing the autonomic system. In: Jonas U, Thon WF, Stief CG, editors. Erectile dysfunction. Springer-Verlag: Berlin; 1991. p. 187–93.
123. Daffertshofer M, Linden D, Syren M, Junemann K-P, Berlit P. Assessment of local sympathetic function in patients with erectile dysfunction. Int J Impot Res. 1994;6(4):213–25.
124. Yiou R, De Laet K, Hisano M, Salomon L, Abbou CC, et al. Neurophysiological testing to assess penile sensory nerve damage after radical prostatectomy. J Sex Med. 2012;9:2457–66.
125. Wagner G, Gerstenberg T, Levin RJ. Electrical activity of corpus cavernosum during flaccidity and erection of the human penis: a new diagnostic method? J Urol. 1989;142:723–5.
126. Djamilian M, Stief CG, Hartmann U, Jonas U. Predictive value of real-time RigiScan monitoring for the etiology of organogenic impotence. J Urol. 1993;149:1269–71.
127. Bhasin S, Cunningham GR, Hayes FJ, et al. Testosterone therapy in men with androgen deficiency syndromes: an endocrine society clinical practice guideline. J Clin Endocrinol Metab. 2010;95(6): 2536–59.
128. Seftel AD, Kathrins M, Niederberger C. Critical update of the 2010 endocrine society clinical practice guidelines for male hypogonadism: a systematic analysis. Mayo Clin Proc. 2015;90(8):1104–15.
129. Corona G, Petrone L, Paggi F, Lotti F, Boddi V, et al. Sexual dysfunction in subjects with Klinefelter's syndrome. Int J Androl. 2010;33:574–80.
130. Maggi M, Buvat J, Corona G, Guay A. Hormonal causes of male sexual dysfunctions and their management (Hyperprolactinemia, thyroid disorders, GH Disorders, and DHEA). J Sex Med. 2012;10:661–77.

131. Fischer C. Cycle of penile erection synchronous with dreaming sleep. Arch Gen Psychiatry. 1965;12:29–45.
132. Karacan I. Clinical value of nocturnal penile erection in the prognosis of impotence. Med Aspects Hum Sex. 1970;4:27.
133. Morales A, Condra M, Heaton JP, Johnston B, Fenemore J. Diurnal penile tumescence recording in the etiological diagnosis of erectile dysfunction. J Urol. 1994;152:1111–4.
134. Bradley WE, Timm GW, Gallagher JM, Johnson BK. New method for continuous measurement of nocturnal penile tumescence and rigidity. Urology. 1985;26:4–9.
135. Allen RP, Smolev JK, Engel RM, Brendler CB. Comparison of RigiScan and formal nocturnal penile tumescence testing in the evaluation of erectile rigidity. J Urol. 1993;149:1265–8.
136. Rosen RC, Cappelleri JC, Smith MD, Lipsky J, Pena BM. Development and evaluation of an abridged, 5-item version of the International Index of Erectile Function (IIEF-5) as a diagnostic tool for erectile dysfunction. Int J Impot Res. 1999;11:319–26.
137. Rosen RC, Riley A, Wagner G, Osterloh IH, Kirkpatrick J, Mishra A. The international index of erectile function (IIEF): a multidimensional scale for assessment of erectile dysfunction. Urology. 1997;49:822–30.
138. Cappelleri JC, Rosen RC, Smith MD, Mishra A, Osterloh IH. Diagnostic evaluation of the erectile function domain on the International Index of erectile function. Urology. 1999;54:346–51.
139. Derby CA, Araujo AB, Johannes CB, Feldman HA, McKinlay JB. Measurement of erectile dysfunction in population-based studies: the use of a single question self assessment in the Massachusetts Male Aging Study. Int J Impot Res. 2000;12:197–204.
140. Cappelleri JC, Siegel RL, Glasser DB, Osterloh IH, Rosen RC. Relationship between patient self-assessment of erectile function and the sexual health inventory for men. Clin Ther. 2001;23:1707–19.
141. Jardin A, Wagner G, Khoury S, et al. Recommendations of the 1st international consultation on erectile dysfunction. In: Jardin A, Wagner G, Khoury S, et al., editors. Erectile dysfunction. Plymouth, U.K: Health Publication Ltd; 2000. p. 711–26.
142. The Process of Care Consensus Panel. A process of care model for evaluation and treatment of erectile dysfunction. Int J Impot Res. 1999;11:11–9.
143. Rosen RC, Cappelleri JC, Gendrano III. N. The international index of erectile function (IIEF): a state-of-the science review. Int J Impot Res. 2002;14(4):226–44.
144. Cella D, Yount S, Rothrock N, Gershon R, Cook K, Reeve B, Ader D, Fries JF, Bruce B, Rose M, PROMIS Cooperative Group. The Patient-Reported Outcomes Measurement Information System (PROMIS): progress of an NIH Roadmapcooperative group during its first two years. Med Care. 2007;45(5 Suppl 1): S3–S11.
145. Weinfurt KP, Lin L, Bruner DW, Cyranowski JM, Dombeck CB, Hahn EA, Jeffery DD, Luecht RM, Magasi S, Porter LS, Reese JB, Reeve BB, Shelby RA, Smith AW, Willse JT, Flynn KE. Development and initial validation of the PROMIS(®) sexual function and satisfaction measures version 2.0. J Sex Med. 2015;12(9):1961–74. doi:10.1111/jsm.12966.. Epub 2015 Sep 7.

13 Treatment of Erectile Disorder

Ezzat A. Ismail and Ahmed I. El-Sakka

Introduction

Erectile dysfunction (ED) is defined as the inability to achieve and/or maintain an erection sufficient to permit satisfactory sexual intercourse. ED may result from psychological, neurologic, hormonal, vascular, or impairment of cavernosal smooth muscle function. The last 3 decades have witnessed a phenomenal improvement in diagnosis and treatment of ED. In the current chapter we review contemporary medical and surgical treatments for ED and novel therapies in development [1], Table 13-1.

Lifestyle Modification

Cardiovascular disease, diabetes, and metabolic syndromes significantly increase the risk of developing ED. Modification of these medical conditions either prevents or decreases the risk of ED development [2].

(a) *Weight reduction*: BMI changes, weight and caloric intake reduction ameliorate ED-associated metabolic syndromes [3].
(b) *Exercise*: there is an evidence of ED improvement in men who practice physical exercise over men with sedentary lifestyle [4]. IIEF score is significantly improved in obese men with no cardiovascular disease after weight reduction and physical exercise [5].
(c) *General habits*: cessation of smoking improves erectile function recovery [6]. Bicycle riders showed improvement of erectile function when they change saddle from conventional to no-nose, probably by decreasing perineal trauma [7]. Current systematic reviews emphasized the role of lifestyle modification in ameliorating sexual function through increasing testosterone level, mood and self-esteem improvement and reduction of cardiovascular risks [2].

Medication Changes

Switching medications or dose reductions might be needed to alleviate their offending effects on erectile function and ultimately may improve potency in some patients [8].

(a) **Antihypertensives**: Nearly all antihypertensives have potential ED as an adverse effect.
   - *Diuretics*: Patients treated with thiazides had a higher rate of ED compared to placebo or atenolol [9].
   - *Beta blockers*: Propranolol and other nonselective beta blockers are associated with increases prevalence of ED; other beta 1-selective agents such as acebutolol have a substantial reduction in ED when compared to nonselective beta blockers [10].
   - *Alpha blockers*: Animal studies showed a beneficial effect of alpha blockers on erectile function, particularly those agents exerting a selective inhibition of alpha 1 receptors by prolongation of cavernous smooth muscle relaxation [11]. Alpha 2 receptors stimulatory drugs such as Clonidine diminish erectile function [12]. Centrally acting drugs such as methyldopa are associated with ED probably by antagonizing hypothalamic alpha 2 receptors [13].
   - *Angiotensin-Converting Enzyme [ACE) Inhibitors:* When compared to other antihypertensive drugs, ACE inhibitors showed no significant effect on erectile function. ACE inhibitors lack any appreciated peripheral or central effect that would interfere with sexual function [12]. Recent studies on angiotensin II Type 1 receptor antagonist [e.g., valsartan, candesartan, losartan) showed a beneficial effect of these agents on potency and reversal of penile vasculature structural changes. They appear to preserve or improve erectile function [14].

W.W. IsHak (ed.), *The Textbook of Clinical Sexual Medicine*, DOI 10.1007/978-3-319-52539-6_13

TABLE 13-1. Options and modalities of ED treatment

1.	Lifestyle modification
	(a) Weight reduction
	(b) Exercise
	(c) General habits
2.	Medication changes
	(a) Antihypertensives:
	• Diuretics
	• Beta blockers
	• Alpha blockers
	• Angiotensin-Converting Enzyme(ACE) Inhibitors
	• Ca channel blockers
	• Aldosterone receptor antagonist
	(b) Psychotropic drugs
	• Antipsychotics
	• Antidepressants
	• Anxiolytics
	• Anticonvulsants
	(c) Antiandrogens
	(d) Miscellaneous
	• Digoxin
	• Statins
	• H2 receptor antagonists
	• Opiates
3.	Oral treatment
	(a) Phosphodiesterase 5 inhibitors (PDE5-I)
	• Conventional PDE5-I
	• Innovative PDE5-I
	• Once daily regimen
	(b) Melanocortin-receptor agonists
	(c) Serotonin-receptor effectors
	(d) Other oral therapies
4.	Intracavernosal Injection (ICI)
5.	Intraurethral suppositories
6.	Vacuum erection device (VED)
7.	Hormonal therapy
	(a) Testosterone replacement
	(b) Alternative hormonal treatments
	(c) Hyperprolactinemia treatments
8.	Evolving modalities
	(a) Soluble guanylate cyclase (sGC) activators
	• BAY 60-2770
	• BAY 41-2272
	• BAY 60-4552
	(b) Stem Cells (SCs)
	• Clinically applicable SCs
	• Investigational SCs
	(c) Low-intensity shockwave therapy (Li-ESWT)
9.	Alternative treatment
	(a) Herbal treatment
	(b) Resveratrol
	(c) Pyrazolopyrimidinone analogues
	(d) Neuromedin B
	(e) Transdermal/topical pharmacotherapy
	(f) Penile vibrators

(continued)

TABLE 13-1. (continued)

	(g) Impulse magnetic-field therapy
	(h) Tissue engineering
	(i) Nanotechnology
	(j) Endovascular tools
10.	Combination therapy
11.	Surgery:
	(a) Reconstructive surgery
	• Arterial revascularization
	• Venous surgery
	(b) Penile prosthesis
12.	Psychosocial Interventions

- Ca *channel blockers:* Ca channel blockers have no adverse effect on erectile function, nevertheless; short-term ejaculatory dysfunction may be elicited when using these agents due to decreased propulsive force of bulbocavernosus muscle [15, 16].
- *Aldosterone receptor antagonist:* Spironolactone has affinity for androgen and progesterone receptors, increasing the likelihood of endocrine adverse effects, including gynecomastia, loss of libido, and impotence. Eplerenone is a second generation antagonist to aldosterone receptor selective for aldosterone receptors only with low affinity for androgen and progesterone receptors [17].

(b) **Psychotropic drugs**

The underlying disorder is ED related rather than medication related and this is due to interrelationship of CNS pathways [18].

- *Antipsychotics:* Sexual dysfunction occurs in 40–70% of patients on antipsychotic drugs [19]. Sexual symptoms are caused by the extrapyramidal side effects of these drugs through beta-blockade, anti-dopaminergic, and anticholinergic action.
- *Antidepressants: Tricyclics* cause orgasmic disorders, and also used to treat premature ejaculation. *MAO inhibitors* have higher rates of orgasmic dysfunction. *SSRIs* cause sexual dysfunction in 50% of patients [20].
- *Anxiolytics:* Benzodiazepines and lithium are associated with sexual dysfunction, while recent anxiolytics such as buspirone are not, and may be used to alleviate sexual dysfunction in such patients [21].
- *Anticonvulsants:* Carbamazepine is a common cause of orgasmic dysfunction and Valproate causes loss of libido [22]. Patients treated with lamotrigine show hypersexuality and improved sexual function [23].

(c) **Antiandrogens:** These agents block androgen action either partially or completely. Effect of androgen deficiency ranges from normal to complete loss of sexual function. Nocturnal erection is androgen-dependent while visual sexual stimulation is not [11]. Finasteride and dutasteride [5 alpha-reductase inhibitors] have the least effect on testosterone level. Medical castration that produces near-complete androgen deprivation that is achieved either by LHRH agonist or antagonist results in significant loss of libido which is accompanied by ED [24].

(d) **Miscellaneous:** based on individual observations rather than controlled trials, the following drugs seem to be associated with ED in men;

- *Digoxin*
- *Statins*
- *receptor antagonists*
- *Opiates*

Oral Treatment

Phosphodiesterase 5 Inhibitors (PDE5-I)

PDE5 inhibitors have been considered as the standard ED treatment since FDA approval of sildenafil citrate in 1998, subsequently; other agents such as vardenafil, tadalafil, and avanafil emerged and gained popularity as an effective oral treatment for ED [25].

PDE5 inhibitors facilitate cavernous smooth muscle relaxation via blockade of cGMP, the catalytic enzyme that involves degradation of nitric oxide (NO). These agents are only effective under the effect of sexual stimulation as their effect is to augment rather than to start penile erection through the release of NO first [26]. Overall, the satisfaction rate of PDE5 inhibitors is approximately 70% [27].

Drug efficacy is enhanced by reduction of food intake that may lag drug absorption. Drug dose escalation and repetition (9–10 times) might be necessary to judge efficacy [28]. Glycemic control, androgen replacement, and dyslipidemic control are also important to potentiate drug efficacy [29].

To avoid PDE5–nitrite interaction, it is absolutely contraindicated to use any form of nitric oxide donors in combination with PDE5I. Hypotension may occur when using PDE5 inhibitors simultaneously with alpha blockers, as they both are vasodilators. Other side effects include headache, dyspepsia, flushing, myalgia, back pain, nasal congestion, and visual disturbances

PDE5 inhibitors have similar modes of action but differ in their pharmacokinetics and pharmacodynamics (Tables 13-2, 13-3, and 13-4).

- Conventional PDE5-I:

Sildenafil (Viagra®, Pfizer) 50 mg is the recommended starting dose, taken 1 h before sexual activity. The maximum recommended frequency is once daily. Drug absorption is impaired by high-fat diet. Sildenafil efficacy has been investigated with other coexisting conditions (e.g., hypertension, spinal cord injury, depression, prostate surgery, diabetes, and

Table 13-2. Comparison of PDE5 inhibitors[a]

	Conventional PDE5 inhibitors	NewPDE5 inhibitors
	Sildenafil, Vardenafil, Tadalafil, Avanafil	*Udenafil, Mirodenafil*
Onset of action (min)	15–120	60–90
Half-life (h)	3–17.5	7.3–12.1
Once daily dose	Tadalafil only	Patients who cannot tolerate PDE5 subtype selectivity of tadalafil
Fatty food	Reduced absorption, but no effect with tadalafil	Reduced absorption
Side effects:		
• Headache	• Yes	• Yes
• Dyspepsia	• Yes	• No
• Facial flushing	• Yes	• Yes
• Backache, myalgia	• Rare, but common with tadalafil	• Rare
• Blurred/blue vision	• Sildenafil only	• No
• Precaution with antiarrhythmics	• Vardenafil only	• No
• Contraindication with nitrates	• Absolutely contraindicated	• Absolutely contraindicated

Udenafil and Mirodenafil are not FDA approved, but approved in Korea.
[a]FDA approval: Sildenafil 1998, Vardenafil and Tadalafil 2003, Avanafil 2012.

Table 13-3. Contraindications and drug interactions to PDE5 inhibitors

Severe (high risk) cardiovascular disease according to Second Princeton Consensus Conference [30, 31]
• left ventricular outflow obstruction
• Impaired control of blood pressure
• Myocardial infarction
• Stroke
• Heart failure
• Coronary artery disease (e.g., unstable angina)
• Extremes of arterial blood pressure (<90/50 mmHg) or (>170/100 mmHg)
• Retinal disorders (retinitis pigmentosa)
• Hepatic impairment (Child-Pugh C)
• End-stage renal disease requiring dialysis
• Dose reduction is needed when used in conjunction with ketoconazole, itraconazole or ritonavir

Table 13-4. Guideline for PDE5 inhibitors therapy

PDE5 inhibitors are contraindicated to be taken with nitrates, but they may be administered by men with coronary disease (not needing nitrates on regular basis) but avoided 1 day before taking a nitrate. Additionally, Initial on-drug exercise testing and blood pressure monitoring is indicated to evaluate the risk of cardiac ischemia with sexual intercourse

Based on data from Ref. 44.

the elderly) [32] with no significant difference in response rates compared to normal cohorts [33–38]. Response rate to sildenafil is significantly diminished in patients who underwent non-nerve sparing radical prostatectomy [36].

Vardenafil (Levitra, Bayer) is a highly selective and potent PDE5 inhibitor. Despite being similar in chemical structure, it is more potent and selective than sildenafil. The recommended starting dose is either 10 or 20 mg oral (Levitra®) or 10 mg sublingual (Staxyn®). Vardenafil has a faster onset of action if compared to other PDE5 inhibitors. Fifty-three percent of patients can obtain erection sufficient for penetration at 25 min. As well as sildenafil, vardenafil absorption is impaired if the drug is taken after a fat meal [39]. Dose-dependent side effects include headache (21%), flushing (13%), and dyspepsia (6%) [40].

Tadalafil (Cialis®, Eli Lilly) has a distinct chemical structure that differs from other PDE5 inhibitors. Recommended on-demand doses are 5, 10, and 20 mg. It is also available at 2,5 and 5 mg as a daily dose medication. Onset of action is within 30–45 min that may last for 24–48 h. Visual side effects encountered with other PDE5 inhibitors are less evident with tadalafil as it has a little inhibitory effect on PDE-6 and it has milder side effects but low back pain is a reported side effect of tadalafil. Drug absorption is not affected by meal or alcohol intake with a unique half-life of 17.5 h, peak plasma concentration of 2, and 36 h duration of action [41].

Avanafil (stendra®, Vivus) has a different chemical structure, fast onset of action and 5–10 h half-life [42]. It shares other PDE5 inhibitors the same side effects [43].

- Innovative PDE5 inhibitors:

TPN729MA is an under-development selective PDE5 inhibitor that has a potent and balanced selectivity for ED treatment. It has a longer duration of action than conventional PDE5 inhibitors in the studied animal models [45].

Preclinical pharmacokinetics of TPN729MA showed promising results that predict its future human application [46].

Udenafil is another new PDE5 inhibitor that acts by modulation of cNOS expression, thus inhibiting cGMP degradation. It compensates diabetes-associated corpus cavernosum changes. Compared to conventional PDE5 inhibitors, udenafil has a comparable safety profile [47].

Mirodenafil is a second generation PDE5 inhibitor that has high affinity and selectivity for PDE5 enzyme compared to conventional PDE5Is with better efficacy for ED treatment. The drug is given in two doses, 50 or 100 mg. Men with ED, hypertension or LUTS due to benign prostatic hyperplasia have adequately tolerated mirodenafil. Similar to other PDE5Is, mirodenafil has mild to moderate side effects (53.7%), commonly flushing (6.7–24.1%) and headache (1.8–14.8%) [48].

- Once daily regimen

Tadalafil once daily regimen is available alternative to on-demand PDE5 inhibitor therapy in ED patients [49]. However, satisfaction and compliance rates are not affected by patient's characteristics or associated comorbidities [50]. More than 68% of men on tadalafil 5 mg once-daily regimen were able to continue this plan for 6 months if they were involved in treatment plan [51]. On the other hand, amelioration of the effect of diabetes on erectile function was achieved by chronic low-dose PDE5 inhibitor administration combined by tight glycemic control [52]. Similarly, endothelial function and insulin sensitivity are enhanced on a 3-months PDE5 inhibitor regimen [18].

Melanocortin-Receptor Agonists

Melanocortin analogues have a central action on melanocortin-4 receptors that modulates erectile function, sexual behavior, food intake and energy. These molecules have shown to improve erectile function in clinical trials [53, 54]. *Bremelanotide* intranasal administration improved erectile function compared to placebo in both control and PDE5I nonresponders. Side effects include flushing and nausea [95, 96]. Nevertheless, melanocortin analogues have not been FDA approved for the treatment of ED due to limited safety profile.

Serotonin-Receptor Effectors

Trazodone (Desyrel) is an antidepressant drug that may cause priapism. This off-label effect promoted trazodone as a possible ED treatment [55]. Its active metabolite acts as an agonist to 5-HT2C receptors promoting erectile function [11]. This drug has limited role in ED treatment given its limited safety profile. Side effects include nausea, vomiting, drowsiness, urine retention, and priapism [56].

Other Oral Therapies

Yohimbine is an alpha 2-blocker that is not indicated in patients with organic ED as it has a marginal effect on erectile function. Studies on non-organic ED patients have shown some response over placebo. Side effects include anxiety, tremors, palpitation and hypertension [57].

Apomorphine (Uprima®) is a dopaminergic (D1/D2 receptors) agonist that is given in a sublingual route. It is a potent emetic drug. It acts as a pro-erectile drug when given in a subcutaneous route in rats and humans. Side effects especially nausea limited its clinical application. Sublingual route is available in Europe, but not FDA approved yet [58].

Phentolamine (Vasomax®) is an oral drug that has been reported to improve erectile function. Its side effects include facial flushing, headache and nasal congestion. It has not been FDA approved yet. [59, 60].

Additional oral drugs have been proposed including L-arginine (nitric oxide precursor amino acid), Limaprost (prostaglandin E1), L-dopa, and Naltrexone (opioid antagonist) [61]. However, role of these drugs remain unclear because they are not thoroughly investigated [25].

Intracavernosal Injection

Intracavernosal injection (ICI) is a very successful line of treatment for severe ED, especially in diabetes-associated ED, following cavernous nerve injury and post-radical prostatectomy patients. Patients who are refractory to PDE5I are also better candidates for ICI programs. Moreover, ICI is a remarkable method in penile rehabilitation during or after RP. It restores natural and spontaneous erection. Nevertheless, several studies are required to validate such perspective. ICI improves endothelial function and hemodynamics of the cavernous smooth muscle by increasing muscle-to-collagen ratio. Despite being a fundamental part in the diagnosis and treatment of ED, the role of ICI is still evolving and still not well defined. Several new ICI materials are currently under clinical investigation [62], Table 13-5.

Satisfaction Rate and Side Effects of ICI

Most patients on ICI are former PDE5I nonresponders. ICI could be offered as a sole second-line treatment or in combination with PDE5I. Satisfactory penile rigidity is restored in 60.2% of patients. Discontinuation of ICI therapy is mainly due to insufficient response (43.1%), poor compliance (18.3%), shift to other treatment (10.7%), loss of desire (6.7%), side effects (5.5%), and return of normal spontaneous erection (2.8%) [80]. Drug withdrawal occurs mainly due to pain. On the other hand, injection anxiety decreases the use of ICI, especially if 'high' injection anxiety is reported, which may be as high as 42% at 4 months [81]. Satisfaction rate seems to be higher in patients who alternate

Table 13-5. Different ICI vasoactive agents

A. Conventional agents	
– *Papaverine* (15 to 60 mg)	Nonspecific phosphodiesterase inhibitor that increases cavernosal tissue levels of cAMP and cGMP [63, 64] Effective in neurogenic and psychogenic ED (80%) compared to vasculogenic (36–50%) Low cost but incidence of priapism is high
– *Phentolamine* (0.5–1 mg)	Competitive alpha blocker. Commonly used in drug combinations. Success rate (63–87%). Side effects are hypotension and tachycardia
– *Caverject* (Alprostadil 5–40 μg/mL)	Administered as a single agent or in combinations with 70–90% efficacy
– *Bimix* (Alprostadil 20 μg/mL + phentolamine 0.5 mg/mL)	
– *Trimix* (Alprostadil 10 μg/mL + papaverine 30 mg/mL + phentolamine + 1.0 mg/mL)	Combination therapy offers maximal erectile response via synergistic effects, especially in patients who have failed monotherapy [25]. In patients with non-vasculogenic ED treatment dose should be titrated [68]
– *Other combinations and doses of vasoactive agents were reported* [25, 27, 65–67]	
B. New ICI agents	
Avanafil	ICI of Avanafil in type II diabetic rats partially improves erectile responses. It may be beneficial for the treatment of type II-associated ED [69]
AVE 0991	Synthetic non-peptide Mas agonist that potentiates erectile response. It is dose-dependent and its effect is antagonized by NO inhibitor (L-NAME) [70]
BAY 41-8543 and *BAY 60-2770*	sGC activator agents that potentiate erectile activity via endogenous and exogenous release of NO [71]. BAY 60-2770 activity is not affected by cavernosal nerve injury or NOS inhibition [72]
PnTx2–6	A toxin that induces priapism in rats, Purified from spider venom (*Phoneutria nigriventer*). It enhances and restores age-related erectile activity via NO pathway [73, 74]
Fibroblast growth factor (FGF)	FGF upregulates mRNA, basic fibroblast growth factor (b-FGF), and nNOS proteins. It improves endothelial function and vasoreactivity of cavernosal tissue [75]
Vascular endothelial growth factor (VEGF)	ICI of VEGF restores cavernosal smooth muscle integrity, promotes extensive neovascularization and ameliorates erectile dysfunction in aged rats [76, 77]
Sodium nitrite (NaNO2)	NaNO2 acts as an NO donor. It increases dose-related erectile activity in rats via increasing IC pressure and decrease systemic blood pressure [78].
Adipose-derived stem cells (ADSCs)	Initial results of ADSCs intra cavernosal injection in animal models showed improvement of erectile response but still under investigation [79]

the use of PDE5I and ICI [82]. Some ED patients prefer ICI even though if they were responding to PDE5I possibly due to better erection quality [83]. Despite being reliable, self-injection is associated with higher rate of penile fibrosis compared to office program [84].

Contraindications to ICI

- Behavioral disorders.
- Risk or history of priapism.
- Unstable cardiovascular disease.
- Severe coagulopathy.
- Reduced manual dexterity (resolved by partner-training).
- Use of MAO inhibitors (precipitates a life-threatening hypertensive crisis [85].

Intraurethral Suppositories

MUSE (Medicated Urethral System for Erection, MEDA Pharmaceuticals, Inc., Somerset, NJ) is a synthetic prostaglandin E1 that is FDA approved in 1996. [86]. It is administered as a semisolid pellet of alprostadil inserted 3 cm from the external urethral meatus. Response rate is approximately 50% [25].

Side effects: MUSE is a less popular option for ED treatment due to its reduced tolerability that includes [87],

- Pain (32%)
- Urethral bleeding (5%)
- Hypotension (3%)
- Dizziness (4%)
- Priapism (0.1%)
- Vaginal burning (5.8%) for female partner

Vacuum Erection Device (VED)

VED act by suction of blood into cavernous spaces. Subsequently, blood is trapped aided by a constriction device applied at the base of the penis. It is an accepted therapy especially for older men. Side effects include bruises, numbness, discomfort, and ejaculatory disorders [25].

VED is not a popular treatment for ED despite being FDA approved since 1982 [53]. However, it has regained some popularity after introduction of penile rehabilitation concept in post RP patients. The mechanism of improving erectile function could be through amelioration of hypoxic, apoptotic, and fibrotic mechanisms encountered in cavernous tissue [88]. In that perspective, VED is now used as a first-line treatment or in combination with PDE5I or ICI in the treatment of post-RP ED [89].

Hormonal Therapy

For men with ED in whom hormonal disturbances are identified, the urologist's role is to treat hyperprolactinemia and primary hypogonadism, while treatment of endocrinopathies is the role of endocrinologists.

Testosterone Replacement

Androgen replacement encompasses monitoring of testosterone level before and after starting treatment. However, clinical response is more important than having a normal androgen level. It is recommended to complete 3-month course of androgen replacement before judging to discontinue the drug [90].

Several testosterone preparations are available for the treatment of hypogonadism, shown in Table 13-6.

TABLE 13-6. Different testosterone preparations

Intramuscular	*Testosterone enanthate, cypionate* (200–250 mg) IM every 2–3 weeks or 100 mg every 7–10 days
	Testosterone propionate 200 mg IM every 2–3 days (shorter half-life)
	Side effects: Mood change and testosterone fluctuations
	Testosterone undecanoate (Nebido) (750 or 1000 mg) IM every 10 weeks. (long acting and maintain normal testosterone level)
Subcutaneous	*Testopel* 75 mg testosterone, 2 6 pellets every 3–6 months (Subcutaneous implantation)
Transdermal	Patch or gel that stimulates normal circadian testosterone levels
	Testoderm TTS 5 mg patch
	Androderm 2.5–5 mg patch
	Side effects: Contact dermatitis and itching
	AndroGel, Testim (1% testosterone gel) contain 50–100 mg of testosterone applied in the morning once daily.
	Axiron (2% testosterone solution) contains 30 mg testosterone applied once daily to each axilla
Buccal	Tablet-Like adhesives (30 mg testosterone), twice daily applied to the gum tissue to allow testosterone absorption through buccal mucosa.
Oral	*Methyltestosterone, fluoxymesterone*
	Limited role due to associated hepatotoxicity. Large doses of oral testosterone (>200 mg/day) needed to overcome first-pass hepatic circulation
	Testosterone undecanoate (120–240 mg) 2–3 times/day[91]

Alternative Hormone Treatments

Dihydrotestosterone (DHT) gel (125–250 mg/day): pure androgen that has no estrogenic effect (not aromatized to estradiol) on the prostate. It produces DHT plasma level that is similar to physiologic testosterone level [92].

Dehydroepiandrosterone (DHEA) has androgen/estrogen-like effects. It has a limited evidence of improving sexual function [93].

Human chorionic gonadotropin (HCG) increases testosterone level by 50%. It would be beneficial to hypogonadal men in a similar manner to testosterone replacement. However, it has no documented improvement on sexual function [94].

Aromatase inhibitors and selective androgen modulators increase testosterone level but they are still investigational. Their therapeutic value and safety profile are still unclear [95].

Hyperprolactinemia Treatments

Treatment of hyperprolactinemia is necessary as regard to insufficiency of testosterone-replacement therapy to ameliorate erectile function. Underlying cause of hyperprolactinemia must be initially identified.

Prolactin-secreting adenoma should be treated medically or surgically if necessary. Bromocriptine (dopamine agonist) reduces prolactin and normalizes testosterone level. It facilitates reduction of adenoma size [96]. Recovery of erectile function is achieved after normalization of serum prolactin elevations [97].

Evolving Modalities

Soluble Guanylate Cyclase (sGC) Activators

- BAY 60-2770

These are new class of molecules that initiate and promote vasodilatation when response to nitric oxide donors and sGC stimulators is attenuated. BAY 60-2770 is an effective molecule in ED treatment in the lack of NO after pelvic nerve injury [72]. These molecules are more effective than sGC stimulators or PDE5 inhibitors when ED is associated with extensive endothelial damage [98]

- BAY 41-2272

BAY 41-2272 acts by direct stimulation of sGC. It increases enzymatic sensitivity to NO and upregulates cGMP by sGC activation independent of NO availability. These mechanisms produce anti-aggregatory, vasodilatory, and antiproliferative effects [99]. Chronically exposed rats to L-NAME showed improved relaxation of corpus cavernosum following 4-week therapy with BAY 41-2272, this indicates the pro-erectile effect of cGMP accumulation into corpus cavernosum [100].

- BAY 60-4552

The acute effect of BAY 60-4552, the soluble guanylate cyclase (sGC) stimulator, and vardenafil was evaluated alone or in combination on erectile responses to electrical stimulation of the cavernous nerve (ES CN) in rats with cavernous nerve (CN) crush injury-induced ED. It was found that combined BAY 60-4552, and vardenafil provides synergistic beneficial effects and might therefore salvage patients who experience treatment failures with PDE5 inhibitors after RP [101].

Stem Cells (SCs)

Stem cell is now an evolving tool to be added to ED treatment armamentarium. SC ability to ameliorate cavernous nerve injury is currently being thoroughly investigated by different researchers. SC is a potential treatment and ultimately a cure to ED [79].

- Clinically applicable SCs

Intracavernosal injection of placental matrix-derived MSCs was investigated on a limited number of patients who failed previous oral therapies. Follow-up for 3 months showed the ability of one patient to achieve spontaneous erection. Further studies on a larger number of patients are needed in this perspective. [102]. On the other hand, ICI of ADSCs produced substantial recovery of erectile function induced by cryoablation of cavernous nerve. This effect thought to be achieved by the increased levels of cavernous tissue neurotrophic factors and the resultant neuroregenerative effects [103]. Patients undergoing radical prostatectomy who develop ED can be treated by ICI of bone marrow mononuclear cells. They show improved cavernous tissue revascularization with no serious side effects [104]. In another setting, structural penile deformity and reduction of Peyronie's-like changes might be corrected by local injection of interferon-labelled ADSC. This effect is thought to be due to decreased expression of metalloproteinases tissue inhibitors [105].

- Investigational SCs

Mesenchymal stem cells (MSCs) and ADSCs showed positive effects on erectile function in animal models of ED. [79] similarly, in another study, human umbilical cord blood MSCs (hUCB-MSCs) showed the ability to ameliorate erectile dysfunction in rat models of cavernous nerve injury [106]. Hepatocyte growth factor-modified ADSCs could potentiate the effect of ADSCs on erection in diabetic rats; this effect may be related to TGFb1down-regulation in the cavernous tissue [107]. Furthermore, Combination of SC and low-intensity extracorporeal shockwave therapy (LI-ESWT) induce cavernous nerve recovery and enhance endothelial function in a rat model of cavernous nerve cryoablation [108].

Low-Intensity Extracorporeal Shockwave Therapy (LI-ESWT)

LI-ESWT has been thoroughly under clinical investigation [109–111]. It can be a newly effective tool to the armamentarium of ED treatment and it may improve erectile function in patients undergoing nerve-sparing radical prostatectomy [112].

Mechanism of how LI-ESWT improves erectile function is not yet clearly understood. Several theories have emerged, including turnover of injured cells, enhancement of cavernous endothelial function and neovascularization on penile tissue of diabetic animal models of ED [113]. However, LI-ESWT is still of limited use due to lack of larger-scale human studies that could clarify its efficacy and safety. There is no consensus on the standardized treatment protocol. Moreover, target population is not yet adequately defined and the action mechanism of LI-ESWT at the histological, molecular, and ultrastructural levels is still not clear [114].

Alternative Treatment

Herbal Treatment

The advantage of herbal treatment is referred to its natural behavior, by which general well-being is maintained. Herbal combinations listed in Table 13-7 have the ability to improve sexual function. Additionally, herbal combinations have become an attractive alternative to western-style medications for treating ED [115].

TABLE 13-7. Common herbal combinations used to improve sexual function

- Korean ginseng
- Panax ginseng (Korean red ginseng)
- Korean mountain ginseng extract
- Rubus coreanus
- *Ginkgo biloba*
- Epimedium koreanum
- Schisandra chinensis
- Male silkworm extract
- *Lepidium meyenii*
- Cuscuta chinensis
- Artemisia capillaris
- Garlic
- Special herbal preparations:
  - Oral combination of ginger, *Paullinia cupana*, L-citrulline, and Muira Puama:

  Comparable to PDE5I efficacy and improve ED-associated histological and functional characteristics especially in aged men [116]
  - Ferula harmonis
  - Enhances erection but reduces fertility with chronic use due to significant decline of testosterone level [117]
  - Kraussianones (polyphenols) [118]
  - Eurycoma longifolia (Tongkat Ali) [119]

[Based on data from Ref. 115].

Resveratrol

It has antioxidative characteristics and upregulates NO. It was found to improve ED in diabetic rats. Additionally, combination of resveratrol with sildenafil has a synergistic effect in ameliorating diabetes-associated ED [120].

Pyrazolopyrimidinone Analogues

Compound-4a is an innovative pyrazolopyrimidinone analogue that may be considered a promising substitute to conventional PDE5Is. This compound has better physicochemical properties and excellent efficacy compared to PDE5Is [121].

Neuromedin B

It was reported that Neuromedin B can ameliorate erectile dysfunction via enhancement of cavernous nerve survival and protection of cavernosal tissue. Therefore, in the near future neuromedin B might be a successfully added tool to the armamentarium of ED treatment specifically in ED-associated cavernosal damage [122].

Transdermal/Topical Pharmacotherapy

These are vasoactive agents topically applied to penile skin that are convenient in promoting penile erection that have several forms (gel or cream). Based on their method of application, simplicity and limited systemic side effects, they are generally appealed. Table 13-8 summarizes some topical preparations for treatment of ED.

Penile Vibrators

Viberect is a penile vibratory stimulator that was FDA approved in 2011. It induces penile erection by stimulation of pudendal nerve branches alongside penile shaft causing reflex parasympathetic activation that induce the release of NO from terminal nerve endings [126, 127].

TABLE 13-8. Topical preparations for ED treatment

- *Nitroglycerin* (NO 2%) paste

  It produces partial tumescence that is insufficient for sexual intercourse, in addition to patient/partner side effects (headache and systemic vasodilatation) [123]
- *Papaverine* gel

  Not currently used due to its large molecular size that precludes transdermal absorption [124]
- Alprostadil 3% combinations, intrameatal application:
  - *Vitaros* (Apricus Biosciences, San Diego, CA)
  - *Alprox-TD* (NexMed, Inc., Robbinsville, NJ).

  More promising with minimal side effects [25]
- Prostaglandin E1 ethyl ester (Prostaglandin E1 prodrug), penile shaft application: produce significant penile rigidity with better skin permeation and less irritation [125]

It is also used for penile rehabilitation to enhance erectile function following nerve-sparing RP. However, despite being an attractive tool for enhancement of penile erection, more studies are required to evaluate long-term outcome in this prospect.

Impulse Magnetic-Field Therapy

Magnetic fields represent a simple and noninvasive method that alleviates ED by increasing cellular oxygen uptake, circulation enhancement, and reversal of penile functional impairment [128]. Efficacy of magnetic-field therapy in ED treatment was postulated in some clinical studies; however, more studies are needed to evaluate its long-term outcome and potential side effects.

Tissue Engineering

With the tremendous advances in current tissue engineering technologies, more pleasant biological substitutions to penile prosthesis seem to be emerging. Since the release of first-known penile reconstruction using bone in 1936, several trials shown the ability to seed and implant bovine chondrocytes into corporeal spaces of animals; there these rods grow and produce penile shaft rigidity [129]. In the same perspective, neo-corpora development has been reported using smooth muscle cell implantation or smooth muscle and endothelial cell implantation onto 3D collagen matrix [130, 131]. However, the clinical application of these technologies has no current real value, but it will be a promising tool in the near future.

Nanotechnology

Topical application of Nanoparticles that vehicle PDE5Is to penile shaft can achieve penile erection, alleviating systemic side effects of PDE5Is. In Experimental studies; Sialorphin, tadalafil, and NO were used as topical nanoparticle gel to produce penile erection. Nanoparticle-vehicled erectogenic materials were utilized in animal studies to produce significant erectile response [132]. Recently, nano-shuttle magnetized ADSCs is now used to stabilize ADSCs inside corpus cavernosum to enhance ADSC therapy in animal models of stem cell therapy for ED [133]. Despite the lack of human studies in the prospect of nanoparticle therapy, this seems to be a promising tool that could revolutionize the therapy for ED but further studies are needed to support this innovative therapy.

Endovascular Tools

For several decades, microsurgical vascular procedures have been continuously tried to alleviate PDE5I-refractory ED due to pudendal artery stenosis. One of the initial trials was the use of *Zotarolimus-Eluting* stent for ED treatment which showed improvement in erectile response with no reported complications [134]. Others reported significant improvement of erectile function following balloon dilatation [135]. In the same perspective, selective endovascular embolization has been evaluated and showed significant efficacy and safety [136]. Similarly, some studies reported the effectiveness aeroblock technique for pelvic vein embolization with aethoxysclerol in the treatment of venous leak. Recently, dorsal penile vein embolization with *N*-butyl-2-cyanoacrylate/ LIPIODOL ULTRA mixture resulted in recovery of erectile response in 88% of patients [137]. These techniques are continuously evolving and promising results are expected in this perspective.

Combination Therapies

Monotherapy for ED does not meet an accepted satisfaction for all patients. About 40% of patients do not respond to single treatment modality for their condition [25]. So, better therapeutic efficacy may be achieved by treatment combinations rather than monotherapy, specifically to overcome its dose-limiting side effects. Different treatment combinations listed in Table 13-9 has met high rates of success.

Safety measures, thorough pretreatment patient evaluation and post-treatment follow-up are strongly recommended to avoid potential complications.

Surgery

Surgical procedures for ED treatment have been evolving since 1902 with the development of dorsal venous ligation and the superficially placed rigid prosthesis to restore sexual function, but with unsatisfactory results [146]. Penile prosthesis is the most successful and effective method for the majority of cases with generally accepted satisfaction rate. Arterial and venous surgeries are only limited to healthy patients with either post-traumatic or congenital ED.

Table 13-9. Different combination therapies for ED

- ICI+VED [138]
- Transurethral pharmacotherapy+VED [139]
- PDE5I+ICI [140]
- Transurethral pharmacotherapy+prosthesis [141]
- PDE5I+transurethral alprostadil [142]
- PDE5I+testosterone replacement [143]
- PDE5I+psychosocial counseling [144]
- PDE5I+VED [145]

Reconstructive Surgery

- Arterial revascularization

ED-associated penile arterial insufficiency results from arteriosclerotic changes that are encountered in diabetic patients and those who have risk factors (e.g., dyslipidemia, smoking, and hypertension). Arterial insufficiency is evaluated by duplex penile ultrasound after Intracavernosal injection of vasoactive agent. There have been many surgical techniques to perform arterial revascularization that have been described [147–150]. Arterial anastomosis to the dorsal penile artery or the deep dorsal vein to the epigastric artery has limited efficacy in restoration of erectile function in 30–50% of patients; however, with improvement of surgical techniques long-term follow-up showed better outcome (>60% improvement) in a subset of patients [150, 151]. Ideal candidates for these operative techniques are post-pelvic trauma young adults with arterial insufficiency [152]. Further, the integration of laparoscopy to these techniques has improved long-term outcome [153]. Side effects include glandular hyperemia (13%), hematoma, infection and thrombosis.

- Venous surgery

Venous leakage is diagnosed by the persistence of end-diastolic flow >5 cm/s in Doppler measurement [154]. It is better visualized using cavernosography and cavernosometry [155]. Venous surgery is only limited to patients with clearly evident venous leak on cavernosogram. The most frequently ligated veins are the crural, cavernosal and deep dorsal veins. Failure of success include advanced patient's age, prolonged duration of ED, multiple leak sites, associated arterial insufficiency, incompetent surgical procedure and formation of collaterals [156, 157].

Penile Prosthesis

For about half century, penile prostheses are being used for the treatment of ED [158]. Unlike other modalities of ED treatment, penile prosthesis offers the best satisfactory and patient-convenient treatment option for ED [159]. Men undergoing prosthetic surgery for ED experience the sense of being "cured," a feeling that is not reported with other treatment modalities for ED [160]. Penile prosthetic surgery involves irreversible alteration of physiologic erection via placement of two rods inside each corpus cavernosum.

- Indications: Failure of conservative therapy, penile fibrosis, Peyronie's disease, post-priapism, and phalloplasty surgery [161].
- Types: Semirigid (malleable) rods or hydraulic pumps (Two or three-piece inflatable). The selection of which depends on operator's experience, patient's preference anatomy and financial situation of the patient [158].
  - Semirigid rods: they are paired cylindrical rods that are inserted in each corpus cavernosum. They may be either malleable or positional (articulating discs). Its main drawback is constant erection that is difficult to conceal and device's inability to increase girth [162].
  - Inflatable prosthesis: designed to mimic normal erectile function with adequate length, girth and permits penile flaccidity when needed. Consists of two hollow cylinders filled with normal saline inserted in each corpus to produce penile rigidity when inflated and deflated after intercourse. Two-piece inflatable prosthesis consists of two cylinders connected to a scrotal pump, while three-piece device consists of two cylinders, reservoir, and a scrotal pump. It is more rigid when inflated, acting like a normal erection.
- Procedures: with improvement of mechanical properties, the three-piece inflatable device is now the most popular one (70%), two-piece device (20%) and semirigid (10%). [163]
- Patient satisfaction:
- With advancement of design and mechanical improvement, patient satisfaction with penile prosthesis is now the highest among all other ED treatment modalities [160]. Current studies reviewed long-term satisfaction rate of inflatable penile prosthesis which was 86.8% [164]. Patient satisfaction primarily depends on his expectations before surgery which necessitates providing the patient with realistic expectations and precise description of the procedure [165]. Factors that affect satisfaction rate include BMI of 30, Peyronie's disease, and history of radical prostatectomy [166]. The most common postoperative complaint is loss of penile length [167].
- Complications:
- Complications can occur during or after surgery;
  - Intraoperative: Include perforation, corporeal or urethral injury, cylinder cross-over and device damage during insertion
  - Postoperative: The most serious complication is Infection (4% with primary implants and 10% with revision implants). It is caused by cutaneous bacteria that attach to the device during implantation (e.g., *Staphylococcus aureus*, *Staphylococcus epidermidis*, and *Candida albicans*) [168, 169].

Despite becoming uncommon with design improvement, Device malfunction can occur, specifically with three-piece device, which includes silicone tube cracking, leak, cylinder aneurysm, pump rupture, and auto-inflation (2.4–11%) [171].

- Other complications include scrotal hematoma, erosion, S-shaped penile deformity, and poor glans support.

Psychosocial Interventions

Psychotherapy and Sex Therapy as described in details in the chapter on Biopsychosocial Treatments.

Conclusions

As an initial step in treatment of ED, physicians should review all drugs potentially worsening erectile function and a thorough consultation should always be carried out. Data acquired during a routine diagnostic workup for ED should be taken into account when choosing the best ED treatment for the individual patient. Various pharmacological, non-pharmacological, and surgical options are safe and effective. The current treatment of ED is still far from ideal; however, there is promising novel technology and innovative modalities to improve the well-established treatments for ED. We expect to witness new drugs and technologies that may revolutionize ED treatment, especially in complex cases. Oral PDE5I and ICI of vasoactive agents may have a remarkable role to prevent and ameliorate cavernosal fibrosis [172, 173]. The dream of ED becoming a curable condition may become true in the near future.

References

1. Ismail EA, El-Sakka AI. Innovative trends and perspectives for erectile dysfunction treatment: a systematic review. Arab J Urol. 2016;14:84–93.
2. Glina S, Sharlip ID, Hellstrom WJG. Modifying risk factors to prevent and treat erectile dysfunction. J Sex Med. 2013;10: 115–9.
3. Esposito K, Ciotola M, Giugliano F, et al. Mediterranean diet improves erectile function in subjects with the metabolic syndrome. Int J Impot Res. 2006;18:405–10.
4. Derby CA, Mohr BA, Goldstein I, et al. Modifable risk factors and erectile dysfunction: can lifestyle changes modify risk? Urology. 2000;56:302–6.
5. Esposito K, Giugliano F, Di Palo C, et al. Effect of lifestyle changes on erectile dysfunction in obese men: a randomized controlled trial. JAMA. 2004;291:2978–84.
6. Bacon CG, Mittleman MA, Kawachi I, et al. A prospective study of risk factors for erectile dysfunction. J Urol. 2006;176:217–21.
7. Schrader SM, Breitenstein MJ, Lowe BD. Cutting off the nose to save the penis. J Sex Med. 2008;5:1932–40.
8. Ralph D, McNicholas T. UK management guidelines for erectile dysfunction. BMJ. 2000;321:499–503.
9. Wassertheil-Smoller S, Blaufox MD, Oberman A, et al. Effect of antihypertensives on sexual function and quality of life: the TAIM Study. Ann Intern Med. 1991;114:613–20.
10. Grimm Jr RH, Grandits GA, Prineas RJ, et al. Long-term effects on sexual function of five antihypertensive drugs and nutritional hygienic treatment in hypertensive men and women. Treatment of Mild Hypertension Study (TOMHS). Hypertension. 1997;29: 8–14.
11. Andersson KE, Wagner G. Physiology of penile erection. Physiol Rev. 1995;75:191–236.
12. Srilatha B, Adaikan PG, Arulkumaran S, et al. Sexual dysfunction related to antihypertensive agents: results from the animal model. Int J Impot Res. 1999;11:107–13.
13. Croog SH, Levine S, Sudilovsky A, et al. Sexual symptoms in hypertensive patients. A clinical trial of antihypertensive medications. Arch Intern Med. 1988;148:788–94.
14. Hannan JL, Smallegange C, Hale TM, et al. Impact of antihypertensive treatments on erectile responses in aging spontaneously hypertensive rats. J Hypertens. 2006;24:159–68.
15. Suzuki H, Tominaga T, Kumagai H, et al. Effects of frst-line antihypertensive agents on sexual function and sex hormones. J Hypertens Suppl. 1988;6:S649–51.
16. Cushman WC, Cohen JD, Jones RP, et al. Comparison of the fxed combination of enalapril/diltiazem ER and their monotherapies in stage 1 to 3 essential hypertension. Am J Hypertens. 1998; 11:23–30.
17. Sica DA. Pharmacokinetics and pharmacodynamics of mineralocorticoid blocking agents and their effects on potassium homeostasis. Heart Fail Rev. 2005;10:23–9.
18. Aizenberg D, Zemishlany Z, Dorfman-Etrog P, et al. Sexual dysfunction in male schizophrenic patients. J Clin Psychiatry. 1995; 56:137–41.
19. Wirshing DA, Pierre JM, Marder SR, et al. Sexual side effects of novel antipsychotic medications. Schizophr Res. 2002;56:25–30.
20. Keltner NL, Mcafee KM, Taylor CL. Mechanisms and treatments of SSRI induced sexual dysfunction. Perspect Psychiatr Care. 2002;38:111–6.
21. Gitlin MJ, Suri R, Altshuler L, et al. Bupropion-sustained release as a treatment for SSRIinduced sexual side effects. J Sex Marital Ther. 2002;28:131–8.
22. Kuba R, Pohanka M, Zakopcan J, et al. Sexual dysfunctions and blood men with focal epilepsy. Epilepsia. 2006;47:2135–40.
23. Gil-Nagel A, Lopez-Munoz F, Serratosa JM, et al. Effect of lamotrigine on sexual function in patients with epilepsy. Seizure. 2006;15:142–9.
24. Basaria S, Dobs AS. Hypogonadism and androgen replacement therapy in elderly men. Am J Med. 2001;110:563–72.
25. Porst H, Burnett A, Brock G, et al. SOP conservative (medical and mechanical) treatment of erectile dysfunction. J Sex Med. 2013;10:130–71.
26. Burnett AL. Phosphodiesterase 5 mechanisms and therapeutic applications. Am J Cardiol. 2005;96:M29–31.
27. Khera M, Goldstein I. Erectile dysfunction. Clin Evid (Online) 2011; Jun 29:1803.
28. Shindel AW. 2009 update on phosphodiesterase type 5 inhibitor therapy, part 2: updates on optimal utilization for sexual concerns and rare toxicities in this class. J Sex Med. 2009;6:2352–64 .quiz 2365–6
29. Sadovsky R, Brock GB, Gutkin SW, et al. Toward a new "EPOCH": optimising treatment outcomes with phosphodiesterase type 5 inhibitors for erectile dysfunction. Int J Clin Pract. 2009;63:1214–30.
30. De Backer G, Ambrosioni E, Borch-Johnsen K, Brotons C, Cifkova R, Dallongeville J, et al. European guidelines on cardiovascular disease prevention in clinical practice. Third Joint Task Force of European and Other Societies on Cardiovascular Disease Prevention in Clinical Practice. Eur Heart J. 2003;24:1601–10.
31. Jackson G, Montorsi P, Adams M, Anis T, El-Sakka A, Miner M, Vlachopoulos C, Kim E. Cardiovascular aspects of sexual medicine. J Sex Med. 2010;7:1608–26.
32. Carson CC, et al. The efficacy of sildenafil citrate (Viagra) in cli update. Urology. 2002;60(2 Suppl 2):12 27.
33. Kloner RA, et al. Effect of sildenafil in patients with erectile dysfunction taking antihypertensive therapy. Sildenafil Study Group. Am J Hypertens. 2001;14(1):70–3.

34. Lombardi G, et al. Ten-year follow-up of sildenafil use in spinal cord-injured patients with erectile dysfunction. J Sex Med. 2009;6(12):3449–57.
35. Seidman SN, et al. Treatment of erectile dysfunction in men with depressive symptoms: results of a placebo-controlled trial with sildenafil citrate. Am J Psychiatry. 2001;158(10):1623–30.
36. Blander DS, et al. Efficacy of sildenafil in erectile dysfunction after radical prostatectomy. Int J Impot Res. 2000;12(3):165–8.
37. Rendell MS, et al. Sildenafil for treatment of erectile dysfunction in men with diabetes: a randomized controlled trial. Sildenafil Diabetes Study Group. JAMA. 1999;281(5):421–6.
38. Wagner G, et al. Sildenafil citrate (VIAGRA) improves erectile function in elderly patients with erectile dysfunction: a subgroup analysis. J Gerontol A Biol Sci Med Sci. 2001;56(2):M113–9.
39. Rajagopalan P, et al. Effect of high-fat breakfast and moderate-fat evening meal on the pharmacokinetics of vardenafil, an oral phosphodiesterase-5 inhibitor for the treatment of erectile dysfunction. J Clin Pharmacol. 2003;43(3):260–7.
40. Montorsi F, et al. Earliest time to onset of action leading to successful intercourse with vardenafil determined in an at-home setting: a randomized, double-blind, placebocontrolled trial. J Sex Med. 2004;1(2):168–78.
41. Forgue ST, et al. Tadalafil pharmacokinetics in healthy subjects. Br J Clin Pharmacol. 2006;61(3):280–8.
42. Jung J, et al. Tolerability and pharmacokinetics of avanafil, a phosphodiesterase type 5 inhibitor: a single- and multiple-dose, double-blind, randomized, placebocontrolled, dose-escalation study in healthy Korean male volunteers. Clin Ther. 2010;32(6): 1178–87.
43. Kyle JA, Brown DA, Hill JK. Avanafil for erectile dysfunction. Ann Pharmacother. 2013;47(10):1312–20.
44. Cheitlin MD, et al. ACC/AHA expert consensus document. Use of sildenafil (Viagra) in patients with cardiovascular disease. American College of Cardiology/American Heart Association. J Am Coll Cardiol. 1999;33(1):273–82.
45. Wang Z, Zhu D, Yang X, Li J, Jiang X, Tian G, et al. The selectivity and potency of the new PDE5 inhibitor TPN729MA. J Sex Med. 2013;10:2790–7.
46. Gao ZW, Zhu YT, Yu MM, Zan B, Liu J, Zhang YF, et al. Preclinical pharmacokinetics of TPN729MA, a novel PDE5 inhibitor, and prediction of its human pharmacokinetics using a PBPK model. Acta Pharmacol Sin. 2015;36:1528–36.
47. Ahn GJ, Chung HK, Lee CH, Kang KK, Ahn BO. Increased expression of the nitric oxide synthase gene and protein in corpus cavernosum by repeated dosing of udenafil in a rat model of chemical diabetogenesis. Asian J Androl. 2009;11:435–42.
48. Cho MC, Paick JS. A review of the efficacy and safety of mirodenafil in the management of erectile dysfunction. Ther Adv Urol. 2016 Apr;8(2):100–17.
49. Kim E, Seftel A, Goldfischer E, Baygani S, Burns P. Comparative efficacy of tadalafil once daily in men with erectile dysfunction who demonstrated previous partial responses to as-needed sildenafil, tadalafil, or vardenafil. Curr Med Res Opin. 2015;31: 379–89.
50. Hatzichristou D, d'Anzeo G, Porst H, Buvat J, Henneges C, Rossi A, et al. Tadalafil 5 mg once daily for the treatment of erectile dysfunction during a 6-month observational study (EDATE): impact of patient characteristics and comorbidities. BMC Urol. 2015;15:111.
51. Buvat J, Hatzichristou D, Boess FG, Büttner H, Gehchan N, Henneges C, et al. Continuation and effectiveness of tadalafil once daily during a 6-month observational study in erectile dysfunction: the EDATE study. Int J Clin Pract. 2014;68:1087–99.
52. Choi WS, Kwon OS, Cho SY, Paick JS, Kim SW. Effect of chronic administration of PDE5 combined with glycemic control on erectile function in streptozotocin-induced diabetic rats. J Sex Med. 2015;12:600–10.
53. Wessells H, Levine N, Hadley ME, et al. Melanocortin receptor agonists, penile erection, and sexual motivation: human studies with melanotan II. Int J Impot Res. 2000;12(Suppl. 4):S74–9.
54. Diamond LE, Earle DC, Rosen RC, et al. Double-blind, placebo-controlled evaluation of the safety, pharmacokinetic properties and pharmacodynamic effects of intranasal PT-141, a melanocortin receptor agonist, in healthy males and patients with mild-to-moderate erectile dysfunction. Int J Impot Res. 2004;16:51–9.
55. Lal S, Rios O, Thavundayil JX. Treatment of impotence with trazodone: a case report. J Urol. 1990;143:819–20.
56. Costabile RA, Spevak M. Oral trazodone is not effective therapy for erectile dysfunction: a double-blind, placebo controlled trial. J Urol. 1999;161:1819–22.
57. Ernst E, Pittler MH. Yohimbine for erectile dysfunction: a systematic review and meta-analysis of randomized clinical trials. J Urol. 1998;159(2):433–6.
58. Heaton JP, et al. Recovery of erectile function by the oral administration of apomorphine. Urology. 1995;45(2):200–6.
59. Gwinup G. Oral phentolamine in nonspecific erectile insufficiency. Ann Intern Med. 1988;109(2):162–3.
60. Zorgniotti AW. Experience with buccal phentolamine mesylate for impotence. Int J Impot Res. 1994;6(1):37–41.
61. Burnett AL. Oral pharmacotherapy for erectile dysfunction: current perspectives. Urology. 1999;54:392–400.
62. El-Sakka AI. What is the current role of intracavernosal injection in management of erectile dysfunction? Int J Impot Res. 2016;1–8.
63. Jeremy JY, et al. Effects of sildenafil, a type-5 cGMP phosphodiesterase inhibitor, and papaverine on cyclic GMP and cyclic AMP levels in the rabbit corpus cavernosum in vitro. Br J Urol. 1997;79(6):958–63.
64. Stief CG, Wetterauer U. Erectile responses to intracavernous papaverine and phentolamine: comparison of single and combined delivery. J Urol. 1988;140(6):1415–6.
65. Zorgniotti AW, Lefleur RS. Auto-injection of the corpus cavernosum with a vasoactive drug combination for vasculogenic impotence. J Urol. 1985;133:39–41.
66. Bennett AH, Carpenter AJ, Barada JH. An improved vasoactive drug combination for a pharmacological erection program. J Urol. 1991;146:1564–5.
67. Floth A, Schramek P. Intracavernous injection of prostaglandin E1 in combination with papaverine: enhanced effectiveness in comparison with papaverine plus phentolamine and prostaglandin E1 alone. J Urol. 1991;145:56–9.
68. Fallon B. Intracavernous injection therapy for male erectile dysfunction. Urol Clin North Am. 1995;22:833–45.
69. Yilmaz D, Bayatli N, Un O, Kadowitz PJ, Sikka SC, Gur S. The effect of intracavernosal avanafil, a newer phosphodiesterase-5 inhibitor, on neonatal type 2 diabetic rats with erectile dysfunction. Urology. 2014;83:e7–e12.
70. da Costa Gonçalves AC, Fraga-Silva RA, Leite R, Santos RA. AVE 0991, a nonpeptide Mas-receptor agonist, facilitates penile erection. Exp Physiol. 2013;98:850–5.
71. Lasker GF, Pankey EA, Allain AV, Dhaliwal JS, Stasch JP, Murthy SN, et al. Analysis of erectile responses to BAY 41-8543 and muscarinic receptor stimulation in the rat. J Sex Med. 2013;10: 704–18.
72. Lasker GF, Pankey EA, Frink TJ, Zeitzer JR, Walter KA, Kadowitz PJ. The sGC activator BAY 60-2770 has potent erectile activity in the rat. Am J Physiol Heart Circ Physiol. 2013;304:H1670–9.
73. Nunes KP, Costa-Gonçalves A, Lanza LF, Cortes SF, Cordeiro MN, Richardson M, et al. Tx2-6 toxin of the *Phoneutria nigriventer* spider potentiates rat erectile function. Toxicon. 2008;51: 1197–206.
74. Nunes KP, Toque HA, Borges MH, Richardson M, Webb RC, de Lima ME. Erectile function is improved in aged rats by PnTx2-6, a toxin from *Phoneutria nigriventer* spider venom. J Sex Med. 2012;9:2574–81.

75. Xie D, Pippen AM, Odronic SI, Annex BH, Donatucci CF. Intracavernosal basic fibroblast growth factor improves vasoreactivity in the hypercholesterolemic rabbit. J Sex Med. 2006;3:223–32.
76. Park K, Ahn KY, Kim MK, Lee SE, Kang TW, Ryu SB. Intracavernosal injection of vascular endothelial growth factor improves erectile function in aged rats. Eur Urol. 2004;46:403–7.
77. Gou X, He WY, Xiao MZ, Qiu M, Wang M, Deng YZ, et al. Transplantation of endothelial progenitor cells transfected with VEGF165 to restore erectile function in diabetic rats. Asian J Androl. 2011;13:332–8.
78. Lasker GF, Matt CJ, Badejo Jr AM, Casey DB, Dhaliwal JS, Murthy SN, et al. Intracavernosal administration of sodium nitrite as an erectile pharmacotherapy. Can J Physiol Pharmacol. 2010; 88:770–6.
79. Soebadi MA, Moris L, Castiglione F, Weyne E, Albersen M. Advances in stem cell research for the treatment of male sexual dysfunctions. Curr Opin Urol. 2016;26:129–39.
80. Sung HH, Ahn JS, Kim JJ, Choo SH, Han DH, Lee SW. The role of intracavernosal injection therapy and the reasons of withdrawal from therapy in patients with erectile dysfunction in the era of PDE5 inhibitors. Andrology. 2014;2:45–50.
81. Nelson CJ, Hsiao W, Balk E, Narus J, Tal R, Bennett NE, et al. Injection anxiety and pain in men using intracavernosal injection therapy after radical pelvicsurgery. J Sex Med. 2013;10:2559–65.
82. Mulhall JP, Simmons J. Assessment of comparative treatment satisfaction with sildenafil citrate and penile injection therapy in patients responding to both. BJU Int. 2007;100:1313–6.
83. Kim SC, Chang IH, Jeon HJ. Preference for oral sildenafil or intracavernosal injection in patients with erectile dysfunction already using intracavernosal injection for 41 year. BJU Int. 2003;92: 277–80.
84. El-Sakka AI. Intracavernosal prostaglandin E1 self-versus office injection therapy in patients with erectile dysfunction. Int J Impot Res. 2006;18:180–5.
85. Sharlip ID. Evaluation and nonsurgical management of erectile dysfunction. Urol Clin North Am. 1998;25:647–59.
86. Padma-Nathan H, Hellstrom WJ, Kaiser FE, et al. Treatment of men with erectile dysfunction with transurethral alprostadil. Medicated Urethral System for Erection (MUSE) Study Group. N Engl J Med. 1997;336:1–7.
87. Guay AT, Perez JB, Velásquez E, et al. Clinical experience with intraurethral alprostadil (MUSE) in the treatment of men with erectile dysfunction. A retrospective study: medicated urethral system for erection. Eur Urol. 2000;38:671–6.
88. Zippe CD, et al. Treatment of erectile dysfunction after radical prostatectomy with sildenafil citrate (Viagra). Urology. 1998;52 (6):963–6.
89. Padma-Nathan H. Efficacy and tolerability of tadalafil, a novel phosphodiesterase 5 inhibitor, in treatment of erectile dysfunction. Am J Cardiol. 2003;92(9A):19M–25M.
90. Bhasin S, Cunningham GR, Hayes FJ, et al. Testosterone therapy in men with androgen defciency syndromes: an Endocrine Society clinical practice guideline. J Clin Endocrinol Metab. 2010;95: 2536–59.
91. Bagatell CJ, Bremner WJ. Androgens in men—uses and abuses. N Engl J Med. 1996;334:707–14.
92. Kunelius P, Lukkarinen O, Hannuksela ML, et al. The effects of transdermal dihydrotestosterone in the aging male: a prospective, randomized, double blind study. J Clin Endocrinol Metab. 2002; 87:1467–72.
93. Morales A, Buvat J, Gooren LJ, et al. Endocrine aspects of sexual dysfunction in men. J Sex Med. 2004;1:69–81.
94. Tsujimura A, Matsumiya K, Takao T, et al. Treatment with human chorionic gonadotropin for PADAM: a preliminary report. Aging Male. 2005;8:175–9.
95. Wang C, Nieschlag E, Swerdloff R, International Society of Andrology (ISA), International Society for the Study of Aging Male (ISSAM), European Association of Urology (EAU), European Academy of Andrology (EAA), American Society of Andrology (ASA), et al. Investigation, treatment, and monitoring of late-onset hypogonadism in males: ISA, ISSAM, EAU, EAA, and ASA recommendations. J Androl. 2009;30:1–9.
96. Gillam MP, Molitch ME, Lombardi G, et al. Advances in the treatment of prolactinomas. Endocr Rev. 2006;27:485–534.
97. Netto Júnior NR, Claro JA. The importance of hyperprolactinemia in impotence. Rev Paul Med. 1993;111:454–5.
98. Estancial CS, Rodrigues RL, De Nucci G, Antunes E, Mónica FZ. Pharmacological characterisation of the relaxation induced by the soluble guanylate cyclase activator, BAY 60-2770 in rabbit corpus cavernosum. BJU Int. 2015;116:657–64.
99. Evgenov OV, Pacher P, Schmidt PM, Haskó G, Schmidt HH, Stasch JP. NO-independent stimulators and activators of soluble guanylate cyclase: discovery and therapeutic potential. Nat Rev Drug Discov. 2006;5:755–68.
100. Claudino MA, da Silva FH, Mónica FZ, Rojas-Moscoso JA, De Nucci G, Antunes E. Long-term oral treatment with BAY 41–2272 ameliorates impaired corpus cavernosum relaxations in a nitric oxide-deficient rat model. BJU Int. 2011;108:116–22.
101. Oudot A, Behr-Roussel D, Poirier S, Sandner P, Bernabé J, Alexandre L, Giuliano F. Combination of BAY 60-4552 and vardenafil exerts proerectile facilitator effects in rats with cavernous nerve injury: a proof of concept study for the treatment of phosphodiesterase type 5 inhibitor failure. Eur Urol. 2011;60(5): 1020–6.
102. Levy JA, Marchand M, Iorio L, Cassini W, Zahalsky MP. Determining the feasibility of managing erectile dysfunction in humans with placental-derived stem cells. J Am Osteopath Assoc. 2016;116:e1–5.
103. Yang R, Fang F, Wang J, Guo H. Adipose-derived stem cells ameliorate erectile dysfunction after cavernous nerve cryoinjury. Andrology. 2015;3:694–701.
104. Yiou R, Hamidou L, Birebent B, Bitari D, Lecorvoisier P, Contremoulins I, et al. Safety of intracavernous bone marrow mononuclear cells for postradical prostatectomy erectile dysfunction: an open doseescalation pilot study. Eur Urol. 2015;. http://dx.doi.org/10.1016/j.eururo.2015.09.026 [Epub ahead of print].
105. Gokce A, Abd Elmageed ZY, Lasker GF, Bouljihad M, Braun H, Kim H, et al. Intratunical injection of genetically modified adipose tissue-derived stem cells with human interferon a 2b for treatment of erectile dysfunction in a rat model of tunica albugineal fibrosis. J Sex Med. 2015;12:1533–44.
106. Song L, Zhu J, Zhang X, Cui Z, Fu Q, Huang J, et al. BDNFhypersecreting human umbilical cord blood mesenchymal stem cells promote erectile function in a rat model of cavernous nerve electrocautery injury. Int Urol Nephrol. 2016;48:37–45.
107. Liu T, Peng Y, Jia C, Fang X, Li J, Zhong W. Hepatocyte growth factor-modified adipose tissue-derived stem cells improve erectile function in streptozotocin-induced diabetic rats. Growth Factors. 2015;33(4):282–9.
108. Jeon SH, Shrestha KR, Kim RY, Jung AR, Park YH, Kwon O, et al. Combination therapy using human adipose-derived stem cells on the cavernous nerve and low-energy shockwaves on the corpus cavernosum in a rat model of post-prostatectomy erectile dysfunction. Urology. 2016;88(226):e1–9.
109. Vardi Y, Appel B, Kilchevsky A, Gruenwald I. Does low intensity extracorporeal shock wave therapy have a physiological effect on erectile function? Short term results of a randomized, double-blind, sham controlled study. J Urol. 2012;187:1769–75.
110. Young S, Dyson M. The effect of therapeutic ultrasound on angiogenesis. Ultrasound Med Biol. 1990;16:261–9.

111. Qiu X, Lin G, Xin Z, Ferretti L, Zhang H, Lue T, et al. Effects of low-energy shockwave therapy on the erectile function and tissue of a diabetic rat model. J Sex Med. 2013;10:738–46.
112. Frey A, Sønksen J, Fode M. Low-intensity extracorporeal shockwave therapy in the treatment of postprostatectomy erectile dysfunction: a pilot study. Scand J Urol. 2016;50:123–7.
113. Liu J, Zhou F, Li GY, Wang L, Li HX, Bai GY, et al. Evaluation of the effect of different doses of low energy shock wave therapy on the erectile function of streptozotocin (STZ)-induced diabetic rats. Int J Mol Sci. 2013;14:10661–73.
114. Abu-Ghanem Y, Kitrey ND, Gruenwald I, Appel B, Vardi Y. Penile low-intensity shock wave therapy: a promising novel modality for erectile dysfunction. Korean J Urol. 2014;55:295–9.
115. Shin YS, Zhao C, Zhang LT, Park JK. Current status and clinical studies of oriental herbs in sexual medicine in Korea. World J Mens Health. 2015;33:62–72.
116. Ferrini MG, Hlaing SM, Chan A, Artaza JN. Treatment with a combination of ginger, L-citrulline, muira puama and *Paullinia cupana* can reverse the progression of corporal smooth muscle loss, fibrosis and veno-occlusive dysfunction in the aging rat. Androl Open Access. 2015;4(1). pii: 131.
117. Ayuob NN, Al-Harbi MS, Abdulhadi SS. Is the chronic use of Ferula harmonis to enhance mice erectile function effective and safe? A histopathological study. Syst Biol Reprod Med. 2014; 60:282–92.
118. Pavan V, Mucignat-Caretta C, Redaelli M, Ribaudo G, Zagotto G. The old made new: natural compounds against erectile dysfunction. Arch Pharm (Weinheim). 2015;348:607–14.
119. Kotirum S, Ismail SB, Chaiyakunapruk N. Efficacy of Tongkat Ali (Eurycoma longifolia) on erectile function improvement: systematic review and meta-analysis of randomized controlled trials. Complement Ther Med. 2015;23:693–8.
120. Bai Y, An R. Resveratrol and sildenafil synergistically improve diabetes associated erectile dysfunction in streptozotocin-induced diabetic rats. Life Sci. 2015;135:43–8.
121. Sawant SD, Lakshma Reddy G, Dar MI, Srinivas M, Gupta G, Sahu PK, et al. Discovery of novel pyrazolopyrimidinone analogs as potent inhibitors of phosphodiesterase type-5. Bioorg Med Chem. 2015;23:2121–8.
122. Nishimatsu H, Suzuki E, Saito Y, Niimi A, Nomiya A, Yamada D, et al. Neuromedin B restores erectile function by protecting the cavernous body and the nitrergic nerves from injury in a diabetic rat model. PLoS ONE. 2015;10:e0133874.
123. Owen JA, Saunders F, Harris C, et al. Topical nitroglycerin: a potential treatment for impotence. J Urol. 1989;141:546–8.
124. Kim ED, el Rashidy R, McVary KT. Papaverine topical gel for treatment oferectile dysfunction. J Urol. 1995;153:361–5.
125. Schanz S, Hauck EW, Schmelz HU, et al. Topical treatment of erectile dysfunction with prostaglandin E ethyl ester. J Dtsch Dermatol Ges. 2009;7:1055–9.
126. Everaert K, de Waard W, Van Hoof T, Kiekens C, Mulliez T, D'Herde C. Neuroanatomy and neurophysiology related to sexual dysfunction in male neurogenic patients with lesions tothe spinal cord or peripheral nerves. Spinal Cord. 2010;48: 182–91.
127. Tajkarimi K, Burnett A. Viberect device use by men with erectile dysfunction: safety, ease of use, tolerability, and satisfaction survey. J Sex Med 2011; 8(Suppl), 441–441.
128. Shafik A, El-Sibai O, Shafik A. Magnetic stimulation of the cavernous nerve for the treatment of erectile dysfunction in humans. Int J Impot Res. 2000;12:137–42.
129. Yoo J, Park H, Lee I, Atala A. Autologous engineered cartilage rods for penile reconstruction. J Urol. 1999;162:1119–21.
130. Kershen R, Yoo J, Moreland R, Krane R, Atala A. Reconstitution of human corpus cavernosum smooth muscle in vitro and in vivo. Tissue Eng. 2002;8:515–24.
131. Chen K, Eberli D, Yoo J, Atala A. Bioengineered corporal tissue for structural and functional restoration of the penis. Proc Natl Acad Sci U S A. 2010;107:3346–50.
132. Han G, Tar M, Kuppam D, Friedman A, Melman A, Friedman J, et al. Nanoparticles as a novel delivery vehicle for therapeutics targeting erectile dysfunction. J Sex Med. 2010;7:224–33.
133. Lin H, Dhanani N, Tseng H, Souza GR, Wang G, Cao Y, et al. Nanoparticle improved stem cell therapy for erectile dysfunction in a rat model of cavernous nerve injury. J Urol. 2016;195:788–95.
134. Rogers JH, Goldstein I, Kandzari DE, Köhler TS, Stinis CT, Wagner PJ, et al. Zotarolimus-eluting peripheral stents for the treatment of erectile dysfunction in subjects with suboptimal response to phosphodiesterase-5 inhibitors. J Am Coll Cardiol. 2012;60:2618–27.
135. Babaev A, Jhaveri R. Angiography and endovascular revascularization of pudendal artery atherosclerotic disease in patients with medically refractory erectile dysfunction. J Invasive Cardiol. 2012;24:236–40.
136. Herwig R, Sansalone S. Venous leakage treatment revisited: pelvic venoablation using aethoxysclerol under air block technique and Valsalva maneuver. Arch Ital Urol Androl. 2015;87:1–4.
137. Aschenbach R, Steiner T, Kerl M, Zangos S, Basche S, Vogl T. Endovascular embolisation therapy in men with erectile impotence due to veno-occlusive dysfunction. Eur J Radiol. 2013;82: 504–7.
138. Chen J, Godschalk MF, Katz PG, et al. Combining intracavernous injection and external vacuum as treatment for erectile dysfunction. J Urol. 1995;153:1476–7.
139. John H, Lehmann K, Hauri D. Intraurethral prostaglandin improves quality of vacuum erection therapy. Eur Urol. 1996;29:224–6.
140. McMahon CG, Samali R, Johnson H. Treatment of intracorporeal injection nonresponse with sildenafl alone or in combination with triple agent intracorporeal injection therapy. J Urol. 1999;162:1992–7.
141. Benevides MD, Carson CC. Intraurethral application of alprostadil in patients with failed inflatable penile prosthesis. J Urol. 2000;163:785–7.
142. Nehra A, Blute ML, Barrett DM, et al. Rationale for combination therapy of intraurethral prostaglandin E (1) and sildenafl in the salvage of erectile dysfunction patients desiring noninvasive therapy. Int J Impot Res. 2002;14(Suppl. 1):S38–42.
143. Shabsigh R, Kaufman JM, Steidle C, et al. Randomized study of testosterone gel as adjunctive therapy to sildenafl in hypogonadal men with erectile dysfunction who do not respond to sildenafl alone. J Urol. 2004;172:658–63.
144. Althof SE, Leiblum SR, Chevret-Measson M, et al. Psychological and interpersonal dimensions of sexual function and dysfunction. J Sex Med. 2005;2:793–800.
145. Canguven O, Bailen J, Fredriksson W, et al. Combination of vacuum erection device and PDE5 inhibitors as salvage therapy in PDE5 inhibitor nonresponders with erectile dysfunction. J Sex Med. 2009;6:2561–7.
146. Wooten JS. Ligation of the dorsal vein of the penis as a cure for atonic impotence. Texas Med J. 1902;18:325–7.
147. Virag R, et al. Investigation and surgical treatment of vasculogenic impotency (author's transl). J Mal Vasc. 1980;5(3):205–9.
148. Breza J, et al. Cavernous vein arterialization for vasculogenic impotence. An animal model. Urology. 1990;35(6):513–8.
149. Goldstein I. Overview of types and results of vascular surgical procedures for impotence. Cardiovasc Intervent Radiol. 1988; 11(4):240–4.
150. Hauri D. Penile revascularization surgery in erectile dysfunction. Urol Int. 2003;70(2):132–40.
151. Zumbe J, et al. Indications for penile revascularization and long-term results. Andrologia. 1999;31(Suppl 1):83–7.
152. Goldstein I. Arterial revascularization procedures. Semin Urol. 1986;4(4):252–8.

153. Lund GO, Winfield HN, Donovan JF. Laparoscopically assisted penile revascularization for vasculogenic impotence. J Urol. 1995;153(6):1923–6.
154. Benson CB, Vickers MA. Sexual impotence caused by vascular disease: diagnosis with duplex sonography. AJR Am J Roentgenol. 1989;153(6):1149–53.
155. Delcour C, et al. Impotence: evaluation with cavernosography. Radiology. 1986;161(3):803–6.
156. Kim ED, McVary KT. Long-term results with penile vein ligation for venogenic impotence. J Urol. 1995;153(3 Pt 1):655–8.
157. Motiwala HG, et al. Experience with penile venous surgery. Urol Int. 1993;51(1):9–14.
158. Small MP, Carrion HM, Gordon JA. Small-Carrion penile prosthesis: new implant for management of impotence. Urology. 1975;5(4):479–86.
159. Mulcahy JJ, et al. The penile implant for erectile dysfunction. J Sex Med. 2004;1(1):98–109.
160. Rajpurkar A, Dhabuwala CB. Comparison of satisfaction rates and erectile function in patients treated with sildenafl, intracavernous prostaglandin E1 and penile implant surgery for erectile dysfunction in urology practice. J Urol. 2003;170(1):159–63.
161. Al-Enezi A, Al-Khadhari S, Al-Shaiji TF. Three-piece inflatable penile prosthesis: surgical techniques and pitfalls. J Surg Tech Case Rep. 2011;3(2):76–83.
162. Montague DK. Penile prosthesis implantation in the era of medical treatment for erectile dysfunction. Urol Clin North Am. 2011;38(2):217–25.
163. Mulcahy JJ, Wilson SK. Current use of penile implants in erectile dysfunction. Curr Urol Rep. 2006;7(6):485–9.
164. Ji YS, Ko YH, Song PH, Moon KH. Long-term survival and patient satisfaction with inflatable penile prosthesis for the treatment of erectile dysfunction. Korean J Urol. 2015 Jun;56(6): 461–5.
165. Kramer Akin-Olugbade O, Parker M, Guhring P, et al. Determinants of patient satisfaction following penile prosthesis surgery. J Sex Med. 2006;3(4):743–8.
166. Akin-Olugbade O, Parker M, Guhring P, et al. Determinants of patient satisfaction following penile prosthesis surgery. J Sex Med. 2006;3(4):743–8.
167. Lee K, Brock G. Strategies for maintaining penile size following penile implant. Transl Androl Urol. 2013;2(1):67–73.
168. Henry GD, Wilson SK, Delk 2nd JR, et al. Penile prosthesis cultures during revision surgery: a multicenter study. J Urol. 2004;172(1):153–6.
169. Wilson SK, Mulcahy JJ. Penile implants. In: Mulcahy J, editor. Male sexual function: a guide to clinical management. 2nd ed. Jersey City, NJ: Humana; 2006. p. 331–79.
170. Bettocchi C, Palumbo F, Spilotros M, et al. Penile prostheses. Ther Adv Urol. 2010;2(1):35–40.
171. Wilson SK, Henry GD, Delk Jr JR, et al. The mentor alpha 1 penile prosthesis with reservoir lock-out valve: effective prevention of auto-inflation with improved capability for ectopic reservoir placement. J Urol. 2002;168(4 Pt 1):1475–8.
172. El-Sakka AI, Yassin AA. Amelioration of penile fibrosis: myth or reality. J Androl. 2010;31:324–35.
173. El-Sakka AI. Alleviation of post-radical prostatectomy cavernosal fibrosis: future directions and potential utility for PDE5 inhibitors. Expert Opin Investig Drugs. 2011;20(10):1305–9.

14 Evaluation of Female Orgasmic Disorder

Stuart Brody

Epidemiology (Incidence/Prevalence)

An important review paper on disorders of orgasm in women noted that orgasm disorder is second only to hypoactive sexual desire disorder in women's sexual disorder prevalence [1]. A recent meta-analysis of studies (limited to English language publications published between 2000 and 2014) on the prevalence of female sexual dysfunction among premenopausal women reported an overall female orgasmic disorder prevalence of 20.9%, increasing to 25.7% when a statistical model meant to adjust for the quality of studies was applied to the analysis [2]. That meta-analysis noted substantial variability in the diagnostic criteria used for ascertaining female orgasmic disorder (including variability in the qualifying period for prevalence) and also reported that prevalence of female orgasmic disorder in Africa was highest, followed by Asia and the Middle East, with the lowest nominal prevalence in Europe and the non-European West. Optimal nationally representative sampling was used in only a minority of studies included in the meta-analyses, which raises issues of selection bias and participation bias in many studies in the review, as well as other studies pertaining to sexual function and sexual dysfunction that were not part of the review. Interestingly, the authors of the meta-analysis concluded that studies of the prevalence of orgasmic dysfunction funded by pharmaceutical companies tended to be of higher quality than other studies [2].

The meta-analysis did not differentiate between orgasm triggers (specifics of the sexual behavior intended to induce orgasm; see discussion of the Sexual Behavior Questionnaire in the Scales section for a list of major orgasm triggers), and unfortunately many, perhaps most, studies also fail to differentiate between orgasm triggers. As should become clear in this chapter, there are substantial psychological, interpersonal, and physiological differences between women's various sexual behaviors and corresponding orgasm triggers [3]. To be optimally supportive of women's health in sexual and other health and interpersonal realms requires respect for these differences and support for the specific sexual behaviors and orgasm triggers most associated with optimal health and intimate relationship quality [4].

One study that did differentiate the orgasm trigger was a large nationally representative survey of Czech women over age 15 [5]. That survey found that only 21.9% of the women had never had a vaginal orgasm (women's orgasm triggered directly by penile–vaginal intercourse, without concomitant clitoral masturbation by either partner for the orgasm), 29.7% of the women had vaginal orgasm consistency (percentage of penile–vaginal intercourse occasions resulting in vaginal orgasm) of 1–25%, 21.7% of the women had vaginal orgasm consistency of 26–50%, 15% of the women had vaginal orgasm consistency of 50–75%, and 11.7% of the women had vaginal orgasm consistency of 75–100% [5]. In another study of a nationally representative sample of Czech women aged 35–65 years, the vaginal orgasm consistency rates were somewhat greater: only 17.0% of the women had never had a vaginal orgasm, 22.3% of the women had vaginal orgasm consistency of 1–25%, 24.4% of the women had vaginal orgasm consistency of 26–50%, 21.1% of the women had vaginal orgasm consistency of 50–75%, and 15.0% of the women had vaginal orgasm consistency of 75–100% [6]. The greater vaginal orgasm consistency rates observed in the older group might reflect some combination of experience, maturity, and cohort effects. Such cohort effects can be due to changes over time in the culture or other aspects of the environment, education, modal experience, nutrition, and other factors (examples of changes over time in the information that is received regarding sex include the widespread availability of pornography over the Internet and promotion of masturbation in many forms of sex education). In the American sample of women with intact marriages collected by Kinsey and colleagues in earlier decades of the twentieth century [7], penile–vaginal intercourse lasting 1–15 min resulted in women's orgasm always or nearly always

W.W. IsHak (ed.), *The Textbook of Clinical Sexual Medicine*, DOI 10.1007/978-3-319-52539-6_14

(90–100% consistency) for the majority of the women. For the women who usually had penile–vaginal intercourse lasting 16 min or longer, two-thirds of the women reported penile–vaginal intercourse orgasms always or nearly always (and only 5.1% of the women in that group reported never having had a penile–vaginal intercourse orgasm) [7]. The issues of the duration of both penile–vaginal intercourse and foreplay will be discussed later in this chapter, but the limiting factor in adequate duration of penile–vaginal intercourse might often be the functioning of the male partner.

Etiology

Genetic and Prenatal Factors

There are indications of genetic and other prenatal contributions to likelihood of female orgasmic disorder [1, 8], as well as to specifically the likelihood of impaired vaginal orgasm [9]. The heritability of women's orgasm from penile–vaginal intercourse has been estimated at 34%, and the heritability of women's orgasm from masturbation has been estimated at 45% [10]. Of note, the latter study found no difference in the proportion of women (monozygotic and dizygotic twins that constituted their research sample) who infrequently or never reached orgasm triggered by penile–vaginal intercourse as compared to orgasm triggered by masturbation [10].

One study of potential prenatal influences on vaginal orgasm [9], as differentiated from other orgasm triggers, relied upon a novel anatomical marker: the tubercle of the upper lip. The presence and shape of the tubercle of the upper lip is likely largely determined during the fetal period and might be associated with more complete prenatal brain development. The presence of a clearly defined tubercle of the upper lip was found to be positively related to vaginal orgasm but was not associated with other orgasm triggers [9].

Family and Other Experiential Factors

In a large sample of Czech women, the majority of women were normally coitally orgasmic (in at least 70% of coital encounters). In statistical analyses, the normally coitally orgasmic majority of women were compared with the women who were rarely (fewer than 30% of encounters) coitally orgasmic, and the latter group was divided into those with and without the presence of sexual distress [11]. Compared with the rarely orgasmic group, the normally coitally orgasmic women were more educated, less likely to have three or more siblings, more likely to be a first-born child, more likely to report a happy childhood, more likely to have had an earlier menarche, more likely to have had an earlier first penile–vaginal intercourse (albeit with a mean age of 18.7 years), more likely to have had more premarital sex partners (albeit with a mean of only 1.3 premarital sex partners), more likely to be having penile–vaginal intercourse at least twice weekly, and less likely to have penile–vaginal intercourse initiated solely by the husband (i.e., they were more likely to either initiate penile–vaginal intercourse themselves or to jointly initiate penile–vaginal intercourse with the husband). The sexually distressed group was more likely to have lost their mother before age six, more likely to have lost their father before age six, more likely to have a higher number of somatic and psychological symptoms, more likely to report a decline in coital orgasm over time, more likely to report that their husband had lower levels of sexual desire, more likely to report that their husband had problems with sexual potency, and less likely to report a happy marriage. The authors of this important study [11] inferred that biological as well as developmental and psychological factors play a role in difficulties in being coitally orgasmic and that being sexually distressed reflects a different group of psychological problems.

The finding in the Czech sample regarding first-born women being more coitally orgasmic [11] is consistent with the findings of earlier studies in other countries [12]. However, a British twin study found that although there were significant genetic and non-shared environmental influences on orgasm, there was little or no role for shared environmental factors, including religion or social class [10].

Women reporting adequate contact with their father in childhood had greater penile–vaginal intercourse orgasm consistency. In contrast, their contact with their mother was not a significant predictor of penile–vaginal intercourse orgasm consistency [12]. These differential associations suggest that women's early experiences with their father shape their sexual development, their sense of men, and capacity for fuller appreciation of penile–vaginal stimulation. It is also possible that there is a role for genetic factors affecting both father–daughter interaction and the daughter's eventual penile–vaginal intercourse orgasm consistency.

In a large representative sample of Czech women, vaginal orgasm consistency was associated with women having been educated in their youth that the vagina is a source of women's orgasm, and the authors observed that a purely clitoral focus (in any formal or informal sex education or in the course of sexual behaviors) can undermine the capacity for vaginal orgasm [5].

Women reporting a history of being sexually abused are more likely to report orgasmic dysfunction than women who were not abused [13, 14], and there is some indication that orgasm might be more affected than other aspects of sexual function by a history of sexual abuse [14].

Age and Parity

In DSM-5, it is stated that, generally, menopausal status is considered not to be associated with orgasmic disorder [15]. In contrast to that statement in DSM-5, some large-scale studies suggest increased rates of orgasm difficulties at older ages [16, 17]. However, it is unclear to what extent those age associations are due to health problems, impaired partner functioning, or possible menopause-associated arousal difficulties. In a Turkish study of women who were not depressed, poorer orgasmic function was associated with being postmenopausal [18]. Of note, some studies have reported that women between 40 and 45 years of age might have the lowest rate of orgasmic dysfunction of any age group [19].

A Turkish study of 40 women found a decline in orgasmic function (as measured by the orgasm domain of the Female Sexual Functioning Index; FSFI) during the third trimester of pregnancy [20]. A British study found that 14% of 796 primiparous women reported difficulty having an orgasm in the year before becoming pregnant, increasing to 33% of the women in the 3 months following childbirth, and recovering partly to 23% at about 6 months after delivery [21]. Although the study did not provide details of the association of orgasm difficulty with mode of delivery, the study did report that dyspareunia was most common among women who had a forceps-assisted vaginal delivery, followed by normal vaginal delivery, with the lowest rate among women who had cesarean delivery [21]. Other studies have obtained mixed results of the effects of parity on orgasmic function.

Intimate Relationship Factors

In a multivariate study, when genetic influences were statistically controlled, relationship satisfaction was shown to be an important correlate of female orgasmic dysfunction [22]. Similarly, marital difficulties were found to be an important correlate of female orgasmic dysfunction in previous studies [23]. Interestingly, in a multivariate analysis, men's sexual satisfaction score was significantly predicted by greater penile–vaginal intercourse frequency and vaginal orgasm of their female partners [24]. There might well be bidirectional effects between relationship satisfaction and penile–vaginal intercourse (frequency and orgasm): women who are more satisfied in their relationship with their partner might be more motivated to have more frequent penile–vaginal intercourse and be more orgasmic with their partner. Similarly, more rewarding penile–vaginal intercourse could lead to greater intimate relationship satisfaction. Similarly, there might be bidirectional effects for the other aspects of satisfaction (life in general, sex life, and personal mental health) associated specifically with penile–vaginal intercourse frequency, vaginal orgasm, and male partner erectile function [6, 25–27].

Scheduling regular sexual activity has itself been found to improve women's orgasm function, which might be due in part to reducing avoidance behavior [28].

In a nationally representative sample of Czechs aged 35–65 years, mean scores on the IIEF-5 (International Index of Erectile Function) measure of erectile function were similar when the scale was completed by men or by their female partner, and the erectile function scores were similarly well correlated with sexual satisfaction, relationship satisfaction, own mental health satisfaction, and life satisfaction for both men and women [26]. Vaginal orgasm consistency is associated with better erectile function [26], which is not surprising, given that adequate erectile function is required for adequate vaginal stimulation during penile–vaginal intercourse. Similarly, in another study (which did not differentiate vaginal orgasm), women whose male partners had erectile dysfunction were less likely to experience orgasm, but for women in that group, orgasm likelihood was improved when the affected male partners were taking a phosphodiesterase type 5 (PDE5) inhibitor for ameliorated erectile function [29].

When presented with the major theoretical models of women's sexual response cycle, women who endorsed a model of progression from excitement/arousal to plateau and orgasm (perhaps including preexisting desire) as representing their own experience had greater FSFI orgasm domain scores and less likelihood of sexual dysfunction than women who endorsed a model in which, rather than necessarily having their own spontaneous sexual desire, women may respond to their partner's desire. The latter group still had greater FSFI orgasm domain scores and less likelihood of dysfunction than women who endorsed none of the presented models of women's sexual response cycle [30, 31].

In a nationally representative sample of Czech women, women's partnered orgasm consistency was associated with duration of penile–vaginal intercourse, but not (in multivariate analyses simultaneously considering both durations) duration of foreplay [32]. This is an important research finding, given the prevalent assertion in sex education and sex therapy that foreplay duration and clitoral focus are supposedly so important for women's orgasm. These findings from the nationally representative Czech sample are also consistent with the (nonrepresentative) American data collected by Kinsey and colleagues, in which foreplay also did not play a major role in women's coital orgasm: the prevalence of women having coital orgasm on 40–100% of occasions ranged from 76.5% for foreplay of 1–10 min to 83.5% for foreplay of greater than 20 min [7].

In a sample of Portuguese women, orgasm from penile–vaginal intercourse was associated with Perceived Relationship Quality Inventory components of satisfaction, intimacy, passion, love, and global relationship quality [33]. In contrast, noncoital partnered sexual behaviors were uncorrelated with the Perceived Relationship Quality Inventory components, and masturbation was associated with both less love and less penile–vaginal intercourse orgasm [33]. In a multivariate analysis of Czech couples' sexual behavior and intimate relationship function, sexual compatibility was independently significantly predicted by greater frequency of penile–vaginal intercourse and greater vaginal orgasm consistency [24].

In the same Czech study, women's sexual satisfaction was significantly predicted by greater vaginal orgasm consistency, greater frequency of the partner providing genital stimulation, and adversely with masturbation [24]. Concordance of the two partner's estimates of vaginal orgasm consistency (hence, men's discernment of their partner's vaginal orgasm) was associated with better dyadic adjustment [24]. Of note, women who often fake orgasm are more likely to have a sexual dysfunction than other women [34].

Metabolic, Nutritional, Substance Use, and Exercise Factors

Women's larger waist (even within the normal, non-obese range) was associated with both lesser likelihood of vaginal orgasm and more likelihood of masturbation [35]. In another study, women's higher body mass index was associated with poorer FSFI orgasm scores (due to the shortcomings of the FSFI, women are not allowed to differentiate vaginal orgasm or coital orgasm from other orgasm triggers) [36]. There might be several pathways underlying the association of impaired orgasm with indices of higher levels of body fat. Both cross-sectional and longitudinal studies have found that adverse characterological factors and psychopathology (including depression, anger, hostility, and less conscientiousness) lead to poorer food choice and to the accumulation of body fat [35, 37, 38]. It was also found that higher levels of personal importance of "junk food" were associated with more use of immature psychological defense mechanisms [39] (see below for a discussion of these psychological processes). Greater levels of body fat can also lead to psychophysiological and physiological dysregulation, which might adversely affect orgasmic function. Experimental animal studies determined that when female mice were fed a diet which led to obesity, they developed both functional sensory nerve conduction deficits and tactile allodynia; this finding suggests that greater body fat levels might reduce pleasurable aspects of penile–vaginal intercourse as well as perhaps increasing the aversiveness of intimate contact [37]. In the context of tactile sensitivity issues, it is noteworthy that women's greater tactile sensitivity is associated with both greater past month likelihood of vaginal orgasm and greater past month penile–vaginal intercourse frequency [40]. It has also been found that women with larger waists tend to have male partners with poorer erectile function (an effect not attributable to age of either partner) [37].

Exercise has been found to decrease depression [41, 42], with effect sizes of the benefits of exercise not significantly different from antidepressant medication or psychological therapy. Exercise is positively correlated with women's orgasm function [43], and at least one form of exercise (Pilates) has been shown to improve women's orgasm function [41].

In an Italian study [44] (which excluded even moderately heavy drinkers, as opposed to the higher alcohol consumption ranges used in a study of British women's personality, alcohol consumption before sexual activity, sexual behaviors, and orgasm function [45]), women who were moderate drinkers of alcohol (11–20 drinks/month) had greater vaginal orgasm incidence (but not greater clitoral orgasm incidence) than women who were lighter drinkers or nondrinkers (71% vs. 52% and 50%) and also had greater penile–vaginal intercourse frequency than women who were lighter drinkers or nondrinkers. Despite the Beck Depression Inventory scores being within the normal range (hence limited statistical variance making detection of effects more difficult), Beck Depression Inventory scores were inversely associated with women's orgasm frequency and intensity, but no association was found between genital vascular function and alcohol consumption [44]. Thus, it is possible that psychological factors (leading to openness to consume moderate amounts of alcohol and/or psychological effects of moderate alcohol consumption) rather than genital blood flow enhancement accounted for the association of moderate alcohol consumption with greater vaginal orgasm incidence.

Some studies which did not differentiate vaginal orgasm from clitoral orgasm found no association between alcohol consumption or other substance use (in a normal population) and orgasm function [46, 47]. However, it might be that an insufficient number of pathological substance (including alcohol) users were included, thus making it difficult to detect statistical significance. In a study in the American city of St. Louis, an association was observed between inhibited orgasm and both alcohol and cannabis use (however, the report did not make it completely clear if that result applied to women or only to men) [48].

In an Italian study, vaginal orgasm was normally experienced by 65% of nonsmokers of cigarettes, 57% of light smokers, and 43% of the heavy smokers [49].

Heroin users report that the use of heroin decreases their orgasm likelihood [50], which is consistent with orgasm being impaired by opiate activity.

Physiological, Psychophysiological, and Hormonal Factors

Physiology and psychology interact to affect the ability to achieve orgasm. In the case of functional muscle-skeletal variations, capacity for vaginal orgasm might be discernable from observing a woman's spontaneous gait. Sexologists trained in the functional–sexological approach to sex therapy observed videotapes of a small sample of healthy young Belgian women and judged the women's orgasmic capacity based solely on observing the women's gait [51]. The research participants were all blind to the experiment hypotheses, and half of the sample had a history of vaginal orgasm. History of vaginal orgasm was assessed correctly by the raters in a statistically significant 81.25% of women. Vaginally orgasmic women had a gait that was physiologically normal for women: the healthy gait was unblocked in the normal pelvic rotation movements and additionally described by the researchers as more energetic, fluid, sensual, and free. Observer ratings of whether the woman was vaginally orgasmic were unrelated to the women's reports of clitoral orgasm with a partner, and the women's history of clitoral orgasm was unrelated to their history of vaginal orgasm. The association between specifically vaginal orgasm and a more natural gait was interpreted as being due to some combination of chronic muscle blocks or excessive muscle flaccidity impairing sexual function by impairing feeling and the discharge of sexual tension (thus, a direct mechanism) and to the psychological factors that led to suboptimal pelvic muscle tone also impairing vaginal orgasm (thus, a clinical sign or correlate) [51].

Studies of the association between greater pelvic floor muscle strength and women's orgasm function have led to mixed results [52, 53]. In a study of 29 patients, abdominal–pelvic adhesions were reported to underlie some cases of women's orgasmic dysfunction, and the impairment attributed to the adhesions was shown to be responsive to a manual physical therapy technique [54].

Women who had a coital orgasm in the past month had greater tactile sensitivity (as measured at the finger), but other orgasm triggers were not associated with tactile sensitivity (a similar pattern was observed for frequency of sexual activities) [40]. In an earlier study that did not differentiate coital orgasm from orgasm triggered by other partnered sexual activities, no association of finger sensitivity with orgasm incidence was detected [55].

Elevated resting levels of prolactin are associated with impairment of many aspects of sexual function, including orgasm. Such elevated prolactin levels might be normal (during lactation) or caused by prolactin-secreting tumors or as a side effect of typical antipsychotic medications [56]. Recent research with a small sample of women suggests that monomeric prolactin and total prolactin levels, but not macroprolactin levels, are associated with impaired orgasm function scores [57] (macroprolactin levels were associated with impaired desire). The mechanism by which prolactin inhibits sexual function might involve not only the well-known inverse relationship with central dopaminergic tone but might also involve peripheral mechanisms [56]. The likely functions of the postorgasmic prolactin surge are to generate some degree of satiety (decreasing immediate desire) and satisfaction and to rebalance central dopaminergic tone. When women's postorgasmic serum prolactin surges following penile–vaginal intercourse were examined in relation to perceived quality of orgasm and resulting sexual satisfaction, it was found that there were strong correlations between prolactin changes and both orgasm quality ($r = 0.85$) and sexual satisfaction ($r = 0.75$). Thus, postorgasmic prolactin surges provide an objective index of orgasm and orgasm quality [56]. Not only did penile–vaginal intercourse orgasm increase prolactin levels greatly, but multiple orgasms led to even greater prolactin increases [56]. For both men and women, orgasm triggered by penile–vaginal intercourse led to an approximately 400% greater prolactin surge compared with orgasm from masturbation (compared with a control condition) [58], suggesting not only one mechanism for penile–vaginal intercourse being more satisfying than masturbation but also perhaps one mechanism by which penile–vaginal intercourse is associated (perhaps causally) with indices of better psychological and psychophysiological health and one mechanism by which masturbation is often associated with indices of poorer psychological and psychophysiological health [3, 58].

Experimental induction of hypogonadism in healthy young women (with depot leuprolide acetate) resulted in a decline in quality of orgasm [59]. Multiple studies with postmenopausal women have found that treatment with testosterone can improve women's orgasm function [1, 60]. This benefit might be due to replacing the testosterone levels that existed before menopause, as testosterone is involved in women's sexual desire, arousal, and orgasm [61]. It has also been observed that menopause-related declines in estrogen might weaken pelvic muscles in some cases [1]. In the case of vulvar or vaginal atrophy attributable to menopause, there can be impairment of several aspects of sexual function, and the selective estrogen agonist/antagonist ospemifene has been shown to improve orgasm function [62].

Personality, Psychopathology, and Iatrogenic Psychopharmacological Issues

In a large sample of women, difficulty having an orgasm during penile–vaginal intercourse was found to be associated with the personality traits of emotional instability (neuroticism), introversion, and being less open to new experiences [63].

Disturbances of the capacity for emotional attachment can be reflected in sexual behavior, including orgasm function. Anxious attachment (involving preoccupations about abandonment) was found to be associated with poorer vaginal orgasm consistency but also with higher frequency of orgasm from vibrator use or receptive anal intercourse. Avoidant attachment (avoidance of closeness in relationships) was found to be associated with higher frequency of orgasm from vibrator use [64]. Thus, secure attachment was associated with better vaginal orgasm consistency and with not using a nonliving object to trigger orgasm.

In a large representative sample of Swedish women, those who had experienced a vaginal orgasm were more satisfied with their mental health than the minority of women who had not experienced vaginal orgasm (regardless of whether the women who had not experienced vaginal orgasm had experienced clitoral orgasm) [27].

In a longitudinal study of Swiss women, orgasmic difficulties were associated with a broad range of psychopathological traits, including anxiety, depression, hostility, obsessive–compulsive features, paranoid ideation, psychoticism, and somatization [65]. Other research studies also found that anxiety and depression were associated with women's orgasmic difficulties [23]. Women's poorer orgasm consistency during penile–vaginal intercourse was also found to be associated with a higher level of neurotic symptoms and with some indications of unstable gender identity [12].

One important link between personality traits and psychopathology is the adaptive level of psychological defense mechanisms that a person uses. Psychological defense mechanisms are processes largely outside of conscious awareness and therefore could be termed either unconscious or implicit, depending on theoretical orientation. Psychological defense mechanisms serve to reduce distress caused by emotional conflict. Maladaptive psychological defense mechanisms involve a distortion of reality and/or impairment of awareness, and they are associated with a variety of indices of poorer mental health and interpersonal relatedness, psychological immaturity, lesser ability to relate intimately with the opposite sex, lack of emotional awareness, and with a variety of psychiatric disorders [3, 66]. Because of their association with some of the normal processes found in small children (as well as with more pathological mechanisms) and the inference that adverse events in childhood can impair the ability to progress to more adaptive and mature levels of emotional development and emotion regulation, maladaptive psychological defenses are also termed immature [3, 66]. Originally a psychodynamic construct, the concept of psychological defenses and their level of adaptiveness or maturity, has become much less bound to a specific theoretical orientation. The previous edition of the Diagnostic and Statistical Manual of the American Psychiatric Association (DSM IV) included the defensive functioning scale (with seven levels of adaptiveness and some useful definitions) as a proposed axis for further study [67]. As is common with the sometimes arbitrary changes of fashion found in subsequent editions of DSM, psychological defenses are mentioned far less in DSM-5 (in which immature defense mechanisms as such are mentioned in the context of dissociative disorders) [15]. In a Portuguese sample [66], vaginal orgasm was associated with less overall use of immature psychological defense mechanisms and with less use of the specific component immature defenses of dissociation, somatization, displacement, autistic fantasy, devaluation, and isolation of affect. Orgasm triggered by clitoral stimulation or by clitoral masturbation (by either partner) concurrent with penile–vaginal intercourse stimulation was not associated with less use of immature defense mechanisms and was actually associated with more use of some immature defense mechanisms. Further analyses revealed that both any masturbation orgasm in the past month and less vaginal orgasm consistency made independent significant contributions to the statistical prediction of immature defense mechanism scores. Similarly, the use of clitoral masturbation by either partner for penile–vaginal intercourse orgasm and lack of any vaginal orgasm made independent significant contributions to the statistical prediction of immature defense mechanism scores. Women who did not have vaginal orgasms had immature defense mechanism scores comparable to those of outpatient psychiatric patients (with diagnoses of depression, social anxiety disorder, panic disorder, and obsessive–compulsive disorder). The results of the study were not confounded by the bias that could be caused by a tendency to distort information in what some people consider a socially desirable manner (social desirability responding) [66]. A replication of this study in another country obtained comparable results: in a sample consisting primarily of British women [45], more use of immature psychological defense mechanisms was associated with lesser vaginal orgasm consistency but also with having an orgasm from clitoral masturbation (by either partner) during penile–vaginal intercourse and with greater frequency of masturbation orgasm. Immature psychological defense mechanisms also statistically explained the association between greater quantity of alcohol consumed before sex and both lack of vaginal orgasm and greater frequency of other sexual behaviors [45]. Of note, the range of alcohol consumed by the British women was far greater than in the aforementioned Italian study of at most moderate drinkers [44], so in the British sample, the higher levels of alcohol consumption might be unhealthy levels. Another study of Dutch women [40] found that women who had a penile–vaginal intercourse orgasm (not explicitly differentiating vaginal orgasm) in the past month, as well as women who ever had a penile–vaginal intercourse orgasm, made less use of immature defense mechanisms. However, in that study, other orgasm triggers were not associated with immature defense mechanisms [40].

Studies have found that depression is associated with masturbation in women and that women with a history of depression have a greater desire to masturbate (but not a greater desire to have penile–vaginal intercourse) than do women without a history of depression [68]. In a sample of mostly British women, poorer emotion regulation traits (use of immature psychological defense mechanisms) were associated with greater frequency of engaging in masturbation, greater frequency of desire to engage in masturbation, and lesser frequency of desire to engage in penile–vaginal intercourse [68].

In a study examining the relationship between sexual behavior, psychological defense mechanisms, and cognitive distortions leading to exaggerated risk perception related to penile–vaginal intercourse, a sample of Scottish women were asked to estimate the total number of women who died from AIDS in Scotland nominally as a result of heterosexual transmission in the United Kingdom from a partner not known to be an injecting drug user, bisexual, or infected through transfusion [69]. The average participant's estimate was 226,000% greater than the official data (the official data itself is likely to overestimate the number in this risk category [69]), and women providing relatively lower estimates made less use of immature psychological defense mechanisms and also had lower frequency of orgasms from clitoral masturbation during penile–vaginal intercourse and from vibrator use. The results imply that people who perceive that "heterosexual transmission" (an unclear term that fails to differentiate penile–vaginal intercourse from anal intercourse [3]) was responsible for many AIDS deaths have poorer psychological functioning and might be less able to respond fully to penile–vaginal intercourse.

In a study of Czech women, a control group of women was compared to groups of women with diagnoses of schizophrenia, bipolar disorder, neurosis, and anorexia nervosa with regard to their experience having had an orgasm during penile–vaginal intercourse. The researchers found that all the clinical groups except the bipolar patients had lower rates of coital orgasm than did the control group [70]. In another Czech study, women diagnosed with neurotic disorders had lower rates of orgasm during penile–vaginal intercourse, but they did not differ from a control group in their likelihood of orgasm triggered by direct clitoral stimulation [71].

Obsessive–compulsive disorder and histrionic personality disorder are also associated with impaired orgasm in women [72]. Studies have also indicated that women with antisocial personality disorders have a higher rate of orgasm dysfunction than do other women [48] and that women with a history of prostitution (who have elevated rates of antisocial and borderline personality disorders) have an elevated rate of impaired orgasm specifically during penile–vaginal intercourse [73, 74].

In a review of issues related to psychiatric disorders and sexual dysfunctions, Waldinger [72] noted that both the disorders themselves, as well as at least some medications used to treat the disorders, can impair sexual function, including women's orgasm. Selective serotonin reuptake inhibitors (SSRIs) are especially notorious for impairing many aspects of sexual function, including women's orgasm. However, other classes of antidepressant medication also carry a risk of causing orgasm impairment, with the exceptions (at a group level) of bupropion, moclobemide, and agomelatine and perhaps mirtazapine, vortioxetine, and amineptine. In some case report studies, adverse effects (including genital anesthesia) of selective serotonin reuptake inhibitors persisted long after discontinuation of their consumption. In a recent study, the SSRI escitalopram did not differ significantly from the supplement S-adenosyl-L-methionine or even placebo with regard to the alleviation of depression, but escitalopram was associated with a significantly higher rate of anorgasmia as an adverse effect [75]. Of course, medication effects can in some cases be a result of interaction of the medication with personality and/or other genetic effects. For example, in a large sample of persons taking the selective serotonin reuptake inhibitor citalopram, orgasmic dysfunction was more likely in those with single nucleotide polymorphisms in glutamatergic genes (GRIA1), with effects also noted for some serotonergic genes [76]. Typical neuroleptic medications given to schizophrenics can impair orgasm and other aspects of sexual function, an effect which is likely due in part to the medication increasing prolactin levels and dopamine blockade. Atypical antipsychotics might carry less risk of orgasm impairment. Waldinger also reviewed studies indicating that adverse sexual effects of psychiatric medication were a major reason for noncompliance with medication [72].

Nonpsychiatric Medical Conditions and Iatrogenesis

Orgasm impairments associated with diseases and medical conditions can be due to any combination of the disease process per se, the treatments, the psychological and interpersonal consequences of the disease or treatment, and perhaps shared causal pathways (although this latter possibility has not been adequately studied). A recent review [50] noted the following medical conditions and treatments as being among the risk factors for women's orgasmic difficulties: hypertension (and antihypertensive medications, which might be a greater risk factor than hypertension per se [23]), heart disease (mixed findings in various studies), thyroid disorders, arthritis, spinal cord injury, multiple sclerosis, obesity, obstructive sleep apnea, fibromyalgia, and stress urinary incontinence. Women with urinary incontinence often have impaired orgasmic function but have been shown to respond to physical therapy and pelvic floor exercises with improved orgasm function [77]. Renal dysfunction (especially when requiring hemodialysis or transplant) is associated with a very high rate of orgasm dysfunction, as well as with a high rate of depression [1]. The presence of Parkinson's disease and markers of its progression are associated with impairment of women's orgasm [78]. Breast cancer treatment has been associated with impaired orgasm, and recent studies indicated that when treatments were compared, women who were treated with breast conserving treatment had less orgasmic dysfunction than women who had a mastectomy [79] and that intermediate orgasm function results were noted for women who had reconstruction at the time of mastectomy

[80]. Similarly, there might be less risk of orgasm impairment when nerve-sparing approaches are used in the treatment of cervical cancer, rather than radical hysterectomy [81]. Even for women with complete spinal cord injuries, orgasm might still be possible because deep vaginal–cervical stimulation (but not clitoral stimulation) conveys signals to the brain via the vagus nerve [82, 83].

Pathophysiology

Female orgasmic disorder can involve disruption of any of the many physiological, psychophysiological, and/or psychological processes involved in orgasm.

Although some women are capable of orgasm from stimulation of nongenital sites (and in some cases from imagery alone) [84], in most cases, orgasm results from clitoral and/or vaginal stimulation. However, vaginal and clitoral stimulation have different neurophysiological pathways, and orgasms triggered by vaginal versus clitoral stimulation also have different psychophysiological, psychological, and interpersonal correlates.

Clitoral stimulation signals are transmitted via the pudendal nerve to the spinal cord and then the brain, but vaginal stimuli (including deep vaginal stimulation of the cervix) are additionally transmitted via the pelvic nerve, pudendal nerve, and hypogastric nerve [3, 82, 85]. There is also evidence that deep vaginal–cervical stimulation (but not clitoral stimulation) sends signals to the brain via the vagus nerve (hence, not relying on the spinal cord) [82, 83]. At the level of the brain, stimulation of the deep vagina and cervix, shallow vagina, and clitoris activate different regions of the somatosensory cortex (there is also a region of overlap) [86].

In addition to spinal and supraspinal circuits, dysregulation of central and peripheral neurotransmission mechanisms (including serotonergic and noradrenergic mechanisms) can be involved in impaired orgasm [87].

Resting heart rate variability is an index of parasympathetic tone as well as an index of integration between the autonomic nervous system and prefrontal brain function. Greater resting heart rate variability (mediated largely by the activity of the vagus nerve) is associated with better emotional regulation and mental health, as well as with better physical health and longevity [88]. In a study which examined the relationship between resting heart rate variability and women having had an orgasm in the past month from 13 different orgasm triggers (and controlled for possible social desirability response bias), only vaginal orgasm was associated with better (greater) resting heart rate variability (orgasm from vaginally focused manual stimulation by a partner missed achieving statistical significance). The authors discussed not only the possibility that the better emotion regulation and relatedness associated with better heart rate variability allows for greater probability of specifically vaginal orgasm but also the possibility that specifically penile–vaginal stimulation and the orgasm that it directly produces might even lead to better parasympathetic tone and other beneficial processes associated with greater resting heart rate variability [88].

Women who are more consistently orgasmic from penile–vaginal intercourse have a very good correlation between laboratory-measured subjective sexual arousal and vaginal pulse amplitude (a measure of vaginal vasocongestion indicative of sexual arousal) responses to erotica. This very good correlation between laboratory-measured subjective sexual arousal and vaginal pulse amplitude is not present for women who are only orgasmically consistent from other partnered sexual activities or from masturbation, but not from penile–vaginal intercourse [89, 90]. These findings suggest that for some reason, women who are not orgasmically consistent from penile–vaginal intercourse are insufficiently aware of their vaginal responses, not integrating their vaginal responses into their sense of arousal or not responding at some level (or some combination of these processes).

Studies prescribing sildenafil for female orgasmic disorder have led to results ranging from mixed to positive [1]. Given that it is women with a history of good penile–vaginal intercourse orgasmic consistency that display evidence of integrating their vaginal vasocongestion responses into their mental sense of sexual arousal [89, 90], future research should examine the possibility that women with a prior history of penile–vaginal intercourse orgasm (or more specifically vaginal orgasm) who have recently developed problems of arousal or orgasm might be more likely to benefit from sildenafil and/or other PDE5 inhibitors than other women [91].

In a nationally representative Czech study, it was found that women who had a male partner with an erect penis length of at least 14.5 cm had greater vaginal orgasm consistency [5]. This finding was replicated in an online convenience sample consisting largely of British women [92]. The British study also found that penis length was not associated with clitoral orgasm [92]. These findings are consistent with the finding in another Czech study that vaginal orgasm consistency was associated with greater sexual arousability from deep vaginal stimulation, but not with sexual arousability from the clitoris or even the shallow or middle vagina [93], because shorter penises would be less likely to adequately stimulate the deep vagina and cervix. These findings are also consistent with different peripheral nerves conducting stimuli from the clitoris and from the deep vagina to the brain, and with the different regions of the somatosensory cortex of the brain activated by stimulation of the clitoris, lower vagina, and cervix [86]. These research findings are also consistent with the result in a large representative sample of Czech women that vaginal orgasm consistency was associated with being mentally focused on specifically vaginal sensations during penile–vaginal intercourse [5].

In contrast to the findings of male partner penis length being associated with greater likelihood of vaginal orgasm [5, 92], one study found that there was no difference in female external genital measurements between women who orgasm from penile–vaginal intercourse usually to always and women who orgasm from penile–vaginal intercourse never to sometimes [94]. However, an Italian study found that the greater the distance between the vagina and the urethra, the more likely a woman is to have experienced vaginal orgasm [95]. The finding that the thickness of the urethrovaginal space was greater in women with vaginal orgasm than in women without vaginal orgasm [95] could be due to some combination of factors, including more vaginal nerves in women with a thicker urethrovaginal space and/or an exercise effect (in which more vaginal orgasms lead to better vaginal tissue tone). At least some women have nitric oxide type 5 phosphodiesterase pathways in the vagina (which might be responsive to phosphodiesterase type 5 inhibitors such as sildenafil), and some women have cavernous or pseudocavernous tissue in the vaginal wall [96].

A physician in the United States reported that in an uncontrolled trial, three sessions of transcutaneous temperature controlled radiofrequency to the vagina, labia, and clitoris of 25 women led to improvements in their orgasmic function. The women enrolled in the study all once had good orgasmic function but had become either anorgasmic or slow to orgasm [97]. That author reported that the women who had developed anorgasmia responded to treatment by becoming orgasmic, and the women who had developed a much longer time to have an orgasm responded to treatment by requiring a shorter time to orgasm [97]. The author implied that the treatment ameliorated vulvovaginal laxity and improved blood flow. Further research with controlled trials would be needed to provide more evidence of this approach.

Receptive anal intercourse has been found to be associated with increased risk of sexual dysfunction (as well as anorectal disorders), which might be due to some combination of psychological and interpersonal factors and possible dysregulation of at least the pudendal nerve induced by receptive anal intercourse [98].

Among the physiological processes differentiating penile–vaginal intercourse from other sexual activities (including stimulation of the vagina with other objects) is the reciprocal pulsation between the penis and vagina. When the penis thrusts in the vagina and against the cervix, the vaginal muscles reflexively grip the lower part of the penis, which might produce a virtuous circle of subtle but differentiating genital responses [99, 100].

Phenomenology/DSM-5 Diagnostic Criteria

The fifth edition of the American Psychiatric Association's Diagnostic and Statistical manual (DSM-5) [15] includes its latest version of their committee criteria for female orgasmic disorder. Diagnosis includes specification of whether the disorder is lifelong or acquired, whether generalized or situational, and whether it is mild, moderate, or severe.

The DSM-5 criteria involve the infrequency or absence of orgasm or greatly reduced sensation of orgasm or greatly increased time needed for orgasm in at least 75% of sexual events (or at least 75% of specified sexual events for the situational variety of the disorder) over the past 6 months. Exclusion criteria for the diagnosis include that the sexual dysfunction is attributable to effects of a substance or medication, to another medical condition or mental disorder (other than a sexual one), or to significant stressors (including relationship distress). It is also recommended in DSM-5 that the diagnosis not be made if the clinician judges that stimulation has been inadequate.

One additional diagnostic criterion in DSM-5 is that the sexual symptoms cause significant distress for the individual (this will be discussed at greater length below) (see Table 14-1).

In the DSM-5 discussion of the diagnosis, reference is also made to some cultural prohibitions against pleasure. The common occurrence of comorbidity of female orgasmic disorder with sexual interest and arousal disorders is appropriately noted.

Some of the statements in the DSM-5 criteria and related diagnostic discussion do not reflect best evidence but instead reflect common biases. The need for clinically significant distress to qualify for a diagnosis, the assertion that orgasm is not strongly correlated with sexual satisfaction, the use of an "always" criterion in mentioning supposedly infrequent orgasm from penile–vaginal intercourse, and the dismissiveness of lack of intercourse orgasm being important are all at odds with best evidence.

Rather than being a valuable index of clinical significance or even seemingly a reaction to a condition, distress might constitute an enduring composite of anxiety and depression that approximates a disorder in itself [101, 102]. In a large sample of Czech women, biological as well as developmental and psychological factors were found to be associated with difficulties in being coitally orgasmic, but it was also found that being sexually distressed reflects a different group of psychological problems [11]. Other developmental factors, early experience, and trauma can strongly shape the likelihood of experiencing sexual distress, as is evidenced by the finding that women who report a history of being sexually abused in childhood do not manifest as clear an inverse

TABLE 14-1. DSM-5 Diagnostic Criteria for Female Orgasmic Disorder. 302.73 (F52.31)

A. The presence of either of the following symptoms and experience on almost all or all (approximately 75–100%) occasions of sexual activity (in identified situational contexts or, if generalized, in all contexts):

1. Marked delay in, marked infrequency of, or the absence of orgasm
2. Markedly reduced intensity of orgasmic sensations

B. The symptoms in criterion A have persisted for a minimum duration of approximately 6 months

C. The symptoms in criterion A cause clinically significant distress in the individual

D. The sexual dysfunction is not better explained by a nonsexual mental disorder or as a consequence of severe relationship distress (e.g., partner violence) or other significant stressors and is not attributable to the effects of a substance/medication or another medical condition

Specify whether:

Lifelong: The disturbance has been present since the individual became sexually active

Acquired: The disturbance began after a period of relatively normal sexual function

Specify whether:

Generalized: Not limited to certain types of stimulation, situations, or partners

Situational: Only occurs with certain types of stimulation, situations, or partners

Specify if:

Never experienced an orgasm under any situation

Specify current severity:

Mild: Evidence of mild distress over the symptoms in criterion A

Moderate: Evidence of moderate distress over the symptoms in criterion A

Severe: Evidence of severe or extreme distress over the symptoms in criterion A

association between better sexual function and less distress as women without a history of such abuse (women who report a history of being sexually abused in childhood also have poorer orgasmic function as measured by the FSFI orgasm domain, with no difference between penetrative and non-penetrative abuse) [13]. Similarly, the correlates of female sexual arousal disorder symptoms differ when a distress criterion is required (those differences include the significant predictors: history of no vaginal orgasm but a history of having engaged in masturbation). However, in cases of female sexual arousal disorder both with and without distress, there is an association of female sexual arousal disorder with lack of attention to vaginal sensations during penile–vaginal intercourse [101]. A focus group with women having difficulties experiencing orgasm found that "distress" was a term rarely used and that the more common term was "frustrated" [103]. This is an important contrast between women's actual experience and the words used in the DSM-5 criteria for female orgasmic disorder. By requiring the presence of a term not best reflecting the experience of women, there is a risk of failing to help women with orgasm problems. An interesting twin study that examined genetic and environmental factors revealed that sexual distress has little to do with sexual dysfunction but a great deal to do with the factors (including obsessive–compulsive symptoms and general anxiety sensitivity) associated with general anxiety in women [104].

There is a curious exceptionalism that applies to DSM-5 diagnosis of many sexual disorders. By requiring the presence of "distress," the clinician risks reinforcing patient denial of a problem, a process that is not routinely promoted for other psychological or medical problems (with the possible exception of overweight).

In contrast to the assertions in DSM-5, research in multiple countries has shown that women's orgasm is indeed associated with women's sexual satisfaction [105, 106].

Unfortunately, DSM-5 is not the only example of consensus guidelines deviating sharply from best evidence regarding female orgasmic disorder evaluation and treatment [4]. Professional resistance to appreciation of the unique role of the vagina in women's orgasm does a disservice to women whose sexual, interpersonal, and global psychological functioning might benefit from more specific education and treatment, rather than the denial of differences between vaginal and clitoral stimulation and corresponding orgasm. Given the associations between better penile–vaginal intercourse (including frequency, vaginal orgasm, and simultaneous orgasm) and multiple measures of women's psychological health, psychophysiological health, and intimate relationship function, the insistence on a distress criterion and the common denial of the special value of penile–vaginal intercourse and vaginal orgasm amount to harm to women's health by many health professionals [4].

Another potential concern in DSM-5 criteria is the presence of other mental disorder being an exclusion criterion. Given that depression is common among sexual disorders [107], and in some cases the pharmacological interventions for depression might be at least as sexually impairing as the depression the medications are intended to treat, one should consider the merit in diagnosing and treating both depression and orgasmic disorder. The fact that the personality features which can predispose to depression also predispose to some orgasmic impairment [12, 40, 45, 63, 66, 71] also argues against at least depression being a simple exclusion criterion. Of note, even within the normal (nonclinical) range of depression scores, Beck Depression Inventory scores were inversely associated with women's orgasm frequency and intensity [44]. In some cases, especially milder forms of depression might reflect personality influences, rather than disease processes.

Members of the DSM-V sexual dysfunctions working group responded [108] to some of the published criticisms on the changes they made from the previous edition of DSM (Diagnostic and Statistical Manual of Mental Disorders, fourth edition, text revision; DSM-IV-TR). However, the serious problems noted in this chapter regarding the DSM-V diagnostic criteria for female orgasmic disorder were not among the issues that they addressed.

Although DSM-5 is widely used (especially in the United States, where its use might be required for insurance claims or to comply with other administrative demands), it is important to understand not only the shortcomings of DSM-5 but also the existence of the much more straightforward diagnosis of female orgasmic dysfunction found in the tenth edition (2016 version) of the World Health Organization's International Statistical Classification of Diseases and Related Health Problems (ICD-10), under the category of sexual dysfunction not caused by organic disorder or disease [109]. The criterion is refreshingly clear: "Orgasm does not occur or is markedly delayed" (http://apps.who.int/classifications/icd10/browse/2016/en#/F52.3).

Implications for Treatment

As the evidence briefly reviewed above indicates, distress is not a legitimate requirement (scientifically or clinically) for men or women to qualify for diagnosis and treatment of their sexual dysfunctions. Obtaining information about other disorders also requiring treatment is important, as is obtaining information regarding medications and physiological states that might be causing or contributing to sexual dysfunction, lifestyle factors, and characteristics of the partner and the partnership.

Many studies have found that vaginal orgasm is associated with indices of better psychological and psychophysiological function, but other orgasm triggers (including masturbation during penile–vaginal intercourse) are associated with poorer psychological and psychophysiological function [3, 64]. These differential findings (multivariate analyses allow for concurrent statistical control of other sexual behaviors, so that observed adverse correlates of masturbation are not simply due to lack of penile–vaginal intercourse) speak not only to differences between sexual behaviors but also raise serious questions regarding the usual approach to treating female orgasmic dysfunction with directed masturbation. It has been noted that for some women, repeated orgasm from clitoral stimulation can interfere with the development of pathways leading to vaginal orgasm [110, 111]. A large representative study of Swedish women found that penile–vaginal intercourse orgasm is inversely associated with masturbation frequency [27], and some smaller studies found no correlation between orgasm consistency triggered by penile–vaginal intercourse and triggered by masturbation [89, 90]. In a large representative sample of women in the Czech Republic, vaginal orgasm consistency was associated with a variety of factors that make vaginal stimulation during penile–vaginal intercourse more thorough or more psychologically salient. These factors include women having been educated in their youth that the vagina is a source of women's orgasm, being mentally focused on vaginal sensations during penile–vaginal intercourse, greater duration of penile–vaginal intercourse, and sufficient male partner penis length [5]. The authors of that study observed that a purely clitoral focus can undermine the capacity for vaginal orgasm. It should be noted that there are effective penile–vaginal intercourse-based treatments for female orgasmic dysfunction [112] and that women should not be directed away from penile–vaginal sensations in the hope that would develop the ability to respond orgasmically to penile–vaginal intercourse. A penile–vaginal intercourse-based treatment that has been shown to be effective at improving women's penile–vaginal intercourse orgasm is the coital alignment technique (also known by its acronym CAT) developed by Eichel. The coital alignment technique involves a synchronized rocking movement by the man and woman during penile–vaginal intercourse, with a riding high variant of the missionary position [112].

Best Practice or Evidence-Based Approach to Diagnosis Including Diagnostic Tests, Instruments, or Rating Scales

Scales

The Female Sexual Function Index (FSFI) [113] might be the most commonly used female sexual function scale. It has one question each (rated on a six-point scale) inquiring about frequency of orgasm, difficulty in reaching orgasm, and satisfaction from the ability to reach orgasm. A serious problem with the FSFI is that it explicitly asks women to not differentiate between penile–vaginal intercourse and other sexual activity. As with some other scales, the use of several conceptually related questions leads to internal statistical consistency (technically termed reliability), but ultimately, the data from the FSFI and similar scales might not be as useful and differentially valid as more objective measures of sexual behaviors and corresponding orgasm frequencies (see below).

The Golombok Rust Inventory of Sexual Satisfaction (GRISS) has one question each (rated on a five-point scale) inquiring about ability to have an orgasm with a partner, finding it impossible to have an orgasm, orgasm from partner stimulating the clitoris during foreplay, and failure to reach orgasm during intercourse [114].

The Arizona Sexual Experience Scale (ASEX) was developed to measure various adverse sexual effects of medication, and the single item for women's orgasm function is rating on a six-point scale how easily one reaches orgasm [115].

The Changes in Sexual Functioning Questionnaire (CSFQ) was also developed to measure medication (or illness)-induced changes in sexual function [116]. It has one question each (rated on a five-point scale) inquiring about frequency of orgasm, ability to reach orgasm when the respondent wants to have an orgasm, and degree of pleasure from orgasm (there is also a question on painful orgasms).

The Sexual Functioning Questionnaire by Quirk et al. [105] was developed for use in clinical trials of treatments of female sexual dysfunctions. It has one question each (rated on a five-point scale plus an option of no activity during the 4-week queried period) inquiring about frequency of orgasm, ease of reaching orgasm, and pleasure experienced from orgasms.

The Patient-Reported Outcomes Measurement Information System (PROMIS) Sexual Function and Satisfaction Measures Version 2.0 [117] has many items on aspects of sexual behavior for both sexes, but only two items on female orgasmic function. One item is how relatively often in the past 30 days the woman has been able to have an orgasm when she wanted an orgasm, and the other is how satisfying her orgasms have been. Both items are rated on a five-point scale from never to always (plus the respective options of not attempted and no orgasm in the past 30 days). Although the overall scale benefitted from several useful methodological features in the course of its development, the authors of the report on the scale observed that additional work is required in the orgasm domain of the scale.

An alternative approach is found in the Sexual Behavior Questionnaire developed by Brody and colleagues [66, 69, 88]. Women report how many days in a recent representative month they (1) engaged in and (2) had an orgasm from various specific sexual activities. The specific sexual activities in the scale typically include penile–vaginal intercourse *without* additional simultaneous clitoral stimulation, penile–vaginal intercourse *with* additional simultaneous clitoral stimulation, clitorally focused masturbation (further differentiated as with or without a vibrator), vaginally focused masturbation (further differentiated as with or without a vibrator), clitorally focused manual stimulation by a partner, vaginally focused manual stimulation by a partner, cunnilingus, and receptive anal intercourse [88]. The scale can also include a further differentiation of partnered noncoital sexual behaviors as occurring with or without penile–vaginal intercourse on the same day. The Sexual Behavior Questionnaire items are usually presented in a matrix format for completion (with instructions to the respondent including that if the answer for an item is either never or zero, to write 0 rather than leaving any item blank). The sexual behavior items can be expanded or reduced as needed. The validity of the Sexual Behavior Questionnaire has been demonstrated both in its associations with various psychological and psychophysiological measures in several of the studies reviewed in this chapter, as well as examination of the role of social desirability response bias, a consideration not often examined in research on sexual behavior. Additional columns can be added to measure age at first engaging in each activity (or indicating that the specific sexual activity was never tried) and age at first having an orgasm from each activity. The approach of the Sexual Behavior Questionnaire provides not only more precise information on specific sexual behaviors and orgasm than more common scales, but the numerator (orgasm) and denominator (times tried in the month) provide additional useful information, as do the ratio (orgasm consistency from the specific activity). This specific quantitative approach is in contrast to the vague relative terms used in other scales. Each of the items in the Sexual Behavior Questionnaire can provide useful information. For example, if the number of days per month of penile–vaginal intercourse is low, the interview can include further questions on what factors led to the low number of days per month (such as partner availability, lack of interest by the woman and/or her partner, illness, etc.). The presence of masturbation, especially if a high number of days per month, can also be examined, as it might suppress pursuit of and/or full response to penile–vaginal intercourse in some cases. Additional subcategories of activities can also be added, such as vaginal orgasm occurring at the same time as male penile–vaginal intercourse orgasm (simultaneous orgasm; in a nationally representative survey of 35–65-year-old Czechs, simultaneous penile–vaginal orgasm was associated with better sexual satisfaction, relationship satisfaction, personal mental health satisfaction, and life satisfaction [6]). The Sexual Behavior

Questionnaire also has a version for use with men, in which an item for fellatio is substituted for the cunnilingus item, all references to clitoral stimulation are removed, and an item for insertive anal intercourse is added [88].

Interview and Best Practice

Many patients do not spontaneously report sexual problems, and many general clinicians do not spontaneously enquire about patient sexual function. Even if one does not have time or need to use a scale, a few minutes of direct calm questioning can elicit some important information. The Sexual Behavior Questionnaire (see above) can save time in gathering quantitative details of specific sexual behavior history and frequency and corresponding orgasm consistency, but further questions regarding medical conditions and the sexual function of partners are also suggested, even in the course of a nonspecialist anamnesis. Although multi-item satisfaction (intimate relationship, sexual, life, mental health, etc.) scales exist, a clinician or even researcher can also simply ask for a rating of the specific domain of satisfaction on a scale from one to six, providing the anchors of one = very unsatisfying and six = very satisfying (such scales are not only time-efficient but valid as well [25]). Information on the degree to which the woman feels sexual desire and experiences sexual arousal and lubrication before and during sex can also provide useful information (even if pre-existing desire is not essential for orgasm), as can information on the degree to which she is able to focus her attention on vaginal sensations during penile–vaginal intercourse [5].

It is important to query women about the sexual function of their partner, because in quite a few cases, the woman's seemingly impaired function might be due to the premature ejaculation or inadequate erectile function of their partner. Similarly, the possibility should also be considered that a woman with a chronic sexual dysfunction (or negative attitude toward sex) might adversely affect the function of their partner. Chronic sexual dysfunction of one partner can create adverse expectations for sexual interaction with at least that partner, which can affect sexual function. Information on partners can include an assessment of intimate relationship satisfaction with their partner, sexual desire for their partner, the presence of premature ejaculation or erectile dysfunction, and whether the woman's orgasm problem also existed earlier in the same intimate relationship or in other intimate relationships. Although scales for the ascertainment of premature ejaculation and erectile dysfunction exist, the clinician might begin assessment of partner sexual function by simply asking the woman if her male partner(s) ejaculate earlier than what might make for an optimal opportunity for her orgasm and if her male partner(s) have difficulty maintaining a sufficiently hard erection during intercourse.

After the diagnosis of female orgasmic disorder is made and the essential aspects of history are obtained (including asking the patient what they have already tried to overcome their orgasm difficulty), one of the first places to start treatment planning is considering whether relatively simple solutions are available. These include evaluating whether any medications or health habits might be changed and evaluating whether the male partner needs an evaluation for his sexual dysfunction. In some cases, assessment of the woman's hormone levels might be indicated. Intimate relationship quality issues might in some cases respond to couples counseling but in other cases might not. Similarly, in some cases, psychological or psychiatric problems might respond to psychological treatment, but in other cases, one might proceed to more direct sexological interventions. At the very least, a woman with orgasmic disorder might benefit from discussion of her focusing attention on vaginal sensations during intercourse and scheduling sex sufficiently frequently (preferably at a time and with an ambience that is optimal for her). As noted above, there are effective penile–vaginal intercourse-based (non-masturbatory) treatments for female orgasmic disorder.

References

1. IsHak WW, Bokarius A, Jeffrey JK, Davis MC, Bakhta Y. Disorders of orgasm in women: a literature review of etiology and current treatments. J Sex Med. 2010;7:3254–68.
2. McCool ME, Zuelke A, Theurich MA, Knuettel H, Ricci C, Apfelbacher C. Prevalence of female sexual dysfunction among premenopausal women: a systematic review and meta-analysis of observational studies. Sex Med Rev. 2016;4:197–212.
3. Brody S. The relative health benefits of different sexual activities. J Sex Med. 2010;7:1336–61.
4. Brody S, Costa RM, Hess U. "Standard Operating Procedures for Female Orgasmic Disorder" is not based on best evidence. J Sex Med. 2013;10:2606–9.
5. Brody S, Weiss P. Vaginal orgasm is associated with vaginal (not clitoral) sex education, focusing mental attention on vaginal sensations, intercourse duration, and a preference for a longer penis. J Sex Med. 2010;7:2774–81.
6. Brody S, Weiss P. Simultaneous penile–vaginal intercourse orgasm is associated with satisfaction (sexual, life, partnership, and mental health). J Sex Med. 2011;8:734–41.
7. Gebhard PH. Factors in marital orgasm. J Soc Issues. 1966; 22:88–95.
8. Burri A, Greven C, Leupin M, Spector T, Rahman Q. A multivariate twin study of female sexual dysfunction. J Sex Med. 2012; 9:2671–81.
9. Brody S, Costa RM. Vaginal orgasm is more prevalent among women with a prominent tubercle of the upper lip. J Sex Med. 2011;8:2793–9.
10. Dunn KM, Cherkas LF, Spector TD. Genetic influences on variation in female orgasmic function: a twin study. Biol Lett. 2005; 1:260–3.
11. Raboch J, Raboch J. Infrequent orgasms in women. J Sex Marital Ther. 1992;18:114–20.
12. Uddenberg N. Psychological aspects of sexual inadequacy in women. J Psychosom Res. 1974;18:33–47.

13. Stephenson KR, Hughan CP, Meston CM. Childhood sexual abuse moderates the association between sexual functioning and sexual distress in women. Child Abuse Negl. 2012;36:180–9.
14. Oberg K, Fugl-Meyer KS, Fugl-Meyer A. On sexual well-being in sexually abused Swedish women: epidemiological aspects. Sex Relat Ther. 2002;17:329–41.
15. American Psychiatric Association. Diagnostic and statistical manual of mental disorders. 5th ed. (DSM-5). Washington, DC: American Psychiatric Association; 2013.
16. Lee DM, Nazroo J, O'Connor DB, Blake M, Pendleton N. Sexual health and well-being among older men and women in England: findings from the English Longitudinal Study of Ageing. Arch Sex Behav. 2016;45:133–44.
17. Aslan E, Beji NK, Gungor I, Kadioglu A, Dikencik BK. Prevalence and risk factors for low sexual function in women: A study of 1,009 women in an outpatient clinic of a university hospital in Istanbul. J Sex Med. 2008;5:2044–52.
18. Verit FF, Verit A, Billurcu N. Low sexual function and its associated risk factors in pre- and postmenopausal women without clinically significant depression. Maturitas. 2009;64:38–42.
19. Hendrickx L, Gijs L, Enzlin P. Age-related prevalence rates of sexual difficulties, sexual dysfunctions, and sexual distress in heterosexual women: results from an online survey in Flanders. J Sex Med. 2015;12:424–35.
20. Aslan G, Aslan D, Kızılyar A, Ispahi C, Esen A. A prospective analysis of sexual functions during pregnancy. Int J Impot Res. 2005;17:154–7.
21. Barrett G, Pendry E, Peacock J, Victor C, Thakar R, Manyonda I. Women's sexual health after childbirth. BJOG. 2000;107: 186–95.
22. Burri A, Spector T, Rahman Q. A discordant monozygotic twin approach to testing environmental influences on sexual dysfunction in women. Arch Sex Behav. 2013;42:961–72.
23. Dunn KM, Croft PR, Hackett GI. Association of sexual problems with social, psychological, and physical problems in men and women: a cross sectional population survey. J Epidemiol Community Health. 1999;53:144–8.
24. Klapilova K, Brody S, Krejcova L, Husarova B, Binter J. Sexual satisfaction, sexual compatibility, and relationship adjustment in couples: the role of sexual behaviors, orgasm, and men's discernment of women's intercourse orgasm. J Sex Med. 2015;12: 667–75.
25. Brody S, Costa RM. Satisfaction (sexual, life, relationship, and mental health) is associated directly with penile–vaginal intercourse but inversely with other sexual behavior frequencies. J Sex Med. 2009;6:1947–54.
26. Weiss P, Brody S. International Index of Erectile Function (IIEF) scores generated by men or female partners correlate equally well with own satisfaction (sexual, partnership, life, and mental health). J Sex Med. 2011;8:1404–10.
27. Brody S. Vaginal orgasm is associated with better psychological function. Sex Relat Ther. 2007;22:173–91.
28. Lorenz TA, Meston CM. Exercise improves sexual function in women taking antidepressants: Results from a randomized crossover trial. Depress Anxiety. 2014;31:188–95.
29. Fisher WA, Rosen RC, Eardley I, Sand M, Goldstein I. Sexual experience of female partners of men with erectile dysfunction: the Female Experience of Men's Attitudes to Life Events and Sexuality (FEMALES) study. J Sex Med. 2005;2:675–84.
30. Sand M, Fisher MA. Women's endorsement of models of female sexual response: The nurses' sexuality study. J Sex Med. 2007; 4:709–20.
31. Nowosielski K, Wrobel B, Kowalczyk R. Women's endorsement of models of sexual response: correlates and predictors. Arch Sex Behav. 2016;45:291–302.
32. Weiss P, Brody S. Women's partnered orgasm consistency is associated with greater duration of penile–vaginal intercourse but not of foreplay. J Sex Med. 2009;6:135–41.
33. Costa RM, Brody S. Women's relationship quality is associated with specifically penile–vaginal intercourse orgasm and frequency. J Sex Marital Ther. 2007;33:319–27.
34. Holla K, Jezek S, Weiss P, Pastor Z, Holly M. The prevalence and risk factors of sexual dysfunction among czech women. Int J Sex Heal. 2012;24:218–25.
35. Costa RM, Brody S. Orgasm and women's waist circumference. Eur J Obstet Gynecol Reprod Biol. 2014;182:118–22.
36. Esposito K, Ciotola M, Giugliano F, Bisogni C, Schisano B, Autorino R, et al. Association of body weight with sexual function in women. Int J Impot Res. 2007;19:353–7.
37. Brody S, Weiss P. Slimmer women's waist is associated with better erectile function in men independent of age. Arch Sex Behav. 2013;42:1191–8.
38. Costa RM, Brody S. Immature psychological defense mechanisms are associated with greater personal importance of junk food, alcohol, and television. Psychiatry Res. 2013;209:535–9.
39. Brody S, Costa RM. Associations of immature defense mechanisms with personal importance of junk food, television and alcohol are independent of age. Psychiatry Res. 2013;210:1327–8.
40. Brody S, Houde S, Hess U. Greater tactile sensitivity and less use of immature psychological defense mechanisms predict women's penile–vaginal intercourse orgasm. J Sex Med. 2010;7:3057–65.
41. Halis F, Yildirim P, Kocaaslan R, Cecen K, Gokce A. Pilates for better sex: changes in sexual functioning in healthy Turkish women after pilates exercise. J Sex Marital Ther. 2016;42:302–8.
42. Cooney GM, Dwan K, Greig CA, Lawlor DA, Rimer J, Waugh FR, et al. Exercise for depression. Cochrane Database Syst Rev. 2013:CD004366.
43. Cabral PU, Canário AC, Spyrides MH, Uchôa SA, Eleutheria Júnior J, Giraldo PC, et al. Physical activity and sexual function in middle-aged women. Rev Assoc Med Bras. 2014;60:47–52.
44. Battaglia C, Battaglia B, Mancini F, Nappi RE, Paradisi R, Venturoli S. Moderate alcohol intake, genital vascularization, and sexuality in young, healthy, eumenorrheic women. A pilot study. J Sex Med. 2011;8:2334–43.
45. Costa RM, Brody S. Immature defense mechanisms are associated with lesser vaginal orgasm consistency and greater alcohol consumption before sex. J Sex Med. 2010;7:775–86.
46. Mondaini N, Cai T, Gontero P, Gavazzi A, Lombardi G, Boddi V, et al. Regular moderate intake of red wine is linked to a better women's sexual health. J Sex Med. 2009;6:2772–7.
47. Smith AM, Lyons A, Ferris JA, Richters J, Pitts MK, Shelley JM, et al. Incidence and persistence/recurrence of women's sexual difficulties: findings from the Australian Longitudinal Study of Health and Relationships. J Sex Marital Ther. 2012;38:378–93.
48. Johnson SD, Phelps DL, Cottler LB. The association of sexual dysfunction and substance use among a community epidemiological sample. Arch Sex Behav. 2004;33:55–63.
49. Battaglia C, Battaglia B, Mancini F, Persico N, Nappi RE, Paradisi R, et al. Cigarette smoking decreases the genital vascularization in young healthy. Eumenorrheic Women J Sex Med. 2011;8:1717–25.
50. McCabe MP, Sharlip ID, Lewis R, Atalla E, Balon R, Fisher AD, et al. Risk factors for sexual dysfunction among women and men: a consensus statement from the Fourth International Consultation on Sexual Medicine 2015. J Sex Med. 2016;13:153–67.
51. Nicholas A, Brody S, de Sutter P, de Carufel F. A woman's history of vaginal orgasm is discernible from her walk. J Sex Med. 2008;5:2119–24.
52. Lowenstein L, Gruenwald I, Gartman I, Vardi Y. Can stronger pelvic muscle floor improve sexual function? Int Urogynecol J. 2010;21:553–6.

53. Gameiro MO, Miraglia L, Gameiro LF, Padovani CR, Amaro JL. Pelvic floor muscle strength evaluation in different body positions in nulliparous healthy women and its correlation with sexual activity. Int Braz J Urol. 2013;39:847–52.
54. Wurn LJ, Wurn BF, King CR, Roscow AS, Scharf ES, Shuster JJ. Increasing orgasm and decreasing dyspareunia by a manual physical therapy technique. MedGenMed. 2004;6:47.
55. Brody S, Fischer AH, Hess U. Women's finger sensitivity correlates with partnered sexual behavior but not solitary masturbation frequencies. J Sex Marital Ther. 2008;34:343–52.
56. Leeners B, Kruger TH, Brody S, Schmidlin S, Naegeli E, Egli M. The quality of sexual experience in women correlates with post-orgasmic prolactin surges: results from an experimental prototype study. J Sex Med. 2013;10:1313–9.
57. Krysiak R, Drosdzol-Cop A, Skrzypulec-Plinta V, Okopien B. Sexual function and depressive symptoms in young women with elevated macroprolactin content: a pilot study. Endocrine. 2016;53:291–8.
58. Brody S, Kruger TH. The post-orgasmic prolactin increase following intercourse is greater than following masturbation and suggests greater satiety. Biol Psychol. 2006;71:312–5.
59. Schmidt PJ, Steinberg EM, Negro PP, Haq N, Gibson C, Rubinow DR. Pharmacologically induced hypogonadism and sexual function in healthy young women and men. Neuropsychopharmacology. 2009;34:565–76.
60. Fernandes T, Costa-Paiva LH, Pinto-Neto AM. Efficacy of vaginally applied estrogen, testosterone, or polyacrylic acid on sexual function in postmenopausal women: a randomized controlled trial. J Sex Med. 2014;11:1262–70.
61. Graziottin A. The biological basis of female sexuality. Int Clin Psychopharmacol. 1998;13:S15–22.
62. Constantine G, Graham S, Portman DJ, Rosen RC, Kingsberg SA. Female sexual function improved with ospemifene in postmenopausal women with vulvar and vaginal atrophy: results of a randomized, placebo-controlled trial. Climacteric. 2015;18:226–32.
63. Harris JM, Cherkas LF, Kato BS, Heiman JR, Spector TD. Normal variations in personality are associated with coital orgasmic infrequency in heterosexual women: A population-based study. J Sex Med. 2008;5:1177–83.
64. Costa RM, Brody S. Anxious and avoidant attachment, vibrator use, anal sex, and impaired vaginal orgasm. J Sex Med. 2011;8:2493–500.
65. Leeners B, Hengartner MP, Rössler W, Ajdacic-Gross V, Angst J. The role of psychopathological and personality covariates in orgasmic difficulties: a prospective longitudinal evaluation in a cohort of women from age 30 to 50. J Sex Med. 2014;11:2928–37.
66. Brody S, Costa RM. Vaginal orgasm is associated with less use of immature psychological defense mechanisms. J Sex Med. 2008;5:1167–76.
67. American Psychiatric Association. Diagnostic and statistical manual of mental disorders. 4th edition, Text Revision ed. Washington, D.C.: American Psychiatric Association; 2000.
68. Brody S, Nicholson S. Immature psychological defense mechanisms are associated with women's greater desire for and actual engaging in masturbation. Sex Relat Ther. 2013;28:419–30.
69. Brody S, Costa RM. Overestimation of heterosexually attributed AIDS deaths is associated with immature psychological defence mechanisms and clitoral masturbation during penile–vaginal intercourse. Int J STD AIDS. 2009;20:869–75.
70. Raboch J. Sexual development and life of psychiatric female patients. Arch Sex Behav. 1986;15:341–53.
71. Kratochvil S. Sexualni stimulace a zensky orgasmus [Sexual stimulation and female orgasm]. Cesk Psychiatr. 1993;89:191–9.
72. Waldinger MD. Psychiatric disorders and sexual dysfunction. In: Vodusek DB, Boller F, editors. Handbook of clinical neurology, Vol. 130 (3rd series), Neurology of sexual and bladder disorders. Amsterdam: Elsevier; 2015. p. 469–489.
73. Nedoma K, Sipova I. Sexualni chovani a reaktivita u prostitutek [Sexual behavior and reactivity in prostitutes]. Cesk Psychiatr. 1972;68:214–7.
74. Brody S, Potterat JJ, Muth SQ, Woodhouse DE. Psychiatric and characterological factors relevant to excess mortality in a long-term cohort of prostitute women. J Sex Marital Ther. 2005;31:97–112.
75. Mischoulon D, Price LH, Carpenter LL, Tyrka AR, Papakostas GI, Baer L, et al. A double-blind, randomized, placebo-controlled clinical trial of S-adenosyl-L-methionine (SAMe) versus escitalopram in major depressive disorder. J Clin Psychiatry. 2014;75:370–6.
76. Perlis RH, Laje G, Smoller JW, Fava M, Rush AJ, McMahon FJ. Genetic and clinical predictors of sexual dysfunction in citalopram-treated depressed patients. Neuropsychopharmacology. 2009;34:1819–28.
77. Sacomori C, Cardoso FL. Predictors of improvement in sexual function of women with urinary incontinence after treatment with pelvic floor exercises: A secondary analysis. J Sex Med. 2015;12:746–55.
78. Jitkritsadakul O, Jagota P, Bhidayasiri R. Postural instability, the absence of sexual intercourse in the past month, and loss of libido are predictors of sexual dysfunction in Parkinson's disease. Parkinsonism Relat Disord. 2015;21:61–7.
79. Aerts L, Christiaens MR, Enzlin P, Neven P, Amant F. Sexual functioning in women after mastectomy versus breast conserving therapy for early-stage breast cancer: a prospective controlled study. Breast. 2014;23:629–36.
80. Öztürk D, Akyolcu N. Assessing sexual function and dysfunction in Turkish women undergoing surgical breast cancer treatment. Jpn J Nurs Sci. 2016;13:220–8.
81. Krychman M, Millheiser LS. Sexual health issues in women with cancer. J Sex Med. 2013;10(suppl 1):5–15.
82. Komisaruk BR, Whipple B. Functional MRI of the brain during orgasm in women. Annu Rev Sex Res. 2005;16:62–86.
83. Komisaruk BR, Whipple B, Crawford A, Liu WC, Kalnin A, Mosier K. Brain activation during vaginocervical self stimulation and orgasm in women with complete spinal cord injury: fMRI evidence of mediation by the vagus nerves. Brain Res. 2004;1024:77–88.
84. Komisaruk BR, Whipple B. Non-genital orgasms. Sex Relat Ther. 2011;26:356–72.
85. Komisaruk BR, Whipple B. Love as sensory stimulation: physiological consequences of its deprivation and expression. Psychoneuroendocrinology. 1998;23:927–44.
86. Komisaruk BR, Wise N, Frangos E, Liu WC, Allen K, Brody S. Women's clitoris, vagina, and cervix mapped on the sensory cortex: fMRI evidence. J Sex Med. 2011;8:2822–30.
87. IsHak WW. The guidebook of sexual medicine. Beverly Hills: A&W; 2007.
88. Costa RM, Brody S. Greater resting heart rate variability is associated with orgasms through penile–vaginal intercourse, but not with orgasms from other sources. J Sex Med. 2012;9:188–97.
89. Brody S, Laan E, van Lunsen RH. Concordance between women's physiological and subjective sexual arousal is associated with consistency of orgasm during intercourse but not other sexual behavior. J Sex Marital Ther. 2003;29:15–23.
90. Brody S. Intercourse orgasm consistency, concordance of women's genital and subjective sexual arousal, and erotic stimulus presentation sequence. J Sex Marital Ther. 2007;33:31–9.
91. Brody S. Phosphodiesterase inhibitors and vaginal intercourse orgasm. Int J STD AIDS. 2009;20:440.
92. Costa RM, Miller GF, Brody S. Women who prefer longer penises are more likely to have vaginal orgasms (but not clitoral orgasms): implications for an evolutionary theory of vaginal orgasm. J Sex Med. 2012;9:3079–88.

93. Brody S, Klapilova K, Krejcova L. More frequent vaginal orgasm is associated with experiencing greater excitement from deep vaginal stimulation. J Sex Med. 2013;10:1730–6.
94. Krissi H, Ben-Shitrit G, Aviram A, Weintraub AY, From A, Wiznitzer A, et al. Anatomical diversity of the female external genitalia and its association to sexual function. Eur J Obstet Gynecol Reprod Biol. 2016;196:44–7.
95. Gravina GL, Brandetti F, Martini P, Carosa E, Di Stasi SM, Morano S, et al. Measurement of the thickness of the urethrovaginal space in women with or without vaginal orgasm. J Sex Med. 2008;5:610–8.
96. D'Amati G, di Gioia CR, Bologna M, Giordano D, Giorgi M, Dolci S, et al. Type 5 phosphodiesterase expression in the human vagina. Urology. 2002;60:191–5.
97. Alinsod RM. Transcutaneous temperature controlled radiofrequency for orgasmic dysfunction. Lasers Surg Med. 2016;48:641–5.
98. Sultan AH, Monga A, Lee J, Emmanuel A, Norton C, Santoro G, et al. An international urogynecological association (IUGA) / international continence society (ICS) joint report on the terminology for female anorectal dysfunction. Neurourol Urodyn. 2017; 36:10–34. DOI: 10.1002/nau.23055
99. Shafik A. Vaginocavernosus reflex. Clinical significance and role in sexual act. Gynecol Obstet Investig. 1993;35:114–7.
100. Shafik A. Cervico-motor reflex: description of the reflex and role in sexual acts. J Sex Res. 1996;33:153–7.
101. Weiss P, Brody S. Female sexual arousal disorder with and without a distress criterion: prevalence and correlates in a representative Czech sample. J Sex Med. 2009;6:3385–94.
102. Balon R, Segraves RT, Clayton A. Issues for DSM-V: sexual dysfunction, disorder, or variation along normal distribution: toward rethinking DSM criteria of sexual dysfunctions. Am J Psychiatry. 2007;164:198–200.
103. Kingsberg SA, Tkachenko N, Lucas J, Burbrink A, Kreppner W, Dickstein JB. Characterization of orgasmic difficulties by women: focus group evaluation. J Sex Med. 2013;10:2242–50.
104. Burri A, Rahman Q, Spector T. Genetic and environmental risk factors for sexual distress and its association with female sexual dysfunction. Psychol Med. 2011;41:2435–45.
105. Quirk FH, Heiman JR, Rosen RC, Laan E, Smith MD, Boolell M. Development of a sexual function questionnaire for clinical trials of female sexual dysfunction. J Womens Health Gend Based Med. 2002;11:277–89.
106. Philippsohn S, Hartmann U. Determinants of sexual satisfaction in a sample of German women. J Sex Med. 2009;6:1001–10.
107. Johannes CB, Clayton AH, Odom DM, Rosen RC, Russo PA, Shifren JL, et al. Distressing sexual problems in United States women revisited: prevalence after accounting for depression. J Clin Psychiatry. 2009;70:1698–706.
108. Binik YM, Brotto LA, Graham CA, Segraves RT. Response of the DSM-V sexual dysfunctions subworkgroup to commentaries published in JSM. J Sex Med. 2010;7:2382–7.
109. World Health Organization. International statistical classification of diseases and related health problems. 10th ed. Geneva: World Health Organization; 2016.
110. Perry JD. The primitive psychology of Alfred Kinsey. Paper presented at the Spring Scientific Meeting of the Maine Psychological Association; Lewiston, Maine. 1984.
111. Kegel AH. The Kinsey report. JAMA. 1953;153:1303–4.
112. Pierce AP. The coital alignment technique (CAT): an overview of studies. J Sex Marital Ther. 2000;26:257–68.
113. Rosen R, Brown C, Heiman J, Leiblum S, Meston C, Shabsigh R, et al. The Female Sexual Function Index (FSFI): a multidimensional self-report instrument for the assessment of female sexual function. J Sex Marital Ther. 2000;26:191–208.
114. Rust J, Golombok S. The GRISS: a psychometric instrument for the assessment of sexual dysfunction. Arch Sex Behav. 1986;15:157–65.
115. McGahuey CA, Gelenberg AJ, Laukes CA, Moreno FA, Delgado PL, McKnight KM, et al. The Arizona Sexual Experience Scale (ASEX): reliability and validity. J Sex Marital Ther. 2000;26:25–40.
116. Clayton AH, McGarvey EL, Clavet GJ. The Changes in Sexual Functioning Questionnaire (CSFQ): development, reliability, and validity. Psychopharmacol Bull 1997;33:731–745.
117. Weinfurt KP, Lin L, Bruner DW, Cyranowski JM, Dombeck CB, Hahn EA, et al. Development and initial validation of the PROMIS ® sexual function and satisfaction measures version 2.0. J Sex Med. 2015;12:1961–74.

15 Treatment of Female Orgasmic Disorder

Margaret Redelman

Introduction

Orgasm, especially female orgasm, has captured human imagination across time.

Komisaruk ([1], Preface) wrote "orgasm is a remarkable phenomenon and one of life's most intriguing experiences" and Bancroft [2] added "of all the various sexual responses, orgasm remains the most mysterious and least well-understood."

This chapter aims to look at female orgasmic function (FOF) and female orgasmic dysfunction (FOD), why understanding and assistance for FOD is important and how to help women with difficulties in achieving the experience they want to have.

Human behaviour is fascinating as it is only rarely without motive. Motivations for sex, which can be culturally determined, can impact on sexual behaviours, arousal and ultimately orgasm and therefore, sexual and relationship satisfaction. Women's sexual autonomy (the extent to which a woman feels that her sexual behaviours are self-determined) [3] is not a given, as is the case with most men. Many of our premises, such as orgasms not being as important to women as to men, may need revisiting.

Humans (sophisticated mammals) appear to be relatively unique among mammals in that both males and females can experience orgasm as a result of sexual activity although chimpanzees, bonobos, and stump-tailed macaques exhibit evidence of female orgasms. However, orgasm occurs much less reliably and consistently for females than for males [4]. Humans also seem to be the first species to elevate sexual activity to a purely recreational form. The female orgasm is an intensely personal experience. Whether other female mammals experience similar degrees of difficulty achieving orgasm or pleasure during partnered sex is uncertain. Reproductive physiologists have not been able to identify all the physiological changes that occur in human females during orgasm. Other female mammals do have a clitoris which seems to suggest that orgasm is potentially possible for them. Masturbation-like behaviour can be observed in both genders in many species and appears to be pleasurable. In the usual primate position, the female presents her rear to the male and intercourse is brief and biologically driven: on the other hand, the human experience has the potential to be vastly different. The emotional understanding of "orgasm" in humans is very broad.

Why the biological ability to achieve orgasm varies between women when given the same cultural and social background is not known and the variable factors are not clearly understood despite substantial research on female orgasm [5, 6]. It is likely that there is a significant genetic component to variations in female orgasmic function [7]. There is no objective "marker" of orgasm, such as ejaculation in men, experienced by women, so research and definitive conclusions must be based on clear definitions of what is being researched. It is not so uncommon for women to have difficulty knowing if an orgasm has even occurred [2] and the clinical diagnosis of difficulty is based on the woman's self-report. The labelling of "good orgasm" or "bad orgasm" is very subjective and mediated by expectations which are often culturally influenced.

There is no clear understanding of what is biologically or socially normal for female orgasmic behaviour. Should all women be orgasmic within a specific time/stimulation framework, much the same as the majority of men are? Is there a normal or healthy frequency of having orgasms? What are the benefits of female orgasm? Why is it that so many species function very well reproductively without females having orgasms? Why evolve now? Is the female orgasm "a work in progress"? If so, what standard of function should the therapeutic fraternity apply to it? In other words, what is medically normal? What is socially normal? What is merely commercially desirable? These considerations impact on our definitions of normal and dysfunctional, inform directions for further research and guide strategies for therapy.

What has now become controversial for many is the quest for pharmacological treatments for female sexual conditions.

W.W. IsHak (ed.), *The Textbook of Clinical Sexual Medicine*, DOI 10.1007/978-3-319-52539-6_15

The debate goes on about medical standards versus profit generating needs creating "conditions for treatment" [8]. The "Hollywood Model" with high romance, young beautiful bodies and loud multiorgasmic experiences for sexual behaviour has created unrealistic expectations for a highly wanted, valued and enjoyable experience. The issue is further complicated in that men have been hugely helped in sexual performance by the development of the phosphodiesterase 5 class of drugs and women now feel entitled to the same help.

Along with increasing longevity of life and many years of relationship beyond menopause, there are increasing expectations for a continuing good sex life in this period. The impact on sexual function of longevity, expected monogamy and normal relationship dynamics are discussed by Schnarch throughout his book [9] and issues such as the dilemma of "wanting sexual diversity for oneself and monogamy for one's partner" ([9], page 360) need to be factored into expectations.

What Is an Orgasm?

The word orgasm possibly comes from the Greek 'orgasmos' meaning to swell with lustful excitement [10]. The subjective experience of orgasm is difficult to describe although it is interesting to find that men and women use similar descriptors for the subjective experience [11]. The subjectivity of the orgasmic experience; difficulty with language and cultural differences result in a collection of definitions. The commonly understood simple meaning for "orgasm" is the experience of the sudden release of muscular and nervous tension at the peak of sexual arousal. It is expected that this event should be pleasurable. However, women find the experience is difficult to describe and there is wide inter- and intra- person variation. Women also have a potential to experience multiple orgasms within a short period of time, without a refractory period, given appropriate mental and physical stimulation wanted by the woman.

There is no consensus on how women should achieve the orgasmic state, with what ease, how often or how it should be experienced. This makes diagnosing a difficulty or dysfunction problematic.

Meston [6] defined orgasm as: "A variable, transient peak sensation of intense pleasure creating an altered state of consciousness, usually accompanied by involuntary, rhythmic contractions of the pelvic striated circumvaginal musculature, often with concomitant uterine and anal contractions and myotonia that resolves sexually induced vasocongestion (sometimes only partially) usually with an induction of well-being and contentment". This definition may not give enough space for the experience of women who become aroused and experience contractions but do not experience the arousal or orgasm as pleasurable and do not experience well-being and contentment post orgasm. The fact that orgasm itself is a disappointment for some women is not often researched.

The debate about differences in sensory quality of orgasm depending on where in the genital system the woman is stimulated still remains unresolved [12]. The differences in sensory quality are most likely due to receiving sensory information from different nerves: clitoris mainly pudendal, vagina and cervix mainly pelvic, cervix and uterus mainly hypogastric and vagus, and breast afferent nerves from sensory neurons. Combined stimulation is probably additive giving a bigger experience.

Different Types of Female Orgasms

In 1966 Masters and Johnson claimed that all orgasms in females were physiologically identical, regardless of the source of stimulation. However, the instrumentation they used for vaginal filming covered areas of the anterior vaginal wall now regarded as sexually sensitive and important in arousal and orgasms [1] and anatomical knowledge of the clitoris was rudimentary [13]. There is now some limited physiological laboratory evidence that different patterns of uterine (smooth muscle) and striated pelvic muscular activity may occur with vaginal anterior wall stimulation, as opposed to clitoral stimulation. Some data suggests that women may not be able to clearly identify clitoris or vagina initiated orgasms [14, 15]. Women tend to classify their orgasms by majority attribution to direct clitoral stimulation or vaginal intercourse. While most women would identify the glans of the clitoris as particularly sensitive to sexual feelings, it is not the only site of sexual arousability as can be seen in individuals with spinal cord injuries [16, 17] and ablation of labia and clitoris [18].

The question needs to be asked, "why should all women have the same 'orgasm' given that there is no clear direct imperative to have this experience for reproduction, child care or survival?". The physiological response of pelvic floor contraction, increased heart rate, perspiration, pupil dilatation etc. can be measured and considered within a normative range. However, the expectation that the subjective perception of the strength and breath of physiological response should be the same through masturbation, partner sex, sex with a good lover as opposed to a incom petent lover, when tired or not tired and all the other psycho-socio-sexual variables is unrealistic. It is troubling because of the pressure it imposes on women to achieve something that may not be achievable. While the 60's sexual liberation was undoubtedly a good thing, for some women having an orgasm, and more recently a particular type of orgasm, has become a duty to be fulfilled [19]. Many women who are unable to conform to today's orgasm imperative, experience negative feelings of inadequacy and failure. Why is it difficult to accept that there are varying pathways comprising mental and physical stimuli, to reaching a threshold of sexual arousal needed for orgasm? In nature there is always a Bell Curve range and women will align on this curve for ease of arousability and range of each woman's individual response. Each woman can then either reach the best of her biological ability, or some point below it, depending on her "conditions for good sex" being met.

Comparing the subjective value of masturbatory orgasms with partner orgasms seems another futile exercise. There is no way a masturbatory orgasm can cuddle, caress, reassure, compliment or validate the woman. There is also little chance of a partner's touch being as responsive as one's own touch to variations in feeling and need as can occur in masturbation. Each activity should be celebrated on its own merits and made the best possible.

What Is Anorgasmia?

Anorgasmia is a primary or secondary situation where a woman experiences a persistent or recurrent reduced intensity, delay, infrequency or absence of sexual orgasm following a normal excitement/arousal phase with adequate stimulation. Hite [20] felt that "anorgasmic" when applied to a woman was quite pejorative and coined the much kinder descriptor "preorgasmic" with its implication of potential. It has been estimated that only about 10% of women are never, or will never be orgasmic [21]. Primary anorgasmia occurs when a woman has never been able to achieve an orgasm either alone or with a partner by any means. Secondary anorgasmia occurs when a woman has been able to achieve orgasms by any means in the past, but is no longer able to do so. DSM classification added that subjective distress about this situation needed to be in place for the diagnosis to be made. Laan [22] reported that in her study more than half of the married women had an arousal or orgasm problem although three quarters reported that they were satisfied with their sexual relationship. Hypo-orgasmia is the situation where there is infrequent or troublesome climaxing or the orgasms are of weak intensity.

Orgasm problems are the second most frequently reported sexual problems in women.

Zietsch [23] casts doubt on the validity of FOD as a psychiatric construct based on the assumption that high rates of orgasm are functional and low rates of orgasm are dysfunctional. He looked at orgasm rates in 2914 female adult Australian twins and concluded that orgasm rates showed high variance across women, substantial heritability, were largely independent of other traits and that masturbation was the easier mode for achieving orgasm.

Evolutionary Theories for Female Orgasm

The theories of evolutionary benefit for female orgasm are based on orgasm being a pinnacle of sexual pleasure and therefore reinforcing for the recurrence of sexual activity, and that this would lead to natural selection. However, women do not always achieve orgasm with partners [24] and orgasm frequency is weakly related to relationship satisfaction except in a recent study [25] of young, short duration couples where the conclusion was "that specifically penile–vaginal intercourse frequency and vaginal orgasm consistency are associated with indices of greater intimate relationship adjustment, satisfaction, and compatibility of both partners" [26]. For many women sexual satisfaction is an important indicator of sexual health and is strongly associated with relationship satisfaction [27] and the frequency and type of orgasm needs to be positioned within the overall relationship satisfaction and personal happiness frame. Pleasure as a sexual motivator [28] has not been sufficiently clarified or defined in previous models of sexual satisfaction [29].

Lloyd [4] looked at the 20 leading theories to explain the rationale for female orgasm, for example: the Poleax Theory that postulates that the female orgasm (with release of oxytocin) evolved to flatten the woman with post coital lassitude and stop her getting up after intercourse to allow sperm to reach the egg; the Upsuck Theory that postulates that fertility is increased by enhanced sperm retention and facilitation to the ovum by the angle and contractions of the uterus during and after orgasm; the Cuddles Theory that female orgasm developed to help couples bond. She argues that the female orgasm has no evolutionary function and endorses the theory put forward by Symons [30] that the female orgasm is a by-product of the common origin of male and female sexual development much as nipples are in men.

More recently a plethora of Health Benefit Theories have been put forward. The endorphin release of orgasm has been touted as beneficial for mental health (sexually active people are less vulnerable to depression and suicide), pain management (oxytocin causes release of endorphins which act as analgesics), immunity (frequent sexual activity boosts levels of white cells), cancer (oxytocin and dehydroepiandrosterone levels affecting breast cancer) and heart disease (good aerobic exercise and burns 200 calories) etc. [1, 31]

Most of these theories are the result of small, unvalidated studies or clinical observations and have as many arguments for as against. Certainly many women who don't enjoy sex have orgasms, dislike their partner and become pregnant and have good sex lives yet become ill. However, the human quest for understanding, explaining and wanting reasons is fascinating.

The most likely psychosocial function of female orgasm today is that of a secondary reinforcer for sexual activity and relationship engagement. That is, reinforcement of partner as a good lover worth keeping.

The Politics of Female Sexual Pleasure

Consideration of female sexual behaviour and pleasure cannot be taken out of context with culture. Presumably before written history in matriarchal societies women's sexuality was freely enjoyed. It would make sense that physically observant people would discover the arousal potential of the clitoris and enjoy the pleasure of orgasm. However, once man understood his role in paternity and wealth/ownership issues arose, literature shows a definite shift to control of women's sexuality/fertility. The influence of organised religion is also very significant with its negative or ambivalent portrayal of women's sexuality. The full implication of this control is not clearly understood across all cultures, as for example, many women in cultures where they are considered little more than chattel are orgasmic and many women in sexually open cultures are not. Certainly, in Anglo-Saxon cultures, by Victorian times, the orgasm was seen as unnecessary, unseemly or perhaps even unhealthy for women.

Freud [32] added a new dimension to the perception of female sexuality when he wrote "with the change to femininity, the clitoris should wholly or in part, hand over its sensitivity and at the same time its importance to the vagina". This idea significantly impacted on female orgasmic potential in the Western world. As a result, for a long time orgasmic difficulties were thought to be caused primarily by psychological and interpersonal issues and women were told they needed to climax primarily through intercourse or be considered dysfunctional and "immature". The focus of management was psychotherapy.

By the 1960's Masters and Johnson [33] made the scientific study of female sexuality more acceptable and the clitoris re-entered the arena. Masters and Johnson claimed that all orgasms were the same irrespective of the sensory input. Masturbation and vibrators became acceptable. Orgasm through outercourse was validated and management focus became more behavioural. The sexual liberation gave permission for women to enjoy sex equally to men. This new view helped some, but certainly not all women, to find sex desirable and enjoyable.

In 1982 Ladas [34] re-described the G spot area and orgasm, and the kind of orgasm a woman could have or should have re-entered the arena. Brody has been particularly vocal on the topic [35] claiming that clitoral orgasms are inferior to vaginal orgasms. Laan [3] points out that we now know that the clitoris is much more than the visible "glans" and that intercourse stimulates the body of the clitoris. Levin [36] said "it is hard to imagine any type of sexual activity, including vaginal intercourse, that does not involve the clitoris". Researchers have since labelled other areas in the genital tract as having increased erotic sensation capable of orgasmic potential in some women.

The political landscape now puts pressure on women to be easily orgasmic in partnered sex with intercourse. This assumes that all women have equal sexual autonomy [37, 38], genetic potential, safe environments, partners with good sexual knowledge and expertise, good health and so on.

There has been much written on whether women value or want orgasms as much as men do. Often the conclusion stated is that women do not need or want orgasms as much as men do, as only about 50% of women with orgasmic difficulties are distressed about them [50]. Unfortunately it is difficult to have this discourse without the cultural filter such as having to please the man to have a partner, family and safety concerns, and the stigma attached to being selfish, aggressive or promiscuous if sexually assertive. There have been very significant cultural changes in attitudes to women, sex and relationships in the last few decades, especially in Western countries, and older research may not be so relevant to today's young woman. With today's expectation to be orgasmic many women feel inadequate [40] when they do not conform with social expectations. This creates further negative conditions for them to achieve orgasm [41]. Researchers have found that women who orgasm more easily are also likely to find sex important [39]. This makes sense in that a woman who values having orgasms but finds it difficult to have them will want to reduce her cognitive dissonance by decreasing her desire for orgasms and activity around the event. Laan [32] points out that it is reasonable that men who orgasm easily through vaginal intercourse should value and want this activity more than women who find it more difficult or inconsistent. She further postulates that "orgasms are important to women's sexual satisfaction and that placing less importance on orgasms is related to women's lesser consistency of orgasm during partnered sexual activity and not to orgasm being less important per se" [3]. Perhaps women's overall greater value attached to partner-related emotional rewards during partnered sexual activity reflect an adaptation to valuing what can be reasonably consistently achieved. If social media is to be credited, then today's young Western woman wants and expects to have orgasms with her partner and at least some of the time through intercourse.

Sexual politics are reflected in the models of sexual function that are used for understanding sexual response at any particular time. The evolution has been from very linear physiological goal directed "male" sympathetic models to more female friendly circular models that acknowledge that many women do not have the robust testosterone driven sex drive that men have and that desire can be either spontaneous or responsive. Motivation for engaging in sexual activity can also be varied with sexual desire being only one option. The desired goal may be different depending on why the woman

TABLE 15-1. Models of female sexual response and orgasm

1966—Masters and Johnson's Sexual Response Model [131]
This linear model focuses on genital and peripheral physiological changes and on the classification of sexual dysfunctions based on designated functional stages. Interest and desire are not included. The implication is that sexual desire and arousal lead to and correlate with orgasmic frequency for men and women. Orgasm is thought to be so intensely pleasurable and self-reinforcing that it maintains the cycle for repetition of sexual activity. This model is more sympathetic with male sexual functioning especially of the younger male and for females with easy arousability and lower threshold for orgasmic attainment
1979—Helen Singer Kaplan's Triphasic Model of Human Sexuality [132]
This linear model introduced desire as the lead-in to sexual behaviour. While more female sympathetic it is still linear with orgasm as the desired successful outcome. Kaplan did note that frequency or ease of women achieving orgasm was often uncorrelated with the degree of physiological arousal or subjective pleasure. Garde & Lunde [133] showed that roughly 30% of women never experience spontaneous desire despite adequate arousal and orgasm
This is a 2 dimensional model of arousal and orgasm thresholds. This model is significant for the introduction of "meanings and feelings for and about" sexual activity, partner and context and how this biofeedback can increase or decrease ability to reach arousal and orgasm thresholds. Emotional satisfaction rather than orgasm can motivate for more sexual behaviour. Stimulus thresholds are very individual, vary over time and with intra and extra-person changes such as health or partner behaviour. Conscious or hormonally driven sexual hunger, possibly very important in masturbation, becomes only one factor for engaging in couple sexual behaviour.
2001—Rosemary Basson's Human Sex-Response Cycle [130]
The earlier linear models have a clear beginning and end. The end of successful sexual behaviour being determined by having an orgasm. The conclusion is then drawn that having difficulty achieving an orgasm or not having an orgasm is a failure to complete the transaction and is deemed a dysfunction that needs treatment. The later "intimacy" driven and circular models of sexuality are more applicable to many women in that they allow women to enter sexual activity at various points for different reasons and integrate "spontaneous" and "responsive" desire. These models also include sexual behaviour incentives and disincentives. The psychological and biological factors are additive and interactive. The physiological sexual health and adequate total sexual stimulation for orgasm is still needed, however, orgasm itself is not the only or main incentive to be sexual or the endpoint goal.

engaged in sexual activity, and not having an orgasm may be the perfect outcome when the goal for the activity was to participate in the partner's need to have an orgasm and her need was to be wanted as a sexual partner and cuddled. This model allows women to be flexible, decreases the cognitive dissonance and increases sexual autonomy (i.e. the extent to which one feels that one's sexual behaviours are self-determined). However, no single model can accurately cover the sexual response of all men and women, and the linear models seem to reflect the sexual response of many younger women and women with higher sex drives or when in more erotically charged situations such as with a new lover or a special occasion with extra aphrodisiacs. The circular models can apply to some men and on some occasions when sexual activity is initiated by the partner and a decision is made to engage. Often, given good conditions for the participation, there is a mental 'catch-up' and erections and orgasm can occur. It is likely that eventually the therapeutic community will accept a number of sexual response patterns as possibilities (Table 15-1).

Female Genital Anatomy

The scientific study of anatomy started during the Renaissance and of necessity focused on males. Although the discipline developed, Victorian morality did not allow for the study of female sexuality/genitalia. The anatomy bible for medical students Gray's Anatomy [42] hardly mentioned the clitoris and the vaginal opening was mostly depicted as a round hole. The result was that women seeing the diagram expected the penis to fit into the "hole". In 1998 O'Connell [13] and subsequently others [43] have presented a fuller understanding of the true size and distribution of the clitoris. The visible glans of the clitoris was shown to be a very small part of the whole clitoris with its two crura running along both sides of the vaginal vault. The fuller understanding of the extent of the clitoral and the pelvic nerve distribution is particularly important in understanding women's orgasmic potential with genital/pelvic surgery such as hysterectomy and post menopausal changes. It also highlights how direct clitoral glans stimulation by mouth, fingers or vibrator, and vaginal penetration with fingers, dildo or penis can lead to stimulation and sexual arousal. It is not possible to have vaginal penetration without clitoral stimulation.

Classification of Female Sexual Dysfunction (FSD)/Female Orgasmic Disorder (FOD)

Classification is important for defining what is a problem; for allowing consistency and comparability in research; and to help generate and guide management/treatment strategies. The classification of female sexual dysfunctions has undergone rethinking in recent years and is still ongoing. Women with FOD experience delay in or absence of sexual

Table 15-2. DSM-5 Diagnostic Criteria for Female Orgasmic Disorder 302.73 (F52.31)

A. Presence of either of the following symptoms and experienced on almost all or all (approximately 75–100%) occasions of sexual activity (in identified situational contexts or, if generalized, in all contexts):
1. Marked delay in, marked infrequency of, or absence of orgasm
2. Markedly reduced intensity of orgasmic sensations
B. The symptoms in Criteria A have persisted for a minimum duration of approximately 6 months
C. The symptoms in Criteria A cause clinically significant distress in the individual.
D. The sexual dysfunction is not better explained by a nonsexual mental disorder or as a consequence of severe relationship distress (e.g., partner violence) or other significant stressors and is not attributable to the effects of a substance/medication or another medical condition
Specify whether:
Lifelong: The disturbance has been present since the individual became sexually active
Acquired: The disturbance began after a period of relatively normal sexual function
Specify whether:
Generalized: Not limited to certain types of stimulation, situations, or partners
Situational: Only occurs with certain types of stimulation, situations, or partners
Specify if:
Never experienced an orgasm under and situation
Specify current severity:
Mild: Evidence of mild distress over the symptoms in Criteria A
Moderate: Evidence of moderate distress over the symptoms in Criteria A
Severe: Evidence of severe or extreme distress over the symptoms in Criteria A

orgasm. The woman has to be distressed by her situation before it can be labelled a dysfunction. DSM-V has included an experiential component with "reduced intensity of orgasm". The difficulty needs to be persistent for some period of time (Table 15-2).

Neurophysiology of Female Orgasm

Arousal and orgasm are attained when thresholds of stimulation are reached from a variable combination of mental and physiological stimulation. At one end of the spectrum are mental/fantasy/dream orgasms with no body/genital stimulation [44] and at the other end of the spectrum are vibrator on clitoris orgasms while having totally non-sexual thoughts. Most women employ a combination of mental and physical stimulation. One of the difficulties experienced by many women is the gradual change post "honey moon phase" of their sexual relationship when decrease in spontaneous mentally driven sexual arousal needs to be compensated for by improved sexual technique and physical stimulation. In consensual sexual activity there is the presumption of willingness to engage in the process. Without the willingness to participate in sexual activity or to be receptive to a partner's initiation, arousal and orgasm will be affected. However, due to anxiety driven activation of brain centres, nonconsensual sexual behaviour (overt as in rape or more subtle as in pressured or obligatory) can also result in orgasm.

Mental arousal (desire) is triggered biologically by androgens and by psychologically meaningful interactions e.g. bonding. There is a bio-feedback interaction so that mental arousal may trigger genital and non-genital peripheral arousal and in turn be triggered by those activities. The quality, quantity and meaningfulness of erotic stimulation is important to reach biological thresholds of arousal and orgasm. Brain studies show increased activation in the paraventricular nucleus of the hypothalamus, periaquaductal gray of the midbrain, hippocampus and the cerebellum at orgasm.

Genital arousal results in the production of vaginal transudate. This is mediated by the neurotransmitter vasointestinal peptide under the "permitting" influence of estrogens. Nitric oxide stimulates the neurogenic congestion of the clitoris and vestibular bulb corpora cavernosa. Androgens are potentiating factors for nitric oxide. At the genital end orgasm is a sensorimotor response that can be triggered by physical and/or mental stimuli. In order to enable a genital orgasm four structures and processes need to be intact: pudendal nerve fibres S2, 3 & 4 and corticomedullary fibres; cavernosal structures with intact nerves; adequate pelvic floor muscle strength; and adequate genital arousal and congestion.

The orgasmic response begins with strong rhythmic contractions of the outer one third of the vagina (the orgasmic platform). These contractions last 5–8 s starting with intervals less than 1 s [45] and then as they become weaker at longer intervals. However, there are different patterns, between women and for women depending on the levels of mental and physical stimulation. Some examples of orgasmic patterns include several small contractions of equal intensity that feel like "a flutter", several stronger contractions of equal intensity and small contractions ending in a strong contraction. Almost at the same time, the uterus begins to contract. The weak contractions start at the top and progress down the uterus. The sphincter muscles of the rectum may also contract.

The "sex flush" on the neck and upper chest becomes more pronounced especially in fair skinned women and may cover a greater percentage of the body. Myotonia may be evident throughout the body, especially in the face, hands and feet and arching of the back. A facial rictus is usual. At the peak of orgasm the entire body may become momentarily rigid. The breathing rate, pulse rate and blood pressure increase and there is a positive Babinski reflex and dilated pupils. Some women hold their breath. There may be involuntary sounds or speech. A few women have "female ejaculation" of what appears to be prostate-like fluid [34, 46]. Continued sexual stimulation may lead to a repeat of the orgasmic response if the woman desires this [47, 48]. Although each woman has a pattern of orgasm usual for her, the intensity, pleasure and meaningfulness will vary with each experience depending on the context, quality and quantity of the sexual stimulation.

Prevalence of FOD

The data suggests that sexual difficulties are very common in women but many question the appropriateness of a dysfunction label when 10–42% [49, 50] of the population is classified as having the dysfunction. The older studies did not use clinical diagnoses, validated questionnaires or measures to assess women's function or distress. Hayes [51] showed how the prevalence of sexual dysfunction declined when validated questionnaires including distress and persistence of the difficulty beyond 6 months were included. The effects of co-morbid conditions also has a significant effect on the prevalence rates of FOD, arousal and desire [52] and need to be included before a sexual dysfunction is diagnosed.

The yardstick for what is normal over a woman's lifespan has yet to be established. Presumably it may be normal to have a sexual difficulty at some time over the lifespan when conditions for good sex are not met or when hormonal levels drop below the physiological levels necessary to maintain function. The element of distress experienced by the woman herself over the difficulty in not achieving orgasms or having orgasms different from those she previously had, needs to be factored into the assessment before applying diagnostic labels. However, the issue of "distress" is itself not without contention as women may accommodate to a "non-distressed" state about no or inconsistent orgasms as a coping mechanism to avoid ongoing anxiety, upset or anger. When "distress" is factored in, the numbers drop very significantly especially in older women. Around 60–80% of women do not reach orgasm reliably during intercourse and approximately 10% of women do not experience orgasm by any means over their lifetime [4, 7, 39, 53].

Richters ([54], page 88) from Australian data reported that 29% premenopausal women experienced FOD and 42% postmenopausal women. Hisasue [55] in Japan reported that 15.2% premenopausal women experienced FOD and 32.2% postmenopausal women. Laumann [49] in USA reported that 24% of his study population of women reported orgasmic difficulties.

Richters [54] also looked at combinations of activities that resulted in orgasms for women. The statistics on the combinations of sexual behaviours and success in terms of orgasm success highlight the fact that intercourse alone may be a more useful activity for achieving pregnancy and stimulating the penis than helping women achieve orgasm. Richter's results showed that only 20% of her sample restricted themselves to intercourse only and of these 50% reached orgasm. Fifty-three percent practiced intercourse and manual stimulation and here 71% reached orgasm. A combination of intercourse, oral and manual stimulation was practiced by 21% and now 86% of women reached orgasm. This confirmed Hite's [56] finding that intercourse is not the most efficient way for women to reach orgasm. Hite [56] surveyed 3000 women and concluded that "most" women do not reach orgasm during intercourse and masturbation is more effective than intercourse for orgasm.

Kinsey [57] reported that 25% of women are totally anorgasmic in the first year of marriage, 10% are never orgasmic with intercourse throughout marriage, that 39% married less than 12 months are almost always orgasmic during intercourse and that 47% women married 20 years are almost always orgasmic during intercourse. Morton Hunt [58] reported that 53% of married women are orgasmic almost all the time and 7% of married women are never orgasmic.

The figures vary depending on the decade at time of research and criteria used. More research is needed over a lifespan and including co-morbid conditions so that normal (albeit undesired states) are not pathologized. This does not mean that women with these normal states should not be helped.

Effects of Menopause on FOD

Worldwide there is an increasing, healthy aging female population who want to maintain the sexual pleasure they enjoyed in younger years and maintain their quality of life. Menopause is a given for all women, usually occurring

TABLE 15-3. Possible changes with Female Androgen Insufficiency Syndrome (FAIS)

1. Diminished sense of well being, dysphoric mood and/or blunted motivation
2. Persistent unexplained fatigue
3. Sexual function changes, including decreased libido, sexual receptivity and pleasure
4. Bone loss
5. Decreased muscle strength
6. Changes in cognition/memory

(Based on data from Ref. [135]).

between the ages of 45–55 years. Menopause is the permanent cessation of menstrual periods that occurs naturally or induced by surgery, chemotherapy or radiation leading due to loss of ovarian follicular activity resulting in a drop in oestrogen and progesterone levels. Most women approaching menopause will have some of the following symptoms: hot flashes, mood swings, fatigue, depression, irritability, sleep disturbances, altered urinary and bowel function, vulval irritation and vaginal dryness. The pelvic changes due to oestrogen loss include reduced pelvic floor tone leading to incontinence and laxity, reduced lubrication and vulval and vaginal dryness causing dyspareunia and possibly secondary vaginismus.

Oestrogen and testosterone have been linked with the physical experience of orgasm [59]. There is usually no significant change in testosterone levels during the menopausal transition. Testosterone and dehydroepiandrosterone sulphate levels fall between the ages of 20 and 45 years [60] but testosterone then shows little further change while dehydroepiandrosterone sulphate continues to fall with age [61]. Lobo [62] presents a full account of the hormones involved in the human female sexual response.

Iatrogenic menopause brought on by pelvic surgery, cancer treatment and conditions/medications that increase Sex Hormone Binding Globulin such as Thyroxine, oral estrogens and pregnancy, seems to have a greater impact on testosterone levels than natural menopause. Oxytocin is another very important neurochemical, involved in moderating interpersonal bonding behaviour and is released with orgasm. Endorphins may certainly be very important in perception of pleasure and the motivation to repeat sexual activity (Table 15-3).

However, there is no reason why the same age related changes that occur in men should not also occur in women. Vascular problems with aging may reduce blood flow to the genital region so that tissues and structures become less engorged during sexual arousal. This may feed into the negative biofeedback loop through decreased perception of arousal and increased anxiety, or less nerve stimulation so that the orgasmic threshold is not reached. Sarrel [63] showed that levels of oestradiol below 50 pg/ml resulted in decreased genital blood flow, sensation and sex drive. Berman [50] showed that genital changes of arousal diminish in older women. Park [64] showed that decreased pelvic blood flow leads to vaginal wall and clitoral smooth muscle fibrosis. Labial swelling and clitoral engorgement are uncommon after age 60. Vaginal lubrication slows from seconds to minutes in women after 40 and the ability of the vagina to elongate, widen and expand is reduced. Berman [50] found that any condition or event that affects the nerves or blood supply to the genitals can have a direct local affect on orgasmic potential. Rako [65] found that ovarian atrophy and fibrosis of the vagina and clitoris can occur after disruption of the uterine vessels.

There are real physiological changes that do occur with menopause and aging, both of which are normal events. Does a pathological classification need to be given so that medical insurance can be claimed? Or can help just be given because the natural outcome is not desirable?

Diagnosis

The first step in diagnosing a sexual dysfunctional is a very extensive medical and psycho-socio-relational-sexual history. Not only does this give information to the clinician for best management but it also usually gives insight into the difficulty to the woman and her partner, so that co-operation and shared responsibility are achieved. The burden of "craziness or abnormality" is also removed when people see that it makes sense for there to be a difficulty given the conditions involved. Ultimately, the diagnosis of FOD is based on the clinician's judgement that the woman's orgasmic capacity is less than would be reasonable for her age, sexual experience and adequacy of the sexual stimulation she has received within the context of her sexual situation. The main criterion for FOD is that there has been a normal sexual excitement phase and whether the woman's self report of this occurring is correct. This subjective experience is difficult to quantify and convey to another person. This can be especially difficult for women with primary anorgasmia who do not know what they need or how that should feel. Clinicians need to be patient with women struggling to explain their feelings and physiological experiences.

The boundary between female sexual arousal disorder and FOD is difficult and there can be a case made for FOD being the extreme end of an arousal disorder. The determination that adequate sexual stimulation has been given is subjective both on the part of the woman and on the clinician.

The order of questioning when taking a history should be from the least threatening and intrusive to the more personal, embarrassing and threatening.

1. **Medical history** includes all general medical systems (especially cardiovascular, chronic systemic diseases and cancer), surgical, endocrine, gynaecological/obstetric (for example perineal tears and number of births), contraception and urinary tract function. Medication history including over the counter medications and recreational drugs, cigarette smoking and alcohol consumption. Menopausal status and symptoms and any medications for these need to be included.
2. **Psychological history** includes general emotional robustness and coping skills including emotional and psychiatric problems. Medication. Depression history. Post natal depression (PND). Self esteem. I always include pain threshold here.
3. **Social history** includes family of origin information, position in family, siblings, family traumas e.g. violence, divorce, deaths etc. Difficulties in social and work situations. Money problems. Communication pattern and skills. Do other family members have known sexual difficulties?
4. **Relational history** includes history of present relationship. Characteristics and attributes of partner. History of past relationships.
5. **Sexual history** includes detailed history of the specific presenting sexual difficulty. Onset i.e. gradual or rapid. Situational or generalised. Any specific pertinent event around time of onset of difficulty. Sexual difficulties in other relationships. A detailed history of personal sexual learning and experiences, and feelings about these. An example may be parent's sexual behaviour and how the woman perceived this. History and style of masturbation. History of sexual trauma. Sexual orientation may be relevant. The content of sexual fantasies may be relevant. Exploring the woman's thoughts during sexual activity is important as distracting or intrusive thoughts interfere in mental processing of erotic cues and are important in preventing arousal and orgasm [66]. Co-morbidity with more than one sexual dysfunction being present should be looked for. Detailed history of how the couple actually make love i.e. the sexual script should be understood in as much detail as possible as often the woman or couple just assume that what they are doing is normal or standard and do not understand the negative implications. The level of partner's lovemaking skills and/or sexual difficulties need to be explored. The assumption that men should have the knowledge and skill that a woman needs for her pleasure needs to be debunked. It is interesting that women's orgasmic ease or regularity is different for straight, bisexual and gay women perhaps indicating technical understanding or maybe patience [67].

The woman/couple should be given the opportunity to elucidate what they think is causing the difficulty, what they have tried in the past and what they think will help. It is pertinent to enquire how much energy is available for effort to change the current situation. Change requires effort and energy from both the woman and the couple and is never achieved without some struggle.

Physical examination may reveal infection, dermatological changes, atrophy, anatomical variations and the woman's attitude to her genitals. If the woman cannot accept her "playground" then relaxed, engaged, enjoyable genital play, arousal and orgasm become difficult to achieve.

Management of FOD

It is important to accept that the management of sexual difficulties is not an exact science. There is no 'best practice' recommendation for the management of FOD. There is 'art' involved on the part of the clinician. The 'fit' in personality and style of practice is often the only difference between two clinicians with the same scientific knowledge. The fit may also include age, gender, race and even qualifications so that individuals who prefer alternate health care may prefer to go to a counsellor or therapist rather than a doctor. However, the high prevalence of FOD and the significant negative effect it has on the quality of life of the woman and possibly the partner and relationship means that it should have enough gravitas for health professional attention and research.

The starting point for management of sexual difficulties is the formation of a therapeutic alliance between the woman, her male or female partner and the Clinician/Therapist. Individuals who come for help with sexual agenda are usually anxious, embarrassed, shy, feel guilty, and generally feel that that is something very wrong with them and that they are defective in a way that most people are not. If the woman is in a relationship then engagement of the partner in the therapeutic situation is very important. Many partners are angry, disappointed or frustrated by the time the woman comes to therapy. Sabotage can occur, especially at home where previously established patterns of interaction are likely to reassert themselves when the situation becomes stressful or change is slow in coming. The change process is difficult for most people, even if they sincerely want the outcome and they understand the processes and changes that must take place to achieve it. Two individuals will see and experience any given situation differently and in order to achieve success, conscious cognitive understanding and alliance to work supportively must be gained. The clinician needs to maintain a position of empathy i.e. understanding that the situation is difficult but must push gently or not so gently for the homework exercises to be done and reluctance overcome if change is to occur. The partner must be factored in and supported through the process. The partner's sexual needs need to be acknowledged and factored into the therapy. Empathy and forward encouragement rather than sympathy are needed.

FIGURE 15-1. Factors IMPORTANT for 'good enough' SEXUAL function [Courtesy of Dr. Margaret Redelman].

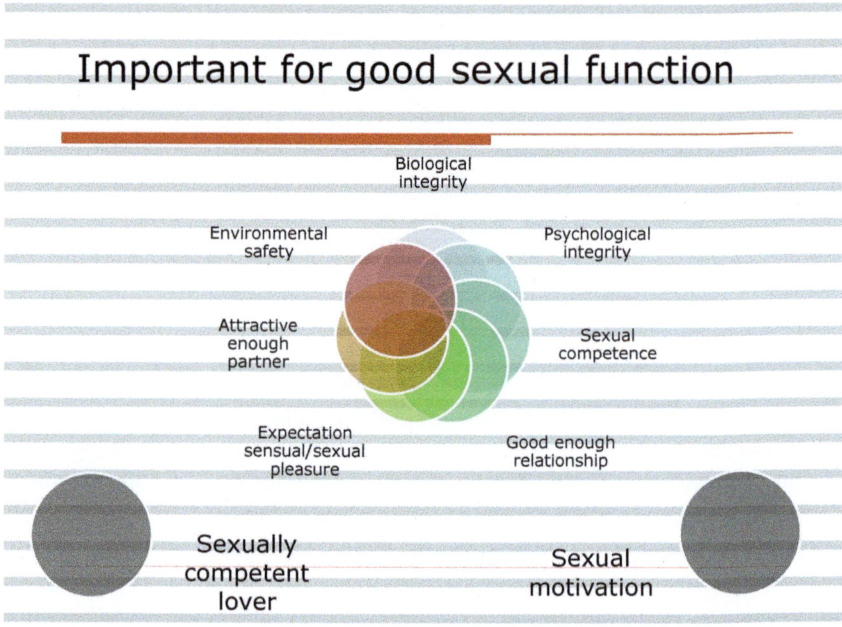

The homework exercises offered must be within the comfort frame of the woman and she must understand that the rate of change is under her control. Encouragement of self exploration may be repugnant for some women and needs empathic discussion. Religious and cultural constraints have to be respected and somehow incorporated and reframed to be part of the homework. It is important to explore the source of beliefs about genitals being unclean, unsafe, not belonging to the woman like other parts of her body, ugly etc. so that they can be worked with and hopefully gradually changed into beliefs that are more helpful to good sexuality. Masturbation, likewise, may be rejected on religious or other personal grounds and needs to be presented as a learning/training exercise and not a goal in itself that takes the woman away from sexuality with her partner or makes her self-reliant sexually. Engagement of a religious cleric important to the woman/couple, who is educated and empathic about sexuality, may be helpful.

Sexual desire disorders and arousal disorders are often precursors to orgasmic disorders. This can be understood from the circular models of female sexual function, with feedback loops involving meaning and emotion and biological/medical functions. Treatment of orgasmic difficulties of necessity often involves treatment of desire and/or arousal difficulties. However, it is pertinent not to over focus on desire or libido as a prerequisite for engaging in sexual behaviour, as waiting for desire to strike, is unpredictable. Rather, it is better to create the best possible sensual, relaxing, exciting and erotic context/environment for the sexual homework i.e. actively make changes and thereby provide the context within which desire may evolve. Desire is not a prerequisite for achieving orgasms.

It is not uncommon for individuals with sexual difficulties, anxieties and insecurities to partner up with individuals who also have sexual difficulties or insecurities, even if they are not consciously aware that the other has issues. The partner's sexual history must be taken to understand his or her function. The partner's sexual script, their sexual responses and ability, their personality characteristics such as empathy, patience, enjoyment of sensuality, creativity will impact on the presenting patient.

Relationship dynamics impact significantly on sexual functioning especially in longer established relationships and this must be understood and included in the therapy management for the orgasmic difficulty. While some women will orgasm occasionally under stressful situations such as rape, the usual situation is that reasonable emotional and physical safety is needed to meet the conditions for arousal to orgasm. Conditions for good enough sexual functioning need to be met (Figure 15-1).

The success rate for treating anorgasmia with cognitive behavioural treatment (CBT) is very good. LoPiccolo [68] found that 95% of 150 previously anorgasmic women were able to achieve orgasm through a directed masturbation program (85% could reach orgasm through manual stimulation by partner and 40% could reach orgasm during coitus). Combining direct clitoral stimulation with coitus improved the rate for coital orgasms. The CBT approach incorporating sensate focus, systematic desensitisation and directed masturbation has received the greatest amount of empirical support for treating FOD. Reported success rates range between 88–90% [69, 70]. However, where orgasmic difficulties are part of severe psychological distress, personality disorder or highly stressed relationship, especially with violence being involved, this treatment strategy may be inappropriate. In post-menopausal situations return to pre-menopausal orgasmic function may not be possible despite various CBT/medication regimes, and counselling to accept the best possible outcome may be needed. Grief counselling for the loss of the past sexual function may need to be undertaken before the patient/client can move forward. No-one likes to lose something that was valued and the phrase "it's not fair" is common.

The most successful treatment outcome will result from the clinician taking a detailed history, conducting appropriate physical examinations and blood tests and constructing an individualised treatment program. An eclectic approach using CBT, psychodynamic and relational strategies is likely to give the best outcome. Realistic outcomes and time frames should be given. Most individuals will respond with appreciation and gratitude to achieving their goals faster, rather than being given unrealistic expectations that are not achievable or not achievable in the time frame given. Engendering further feelings of failure is to be avoided.

If possible all medical treatments should be initiated before starting the CBT to set up the best chance of success. These may include treatment for depression, pain management, revision of episiotomy scars, change or modification of medication regime, hormone replacement therapy and so on. Individual psychopathologies and psychiatric conditions should be treated separately with medical treatment and psychotherapy either before couple's work or concurrently as appropriate.

Relationship counselling may be very relevant to help resolve festering resentments and unresolved issues. Anger management for the partner may be necessary as freedom from fear is important for most women. The teaching of intimate communication skills needs to be included as it is very difficult for many women to say "I love you and want to make love with you, but the way my clitoris is being rubbed is causing irritation. I would love it if my clitoris could be touched this way … ". Very few individuals are taught these intimate communication skills by their family of origin or educational institutions. (Table 15-4)

Comorbidity

FOD has a very high likelihood of other sexual and non-sexual co-morbid conditions. Low sexual interest and/or arousal disorder will lead to an orgasmic difficulty unless the woman has a very low biological threshold for orgasm. Depression leading to low sexual interest and anhedonia is also commonly associated with FOD. There is a bio-feedback between all conditions that decrease the good conditions needed for orgasm and orgasmic potential. Laan [22] reported that 31% of women diagnosed with FOD also had an arousal disorder, 50% had problems with lubrication, desire, pain or vaginismus, 25% had anxiety and more than 50% met the criteria for depression (Tables 15-5 and 15-6).

Pelvic floor muscles act as a sling for keeping the pelvic organs within the pelvis, enable controlled behaviour around urination and defecation and in intact women account for the major experience of orgasm when the muscles contract as a result of sexual tension build-up. Age, childbearing, constipation, obesity, heavy lifting, chronic coughing and menopause all effect the robustness of the pelvic floor muscles and

TABLE 15-4. Three Point system for difficult communication

1. Say something nice, complimentary or empathic
   - to engage the recipient
   - make sure that body language is open and positive
   - make sure that verbal and non-verbal communication is syntonic
2. Give information about what is happening for you using personal "I" language
   - no "you" or "we"
   - just information giving re your personal experience, feelings, beliefs
   - hopefully partner will be curious why you feel this way etc.
3. (a) Say what you want or think will improve things for you
   - this does not have to be the perfect definitive solution
   - starting point for negotiation (often compromise)
   - negotiated compromise has to be acceptable to both

   (b) If the partner has not taken up the suggestion or rescinded back to previous behaviour then the consequence for you if behaviour continues needs to be presented
   - once again using "I" language state what may happen for you if the current behaviour continues

Example if the amount of clitoral stimulation is inadequate

1. I love you being my lover
2. and get aroused when you rub my clitoris but then lose arousal and get frustrated when the stimulation stops sooner than I want
3. (a) I'd love it to go for 5 min longer with some lubrication. Is that possible?
   (b) and I'm scared if it continues like this I'll lose interest in making love

[Courtesy of Dr. Margaret Redelman].

TABLE 15-5. Some predisposing factors for FOD flowing from Figure 15-1

1. Difficulty and shyness communicating about sexual issues
2. Partner factors i.e. partner's sexual function/dysfunction, health, personality or generosity
3. Relationship factors i.e. poor communication both general and specifically sexual, aggression, violence, control, desire discrepancy
4. Individual vulnerability i.e. poor body image, history of emotional, physical or sexual abuse, psychiatric co-morbidity e.g. depression, anxiety, guilt about sexual feelings or content of sexual fantasies
5. Stressors e.g. job loss, bereavement, affairs, lack of physical safety or privacy for sexual activity, guilt about time takes to become aroused or have orgasm
6. Cultural/religious factors or conservatism i.e. prohibitions against sexual activity e.g. masturbation, pre-marital sex, attitudes towards sexuality, role stereotypes
7. Medical factors i.e. hormonal changes, chronic conditions such as metabolic syndrome, obesity, cardiovascular disease, obstructive sleep apnoea, diabetes, multiple sclerosis, pelvic nerve damage from radical hysterectomy, spinal cord injury, SSRIs, vulvovaginal atrophy

TABLE 15-6. Some maintaining factors for FOD

1. Lack of good will or motivation
2. Ongoing poor communication
3. Continuing affair/s
4. Rigid role stereotyping
5. Rigid religious adherence
6. Continuing violence
7. External environmental factors such as war, famine, earthquakes

can result in prolapse of bladder and/or rectum, incontinence and changes in orgasmic potential either in difficulty reaching the threshold to climax or in decreased perception of strength of orgasmic contractions which leads to subjective disappointment. In an increasingly aging population pelvic floor muscle weakness is a growing problem.

Women need to be taught about the need for good pelvic floor health and encouraged to do the daily exercises necessary for rehabilitation [71, 72]. In general women stop doing their pelvic floor exercises within days or weeks of leaving the maternity hospital. The exercises are free, painless and can be done anywhere at any time. They help prevent or ameliorate incontinence, help with becoming orgasmic, help with experiencing stronger orgasms and even with becoming multiorgasmic. There are various regimes recommended by pelvic floor physiotherapists. I recommend 120 contractions daily: five lots of 20 quick contracts and 20 slow contractions with deep diaphragmatic breathing to the count of four i.e. a slow deep breath in to the count of four while pulling the pelvic floor up as much as possible, holding the breath and pelvic floor for the count of four and then a slow controlled release of breath and pelvic floor. These can be done throughout the day while waiting at traffic lights, during commercial breaks on the TV while chatting to friends or sitting on the train. The point is to incorporate them into daily living.

Behavioural Treatment of FOD

As FOD is a multifactorial condition the treatment must be tailored to the woman/couple as understood by the clinician from the history and examination.

Any underlying medical condition and physical impediment-needs to be addressed first before instigating the sex therapy. No one model of psychosocial intervention meets the specific needs of each case and to a large extent integration of models has the best outcome. Clinician flexibility and responsiveness to the patient is important rather than fitting the patient into a preordained model, that is, integration of psychodynamic therapy with behavioural and cognitive interventions depending on the individual needs of each case. Psychodynamic therapy is useful when the woman/couple are stuck in maladaptive behaviours that prevent them being able to engage with the behavioural homework tasks that the clinician recommends. Understanding the unconscious meanings and defences that evolved due to their particular life experiences may enable them to engage more appropriately in the present. Not all patients need psychodynamic interventions which are often costly and protracted. Behavioural and cognitive interventions such as psychosexual education, sensate focus, teaching of responsible selfishness and erotic self-focus, directed masturbation, teaching the transferring of skills from masturbation to partner sex, encouragement to explore erotica and to expand boundaries of sexual behaviour within the context of giving approval and permission to be sexual and to enjoy sexuality are the cornerstones of Cognitive Behavioural Sex Therapy (CBT) in anorgasmia. While many women/couples may desire to be synchronously multiorgasmic with intercourse, this may not be an achievable goal. Realistic goals and a continuum of possibilities need to be discussed. Possibilities may be: becoming orgasmic with masturbation alone, self masturbation with the partner present; with partner masturbation by hand or vibrator; with intercourse assisted by self masturbation; or partner clitoral stimulation or concurrent use of a vibrator during intercourse. All options need to be presented as good options.

Deconstructing the importance of achieving orgasm for validation of self, partner as lover, relationship quality and being in love may paradoxically enable more freedom and spontaneity in sexual expression and capacity for fun and enjoyment in the lovemaking.

Research evidence for treatment efficacy is mainly available for cognitive behavioural and pharmacological therapies [73]. Mindfulness-based therapies have shown positive responses to improving sexual desire and subsequently arousal and orgasm [74].

Management of Primary Anorgasmia

History will give insight into whether an intrinsic low biological sex drive, timid personality, repressive sexual environment ± poor sexual knowledge, abusive experiences, poor love-making style, troubled relationship/s or medical problems are major factors in the anorgasmia. Psychological factors including sexual inexperience, lack of sexual knowledge on how to achieve sufficient stimulation and sexual shyness are more common than medical factors in primary anorgasmia. For some women with busy lives, serious goals and a need to stay in control has meant that sexuality has never been prioritised or valued enough to spend the time to explore the potential. The possibility of loss of control may be too frightening. Entitlement to sexual pleasure may also be an issue.

Normalising the FOD is often the first step. Libido and ease of orgasm (threshold) fall on a Bell Curve continuum. As such, there will be women who are at the low end of libido and never had enough sexual interest or motivation to explore their own genitals and/or masturbate to relieve any sexual tension. Sexually repressive environments will exacerbate these states. At the other end of the Bell Curve are women with naturally high libidos who will discover masturbation despite repressive environments. Women with lower thresholds for orgasm may learn to masturbate to orgasm more easily than women who have high thresholds who need specific conditions or high levels of stimulation such as use of a vibrator for an extended time.

How the first sexual experience occurred may be relevant for subsequent orgasmic ease. An unpleasant or painful first sexual experience may colour all future experiences so that the woman never allows herself to stop being vigilant and self-protective. The partner's skill, preferences and sexual performance need to be assessed as premature ejaculation is a very common male sexual condition, especially in younger men who are the most likely partners for younger women. The partner's knowledge about women's needs for sexual stimulation to reach orgasm needs to be explored. Many men assume that if they enjoy something their female partner will also enjoy it. A common refrain from men is "she takes too long". It is important to explore what this means i.e. partner just lies there and gives no feedback, he has no interest in her satisfaction, he doesn't understand that 10–15 min is not unusual and so on. Often, the woman herself feels she is taking too long and will move sexual activity onto intercourse thereby guaranteeing that her arousal level is inadequate for orgasm. Many older women with primary anorgasmia have never really explored their sexual response enough to learn what they need to reach orgasm given the mores of their culture/time. A relationship where the woman's sexual pleasure is irrelevant or secondary is unlikely to provide an environment for exploring the woman's potential.

Women with intellectual or physical disabilities may not have been given the opportunity, permission or privacy to learn about their sexual responses and will need more targeted strategies of management. With younger women and those in care, the carers may need to be educated and brought on board so that permission and space to be sexual in a safe way is allowed.

Directed masturbation [75] is the cornerstone of therapy for primary anorgasmia as presented by Julia Heiman and Jo LoPiccolo [76] in 1988 although the research is soft. However, most clinicians see positive outcomes with this behavioural strategy. (Table 15-7)

TABLE 15-7. Management of FOD

1. Assess and treat co-morbid factors where possible
2. Normalise given the predisposing and maintaining conditions present
3. Educate about sexual anatomy and function
4. Improve self-confidence and teach assertiveness
5. Educate about normal range of adult sexual behaviour and entitlement to adult sexuality
6. Encourage self-exploration of whole body and genitals. Sensate focus and systemic desensitization through repetition in the best environment possible
7. Teach acceptance and appreciation of genitals i.e. become "friends" so can "play" together
8. Reduce spectatoring (critically observing oneself is not an erotic activity)
9. Teach positive erotic focusing skills e.g. fantasy, reading erotica, mindfulness. Enhance mental arousal using senses and fantasy to create sensual ambiance and variety
10. Give permission to be sexually selfish (i.e. the woman is allowed to consider herself and her sexual needs first some of the time)
11. Deal with specific sexual fears and fear of orgasm. Practice extreme role-play orgasms. Relaxation techniques may be necessary
12. Teach pelvic floor exercises (daily, lifelong asset for good sexuality)
13. Directed masturbation exercises as per Heiman's [75] masturbation program. All genital touch to be with lubricant. Encourage persistence and patience to practice at least three times a week for 30 min
14. Vibrator use if more stimulation needed
15. Transfer masturbation skills to couples situation. Coitus alone is an inefficient method of eliciting female orgasm so couple need to be taught to broaden sexual scripts to include manual (self and partner), oral and vibrator stimulation before and/or during penile penetration. Explore specific positions that allow clitoral stimulation during penetration. Couples therapy may be needed

Management of Secondary Anorgasmia

In this situation the woman has been satisfactorily orgasmic previously but now cannot orgasm, orgasms infrequently or the orgasms are unsatisfactory.

Sudden or rapid onset of orgasmic difficulties may have a biological cause whereas a more gradual onset a more relational social cause. Overt or covert resentment and anger at the partner can often be expressed as loss of sexual interest and orgasmic potential with that partner. The expression "everything in our relationship/life is perfect apart from this" is often not true and individuals do not see or understand the dynamics operating in the relationship. David Schnarch [9, 77] presents how couples' dynamics play out in the sexual arena and how to address them.

Good history taking will highlight possible causes for the loss of the orgasmic potential previously had. In younger women the causes are more likely to be due to lifestyle issues, stress and tiredness, relationship difficulties, poor sexual scripts and health issues such as depression and infections. Anger and/or resentment at a partner are especially common around negotiating equitable domestic and child caring roles. Frustration over lost career opportunities or loss of family and friends with partner's job moves are common issues. Contraceptive dilemmas, traumatic birth or fear of pregnancy may also inhibit sexual expression. Desire discrepancy with conflict over the frequency and type of sex in the relationship is very common and can be a significant causative factor in a woman losing orgasmic potential due to feeling pressured to perform sexually beyond her desire to do so. Schnarch argues that any relationship of two individuals is primed for desire discrepancy in a longer term relationship because it is unreasonable to expect people to be totally synchronised over a long period. We don't expect this for the type and amount of food we want or books we want to read. Yet when our partner does not want the same type or frequency of sex it becomes a personal reflection. Pathologising either the higher sex drive or the lower sex drive partner further de-eroticises the sexual relationship.

Fertility issues often result in sexual difficulties as do the management regimes for the infertility and need to be considered with these couples. Fertility issues are on the increase with the age of having the first child increasing and obesity becoming an epidemic.

In older women, health issues, medications and menopause are more often responsible. Entrenched lovemaking patterns sometimes limit people when changes occur and help has to given to expand sexual repertoires and build resilience. Sexual boredom and taking one's partner for granted are common patterns seen in longer relationships. Desire discrepancy where the woman is the lower sex drive partner can create a feeling that sex is wanted rather than that she is wanted. Most women do not find this attractive, desirable or a turn-on. Sex is not inherently intimate and many women find sex without emotional intimacy in a long term relationship a turn off. Depression can occur with life stage changes inhibiting sexuality especially for women who built their self-esteem on their domestic role. Society has always focused on women's physical attractiveness as a sexual cue however, with the empowerment of women the issue of male attractiveness also arises. Where the partner has gained excessive weight, changed grooming care, drinks, smokes etc. the way he is viewed as a sexual partner can be affected.

Acute accidents such as sporting and motor vehicle accidents and cardiovascular events can rapidly create changes that most individuals cannot cope with. The focus needs to be on compensating for losses and changes and encouraging looking at what is able to be done and enjoyed rather than what has been lost. The same focus needs to be kept with chronic conditions such as severe diabetes, Parkinson's Disease, multiple sclerosis, cancers and so on. An important predictor of successful sexual rehabilitation is the pre-injury sexual health of the individual and couple.

Teaching women patience and persistence is a crucial factor for success in learning how to orgasm or regain orgasmic ability. A holistic framework is helpful reminding women (and often their partners) that sexual satisfaction and relationship satisfaction are not necessarily correlated with orgasmic experience i.e. many women report high levels of happiness with their partner and their lovemaking even though they rarely or never experience orgasm. Conversely being easily orgasmic does not make some women want to engage in lovemaking more.

For many women, especially as they get older and are in longer term relationships, desire or lust are not the only or main drivers for sexual activity. Women can want and participate happily in sexual activity because they want intimate connection with their partner, physical comfort, closeness, validation, to be generous for partner's needs, to give and receive love etc.

Another common presentation is the woman being able to reach orgasm on her own but not with a partner. The usual personality, relationship dynamics and partner sexual history need to be explored. However, particular interest needs to be directed at the woman's masturbation style. It needs to be understood so that the expertise she already has, can be extended into the lovemaking situation or an idiosyncratic masturbation style can be modified to enable couple enjoyment. It is not unusual for women to discover orgasms through such behaviours as rocking face down on the bed with legs crossed and bearing down. There is nothing wrong with this but it does not allow for much partner participation. Broadening of the woman's sexual script needs to occur if she wants to be able to orgasm with a partner.

Biological Treatment of FOD

Medical Treatments

There are very few approved medications specifically for FOD. Medications act generally in the arena of wellbeing, increased sexual interest and ability for erotic focus, genital comfort and increased lubrication. As the condition is multifactorial, art and science have to be combined for the best outcome possible for the woman.

Hormones

The human endocrine system is quite complex and diabetes, thyroid imbalances, high prolactin levels and sex hormones should be investigated before addressing the FOD. If there is suspicion of early onset menopause or natural menopause then responsible replacement of oestrogen/progesterone/testosterone should be discussed with the woman if the symptoms warrant this management and the sexual function changes are causing distress. Many women (and clinicians) became scared of using Hormone Replacement Therapy (HRT) following release of the Women's Health Initiative data [78]. A more balanced position seems to be in place now. The woman's health status and cardiovascular risk factors are factored more holistically in with her quality of life and personal informed choice. The three hormones of particular relevance at menopause are oestrogen, progesterone and testosterone. Menopausal symptoms are created by changes in the levels of oestrogen and progesterone and their relative balance with testosterone. HRT is the medical replacement of these hormones and requires the fine tuning of dosage to give the woman the best possible alleviation of symptoms at the lowest dose of hormones.

Davis [79] has summarized the literature regarding the potential role of testosterone therapy for women and randomized placebo-controlled trials. Research shows that transdermal testosterone therapy improves sexual desire, arousal, orgasm frequency and satisfaction in premenopausal and postmenopausal women presenting with sexual desire/arousal problems. No adverse metabolic effects have been observed in these studies. It would be medically negligent to prescribe doses of testosterone that result in masculinisation. A good starting dose for a woman with symptoms of androgen deficiency and sexual difficulties is 300 μg daily and then to retest and titrate dose. Dosage must be individualised up or down as no accepted standards exist. Off label medication treatment must be given with full disclosure and agreement of the patient. Van Anders [59] showed that free testosterone levels were correlated with the subjective experience of orgasm and oestrogen with the physical experience of orgasm. This makes sense given that testosterone is a 'feel good' drug which makes women feel more positive, energetic and enthusiastic, more open to advances by the partner, better able to engage with erotica and maintain erotic focus and to lubricate and become aroused more easily. Tibolone is a synthetic steroid with estrogenic, androgenic and progestagenic properties which wins in the convenience stakes. Tibolone reduces sex hormone binding globulin and, hence, increases bioavailable testosterone, estradiol and dehydroephiandrosterone-sulphate [80]. The aesthetic delivery of once daily oral tablet makes this preparation attractive.

IsHak et al. [81] have an excellent literature review of trials using drugs such as Alprostadil, ArginMax, Bupropion, Estrogens, Ginko bilboa, Sildenafil, Testosterone, Tibolone, Mianserin, Yohimbine, Zestra and others which have shown a positive effect on arousal and orgasmic potential.

Oxytocin

Human sexual behaviour is a cognitively mediated part of interpersonal relationships. Research into the neurophysiology of attachment, love and sexual bonding in rodents whose subcortical systems are similar to humans indicates that the neuropeptides oxytocin and vasopressin, secreted from the pituitary gland, have a vital role in partner preference and copulation. Oxytocin inhibits the secretion of glucocorticoids, and is needed for smooth muscle contractions of the uterus after parturition and pulsatile release is crucial for lactation. Oxytocin is necessary for subjective pleasure during arousal and orgasm and is regulated by oestrogen [82].

Carmichael [83] reported significant temporal patterns of increase in plasma oxytocin levels in women and men from baseline, through stimulation, to ejaculation/orgasm and for 5 min post orgasm. In 1994 Carmichael [84] found a significant correlation between increases in oxytocin levels and intensity of muscular contractions during orgasm. He suggested that oxytocin may influence orgasm by facilitating the vasocongestion associated with sexual arousal, and by acting on smooth muscles in the genital area to induce contractions.

Muin [85] conducted a 22 week cross-over trial of intranasal oxytocin and placebo in 30 pre- and postmenopausal women. He concluded that intranasal oxytocin was not superior to placebo for any of the outcomes under investigation and that generally the up to 40% placebo effect seen in management of female sexual dysfunctions comes from the extra mindfulness by the woman on herself and her sexuality and possibly the relationship and sexual scripts.

Oxytocin needs further research especially in women and for FSD and FOD before any conclusions can be reached re its efficacy in this area beyond placebo and bonding/liking feelings towards the partner.

PDE5 Drugs

The PDE5 drugs such as sildenafil, tadalafil, vardenafil etc treat erectile dysfunction in men by inhibiting the enzyme nitric oxide synthase to improve blood flow to the penis. It is not unreasonable to postulate that the same vascular pathology and mechanisms operate in the female clitoris and pelvic structures [86].

Berman's [87] study on 35 women showed improved sensation and ability to reach orgasm with increased blood flow following sildenafil. The PDE5 female trials are often ambivalent but it could be that only a specific population of women benefits from increased genital blood flow if other factors are not an issue. Older women with vascular disease may respond in the same way that men do to the PDE5 drugs. Of course the same contra-indications apply. I prefer the daily dosing routine divorced from sexual activity and recommend 2.5 mg daily tadalafil (of label). With women and especially older women who have lost their previous routine of sexual activity, I stress the "habit" of regular weekly or bi-weekly genital activity within an erotic environment as a PDE5 alone will not achieve much change.

Antidepressant Medication

Depression and sexual difficulties are known to be bi-directional [88]. That is, having a sexual difficulty can cause depression and having depression can cause a sexual difficulty and the treatment for depression can cause sexual difficulties.

Sexual dysfunction, especially loss of desire, difficulty reaching orgasm and anorgasmia, is recognized as being associated with selective and nonselective serotonin reuptake inhibitor antidepressants which are the most common first line drugs used for depression. A change to a different antidepressant with decreased sexual side effects and increased dopaminergic activity [89–92] is one option. Another is to add a PDE5 to the regime. Most of the trials have small numbers, are of short duration and Pharmacology industry sponsored, however, modest improvements which are clinically significant are reported [93]. Given the distress with loss of sexual function with antidepressants and cost to patients stopping their medication to avoid the sexual side effects, the PDE5s are well worth a try. This is especially so since sildenafil has came off patent. However, I have found tadalafil 2.5mg daily a nicer option for women with separation of pill taking with sexuality and less nasal congestion and facial flushing.

Bupropion

Bupropion, is an antidepressant of the aminoketone class, which is not related to tricyclics and selective serotonin reuptake inhibitors. It has no direct serotonergic action and acts as an agonist on dopamine and norepinephrine which together with its antidepressant activity probably accounts for its pro-sexual effects. Helen Kaplan [99] recommended Bupropion as an adjunct to the treatment of female sexual problems. Bupropion focused studies show positive effects on orgasmic function [100, 101]. However, more studies are needed to understand if bupropion acts by not having the sex-negative seratonergic effects or an actual sex-positive affect mediated by the dopaminergic action. It is worth trying as an antidepressant alternative for a woman with depression, lowered libido and inhibition of orgasm due to an SSRI.

Flibanserin

Flibanserin [94] is thought to work by increasing the release of the neurotransmitter hormones dopamine and norepinephrine, while decreasing serotonin release in the area of the brain that regulates sexuality. The improvement in satisfying sexual events was very small but time and more research will show whether there is a specific group of women who can benefit from this medication.

Ospemifene

Ospemifene is an estrogen agonist and antagonist which has agonistic effects on the endometrium and was approved in 2013 by the U.S. Federal Drug Administration for the treatment of moderate to severe dyspareunia, a symptom of vulvar and vaginal atrophy, due to menopause. Ospemifene increases therapeutic options when added to the other symptom-based therapies—nonhormonal vaginal lubricants, vaginal moisturizers, topical estrogen and systemic estrogen. A progestin should be considered in a woman with an intact uterus to reduce the risk of endometrial cancer. The dose is one 60 mg tablet with food once daily.

Vulvovaginal atrophy (VVA) is a common problem experienced by postmenopausal women and often leads to avoidance of sexual activity due to dyspareunia and then loss of orgasmic producing behaviours and attitudes. Several studies have evaluated the effects of ospemifene on VVA and dyspareunia and indicate an improvement in subjective findings [95–97]. However, randomised placebo controlled trials are needed especially for duration of efficacy [98].

Mechanical Devices

The sexual revolution has spawned a whole industry of mechanical devices to help women with sexual activity and pleasure. Particularly in the last decade dildoes and vibrators have become increasingly attractive and female friendly with surgical grade silicon, lovely colours and interesting shapes. Curved dildoes for anterior wall stimulation, ergonometric shapes and handles, remote controls with a range of vibratory settings and couples use vibrators like wi-vibe have "normalised" the inclusion of extra stimulation for self and with partner activity.

The Eros-Clitoral Therapy Device is the only device approved by the FDA for FOD. It was designed to increase blood flow to the clitoris to maintain clitoral engorgement while facilitating arousal and orgasm in women. The battery operated device provides three levels of gentle vacuum suction when applied to the glans clitoris. The device has been shown to improve genital sensation, vaginal lubrication, orgasm, and overall sexual satisfaction when used three times a week for 3–5 min [102]. The Satisfyer Pro 2 is a friendly clitoral vacuum vibrator and waterproof that gives very effective stimulation.

Topical Lubricants and Vaginal Moisturizers

The use of lubricants must be stressed as any perceived irritation or discomfort with genital touch will distract the woman from focusing on pleasurable excitatory sensations. This is particularly relevant for post-menopausal women with tissue thinning and drying. Spectatoring to locate the source of discomfort or to modify behaviour to limit discomfort will decrease arousal and possibility of orgasm. Lubrication must be used from first touch as applying lubrication to already irritated tissue is not beneficial. Saliva is also a good moisturizer even if not as slippery as lubricants. When lubricants become dry and tacky they can be re-wet with saliva. Oil-based lubricants are not recommended for use with condoms because they can cause them to break down. Silicone lubricants are not absorbed by the skin so stay fluid longer. Adriaens [103] found that the osmolality of the product was an important determinant of mucosal tolerability so not all "water-based" lubricants are equal. If a woman experiences discomfort with the use of a particular lubricant, a similar product may be tolerated better.

Replens is a vaginal moisturizer inserted into the vagina twice a week. It contains polycarbophil, which has the capability of retaining up to 60 times its weight in water. The gel produces a moist film over the vaginal tissues and attaches to the epithelial surface. As the epithelial cells regain moisture, elasticity is restored, and the vaginal tissues are rejuvenated. The hydration of the epithelium reduces the incidence of vaginal itching, irritation, and dyspareunia [104]. Although Replens should make intercourse more comfortable, a lubricant is often still needed especially on the labia and at insertion of fingers or penis. Replens should be used at least every 3 days, depending on the severity of the dryness. It is safe to use daily.

Fractional CO_2 Treatment for Vulvo-Vaginal Atrophy (VVA)

VVA is a progressive, chronic condition that manifests as involution of the vulvo-vaginal mucous membranes and tissues due to the menopausal drop in oestrogen levels. The clitoris can become atrophic. Fractional CO_2 laser treatment seems to be effective as it induces the topical remodelling of connective tissue and the production of collagen and elastic fibres. The treatment is easy to administer and relatively comfortable with few side effects. Three treatments over 12 weeks seems to be the standard with annual top-ups [105, 106].

While not a specific treatment for secondary anorgasmia, fractional CO_2 laser treatment appears to be a very reasonable option for repairing genital tissue if a major contributor to the anorgasmia is genital discomfort and decreased sensitivity. The use of fractional CO_2 laser treatment may be particularly helpful for women not able to use HRT as for example breast cancer survivors [93, 107].

Other Items for Consideration

G Spot and Female Ejaculation

The G-spot is an ill-defined region said to be located on the anterior vaginal wall, in its upper outer third [12]. This area is sensitive to tactile touch in some women and this touch is claimed to result in an intense orgasm different from a clitoral orgasm. The G-spot is thought to be the vaginal component of the posterior part of the "female prostate gland", which, when stimulated, results in expulsion of fluid during orgasm. Levin [108] postulated that it is more sensible to call the whole urethra-clitoral-G area-Halban's fascia area which has the potential for sensual sensory input, the "anterior wall erogenous complex" as there is no identified discrete area. Jannini [109] named the area triggering a vaginally activated orgasm the clito-urethral-vaginal complex.

Female ejaculation was defined by Grafenberg in 1950 [110] as a propulsive emission of fluid during orgasm. The source of the emitted fluid is proposed to be the female para-urethral glands, also known as the female prostate or Skene's glands [110–112]. What is still unclear is whether the released fluid is excessive vaginal lubrication, urinary incontinence or some prostate homologue fluid [113, 114] although there is some evidence for the presence of prostatic acid-phosphatase in some of the studied ejaculates.

The incidence of female ejaculation in the community is currently unknown although the increased media reporting and increased validation of the experience as a "value added" event for lovemaking may make it easier to research. The embarrassment of "wetting the bed" may have led to silence on the matter and in some women suppression of orgasm to prevent it. Wimpissinger [115] conducted on on-line study over a period of 18 months of 320 women from all over the world. He reported that most women ejaculated a few times a week with a volume of approximately 57 g of clear water-like fluid although there was quite a range. He concluded from his study that the perceived female ejaculation occurs in women of all ages. Most women who ejaculate do so on a regular basis and the experience enriches their sexual lives.

Validating the woman's experience, and once any medical cause such as incontinence are excluded, normalising it, is all that is needed. A rubberised cot liner or towel depending on the volume of fluid that the individual women expels can be suggested.

Tantric Practices

The contemporary popularization of "tantra" in Western cultures has focused on some of its specific procedures for improving intimacy, enriching sexual satisfaction and enhancing orgasmic experience [116]. Tantra itself is a spiritual tradition, a belief system that incorporates sexuality and spirituality although not all varieties of tantric practice involve sexual activity. Certain methods and procedures derived from tantric spiritual practices are being applied to enhance erotic connections, and heal sexual distress and disability. However, participants need to be somewhat open to the concept of "energies" flowing and being shared. Tantra teaches that erotic life and emotional life are part of spiritual being and must be honouring and reverential. A description of tantric orgasms and possible tantric application to specific sexual conditions are provided by Lousada and Angel [117]. While tantric concepts can seem very foreign, the mindfulness, slowness and respect combined with focused breathing provide a different way of dealing with our sexual selves.

Pleasure Dissociative Orgasmic Disorder/Orgasmic Anhedonia

This is defined as "a secondary or acquired orgasmic condition where the individual is aware of having an orgasm but there is no ability to experience the same sense of pleasure from the orgasm as previously experienced " [118]. It is thought that women with pleasure dissociative orgasmic disorder or orgasmic anhedonia have a dysfunction in regulation of the brain neurochemical dopamine in the region of the brain's reward centre, the nucleus accumbens.

This uncommon condition may be caused by psychological issues such as depression, drug addiction, high levels of prolactin, low levels of testosterone, medications such as SSRI antidepressants, oral contraceptives, spinal cord injury and chronic medical problems such as chronic fatigue syndrome.

A full history needs to be taken to try to identify any potential factors that can be treated as in depression or medications that can be changed. A physical examination should be done to exclude any possible genital pathology such as lichen sclerosis of the clitoris or vulvovaginal atrophy but most importantly to reassure the woman that you are taking her difficulty seriously and are able to say that her genitals are normal. Blood tests for sex hormone (testosterone, sex hormone binding globulin, dihydrotestosterone, LH, FSH, oestradiol and progesterone), prolactin, TSH and BSL and FBC should be taken.

All negative psychological issues should be explored and best conditions for sexual activity implemented. Mindfulness may be particularly useful to help the woman focus on any sensations she is perceiving and then interpreting them positively. Pelvic floor strengthening and awareness exercises may be helpful. Medications that may help with orgasm function include dopamine agonists, oxytocin, phosphodiesterase type 5 inhibitors and alpha-2 receptor blockers such as yohimbine hydrochloride [119]. Yohimbine has been studied as a potential treatment for erectile dysfunction but there is insufficient evidence to rate its effectiveness and it is not FDA approved. Use in women is still experimental with few validated reproducible studies [120].

Faking Orgasms

There has been little research on motives for faking orgasm [121–123]. Following other research on reasons for having sex, faking orgasm for positive reasons such as for love or intimacy may have beneficial sexual and/or relationship outcomes. Faking orgasms for negative effective reasons such as insecurity may have the opposite effect. Women are more likely to report pretending orgasm during intercourse than are men [56, 121, 124] with rates of 50–67% [14, 123].

The positive reasons for faking orgasm include wanting to appear sexually competent or sophisticated, wanting to validate the partner's lovemaking skills, wanting to make the partner happy and wanting to keep the partner. The negative reasons may be to avoid the partner being upset or derisive over lack of sexual response. It may be that association of orgasm with satiety or completion may be being used to communicate the desire to end sexual behaviour with the partner [14] or that the orgasm was unlikely or taking too long [124]. Cooper [125] created a scale with four primary motivations for women to fake orgasm: altruistic deceit (faking orgasm out of concern for partner's feelings); fear and insecurity (faking orgasm to avoid emotions); elevated arousal (faking orgasm to increase own arousal); and sexual adjournment (faking orgasm to quickly end sexual intercourse). Seguin [126] found that women's motives for faking orgasm varied between sexual episodes and partners and that about 40% occasionally pretended orgasm within a committed relationship.

Faking orgasms also complies with meeting the expected sexual scripts normalised by social media, such as normal time frame for achieving an orgasm, that women should experience an orgasm during intercourse, that sexual activity should end in an orgasm, that both partners should have an orgasm i.e. that sexual activity should be fair and reciprocal.

Whatever the original or maintaining factors for faking orgasm it is stressful to bring this out in an established relationship, as there is initially loss of trust due to exposure of the lie. However, it is extremely difficult to invite change in the lovemaking script without giving a valid reason. The woman may need individual help to formulate in her mind how she will introduce this to her partner. Putting a positive spin on the invitation for change is more likely to be met with less resistance i.e. " I love you and want us to have a great sex life together but I've been having difficulties becoming aroused and/or having orgasms lately and ask if you could help me regain lost ground. I think................. may make it better for me. What do you think ...". Partner's anger or disappoint may be ameliorated by "I understand that you're hurt by what I've disclosed but I'm saying it now because I love and trust you and really want to have a great sex life together ...".

Research

Research is very expensive and is mainly driven by financial gain possibilities. The medical treatment of FSD and FOD is a potential gold-mine. The psycho-socio-relational factors confound medication use but there are neurotransmitter and hormonal components involved in FOD that are available for manipulation.

Belkin [127] discusses drugs such as intranasal testosterone, sublingual testosterone, sildenafil, topical alprostadil and intravaginal dehydroepiandrosterone that are in early clinical development. Bremelanotide [128, 129] seems to promise benefits for women but has not been refined for clinical use yet.

Conclusion

Having orgasms has become a socially valued and desired activity. It is unclear whether female orgasm has any beneficial evolutionary benefit and what rates or ease of attaining orgasm are normative or healthy. Given these questions it seems interesting to take difficult or absent orgasms as the principal criterion for having a psychiatric disorder such as FOD [23]. At the same time the natural distress experienced by women who do not want to miss out on a valued experience or who have lost what they once had, should be treated as worthwhile and with respect. Sexual medicine should develop the best possible advice, therapies and medications to help these women and by extension their partners [81].

The past focus on "non-organic" aspects of FOD no doubt reflected our level of knowledge of female sexual function and physiology, and availability of medical solutions. It is not so long ago that we were telling men that erectile dysfunction was mostly a psychological problem [131]. HRT has not had an easy time of late and Testosterone Replacement Therapy for women is not totally approved. The importance of better surgical techniques to spare pelvic nerves (in line with nerve sparing prostatectomy) needs to be stressed to surgeons and gynaecologists. However, all solutions do not have to come from pills. Basson's [130] circular biofeedback interactive model clearly shows how important are the psycho-socio-relational aspects of a woman's sex life. The best results will be gained by seeing the whole big picture affecting any one individual woman and tailoring a program for her from all available treatment modalities. CBT which relies on maximising stimulation (mental and physical) and minimising the inhibitors has a proven positive record.

However, our expectations for good healthy sexual functioning are perhaps unrealistic if we are stressed, obese, smoke, don't exercise, don't do pelvic floor exercises every day, are ignorant of how to get the best out of our bodies and do nothing to make sexual activity "fun". The twentieth and twenty-first centuries have seen many changes in terms of timing of first sexual experiences, increased number of sexual partners prior to marriage, increasing expectation of sexual activity as a pleasurable recreation and expectation of continuing interest and participation in sexual activity past reproductive ability.

While women can and do engage in lovemaking for reasons other than orgasm e.g. emotional closeness, bonding, commitment, skin hunger, validation, to please the partner, showing love etc. if a woman wants to learn to orgasm or to regain orgasmic ability then she should be assisted as much as possible.

Finally, it is important to maintain a sense of humour about the human sexual experience. Once sexual activity becomes a chore, a duty, an obligation or a goal to be achieved then recreational sexuality becomes impossible.

References

1. Komisaruk BR, et al. The science of orgasm. Baltimore, MD: John Hopkins University Press; 2006.
2. Bancroft J. Human sexuality and its problems. 3rd ed. Edinburgh: Churchill Livingston/Elsevier; 2009. p. 84.
3. Laan E, Rellini AH. Can we treat anorgasmia in women? The challenge to experiencing pleasure. Sex Relat Ther. 2011;26(4): 329–41.
4. Lloyd EA. The case of the female orgasm: bias in the science of evolution. Cambridge, MA: Harvard University Press; 2005.
5. Mah K, Binik YM. Are orgasms in the mind or the body? Psychosocial versus physiological correlates of orgasmic pleasure and satisfaction. J Sex Marital Ther. 2005;31(3):187–200. [Internet] Available from: http://www.ncbi.nlm. nih.gov/pubmed/16020138.
6. Meston CM, Levin RJ, Sipski ML, Hull EM, Heiman JR. Women's orgasm. Annu Rev Sex Res. 2004;15(November):173–257. [Internet] Available from: papers://60fb8def-f376-4893-9200-0f8da574d9e1/Paper/p87.
7. Dawood K, Kirk K, Bailey J, Al E. Genetic and environmental influences on the frequency of orgasm in women. Twin Res Hum Genet. 2005;8:27–33.
8. Tiefer L, Hall M, Travis C. Beyond dysfunction: a new view of women's sexual problems. J Sex Marital Ther. 2002;28(s): 225–32.
9. Schnarch D. Constructing the sexual crucible: an integration of sexual and marital therapy. New York: Norton; 1991.
10. Wain H. The story behind the word. Springfield, IL; 1958. 229 p.
11. Vance EB, Wagner NN. Written descriptions of orgasm: a study of sex differences. Arch Sex Behav. 1976;5:87–98.
12. Ladas A, Whipple B. Perry J. The G Spot and other discoveries about human sexuality: New York Owl Books; 2005.
13. O'Connell H, Anderson C, Plenter R. Anatamical relationship between the urethra and clitoris. J Urol. 1998;159:1892–7.
14. Prause N. The human female orgasm: critical evaluations of proposed psychological sequelae. Sex Relat Ther. 2011;26:315–28.
15. Levin R. The human female orgasm: a critical evaluation of its proposed reproductive functions. Sex Relat Ther. 2011;26(4): 301–14.
16. Kreuter M, Taft C, Siosteen A, Al E. Women's sexual functioning and sex life after spinal cord injury. Spinal Cord. 2011;49: 154–60.
17. Komisaruk BR, Whipple B, Crawford A, et al. Brain activation during vaginocervical self-stimulation and orgasm in women with complete spinal cord injury. Brain Res. 2004;1024:77–88.
18. Lightfoot-Klein H. The sexual experience and marital adjustment of genitally circumcised and infibulated females in the Sudan. J Sex Res. 1989;26:375–92.
19. Tiefer L. Sex is not a natural act and other essays. Boulder, CO: Westview; 1995.
20. Hite S. The Hite Report. New York: Macmillan; 1976.
21. Spector IP, Carey MP. Incidence & prevalence of sexual dysfunctions: a critical review. Arch sex Behav. 1990;19:389–408 .New York: Macmillan
22. Laan E, Rellini AH, Barnes T. Standard operating procedures for female orgasmic disorder: consensus of the International Society for Sexual Medicine. J Sex Med. 2013;10(1):74–82.
23. Zietsch BP, Miller GF, Bailey JM, Martin NG. Female orgasm rates are largely independent of other traits: Implications for "female orgasmic disorder" and evolutionary theories of orgasm. J Sex Med. 2011;8(8):2305–16.
24. Laumann E, Paik A, Rosen R. Sexual dysfunction in the United States: prevalence, predictors and outcomes. J Am Med Assoc. 1999;281(6):537–44.
25. Klapilová K, Brody S, Krejcová L, et al. Sexual satisfaction, sexual compatibility, and relationship adjustment in couples: the role of sexual behaviors, orgasm, and men's discernment of women's intercourse orgasm. J Sex Med. 2015;12:667–75.
26. Weiss P, Brody S. Women's partnered orgasm consistency is associated with greater duration of penile-vaginal intercourse but not of foreplay. J Sex Med. 2009;6(1):135–41.
27. Pascoal C, Narciso I. What is sexual satisfaction? Thematic analysis of lay people's definitions. J Sex Res. 2014;51(1):22–30.
28. Meston C, Buss DM. Why humans have sex. Arch Sex Behav. 2007;36(4):477–507.
29. Basson R. The female sexual response: a different model. J Sex Marital Ther. 2000;26(1):51–65.
30. Symons D. The evolution of human sexuality. Oxford, UK: Oxford University Press; 1979.
31. Whipple B, Knowles J, Davis J. The health benefits of sexual expression. White paper. New York: Katherine Dexter McCormick Library, Planned Parenthood Federation of America; 2003.
32. Freud S. Introductory lectures on psychoanalysis. Digireads.com; 2013.
33. Masters EH, Johnson VE. Human sexual response. Boston, MA: Little Brown; 1966.
34. Ladas AK, Whipple B, Perry JD. The G-spot and other discoveries about human sexuality. New York: Holt, Rinehart & Winston; 1982.
35. Brody S, Weiss P. Vaginal orgasm is associated with vaginal (not clitoral) sex education, focusing mental attention on vaginal sensations, intercourse duration, and a preference for a longer penis. J Sex Med. 2010;7(8):2774–81.
36. Levin R. The G-spot – reality or illusion? Sex Relat Ther. 2003; 18(1):117–9.
37. Sanchez D, Crocker J, Boike K. Doing gender in the bedroom: investing in gender norms and sexual experience. Personal Soc Psychol Bull. 2005;31:1445–55.
38. Sanchez D, Kiefer A, Ybarra O. Sexual submissiveness in women: costs for sexual autonomy and arousal. Personal Soc Psychol Bull. 2006;32:512–24.
39. Graham CA. The DSM diagnostic criteria for female orgasmic disorder. Arch Sex Behav. 2010;39(2):256–70.
40. Wade L, Kremer E, Brown L. The incidental orgasm: the presence of clitoral knowledge and the absence of orgasm for women. Women Health. 2005;42:117–38.
41. Birnbaum G. The meaning of heterosexual intercourse among women with female orgasmic disorder. Arch Sex Behav. 2003;32: 61–71.
42. Gardener E, Gray DJR, O'Rahilly R. Anatomy: a regional study of human structure. Philadelphia: W.B. Saunders; 1963. p. 608–22.
43. Pauls R. Anatomy of the clitoris and the female sexual response. Clinical anatomy. New York: Alan R. Liss, Inc.; 2015. p. 376–84.
44. Henton C. Nocturnal orgasm in college women: its relation to dreams and anxiety associated with sexual factors. J Genet Psychol. 1976;129:245–51.
45. Reinisch JM. The Kinsey Institute New Report on Sex. New York: The Kinsey Institute; 1990.
46. Cartwright R, Elv S, Cardozo L. Do women with female ejaculation have detrusor overactivity? J Sex Med. 2007;4(6):1655–8.
47. Levin R. Sexual activity, health and well-being: the bneficial roles of coitus and masturbation. Sex Relat Ther. 2007;22(1):135–48.
48. Levin R. Revisiting post-ejaculation refractory time: what we know and what we do not know in males and females. J Sex Med. 2009;6(9):2376–89.
49. Laumann EO, Paik A, Rosen RC. Sexual dysfunction in the United States: prevalence and predictors. JAMA. 1999;281: 537–44.

50. Berman JR, Goldstein I. Female sexual dysfunction. Urol Clin North Am. 2001;28:405–16.
51. Hayes RD, Dennerstein L, Bennett CM, et al. What is the "true" prevalence of female sexual dysfunction and does the way we assess these conditions have an impact? J Sex Med. 2008; 5:777–87.
52. Johannes C, Clayton A, Odom D, et al. Distressing sexual problems in United States women revisited: prevalence after accounting for depression. J Clin Psychiatry. 2009;70:1698–706.
53. Burri A. Heinrichs m, Schedlowski M, al et. The acute effects of intranasal oxytocin administration on endocrine and sexual function in males. Psychoneuroendocrinology. 2008;33:591–600.
54. Richters J, Rissel C. Doing it down under: the sexual lives of Australians. NSW, Australia: Allen & Unwin; 2005.
55. Hisasue S, Kumamoto Y, Sato Y, et al. Prevalence of female sexual dysfunction symptoms and its relationship to quality of life: a Japanese female cohort study. Urology. 2005;65(1):143–8.
56. Hite S. Hite Report: a nationwide study of female sexuality. New York: Dell; 1976.
57. Kinsey AC, Wardell BP, Martin CE. Sexual behaviour in the human female. New York: Pocket Books Inc; 1965.
58. Hunt M. Sexual behaviour in the 1970s. New York: Dell Publishing Co.; 1974.
59. van Anders S, Dunn E. Are gonadal steroids linked with orgasm perceptions and sexual assertiveness in women and men? Horm Behav. 2009;56:206–13.
60. Davison S, Bell R, Donath S, et al. Androgen levels in adult females: changes with age, menopause and oophorectom. J Clin Endocrinol Metab. 2005;90:3847–53.
61. Burger H, Dudley E, Cui J, Al E. A prospective longitudinal study of serum testosterone dehydroepiandrosterone sulphate and sex hormone binding globulin levels through the menopause transition. J Clin Endocrinol Metab. 2000;85:2832–938.
62. Lobo RA. Treatment of postmenopausal women. Boston, MA: Lippincott; 1999.
63. Sarrel PM. Sexuality and menopause. Obs Gynaecol. 75:26s–30s.
64. Park K, Goldstein I, Andry C, Al E. Vasculogenic female sexual dysfunction: the haemodynamic basis for vaginal engorgement insufficiency and clitoral erectile insufficiency. Int J Impot Res. 1997;9:27–37.
65. Rako S. Testosterone deficiency and supplementation for women: matters of sexuality and health. Psychiatr Ann. 1999;29:23–6.
66. Elliott A, O'Donohue W. The effects of anxiety and distraction on sexual arousal in a nonclinical sample of heterosexual women. Arch Sex Behav. 1997;26(6):607–24.
67. Garcia J, Lloyd E, Wallen K, Al E. Variation in orgasm occurrence by sexual orientation in a sample of U.S. singles. J Sex Med. 2014;11:2645–52.
68. LoPiccolo J, Stock WE. Treatment of sexual dysfunction. J Consult Clin Psychol. 1986;54:158–67.
69. Meston C, Frolich P. Update on female sexual function. Curr Opin Urol. 2001;11:603–9.
70. Heiman JR, Meston CM. Empirically validated treatment for sexual dysfunction. Annu Rev Sex Res. 1997;8:148–94.
71. Schvartzman R, Bertotto A, Schvartzman L, Al E. Pelvic floor muscle activity, quality of life, and sexual function in peri- and recently postmenopausal women with and without dyspareunia: a cross-sectional study. J Sex Marital Ther. 2014;40(5):367–78.
72. Martinez C, Ferreira F, Castro A, Al E. Women with greater pelvic floor muscle strength have better sexual function. Acta Obstet Gynecol Scand. 2014;93:497–502.
73. Heiman J. Orgasmic disorders in women. In: Leiblum S, Rosen R, editors. Principles and practice of sex therapy. 3rd ed. New York: Guilford; 2000.
74. Brotto L, Basson R. Group mindfullness-based therapy significantly improves sexual desire in women. Behav Res Ther. 2014; 57:43–54.
75. Ter Kuile M, Both S, Van Lankveld J. Sexual dysfunctions in women. In: Sturmey P, Hersen M, editors. Handbook of evidence-based practice in clinical psychology. Vol 2: Adu. New York: Hoboken/Wiley; 2012. p. 413–36.
76. Heiman JR, LoPiccolo J. Becoming orgasmic: a sexual and personal growth program for women. New York: Prentice Hall; 1988.
77. Schnarch D. Passionate marriage. New York: Norton; 1997.
78. Manson J, Chlebowski R, Stefanick M, et al. Menopausal hormone therapy and health outcomes during the intervention and extended poststopping phases of the Women's Health Initiative randomized trials. JAMA. 2013;310(13):1353–68.
79. Davis SR. Androgen therapy in women, beyond libido. Climacteric. 2013;16(Suppl 1):18–24.
80. Doren M, Rubig A, Coelnigh Bennink H, et al. Differential effects on the androgen status of postmenopausal women treated with tibolone and continuous combined estradiol and norethindrone acetate replacement therapy. Fertil Steril. 2001;75:554–9.
81. IsHak WW, Bokarius A, Jeffrey JK, Davis MC, Bakhta Y. Disorders of orgasm in women: a literature review of etiology and current treatments. J Sex Med. 2010;7(10):3254–68.
82. Hillier J. Speculation on the links between feelings, emotions and sexual behaviour: are vasopressin and oxytocin involved? Sex Relat Ther. 2004;19(Nov):393–412.
83. Carmichael M, Humbert R, Dixon J, Al E. Plasma oxytocin release in the human sexual response. J Clin Endocrinol Metab. 1987;64:27–31.
84. Carmichael M, Warburton V, Dixen J, et al. Relationships among cardiovascular, muscular and oxytocin responses during human sexual activity. Arch Sex Behav. 1994;23:59–79.
85. Muin D, Wolzt M, Marculescu R, et al Effect of longterm intranasal oxytocin on sexual dysfunction in premenopausal and postmenopausal women: A randomised trial. Fertil Steril. 2015;104(3): 715–23.e4
86. Berman JR, Berman LA, Lin H, et al. Effect of Sildenafil on subjective and physiologic parameters of the female sexual response in women with sexual arousal disorder. J Sex Marital Ther. 2001;27:411–20.
87. Berman J. Women too may benefit from Viagra. J Women's Health. 1998;7(7):795–6.
88. Lankveld JJ, Grotiohann Y. Psychiatric comorbidity in heterosexual couples with sexual dysfunction assessed with the composite international diagnostic interview. Arch Sex Behav. 2000;29: 478–9.
89. Werneke U, Northey S, Bhugra D. Antidepressants and sexual dysfunction. Acta Psychiatr Scand. 2006;114:384–97.
90. Bostwick J. A generalist's guide to treating patients with depression with an emphasis on using side effects to tailor antidepressant therapy. Mayo Clin Proc. 2010;85:538–50.
91. Williams V, Baldwin D, Hogue S, Al E. Estimating the prevalence and impact of antidepressant induced sexual dysfunction in 2 European countries: a cross-sectional patient survey. J Clin Psychiatry. 2006;67:204–10.
92. Clayton A, Pradko J, Croft H, Al E. Prevalence of sexual dysfunction among newer antidepressants. J Clin Psychiatry. 2002;63: 357–66.
93. Nurnberg H, Hensley P, Heiman J. Sildenafil treatment of women with antidepressant-associated sexual dysfunction a randomized controlled trial. JAMA. 2008;300(4):395–404.
94. Gallad W, Flynn K, Alexander G. Evaluation of flibanserin: science and advocacy at the FDA. JAMA. 2015;314(9):869–70.

95. McLendon A, Clinard V, Woodis C. Ospemifene for the treatment of vulvovaginal atrophy and dyspareunia in postmenopausal women. Pharmacotherapy. 2014;34(10):1050–60.
96. Goldstein S, Bachmann G, Koninckx P, Ospemifene Study Group, et al. Ospemifene 12-month safety and efficacy in postmenopausal women with vulvar and vaginal atrophy. Climacteric. 2014;17:173–82.
97. Portman D, Bachmann G, Simon J, Ospemifene Study Group. Ospemifene, a novel selective estrogen receptor modulator for treating dyspareunia associated with postmenopausal vulvar and vaginal atrophy. Menopause. 2013;20:623–30.
98. Salvatore S, Athanasiou S, Candiani M. The use of pulsed CO2 lasers for the treatment vulvovaginal atrophy. Curr Opin Obstet Gynecol. 2015;27(6):504–8.
99. Wagner G, Kaplan H. The new injection treament for impotence. New York: Brunner/Mazel; 1993.
100. Modell J, May R, Katholi C. Effect of bupropion-SR on orgasmic dysfunction in nondepressed subjects: a pilot study. J Sex Marital Ther. 2000;26:231–40.
101. Taylor M, Rudkin L, Bullemor-Day P, et al. Strategies for managing sexual dysfunction induced by antidepressant medication. Cochrane Database Sys Rev. 2013;5(CD003382)
102. Wilson S, Delk J, Billups K. Treating symptoms of female sexual arousal disorder with the eros-clitoral therapy device. J Gender-Specific Med. 2001;4(2):54–8.
103. Adriaens E, Remon J. Mucosal irritation potential of personal lubricants relates to product osmolality as detected by slug mucosal irritation assay. Sex Transm Dis. 2008;35(5):512–6.
104. van der Laak J, de Bie L, de Leeuw H, et al. The effect of Replens® on vaginal cytology in the treatment of postmenopausal atrophy: cytomorphology versus computerised cytometry. J Clin Pathol. 2002;55:446–51.
105. Salvatore S, Nappi R, Parina M, et al. Sexual function after fractional microablative CO2 laser in women with valvovaginal atrophy. Climacteric. 2014;17:1–7.
106. Perino A, Calligaro A, Forlani F, et al. Vulvo-vaginal atrophy: a new treatment modality using thermo-ablative fractional CO2 laser. Mauritas. 2015;80(3):296–301.
107. Pieralli A, Fallani M, Becorpi A, Al E. Fractional CO^2 laser for valvovaginal atrophy (VVA) dyspareunia relief in breast cancer survivors. Arch Gynecol Obstet. 294(4):841–6.
108. Levin R. The G spot - reality or illusion? Sex Relat Ther. 18:117–9.
109. Jannini E, Gravina G, Buisson O, et al. A letter to the editoron the article by Burri et al. J Sex Med. 2010;7:2289–92 .Author reply 2292–4
110. Gräfenberg E. The role of the urethra in female orgasm. Int J Sexol. 1950;3:145–8.
111. Tepper S, Jagirdar J, Heath D, et al. Homology between the female paraurethral (Skene's) glands and the prostate. Immunohistochemical demonstration. Arch Pathol Lab Med. 1984;108:423–5.
112. Darling CA, Davidson JKS, Conway-Welch C. Female ejaculation: perceived origins, the Grafenberg spot/area, and sexual responsiveness. Arch Sex Behav. 1990;19:29–47.
113. Belzer J. Orgasmic expulsions of women: a review and heuristic inquiry. J Sex Res. 1981;17:1–12.
114. Goldberg D, Whipple B, RE F, et al. The Grafenberg spot and female ejaculation: a review of initial hypotheses. J Sex Marital Ther. 1983;9:27–37.
115. Wimpissinger F, Springe C, Stackl W. International online survey: female ejaculation has a positive impact on women's and their partners' sexual lives. BJU Int. 2013;112:E177–85.
116. Barratt B, Rand M. On the relevance of tantric practices for clinical and educational sexology. Contemp Sex. 2007;41(2):7–12.
117. Lousada M, Angel E. Tantric orgasm: beyond Masters and Johnson. Sex Relat Ther. 2011;26(4):389–402.
118. Wylie K, Levin R. A self-treated case of female Pleasure Dissociative Orgasmic Disorder (PDOD). Sex Relat Ther. 2013;28(3):294–8.
119. Perelman M. Orgasmic anhedonia/PDOD overview [Internet]. 2010. Available from: https://sexualmed.org/known-issues/anhedonia
120. Meston C, Worcel M. The effects of yohimbine plus L-arginine glutamate on sexual arousal in postmenopausal women with sexual arousal disorder. Arch Sex Behav. 2002;31(4):323–32.
121. Darling CA, Davidson J. Enhancing relationships: understanding the feminine mystique of pretending orgasm. J Sex Martial Ther. 1986;12:182–96.
122. Dove N, Wiederman M. Cognitive distraction and women's sexual functioning. J Sex Marital Ther. 2000;26(1):67–78.
123. Wiederman M. Pretending orgasm during sexual intercourse: correlates in a sample of young women. J Sex Marital Ther. 1997;23(2):131–9.
124. Muehlenhard CL, Skippee SK. Men's and women's reports of pretending orgasm. J Sex Res. 2010;47:552.
125. Cooper E, Fenigstein A, Fauber R. The faking orgasm scale for women: psychmetric properties. Arch Sex Behav. 2014;43(3):423–35.
126. Seguin L, Milhausen R, Kukkonen T. The development and validation of the motives for feigning orgasms scale. Can J Hum Sex. 2015;24(1):31–48.
127. Belkin Z, Kragf J, Goldstein A. Drugs in early clinical development for the treatment of female sexual dysfunction. Expert Opin Investig Drugs. 2015;24:159–67.
128. Pfaus J, Giuliano F, Gelez H. Bremelanotide: an overview of preclinical CNS effects on female sexual function. J Sex Med. 2007;4(Suppl 4):269–79.
129. Diamond L, Earle D, Heiman J. An effect on the subjective sexual response in premenopausal women with sexual arousal disorder by bremelanotide (PT-141), a melanocortin receptor agonist. J Sex Med. 2006;3:628–38.
130. Basson R. Human sex-response cycles. J Sex Marital Ther. 2001;27:33–43.
131. Masters Johnson VEWH. Human sexual inadequacy. Boston: Little Brown; 1970 .p. 252
132. Kaplan HS. The new sex therapy. London: Balliere Tindal; 1974.
133. Garde I, Lunde I. Female sexual behaviour - a study in a random sample of 40-year-old women. Maturitas. 1980;2:240–55.
134. American Psychiatric Association. DSM-V: Diagnostic and Statistical Manual of Mental Disorders (Fifth ed.). Arlington, VA: American Psychiatric Publishing; 2013. p. 5–25.
135. Bachmann GA, Bancroft J, Braunstein G, et al. Female androgen insufficiency: The Princeton consensus statement on definition, classification and assessment. Fertil Steril. 2002;77:660–5.

16 Evaluation of Delayed Ejaculation

David L. Rowland

Chapter Goals In this chapter, we:

A. Review the sexual response cycle and the role of ejaculation
B. Define and describe delayed ejaculation (DE), and review its prevalence
C. Include information on models of sexual arousal and orgasm
D. Discuss physiogenic, psychorelational, and cultural risk factors for DE
E. Provide definitional and diagnostic criteria for DE, while also giving a brief view of the lived experiences of men with delayed ejaculation
F. Emphasize the need for taking an integrated approach in evaluation
G. Elaborate on the steps involved in carrying out a biopsychosocial evaluation
H. Summarize major issues and points

Introduction

Scope of the Chapter

Men may suffer from a number of possible ejaculatory difficulties, including premature ejaculation, delayed ejaculation, inhibited ejaculation, retrograde ejaculation, partial ejaculatory incompetence (diminished volume, force, or sensation), anorgasmia (when ejaculation occurs without orgasm), and painful ejaculation. This chapter focuses on one such ejaculatory problem, namely *delayed* or *inhibited ejaculation.* Many men suffering from this condition can be treated successfully and achieve or regain a satisfying sexual life.

Herein we provide information about the definition, prevalence, possible etiology, and diagnosis of this disorder. We encourage taking a holistic approach to delayed ejaculation—fully considering biological, psychological, relationship, and cultural issues—yet we also recognize that various conceptual and methodological approaches may be more suited to or preferred by some patients and health care providers than others. Nevertheless, in order to provide an evaluation strategy that is both effective and results in patient satisfaction, a broad understanding of the problem is helpful.

Taking an integrated approach to the treatment of delayed/inhibited ejaculation requires that the clinician recognize that sexual response and dysfunction are influenced by many factors. Therefore, evaluation and, later, effective treatment will most likely involve an integrated biopsychosocial approach, one that requires the clinician to have at least a rudimentary understanding of the multiple factors that impinge on sexual problems and healthy sexual relationships.

The Sexual Response Cycle: From Desire to Arousal to Orgasm/Ejaculation

Within the framework of the sexual response cycle, orgasm (and ejaculation) in men is both a biological (reproductive) and psychological (reward) endpoint [1]. Arousability and arousal—distinct but interrelated constructs—are precursors to this endpoint. Arousability and sexual interest/desire are psychological constructs used to explain variability in the intensity and frequency of sexual response, and they might best be conceptualized as the person's readiness to respond, a condition that in men usually depends on both internal (hormonally "primed" diencephalic brain structures) and external (appropriate partner and situation) stimulus conditions. Sexual arousal or excitement—the person's actual response to the sexual stimulus conditions—represents both a subjective/cerebral state of autonomic activation and a peripheral physiological response (erection) that prepares the man for sexual activity. During sexual activity, increasing levels of sexual arousal reach a threshold that triggers the ejaculatory response, which then typically terminates the sexual episode for the male. The subjective (brain) perception of urethral distension and bladder neck closure of the emission phase of ejaculation is associated with the sensation experienced as "ejaculatory inevitability." The perception of

W.W. IsHak (ed.), *The Textbook of Clinical Sexual Medicine*, DOI 10.1007/978-3-319-52539-6_16

the striated muscle contractions responsible for semen expulsion during ejaculation, mediated through sensory neurons in the pelvic region, gives rise to the experience of orgasm.

Although ejaculation and orgasm in men are concomitant events, they are not synonymous. Ejaculation is a spinal and peripherally mediated neural response, whereas orgasm is a brain-mediated response—that is, orgasm is a centrally mediated perception of the peripheral ejaculatory response. In men, these two events, because they nearly always coincide, are often presumed to be one and the same. However, rare instances occur whereby these events become dissociated. Ejaculation may occur without the experience of orgasm, and/or orgasm may occur in the absence of ejaculatory contractions. But because such dissociations are rare, in this chapter difficulties with orgasm are dealt with as if they were difficulties with ejaculation.

Epidemiology

Nomenclature

Sometimes referred to as retarded or inhibited ejaculation, herein we categorize all situations where men have difficulty reaching orgasm/ejaculation—whether merely delayed or fully inhibited—under the nomenclature of *delayed ejaculation*, recognizing that in some circles, inhibited ejaculation refers specifically to the complete inability to ejaculate. The prevalence of inhibited ejaculation is unclear (see Sect. "Prevalence"), as there is a dearth of data defining the duration of "normal" ejaculatory latency, particularly regarding the right tail of the distribution (i.e., beyond the median latency to ejaculation). Furthermore, larger epidemiologic studies have not subdivided men into various types of delayed ejaculation—for example, the continuum (and/or overlap) from delayed to inhibited ejaculation has not been adequately delineated, nor has the prevalence of delayed vs. inhibited ejaculation been enumerated.

Prevalence

Some time ago, DE was considered to be rare, typically occurring in only about 3–5% of men [2–4]; thus it had been viewed as clinically uncommon and thus perhaps less worthy of medical attention than erectile dysfunction or premature ejaculation. However, more recent estimates based on clinical experiences suggest a higher prevalence, perhaps somewhere in the range of 5–15% [5–9].

The prevalence of DE appears to be moderately and positively related to age—not surprising in view of the fact that sexual and ejaculatory function as a whole tends to diminish over the lifespan. For example, not only may the latency to ejaculation increase, but the force of contractions and volume of semen decreases. Part of the age effect may result from diminished sensitivity of penile receptors [10], but decline in other physiological systems probably contribute as well (e.g., decreases in autonomic function or somatic contractions of the bulbocavernosus muscle). Indeed, whether the recent uptick in prevalence is a function of an aging male population in the USA, an increased use of medications for chronic disease that dampen the ejaculatory reflex, or simply greater awareness and open discussion about sexual problems is unknown. No large-scale studies have systematically investigated how such factors as age and general health status impact men's capacity to reach orgasm.

Lifelong vs. Acquired DE

As qualified in DSM-5, health care providers may distinguish between lifelong and acquired DE. That is, failure to ejaculate can be a lifelong (or primary) condition (e.g., congenital anorgasmia) or an acquired (secondary) condition. It can be global, occurring in every sexual encounter, or it may be intermittent and/or linked to specific situations or partners. Although normative data from large samples of DE men have not been available, a recent analysis identified 25% of a clinical sample suffering from lifelong/primary DE, with the remainder reporting an acquired/secondary problem [11]. While primary DE is frequently the treatment driver (especially for extremely religious individuals referred for fertility problems), heterosexual men may also seek treatment when distressed by their inability to achieve orgasm in response to manual, oral, or vaginal stimulation by their partner. Data available on homosexual men are limited, but distress/frustration associated with not being able to ejaculate by any desired/chosen mode of stimulation remains fairly constant across all men, regardless of sexual orientation [11].

Acquired/secondary DE occurs after some period of normal function and typically results from pathophysiological, psychological, or relationship changes. Many men with secondary DE can masturbate to orgasm but have difficulty reaching orgasm during partnered sex. Approximately 75% of one clinical sample of DE men could reach orgasm through masturbation, while the remainder either would not or could not [12]. Interestingly, correlational evidence suggests that masturbatory frequency and style may be predisposing factors for DE, since a substantial portion of men who present with coital (secondary) DE report high levels of masturbatory activity with an idiosyncratic style [13–15].

Etiology, Physiology, and Pathophysiology

Models of Sexual Arousal and Orgasm: Excitatory and Inhibitory Factors

Sexual arousal and orgasm may be viewed as a process that involves both excitation and inhibition [16–18]. In these models excitatory factors may be individual, relational, and contextual—they include both neurobiological and psychosociocultural factors (which ultimately act upon neurobiological substrates). For example, a strong endogenous drive for sexual activity, the desire and attraction to one's partner, and the value of sexual intimacy and a satisfying relationship represent relevant excitatory elements. Inhibitory factors —ones that are likely to interfere with sexual response—also include both individual and psychosociocultural components. Inhibitory factors might include specific neurobiological predispositions for anxiety, medical conditions, relationship conflict that suspends sexual advances, or cognition/assessment of risk factors resulting from infectious disease, inappropriate (and sometimes illegal) objects of desire, and so on.

Perelman's variant of the excitation-inhibition approach [11, 16], referred to as the Sexual Tipping Point Model, assumes a threshold that must be exceeded in order for ejaculation to occur, which depends on a mix of psychogenic and organic factors. According to this model, the specific threshold for the sexual response is determined by these multiple factors for any given moment or circumstance, with certain factors dominating and others receding in importance. For instance, every man, whether experiencing a "normal" ejaculatory latency, or premature or delayed ejaculation, has a multidimensional predetermined "ejaculatory tipping point." Perelman's model leads to the assumption that appropriate assessment requires an appreciation of the interdependent influence of all these factors on the endpoint dysfunction (DE) for a particular individual, at a particular moment in time.

Less directly related to orgasmic function, Barlow's model [18] focuses on performance anxiety related to male and female sexual arousal (erection in men, psychosexual arousal in women). Barlow proposed a cognitive-affective process that distinguished functional men from dysfunctional men through a series of feedback loops. According to this widely referenced model, functional men progress through a series of stages during a sexual situation that lead to stepwise increases in autonomic arousal, subsequent functional performance, and future approach toward similar situations. In contrast, dysfunctional men progress through similar stages, yet due to low expectancies, self-efficacy, perception of control, and attention on consequences of failure rather than on erotic cues, these variant stages lead to autonomic arousal/anxiety, dysfunctional performance, and avoidance in future situations. Although this descriptive model has been used mainly to understand anxiety's role in erectile problems, general aspects of the model are also applicable to understanding anxiety's role in delayed ejaculation.

With respect to DE, the models above help identify potential areas of risk that warrant exploration in men having difficulty reaching orgasm. At the same time, the models identify potential excitatory factors that may enhance arousal and thereby counter inhibitory factors operating on the ejaculatory process. Given that successful expression of sexual response (desire, arousal, and orgasm) represents the predominance of excitatory over inhibitory factors, the health care provider might broadly frame the remediation of DE as a process that increases excitatory factors while mitigating inhibitory factors.

The Physiology of Ejaculation

The precise mechanism of ejaculation is much less firmly established than the physiology of erection, and for this reason, the physiology of ejaculatory disorders is less understood than that of ED. For conceptual convenience, normal ejaculation is identified by its two continuous phases, emission and expulsion, with each representing distinct events regulated by separate neural pathways [19]. Specifically, after a variable period of penile sensory stimulation accompanied by psychosexual arousal, a rapid, involuntary sequence of events ensues [2, 20]. The emission phase, under the control of the sympathetic nervous system, begins with closure of the bladder neck to prevent urinary contamination followed by deposition of semen from the seminal vesicles and prostate into the posterior urethra. A sensation experienced as "ejaculatory inevitability" arises from this urethral distension which, in turn, stimulates rhythmic contractions of the bulbocavernous and ischiocavernous muscles responsible for semen expulsion (hence, the expulsion phase)—a process under probable autonomic control but with both smooth and somatic muscle endpoints [20].

The ejaculatory reflex is mediated through the spinal control center, sometimes also referred to as the spinal ejaculation generator, spinal pattern generator, or spinal pacemaker. A combination of sensory input from the pudendal nerve (dorsal nerve of the penis) and descending cerebral pathways activates the spinal ejaculation generator, which coordinates the sympathetic, parasympathetic, and somatic motor outflow needed to induce emission and expulsion [19, 20]. As with other spinal reflex processes (e.g., urination), cerebral control is presumed to supersede spinal control of the ejaculatory response.

General Perspective Regarding Etiology

In some instances, a somatic condition may account for DE, and indeed, any procedure or disease that disrupts sympathetic or somatic innervation to the genital region has the potential to affect ejaculatory function and orgasm. Nevertheless, a sizable portion of men with DE exhibit no clear somatic factors that account for the disorder. These men neither ejaculate—or do so only with great difficulty—nor experience orgasm in response to varying forms of sexual stimulation. Men whose problem cannot be linked to a specific somatic or pathophysiological etiology are frequently assumed, though perhaps in error, to have a psychogenic etiology. Just as a pathophysiological etiology should not be assumed without a thorough medical investigation, a psychogenic etiology should not be assumed without an appropriate psychosexual history. Of course, psychological and somatic etiologies are neither independent nor mutually exclusive classifications—not only do the categories themselves overlap (e.g., is a problem of diminished sympathetic arousal a psychogenic or physiological classification?), but the causes of sexual dysfunctions often include a mix of factors involving both domains. In fact, most cases of DE are unlikely to result from a simple or single set of causal factors.

TABLE 16-1. Putative negative effects of various medications on erectile/arousal and ejaculatory function in men

Substance type	Examples	Arousal and/or erection	Orgasmic function
Antihypertensives	α- and β-blockers, sympathetic inhibitors	x	x
Antidepressants	SSRIs, MAOIs, tricyclics	x	x
Antipsychotics	Phenothiazines, thioxanthenes	x	x
Antiepileptics	Gabapentin, topiramate, etc.	x	x
Anxiolytics/ tranquilizers	Benzodiazepines	x	
Hypnotics/sedatives	Barbiturates, alchohol	x	x
Muscle relaxants	GABA β receptor agonists	–	x
Cancer treatments	GRH agonists	x	–
Immunosuppressive	Sirolimus, everolimus	x	–
Antiandrogens	Finasteride, cyproterone acetate, etc.	x	x
Steroids	Prednisone	x	?
Analgesics	Opiods, methadone		x
Other	Antihistamines, pseudoephedrine, recreational	x	?

Based on data from Refs. [11, 24].

Physiological and Pathophysiological Factors

Biological/somatic risk factors may be either physiological *or* pathophysiological. Physiological risk factors refer to those inherent to the system—part of the person's hardwired neurophysiology. Pathophysiological risk factors, on the other hand, represent disruption of normal biological processes, and include disease, trauma, aging, medication, and other biological conditions.

No clear *physiological* factors are known to account for DE in men with a lifelong (or primary) condition. However, natural variation occurs in ejaculatory latencies among men, with some consistently falling toward the right tail of a presumably positively skewed distribution. Yet the reason why some men appear to have naturally higher thresholds and/or latencies to ejaculation than others is unknown. Multiple physiological systems ranging from lower penile sensory receptor sensitivity, to neurochemical production, utilization, and degradation in the neural reflex pathways, to the neuromuscular response involved in seminal emission and expulsion could all contribute to such individual variation, but strong evidence suggesting a significant role for any particular component or system in the ejaculatory process is lacking.

Men with DE based on a *pathophysiological* condition most likely have *acquired* (or secondary) DE, a fact that would typically emerge through a medical history and examination. Specifically, any procedure, disease, or condition that disrupts sympathetic or somatic innervation to the genital region has the potential to affect ejaculatory function and orgasm. Thus, spinal cord injury, multiple sclerosis, pelvic-region surgery, severe diabetes, lower urinary tract symptoms (LUTS), and medications that inhibit α-adrenergic innervation of the ejaculatory system have been associated with DE [21–23]. As examples, surgical therapy for prostatic obstruction is likely to disrupt bladder neck competence during emission, and pathologic lesions of the sympathetic innervation of the coordinated ejaculatory reflex may have variable effects on the quality of ejaculation or orgasm. Furthermore, a wide range of medications are known to inhibit ejaculatory response, many of which may be prescribed as treatment for chronic or long lasting diseases (e.g., hypertension and depression). A list of common medications is provided in Table 16-1, but also included are medications that interfere with the erectile process, as DE may sometimes be secondary to problems (or worry about) maintaining an erection for sufficient duration to reach ejaculation.

As mentioned previously, most ejaculatory problems increase with aging, not only those associated with longer latencies. This increase may be due not only to an overall decrease in health and stamina, but also to increased prevalence of specific diseases. For example, the severity and frequency of lower urinary tract symptoms (LUTS) increases with age, yet this condition also exerts effects on ejaculatory function beyond (i.e., independent of) those of just aging [25, 26]. Diminished penile sensitivity associated with aging, diabetes, and various chronic diseases may also reduce the efficacy of penile stimulation, and when coupled with diminished stimulation from an aging partner (e.g., loss of vaginal elasticity that occurs with aging), the amount and intensity of genital stimulation may be insufficient to reach ejaculation [10, 27]. Nevertheless, reduced penile sensitivity is unlikely to be a primary cause for DE; more likely, ejaculatory latency is influenced more by central (cognitive-affective-arousal) processes than peripheral hardwiring of spinal reflexes [20].

More difficult to assess is whether the man may have lost physical stamina or endurance over the years as the result of general health issues and/or aging. Lack of stamina may result in physical and mental fatigue, distraction, less vigorous thrusting, and thus sooner abandonment of the effort. For comparison, about 125–150 calories are burned during 30 min of sexual intercourse for 155 lb man, with a typical heartrate reaching 110–120 bpm during orgasm [28][1]. Caloric use during sex is equivalent to about 30 min of leisure cycling, kayaking, low-medium impact aerobics, or brisk pace walking, although this use increases by about 15% for a man weighing 180 lbs, and 30% for a man weighing 200 lbs. Heart rate during moderate cycling may typically range from 95–120 bpm. Thus, men lacking sufficient stamina may, for example, need to devise creative ways with their partners to achieve levels of arousal sufficient for orgasm that preclude vigorous physical exertion.

From the clinician's perspective, pathophysiological and physiological factors have three important implications. First, any man having recently (or over a period of time) acquired DE should be referred for a medical exam that might include attention to the pelvic area, recent medications, or other disease states. Second, if no obvious pathophysiology is identified, then psychological and relationship factors warrant careful exploration. And third, the clinician might use the opportunity to educate the patient and his partner regarding possible inherent (and naturally occurring) biological differences in the hardwiring of ejaculatory response and latencies, thereby removing some of the burden of guilt and responsibility often associated with this sexual dysfunction.

Cultural Factors

Culturally derived expectations may contribute to DE in some men. A relationship between religious orthodoxy and DE was first proposed in Masters and Johnson's *Human Sexual Inadequacy* [3] where the authors suggested that certain beliefs may inhibit normal ejaculatory response or limit the sexual experience necessary for developing control over ejaculation. Consistent with this notion, Perelman [8] reported that in a clinical sample of 75 DE men, about 35% scored high on religious orthodoxy. Some such men tended to have limited sexual knowledge and, perhaps due to religious strictures, had masturbated minimally or not at all. Others, similar to their less religious counterparts, had masturbated for years, but due to their particular religious upbringing or restrictive household attitudes toward sex, they had experienced guilt and anxiety about this sexual outlet, which in turn resulted in DE [8]. As religious taboos and health concerns about masturbation have waned in Western cultures over the past half century, the effects of these specific cultural factors have undoubtedly become less significant among younger men. Despite the lack of supporting data, however, one might imagine that men from cultures or developmental environments that forbid masturbation or reinforce negative attitudes about sexuality in general, and "spilling seed" in particular, might well experience problems with DE.

Psychological and Relationship Factors

Psychological and relationship factors are often involved in long or increasing ejaculatory latencies in some men. In such men, the problem may evolve gradually over a period of time—sometimes years—but not reach levels of concern until a particular need is unfulfilled (e.g., to start a family) or unless the sexual activity involves the partner.

Psychological factors may include specific emotions and cognitions tied to the evaluative/performance aspects of sex with a partner [29]. Self and perceived partner expectations can lead to "sexual performance anxiety" which may then contribute to DE. Such anxiety typically stems from the individual's lack of confidence to perform adequately, to appear and feel attractive (body image), to satisfy his partner sexually, to experience an overall sense of self-efficacy—in some respects to measure up to the "competition" [30, 31]. The impact of this anxiety on men's sexual response varies depending on the individual and the situation. But in some men, it may interfere with the ability to respond adequately and it may, as a result, generate a number of maladaptive responses (e.g., setting unrealistic expectations). With respect to DE, anxiety surrounding the difficulty of ejaculating may draw the man's attention away from erotic cues that normally serve to enhance arousal. Accordingly, Apfelbaum [32] has emphasized the need to remove the "demand" (and thus anxiety-producing) characteristics of the situation, noting that men with DE may be overly conscientious about pleasing their partner. This "ejaculatory performance"

[1] For caloric expenditure: http://www.nutristrategy.com/caloriesburned.htm

For heartrate: https://www.nhlbi.nih.gov/files/docs/public/heart/phy_active.pdf

anxiety interferes with the erotic sensations of genital stimulation, resulting in levels of sexual excitement and arousal that are insufficient for climax although more than adequate to maintain an erection.

Relationship factors may be associated with current interpersonal dynamics or with longer term relationship developmental changes. In some instances, sex with the partner may become insufficiently arousing for the man to reach ejaculation, a situation that may involve any number of factors operating individually or together. For example, some men may have a strong "autosexual" orientation that involves an idiosyncratic and vigorous masturbation style—carried out with high frequency—which does not "match" vaginal stimulation [11]. As a result, the stimulation generated from vaginal thrusting may no longer be sufficiently arousing/intense for the man to reach ejaculation or, in other words, the vagina is unable to compete with the habitual strokes and tighter grip of the moving hand. In other instances, disparity between the reality of sex with the partner and the man's sexual fantasy (whether or not conventional) used during masturbation is another potential cause of DE [11]. At a time when explicit sexual/erotic materials can be accessed easily, in complete privacy (sometimes secrecy), and at little or no cost, such disparity between expected/fantasized sex and actual sex may be increasing in frequency. These disparities may involve a number of different factors, such as the partner's attractiveness and body type (relative to that of, say, a porn star), homosexual or heterosexual attraction, and the specific sex activity performed (e.g., oral vs. anal vs. vaginal), with each having the potential to diminish arousal cues during partnered sex. In most instances, these men fail to communicate their preferences to their partners because of shame, embarrassment, or guilt. Yet such behavioral and cognitive patterns may well predispose men to experience problems reaching ejaculation—these men are simply not sufficiently aroused during coitus (as they might be during masturbation) to achieve orgasm.

The above issues suggest then that DE men may lack sufficient levels of physical and/or psychosexual arousal during coitus: their arousal response to their partner cannot match their response to self-stimulation, self-generated fantasy, and/or pornography. Support for this idea has been provided by several observations. First, psychophysiological investigation of men with DE has demonstrated that although they attain erectile responses comparable to or better than sexually functional controls during visual and penile psychosexual stimulation, they report far lower levels of psychosexual arousal [13, 33]. Apfelbaum [32] has suggested that during partnered sex the couple interprets the (DE) man's strong erectile response as erroneous evidence that he is ready for sex, highly aroused, and capable of achieving orgasm. Second, inadequate arousal may also be responsible for increased anecdotal clinical reports of DE for men using oral medications such as PDE-5 inhibitors (e.g., Viagra) for the treatment for ED [34, 35]. While most men using PDE-5 inhibitors experience restored erections and coitus with ejaculation, others experience erection in the absence of comparable psychoemotional arousal, confusing their erect state as an indication of sexual arousal when it primarily indicated vasocongestive success [36].

As the clinician might surmise, discussions about masturbation style and frequency, attractiveness of the partner, sexual fantasies (either conventional or unconventional), and the use of pornography are extremely sensitive topics and most men would feel shame and embarrassment discussing such topics openly with the clinician (or with their partner). Such topics could only be broached after an atmosphere of openness is reinforced and a sense of trust between clinician and patient has been well established (see Sect. "Steps in the evaluation process of DE").

From the health care provider's perspective, an understanding of the man's personal experience and interpretation of his impairment is important—how it makes him feel, how it affects his thoughts and feelings, how it affects his relationship with his partner, and so on. Furthermore, evaluating both the man and his partner to determine the impact of DE on the couple's relationship may be helpful. Since effective treatment of DE usually requires the cooperation of the partner, including the partner in the evaluation process can help establish the precedent that remediation of DE will require both partners working as a team. In addition, engaging the man and his partner early in the process can help address both sexual and nonsexual relationship issues—often intertwined—which may result in more positive outcomes regarding overall sexual satisfaction than merely focusing on narrow response sets such as ejaculatory latency.

Defining and Diagnostic Criteria

Defining Delayed Ejaculation

Delayed ejaculation is listed among the sexual dysfunctions in the Diagnostic and Statistical Manual of Mental Disorders, Fifth Edition (DSM-5: 302.74) [37]. It is characterized as a marked delay or infrequency of ejaculation occurring in about 75–100% of partnered sexual activity, accompanied by a desire *not* to delay the ejaculation—indicating that the delay is neither intentional nor wanted. In addition, the DSM-5 definition assumes that the condition is accompanied by clinically significant distress and that it has persisted for at least 6 months. The International Classification of Diseases ((ICD-10 Version 2016: www.who.int/classifications/icd/en/) [38], the standard diagnostic tool used to monitor the incidence and prevalence of diseases and other health problems, also includes a code for delayed ejaculation under the nomenclatures of "inhibited orgasm" and "psychogenic anorgasmy;" (F52.3, Orgasmic Dysfunction: Inhibited Orgasm [male][female]), the latter suggesting a condition of orgasmic absence distinguished by its psychological origin. Neither the DSM-5 nor ICD-10 classification is fully inclusive, comprehensive, or clear in meaning. For example, DSM-5 neither temporally defines "delay" nor specifies situations of inadequate arousal or severe relationship distress in the classification. ICD-10, on the other hand, does not elaborate upon its coding categories to differentiate orgasm from ejaculation, or inhibited orgasm from psychogenic anorgasmy; and it too provides no temporal parameters for "delay," stating only that orgasm "does not occur or is markedly delayed." To its credit, DSM-5 includes relevant qualifiers such as "acquired" or "lifelong" (see Sect. "Lifelong vs. acquired DE"), and "generalized" or "situational," along with designation of "mild, moderate, or severe." In addition, DSM-5 notes the importance of considering five other factors: (1) partner, (2) relationship, (3) individual vulnerability (e.g., history of abuse), psychiatric comorbidity (e.g., depression), and stressors, (4) cultural/religious influences, and (5) medical factors. The relevance of these risk/qualifying factors were discussed in detail in Sect. "Etiology, Physiology, and Pathophysiology," of this chapter (see Table 16-2).

There are no clearly specified parameters as to when a man actually meets the conditions for DE, as operationalized criteria do not exist. Perhaps a simplified strategy is to use an approach that parallels that of another male orgasmic disorder—namely premature ejaculation—in which three criteria are considered: ejaculatory latency, self-efficacy, and level of distress or bother [1, 39]. The first criterion regarding ejaculatory latency for men with DE can be based on findings that the median ejaculation time for most men is around 6–10 min (standard deviation = ± 3–4) [40, 41]. Therefore, those men who meet the following three criteria might be considered candidates for a DE diagnosis.

- The man takes more than 16–20 min (i.e., ≥ about 2 standard deviations above the mean/median) to reach ejaculation or, alternatively, terminates intercourse due to frustration or exhaustion after prolonged stimulation;
- The man is unable to advance his ejaculatory response, that is, he is not prolonging intercourse purposefully (a measure of self-efficacy);
- The man is distressed or bothered by the situation, and/or his partner is bothered or dissatisfied by the condition.

The above characteristics, together with the fact that a man and/or his partner are sufficiently concerned or upset by the condition that they have decided to seek help for the problem, are grounds for considering a DE diagnosis.

TABLE 16-2. DSM-5 Diagnostic Criteria for Delayed Ejaculation 302.74 (F52.32)

A. Either of the following symptoms must be experienced on almost all or all occasions (approximately 75–100%) of partnered sexual activity (in identified situational contexts or, if generalized, in all contexts), and without the individual desiring delay:
   1. Marked delay in ejaculation
   2. Marked infrequency or absence of ejaculation

B. The symptoms in Criterion A have persisted for a minimum duration of approximately 6 months

C. The symptoms in Criterion A cause clinically significant distress in the individual

D. The sexual dysfunction is not better explained by a nonsexual mental disorder or as a consequence of severe relationship distress or other significant stressors and is not attributable to the effects of a substance/medication or another medical condition

Specify whether:

Lifelong: The disturbance has been present since the individual became sexually active

Acquired: The disturbance began after a period of relatively normal sexual function

Specify whether:

Generalized: Not limited to certain types of stimulation, situations, or partners

Situational: Only occurs with certain types of stimulation, situations, or partners

Specify current severity:

Mild: Evidence of mild distress over the symptoms in Criterion A

Moderate: Evidence of moderate distress over the symptoms in Criterion A

Severe: Evidence of severe or extreme distress over the symptoms in Criterion A

The Lived Experiences of Men with Delayed Ejaculation

Delayed ejaculation has not attracted the same level of attention in the media as erectile dysfunction (ED) and premature ejaculation (PE). No FDA approved medication is available for the treatment of DE (as is the case for ED), and unlike PE, pharmaceutical companies have not vigorously studied and pursued biomedical treatments for delayed ejaculation. As a result, men whose sexual relationships are disrupted by their difficulty or inability to ejaculate remain somewhat hidden from view, receiving little or no attention from the popular press and, more disconcertingly, from close and sustained investigation by the research community [11, 42]. As a result, we know little about the etiology of DE based on large study samples—for example, whether these men have always had difficulty reaching ejaculation or whether they typically develop the problem after a period of more typical ejaculatory latencies; we have little empirically based information regarding etiological factors for those men who have had a lifelong problem with reaching ejaculation; we have little understanding of the level of distress these men experience about their condition—for example, whether the difficulty or inability to reach orgasm results in levels of distress comparable to men experiencing erectile dysfunction [43] or premature ejaculation [44, 45]; and we have little insight into how the problem affects their sexual relationship.

On the other hand, sufficient numbers of men do seek help for DE to suggest that the inability to ejaculate imparts a number of psychobehavioral consequences, including diminished sexual satisfaction, low self-efficacy, and a lack of self-confidence [13, 16]. Furthermore, such men typically report a history of unsatisfying sexual relationships and, in some instances, a preference for masturbation over intercourse [14, 46]. In those instances where procreation and having a family are among the couple's goals of sexual intercourse, delayed and/or inhibited ejaculation may be particularly troubling and frustrating to one or both partners.

Similar to men with other types of sexual dysfunction, men with DE indicate high levels of relationship distress, sexual dissatisfaction, anxiety about their sexual performance, and general health issues—significantly higher than sexually functional men. In addition, along with other sexually dysfunctional counterparts, men with DE typically report lower frequencies of coital activity [13]. A distinguishing characteristic of men with DE—and one that has implications for treatment—is that they usually have little or no difficulty attaining or keeping their erections—in fact they are often able to sustain erections for prolonged periods of time. But despite their good erections, they report lower levels of psychosexual arousal, at least compared with sexually functional men [33].

Best Practices Regarding Diagnosis

Taking an Integrated Biopsychosocial Approach

Comprehending the array of factors that account for variation in latency to ejaculation following vaginal intromission is key to understanding any sexual problem. As with many other biobehavioral responses, variation in ejaculatory latency is under the influence of both biological and psychological-behavioral factors. One contemporary way of conceptualizing the interaction of these systems has been proposed by those who study evolutionary psychology [47]. The ejaculatory latency *range* for each individual may be predisposed or biologically set (e.g., via genetics), but the actual timing or moment of ejaculation within that range depends on a variety of contextual, psychological-behavioral, and relationship-partner variables [16, 48]. Such thinking is clearly supported by the fact that ejaculatory latency in men with ejaculatory disorders (either premature or delayed ejaculation) is often quite different during coitus than during masturbation [49].

The most useful approach to understanding biobehavioral responses is that of integrating—rather than isolating—the biological and psychological-behavioral components, with the goal of identifying those organismic elements—peripheral and/or central—that contribute to and explain variation in the response. Undoubtedly, some components of the ejaculatory response that influence latency are hardwired and not easily modified, with individual differences accounted for by gene-regulated processes (membrane receptors; biodynamics of neurotransmitter synthesis, activation, modulation, and degradation; androgenic and estrogenic hormones, etc.). Such genetically regulated predispositions are likely to impact the typical speed and ease of ejaculation for any particular organism. Yet some aspects of the ejaculatory response are "soft wired," that is, they are influenced by the past experiences and present contexts in which the response is occurring [48]. In the human, most such processes are central and/or cerebral and, although no less biological in nature than the hardwired system, allow for flexibility as the organism responds to the demands of the particular situation. As noted previously, the fact that men who have DE during intercourse often do not have similar problems during masturbation is strong testimony to the relevance of these contextual factors. These soft-wired biological processes give rise to subjective experiences that are then identified and studied as psychological-behavioral constructs that carry both descriptive (naming) and explanatory meaning for men and women. Thus, emotion, anxiety, motivation, arousal, and learning represent constructs—all underlain by biological events—used by biopsychosocial scientists to help explain variation in the intensity, speed, frequency, latency, and duration of a response. Such constructs—the values of which vary over time and situations—play an important role in determining ejaculatory latency. Realizing this, the clinician (and patient) is in a better position to understand DE as an endpoint/response that represents the interaction of biological, psychological, and relationship factors over the course of a man's life cycle.

Steps in the Evaluation Process of DE

The evaluation of DE consists of a number of exploratory steps designed for three overarching purposes: (1) ascertaining that the problem is best classified as delayed ejaculation; (2) broadly identifying excitatory and inhibitory factors related to sexual arousal and orgasm in the patient; and (3) systematically eliminating various risk factors in order to identify the most probable cause of the DE. An outline of this process is provided below and summarized in Table 16-3.

TABLE 16-3. Typical steps in the evaluation of DE

Step	Goal	Information/procedure examples
Setting the tone	Establish openness and trust	Normalizing and destigmatizing the problem
Differential diagnosis	Rule out other sexual problems	Verify problem of inhibited ejaculation • Typical ejaculatory latency • Inability to affect ejaculatory latency • Significant distress
History and scope of the problem	Obtaining detailed parameters about development of the problem	Lifelong, acquired; onset, duration, situation, exacerbation, self-management, motivation for change;
Medical history and exam	Pathophysiological etiology	Physical exam, review of illnesses, surgeries, medications, injuries, drug use, etc. including general life stressors/transitions that are job-related, financial, family based, etc.
Psychosexual evaluation	Identify possible psychological and relationship predisposing factors	Current sexual practices and activities in contexts: • Predisposing religious and cultural issues, including sexual knowledge and beliefs • Masturbatory and coital activities including fantasy, use of erotic materials, etc. • Relationship parameters involving quality and intimacy, communication, partner attractiveness and dysfunction
Summary of relevant factors to review with patient (and partner)	Gain patient acceptance of the problem, its etiology, and encourage value/motivation for change	Verify and align clinical notes with patient and partner self-report and perceptions.

Setting the Tone

Most men and women have difficulty discussing sexual issues openly, and many clinicians who are not sexual specialists share a similar reluctance about discussing details of a patient's sexual problems. Therefore, one of the most important elements of the evaluation process is overcoming the potential anxiety and embarrassment associated with direct discussion of sexual details. The clinician plays the primary role in establishing an atmosphere of normalcy, trust, and openness—critically important for obtaining detailed and honest information from the patient (and his partner) about issues that are extremely private and often stigmatized when perceived as being a bit unconventional. We offer two examples of the kinds of approach that might be used to begin a conversation or respond to an inquiry—there are, of course, infinite variations that individual clinicians may find more effective.

- The clinician may, for example, take the initiative by broaching the topic, asking the patient about any recent sexual issues, while informing the patient that often a sexual problem serves as a good marker for possible other "more serious" problems. For example, erectile problems may be indicative of cardiovascular or diabetic disease, ejaculatory problems may be associated with LUTS or pelvic trauma, etc. Such a conversation can help normalize the condition and thus destigmatize the problem. The clinician may also use this conversation as an opportunity to discuss the sexual response cycle with the patient, to help pinpoint the problem, and to discuss various preliminary steps that might be considered (see next Sect. "The differential diagnosis")
- If the patient himself raises the issue, the clinician can respond with a positive and acknowledging response, such as, "I'm glad that you brought this up, as a healthy sexual life is not only important to one's overall well-being, but issues with sexuality may indicate a possible 'more serious' problem, such as developing cardiovascular or diabetic response." The clinician can then follow the subsequent steps outlined in the first scenario designed to normalize and further reassure the patient.

Each clinician will have his/her own style, but because this initial conversation sets the tone for future ongoing clinician-patient communication regarding DE, establishing normalcy, openness, trust, reassurance, and a sense of support at the outset is key.

The Differential Diagnosis

The differential diagnosis is intended: (1) to ascertain the problem is really one affecting the ejaculatory phase of the sexual response; and if so, (2) to help determine whether the delayed ejaculation is primary or, alternatively, secondary to some other medical, physical, or psychological factor that needs to be addressed first. A flowchart indicating steps in this process is provided in Figure 16-1.

Regarding the first purpose of the differential diagnosis, eliminating a lack of sexual desire/interest and pain as possible mediating factors is necessary. Furthermore, as noted previously, insufficient psychological-sexual arousal is often

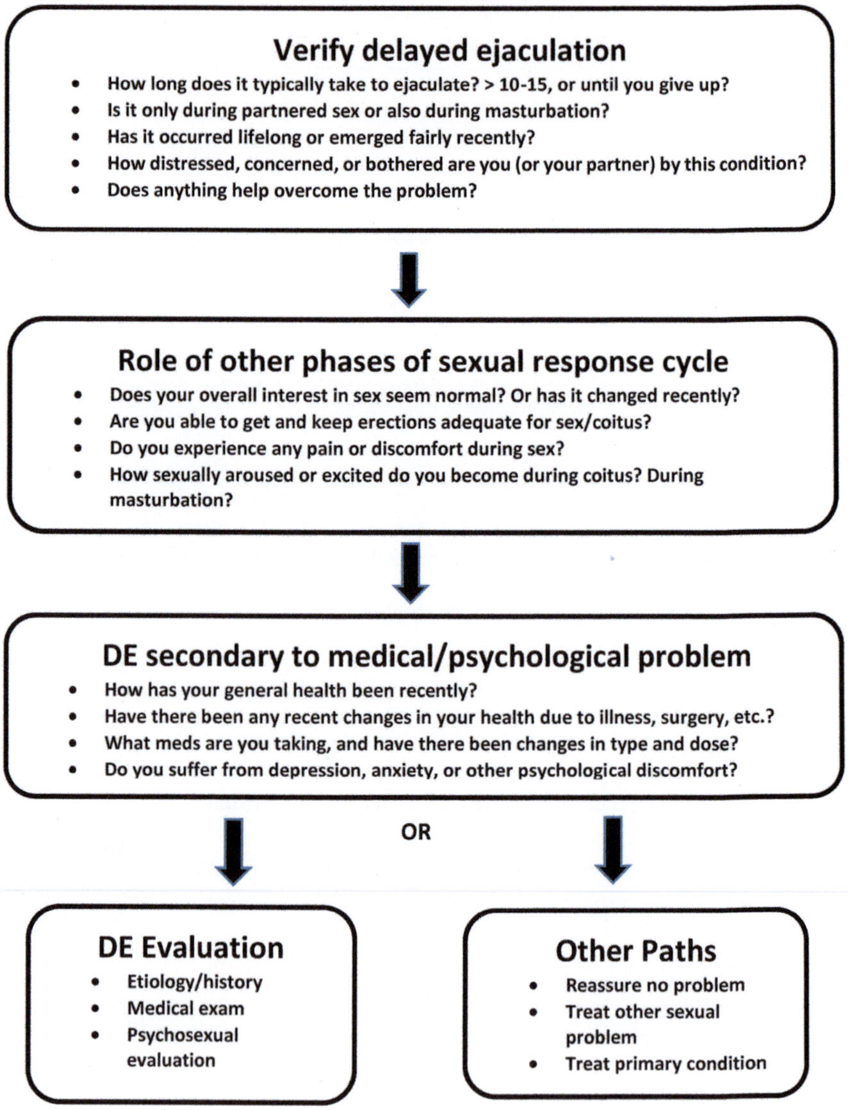

FIGURE 16-1. Sample queries for the differential diagnosis of delayed ejaculation.

a major factor contributing to DE; neither DSM-5 nor ICD exclude men from a DE diagnosis based on insufficient arousal (as is the case for Female Orgasmic Disorder), so such men—even though technically having difficulty with the arousal rather than orgasm phase—may be considered as having DE. Even though these men may have little or no difficulty getting and sustaining an erection of significant duration for penetration and thrusting [13, 33], their level of subjective/psychosexual arousal (i.e., being "turned on") may be insufficient to activate sympathetically mediated ejaculation.

A brief attempt to obtain information regarding the three criteria for DE discussed in the Sect. "Defining delayed ejaculation," should also be undertaken to ensure: (1) that the latency to ejaculation is more than average, that is, more than about 15 min or of sufficient duration such that the man abandons hope of ejaculating; (2) that the patient has been unable to shorten this latency; and (3) that the man and/or his partner are distressed by the situation.

Regarding the second purpose of a differential diagnosis, if the man is having difficulty reaching orgasm, good clinical practice first necessitates treatment (to the extent that it is possible) of any medical condition to which the DE is secondary on the assumption that such treatment will likely ameliorate the DE. For example, if LUTS, or depression, or significant relationship conflict are probable etiological factors, such conditions should be discussed and first considered for remediation.

Understanding the History and Scope of the Problem

The clinician should obtain a history of the problem along with other aspects of general psychosexual functioning. For example, the following types of questions might be asked: Has the problem been lifelong? Recent? Developed over a period of time? Related to any other life events? Situation

Table 16-4. Examples of potentially useful instruments for assessing sexual problems and relationship issues

Medical and psychological sexual assessments	
International Index of Erectile Function (IIEF)	A widely used 15-item instrument having subscales related to erectile function, orgasmic function, sexual desire, intercourse satisfaction, and overall satisfaction ([50]; http://urologyspecialists.net/print/iief.html)
Promis® (Patient Reported Outcomes Measurement Information Systems): Physical Health Measures on Sexual Function and Satisfaction	Provides validated assessment items for a range of sexual problems, including but not limited to: global satisfaction (7 items), interfering factors (10 items), orgasm (3 items), and orgasm pleasure (3 items). Promis is registered to the US Department of Health and Human Services/NIH. ([51]: link to: http://www.healthmeasures.net/explore-measurement-systems/promis/intro-to-promis; and https://www.assessmentcenter.net/documents/Sexual%20Function%20Manual.pdf
Sexual Health Inventory for Men (SHIM) or IIEF-5	A shortened version of the IIEF using 5-items for screening and diagnosis of erectile dysfunction (ED) and its severity in clinical practice and research. ([52]; can be found at http://rohbaltimore.com/SHIM.pdf)
Male Sexual Health Questionnaire (MSHQ)	25-item questionnaire measuring erection, ejaculation, and satisfaction with a focus on ejaculatory function. Elevated cultural sensitivity compared to many other tools. (Can be found in [53])
Relational assessments	
Dyadic Adjustment Scale (DAS)	Self-report measure of relationship adjustment, and both partner's perception of satisfaction. [54] http://trieft.org/wp-content/uploads/2010/09/DAS + 1.pdf
Golombok Rust Inventory of Sexual Satisfaction (GRISS)	28-item questionnaire. Assessment of sexual satisfaction and dysfunction; beneficial to identify the extent of improvement over time as the result of medication or therapy. [55] http://www.psychometrics.cam.ac.uk/productsservices/psychometric-tests/GRISS
Self-Esteem and Relationship Questionnaire (SEAR)	The SEAR questionnaire possesses strong psychometric properties that support its validity and reliability for measuring sexual relationship, confidence, and self-esteem. [56] http://www.nature.com/ijir/journal/v16/n1/fig_tab/3901095 t1.html

specific? Or more generalized? Can the man masturbate to orgasm? Has there been a noticeable increase in ejaculatory latency during masturbation? What are the patient's current sexual practices, in terms of coital and masturbation frequency, and under what conditions is the man able to ejaculate with the partner (e.g., with masturbation, with the partner's hand or mouth stimulation, in specific coital positions) and during masturbation (using erotic materials, specific fantasies, etc.). If orgasmic attainment had been possible previously, the clinician should review the life events/circumstances temporally related to orgasmic failure—events in question might include the use of pharmaceuticals, illness, life stressors and/or other psychological factors previously highlighted in the section on etiology.

Medical History

At some point toward the outset of the evaluation process, a genitourinary examination and medical history may help identify physical anomalies associated with ejaculatory dysfunction. In addition, concomitant or contributing neurologic, endocrinologic, pain, or erectile disorders can be explored and identified. Reversible urethral, prostatic, epididymal, and testicular infections need to be addressed. Particularly with secondary (acquired) DE, side effects to specific medications (Table 16-1) should be evaluated, discussed, and possibly ruled out.

Psychosexual Evaluation

A focused sexual history and psychosexual evaluation are important to a full understanding of DE, independent of whether the etiology is primarily pathophysiological or presumed psychogenic [1]. Psychological factors (e.g., anxiety) can exacerbate somatically caused DE, just as somatic factors (e.g., aging) can exacerbate psychobehavioral DE. Although no specific format is essential, domains related to the psychological and relationship issues commonly associated with DE (identified in the previous section) require investigation, with a complete exploration identifying predisposing, precipitating, and maintaining factors for the dysfunction. Although no standardized assessment form for evaluating DE is available, a list of ancillary assessment forms that might be helpful in this evaluation is included in Table 16-4.

Psychosexual issues might fall into three general categories as noted below. Because of the extremely personal and potentially embarrassing nature of some of these issues, these are usually best explored first individually with the patient and then, with the patient's approval and clinician's encouragement, in a follow up session that includes the partner.

- Predisposing issues of religiosity, restrictive attitudes, and other cultural factors that may have played a formative role in the patient's sexual development.
- Partnered and masturbatory sexual activity, including frequency and manner of masturbation and partnered sex, use of erotic supplementary materials during self and partnered sex, use of sexual fantasies during self and partnered sex, and anxiety/pressure surrounding performance. Included is discussion of variables and situations that either improve or worsen the DE, as well as assessment of psychosexual arousal related to various types and situations of sexual activity.
- The nature of the sexual relationship, including types of sexual activities, communication about needs, attractive

value of the partner, feelings of sexual and physical intimacy, satisfaction, and so on. Important to this discussion is the potential for disparity in arousal and satisfaction during masturbation relative to partnered sex.

Since many men having sexual problems attempt their own remedies, the patient's previous approaches to improving ejaculatory response (shortening the latency) should be investigated, including the use of herbal or folk therapies, prior treatments, and home remedies (e.g., using particular cognitive or behavioral strategies).

Summary of Clinical Observations

Once the clinician has gathered and sorted through clinical notes and observations—assuming a frank and open conversation with the patient (and when possible his partner) has taken place—he/she will want to share relevant clinical assessments in a nonjudgmental manner regarding any factors that might be responsible for or contributing to the DE. It may well be that no one specific cause/etiology is readily identified, but an understanding of the biopsychosocial context of the problem can help both the patient and clinician know how best to approach the problem for eventual treatment. For example, if the problem results from a pathophysiological condition, then treatment would first need to focus on ameliorating that condition. On the other hand, if the problem results from a lack of allocated time for sex (e.g., the man believes that with more time, he would eventually ejaculate), diminished partner attraction, or decreased functioning due to aging, an approach that focuses on stimulation enhancement might be undertaken. Or if the problem results from a strong autosexual preference over partnered sex, a reorientation back to an arousing and satisfying partnered experience might be the focus. No matter the possible cause, supportive and reassuring language continues to be important. As an example, in situations where the cause may be related to a strong autosexual orientation—a potentially embarrassing situation for most men—Perelman [8] suggests using supportive language such as "the difficulty is merely a reflection of not rehearsing for the part you're wanting to play" in sex with your partner. Such language can once again assist in minimizing the stigma associated with the problem and in engaging the patient and his partner in the therapeutic process. Important to this summary is communication to the patient (and partner) that with sufficient motivation, coaching, and partner support, many men are successful in overcoming the DE. Once this body of knowledge is complete, an appropriate treatment plan, developed in conjunction with the couple, can be implemented, as detailed in Chap. 17, Treatment of Delayed Ejaculation.

Concluding Remarks and Notes

Several final points regarding the evaluation of any sexual dysfunction, including DE, are worth noting and/or reiterating when working with men who report having difficulty reaching ejaculation.

- *Most people, especially men, have difficulty talking about their sexual problems*, so it is incumbent upon the clinician to create an atmosphere of comfort and openness. The clinician should support the patient's attempts to communicate concerns related to his sexual life.
- *The typical male patient has little or no concept of the sexual response cycle* as understood by clinicians and often noted in textbooks. The therapist should discuss the problems with the patient in familiar language while concomitantly using this conversation to specify the precise nature of the problem—for example, is the problem one of low interest or desire to have sex? Of inadequate arousal? Of the inability to keep an erection because of ejaculating too quickly?
- *Men often focus heavily on their genital response.* The clinician should broaden the conversation to include the man's individual experience of the problem, his partner's perspective, general relationship concerns, and other dimensions beyond just the physical.
- *DE may result from organogenic/somatic and psychogenic factors, or both.* Lifelong vs. acquired DE may have different origins, but the evaluation process needed to explore either of these runs, to a large extent, a similar course.
- *An understanding of the physiological, psychological, relational, and sociocultural contribution to the sexual problem is warranted.* The clinician should explore each of these domains at least briefly to determine whether deeper issues need to be addressed and/or how they contribute to the DE problem.
- *Medical issues should be investigated.* The clinician should carry out a physical exam, or if not qualified to do so, refer the patient to a physician for a check-up, with advance notation to the physician about the sexual problem. A sexual problem is sometimes a manifestation of a broader health issue.
- *Communication between sexual partners is important to sexual, partner, and relationship satisfaction.* The clinician should encourage the inclusion of the partner in conversations in the evaluation process (when the time is appropriate), so the couple is already working as a team as they strategize and select treatment options.
- *Treatment success for DE based on psycho-behavioral patterns tends to be high.* Even within the context of the evaluation process, it is important for the clinician to

point out the potential for remediation of the problem, and reassure the patient and partner that therapy for sexual problems usually need not be extensive. Nevertheless, the clinician must, at the same time, realize that not all men or couples want to undertake the changes necessary for improving their sex life.

References

1. Rowland DL. Sexual dysfunction in men: advances in psychotherapy-evidence based practice. Cambridge, MA: Hogrefe Publishing; 2012 .p. 1–5
2. Masters WH, Johnson VE. Human sexual response. Boston: Little, Brown & Co; 1966. p. 210–22.
3. Masters WH, Johnson VE. Human sexual inadequacy. Boston: Little, Brown & Co; 1970. p. 116–36.
4. Kaplan H. The evaluation of sexual disorders: psychologic and medical aspects. New York: Brunner/Mazel; 1983. p. 139–49.
5. Lauman EO, Paik A, Rosen RC. Sexual dysfunction in the United States: prevalence and predictors. JAMA. 1999;281:537–44.
6. Lewis RW, Fugl-Meyer KS, Corona G, Hayes RD, Laumann EO, Moreira Jr ED, Rellini AH, Segraves T. Definitions/epidemiology/risk factors for sexual dysfunction. J Sex Med. 2010;7:1598–607.
7. Simons J, Carey MP. Prevalence of sexual dysfunctions: results from a decade of research. Arch Sex Res. 2001;30(2):177–219.
8. Perelman M. Retarded ejaculation. Curr Sex Health Rep. 2004;1(3):95–101.
9. Mercer CH, Fenton K, Johnson AM. Sexual problems and health seeking behavior in Britain: probability sample survey. Br Med J. 2003;327:426–7.
10. Rowland DL. Penile sensitivity in men: an overview of recent findings. Urology. 1998;52:1101–5.
11. Perelman M., Rowland, DL. Retarded or inhibited ejaculation (male orgasmic disorder). In: Rowland DL, Incrocci L, editors. Handbook of sexual and gender identity disorders. New York: Wiley Press; 2008. p. 100–21.
12. Perelman, M. Combination therapy: integration of sex therapy and pharmacotherapy. In: Balon R, Seagraves R, editors. Handbook of sexual dysfunction. New York: Marcel Dekker Inc.; 2005. p. 13–41.
13. Rowland DL, van Diest S, Incrocci L, Slob AK. Psychosexual factors that differentiate men with inhibited ejaculation from men with no dysfunction or another sexual dysfunction. J Sex Med. 2005;2:383–9.
14. Perelman M. Idiosyncratic masturbation patterns: a key unexplored variable in the treatment of retarded ejaculation by the practicing urologist. J Urol. 2005;173(4):Abstract 1254.
15. Perelman M, McMahon C, Barada J. Evaluation and treatment of ejaculatory disorders. In: Lue TF, editor. Atlas of male sexual dysfunction. Philadelphia, PA: Current Medicine LLC; 2004. p. 127–57.
16. Perelman M. Delayed ejaculation. In: Binik YM, Hall KS, editors. Principles and practice of sex therapy, 5th ed. New York: The Guilford Press; 2014. p. 138–55.
17. Bancroft J, Janssen E. The dual control model of sexual response: a theoretical approach to centrally-mediated erectile dysfunction. Neurosci Biobehav Rev. 2000;24:571–9.
18. Barlow DH. Causes of sexual dysfunction: the role of anxiety and cognitive interference. J Consult Clin Psychol. 1986;54(2):140–8.
19. Giuliano F, Clément P. Physiology of ejaculation: emphasis on serotonergic control. Eur Urol. 2005;48(3):408–17.
20. Motofei IG, Rowland DL. The neurophysiology of ejaculation: developing perspectives. Br J Urol Int. 2005;96:1333–8.
21. Vale J. Ejaculatory dysfunction. Br J Urol Int. 1999;83:557–63.
22. Witt MA, Grantmyre JE. Ejaculatory failure. World J Urol. 1993;11:89–95.
23. Master VA, Turek PJ. Ejaculatory physiology and dysfunctions. Urol Clin North Am. 2001;28:363–75.
24. Conaglen HM, Conaglen JV. Drug induced sexual dysfunction in men and women. Aust Prescr. 2013;36(2):42. –45, 2013.
25. Blanker MH, Bosch JL, Broeneveld FP, Bohnen AM, Prins A, Thomas S, et al. Erectile and ejaculatory dysfunction in a community-based sample of men 50 to 78 years old: prevalence, concern, and relation to sexual activity. Urology. 2001;57:763–8.
26. Rosen R, Altwein J, Boyle P, Kirby RS, Lukacs B, Meuleman E, et al. Lower urinary tract symptoms and male sexual dysfunction: the Multinational Survey of the Aging Male (MSAM-7). Eur Urol. 2003;44:637–49.
27. Paick JS, Jeong H, Park MS. Penile sensitivity in men with early ejaculation. Int J Impot Res. 1998;10:247–50.
28. Nemec ED, Mansfield L, Kennedy JW. Heart rate and blood pressure responses during sexual activity in normal males. Am Heart J. 1976;92(3):274–7.
29. Rowland DL, van Lankveld J, Tempel A, Kostelyk K. Anxiety in sex, sport, and stage: identifying common ground. J Sex Res. Under review.
30. Zilbergeld B. The new male sexuality. New York: Bantam Books; 1993. p. 1–14.
31. Althof SE, Lieblum SR, Chevert-Measson M, Hartmann U, Levine SB, McCabe M et al. Psychological and interpersonal dimensions of sexual function and dysfunction. In: Lue TF, Basson R, Rosen R, et al., editors. Sexual medicine: sexual dysfunctions in men and women. 2nd International Consultation on Sexual Dysfunctions: Paris, France; 2004. p. 73–116. www.icud.info/sexualdysfunctions.html
32. Apfelbaum B. Retarded ejaculation, a much-misunderstood syndrome. In: Lieblum SR, Rosen RC, editors. Principles and practice of sex therapy, 2nd ed. New York: Guilford Press; 2000. p. 205–41.
33. Rowland DL, Keeney C, Slob AK. Sexual response in men with inhibited or retarded ejaculation. Int J Impotence Res. 2004;16:270–4.
34. Perelman M. Sildenafil, sex therapy, and retarded ejaculation. J Sex Educ Ther. 2001;26:13–21.
35. Perelman M. Regarding ejaculation: delayed and otherwise [letter]. J Androl. 2003;24:496.
36. Perelman M. Integrating sildenafil and sex therapy: unconsummated marriage secondary to ED and RE. J Sex Educ Ther. 2001;26(1):13–21.
37. American Psychiatric Association. Diagnostic and statistical manual of mental disorders, 5th ed. (DSM-5). Washington DC: American Psychiatric Association; 2013, p. 424–426.
38. World Health Organization. ICD-10: International statistical classification of diseases and related health problems. 10th rev. ed. New York, NY. 2002., http://www.who.int/classifications/icd/en/. Accessed May 23, 2016.
39. McMahon C, Abdo C, Incrocci L, Perelman M, Rowland D, Waldinger M, et al. Disorders of orgasm and ejaculation in men. J Sex Med. 2004;1:58–65.
40. Patrick DL, Althof SE, Pryor JL, Rosen R, Rowland DL, Ho KF, et al. Premature ejaculation: an observational study of men and their partners. J Sex Med. 2005;2:358–67.
41. Waldinger MD, Quinn P, Dilleen M, Mundayat R, Schweitzer DH, Boolell M. A multinational population survey of intravaginal ejaculation latency time. J Sex Med. 2005;2:492–7.
42. Hartmann U, Waldinger M. Treatment of delayed ejaculation. In: Leiblum SR, editor. Principles and practice of sex therapy. New York: Guilford Press; 2007. p. 252–63.

43. Sanchez-Cruz JJ, Cabrera-Leon A, Martin-Morales A, Fernandez A, Burgos R, Rejas J. Male erectile dysfunction and health-related quality of life. Eur Urol. 2003;44:245–53.
44. Rowland DL, Patrick DL, Rothman M, Gagnon DD. The psychological burden of premature ejaculation. J Urol. 2007;177:1065–70.
45. Rowland DL. Psychological impact of premature ejaculation and barriers to its recognition and treatment. Curr Med Res Opin. 2011;27:1509–18.
46. Robbins-Cherry SA, Hayter M, Wylie KR, Goldmeier D. The experiences of men living with inhibited ejaculation. Sex Rel Ther. 2011;26:242–53.
47. Gaulin SJC, McBurney DH. Evolutionary psychology. 2nd ed. Upper Saddle River, NJ: Pearson Prentice Hall; 2004. p. 1–24.
48. Rowland DL, Motofei I. The aetiology of premature ejaculation and the mind-body problem: implications for practice. Int J Clin Pract. 2007;61(1):77–82.
49. Rowland DL, deGouvea Brazao C, Strassberg D, Slob AK. Ejaculatory latency and control in men with premature ejaculation: a detailed analysis across sexual activities using multiple sources of information. J Psychosom Res. 2000;48:69–77.
50. Rosen RC, Riley A, Wagner G, Osterloh IH, Kirkpatrick J, Mistra A. The international index of erectile function (IIEF): a multidimensional scale for assessment of erectile dysfunction. Urology. 1997;49(6):822–30.
51. Weinfurt KP, Lin L, Bruner DW, Cyranowski JM, Dombeck CB, Hahn EA, Jeffery DD, Luecht RM, Magasi S, Porter LS, Reese JB, Reeve BB, Shelby RA, Smith AW, Willse JT, Flynn KE. Development and initial validation of the PROMIS® sexual function and satisfaction measures version 2.0. J Sex Med. 2015;12:1961–74.
52. Rosen RC, Cappelleri JC, Smith MD, Lipsky J, Pena BM. Development and evaluation of an abridged, 5-item version of the International Index of Erectile Function (IIEF-5) as a diagnostic tool for erectile dysfunction. Int J Impot Res. 1999;11:319–26.
53. Rosen RC, Catania J, Pollack L, Althof S, O'Leary M, Seftel A. Male sexual health questionnaire (MSHQ): scale development and psychometric validation. J Urol. 2004;64(4):777–82.
54. Spanier GB. Dyadic adjustment scale manual. Multi-Health Systems: North Tonawanda, NY; 1989.
55. Rust J, Golombok S. The Golombok-Rust inventory of sexual satisfaction (GRISS). Br J Clin Psychol. 1985;24:63–4.
56. Cappelleri JC, Althof SE, Siegel RL, Shpilsky A, Bell SS, Duttagupta S. Development and validation of the self-esteem and relationship (SEAR) questionnaire in erectile dysfunction. Int J Impot Res. 2004;16:30–8.

17 Treatment of Delayed Ejaculation

Michael J. Butcher and Ege Can Serefoglu

Introduction

As Masters and Johnson [1] originally proposed, the stages of normal male sexual cycle are: desire, arousal, orgasm, and resolution. Each of these stages is associated with distinct physiological changes in the male. Ejaculation, which normally occurs during the orgasm phase, involves highly complex neurological and hormonal mechanisms (Figure 17-1). Ejaculation disorders, which are the most common type of male sexual dysfunction [2, 3], can be detrimental to men on their relationships and quality of life [4]. In a survey of 12,815 US and European men aged 50 years or older, the authors found that ejaculatory disorders affect 30.1% of men between 50 and 59 years of age. A majority (50.2%) of these affected men reported bother, or lower sexual satisfaction scores due to their ejaculatory problems [4]. Although there is an increased interest on erectile dysfunction since the development of oral treatment alternatives, ejaculatory problems are almost as common and should be equally treated by the clinicians, who should be trained on how to manage patients with these ejaculatory disorders.

Introduction of dapoxetine, which is the first oral compound developed specially for the treatment of premature ejaculation in 2006 [5], unveiled the unknowns regarding this common problem; however, our understanding regarding the disorder of delayed ejaculation (DE) remained limited, probably due to the rareness of this condition.

DE is a disorder which negatively affects men for which many practitioners do not understand [6, 7]. In part, this misunderstanding is due to the complex pathologies and various treatment options which are also not well known. Randomized, placebo-controlled, blinded studies on this topic are rare, leaving only case studies, small cohorts, consensus, and expert opinions for treatment recommendations. This section reviews the etiologies, diagnosis, and treatments for conditions that lead to or are affiliated with DE.

Terminology

In order to better understand the phenomenon of DE, it is imperative that lexicon used to describe the disorder is clearly understood. Delayed ejaculation, inhibited ejaculation, and the debasing term retarded ejaculation are all synonymous terms referring to persistent or recurrent delay or difficulty in achieving an ejaculation despite appropriate stimulation which in turn causes a degree of distress to the patient [8, 9] In addition to these terms, ejaculatory overcontrol, impaired ejaculation, impaired orgasm, deficient ejaculation, ejaculatory incompetence, and inhibited male orgasm have all been used and mean essentially the same clinical entity. DE is the current preferred term in the literature and will be used as the term in this chapter.

The American Psychiatric Association describes DE as requiring one of two symptoms which is: marked delay, infrequency, or absence of ejaculation on 75–100% of occasions that persists for at least 6 months [10]. DE is a medical and/or psychological condition that is not associated with other types of psychiatric diagnosis (paraphilias, psychotic disorders, etc.). The Sexual Medicine Society of North America defines DE as difficulty achieving an ejaculation despite sufficient stimulation, good erection, and arousal [11]. The International Society for Sexual Medicine, describes DE as ejaculations that take longer than a man would like despite him having a full erection and good arousal and stimulation [12]. The European Urology Association define DE as an abnormal stimulation of the erect penis that is needed to have an orgasm and ejaculation [13]. This definition is paramount to understanding the psychologic implications and treatment strategies that are reviewed later in this chapter.

The accepted standard time it takes to have an ejaculation is not directly defined for DE. The median intravaginal ejaculation latency time (IELT) is 5.4 min in normal subjects from around the world with a range of 4–10 min following intromission [14]. Men who report distress or cease sexual activity due to fatigue or irritation after two standard deviations

W.W. IsHak (ed.), *The Textbook of Clinical Sexual Medicine*, DOI 10.1007/978-3-319-52539-6_17

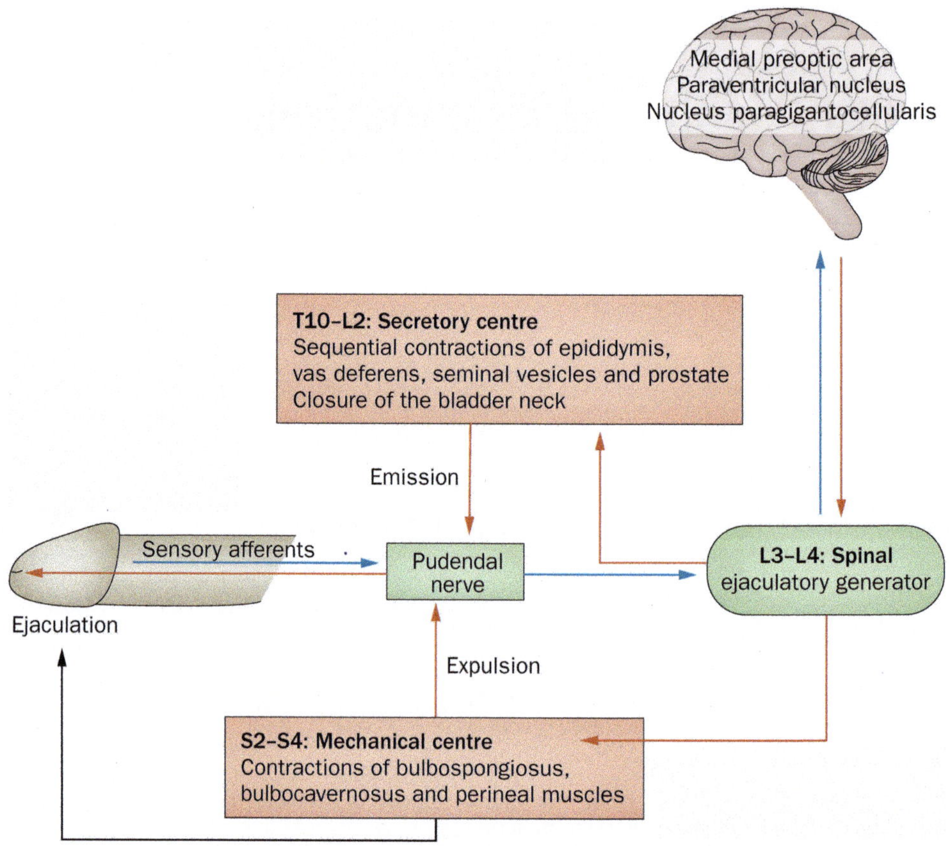

FIGURE 17-1. Physiology of ejaculation. The ejaculation reflex and ejaculatory control. Ejaculation is the result of the coordinated contractile activity involving different ejaculatory organs organized by the spinal ejaculatory generator, located at the T12–L1–L2 level of the spinal cord. Afferent information is received by the spinal ejaculatory generator, which coordinates sympathetic, parasympathetic, and motor outflow for the two phases of ejaculation-emission and expulsion. The SEG integrates these inhibitory and excitatory influences from supraspinal sites, as well as inputs conveying biochemical or mechanical information from the accessory sex organs. Emission of semen involves the sympathetic efferent fibres of the "secretory center" (T10-L2) coordinating sequential contractions of the epididymis, vas deferens, seminal vesicles, and prostate with associated closure of the bladder neck. Expulsion of semen is then initiated somatically by the "mechanical center" of the sacral spinal cord (S2-S4) via the pudendal nerve, which induces contractions of the bulbospongiosus, bulbocavernous, and perineal muscles, which, in turn, rhythmically force the ejaculate through the distal urethra. Abbreviation: *SSRI* selective 5-hydroxytrypomine reuptake inhibitor. Reprinted from Saitz TR, Serefoglu EG. Advances in understanding and treating premature ejaculation. Nat Rev Urol. 2015;12: 629–40. With permission from Nature Publishing Group.

of the mean IELT (21–23 min) and would be considered pathologic [15].

Other ways to define DE is based on the time that the disorder first presented, in a chronologic sense, which too can have multiple terms used to describe the same entity. Primary DE has also been known as congenital DE, lifelong DE, or global DE which occurs from the first sexual experience and throughout a person's life [9]. Secondary DE or acquired DE is intermittent or situational. Secondary DE refers to different responses to sexual stimulation which may or may not result in an ejaculation [16]. This often is seen as an ability to have an ejaculation with masturbation but not with partnered coitus. This form of DE has a high preponderance of psychologic influence as will be discussed later in further detail.

Epidemiology

The true incidence and prevalence of DE is likely underreported due to its varied etiologies and incomplete sexual histories. DE occurred in 2–11% in the general heterosexual population [2, 17–21], and upward of 20–39% in homosexual and HIV-infected males [20, 22–24]. A study of 100 couples in the late 1970s found that upwards of 17% of men presenting to a sexual therapist had inhibited ejaculation [25]. A more recent study found an incidence of 2.5% of the general male population in London, England was unable to have an ejaculation ≥75% of the time according to ICD-10 codes (F 52.3) by general practitioners [26]. The National Health and Social Life Survey (NHSLS) in the USA that included 1246 men aged 18–59 found an incidence of 7.78%

who reported they had been unable to have a climax or ejaculation for a 2-month period over 1 year [2]. In an international study of men and women aged 40–80 years old from 29 countries with over 13,000 male participants who reported up to 2.8% rates of DE or inability to reach orgasm [3]. Although study methods varied, the incidence of DE is high enough in the general population to be found on a regular basis.

Men are living longer, on more medications that affect ejaculation, and have more comorbidities. An American study of 1455 men aged 57–80 who reported a 20% rate of inability to have a climax which bothered 73% of respondents as they got older [27]. Some experts feel that the prevalence of DE is even higher in older men [16, 28]. Comorbidities also contribute to DE incidence. A cross-sectional study of 331 heterosexual Australian men aged 18–65 found those with medical conditions (hypertension, diabetes, obesity, hyperlipidemia, tobacco use, mood disorders, alcohol abuse, etc.) had one or more sexual disorders (low libido, premature ejaculation, DE, erectile dysfunction) [29]. These medical conditions were highly associated with DE and low libido. Low libido has been associated with a 50% incidence of DE [30].

Clinical Impact

The impact of DE on men can be quite detrimental and can easily increase psychologic stress for a man and couple [2]. Sexual dissatisfaction, anxiety, depression, performance anxiety, relationship distress, shame, low self-image, intimacy avoidance, and relationship dissatisfaction have all been implicated in contributing to DE [6, 16, 31–34]. DE impacts both the patient and the partner. This condition, therefore, necessitates cooperation of both parties in the treatment for mutually satisfying sexual experiences. Perhaps this is partly why the sexual bother of DE can range from 50–73% [4, 27].

Etiology

The complexity of DE and the medical condition causing the pathologic etiologies are varied. Genetically predetermined ejaculatory thresholds in combination with psychosocial, biologic, behavioral, and cultural influences contribute to DE [16, 35–37]. Age, congenital, anatomic, neurogenic, infection/inflammation, endocrine, pharmacologic, and psychological issues all play causative roles in DE development (see Table 17-1 [9]).

Table 17-1. Etiological causes of delayed ejaculation, anejaculation, and anorgasmia

Ageing male psychogenic	Degeneration of penile afferent nerves inhibited ejaculation
Congenital	Mullerian duct cyst Wolfian duct abnormalities Prune Belly Syndrome Imperforate Anus Genetic abnormalities
Anatomic causes	Transurethral resection of prostate Bladder neck incision Circumcision
Neurogenic causes	Diabetic autonomic neuropathy Multiple sclerosis Spinal cord injury Radical prostatectomy Proctocolectomy Bilateral sympathectomy Abdominal aortic aneurysmectomy Para-aortic lymphadenectomy
Infective/inflammation	Urethritis Genitourinary tuberculosis Schistomsmiasis Prostatitis Orchitits
Endocrine	Hypogonadim Hypothryoidism Prolactin disorders
Medication	See additional table
Psychological	Acute psychological distress Relationship distress Psychosexual skill deficit Disconnect between arousal and sexual situations Masturbation style

Adapted from Butcher MJ, Brannigan RE. Ejaculatory disorders. In: Köhler TS, McVary KT (editors). Contemporary treatment of erectile dysfunction: a clinical guide. Switzerland: Springer; 2016: 335–359. With permission from Springer International Publishing.

Age

As men age, there are changes to their bodies and sexual response. Changes in the nervous systems are thought to be responsible for neurogenic pathologies resulting in decreased signal transduction with age (signal transduction delays, dermal atrophy, nerve changes) [38–42]. Older patients also tend to have more comorbid diseases that contribute to DE. Depression, peripheral vascular disease, diabetes, late onset hypogonadism, increased body mass index, and psychiatric pathology seem to contribute to DE in older patients [43, 44]. Lifestyle factors such as smoking, obesity, alcohol use, inactivity, and loneliness (such as loss of a spouse which is more common with age) can be potent inhibitors of ejaculation and overall sexual function and satisfaction [45, 46]. As a result, IELT typically increases in older men [14].

Congenital

Genetic disorders and birth defects can result in ejaculatory disorders but it is unclear how this directly relates to DE. Ejaculatory failure has been seen in those born with imperforate anus who have undergone repair [47, 48]. This is often attributed to nerve damage from surgery [38].

There are hypotheses regarding the existence of a genetically predetermined threshold that regulates ejaculation [36]. Some have demonstrated that hyposensitivity and hypoexcitability of the penile shaft skin may result in primary DE [49]. Nerve density and migration of dermal nerve units would all play a part of this genetic/congenital disorder; however, no studies have been done to evaluate this notion to date.

Anatomic/Trauma

Genital tract and pelvic surgical procedures are done on many men to deal with certain disease states that can affect the ejaculatory process. Treatment with transurethral resection of the prostate, transurethral incision of the bladder neck and prostate can cause ejaculatory disorders [50]. A post-ejaculatory urine is needed to distinguish between the retrograde ejaculation and anejaculation. Prostate surgery for cancer removes the seminal vesicles and no ejaculation will occur. Other deep pelvic surgeries like rectal and perineal resections can affect sexual functions through disruption of pelvic ganglia [51, 52]. Retroperitoneal lymph node dissection results in problems in emission from disruption of the sympathetic chain [53, 54]. Likewise, low spine surgery can have similar effect on the pelvic plexus resulting in sympathetic and parasympathetic disorders which in turn effect ejaculation [52]. Abnormal midline prostatic cysts and Zinner syndrome (congenital ipsilateral renal agenesis, ejaculatory duct obstruction, and seminal vesical cysts), can both result in painful ejaculation which may contribute to DE [55, 56].

Circumcision has also been postulated to be a cause of DE. An interesting study recently reported that there could be a connection between circumcision and sexual dysfunction including that of DE [57]. This retrospective study was conducted using a telephone survey of men asking about their sexual function before and after a circumcision. The study reported a delay in orgasm at baseline 11.3%, and after circumcision this increased to 48.4% [57]. A large-scale Danish study looked at the sexual experiences of men and women who had sex with men that were circumcised or not [58]. This study found that there was a 3.12 odds ratio of having delayed orgasm in circumcised men vs. uncircumcised men. It has also been found that the IELT increases by about 2.76 ms based on pudendal evoked potentials between uncircumcised and circumcised males which may lead to DE [59]. Whether this increased pudendal evoked potential causes a clinical difference is not yet known despite the statistical findings. A study looking at sensitivity loss of the penis after circumcision showed no clinical or statistical difference [60], thus the association between the circumcision and sexual functions requires future studies to be elucidated.

Neurogenic

Examination of the neurogenic causes of DE can be divided into medical disease states and trauma. Multiple sclerosis and diabetes are strongly associated with DE [61–64]. A survey of male multiple sclerosis patients demonstrated up to 45% incidence DE [65]. DE and problems with emission and ejaculation can occur in up to 33% of diabetic men [66]. Ninety-five percent of men with complete upper motor neuron lesions are not able to ejaculate [67]. The ability to ejaculate increases progressively with descending spinal injuries [68]. Ejaculatory dysfunction can occur with damage to sympathetic ganglia from para-aortic lymphadenectomy but antegrade ejaculation is preserved in 97% of patients [69].

Men who have primary DE may also have a degree of hyposensitivity to the glans penis and overall decreased excitability perhaps secondary to decreased nerve density and/or deposition in sexual organs. Men with primary DE have much greater success ejaculating with masturbation than with partnered sex [49]. Masturbation was found to have less DE and less premature ejaculation in another study of 21 men with mixed pathology, but does demonstrate that different sexual encounters/experiences can lead to improvement in these types of ejaculatory disorders [70].

Infective/Inflammation

When patients have pain with ejaculation this can lead to DE as a result of psychologic interplay. Orchitis, epididymitis, and severe prostatitis can all lead to DE because of infectious painful ejaculation [71].

Endocrine

The hormonal milieu required for normal ejaculation can be complex, yet can play a definitive role in the normal ejaculatory process. In a group of over 2400 men, a 26% rate of DE was comorbid with hypogonadism [72]. It is important to understand that androgen receptors are present throughout the whole body including the areas of the brain associated with orgasm and arousal [73, 74]. Testosterone levels are related to ejaculatory disturbances where higher levels can be found in those with premature ejaculation and lower levels in DE [75]. This hormonal mismatch was thought to be associated with DE resulting in decrease quality of life, but did not improve in a randomized controlled trial of testosterone replacement [44].

Thyroid hormones are also believed to help control the contractions of the seminal vesicles and ejaculatory musculature. Hyperthyroidism is associated with premature ejaculation and hypothyroidism is associated with DE [76]. Thyroid hormones can change the production of sexual hormone binding globulin which is strongly bound to testosterone and decrease the percentage of bioavailable testosterone. Whether there is a direct effect from thyroid hormone on ejaculatory process or this is a precursor to secondary effects of testosterone is unknown and certainly could be a combination of both pathologies.

Prolactin may be a surrogate marker of serotonergic activity, hence elevated prolactin levels limits ejaculatory function [77, 78]. Prolactin and dopamine are inversely related [75]. As dopamine rises (as what happens with climax and orgasm) prolactin is suppressed. After orgasm, prolactin spikes while dopamine is suppressed. Prolactin is thought to be partly responsible for the refractory period in men after orgasm [78, 79]. Routine hormonal testing investigating perturbations of testosterone, prolactin, and thyroid levels should be performed in patients with ejaculatory dysfunction and corresponding disease symptomatology (see Figure 17-2 for suggested treatment algorithm [80]).

Pharmacology

Certain medications may also cause DE. For example, the most well known and most common side effect of the SSRIs is DE, with a sevenfold increased risk. It is currently thought that the sexual side effects of SSRIs are from their inhibitory effect on dopamine primarily, along with the increase in overall 5-HT levels and how these affect the brain's sex circuitry [81]. As a result, SSRIs are recommended for the treatment for premature ejaculation [82]. IELT is delayed with these drugs due to the serotonergic tone and receptor activation on the central nervous system [14]. There are many other medications that can result in DE which are not SSRIs (Table 17-2) [9, 83].

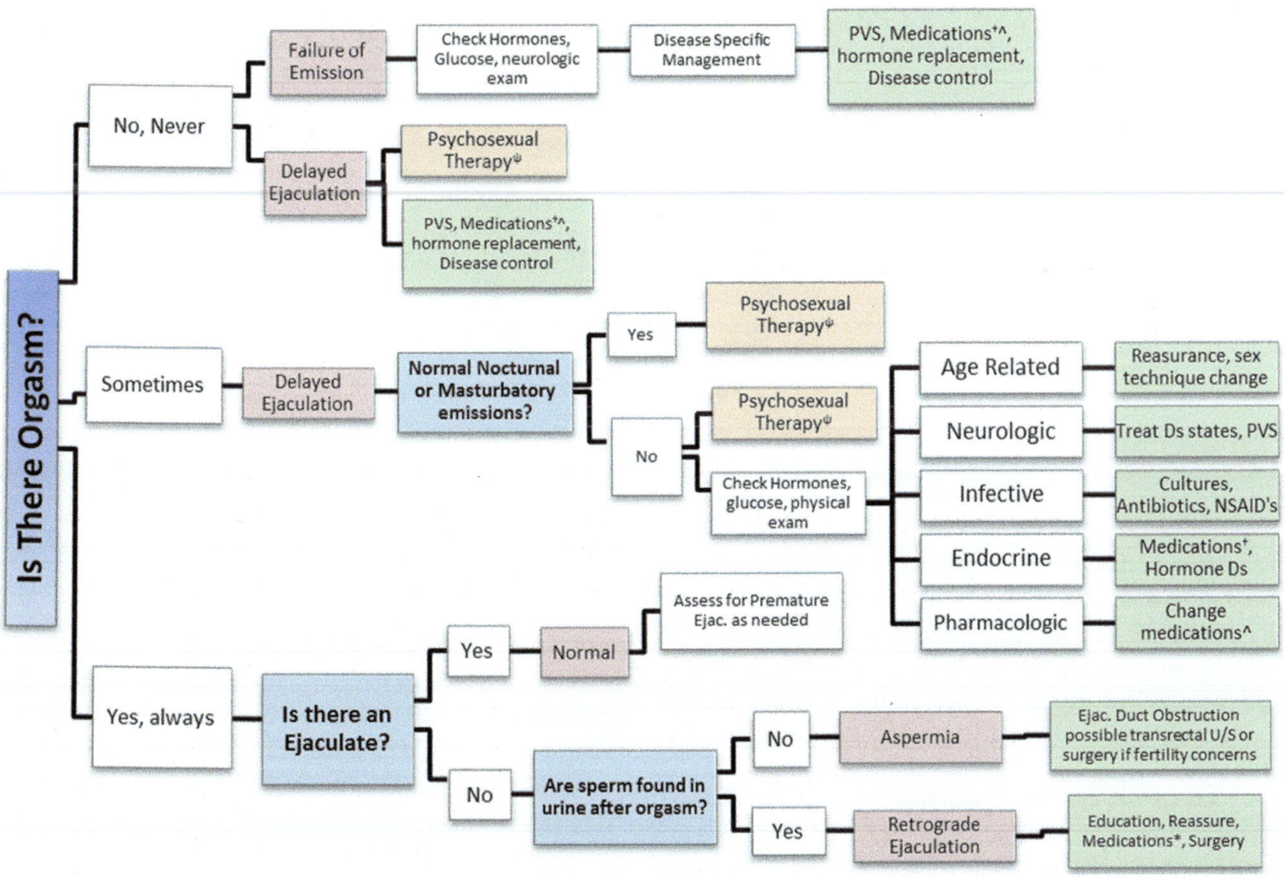

FIGURE 17-2. Algorithm of Disordered Ejaculation in Men. Ψ = See Collaboration of Clinician and Sexual Therapist (Figure 17-3). * = Medications in Table 17-3 can be tried in treatment of Retrograde Ejaculation (see Table 17-3). ^ = If patient on SSRI consider use of SSRI Antidote types of medications (see Table 17-3). † = Medications in Table 17-3 can be used for Prolactin abnormalities (see Table 17-3). Reprinted from Sadowski DJ, Butcher MJ, Köhler TS. Delayed ejaculation: medical and psychological treatments and algorithm. Curr Sex Health Rep. 2015; 7(3): 170–9. With permission from Springer Science + Business Media.

TABLE 17-2. Medications known to effect male ejaculation

Alcohol	Clomipramine	Lorazepam	Phentolamine
Alprazolam	Desmethylimipramine	Mirtazapine	Phenylzine sulphate
Aminocaproic acid	Fluoxetine[a]	Mesoridazine	Prazosin
Amitriptyline	Fluvoxamine	Methadone	Protriptyline
Amoxapine	Guanadrel	Methyldopa	Reserpine
Baclofen	Guanethidine	Naproxen	Sertraline[a]
Bethanidine	Haloperidol	Nortriptyline	Thiazide diuretics
Butaperazine	Hexamthonium	Pargyline	Thioridazine
Chlordiazepoxide	Imiprimine	Paroxetine[a]	Trazadone
Chlorimipramine	Iproniazid	Perphenazine	Trifluoperazine
Chlorpromazine	Isocarboxazid	Phenothiazine	
Chlorprothixine	Labethanol	Phenoxybenzamine	

[a]All selective serotonin reuptake Inhibitors (SSRI's).

Adapted from Butcher MJ, Brannigan RE. Ejaculatory disorders. In: Köhler TS, McVary KT (eds.). Contemporary treatment of erectile dysfunction: a clinical guide. Switzerland: Springer; 2016: 335–59. With permission from Springer International Publishing.

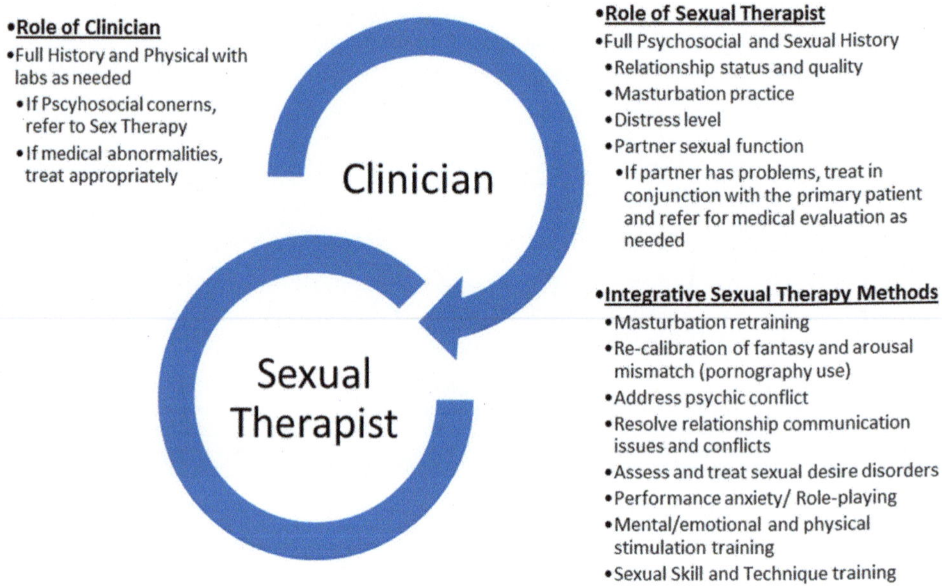

FIGURE 17-3. Collaboration of clinician and sexual therapist. Reprinted from Sadowski DJ, Butcher MJ, Köhler TS. Delayed ejaculation: medical and psychological treatments and algorithm. Curr Sex Health Rep. 2015;7(3): 170–9. With permission from Springer Science + Business Media.

Psychological

The effects of dissatisfaction, performance anxiety, and relationship distress can be causes of DE [6, 7, 35]. It is not uncommon for men to fake orgasm to help their partner feel accepted and secure when in fact, the man is actually dealing with DE. Distress increases when dealing with DE in cases of infertility and can have deleterious consequences in relationships [35].

Proposed psychological underpinnings of DE include: suppressed anger, fear of pregnancy, fear of "defiling" a partner through ejaculation, or unwillingness/inability to accept pleasure [16, 35]. Four different psychological theories leading to DE which are also based on empirical support include: (1) subtle desire disorder concealed as ejaculatory dysfunction (autosexual orientation, partner's touch is inhibiting, compulsion to satisfy partner, etc.), (2) psychic conflict (fear, anxiety, guilt from religious upbringing, loss of self with ejaculation, etc.), (3) insufficient stimulation (mental and physical), and (4) masturbation (too frequent, idiosyncratic style, and incongruence between fantasy and reality) [84] (see Figure 17-3 for sexual therapies [80]).

Subtle desire disorder is a collection of disorders that mimic other diagnosis making the treatment more difficult. An example of this would be a man with DE who enjoys self-sex more than partnered sex known as autosexual orientation. These individuals are inhibited by partners' touch and/or may feel the need to please their partners due to the diminutive effect of partnered sex compared to autoarousal and ejaculation [84]. It has also been proposed that a hyper-control psycho-configuration is the reason for DE and not alexithymia which is commonly comorbid with other male sexual dysfunctions [85] Alexithymia is a multifactorial personality construct that leads to inability to regulate emotions.

Psychic conflict is a cluster of issues that causes psychological opposition to ejaculation mostly from fear. Fear of becoming a father, fear that the female genitals may harm them, shame from religious beliefs, or fear of hurting or anger towards their partner can all manifest in DE and sexual dysfunction [84]. Anxiety disorders and loss of sexual confidence can occur in these individuals.

Physical and mental/emotional stimulation are important components of the normal male sexual cycle. DE can result if appropriate/sufficient stimulation is not achieved in both of these areas. In one study of malleable penile prosthesis there was a 10% incidence of DE [86]. Despite the overly simplistic misconception that male sexual arousal is defined solely by erectile quality, a pathologic disconnect between quality of mechanically induced erections (from VED, penile injections or penile implants) and cognitive arousal often exists.

Masturbation is a good example of the psychologic and physical states combining to result in a sexual experience. This non-partnered practice can be a root cause of DE at times. In a recent US epidemiology study by the Global Online Sexuality Survey, 76.1% of men admitted to masturbation [87]. Other studies indicate 92% of all men masturbate [20, 88]. Although the common practice of masturbation has not been linked to any significant problems for the general population; the frequency, intensity, style, and fantasy associated with the practice has been attributed to ejaculatory problems. Idiosyncratic masturbation style refers to a technique that involves pressure, speed, duration, and intensity needed to achieve an ejaculation and orgasm which is not reproducible with a partner using hands, mouth, or vagina [84, 89]. Men who practice this type of masturbation have more sexual dysfunction [88, 90]. The popular media has proposed masturbation with pornography use/addiction subsequently leads to sexual dissatisfaction and DE [91]. More recent studies have demonstrated that pornography-related masturbation in coupled men is associated with decreased sexual desire [92]. This could potentially lead to DE based on lack of mental/emotional stimulation.

Assessment

Patients should have a full medical and sexual history performed along with a detailed physical exam when evaluating for DE. It is not uncommon for clinicians to feel uncomfortable with the level of sexual information that is warranted in obtaining a full sexual history. Understanding the details of the ejaculatory response, sensation, frequency, and sexual activity/techniques; cultural context and history of the disorder; the quality of the sexual response cycle (desire, arousal, ejaculation, orgasm, and refractory period); the partners' assessment of the disorder and if the partner suffers from any sexual dysfunction her/himself; and the overall satisfaction of the sexual relationship are all important to garner during history taking [93]. Investigation by a sexual therapist is often required to help get a complete psychological evaluation. It is incumbent for the clinician to diagnose medical pathologies that cause or contribute to DE, such as assessing the hormonal milieu, anatomy, and overall medical conditions. Good communication between sexual therapist and medical practitioner is vital to successful diagnosis and treatment of DE. Figure 17-2 shows an algorithm used to help guide in assessment and treatment of ejaculatory disorders, while Figure 17-3 shows the integration of mental health and medical providers [80].

Treatment

Based on the definition and etiology of DE; workup and treatment are geared towards the underlying issues. An example of this focused evaluation and treatment would be looking into a patient's medications and evaluating the quality of his sexual relationship with his partner along with evaluation of the partner's health especially if the patient presented with secondary DE. The partner's health is an important factor as DE may be caused by fear of hurting her/him or a decrease in sexual attractiveness if she has had a mastectomy, hysterectomy, or other types of disfigurements. Patients with anatomical abnormalities (unilateral or bilateral absences of vas for example) may need additional imaging studies looking for corresponding renal abnormalities or transrectal ultrasounds to evaluate for ejaculatory structure defects. Signs of infection (prostatitis, hematospermia) and lower urinary tract symptoms should be evaluated with treatment of underlying medical conditions. Similarly, neurologic conditions such as spinal cord injury or multiple sclerosis should be addressed [15]. If a man is only able to ejaculate with masturbation, it would be important to assess for an idiosyncratic masturbatory style [35].

A recent study by Teloken and Mulhall shows the importance and relative success with goal directed medical therapy targeted towards etiologies of DE [94]. Rates of men with secondary DE from SSRIs were 34%, of which 82% recovered normal ejaculations after cessation of the drug and 34% improved with medication adjustments. The study also found that 35% had abnormal penile sensation and after the use of penile vibratory stimulations treatments, 60% of men improved. Fifteen percent were hypogonadal and 24% of them improved with hormonal treatment. Psychogenic causes were found in 16% of men with DE [94]. Of note, when a psychogenic cause is found, sexual therapy traditionally has had a much higher success rate than treatment of non-psychogenic causes [16, 35].

Treatments for DE can be broken down into pharmacotherapy, penile vibratory stimulation, psychological (sexual therapy, masturbation retraining, etc.), and the "sexual tipping point" model that incorporates the balancing of the biologic, psychological, social, and behavioral aspects that contribute to the disorder.

The treatment of DE should be considered in those who are suffering negative consequences of the condition. Treatment is directed towards the suspected etiology. The following section will detail treatment options based on suspected etiology that have been tried. However, few of the studies are randomized, controlled, blinded or placebo controlled. Nonetheless, certain medications have been used and their uses published in peer-reviewed journals as potential options as detailed below.

Pharmacotherapy

Pharmacologic agents have been used to treat DE with varied success. Unfortunately, there is no Food and Drug Administration (FDA) approved medications to treat DE, as the majority of cited research is based on case-cohort studies that have not been randomized, blinded, or placebo controlled. Many drugs have been used as both primary treatments and/or as antidotes to other medications that can cause DE. A recent survey of sexual health providers demonstrated an overall treatment success of 40% percent with most providers commonly using cabergoline, bupropion, and oxytocin for treatments [95]. However, this survey measured anecdotal results of practitioners and there was no proven efficacy or superiority of any drug due to a lack of placebo-controlled, randomized, blinded, comparative trials. Table 17-3 [80] will show medications that have been suggested for therapeutic intervention for DE along with suggested DE dosing, the overall indication of the agent and the side effects of these medications [8, 15, 38, 66, 93, 96–99].

Cyproheptadine

Cyproheptadine 4–12 mg take 3–4 h prior to sex.

This is a 5-HT antagonist and antihistaminic used to treat allergic rhinitis and anorexia nervosa [100]. In male rats, it has demonstrated shorter refractory periods and increased sexual activity [101]. Cyproheptadine was successfully used as an antidote at doses of 2–16 mg as needed or chronically

Table 17-3. Drug therapy for delayed ejaculation

Drug Generic/(Trade)	Delayed ejaculation dosage (Not FDA approved) As needed	Daily	Indication (FDA approved)	Side effects (At therapeutic FDA indication dose)
Cyproheptadine^ (Periactin)	4–12 mg po (3–4 h prior to sex)	–	• Allergic rhinitis • Urticarial • Anorexia nervosa	**Nausea, dizziness, urinary retention, photosensitivity, rash, abdominal pain, fatigue,** agranulocytosis, thrombocytopenia, heat stroke
Oxytocin† (Pitocin)	24 IU intranasal during sex or SL prior to sex	–	• Labor induction • Abortion adjunct • Postpartum hemorrhage	**Nausea, vomiting,** hypertension, afibrinogenemia, SAIDH **Not for elective labor induction
Pseudoephedrine* (Sudafed)	60–120 mg po (120–150 min prior to sex)	–	• Nasal congestion	**Insomnia, anxiety, nausea, insomnia, tremor, urinary retention, headache, palpitations,** arrhythmias, hypertension
Ephedrine*	15–60 mg po (1 h prior to sex)	–	• Acute bronchospasm • Hypotension	**Nausea, headache, dizziness, insomnia, hypertension, tremor, urinary retention, anxiety, palpitations,** arrhythmias, stroke, seizures, MI, nephrotoxicity, hepatotoxicity
Midodrine* (Orvaten, ProAmatine)	5-40 mg po daily (30–120 min. Prior to sex)	–	• Orthostatic Hypotension	**Dysuria, paresthesia, rigors, pruittus, piloerection, rash,** bradycardia, erythema multiforme, visual field defect ** Supine Elevated Blood Pressure
Apomorphine (Apokyn)	0.5–1.5 mg Intranasal (20 min before sex)	–	• Parkinson Ds	**Yawning, dyskinesia, rhinorrhea, hallucinations, anxiety, UTI, chest pain, diaphoresis,** hypotension, syncope, MI, Priapism, abuse potential, hallucinations
Bethanechol^ (Urecholine)	20 mg po (1–2 h prior to sex)	–	• Urinary retention • Neurogenic bladder • GERD • TCA adjunct treatment • Phenothiazine adjunct Tx	**Abdominal pain, nausea, diarrhea, headache, urinary urgency, malaise, flushing, miosis,** broncospasm, hypotention, tachycardia, seizures

(continued)

TABLE 17-3. (continued)

Drug Generic/(Trade)	Delayed ejaculation dosage (Not FDA approved) As needed	Daily	Indication (FDA approved)	Side effects (At therapeutic FDA indication dose)
Amantadine^ (Symmetrel)	100–400 mg po (for 2 days prior to sex)	75–100 mg po BID or TID	• Influenza A Tx and Prophylaxis • Extrapyramidal sx • Parkinsonism	**Nausea, dizziness, depression, anorexia, halluncinations, compulsivity, hypotension, abnormal dreams, headache, constipation/diarrhea**, arrhythmias, psychosis, coma, impaired vision, pulmonary edema, neutropenia, seizure, heat stroke
Bupropion^ (Wellbutrin, Zyban, Budeprion, Forfivo)	–	75 mg po BID or TID	• Major depressive disorder • Seasonal affective disorder • Smoking cessation • Attention deficit-hyperactivity disorder (ADHD)	**Palpitations, urinary frequency, blurred vision, chest pain**, agitation, psychosis, hallucinations, seizures, hepatotoxicity, HTN, arrhythmias **Suicidality, Neuropsychiatric symptoms
Buspirone^ (BuSpar)	–	5–15 mg po BID	• Anxiety	**Dizziness, nausea, headache, fatigue, blurred vision, numbness, weakness, abdominal pain, insomnia**, serotonin syndrome, tardive dyskinesia, sytonia, hositity, depression
Yohimbine (Yocon)	–	5.4 mg po TID	• Impotence	**Urinary retention, hyperglycemia, tachycardia, irritability, tremor, nausea, dizziness, headache, flushing, diaphoresis, hypertension**, respiratory depression
Cabergoline† (Dostinex)	–	0.25–2 mg po twice a week	• Hyperprolactinemia	**Nausea, dizziness, fatigue, abdominal pain, somnolence, anxiety, vertigo hot flashes, flatulence, breast pain, compulsivity**, orthostatic hypotension, pleural effusion, retroperitoneal fibrosis, depression, psychosis, pulmonary and pericardial fibrosis
Loratadine^ (Claritin, Alavert)	–	10 mg po daily	• Allergic rhinitis • Chronic idiopathic urticaria	**Drowsiness, fatigue, headache, dry mucous membranes, pharyngitis**, bronchospasm, hepatotoxicity, syncope, seizures, thrombocytopenia
Roboxetine (not available in USA)	–	4–8 po mg	• Major depressive disorder • Panic Disorder • Attention deficit-hyperactivity disorder (ADHD)	**Insomnia, nausea, excessive sweating, constipation, urinary tract infection, dysuria, urinary retention, ejaculatory pain**, tachycardia, blood pressure changes
Imipramine* (Tofranil)	–	25–75 mg po daily	• Depression • Chronic pain	**Drowsiness, dizziness, blurred vision, palpitations, increase appetite, weakness, confusion, anxiety, impotence, galactorrhea, gynecomastia, photosensitivity, change in libido**, hypotension, syncope, QT Prolongation, AV block, MI, stroke, seizures, ataxia, leukopenia, hallucinations, depression, hepatitis, angioedema, heat stroke, psychosis, withdrawal symptoms **Suicidality

Bold terms represent more common reactions and un-bolded terms represent serious reactions

^ Works in part as a possible antidote for SSRI and SSNRI for sexual side effect of DE

† May help when abnormalities of Prolactin or other hormonal issues considered

* Known to help with retrograde ejaculation

** Black Box Warning

None of these drugs are FDA approved for delayed ejaculation

Adapted from Sadowski, DJ, Butcher MJ, Köhler TS. Delayed ejaculation: medical and psychological treatments and algorithm. Curr Sex Health Rep. 2015;7(3): 170–9. With permission from Springer Science + Business Media.

to help tamper the effects of SSRIs in humans [102]. In non-controlled case studies, cyproheptadine may reverse the sexual side effects of DE or anorgasmia of the following drugs: citalopram, nortryptylline, fluoxetine, fluvaoxatmine, imipramine, and clomipramine [103–106]. The drug's most frequent side effects include somnolence and poor tolerability. In addition, it may reverse the effects of the antidepressant and/or anti-obsessive properties of SSRIs [107].

Alpha-1-Adrenergic Agonists

Pseudophedrine 60–120 mg 2–3 h prior to sex.
Ephedrine 15–60 mg 1 h prior to sex.
Midodrine 5–40 mg 30–120 min prior to sex.

Medications that act as agonists to the alpha-1-adrenergic receptors have typically been used for nasal congestion, hypotension, and acute bronchospasm. Pseudoephedrine, ephedrine, and midodrine have been shown to aid in the emission process and result in antegrade ejaculation [99, 108–110]. Stimulation of the sympathetic tone and closure of the bladder neck is thought to be the mechanism of action of these agents. Midodrine was shown to have nearly 60% efficacy in treating and/or reversing anejaculation [108]. Patients with multiple sclerosis had the greatest response whereas those with bilateral sympathectomies had the worse response [108].

Amantadine

Amantadine 100–400 mg daily starting 2 days prior to sex OR 75-100 mg 2–3 times a daily.

This central dopaminergic agonist is used to treat the flu, Parkinsonism, and extrapyramidal symptoms [100]. Chronic amantadine administration induced shorter refractory periods and increased sexual frequency with no change in arousal in rats [111]. Taking this drug 5–6 h before sex in humans has been suggested to help treat DE caused by SSRIs at a dose of 100 mg [15, 112].

Cabergoline

Carbergoline 0.25–2 mg twice a week.

Cabergoline is a dopamine-2 agonist which inhibits prolactin secretion and is used for treating hyperprolactinemia [100]. It was shown to enhance erections and orgasms with a decrease in refractory period in those with Parkinson's disease [113]. Cabergoline decreased the refractory period and lowered prolactin levels in a single-blinded, placebo-controlled, crossover study comparing protirelin (prolactin stimulant) and cabergoline [114]. Improvements in both ejaculation and libido were also demonstrated in this study. Other authors have found similar outcomes with anorgasmic men [99]. Some providers have described greater anecdotal success with cabergoline [115]. It is hypothesized that when prolactin levels were high or high normal at baseline carbergoline can be a good first choice. Low or normal prolactin levels prompt some providers to then use oxytocin as their first line agent.

Oxytocin

Oxytocin 24 IU Intranasal 2–10 min prior to desired orgasm or sublingual 10–20 min prior to desired orgasm.

Oxytocin is a peptide hormone that has been shown to have effect in many areas in men, such as increasing ejaculation frequency, paternal nurturing, long-term romantic bonds and attachments, stimulation of sexual desire and conditioning of the sexual experience in preparation of ejaculation and orgasm [116]. Oxytocin surges during male ejaculation, orgasm and detumescence returning to baseline by 10 min after surge [75, 77]. Oxytocin has also been associated with smooth muscle relaxation with an estrogenic effect in the penis which contribute to detumesence after orgasm in rabbits [117]. The use of oxytocin as a nasal or sublingual administration have been tried with various success [118–120].

Buproprion

Buproprion 75 mg 2–3 times a daily.

This is a dopamine and norepinephrine reuptake inhibitor that is used to treat depression, smoking addiction, and attention-deficient-hyperactivity disorder [100]. It can be used as an antidote to the side effects of sexual dysfunction and DE associated with SSRIs and has been shown effective in humans [107, 121]. In 66–69% of patients on SSRIs, daily or as needed buproprion resulted in complete reversal or improvement of negative sexual side-effects [122].

Buspirone

Buspirone 5–15 mg twice daily.

The anxiolytic, buspirone binds to 5-HT and dopamine-2 receptors [100]. It has been used to treat the side effects of sexual dysfunction associated with SSRIs [123]. Buspirone was shown to be effective in patients with generalized anxiety and sexual dysfunction in ranges of 16–60 mg daily [96]. There tends to be a little less sexual side effects with the use of buspirone compared to SSRIss [81].

Yohimbine and Herbal Supplements

Yohimbine 5.4 mg three times daily.

Yohimbine is an herbal supplement that is commonly suggested for use in those who have decreased libido and ejaculatory dysfunction [124]. Rat models of ejaculatory exhaustion demonstrated diminishment of refractory periods and reinitiating of the ejaculation motor reflex after intravenous yohimbine administration [125]. In another study, men treated with fluoxetine for 2 years were given yohimbine which seemed to have countered the effect of this SSRI on orgasm and ejaculation [126]. Multiple studies in human have found yohimbine to help treat ejaculatory and orgasmic dysfunction along with other sexual dysfunction; however, they have not been performed in large blinded, randomized, or placebo-controlled fashion [102, 124].

Similar to yohimbine horney goat weed, MACA root, *Tribulus terrestris*, and saffron are all ancient herbal medicines that have been used for thousands of years in Chinese, Indian, ancient Egyptian, Roman, and Greek cultures to help treat all forms of ejaculatory and erectile dysfunction. The use of these particular medications have been tested in animal models and some in humans which has shown evidence towards decreased ejaculatory latency periods [127].

Bethanechol

Bethanechol 20 mg 1–2 h prior to sex.

Bethanechol, is a cholinergic agonist that increases detrusor and gastrointestinal motility [100]. It is FDA approved drug for urinary retention, gastroesophogeal reflux disease, and adjuvant for tricyclic antidepressants and pheothiazines [100]. Behtanechol is given to help reverse DE which is a result of the adverse side effect of protiptyline, amoxapine, and imipramine [38, 128, 129].

Apomorphine

Apomorphine 0.5 1.5 mg intranasal 20 min prior to sex.

Apomorphine is a central and a peripheral stimulator of post-synaptic dopamine-2 receptors used for hypomobility in Parkinson disease [100, 130]. Apomorphine has been shown to excite the nerve patterns in the lumbosacral plexus associated with ejaculation and is used for treatment of sexual dysfunction and ejaculatory dysfunction in parkinsonism patients [131]. Rat studies showed increased activity of the sympathetic branches of the hypogastric nerve innervating the vas deferens resulting in neuronal activity that occurs during sexual climax [132–134]. Although the drug is commonly administered subcutaneously, it seems to have equal efficacy on sexual function intra-nasally in experiments [135]. Episodic doses in humans have been successful in patients who were using it for sexual dysfunction including erectile dysfunction [136].

Others

Loratadine 10 mg daily or 3–4 h prior to sex.
Roboxetine 4–8 mg dialy (not available in the USA).
Imipramine 25–75 mg daily.

The intermittent use of other drugs may help reverse the DE effect of SSRIs, which include amphetamines [137] and loratadine (10 mg daily) [98]. Reboxetine is a selective noradrenaline reuptake inhibitor that can be used as an alternative to SSRI for depression which has been reported to have less sexual side effects of DE, however there are reports of spontaneous ejaculation with this drug [138–140]. Alterations of SSRI dosages with and without additional medications to use as antidotes can be effective in treatment of DE [141, 142]. It has been proposed that the following drugs may also help in treatment of DE and sexual dysfunction based on human and/or rat models: ropinirole, cocaine, flibanserin, and anandamide [97, 143–146].

Penile Vibratory Stimulation (PVS)

Electro-ejaculation techniques have been used for many years to treat ejaculatory problems in neurogenic patients who present for infertility[147, 148]. Ejaculation can be obtained via stimulation to the pudendal nerves which helps to initiate the ejaculatory reflex [149, 150]. In DE patients, PVS has been used on the frenulum for certain time periods to help increase the sensation to the penis allowing for the ejaculatory reflex to be triggered [151]. It has been shown to work with secondary DE at a rate of 72% [152]. For men with multiple sclerosis, PVS has also been shown to be helpful [153]. Combining PVS with medical therapy increases efficacy of DE treatment [154]. However, to date there have been no studies that are either placebo-controlled or randomized [97].

Psychological

Psychological treatments include but are not limited to: increased genital specific stimulation; sexual education; role-playing on his own and in front of his partner; retraining masturbatory practices; anxiety reduction on ejaculation and performance; and recalibrating the mismatch of sexual fantasies with arousal (such as with pornography use and fantasy stimulation compared to reality) [93]. A basic understanding of the sexual cycle for their respective partners can assist men and women to manage expectations and evaluate their own sexual practices. Masturbation techniques that are either solo or partnered can be considered practice for the "real performance" which can result in greater psychosexual arousal and orgasm for both parties [16]. Although masturbation with fantasy can be harmful when not associated with appropriate sexual arousal and context, fantasy can be quite supportive if it allows blockage of critical thoughts that may be preventing orgasm and ejaculation. Techniques geared towards reduction of anxiety is an important skill that can help overcome the performance anxiety as this can often interrupts the natural erectile through orgasmic progression [155]. A well-trained sexual therapist can be invaluable for these treatments to work. Other addressable psychopathologies that may be masquerading or comorbid with DE can be uncovered via sex therapy. Female sexual dysfunction can contribute to DE in men so evaluation of this is a critical part of treatment. Referral to proper therapist, psychiatrist or psychologist is appropriate and often times warranted (see Figures 17-2 and 17-3).

Sexual Tipping Point Model

Considering the multifactorial etiology of DE and "The Ejaculatory Tipping Point", Perelman theorizes that every man has a multidimensional predetermined ejaculatory threshold that will result in tipping the "scale" of balancing factors towards ejaculation and orgasm [37]. In his model, he has a scale balancing the excitatory and inhibitory factors between the physiologic and organic issues and the psychosocial and behavior issues [16]. Deciphering between the biogenic and psychosocial factors is the goal of both the patient and the clinician in helping achieve the desired outcome whether they suffer from premature ejaculation, DE, or anorgasmia [16, 155]. The sexual tipping point has been embraced as a more holistic approach to ejaculatory dysfunctions as it incorporates all aspects of the disorder to help find solutions [97]. It is also a good diagnostic model to help coordinate care between psychologist and clinician. If both parties have an understanding of the complicated and multifactorial issues involved in DE, they are apt to be able to help more clients/patients cope and recover from the deleterious effects of DE with success.

Prognosis

Due to the complex conditions associated with diagnosis, etiology and treatment options, there has been no consensus on best treatment options for DE. There was a survey done that asked practitioners who were members of The Sexual Medicine Society of North America what their success rates were for treatment of DE. Sixty percent of clinicians reported either seldom (49%) or never (11%) having successful treatment for their patients [95]. We need further studies to evaluate the various treatment modalities and prescriptions as mentioned above. Overall, success is limited, but this may be from lack of understanding of the disease state or treatment options as an appreciation of the diagnosis of DE is limited.

Conclusions

The physiology of ejaculation is highly complex and relies on sympathetic and parasympathetic neural pathways. Ejaculatory dysfunction is fairly common and is a source of significant bother for many of those affected. Unlike premature ejaculation, DE is a rare clinical entity and there is no consensus regarding its etiology and/or management. However, patients with DE should be evaluated through a thorough medical history, physical examination, and laboratory testing to help ensure proper diagnosis. Finally, with directed therapy, many DE patients can be successfully treated. Additionally, integrative models of psychotherapy with clinical integration have been shown to be beneficial. The efficient use of these potential treatments may assist in better diagnosis and treatment of patients affected with DE.

References

1. Masters WH, Johnson VE. Human sexual response. Boston, MA: Little, Brown and Company; 1966.
2. Laumann EO, Paik A, Rosen RC. Sexual dysfunction in the United States: prevalence and predictors. JAMA. 1999;281(6):537–44.
3. Laumann EO, et al. Sexual problems among women and men aged 40-80 y: prevalence and correlates identified in the Global Study of Sexual Attitudes and Behaviors. Int J Impot Res. 2005;17(1):39–57.
4. Rosen R, et al. Lower urinary tract symptoms and male sexual dysfunction: the multinational survey of the aging male (MSAM-7). Eur Urol. 2003;44(6):637–49.
5. Pryor JL, et al. Efficacy and tolerability of dapoxetine in treatment of premature ejaculation: an integrated analysis of two double-blind, randomised controlled trials. Lancet. 2006;368(9539):929–37.
6. Abdel-Hamid IA, Saleh S, et al. Primary lifelong delayed ejaculation: characteristics and response to bupropion. J Sex Med. 2011;8(6):1772–9.
7. Rowland D, et al. Psychosexual factors that differentiate men with inhibited ejaculation from men with no dysfunction or another sexual dysfunction. J Sex Med. 2005;2(3):383–9.
8. Lue, T.F., et al. Chapter 13: Disorders of orgasm and ejaculation in men. In: McMahon CG, et al. editors. Sexual medicine: sexual dysfunctions in men and women. Plymouth, MA: Health; 2004. p. 409–68.
9. Butcher MJ, Kohler T. AUA update series 2015: delayed ejaculation: a condition whose time has come. Linthicum, MD: American Urologic Association Education and Research Inc.; 2015. p. 157–67.
10. American Psychiatric Publishing. Diagnostic and statistical manual of mental disorders. 5th ed. Arlington, VA.: xii 370 pAmerican Psychiatric Publishing; 2013.
11. The Sexual Medicine Society of North America. Overview – Delayed ejaculation. 2016. http://www.sexhealthmatters.org/delayed-ejaculation/overview-delayed-ejaculation. Cited 16 Apr 2016
12. The International Society for Sexual Medicine. What is delayed ejaculation? 2016. http://www.issm.info/education-for-all/sexual-health-qa/what-is-delayed-ejaculation. Cited 16 Apr 2016
13. Colpi G, et al. EAU guidelines on ejaculatory dysfunction. Eur Urol. 2004;46(5):555–8.
14. Waldinger MD, et al. A multinational population survey of intravaginal ejaculation latency time. J Sex Med. 2005;2(4):492–7.
15. McMahon CG, et al. Standard operating procedures in the disorders of orgasm and ejaculation. J Sex Med. 2013;10(1):204–29.
16. Perelman MA, Rowland DL. Retarded ejaculation. World J Urol. 2006;24(6):645–52.
17. Rowland DL, Keeney C, Slob AK. Sexual response in men with inhibited or retarded ejaculation. Int J Impot Res. 2004;16(3):270–4.
18. Nathan SG. The epidemiology of the DSM-III psychosexual dysfunctions. J Sex Marital Ther. 1986;12(4):267–81.
19. Spector IP, Carey MP. Incidence and prevalence of the sexual dysfunctions: a critical review of the empirical literature. Arch Sex Behav. 1990;19(4):389–408.
20. Kinsey AC, et al. Sexual behavior in the human male. Philadelphia.: xv 804 pW. B. Saunders Co.; 1948.
21. Frank E, Anderson C, Rubinstein D. Frequency of sexual dysfunction in "normal" couples. N Engl J Med. 1978;299(3):111–5.

22. Catalan J, et al. The psychosocial impact of HIV infection in men with haemophilia: controlled investigation and factors associated with psychiatric morbidity. J Psychosom Res. 1992;36(5):409–16.
23. Catalan J, et al. The psychosocial impact of HIV infection in gay men. A controlled investigation and factors associated with psychiatric morbidity. Br J Psychiatry. 1992;161:774–8.
24. Rosser BR, et al. Sexual difficulties, concerns, and satisfaction in homosexual men: an empirical study with implications for HIV prevention. J Sex Marital Ther. 1997;23(1):61–73.
25. Frank E, Anderson C, Kupfer DJ. Profiles of couples seeking sex therapy and marital therapy. Am J Psychiatry. 1976;133(5):559–62.
26. Nazareth I, Boynton P, King M. Problems with sexual function in people attending London general practitioners: cross sectional study. BMJ. 2003;327(7412):423.
27. Lindau ST, et al. A study of sexuality and health among older adults in the United States. N Engl J Med. 2007;357(8):762–74.
28. Parelman MA. Regarding ejaculation, delayed and otherwise. J Androl. 2003;24(4):496.
29. McCabe MP, Connaughton C. Psychosocial factors associated with male sexual difficulties. J Sex Res. 2014;51(1):31–42.
30. Corona G, et al. Risk factors associated with primary and secondary reduced libido in male patients with sexual dysfunction. J Sex Med. 2013;10(4):1074–89.
31. Jannini EA, Simonelli C, Lenzi A. Sexological approach to ejaculatory dysfunction. Int J Androl. 2002;25(6):317–23.
32. Montorsi F, et al. Summary of the recommendations on sexual dysfunctions in men. J Sex Med. 2010;7(11):3572–88.
33. Masters WH, Johnson VE. Human sexual inadequacy. London: Churchill; 1970. p. xi- 467.
34. Apfelbaum, B. Retarded ejaculation: a much-misunderstood syndrome. In: Lieblum S, Rosen R, editors. Principles and practices of sex therapy. New York: Guilford; 2000. p. 205–41
35. Binik, Y.M. and K.S.K. Hall. Chapter 6: Delayed ejaculation. In: Perelman MA, editor. Principles and practice of sex therapy. 5th ed. New York: The Guiford Press; 2014. p. 138–55
36. Waldinger MD. Toward evidence-based genetic research on lifelong premature ejaculation: a critical evaluation of methodology. Korean J Urol. 2011;52(1):1–8.
37. Perelman MA. The sexual tipping point: a mind/body model for sexual medicine. J Sex Med. 2009;6(3):629–32.
38. Richardson D, Nalabanda A, Goldmeier D. Retarded ejaculation – a review. Int J STD AIDS. 2006;17(3):143–50.
39. Halata Z, Munger BL. The neuroanatomical basis for the protopathic sensibility of the human glans penis. Brain Res. 1986;371(2):205–30.
40. Johnson RD, Murray FT. Reduced sensitivity of penile mechanoreceptors in aging rats with sexual dysfunction. Brain Res Bull. 1992;28(1):61–4.
41. Edwards AE, Husted JR. Penile sensitivity, age, and sexual behavior. J Clin Psychol. 1976;32(3):697–700.
42. McMahon CG, et al. Disorders of orgasm and ejaculation in men. J Sex Med. 2004;1(1):58–65.
43. Paduch DA, et al. Clinical and demographic correlates of ejaculatory dysfunctions other than premature ejaculation: a prospective. Observational study. J Sex Med. 2015;12(12):2276–86.
44. Paduch DA, et al. Testosterone replacement in androgen-deficient men with ejaculatory dysfunction: a randomized controlled trial. J Clin Endocrinol Metab. 2015;100(8):2956–62.
45. Latini DM, et al. Clinical and psychosocial characteristics of men with erectile dysfunction: baseline data from ExCEED. J Sex Med. 2006;3(6):1059–67.
46. Gierveld Jde J, et al. Quality of marriages in later life and emotional and social loneliness. J Gerontol B Psychol Sci Soc Sci. 2009;64(4):497–506.
47. Holt B, Pryor JP, Hendry WF. Male infertility after surgery for imperforate anus. J Pediatr Surg. 1995;30(12):1677–9.
48. Negri L, et al. Aspermia and chronic testicular pain after imperforate anus correction. Cryopreservation of sperm cells extracted from whole orchiectomized testis: case report. Hum Reprod. 2002;17(11):2935–7.
49. Xia JD, et al. Clinical characteristics and penile afferent neuronal function in patients with primary delayed ejaculation. Andrology. 2013;1(5):787–92.
50. Marra G, et al. Systematic review of lower urinary tract symptoms/benign prostatic hyperplasia surgical treatments on men's ejaculatory function: time for a bespoke approach? Int J Urol. 2016;23(1):22–35.
51. Liu Z, et al. Prognosis and postoperative genital function of function-preservative surgery of pelvic autonomic nerve preservation for male rectal cancer patients. BMC Surg. 2016;16(1):12.
52. Liu Y, et al. Anatomical basis and clinical research of pelvic autonomic nerve preservation with laparoscopic radical resection for rectal cancer. J Huazhong Univ Sci Technolog Med Sci. 2016;36(2):211–4.
53. Kenney PA, Tuerk IA. Complications of laparoscopic retroperitoneal lymph node dissection in testicular cancer. World J Urol. 2008;26(6):561–9.
54. Jacobsen KD, et al. Ejaculation in testicular cancer patients after post-chemotherapy retroperitoneal lymph node dissection. Br J Cancer. 1999;80(1–2):249–55.
55. Kilinc M, et al. Midline prostatic cyst marsupialization using holmium laser. Case Rep Urol. 2015;2015:797061.
56. Sundar R, Sundar G. Zinner syndrome: an uncommon cause of painful ejaculation. BMJ Case Rep. 2015;2015.
57. Dias J, et al. Adult circumcision and male sexual health: a retrospective analysis. Andrologia. 2014;46(5):459–64.
58. Frisch M, Lindholm M, Gronbaek M. Male circumcision and sexual function in men and women: a survey-based, cross-sectional study in Denmark. Int J Epidemiol. 2011;40(5):1367–81.
59. Senol MG, et al. The effect of male circumcision on pudendal evoked potentials and sexual satisfaction. Acta Neurol Belg. 2008;108(3):90–3.
60. Collins S, et al. Effects of circumcision on male sexual function: debunking a myth? J Urol. 2002;167(5):2111–2.
61. DasGupta R, Fowler CJ. Sexual and urological dysfunction in multiple sclerosis: better understanding and improved therapies. Curr Opin Neurol. 2002;15(3):271–8.
62. Enzlin P, et al. Prevalence and predictors of sexual dysfunction in patients with type 1 diabetes. Diabetes Care. 2003;26(2):409–14.
63. Lew-Starowicz M, Rola R. Sexual dysfunctions and sexual quality of life in men with multiple sclerosis. J Sex Med. 2014;11(5):1294–301.
64. Corona G, et al. Sexual dysfunction at the onset of type 2 diabetes: the interplay of depression, hormonal and cardiovascular factors. J Sex Med. 2014;11(8):2065–73.
65. Minderhoud JM, et al. Sexual disturbances arising from multiple sclerosis. Acta Neurol Scand. 1984;70(4):299–306.
66. Jannini EA, Simonelli C, Lenzi A. Disorders of ejaculation. J Endocrinol Investig. 2002;25(11):1006–19.
67. Comarr AE. Sexual function among patients with spinal cord injury. Urol Int. 1970;25(2):134–68.
68. Courtois F, Charvier K. Sexual dysfunction in patients with spinal cord lesions. Handb Clin Neurol. 2015;130:225–45.
69. Beck SD, et al. Ejaculatory status and fertility rates after primary retroperitoneal lymph node dissection. J Urol. 2010;184(5):2078–80.
70. Rowland DL, et al. Ejaculatory latency and control in men with premature ejaculation: an analysis across sexual activities using multiple sources of information. J Psychosom Res. 2000;48(1):69–77.
71. Kul'chavenia EV, et al. Ejaculatory disorders in some regions of the Russian Federation. Urologia. 2010;3:49–52.

72. Corona G, et al. Different testosterone levels are associated with ejaculatory dysfunction. J Sex Med. 2008;5(8):1991–8.
73. Davidson JM. Neurohormonal bases of male sexual behavior. Int Rev Physiol. 1977;13:225–54.
74. Perez-Pouchoulen M, et al. Androgen receptors in Purkinje neurons are modulated by systemic testosterone and sexual training in a region-specific manner in the male rat. Physiol Behav. 2016;156:191–8.
75. Corona G, et al. The hormonal control of ejaculation. Nat Rev Urol. 2012;9(9):508–19.
76. Carani C, et al. Multicenter study on the prevalence of sexual symptoms in male hypo- and hyperthyroid patients. J Clin Endocrinol Metab. 2005;90(12):6472–9.
77. Kruger TH, et al. Specificity of the neuroendocrine response to orgasm during sexual arousal in men. J Endocrinol. 2003;177(1):57–64.
78. Kruger TH, Hartmann U, Schedlowski M. Prolactinergic and dopaminergic mechanisms underlying sexual arousal and orgasm in humans. World J Urol. 2005;23(2):130–8.
79. Fitzgerald P, Dinan TG. Prolactin and dopamine: what is the connection? A review article. J Psychopharmacol. 2008;22(2 Suppl):12–9.
80. Sadowski DJ, Butcher MJ, Köhler TS. Delayed ejaculation: medical and psychological treatments and algorithm. Curr Sex Health Rep. 2015;7(3):170–9.
81. Bijlsma EY, et al. Sexual side effects of serotonergic antidepressants: mediated by inhibition of serotonin on central dopamine release? Pharmacol Biochem Behav. 2014;121:88–101.
82. Althof SE, et al. An update of the International Society of Sexual Medicine's guidelines for the diagnosis and treatment of Premature Ejaculation (PE). Sex Med. 2014;2(2):60–90.
83. Sadowski D, Butcher MJ, Kohler T. A review of pathophysiology and management options for delayed ejaculation. Sex Med Rev. 2016;4(2):167–76.
84. Althof SE. Psychological interventions for delayed ejaculation/orgasm. Int J Impot Res. 2012;24(4):131–6.
85. Michetti PM, et al. Delayed ejaculation and alexithymia: what is the relationship? F1000Res. 2013;2:81.
86. Fathy A, et al. Experience with tube (promedon) malleable penile implant. Urol Int. 2007;79(3):244–7.
87. Shaeer O. The global online sexuality survey (GOSS): The United States of America in 2011 Chapter III – Premature ejaculation among English-speaking male Internet users. J Sex Med. 2013;10(7):1882–8.
88. Bronner G, Ben-Zion IZ. Unusual masturbatory practice as an etiological factor in the diagnosis and treatment of sexual dysfunction in young men. J Sex Med. 2014;11(7):1798–806.
89. Perelman M. Idiosyncratic masturbation patterns: a key unexplored variable in the treatment of retarded ejaculation by the practicing urologist. J Urol. 2005;**173**:340 .Abstract 1254
90. Sank LI. Traumatic masturbatory syndrome. J Sex Marital Ther. 1998;24(1):37–42.
91. Rothbart, D., He's just not that into anyone. (cover story). New York. 7 Feb 2011:38–88 5.
92. Carvalheira A, Traeen B, Stulhofer A. Masturbation and pornography use among coupled heterosexual men with decreased sexual desire: how many roles of masturbation? J Sex Marital Ther. 2014;1–10.
93. Rowland D, et al. Disorders of orgasm and ejaculation in men. J Sex Med. 2010;7(4 Pt 2):1668–86.
94. Teloken P, Nelson C, Mullhall J. Outcomes with medical treatment of secondary delayed orgasm proposal of a clinical care pathway. J Urol. 2012;**187**(4, Supplement 1496):e606.
95. Butcher MJ, et al. How is delayed ejaculation defined and treated in North America? Andrology. 2015;3(3):626–31.
96. Porst, H., J. Buvat, and Standards Committee of the International Society for Sexual Medicine, Chapter 16: Ejaculatory disorders In: McMahon CG, et al. editors. Standard practice in sexual medicine. Malden, MA, Oxford: Blackwell; 2006. p. 188–209.
97. Mulhall, J.P. and W. Hsiao, Chapter 9: Delayed ejaculation and orgasm. In: Nelson CJ, Brock D, Dean RC, editors. Men's sexual health and fertility: a clinician's guide. New York: Springer; 2014.
98. Aukst-Margetic B, Margetic B. An open-label series using loratadine for the treatment of sexual dysfunction associated with selective serotonin reuptake inhibitors. Prog Neuro-Psychopharmacol Biol Psychiatry. 2005;29(5):754–6.
99. Shin D, Spitz A. The evaluation and treatment of delayed ejaculation. Sex Med Rev. 2014;**2**(3–4):121–33.
100. Epocrates Plus Version 16.3 – Medication management application for iPhone and Android. BMJ Publishing Group Ltd. Computer program for medication management; 2016.
101. Menendez Abraham E, et al. Modifications of the sexual activity in male rats following administration of antiserotoninergic drugs. Behav Brain Res. 1988;30(3):251–8.
102. Ashton AK, Hamer R, Rosen RC. Serotonin reuptake inhibitor-induced sexual dysfunction and its treatment: a large-scale retrospective study of 596 psychiatric outpatients. J Sex Marital Ther. 1997;23(3):165–75.
103. Lauerma H. Successful treatment of citalopram-induced anorgasmia by cyproheptadine. Acta Psychiatr Scand. 1996;93(1):69–70.
104. Steele TE, Howell EF. Cyproheptadine for imipramine-induced anorgasmia. J Clin Psychopharmacol. 1986;6(5):326–7.
105. Sovner R. Treatment of tricyclic antidepressant-induced orgasmic inhibition with cyproheptadine. J Clin Psychopharmacol. 1984;4(3):169.
106. McCormick S, Olin J, Brotman AW. Reversal of fluoxetine-induced anorgasmia by cyproheptadine in two patients. J Clin Psychiatry. 1990;51(9):383–4.
107. DeBattista C, et al. A placebo-controlled, randomized, double-blind study of adjunctive bupropion sustained release in the treatment of SSRI-induced sexual dysfunction. J Clin Psychiatry. 2005;66(7):844–8.
108. Safarinejad MR. Midodrine for the treatment of organic anejaculation but not spinal cord injury: a prospective randomized placebo-controlled double-blind clinical study. Int J Impot Res. 2009;21(4):213–20.
109. Chehensse C, et al. The spinal control of ejaculation revisited: a systematic review and meta-analysis of anejaculation in spinal cord injured patients. Hum Reprod Update. 2013;19(5):507–26.
110. Arafa M, El Tabie O. Medical treatment of retrograde ejaculation in diabetic patients: a hope for spontaneous pregnancy. J Sex Med. 2008;5(1):194–8.
111. Ferraz MM, et al. Chronic amantadine treatment enhances the sexual behaviour of male rats. Pharmacol Biochem Behav. 2007;86(4):616–21.
112. Balon R. Intermittent amantadine for fluoxetine-induced anorgasmia. J Sex Marital Ther. 1996;22(4):290–2.
113. Wittstock M, Benecke R, Dressler D. Cabergoline can increase penile erections and libido. Neurology. 2002;58(5):831.
114. Kruger TH, et al. Effects of acute prolactin manipulation on sexual drive and function in males. J Endocrinol. 2003;179(3):357–65.
115. Butcher, M., et al., Delayed ejcaultion remains a recalcitrant condition: Results of a SMSNA survey. 20th Annual Fall Scientific Meeting of SMSNA, November 20–23, 2014 Program Book, 2014(Abstract 041): p. 70.
116. Veening, J.G., et al., The role of oxytocin in male and female reproductive behavior.. Eur J Pharmacol, 2014.
117. Vignozzi L, et al. Oxytocin receptor is expressed in the penis and mediates an estrogen-dependent smooth muscle contractility. Endocrinology. 2004;145(4):1823–34.

118. Burri A, et al. The acute effects of intranasal oxytocin administration on endocrine and sexual function in males. Psychoneuroendocrinology. 2008;33(5):591–600.
119. IsHak WW, Berman DS, Peters A. Male anorgasmia treated with oxytocin. J Sex Med. 2008;5(4):1022–4.
120. MacDonald K, Feifel D. Dramatic improvement in sexual function induced by intranasal oxytocin. J Sex Med. 2012;9(5):1407–10.
121. Labbate LA, et al. Bupropion treatment of serotonin reuptake antidepressant-associated sexual dysfunction. Ann Clin Psychiatry. 1997;9(4):241–5.
122. Ashton AK, Rosen RC. Bupropion as an antidote for serotonin reuptake inhibitor-induced sexual dysfunction. J Clin Psychiatry. 1998;59(3):112–5.
123. Landen M, et al. Effect of buspirone on sexual dysfunction in depressed patients treated with selective serotonin reuptake inhibitors. J Clin Psychopharmacol. 1999;19(3):268–71.
124. Adeniyi AA, et al. Yohimbine in the treatment of orgasmic dysfunction. Asian J Androl. 2007;9(3):403–7.
125. Carro-Juareza M, Rodriguez-Manzo G. Yohimbine reverses the exhaustion of the coital reflex in spinal male rats. Behav Brain Res. 2003;141(1):43–50.
126. Jacobsen FM. Fluoxetine-induced sexual dysfunction and an open trial of yohimbine. J Clin Psychiatry. 1992;53(4):119–22.
127. Melnyk J, Marcone M. Aphrodisiacs from plant and animal sources—A review of current scientific literature. Food Res Int. 2011;44:840–50.
128. Segraves RT. Reversal by bethanechol of imipramine-induced ejaculatory dysfunction. Am J Psychiatry. 1987;144(9):1243–4.
129. Yager J. Bethanechol chloride can reverse erectile and ejaculatory dysfunction induced by tricyclic antidepressants and mazindol: case report. J Clin Psychiatry. 1986;47(4):210–1.
130. Passamonti L, et al. Dopamine-transporter levels drive striatal responses to apomorphine in Parkinson's disease. Brain Behav. 2013;3(3):249–62.
131. Bronner G, Vodusek DB. Management of sexual dysfunction in Parkinson's disease. Ther Adv Neurol Disord. 2011;4(6):375–83.
132. Stafford SA, Coote JH. Activation of D2-like receptors induces sympathetic climactic-like responses in male and female anaesthetised rats. Br J Pharmacol. 2006;148(4):510–6.
133. Sanna F, et al. Role of dopamine D4 receptors in copulatory behavior: studies with selective D4 agonists and antagonists in male rats. Pharmacol Biochem Behav. 2015;137:110–8.
134. Sanna F, et al. Dopamine is involved in the different patterns of copulatory behaviour of Roman high and low avoidance rats: studies with apomorphine and haloperidol. Pharmacol Biochem Behav. 2014;124:211–9.
135. Lu W, et al. Modulation of brain delivery and copulation by intranasal apomorphine hydrochloride. Int J Pharm. 2008;349(1–2): 196–205.
136. Kendirci M, Hellstrom WJ. Intranasal apomorphine. Nastech Pharmaceutical Drugs. 2004;7(5):483–8.
137. Bartlik BD, Kaplan P, Kaplan HS. Psychostimulants apparently reverse sexual dysfunction secondary to selective serotonin re-uptake inhibitors. J Sex Marital Ther. 1995;21(4):264–71.
138. Haberfellner EM. Sexual dysfunction caused by reboxetine. Pharmacopsychiatry. 2002;35(2):77–8.
139. O'Flynn R, Michael A. Reboxetine-induced spontaneous ejaculation. Br J Psychiatry. 2000;177:567–8.
140. Sivrioglu EY, et al. Reboxetine induced erectile dysfunction and spontaneous ejaculation during defecation and micturition. Prog Neuro-Psychopharmacol Biol Psychiatry. 2007;31(2):548–50.
141. Taylor MJ. Strategies for managing antidepressant-induced sexual dysfunction: a review. Curr Psychiatry Rep. 2006;8(6):431–6.
142. Schweitzer I, Maguire K, Ng C. Sexual side-effects of contemporary antidepressants: review. Aust N Z J Psychiatry. 2009;43(9):795–808.
143. Rodriguez-Manzo G, Canseco-Alba A. Anandamide reduces the ejaculatory threshold of sexually sluggish male rats: possible relevance for human lifelong delayed ejaculation disorder. J Sex Med. 2015;12(5):1128–35.
144. Gelez H, et al. Flibanserin treatment increases appetitive sexual motivation in the female rat. J Sex Med. 2013;10(5):1231–9.
145. Ferrari F, Giuliani D. Involvement of dopamine D2 receptors in the effect of cocaine on sexual behaviour and stretching-yawning of male rats. Neuropharmacology. 1997;36(6):769–77.
146. Moll JL, Brown CS. The use of monoamine pharmacological agents in the treatment of sexual dysfunction: evidence in the literature. J Sex Med. 2011;8(4):956–70.
147. Fode M, Ohl DA, Sonksen J. A step-wise approach to sperm retrieval in men with neurogenic anejaculation. Nat Rev Urol. 2015;12(11):607–16.
148. Utida C, et al. Male infertility in spinal cord trauma. Int Braz J Urol. 2005;31(4):375–83.
149. Sonksen J, Ohl DA, Wedemeyer G. Sphincteric events during penile vibratory ejaculation and electroejaculation in men with spinal cord injuries. J Urol. 2001;165(2):426–9.
150. Tajkarimi K, Burnett AL. The role of genital nerve afferents in the physiology of the sexual response and pelvic floor function. J Sex Med. 2011;8(5):1299–312.
151. Wheeler Jr JS, et al. Idiopathic anejaculation treated by vibratory stimulation. Fertil Steril. 1988;50(2):377–9.
152. Nelson CJ, et al. Assessment of penile vibratory stimulation as a management strategy in men with secondary retarded orgasm. Urology. 2007;69(3):552–5 .discussion 555-6
153. Previnaire JG, et al. Sexual disorders in men with multiple sclerosis: Evaluation and management. Ann Phys Rehabil Med. 2014;57(5):329–36.
154. Jenkins LC, Mulhall JP. Delayed orgasm and anorgasmia. Fertil Steril. 2015;104(5):1082–8.
155. Perelman MA. A new combination treatment for premature ejaculation: a sex therapist's perspective. J Sex Med. 2006;3(6): 1004–12.

18 Evaluation of Premature Ejaculation

Marcel D. Waldinger

Introduction

Since its first description in medical literature in 1887, premature ejaculation (PE) has given rise to various and sometimes highly contrasting theories, approaches, and treatments [1, 2]. Although PE was initially considered as nothing more than a peculiar anomaly, it was believed to be mainly a psychological disorder for the first half of the twentieth century [3]. After the first psychoanalytic publications of Sandor Ferenczi and Karl Abraham in 1908 and 1917, respectively, PE was regarded as a symptom of a neurosis that had to be treated by psychoanalysis in order to solve the unconscious conflicts that were assumed to have caused the neurosis [3]. This purely psychoanalytical theory was later challenged by Bernard Schapiro, an originally German but later American endocrinologist, who in 1943 postulated that PE was not a neurotic but a psychosomatic disorder [4]. Years ahead of his time, Schapiro advocated oral and local anesthetic drug treatment to delay ejaculation [4, 5]. Bernard Schapiro should be regarded as the most important pioneer in the research and treatment of PE [6].

First PE Classification of Schapiro

It has been the great merit of Bernard Schapiro who in 1943 for the first time distinguished two subtypes of PE [4]. Based on his long experience with men with PE, Schapiro distinguished Type B or "*the sexually hypertonic or hypererotic type*" and Type A or the "*hypotonic type*" [4]. Both types were later called lifelong PE and acquired PE, respectively [7]. Schapiro noted that in Type B (lifelong PE) "*premature ejaculation, from the very first act of coitus, was continually present*" [4]. But also that "*careful questioning elicited the information that relatives of the patient (father or brother) with type B suffered from the same disorder*" [4]. Therefore, Schapiro assumed that "*in type B (lifelong PE) heredity may play a part in the etiology*" [4]. In addition, Schapiro noted that in type B "*libido and erection were rather overstrong, and erection was provoked by even mild sexual stimulation*", which phenomenon he called "*erectio praecox*" [4]. Schapiro also noted that in type B men, PE was associated with "*abnormally high sexual tension*", which he called a "*hypertonus of the entire sex apparatus*" [4]. Schapiro emphasized that the characteristics of men with type B or lifelong PE were "*entirely different*" than those of men with "type A" or "acquired PE", who did not have family members with PE and in which erectio praecox and hypertonus was not part of the subtype [4].

Unfortunately, the classification and arguments of Schapiro were completely ignored by clinicians and sexologists for nearly 50 years until Godpodinoff [7] distinguished lifelong and acquired PE, which actually were Type B and Type A of Schapiro, respectively. But erectio praecox remained ignored, and actually completely forgotten, until Waldinger mentioned it again in 2002 [2]. Similarly, Schapiro's terms hypertonic and hypotonic have been completely forgotten, until 2014, when Waldinger reintroduced both terms and explained their clinical importance [8].

Psychoanalytic, Behavioristic, and Drug Treatment Approach of PE

Psychoanalytic treatment, mainly conducted by psychiatrists, prevailed throughout the 1940s and 1950s, but unfortunately, very little information of this treatment has been documented in the literature [6]. In contrast to the psychoanalytic, psychosomatic, and urological approach of PE, William Masters and Virginia Johnson stated in 1970 that PE was the result of self-learned behavior and that behavioral treatment in the form of the so-called squeeze technique could cure PE [9]. Their treatment was a modification to the stop-start technique, a masturbation technique, described in 1956 by James Semans, an English urologist [10]. However, there is a dramatic paucity of evidence-based studies demonstrating its efficacy to delay ejaculation in men who ejaculate within seconds [3]. In the mid-1990s, the introduction of the

W.W. IsHak (ed.), *The Textbook of Clinical Sexual Medicine*, DOI 10.1007/978-3-319-52539-6_18

selective serotonin reuptake inhibitors (SSRIs) brought about a revolutionary change in the understanding and treatment of PE [2]. Their efficacy in delaying ejaculation together with the increasing interest of neuroscientists, in investigating sexual behavior in laboratory male rats led to the end of the supremacy of the behavioristic approach of PE that prevailed in the 1970s and 1980s and marked the beginning of the neurobiological view and drug treatment approach of the 1990s [6]. Animal studies and the use of stopwatch assessment of the intravaginal ejaculation latency time (IELT) [11] both during a baseline period and during drug treatment led to a more evidence-based approach of drug treatment trials but also formed the basis of a new classification of PE into four PE subtypes. It should be noted that during the 1990s and around the millennium the evidence-based methodology of investigating drug treatment of PE has been developed by clinical researchers independently of the pharmaceutical industry as in the 1990s SSRI manufacturers have not been interested in official registration of SSRIs for the treatment of PE [6, 12]. However, this very important period in the history of academic interest in PE ended in 2004 when some pharmaceutical companies became interested in PE and an increasing number of clinicians with no previous experience in PE research became involved or participated in PE research of the pharmaceutical industry with its own ideas on how to conduct PE research.

Second PE Classification of Waldinger

In 1994, Waldinger introduced the intravaginal ejaculation latency time (IELT) as a scientific measure of the ejaculation time [11]. The IELT was defined as the time between vaginal intromission and intravaginal ejaculation [11]. Particularly by using a stopwatch—the most accurate tool to measure time—for IELT measurement, it became unambiguously clear that about 85% of men with lifelong PE ejaculate within 1 min after vaginal penetration [13]. In other words, lifelong PE appeared to be a matter of seconds, which was in support of an old psychoanalytic view of PE, whereas later studies provided indications—although less convincing—that acquired PE was a matter of seconds to 3 min [14].

Due to epidemiological stopwatch research of the IELT in the general population in five countries [15, 16], it became no longer tenable to claim that there are only two types of PE. Therefore, Waldinger and Schweitzer postulated the existence of two other PE subtypes: Subjective PE and Variable PE [17–21]. This new classification into four PE subtypes is based on differences in the duration of the IELT, the course of the IELT duration throughout life, the frequency of occurrence of short IELTs, and the cognitive and subjective experience of the IELT [17–21]. Moreover, the etiology and pathogenesis of the four PE subtypes is different [20]. Men with lifelong PE suffer from IELTs that have been consistently less than 1 min since puberty or adolescence [13]. In contrast, acquired PE may be caused by erectile dysfunction, thyroid disorders, acute prostatitis or relationship problems [14, 22–25]. In Subjective PE men have a normal or even long IELT duration but still perceive themselves as having PE. In Variable PE the IELT is only sometimes very short [21]. In other words, according to Waldinger [17–21] there is a natural variation of the IELT in men with Variable PE, and therefore this PE subtype is not based on (psycho)pathology, whereas Subjective PE is mainly related to psychological and cultural factors [17–21]. In contrast, lifelong PE is related to neurobiological and genetic factors, whereas acquired PE is related to mainly medical factors [26, 27]. A clear advantage of this new classification into four subtypes is that any man with a complaint of early ejaculation can be classified into one of the four PE subtypes [21, 28].

Diagnosis of the Four PE Subtypes

Each of the four PE subtypes has its own specific etiology, (patho)genesis and treatment. They are recognizable by taking a brief medical and sexual history with special attention to the duration of the IELT, the frequency of occurrences and the course since the first sexual encounters [6]. In daily clinical practice, diagnosis of the four PE subtypes is not difficult and therefore evaluation with (validated) questionnaires or the use of a stopwatch is not required. However, for drug treatment trials, genetic and epidemiological research, stopwatch assessment of the IELT is a prerequisite [6, 26, 29].

Complaint Versus Disorder

A major misconception in the literature on PE is the idea that PE always represents a male sexual "disorder" [20, 29]. This misconception is blurring an accurate view on diagnosis, classification, epidemiology, genetics, and treatment of PE [6]. In 2006, Waldinger and Schweitzer emphasized the relevance of distinguishing between PE as a "complaint" versus PE as a "syndrome" or "disorder" [17, 18]. PE as a "complaint" may belong to the *norma*l variation of ejaculatory performance in a certain number of men, but may also be the manifestation of medically or psychologically determined *pathological* ejaculatory performance [6]. A "syndrome" is defined as a cluster of symptoms and may give rise to a cluster of various complaints that is similar in a large group of men [6]. In contrast, there are also men who complain of PE but lack the whole symptomatology of men with lifelong PE. They report experiencing early ejaculations only occasionally. In other words, the latter men have "complaints" of PE which are not part of an underlying syndrome or disorder. It should be emphasized that a nondistinction between complaint and disorder leads to misunderstanding of for example the epidemiology of PE [29]. For example, it has become customary to start an article on PE with the following introduction: "PE is the most prevalent male sexual *disorder* affecting some 20-30% of men." This sentence mirrors a general belief that PE always represents a male sexual disorder. However, if one distinguishes PE as a "complaint" versus PE as a "disorder", it appears more appropriate to state "PE is the most prevalent male sexual complaint affecting some 20-30% of men. The prevalence of PE as a sexual disorder, in case of lifelong and acquired PE, in the general male population is 2-3% and 4-5%, respectively" [6].

Lifelong PE

Lifelong PE is a syndrome characterized by the cluster of the following core symptoms: (1) ejaculation occurs too early at nearly every intercourse, (2) with (nearly) every woman, (3) from about the first sexual encounters onwards, (4) in the majority of cases (90%) the male ejaculates intravaginally within 30–60 s, or in a minority of cases (10%) between 1 and 2 min, (5) the early ejaculation remains the same throughout life (70%) or can even aggravate during aging (30%) and, (6) the ability to delay ejaculation, i.e., to withhold ejaculation at the moment of imminent ejaculation may be diminished or lacking [6]. Moreover, as soon as men with lifelong PE get engaged in an erotic or sexual situation they are overwhelmed by an acute hypertonic or hypererotic state that is characterized by an early erection (erectio praecox), an early ejaculation (ejaculatio praecox), and an early penile detumescence (detumescentia praecox) [8]. Some men already get an ejaculation during foreplay, before penetration (ejaculatio ante portas), or as soon as their penis touches the vagina (ejaculatio intra portam). It should be noted that there are no indications that lifelong PE can be cured, neither by drug treatment nor by psychotherapy [6]. In other words, lifelong PE is a chronic ejaculatory dysfunction. However, drug treatment may prolong the IELT as long as the drug is taken [6].

Acquired PE

The complaints of acquired PE differ in relation to the underlying somatic or psychological problem. It is characterized by the following symptoms. (1) Early ejaculation occurs at some point in a man's life, (2) the man has usually had normal ejaculation experiences before the start of complaints, (3) there is either a sudden or gradual onset, (4) men ejaculate within seconds or within 3 min, (5) the ability to delay ejaculation, i.e., to withhold ejaculation at the moment of imminent ejaculation may be diminished or lacking, (5) the dysfunction may be due to urological dysfunctions like erectile dysfunction or acute prostatitis, thyroid dysfunction, and psychological or relationship problems [6]. During sexual activity, there usually is a hypotonic state [8]. Erectio praecox and detumescentia praecox do not occur in acquired PE. In contrast to lifelong PE the acquired form of PE can be cured by treatment of the underlying cause.

Subjective PE

Men with subjective PE experience or complain of early ejaculations while the IELT is in the normal range, i.e., around 3–6 min, and may even be of long duration, i.e., between 5 and 25 min. This type of PE should not be regarded as a symptom or manifestation of true medical pathology [6]. Psychological and/or relationship problems may underlie the complaints. The syndrome is characterized by the following symptoms. (1) Subjective perception of consistent or inconsistent early ejaculation during intercourse. (2) Preoccupation with a perceived early ejaculation or lack of control of ejaculation. (3) The actual IELT is in the normal range or may even be of longer durarion. (4) The ability to delay ejaculation, i.e., to withhold ejaculation at the moment of imminent ejaculation may be diminished or lacking. During sexual activity there is a normal tonic state. Erectio praecox and detumescentia praecox do not occur in subjective PE. In contrast to lifelong PE the subjective form of PE can theoretically be cured by treatment of the underlying cause.

Variable PE

In variable PE, men only coincidentally and situationally experience early ejaculations. This type of PE should not be regarded as a symptom or manifestation of true pathology but of normal variation in sexual performance [6]. Variable PE is characterized by the following symptoms. (1) Early ejaculations are inconsistent and occur irregularly, (2) the ability to delay ejaculation, i.e., to withhold ejaculation at the moment of imminent ejaculation may be diminished or lacking, (3) experiences of diminished ability to delay ejaculation go along with either a short or normal IELT [6]. During sexual activity there is a normal tonic state [8]. Erectio praecox and detumescentia praecox do not occur in variable PE. Similar to lifelong PE there are no indications that the variable form of PE can be cured by drug or psychological treatment.

Epidemiology: Incidence and Prevalence of Four PE Subtypes

Due to a fundamental misunderstanding and disregard of PE in terms of being a complaint or disorder, and therefore also in the responses to questionnaires in epidemiologic studies together with inadequate definitions of PE, large conflicting prevalence rates have been reported in literature. In addition to the lack of a standardized definition and operational criteria, the method of recruitment for study participation and method of data collection have contributed to the broad range of reported prevalence rates [30]. Waldinger and Schweitzer were the first to postulate that the true prevalence of patients actually seeking treatment for lifelong PE was much less than the previously reported high prevalence rates [17, 18]. They also stated that the prevalence rate of lifelong PE in the general population is very low, whereas the prevalence rate of subjective PE in the general population is probably the highest of the four PE subtypes [17, 18]. Their predictions were confirmed by the epidemiologic studies of Serefoglu [31, 32], Zhang et al. [33] and Gao et al. [34].

Serefoglu et al. [31, 32] were the first to investigate and confirm the existence of the four PE subtypes in a urological clinic in Turkey [31] and in the general Turkish male population [32]. Also Zhang et al. [33] and Gao et al. [34] confirmed the existence of the four PE subtypes in an andrologic clinic in China [33] and in the general male population of a Chinese province [34]. Interestingly, the prevalence rates of the PE subtypes in both countries were remarkably similar. A relatively high proportion of men—20.0% in Turkey and 25.8% in China—reported a concern with ejaculating too early [32, 34], and in line with the classification of Waldinger and Schweitzer [17–21], these men could be distinguished into four PE subtypes. Both studies confirmed the prediction of Waldinger and Schweitzer [17–21] that the percentage of men with lifelong PE in the general male population is small, but relatively high in a clinical sample. In the general male population, it was found by Serefoglu et al. [32] that the prevalence of lifelong PE was 2.3% in Turkey. Gao et al. [34] reported a prevalence of 3% in China. In addition, the prevalence of acquired PE was 3.9% in Turkey [32] and 4.8% in China [34]. Similarly, the prevalence of Variable PE was 8.5% in Turkey and 11% in China, and the prevalence of Subjective PE was 5.1% in Turkey and 7% in China [32, 34]. In other words, among men in the general male population who complain of early ejaculation or are not satisfied with their ejaculation time duration, the percentage of men with Variable PE and Subjective PE is twice as high as the percentage of men with Lifelong PE and Acquired PE.

Mathematical Formula for the Prevalence of Lifelong PE

The similar method and design of two prospective stopwatch studies of the IELT in the general population of five countries [15, 16] and in a cohort of men with lifelong PE [13] enabled the formulation of a mathematical formula to calculate the prevalence of any IELT values in any Western Caucasian male population. This idea has recently been proposed and elaborated by Janssen et al. [35]. Janssen et al. [35] introduced a new method in which the fitness of various well-known mathematical probability distributions are compared with the IELT distribution of two previous stopwatch studies of the Caucasian general male population [15, 16] and a stopwatch study of Dutch Caucasian men with lifelong PE [13]. It appeared that the IELT distribution of the three studies was a gamma distribution. Moreover, it was found that the Lognormal Distribution of the gamma distribution most accurately fitted the IELT distribution of 965 men in the general population, with a GOF of 0.057. The Gumbel Max Distribution most accurately fitted the IELT distribution of 110 men with lifelong PE with a GOF of 0.179. Notably, by the Kolmogorov-Smirnov test the accuracy of fitness is expressed by the Goodness of Fit (GOF). The study of Janssen et al. [35] showed that there are more men with lifelong PE ejaculating within 30 and 60 s than can be extrapolated from the probability density curve of the Lognormal IELT distribution of men in the general population. In other words, it was shown that men with lifelong PE have a separate IELT distribution, e.g., a Gumbel Max IELT distribution, that can only be retrieved from the general male population Lognormal IELT distribution when thousands of men would participate in a IELT stopwatch study. As this will always be difficult to perform, the mathematical formula of the Lognormal IELT distribution, as calculated by Janssen et al. [35] appears to be useful for epidemiological research of the IELT at least when the number of men in a specific population is known. Moreover, the mathematical formula of the Gumbel Max IELT distribution of men with lifelong PE is useful for epidemiological research of the IELT among men with lifelong PE, when the number of men with lifelong PE is known. The study of Janssen et al. [35] provided also indications that the prevalence of lifelong PE in Western countries may be as low as about 1%. Such a low prevalence of lifelong PE is probably a better explanation than the existing taboo to talk about PE for the fact that worldwide a very low number of men are actually seeking medical treatment for lifelong PE.

Neurobiological and Genetic Hypothesis of Lifelong PE

Based on in vivo animal research of the 1980s [36–38], Waldinger et al. [26] postulated in 1998 that lifelong PE in terms of an IELT of less than 1 min is related to genetic factors and to diminished central 5-HT neurotransmission and/or a hyperfunction of 5-HT_{1A} receptors and a hypofunction of 5-HT_{2C} receptors. Notably, due to an absence of selective 5-HT_{1A} and 5-HT_{2C} receptor ligands for safe human usage, Waldinger noted that it currently is impossible to explore and confirm his hypothesis in men with lifelong PE [39].

The hypothesis of Waldinger et al. [26] on genetic and central serotonin neurotransmission and receptor involvement does not mean that lifelong PE is a classical Mendelian inheritable disorder affecting all male members of a family [8, 28]. Also in 1943, Schapiro [4] did not think that lifelong PE was a genetic disorder. Instead he assumed that *"heredity may play a part in the etiology*" of lifelong PE [4]. In line with this view, Waldinger et al. [40] reported indications of a familial, but not genetic hereditary, occurrence of lifelong PE in first degree relatives of some male patients with lifelong PE.

Genetic Polymorphisms and Lifelong PE

In 2009, Janssen et al. [41] published the first stopwatch study on the influence of 5-HTTLPR polymorphism on IELT duration in 89 Dutch men with lifelong PE. Of these men 83 men ejaculated within 1 min after vaginal penetration, whereas 6 men ejaculated between 1 and 2 min. In this group of men, those with LL genotype ejaculated within 13.2 s, expressed in geometric mean IELT, whereas men with SL and SS genotype ejaculated within 25.3 and 26.0 s, respectively ($p < 0.05$) [41]. In other words, men with LL genotype ejaculated 100% faster than men with SS genotype and 90% faster than men with SL genotype [41]. Notably, there were no significant differences between these men and a control group of 92 Dutch Caucasian men in 5-HTT polymorphism alleles and genotypes [41]. Using the same stopwatch methodology, Janssen et al. [42] investigated 54 men with respect to the role of the C(1019)G polymorphism of the 5-HT_{1A} receptor gene on the IELT duration. It was shown that men with CC genotype ejaculated within 14.5 s, whereas men with CG and GG genotype ejaculated within 27.7 s, and 36.0 s, respectively [42]. Therefore, it was concluded that men with CC genotype ejaculated 250% earlier than men with GG genotype [42]. Similarly, Janssen et al. [43] investigated the role of the Cys23Ser polymorphism of the 5-HT2c receptor on the IELT duration. It was shown that the wild types (CysCys) had an IELT of 22.6 s, whereas the mutants (Ser/Ser) had an IELT of 40.4 s [43]. Thus, the men with CysCys genotype ejaculated 79% faster than the monozygote mutant (Ser/Ser) men [43].

Importance of Hardy Weinberg Equilibrium

Unfortunately, up to now other researchers have not used the stopwatch methodology and exact study design of Janssen et al. [41–43] in the investigation of the relationship between polymorphisms of 5-HTT and 5-HT receptor genes and the duration of the IELT. However, a few clinicians have investigated the relationship between genetic polymorphisms in men with lifelong PE. For example, two questionnaire studies confirmed that there is no association in the 5-HTTLPR polymorphism between men with lifelong PE and a control group [44, 45]. In contrast, there have been three other studies of men with lifelong PE showing they have a higher SS genotype frequency compared with a control group [46–48]. But as the latter three studies were not in Hardy–Weinberg equilibrium (HWE)—most probably due to technical laboratory insufficiencies—their results are not considered to be reliable [49]. Interestingly, an association of the 5-HT_{1A} receptor gene polymorphism had been previously also found by a questionnaire study of the ELT (and not IELT) in a Finnish cohort of twins [50]. The relatively few aforementioned studies might indicate—at least in men with lifelong PE who ejaculate within 1 min—that the duration of the IELT is associated with polymorphism of the 5-HTTLPR gene, the C(1019)G polymorphism of the 5-HT_{1A} receptor, and the (HTR2C)- CysSer polymorphism of the 5-HT_{2C} receptor. However, more studies are needed in a large cohort of men with lifelong PE and a control group with well controlled polymerase chain reaction analysis and which are in Hardy Weinberg equilibrium in order to confirm the robustness of these indications of a possible link between the aforementioned gene polymorphism and the duration of the IELT in men with lifelong PE. Indeed, Genome Wide Association Studies (GWAS) may represent the best available approach to finding candidate genes related to the IELT and lifelong PE. Nevertheless, it is interesting to note that both the studies of Janssen et al. [41–43] and the animal studies [36–38] that formed the basis for the neurobiological genetic hypothesis of Waldinger et al. [26] provide indications that the short IELT of men with lifelong PE may be associated with central 5-HT neurotransmission, 5-HT_{1A} and 5-HT_{2C} receptor functioning. Although speculative, Waldinger does not exclude the possibility that environmental (maternal and non-maternal) factors that affect gene expression prenatally, shortly after birth or later in life may be associated with the persistent short IELTs in men with lifelong PE [8, 26]. Such epigenetic studies should also be conducted in men with lifelong PE [8, 28].

The IELT in ISSM and DSM-5 Definition of Lifelong and Acquired PE

The aforementioned characteristic features of lifelong PE (see "Lifelong PE" section of this chapter) are not described in such detail in the ISSM definition of lifelong PE [14, 51] nor in the DSM-5 definition of PE [52] as, in general, a definition of a disorder cannot encompass all the detailed features of the disorder (see Table 18-1).

According to the ISSM definition, lifelong PE is defined as "a male sexual dysfunction characterized by ejaculation that always or nearly always occurs prior to or within about 1 min of vaginal penetration and the inability to delay ejaculation on all or nearly all vaginal penetrations, which results in negative personal consequences, such as distress, bother, frustration, and/or the avoidance of sexual intimacy [14, 51]. In contrast, in DSM 5 lifelong PE is not separately defined but PE is defined as "a persistent or recurrent pattern of ejaculation occurring during partnered sexual activity within

TABLE 18-1. DSM-5 Diagnostic Criteria for Premature Ejaculation 302.75 (F52.4)

A. A persistent or recurrent pattern of ejaculation occurring during partnered sexual activity within approximately 1 min following vaginal penetration and before the individual wishes it.
 Note: Although the diagnosis of premature (early) ejaculation may be applied to individuals engaged in nonvaginal sexual activities, specific duration criteria have not been established for these activities.
B. The symptom in Criterion A must have been present for at least 6 months and must be experienced on almost all or all (approximately 75–100%) occasions of sexual activity (in identified situational contexts or, if generalized, in all contexts).
C. The symptom in Criterion A causes clinically significant distress in the individual.
D. The sexual dysfunction is not better explained by a nonsexual mental disorder or as a consequence of severe relationship distress or other significant stressors and is not attributable to the effects of a substance/medication or another medical condition.

Specify whether:

Lifelong: The disturbance has been present since the individual became sexually active.

Acquired: The disturbance began after a period of relatively normal sexual function.

Specify whether:

Generalized: Not limited to certain types of stimulation, situations, or partners.

Situational: Only occurs with certain types of stimulation, situations, or partners.

Specify current severity:

Mild: Ejaculation occurring within approximately 30 seconds to 1 min of vaginal penetration.

Moderate: Ejaculation occurring within approximately 15–30 s of vaginal penetration.

Severe: Ejaculation occurring prior to sexual activity, at the start of sexual activity, or within approximately 15 s of vaginal penetration.

approximately 1 min following vaginal penetration and before the individual wishes it" [52]. Therefore the DSM-5 definition may perhaps erroneously indicate that also acquired PE occurs within about 1 min.

Erectio Praecox (Premature Erection) and Lifelong PE

Erectio praecox or premature erection is a clinically important and specific clinical feature of lifelong PE [4]. Men with erectio praecox get an erection "too early". This subtle symptom of lifelong PE has never been quoted in sexological literature until 2002, when Waldinger [2] reintroduced the term, thereby noting that many men with lifelong PE report this phenomenon either spontaneously or when asked for it. The phenomenon is so subtle, that men with lifelong PE may not be aware of it. It is not strange that it is noted by their female partner when she has had previous sexual experiences with men who did not have lifelong PE. However, until now there has not been any evidence based research into this remarkable and completely underreported clinical phenomenon, although we are currently investigating its occurrence in men with lifelong PE.

The Hypertonic Type Versus the Hypertonic State and Lifelong PE

Schapiro denoted Type B with erectio praecox as "*the sexually hypertonic or hypererotic type*" [4]. In contrast, he reported that Type A or "*the hypotonic type*" was often accompanied by erectile dysfunction [4].

Recently, Waldinger [8] noted that many men with lifelong PE report a very sudden increased arousal, facilitated erection and facilitated ejaculation as soon as they are engaged in erotic or intimate circumstances. Therefore, Waldinger preferred the word hypertonic "state" for this phenomenon, which is characteristic for the inner mental state of men with lifelong PE [8]. As soon as these men get involved in an erotic intimate situation, they are overwhelmed by an acute hypertonic state that starts with a facilitated erection (erectio praecox) and leads to an early ejaculation (ejaculatio praecox). The hypertonic or hypererotic state should not be confused with hypersexuality [8]. Hypersexuality is not a symptom of lifelong PE. The hypertonic or hypererotic state is a rather acute occurring physical sexual state that only occurs in situations of eroticism or making love.

Detumescentia Praecox (Premature Detumescence) and Lifelong PE

Recently, Waldinger [8] also noted a so far unknown clinical symptom in men with lifelong PE. He reported that a substantial number of men with lifelong PE experience a rather immediate and/or complete detumescence of the penis after an ejaculation [8]. Analogous to "ejaculatio praecox" and "erectio praecox", Waldinger denoted this as "detumescentia praecox" or "premature detumescence" [8]. Notably, he also reported that a substantial number of men with lifelong PE report difficulties in attaining a second erection after a premature ejaculation preventing them from a second intercourse [8]. It is as if they have difficulties becoming sexually aroused for the second time. This may be related to the psychological impact of disappointment and irritation from their early ejaculation, as is often thought by sexologists, but Waldinger suggested that this impairment is probably more related to a so far unknown underlying neurobiological mechanism that is related to the underlying neurobiological cause of the acute hypertonic state [8]. Interestingly, Waldinger also noted that daily use of 20 mg paroxetine in some men delays the penile detumescence in such a way that they are still able to thrust with a gradual diminishing erection [8]. In other words, in these men with lifelong PE 20 mg paroxetine does not lead to erectile dysfunction but prolongs erection for a very short time.

Classification into Four PE Subtypes According to Genital Tonus

By including the hypertonic state, erectio praecox and detumescentia praecox into the Four PE Subtype Classification, the separate characteristics of the four PE subtypes become more delineated. Lifelong PE is characterized by a hypertonic state. Acquired PE is characterized by a hypotonic state and Variable PE and Subjective PE are characterized by a normotonic state [28, 53]. Figure 18-1 shows the historical development of the classification of PE into four PE subtypes.

Adaptation of the Neurobiological Hypothesis

In 2014, Waldinger [8] noted that the new triad of "ejaculatio praecox", "erectio praecox" and "detumescentia praecox" as part of the acute "hypertonic or hypererotic" state of lifelong PE necessitates an adaptation of his neurobiological hypothesis of 1998 [26]. The hypertonic state indicates that lifelong PE is not only characterized by a diminished serotonergic neurotransmission and a disturbance of 5-HT_{1A} and 5-HT_{2C} receptor functioning causing a disturbed serotonergic modulation of the IELT [8]. Based on currently available neurobiological knowledge on ejaculation, erectile functioning, and sexual arousal, Waldinger speculated that lifelong PE—when characterized by an acute hypertonic phenotype—is mediated by a more complex interaction of the central nervous system, the peripheral nervous system and the endocrinological system [8, 28]. Therefore, it would have to include serotonergic and other neurotransmitter and endocrinological processes—e.g., increased oxytocinergic, and/or increased dopaminergic neurotransmission, decreased prolactinergic functioning and increased activity of gonadotrophic factors [8, 28]. Also involved is the peripheral nervous system, e.g., the sympathetic and parasympathetic nervous system [8, 28]. What needs to be investigated is any interaction between all these factors which may give rise to a very rapidly occurring "overactivated" or "hypertonic" state of the genital area in relation to the sense organs [8]. New neurobiological and pharmacological research is required to unravel the factors mediating this hypertonic state of lifelong PE. The remarkable phenomenon that SSRIs induce much less erectile dysfunction and decreased libido in men with lifelong PE compared to depressed patients without lifelong PE, may well be related to the fact that these drugs diminish the hypertonus state of erection, ejaculation and arousal toward a more "normal" state represented by "normal" sexual functioning [8].

In recent years, research into oxytocinergic, dopaminergic, and endocrinological factors related to PE has been conducted by a number of research groups [25, 54–58]. However, their attention has not been directed to the hypertonic state of lifelong PE. But hopefully, the integration of neurobiological

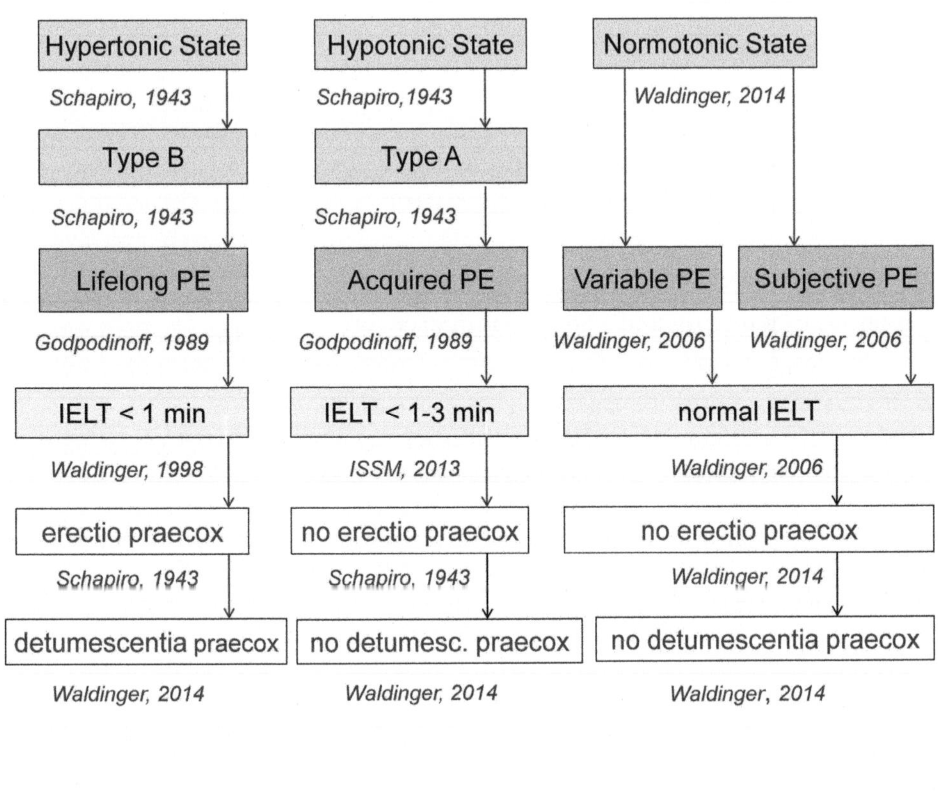

FIGURE 18-1. Classification of Four PE Subtypes. The classification by Waldinger [6, 8] is an extension of the original classification of Schapiro [4] and includes erectio praecox, that was originally reported by Schapiro but has been ignored for many decades. In this classification the hypertonic and hypotonic types of Schapiro have been renamed hypertonic state and hypotonic state. The two new subtypes Variable PE and Subjective PE are examples of a normotonic state with normal IELT values.

and endocrinological knowledge to elucidate the acute co-occurrence of premature ejaculation, premature erection, premature detumescence, and the acute hypererotic state, will become a new focus of research in the current decade [8].

Oxytocin, Erection, Ejaculation and Penile Detumescence

Although other factors may be involved, there are preliminary indications that the rather unknown phenomena of facilitated erection, premature ejaculation, and rapid penile detumescence are associated with an increased release of and/or increased receptor sensitivity to oxytocin [8].

Erection

The release of oxytocin from centrally projecting parvocellular neurons is well known to influence erection and, less clearly, ejaculation (for review see [54]). Increased oxytocinergic neurotransmission in the paraventricular hypothalamic nucleus (PVH) or hippocampus induces either an increase in the number of penile erections or an increase in intracavernous pressure, which is an indication of erection [54, 55].

Detumescence

On the other hand, some evidence indicates that peripherally injected oxytocin might have an inhibiting rather than stimulating effect on erection [54]. For example, systemic oxytocin treatment inhibited the increase in intracavernous pressure elicited by electrical stimulation of the cavernous nerve in rats, which could be prevented by an oxytocin antagonist [57]. It therefore appears that peripheral oxytocin receptors in the corpus cavernosum are involved in penile detumescence [54].

Ejaculation

After ejaculation, oxytocin levels are raised in the blood plasma in rabbits [59] and in the cerebrospinal fluid in rats [60].

Preliminary Pathophysiology of Premature Erection, Ejaculation and Penile Detumescence

In men, plasma oxytocin levels are elevated during sexual arousal, erection, and at the time of orgasm, although the degree of the elevation varies between different studies [61–64]. Taking together animal and human studies, oxytocin appears to play at least a modulating role in erection and ejaculation [65], and in male sexual behavior both peripheral and central oxytocin release seems to be involved [65]. In 2002, Waldinger et al. [2] hypothesized that erectio praecox in the context of lifelong PE may be associated with increased central oxytocin release during coitus as oxytocin facilitates erection and ejaculation. It may further be postulated that an increased peripheral release of oxytocin during ejaculation in men with lifelong PE may be associated with a quick penile detumescence [8].

Rating Scales

The diagnosis of PE and the diagnosis of the four PE subtypes are not difficult as long as one is interested in diagnosing PE and spend time (at least 30 min) to talk with the patient. Questionnaires on PE should never replace the face to face contact of the physician and his PE patient.

So far, five validated questionnaires have been developed and published to date [66]. Currently, there are two questionnaires that have extensive databases meeting most of the criteria for test development and validation: The Premature Ejaculation Profile (PEP) [67] and the Index of Premature Ejaculation (IPE) [68]. A third brief diagnostic measure (PEDT) has also been developed, has a modest database and is available for clinical use [69, 70]. Two other measures, The Arabic Index of Premature Ejaculation and Chinese Index of Premature Ejaculation [71, 72] have minimal validation or clinical trial data available [66]. Importantly, the aforementioned questionnaires are sensitive for complaints of PE, but are inadequate to diagnose any of the four PE subtypes. Therefore, new research for the development of PE Subtype specific questionnaires is warranted.

Premature Ejaculation Profile (PEP)

The PEP is a 4-question patient reported outcome (PRO) that asks a respondent about his subjective sense of control over ejaculation, distress related to PE, interpersonal difficulty and satisfaction with sexual intercourse [66]. Each question is answered on a 5-point Likert-type scale and an index score is derived by averaging the responses to the four questions. A limitation of the PEP is that the original validation of the PEP was based on the DSM-IV-TR PE criterion, which did not have an ejaculation time criterion. The authors of the PEP defined PE in terms of an IELT of less than 2 min [66].

Index of Premature Ejaculation (IPE)

The 10-item IPE was developed as a measure to evaluate sexual satisfaction, control and distress in men with PE [66]. Like the PEP, the initial validation of the IPE used men with a stopwatch assessed IELT of 2 min or less [66].

Premature Ejaculation Diagnostic Tool (PEDT)

The PEDT is a 5-item tool developed to systematically apply the DSM-IV-TR criteria in diagnosing the presence or absence of PE [66]. By employing a three tiered cutoff score it diagnoses PE (score < 8), possible PE (9 or 10), and no PE (>11). The PEDT works best as a screener for PE [66].

Dangers That Threaten Scientific Research of Lifelong PE

Ignoring the PE classification of Bernard Schapiro in lifelong and acquired PE is not solely a tragic phenomenon of the past. Even today the danger exists that long standing hard characteristics of lifelong PE and its accurate research are ignored or become distorted. For example, a cohort of men with lifelong PE usually includes about 90% of males who ejaculate within 1 min and about 10% of males who ejaculate within 1–2 min [13]. A distortion of these percentages will be formed by studies of lifelong PE in which substantially more than 10% of men ejaculate within 1–2 min and less than 90% ejaculate within 1 min. Therefore it is better for scientific research to only include men who ejaculate within about 1 min, on the condition that IELT is measured by a stopwatch. Another danger for scientific research of lifelong PE is formed when one only uses validated or non-validated questionnaires to measure the IELT. For example, recently Ventus et al. [73] argued on the basis of a retrospective questionnaire study among a very small sample of Finnish twins and patients that the term lifelong PE is probably inappropriate as very few participants subjectively reported a bit longer IELT duration on a questionnaire than at baseline questionnaire measurement ignoring the subjective and inaccurate way of their IELT assessment. The consequences of such attempts to ignore or distort the existence of lifelong PE extremely threatens the scientific research of PE in general and will enormously harm the patient with lifelong PE [74].

In an editorial, Waldinger [74] has recently expressed his concern on current research of Lifelong PE, noting that PE research seems more and more to become performed by clinically inexperienced individuals who do not talk to or see patients with PE, do not have clinical experience with PE patients, but who sit behind their PCs, play with statistical programs, try to intimidate clinicians and reviewers with validated questionnaires, selectively choose references, and omit or ignore important information that does not support their view. Particularly, ignoring the necessity of using a stopwatch for accurate IELT research, ignoring the IELT cutoff point of 1 min for inclusion of men with lifelong PE in a study, and with regard to genetic research ignoring the importance of Hardy Weinberg equilibrium endangers the evidence based clinical, pharmacological and genetic research of lifelong PE.

But not only that. Research of lifelong PE that is solely performed by validated questionnairs without face to face contact with a patient with lifelong PE ought to be discouraged [74]. Particularly, studies in which anonymous men are recruited by Internet and are solely investigated by validated questionnaires and become diagnosed as lifelong PE endanger objective research of lifelong PE.

The study of Ventus et al. [73] and the study of Zhu et al. [75] are good examples to which erroneous but catastrophic conclusions such studies can lead. For example, according to the study of Ventus et al. [73] the authors suggest that lifelong PE is an inappropriate diagnosis. And according to Zhu et al. [75] 5-HTTLPR is associated with lifelong PE and L alleles might protect the male against lifelong PE.

Fortunately, the serious limitations and erroneous conclusions of these studies have been reported by other authors [49, 74]. But nevertheless, research of lifelong PE remains endangered by studies that only use validated questionnaires, include anonymous patients, ignore the stopwatch and objective real-time measurement of the IELT.

In order to avoid publication of such potentially harmful articles, Waldinger [74] strongly advised clinicians, reviewers, and editors not to succumb to pressure of technocrats using statistics and questionnaires to understand patients.

Conclusion

For many years it has been thought that lifelong PE is only characterized by complaints of persistent early ejaculations. Both in vivo animal research and neurobiological, genetic, and pharmacological research in men with lifelong PE have much contributed to a better understanding of how the central and peripheral nervous system mediate ejaculation and contribute to persistent early ejaculations. However, our current understanding of the mechanisms behind early ejaculations is far from complete. The new classification of PE into four PE subtypes has much contributed to a better delineation of lifelong PE against acquired PE, subjective PE and variable PE. It has been shown that the symptomatology of lifelong PE strongly differs from the three other PE subtypes. The phenotype of lifelong PE and therefore also the pathophysiology of lifelong PE is much more complex than the phenotype of the three other PE subtypes. A substantial number of men with lifelong PE not only has premature ejaculation, but also premature erection and premature penile detumescence as part of an acute hypertonic or hypererotic state when engaged in an erotic situation or when making love. As both erectio praecox, ejaculatio praecox, detumescentia praecox, and the hypererotic state are part of the phenotype lifelong PE, it is argued that lifelong PE is not only a disturbance of the timing of ejaculation but also a disturbance of the timing of erection, penile detumescence and arousal. Since 1998, the pathophysiology of lifelong PE was thought to be mainly mediated by the central serotonergic system in line with genetic polymorphisms of certain serotonergic genes. However, by accepting that lifelong PE is not only a matter of a short IELT, but also characterized by a facilitated erection and facilitated penile detumescence as part of an acute but reversible hypertonic state, the hypothesis of mainly serotonergic dysfunction is no longer tenable. Instead, it has been postulated that the pathophysiology of lifelong PE is mediated by a very complex interplay of central and peripheral serotonergic, dopaminergic, oxytocinergic, endocrinological, genetic, and probably also epigenetic factors. The classification of PE into four PE subtypes is relevant for pharmacotherapy and counseling of men with complaints of PE. Progress in research of lifelong PE can only be accomplished when a stopwatch is used to measure the IELT and the cut-off point of 1 min for the definition of lifelong PE is maintained. Current use of validated questionnaires, neglect of stopwatch research, clinically inexperienced investigators, and inclusion of anonymous men in a study performed by the Internet endanger the continuation of objective research of lifelong PE and ought to be discouraged.

References

1. Gross S. Practical treatise on impotence and sterility. Edinburgh: YJ Pentland; 1887.
2. Waldinger MD. The neurobiological approach to premature ejaculation. J Urol. 2002;168:2359–67.
3. Waldinger MD. Lifelong premature ejaculation: from authority-based to evidence-based medicine. BJU Int. 2004;93:201–7.
4. Schapiro B. Premature ejaculation, a review of 1130 cases. J Urol. 1943;50:374–9.
5. Schapiro B. Präjaculin. Kombiniertes Epiphysen-Präparat gegen Reizzustände am Genitale und Hypererotismus. Hamburg: Chemische Farbrik Promonta G.m.b.H; 1932.
6. Waldinger MD. Recent advances in the classification, neurobiology and treatment of premature ejaculation. In: Balon R, editor. Sexual dysfunction. The brain-body connection. Advances in psychosomatic medicine, vol. 29. Basel: Karger; 2008. p. 50–69.
7. Godpodinoff ML. Premature ejaculation: clinical subgroups and etiology. J Sex Marital Ther. 1989;15:130–4.
8. Waldinger MD. Ejaculatio praecox, erectio praecox, and detumescentia praecox as symptoms of a hypertonic state in lifelong premature ejaculation: a new hypothesis. Pharmacol Biochem Behav. 2014;121:189–94.
9. Masters WH, Johnson VE. Premature ejaculation. In: Masters WH, Johnson VE, editors. Human sexual inadequacy. Boston: Little, Brown; 1970. p. 92–115.
10. Semans JH. Premature ejaculation: a new approach. South Med J. 1956;49:353.
11. Waldinger MD, Hengeveld MW, Zwinderman AH. Paroxetine treatment of premature ejaculation: a double-blind, randomized, placebo-controlled study. Am J Psychiatry. 1994;151:1377–9.
12. Waldinger MD. Towards evidence-based drug treatment research on premature ejaculation: a critical evaluation of methodology. Int J Impot Res. 2003;15:309–13.
13. Waldinger MD, Hengeveld MW, Zwinderman AH, Olivier B. An empirical operationalization study of DSM-IV diagnostic criteria for premature ejaculation. Int J Psychiatry Clin Pract. 1998;2:287–93.
14. Serefoglu EC, McMahon CG, Waldinger MD, Althof SE, Shindel A, Adaikan G, Becher EF, Dean J, Giuliano F, Hellstrom WJ, Giraldi A, Glina S, Incrocci L, Jannini E, McCabe M, Parish S, Rowland D, Segraves RT, Sharlip I, Torres LO. An evidence- based unified definition of lifelong and acquired premature ejaculation: report of the second International Society for Sexual Medicine Ad Hoc Committee for the Definition of Premature Ejaculation. J Sex Med. 2014;11:1423–41.
15. Waldinger MD, Quinn P, Dilleen M, Mundayat R, Schweitzer DH, Boolell M. A multi-national population survey of intravaginal ejaculation latency time. J Sex Med. 2005;2:492–7.
16. Waldinger MD, McIntosh J, Schweitzer DH. A five-nation survey to assess the distribution of the intravaginal ejaculatory latency time among the general male population. J Sex Med. 2009;6:2888–95.
17. Waldinger MD, Schweitzer DH. Changing paradigms from an historical DSM-III and DSM-IV view towards an evidence based definition of premature ejaculation. Part I: validity of DSM-IV-TR. J Sex Med. 2006;3:682–92.
18. Waldinger MD, Schweitzer DH. Changing paradigms from an historical DSM-III and DSM-IV view towards an evidence based definition of premature ejaculation. Part II: proposals for DSM-V and ICD-11. J Sex Med. 2006;3:693–705.
19. Waldinger MD, Schweitzer DH. The use of old and recent DSM definitions of premature ejaculation in observational studies: a contribution to the present debate for a new classification of PE in the DSM-V. J Sex Med. 2008;5:1079–87.
20. Waldinger MD. Premature ejaculation: different pathophysiologies and etiologies determine its treatment. J Sex Marital Ther. 2008;34:1–13.
21. Waldinger MD. History of premature ejaculation. In: Jannini EA, McMahon CG, Waldinger MD, editors. Premature ejaculation. From etiology to diagnosis and treatment. Italia: Springer-Verlag; 2013. p. 5–24.
22. Jannini EA, Lombardo F, Lenzi A. Correlation between ejaculatory and erectile dysfunction. Int J Androl. 2005;28(Suppl 2):40–5.
23. Carani C, Isidori AM, Granata A, Carosa E, Maggi M, Lenzi A, Jannini EA. Multicenter study on the prevalence of sexual symptoms in male hypo- and hyperthyroid patients. J Clin Endocrinol Metab. 2005;90:6472–9.
24. Screponi E, Carosa E, Di Stasi SM, Pepe M, Carruba G, Jannini EA. Prevalence of chronic prostatitis in men with premature ejaculation. Urology. 2001;58:198–202.
25. Corona G, Jannini EA, Vignozzi L, Rastrelli G, Maggi M. The hormonal control of ejaculation. Nat Rev Urol. 2012;9:508–19.
26. Waldinger MD, Berendsen HHG, Blok BFM, Olivier B, Holstege G. Premature ejaculation and serotonergic antidepressants-induced delayed ejaculation: the involvement of the serotonergic system. Behav Brain Res. 1998b;92:111–8.
27. Olivier B, van Oorschot R, Waldinger MD. Serotonin, serotonergic receptors, selective serotonin reuptake inhibitors and sexual behaviour. Int Clin Psychopharmacol. 1998;13(Suppl 6):S9–S14.
28. Waldinger MD. The pathophysiology of lifelong premature ejaculation. Transl Androl Urol. 2016;5:424–33.
29. Waldinger MD. Premature ejaculation: state of the art. Urol Clin North Am. 2007;34:591–9.

30. Saitz TR, Serefoglu EC. The epidemiology of premature ejaculation. Transl Androl Urol. 2016;5:409–15.
31. Serefoglu EC, Cimen HI, Atmaca AF, Balbay MD. The distribution of patients who seek treatment for the complaint of ejaculating prematurely according to the four premature ejaculation syndromes. J Sex Med. 2010;7:810–5.
32. Serefoglu EC, Yaman O, Cayan S, Asci R, Orhan I, Usta MF, Ekmekcioglu O, Kendirci M, Semerci B, Kadioglu A. The comparison of premature ejaculation assessment questionnaires and their sensitivity for the four premature ejaculation syndromes: results from the Turkish society of andrology sexual health survey. J Sex Med. 2011;8:1177–85.
33. Zhang X, Gao J, Liu J, Xia L, Yang J, Hao Z, Zhou J, Liang C. Distribution and factors associated with four premature ejaculation syndromes in outpatients complaining of ejaculating prematurely. J Sex Med. 2013;10:1603–11.
34. Gao J, Zhang X, Su P, Liu J, Xia L, Yang J, Shi K, Tang D, Hao Z, Zhou J, Liang C. Prevalence and factors associated with the complaint of premature ejaculation and the four premature ejaculation syndromes: a large observational study in china. J Sex Med. 2013;10:1874–81.
35. Janssen PKC, Waldinger MD. The mathematical formula of the intravaginal ejaculation latency time (IELT) distribution of lifelong premature ejaculation differs from the IELT distribution formula of men in the general male population. Investig Clin Urol. 2016;57:119–28.
36. Ahlenius S, Larsson K, Svensson L, Hjorth S, Carlsson A, Lindberg P, Wilkstrom H, Sanchez D, Arvidsson LE, Hacksell U, Nilsson JL. Effects of a new type of 5-HT receptor agonist on male rat sexual behavior. Pharmacol Biochem Behav. 1981;15:785–92.
37. Berendsen HH, Broekkamp CL. Drug-induced penile erections in rats: indications of serotonin1B receptor mediation. Eur J Pharmacol. 1987;135:279–87.
38. Foreman MM, Love RL, Hall JL. Effects of LY237733, a selective 5-HT2 receptor antagonist, on copulatory behavior of male rats. Soc Neurosci Abstr. 1988;14:374.
39. Waldinger MD. Risk factors in premature ejaculation: the genetic risk factor. In: Jannini EA, McMahon CG, Waldinger MD, editors. Premature ejaculation. From etiology to diagnosis and treatment. Italia: Springer-Verlag; 2013. p. 111–23.
40. Waldinger MD, Rietschel M, Nothen MM, Hengeveld MW, Olivier B. Familial occurrence of primary premature ejaculation. Psychiatr Genet. 1998c;8:37–40.
41. Janssen PK, Bakker SC, Réthelyi J, Zwinderman AH, Touw DJ, Olivier B, Waldinger MD. Serotonin transporter promoter region (5-HTTLPR) polymorphism is associated with the intravaginal ejaculation latency time in Dutch men with lifelong premature ejaculation. J Sex Med. 2009;6:276–84.
42. Janssen PKC, van Schaik R, Zwinderman AH, Olivier B, Waldinger MD. The 5-HT$_1$A receptor C(1019)G polymorphism influences the intravaginal ejaculation latency time in Dutch Caucasian men with lifelong premature ejaculation. Pharmacol Biochem Behav. 2014; 121:184–8.
43. Janssen PKC, van Schaik R, Olivier B, Waldinger MD. The 5-HT$_{2C}$ receptor gene Cys23Ser polymorphism influences the intravaginal ejaculation latency time in Dutch Caucasian men with lifelong premature ejaculation Asian J Androl 2014;16:607–10.
44. Jern P, Eriksson E, Westberg L. A reassessment of the possible effects of the serotonin transporter gene linked polymorphism 5-HTTLPR on premature ejaculation. Arch Sex Behav. 2013;42:45–9.
45. Zuccarello D, Ghezzi M, Pengo M, Forzan M, Frigo AC, Ferlin A, Foresta C. No difference in 5-HTTLPR and Stin2 Polymorphisms frequency between premature ejaculation patients and controls. J Sex Med. 2012;9:1659–68.
46. Safarinejad MR. Polymorphisms of the serotonin transporter gene and their relation to premature ejaculation in individuals from Iran. J Urol. 2009;181:2656–61.
47. Ozbek E, Tasci AI, Tugcu V, Ilbey YO, Simsek A, Ozcan L, Polat EC, Koksal V. Possible association of the 5-HTTLPR serotonin transporter promoter gene polymorphism with premature ejaculation in a Turkish population. Asian J Androl. 2009;11:351–5.
48. Luo SW, Wang F, Xie ZY, Huang XK, Lu YP. Study on the correlation of the 5-HTTLPR polymorphism with premature ejaculation in Han Chinese population. Beijing Da Xue Xue Bao. 2011;43:514–8.
49. Janssen PKC, Olivier B, Zwinderman AH, Waldinger MD. Measurement errors in polymerase chain reaction are a confounding factor for a correct interpretation of 5-HTTLPR polymorphism effects on lifelong premature ejaculation: a critical analysis of a previously published meta-analysis of six studies. PLoS One. 2014 Mar 3;9(3):e88031.
50. Jern P, Westberg L, Johansson A, Gunst A, Eriksson E, Sandnabba K, Santtila P. A study of possible associations between single nucleotide polymorphisms in the serotonin receptor 1A, 1B, and 2C genes and self-reported ejaculation latency time. J Sex Med. 2012;9:866–72.
51. McMahon CG, Althof S, Waldinger MD, Porst H, Dean J, Sharlip I, Adaikan PG, Becher E, Broderick GA, Buvat J, Dabees K, Giraldi A, Giuliano F, Hellstrom WJ, Incrocci L, Laan E, Meuleman E, Perelman MA, Rosen R, Rowland D, Segraves R. An evidence-based definition of lifelong premature ejaculation: report of the International Society for Sexual Medicine (ISSM) ad hoc committee for the definition of premature ejaculation. J Sex Med. 2008;5:1590–606.
52. American Psychiatric Association. Diagnostic and Statistical Manual of Mental Disorders (5th edition) (DSM-5). Washington, DC: American Psychiatric Association; 2013.
53. Waldinger MD. Pharmacotherapy for premature ejaculation. Expert Opin Pharmacother. 2015;16:2615–24.
54. de Jong TR, Veening JG, Olivier B, Waldinger MD. Oxytocin involvement in SSRI-induced delayed ejaculation: a review of animal studies. J Sex Med. 2007;4:14–28.
55. Melis MR, Argiolas A, Gessa GL. Oxytocin-induced penile erection and yawning: site of action in the brain. Brain Res. 1986;398:259–65.
56. Peeters M, Giuliano F. Central neurophysiology and dopaminergic control of ejaculation. Neurosci Biobehav Rev. 2008;32:438–53.
57. Chen K, Chang LS. Oxytocinergic neurotransmission at the hippocampus in the central neural regulation of penile erection in the rat. Urology. 2001;58:107–12.
58. Zhang XH, Filippi S, Vignozzi L, Morelli A, Mancina R, Luconi M, Donati S, Marini M, Vannelli GB, Forti G, Maggi M. Identification, localization and functional in vitro and in vivo activity of oxytocin receptor in the rat penis. J Endocrinol. 2005;184:567–76.
59. Stoneham MD, Everitt BJ, Hansen S, Lightman SL, Todd K. Oxytocin and sexual behaviour in the male rat and rabbit. J Endocrinol. 1985;107:97–106.
60. Hughes AM, Everitt BJ, Lightman SL, Todd K. Oxytocin in the central nervous system and sexual behaviour in male rats. Brain Res. 1987;414:133–7.
61. Uckert S, Becker AJ, Ness BO, Stief CG, Scheller F, Knapp WH, Jonas U. Oxytocin plasma levels in the systemic and cavernous blood of healthy males during different penile conditions. World J Urol. 2003;20:323–6.
62. Kruger TH, Haake P, Chereath D, Knapp W, Janssen OE, Exton MS, Schedlowski M, Hartmann U. Specificity of the neuroendocrine response to orgasm during sexual arousal in men. J Endocrinol. 2003;177:57–64.
63. Carmichael MS, Humbert R, Dixen J, Palmisano G, Greenleaf W, Davidson JM. Plasma oxytocin increases in the human sexual response. J Clin Endocrinol Metab. 1987;64:27–31.
64. Murphy MR, Seckl JR, Burton S, Checkley SA, Lightman SL. Changes in oxytocin and vasopressin secretion during sexual activity in men. J Clin Endocrinol Metab. 1987;65:738–41.

65. Waldinger MD. Premature ejaculation: definition and drug treatment. Drugs. 2007;67:547–68.
66. Althof SE. Patient reported outcomes in the assessment of premature ejaculation. Transl Androl Urol. 2016;5:470–4.
67. Patrick DL, Giuliano F, Ho KF, et al. The premature ejaculation profile: validation of self-reported outcome measures for research and practice. BJU Int. 2009;103:358–64.
68. Althof S, Rosen R, Symonds T, et al. Development and validation of a new questionnaire to assess sexual satisfaction, control, and distress associated with premature ejaculation. J Sex Med. 2006;3: 465–75.
69. Symonds T, Perelman MA, Althof S, et al. Development and validation of a premature ejaculation diagnostic tool. Eur Urol. 2007; 52:565–73.
70. Symonds T, Perelman M, Althof S, et al. Further evidence of the reliability and validity of the premature ejaculation diagnostic tool. Int J Impot Res. 2007;19:521–5.
71. Arafa M, Shamloul R. Development and evaluation of the Arabic Index of Premature Ejaculation (AIPE). J Sex Med. 2007;4:1750–6.
72. Yuan YM, Xin ZC, Jiang H, et al. Sexual function of premature ejaculation patients assayed with Chinese Index of Premature Ejaculation. Asian J Androl. 2004;6:121–6.
73. Ventus D, Ristila M, Gunst A, Karna A, Arver S, Piha J, Jern P. A longitudinal analysis of premature ejaculation symptoms raises concern regarding the appropriateness of a "lifelong" subtype. Eur Urol Focus. 2017 (in press).
74. Waldinger MD. Editorial. The danger that threatens current research of premature ejaculation: use of validated questionnaires, performing cnjuring tricks with statistics, and refusing to use real-time stopwatch measurements of the IELT. 2017 (in press).
75. Zhu L, Mi Y, You X, Wu S, Shao H, et al. A meta-analysis of the effects of the 5-hydroxytryptamine transporter gene-linked promoter region polymorphism on susceptibility to lifelong premature ejaculation. PLoS One. 2013;8(1):e54994.

19 Treatment of Premature Ejaculation

Marcel D. Waldinger

Introduction

In the 1920s, Bernard Schapiro developed Präjaculin, which was the first oral drug for the treatment of lifelong PE [1]. Präjaculin was produced by the German company Promonta in Hamburg from 1932 until the mid-1960s [1]. Therefore it is important to know that oral drug treatment for PE has been available since the first publications of PE in medical literature, even more than a decade before the first review article on PE was published by Schapiro in 1943 [2] and long before behavioral treatments were advocated as the first choice of treatment [3]. However, case reports of potential new drugs to delay ejaculation, such as monoamine oxidase inhibitors (MAOIs), mellaril, and clomipramine, started only to appear in the 1970s and 1980s. It was only after the introduction of the selective serotonin reuptake inhibitors (SSRIs) in the early 1990s that drug treatment of PE became revolutionized [4]. In those days, a lack of an operationalized definition of PE and the absence of an objective measure of the ejaculation time hampered a truly scientific approach to investigate the efficacy of drugs in delaying ejaculation.

Evidence-Based Approach to Treatment

Therefore, and in order to develop an evidence-based methodology and design of drug treatment research, Waldinger et al. [5] introduced in 1994 the intravaginal ejaculation latency time (IELT) as a standardized measure of the ejaculation time. The IELT was defined as the time between the start of intravaginal penetration and intravaginal ejaculation [5]. By definition the IELT of an ejaculation outside the vagina (ejaculatio ante portam) is zero. The most objective way to measure the IELT is the use of a stopwatch, handled by the female partner [6]. In order to compare the extent of ejaculation delay, it is required to measure the IELT with a stopwatch at each coitus in a baseline period for a few weeks when no medication is used and to measure it as well at each coitus in an active drug treatment period of a few weeks. By comparing the IELT values of both periods the extent of ejaculation delay is calculated. As the IELT values of one person may have outliers, the statistically best way to calculate this difference is to calculate the geometrical mean IELT of both the baseline period and the active treatment period [7]. After having calculated the geometric mean IELT of both periods, it is easy to finally calculate the fold-increase of the geometric mean IELT. The fold-increase (FI) of the geometric mean IELT = geometric mean IELT value at end of drug treatment/geometric mean IELT value at baseline [5].

A fold increase of 1 means that there is no ejaculation delay induced by a drug. Placebo-controlled studies have shown that a fold-increase of 1 to 2 is a placebo response [8]. Clinically relevant ejaculation delay usually occurs between a fold-increase of 4 to 5. But a fold-increase higher than 7 means a really relevant ejaculation delay [8].

Apart from this prospective stopwatch-mediated methodology to measure the IELT, the design of such drug treatment studies is only evidence-based when one performs a randomized, double-blinded, placebo-controlled research protocol [4]. And of course it is required that the participants of such a study are quite similar. For example, they should not drink alcohol before intercourse, they should not use other drugs that may affect ejaculation, and they should fulfill to a lot of other inclusion and other exclusion criteria.

Drug Treatment of PE

There are six major treatments of premature ejaculation; (1) daily use of SSRIs, (2) on-demand use of dapoxetine, (3) on-demand use of clomipramine, (4) on-demand use of topical local anesthetics, (5) on-demand use of tramadol, and (6) on-demand use of phophodiesterase type-5 inhibitors [8].

With the exception of dapoxetine, all these treatments are off-label [8]. Although daily SSRI treatment very effectively

W.W. IsHak (ed.), *The Textbook of Clinical Sexual Medicine*, DOI 10.1007/978-3-319-52539-6_19

delays ejaculation, none of the companies producing the SSRIs (paroxetine, fluoxetine, sertraline, citalopram, and escitalopram) has been interested to get a Food and Drug Administration (FDA) or European Medicine Agency (EMA) registration for the treatment of PE, as it was argued that it would acknowledge an unwanted sexual side effect of their antidepressant drug [9]. In 2005 the EMA has registered dapoxetine 30 mg and 60 mg, a fast acting SSRI, for the on-demand treatment of PE [10].

Daily Treatment with SSRIs

In scientific studies—but not in daily practice—the IELT has to be measured with a stopwatch. A substantial number of randomized, double-blind, placebo-controlled studies have shown the efficacy of daily SSRIs treatment in mentally healthy men with complaints of PE [8]. With exception of fluvoxamine the SSRIs exert a clinically relevant ejaculation delay [8].

A meta-analysis of daily SSRI treatment studies [8] revealed a rather low placebo-effect, e.g., a geometric mean 1.4-fold IELT increase (95% CI: 1.2–1.7). The meta-analysis also demonstrated a rank order of efficacy: (a) paroxetine 8.8 FI (95% CI: 5.9–13.2); (b) clomipramine 4.6 FI (3.0–7.4); (c) sertraline 4.1 FI (2.6–7.0), and (d) fluoxetine 3.9 FI (3.0–5.4). Thus, in general, daily SSRI treatment studies generate a 2.6–13.2 geometric mean IELT fold increase, dependent on the type of SSRI [8]. Moreover, of all SSRIs, daily use of 20 mg paroxetine exerts the strongest ejaculation delay in the investigated males. The meta-analysis also demonstrated that compared to stopwatch studies measuring the IELT, open and single-blind studies lead to exaggerated IELT values and that retrospective assessment of the IELT by a questionnaire or subjective report lead to far more variability of the IELTs [8].

The outcome data of the SSRI treatment studies published between 2003 and 2014 hardly distort the findings of the meta-analysis of 2004 and therefore its conclusions are still valid today [9, 11, 12].

Dosages of Daily SSRI Treatment

Daily treatment can be performed with paroxetine 20 mg, clomipramine 10–40 mg, sertraline 50–100 mg, fluoxetine 20 mg, citalopram 20 mg, and escitalopram 20 mg [13]. Ejaculation delay usually starts a few days after intake. However, a clinically relevant effect only gradually occurs within 1–3 weeks. Most often the delay continues to exist for years, as long as the SSRI is used, but sometimes it may disappear after 6–12 months. The cause of this tachyphylaxis has not yet been clarified [9, 12].

Daily SSRI treatment is effective in delaying ejaculation, but it does not delay ejaculation in every patient and in the same extent. Ejaculation delay occurs in 70–80% of men. In about 20% of men with lifelong PE, SSRIs do not have relevant ejaculation delaying effect. In such cases one may switch to another SSRI, but other SSRIs may not have an ejaculation-delaying effect either [12].

Advantages and Disadvantages of Daily SSRI Treatment

A clear advantage of daily SSRI treatment is that there is a delayed ejaculation at every spontaneous sexual event. Daily intake does not interfere with the spontaneity of sexual activity. However, a disadvantage is the risk of specific side effects on the short and long term, the risk of a discontinuation syndrome [14, 15], very rare side effects such as bleeding [16] and priapism [17, 18], effects on spermatozoa [19, 20] and very rare side effects such as restless genital syndrome (ReGS) in the male [21], and the extremely rare post SSRI sexual dysfunction (PSSD) [22, 23].

SSRI-Induced Side Effects

Side Effects on the Short Term

On the short-term fatigue, yawning, mild nausea, loose stools, or perspiration may occur. These side effects are usually mild, start in the first 1–2 weeks of treatment, and most often gradually disappear within 2–3 weeks [9, 12]. Although a head-to-head comparative study has not yet been performed, drug treatment studies seem to indicate that in contrast to the side-effects in depressed patients, diminished libido and erectile dysfunction occur less frequently and also to a lesser extent in healthy non-depressed men with lifelong PE [9, 12].

Side Effects on the Long Term

On the long term weight gain may occur, and sexual side effects. These sexual side effects are reversible, but in extremely rare cases they are irreversible [9].

SSRI Discontinuation Syndrome

Patients should be advised not to stop taking the SSRI acutely in order to prevent the occurrence of an SSRI discontinuation syndrome, which is characterized by symptoms like tremor, shock-like sensations when turning the head, nausea and dizziness [15]. One should inform the patient at the beginning that discontinuation of the treatment should be carried out very gradually within about 2 and sometimes even 3 months.

Interaction with Other Drugs of Substances

It is recommended that patients should diminish their use of alcohol particularly in the first weeks of SSRI treatment, as SSRIs may facilitate a "typsi" state [9]. Young men should be informed not to use XTC while taking an SSRI [9]. Its interaction may cause the potentially life-threatening serotonergic syndrome. Older men should be informed not to take tramadol as its interaction with an SSRI may also lead to a serotonergic syndrome. One should not prescribe SSRIs to men <18 years, and to men known with depressive disorder particularly when associated with suicidal thoughts. In those cases, referral to a psychiatrist is indicated.

Negative Effects of SSRIs on Spermatozoa

Particularly in young patients, one should inform the patients that hardly anything is known about the effect of SSRIs on spermatozoa, as research on this topic has hardly been performed [9]. However, a few small studies have shown potential harmful effects of SSRIs on spermatozoa [19, 20]. It is recommended that in case of a wish for pregnancy the male should not start SSRI treatment or when he is already using an SSRI for PE to gradually diminish the dosage of the SSRI and stop taking the drug for 3–4 months [9, 12]. As it takes quite some time for spermatozoa to be renewed, it is advised to make love with a condom for 3 to 4 months after discontinuation of the drug, after which pregnancy is allowed. Notably, this advice is not based on any hard evidence, but only to prevent possible problems in the future when it may perhaps appear that SSRIs used by the male, affect fertility or even may lead to congenital disorders.

Restless Genital Syndrome (ReGS) in the Male

In rare cases, decreasing the dosage of an SSRI or discontinuation of an SSRI may give rise to the Restless Genital Syndrome (ReGS) [21]. In males, ReGS is presumably caused by a sensoric neuropathy of the dorsal nerve of the penis, which is an end branch of the pudendal nerve [21]. ReGS in the male is characterized by persistent, unwanted, disturbing penile sensations of ejaculatory urgency, usually at the basis and top of the penis, in the absence of erection, sexual desire, and/or sexual arousal. However, often these men also report some sort of penile sexual arousal.

Post SSRI Sexual Dysfunction (PSSD)

Usually SSRI-induced sexual side effects are reversible, e.g., their intensity diminishes with dose reduction and they disappear within a few days after SSRI discontinuation. However, in extremely rare cases the sexual side effects are irreversible, e.g., after SSRI discontinuation they do not disappear [22, 23]. Recently, Waldinger distinguished two types of PSSD [23]. Characteristic of both types is the occurrence of penile anesthesia or numbness of the penis, which may be the first symptom of PSSD. Therefore, patients using SSRIs should be informed to stop taking the SSRI as soon as the patient experiences genital anesthesia [23]. PSSD may start within a few days to a few weeks after the start of SSRI treatment with complaints of sudden complete loss of libido, arousal, erection, and ejaculation with genital anesthesia, or it may become manifest after SSRI discontinuation as an aggravation of already existing moderate sexual side effects [23]. So far the pathophysiology and treatment of PSSD remains unclear.

On-Demand Treatment with Oral Drugs and Topical Anesthetics

On-demand treatment with oral drugs may also give rise to side effects or interactions with other drugs. Patients should be informed about the risk of a serotonergic syndrome in case serotonergic drugs (dapoxetine/tramadol) are taken together with other serotonergic drugs [9, 12].

Advantages and Disadvantages of On-Demand Drug Treatment

A clear advantage of on-demand oral drug treatment is that there is no risk of getting the side effects of long term drug treatment. Another advantage is that one can use the drug only when it is required for a better sexual performance. However a disadvantage is that on-demand oral drug treatment may negatively interfere with the spontaneity of sexual activity, particularly when one is inclined to have sex at the spur of the moment [9].

On-Demand Treatment with Dapoxetine

Dapoxetine hydrochloride is a short-acting SSRI. It inhibits serotonin reuptake in the synapse similar to all other SSRIs. However, this mechanism of action occurs faster after intake. Dapoxetine is the first drug that is registered by the EMA for on-demand treatment of PE [10, 24–28]. Dapoxetine (either 30 mg or 60 mg), should be taken 1–3 h prior to intercourse. Its efficacy and side effects have been investigated in more than 6000 patients. Although the extent of ejaculation delay is usually rather small, studies have shown a 3.6–4.5-fold increase, reporting also that dapoxetine may lead to satisfaction and more feelings of control in men with lifelong and acquired PE. In the studies performed dapoxetine showed a good safety profile and a reasonable prevalence of dose-dependent side effects. The most common side effects include nausea, dizziness and headache. Importantly, no SSRI discontinuation syndrome following abrupt withdrawal has been reported [28].

On-Demand Treatment with Clomipramine

On-demand use of clomipramine 10–40 mg is known to delay ejaculation in men with PE. Its efficacy has been investigated in a few studies [8]. Effective ejaculation delay occurs 6 hours after drug intake and also lasts about 6 h, e.g. until about 12 h after drug intake. The most common side effects include dry mouth, blurred vision, constipation and nausea. However, with on-demand treatment these side effects disappear within 1–2 days.

On-Demand Treatment with Topical Local Anesthetics

The use of topical local anesthetics is well established and is effective in delaying ejaculation in men with lifelong and acquired PE [29–34]. By diminishing the glans penis sensitivity it is argued that the spinal and cerebral input of sexually arousable impulses is reduced. However, unequivocal hard evidence for this hypothesis is not yet available.

Two recent meta-analyses confirmed the efficacy and low side effect profile of topical anesthetics [29, 30]. Too much application may cause penile hypesthesia, numbness or erectile difficulties. Transfer of the cream to the female partner may lead to vaginal numbness. To avoid such transfer, the use of a condom is recommended. Analysis of eight trials has shown the efficacy and safety of topical anesthetic treatment for lifelong PE [29, 30]. But despite these trials, a substantial number of men with lifelong PE and with IELTs of 5–30 s complain that local anesthetic sprays have not been effective in delaying ejaculation. These men may need stronger ejaculation delaying drugs such as daily or on-demand SSRIs or clomipramine. Particularly for men with subjective PE, the use of topical local anesthetics might be a good drug to delay ejaculation [9].

Currently, there are four local anesthetics for the treatment of PE: EMLA cream, TEMPE spray, Stud-100 spray and Promescent spray. However, these local anesthetics are not (yet) available in all countries of the world.

EMLA Cream

Eutectic Mixture of Local Anesthetics or EMLA cream is a local anesthetic cream containing 2.5% each of lidocaine and prilocaine. In order to reduce penile sensibility, EMLA cream should be applied approximately 20 min before sexual intercourse [31]. In order not to transfer the cream to the vagina it is advised to also use a condom.

TEMPE Spray

Topical Eutectic Mixture for Premature Ejaculation or TEMPE is a spray containing lidocaine and prilocaine in a metered-dose aerosol-transfer system specifically intended for the treatment of PE. The spray delivers 7.5 mg lidocaine and 2.5 mg prilocaine base per actuation, with three actuations being a standard dose. Patients have to apply the spray to the glans penis 10–15 min before intercourse. As the content of the spray rapidly penetrates the skin the use of a condom is not really necessary. Three randomized, double-blind, and placebo-controlled studies have shown its efficacy to delay ejaculation [32–34].

Stud 100 Spray

Being introduced in 1970, Stud 100 is the oldest topical anesthetic spray which is still on the market as an over the counter product. Stud Spray contains 9.6% w/w lidocaine presented as a metered aerosol spray delivering a dose of 7.7 mg lidocaine base per spray. The recommended dosage is three or more metered sprays with a maximum dose of 8 sprays (62 mg lidocaine).

Promescent Spray

Promescent is a lidocaine spray in a metered-dose delivery system. It is available in the USA and in Europe as an over the counter product. Each spray contains 10 mg of lidocaine in 130 microliters of product with three sprays being a standard dose and ten sprays as a maximal dose. The spray has to be applied at the glans penis 10–15 min before intercourse.

On-Demand Treatment with Tramadol

Three meta-analyses, albeit on a low number of studies, have supported the ejaculation delaying effect of on-demand use of tramadol 25 and 50 mg compared to placebo [35–37]. However, because of the potential risk of opioid addiction, one has to be very cautious for its use as treatment for PE.

On-Demand Treatment with Phosphodiesterase Type-5 Inhibitors

Phosphodiesterase type-5 (PDE-5) inhibitors are registered for the treatment of erectile dysfunction. Their use for the treatment of PE is controversial. According to a recent meta-analysis [38] the method and designs of studies are too insufficient hampering a generalized conclusion of their efficacy to delay ejaculation. However, in case of acquired PE due to erectile difficulties, the erectile dysfunction should be treated with a PDE-5 inhibitor [9].

Ejaculation Delaying Drugs Versus Drugs for Treatment of Premature Ejaculation

The prevalence data of the four PE subtypes has shown that only a minority of men who are not satisfied with their ejaculation suffer from lifelong and acquired PE. The rest are men with subjective and variable PE. Comparison of the ejaculation delaying properties of SSRIs and other drugs has become successful by using an often common methodology and design of studies, e.g., baseline measurements of the IELT, inclusion of men with an IELT of less than 1 min, stopwatch assessment of the IELT, calculation of the geometric mean IELT, and a randomized, placebo-controlled strategy [8]. The very short IELT of men with lifelong and acquired PE necessitated the use of a strict design as both oral and local anesthetic drugs have to show a high fold-increase in order to clinically relevantly delay ejaculation in these men [9]. As a result these drugs have been shown to be “drugs for the treatment of premature ejaculation”. They disrupt the 5-HT equilibrium at the synapse of central serotonergic neurons. However, Waldinger [9] recently argued that as men with subjective and variable PE experience normal IELT values, it should not be required for a drug—meant for these men—to possess the same strong pharmacological ability for producing a very high fold-increase of the baseline IELT, as is required for a drug for lifelong and acquired PE. Accepting this pharmacological view means that the methodology and design of studies for drugs for subjective and variable PE may differ from those of lifelong and acquired PE. This may also become illustrated when one starts to use the term "ejaculation delaying drugs" to differentiate them from "drugs for the treatment of PE", as both subjective and variable PE with normal IELTs significantly differ from the short IELT of lifelong and acquired PE IELTs [8]. Moreover, and importantly, Waldinger [9] argued that ejaculation delaying drugs should be investigated in men with normal IELT values, for example in men with subjective or variable PE but also in male volunteers with normal IELTs. This item has not yet had the required attention of both clinicians and pharmaceutical companies, probably because only lifelong PE and acquired PE are officially recognized as PE disorders by the DSM 5.

Still, there is a need for ejaculation delaying drugs for men with normal IELT values who wish to have a more pleasurable sexual performance. For example, in an epidemiological stopwatch study in five countries, a considerable number of men with normal IELT values who did not have sought medical treatment for PE and had no complaints of PE wanted to delay their ejaculation by medication, when available [39]. These men may have subjective PE or variable PE or even no PE but a desire to just have more control over their ejaculation. So far, hardly any research has been performed in the latter men, as they do not seek medical treatment.

Psychosocial Treatment

In 1956, James Semans described a behavioral intervention, the so-called stop-start technique, to control premature ejaculation [40]. By this technique sexual stimulation of the penis is paused at impeding ejaculation.

In 1970, Masters and Johnson offered a slight variation of Semans technique, which they called the squeeze technique [41]: withdrawal and squeeze of the frenulum of the penis, resulting in a partial loss of erection and total loss of the urge to ejaculate.

In both techniques the man is first sexually stimulated, and then just before ejaculation either the stimulation is halted (Semans) or the penis is squeezed below the frenulum (Masters and Johnson). Both techniques are usually applied in a graduated fashion, starting with masturbation and proceeding through manual stimulation by a partner to active thrusting during intercourse. For many years this was the most common approach to treat PE. Other therapeutic techniques, such as sensate focus exercises, communication training, education, reducing distracting cognitions, and reducing performance demands, have also been used. However, the explanations for the mechanisms by which these techniques are believed to delay ejaculation are vague. Moreover, evidence based studies of the level of the many drug treatment studies have hardly been performed on the behavioral techniques used to treat PE and have not shown a similar objective outcome of ejaculation delay. Nevertheless, psycho-education and counseling are essential for every patient who seeks medical treatment.

Conclusion

The classification of PE into four PE subtypes is relevant for pharmacotherapy, psycho-education and counseling of men with complaints of PE. Various drugs are currently available for the treatment of PE, but all of them, except dapoxetine, are off-label. Of all drugs, daily use of paroxetine 20 mg exerts the strongest ejaculation delay. However, daily use of SSRIs has various side effects, and particularly the irreversible but extremely rare side effect of PSSD should make one cautious with their off-label use to treat lifelong or acquired PE. On the other hand, one may use on-demand oral drugs. Of those, clomipramine 20–30 mg taken 6 h prior to sexual activity seems to be quite effective in delaying ejaculation. For subjective PE that is characterized by normal IELT values, topical local anesthetics seem to become the first choice of treatment. And obviously, any drug treatment of PE requires that prior to prescription the patient is informed about all possible side effects of the various drugs including the very rare side effects.

References

1. Schapiro B. Präjaculin. In: Kombiniertes Epiphysen-Präparat gegen Reizzustände am Genitale und Hypererotismus. Hamburg: Chemische Farbrik Promonta G.m.b.H; 1932.
2. Schapiro B. Premature ejaculation, a review of 1130 cases. J Urol. 1943;50:374–9.
3. Waldinger MD. Commentary: underlying principles in ejaculatory and orgasmic function and dysfunction in the male. In: Lipshultz LI, Pastuszak AW, Goldstein AT, Giraldi A, Perelman MA, editors. Management of sexual dysfunction in men and women: an interdisciplinary approach. New York: Springer Science + Business Media; 2016. p. 133–37.
4. Waldinger MD. The neurobiological approach to premature ejaculation. J Urol. 2002;168:2359–67.
5. Waldinger MD, Hengeveld MW, Zwinderman AH. Paroxetine treatment of premature ejaculation: a double-blind, randomized, placebo-controlled study. Am J Psychiatry. 1994;151:1377–9.
6. Waldinger MD, Hengeveld MW, Zwinderman AH, Olivier B. An empirical operationalization study of DSM-IV diagnostic criteria for premature ejaculation. Int J Psychiatry Clin Pract. 1998;2:287–93.

7. Waldinger MD, Zwinderman AH, Olivier B, Schweitzer DH. Geometric mean IELT and premature ejaculation: appropriate statistics to avoid overestimation of treatment efficacy. J Sex Med. 2008;5:492–9.
8. Waldinger MD, Zwinderman AH, Schweitzer DH, et al. Relevance of methodological design for the interpretation of efficacy of drug treatment of premature ejaculation: a systematic review and meta-analysis. Int J Impot Res. 2004;16:369–81.
9. Waldinger MD. Pharmacotherapy for premature ejaculation. Expert Opin Pharmacother. 2015;16:2615–24.
10. Pryor JL, Althof SE, SteidLE C, et al. Dapoxetine Study Group. Efficacy and tolerability of dapoxetine in treatment of premature ejaculation: an integrated analysis of two double-blind, randomised controlled trials. Lancet. 2006;368(9539):929–37.
11. Waldinger MD. The pathophysiology of lifelong premature ejaculation. Transl Androl Urol. 2016;5:424–33.
12. Waldinger MD. Premature ejaculation: definition and drug treatment. Drugs. 2007;67:547–68.
13. Althof SE, McMahon CG, Waldinger MD, Serefoglu EC, Shindel AW, Adaikan PG, Becher E, Dean J, Giuliano F, Hellstrom WJ, Giraldi A, Glina S, Incrocci L, Jannini E, McCabe M, Parish S, Rowland D, Segraves RT, Sharlip I, Torres LO. An update of the international society of sexual medicine's guidelines for the diagnosis and treatment of premature ejaculation (PE). J Sex Med. 2014 Jun;2(2):60–90.
14. Ditto KE. SSRI discontinuation syndrome; awareness as an approach to prevention. Postgrad Med. 2003;114:79–84.
15. Black K, Shea C, Dursun S, Kutcher S. Selective serotonin reuptake inhibitor discontinuation syndrome: proposed diagnostic criteria. J Psychiatry Neurosci. 2003;25:255–61.
16. Weinrieb RM, Auriacombe M, Lynch KG, Lewis JD. Selective serotonin re-uptake inhibitors and the risk of bleeding. Expert Opin Drug Saf. 2005;4:337–44.
17. Ahmad S. Paroxetine-induced priapism. Arch Intern Med. 1995;155:645.
18. Rand EH. Priapism in a patient taking sertraline. J Clin Psychiatry. 1998;59:538.
19. Koyuncu HH, Serefoglu EC, Yencilek E, Atalay H, Akbas N, Sarica K. Escitalopram treatment for premature ejaculation has a negative effect on semen parameters. Int J Impot Res. 2011;23:257–61.
20. Koyuncu H, Serefoglu EC, Ozdemir AT, Hellstrom WJ. Deleterious effects of selective serotonin reuptake inhibitor treatment on semen parameters in patients with lifelong premature ejaculation. Int J Impot Res. 2012;24:171–3.
21. Waldinger MD, Venema PL, van Gils AP, de Lint GJ, Schweitzer DH. Stronger evidence for small fiber sensory neuropathy in restless genital syndrome: two case reports in males. J Sex Med. 2011 Jan;8(1):325–30.
22. Csoka AB, Bahrick AS, Mehtonen OP. Persistent sexual dysfunction after discontinuation of selective serotonin reuptake inhibitors (SSRIs). J Sex Med. 2008;5:227–33.
23. Waldinger MD, van Coevorden RS, Schweitzer DH, Georgiadis J. Penile anesthesia in Post SSRI Sexual Dysfunction (PSSD) responds to low-power laser irradiation: a case study and hypothesis about the role of transient receptor potential (TRP) ion channels. Eur J Pharmacol. 2015;753:263–8.
24. Buvat J, Tesfaye F, Rothman M, et al. Dapoxetine for the treatment of premature ejaculation: results from a randomized, double-blind, placebo-controlled phase 3 trial in 22 countries. Eur Urol. 2009; 55:957–67.
25. McMahon C, Kim SW, Park NC, et al. Dapoxetine 3003 Study Investigators. Treatment of premature ejaculation in the Asia-Pacific region: results from a phase III double-blind, parallel-group study of dapoxetine. J Sex Med. 2010;7(1 Pt 1):256–68.
26. Kaufman JM, Rosen RC, Mudumbi RV, et al. Treatment benefit of dapoxetine for premature ejaculation: results from a placebo-controlled phase III trial. BJU Int. 2009;103:651–8.
27. McMahon CG, Althof SE, Kaufman JM, et al. Efficacy and safety of dapoxetine for the treatment of premature ejaculation: integrated analysis of results from five phase 3 trials. J Sex Med. 2011;8:524–39.
28. Mirone V, Arcaniolo D, Rivas D, et al. PAUSE study team. Results from a prospective observational study of men with premature ejaculation treated with dapoxetine or alternative care: the PAUSE study. Eur Urol. 2014;65:733–9.
29. Xia JD, Han YF, Zhou LH, Chen Y, Dai YT. Efficacy and safety of local anaesthetics for premature ejaculation: a systematic review and meta-analysis. Asian J Androl. 2013 Jul;15(4):497–502.
30. Pu C, Yang L, Liu L, et al. Topical anesthetic agents for premature ejaculation: a systematic review and meta-analysis. Urology. 2013;81:799–804.
31. Busato W, Galindo CC. Topical anaesthetic use for treating premature ejaculation: a double-blind, randomized, placebo-controlled study. BJU Int. 2004;93:1018–21.
32. Dinsmore WW, Hackett G, Goldmeier D, et al. Topical eutectic mixture for premature ejaculation (TEMPE): a novel aerosol-delivery form of lidocaine-prilocaine for treating premature ejaculation. BJU Int. 2007;99:369–75.
33. Dinsmore WW, Wyllie MG. PSD502 improves ejaculatory latency, control and sexualsatisfactionwhenappliedtopically 5minbeforeintercourse in men with premature ejaculation: results of a phase III, multicentre, double-blind, placebo-controlled study. BJU Int. 2009;103:940–9.
34. Carson C, Wyllie M. Improved ejaculatory latency, control and sexual satisfaction when PSD502 is applied topically in men with premature ejaculation: results of a phase III, double-blind, placebo-controlled study. J Sex Med. 2010;7:3179–89.
35. Wu T, Yue X, Duan X, Luo D, et al. Efficacy and safety of tramadol for premature ejaculation: a systematic review and meta-analysis. Urology. 2012;80:618–24.
36. Yang L, Qian S, Liu H, Liu L, Pu C, Han P, Wei Q. Role of tramadol in premature ejaculation: a systematic review and meta-analysis. Urol Int. 2013;91(2):197–205.
37. Martyn-St James M, Cooper K, Kaltenthaler E, Dickinson K, Cantrell A, Wylie K, Frodsham L, Hood C. Tramadol for premature ejaculation: a systematic review and meta-analysis. BMC Urol. 2015;15(1):6.
38. Asimakopoulos AD, Miano R, FinazziAgrò E, et al. Does current scientific and clinical evidence support the use of phosphodiesterase type 5 inhibitors for the treatment of premature ejaculation? A systematic review and meta-analysis. J Sex Med. 2012;9:2404–16.
39. Waldinger MD, Schweitzer DH. The use of old and recent DSM definitions of premature ejaculation in observational studies: a contribution to the present debate for a new classification of PE in the DSM-V. J Sex Med. 2008;5:1079–87.
40. Semans JH. Premature ejaculation: a new approach. South Med J. 1956;49:353–7.
41. Masters WH, Johnson VE. Premature ejaculation. In: Masters WH, Johnson VE, editors. Human sexual inadequacy. Boston: Little, Brown; 1970. p. 92–115.

20 Evaluation of Genito-Pelvic Pain/Penetration Disorder

Alessandra Graziottin and Dania Gambini

Introduction

Doctor, I can't have intercourse because it hurts! This complaint, with different wordings, is reported by 14% of European women, up to 21% of USA. This means that every day, every gynaecologist or sexual health provider worldwide consults at least 2–4 women complaining of pain at intercourse (or coital pain). Physicians used to define it as "*dyspareunia*," from the Greek: *painful intercourse*.

According to the vaginal site where coital pain is elicited/perceived, the classic medical wording is "*introital dyspareunia*" when pain is perceived at the entrance of the vagina, and "*deep dyspareunia*" when pain is felt more intense deep in the vagina.

Current definitions have changed into genito-pelvic pain/penetration disorder (GPPPD) [1], more comprehensive from the descriptive point of view but too complicated in the clinical dialog with the patient. A more simple "painful intercourse" is easier and direct to the point [2, 3].

Unfortunately this complaint is still neglected or dismissed as a minor nuisance in too many clinical consultations. Women are told that pain is usually in their head and that they should consult a psychologist or a psychosexologist.

Opposite to this wrong belief, pain is rarely purely psychogenic, and coital pain/dyspareunia is no exception. Like all pain syndromes, it usually has one or more biological etiologic factors that can be differentiated according to the woman's hormonal status and the site of pain. The etiology of dyspareunia is complex [4, 5]. Coital pain can be understood as the pain-dominated perception of a mosaic of interacting factors. Sexual pain disorders can therefore be considered as multifactorial, multisystemic, and complex :

Multifactorial: biological, psychosexual, and relational factors can coexist in a woman complaining of coital pain. Over time, these different factors may act as predisposing, precipitating, or perpetuating sexual pain disorders. The multifactorial nature of dyspareunia implies the need for a "dynamic" diagnosis, considering both the natural history of the sexual complaint and interacting factors. Listening carefully to the woman's report and narrative of her sexual pain complaint will prove extremely rich of insights into the etiology and pathophysiology of pain, provided that the physician, while listening, keeps very activated the pertinent diagnostic "files" [6–10].

Multisystemic: sexual function involves the nervous, endocrine, vascular, muscular, and immunological systems and the integrity of the vaginal ecosystem. Thus the pathophysiology of coital pain also involves these various biological systems [11, 12].

Complex: the overall experience of satisfying sexual function is greater than the sum of each physical or emotional factor. Similarly, the experience of coital pain is greater than the simple peripheral tissue damage that may initially trigger the nociceptive component (experienced through pain receptors) of coital pain. When GPPPD becomes chronic, the pathophysiology of pain may gradually shift from nociceptive, a friend signal that should induce self protection and defense, to neuropathic, a disease of the pain system per se, with a progressive involvement of the central nervous system [13–15].

Definition of Different Conditions Contributing to GPPPD

Pain at intercourse or GPPPD is frequently the symptomatic sexual tip of the iceberg of vulvar pain (**vulvodynia**) that can involve all the organ vulva or part of it.

When pain at intercourse is complained of at the entrance (*vestibulum*, in Latin) of the vagina the descriptive term is "provoked vestibulodynia," while the term "vulvar vestibulitis" is more descriptive of its inflammatory component.

When pain is referred at clitoral level, "clitoralgia" or "clitorodynia" are the most frequently used descriptive terms.

W.W. IsHak (ed.), *The Textbook of Clinical Sexual Medicine*, DOI 10.1007/978-3-319-52539-6_20

Table 20-1. Degree of vaginismus, evaluated in a gynecological setting (grades)

Severity of vaginismus (grades)	
I	Spasm of the levator ani, that disappears with patient's reassurance
II	Spasm of the levator ani, that persists during the gynecologic examination
III	Spasm of the levator ani and buttock's tension at any tentative of gynecologic examination
IV	Mild neurovegetative arousal, spasm of the elevator, dorsal arching, thighs adduction, defense and retraction
VO	Extreme defense and neurovegetative arousal, with refusal of the gynecologic examination

[Based on data from Lamont JA, Vaginismus. Am J Obstet Gyn. 1978; 131: 632].

Table 20-2. Biological factors contributing to maintain vaginal "habitability"

- Normal trophism, i.e., healthy introital mucosa and vulvar skin
- Adequate hormonal impregnation, with estrogen (vagina) and testosterone (vulva and vagina)
- Normal tonicity of the perivaginal muscles, levator ani first
- Vascular, connective, and neurological integrity
- Normal local immune response
- No signs or symptoms of inflammation, particularly at the introitus

[Modified from Graziottin A, Murina F. Vulvodynia and Dyspareunia - How Should they be Addressed? In: Graziottin A, Murina F (eds). Vulvodynia tips and tricks. Milan, Italy: Springer-Verlag; 2011: 15–27. With permission from Springer Verlag].

Vulvodynia is a diagnostic term referring to chronic pain in the vulvar area of at least 3–6 months duration. This comprehensive word includes heterogeneous vulvar conditions, with different etiologies and pathophysiologies, and a common symptom: an invalidating, chronic vulvar pain.

Definitions of vulvodynia have varied widely, mirroring the difficulties in understanding and substantiating the biological truth and pathophysiology behind vulvar pain. Vulvodynia (vulvar pain) and dyspareunia (painful intercourse) are closely related: for anatomic, functional, pathophysiologic, emotional, and relational reasons. Definitions of dyspareunia and vaginismus, also named "sexual pain disorders" have varied in the last years [16].

Dyspareunia defines the persistent or recurrent pain with attempted or complete vaginal entry and/or penile vaginal intercourse.

Vaginismus indicates the persistent or recurrent difficulties of the woman to allow vaginal entry of a penis, a finger, and/or any object, despite the woman's expressed wish to do so. There is often (phobic) avoidance and anticipation/fear/experience of pain, along with variable involuntary pelvic muscle contraction (Table 20-1). Structural or other physical abnormalities must be ruled out/addressed.

Vaginal receptiveness is a prerequisite for intercourse, and requires anatomical and functional tissue integrity, both in resting and aroused states. Necessary biological conditions to guarantee vaginal "habitability" are indicated in Table 20-2. Vaginal receptiveness may be further modulated by psychosexual, mental, and interpersonal factors, all of which may result in poor arousal with vaginal dryness [16].

Fear of penetration, and a general muscular arousal secondary to anxiety, may cause a defensive contraction of the perivaginal muscles, leading to lifelong vaginismus.

Classification of Vulvar Pain

For more than a decade it was used the 2003 International Society for the Study of Vulvovaginal Disease (ISSVD) terminology as a guide to diagnosing vulvar pain (see Table 20-3) [1].

Table 20-3. 2003 ISSVD terminology and classification of vulvar pain

A. Vulvar pain related to a specific disorder
  1. Infectious (candidiasis, herpes, etc.)
  2. Inflammatory (lichen planus, immunobullous disorders, etc.)
  3. Neoplastic (Paget disease, squamous cell carcinoma, etc.)
  4. Neurologic (herpes neuralgia, spinal nerve compression, etc.)

B. Vulvodynia
  1. Generalized
     (a) Provoked (sexual, nonsexual, or both)
     (b) Unprovoked
     (c) Mixed (provoked and unprovoked)
  2. Localized (vestibulodynia, clitorodynia, hemivulvodynia, etc.)
     (a) Provoked (sexual, nonsexual, or both)
     (b) Unprovoked
     (c) Mixed (provoked and unprovoked)

[Reprinted from Bornstein J, Goldstein AT, Stockdale CK, Bergeron S, Pukall C, Zolnoun D, Coady D; consensus vulvar pain terminology committee of the International Society for the Study of Vulvovaginal Disease (ISSVD).; International Society for the Study of Women's Sexual Health (ISSWSH).; International Pelvic Pain Society (IPPS). 2015 ISSVD, ISSWSH, and IPPS Consensus Terminology and Classification of Persistent Vulvar Pain and Vulvodynia. J Sex Med.2016;13(4): 607–12. With permission from Elsevier].

The 2003 terminology divides vulvar pain into the following two overarching categories: vulvar pain related to a specific disorder, and vulvodynia, defined as "vulvar discomfort, most often described as burning pain, occurring in the absence of relevant visible findings or a specific, clinically identifiable, neurologic disorder".

Since 2003, the category of "identifiable causes" for vulvar pain has evolved substantially, as have factors "potentially associated" with vulvodynia. Vulvodynia is likely not one disease but a constellation of symptoms of several (sometimes overlapping) disease processes, which will benefit best from a range of treatments based on individual presentation [17, 18]. The vulvar organ can therefore be differently affected.

In 2015, the International Society for the Study of Vulvovaginal Disease, the International Society for the Study of Women's Sexual Health, and the International Pelvic Pain Society adopted a new vulvar pain and vulvodynia terminology

TABLE 20-4. 2015 Consensus terminology and classification of persistent vulvar pain and vulvodynia

A. Vulvar pain caused by a specific disorder[a]
- Infectious (e.g., recurrent candidiasis, herpes)
- Inflammatory (e.g., lichen sclerosus, lichen planus, immunobullous disorders)
- Neoplastic (e.g., Paget disease, squamous cell carcinoma)
- Neurologic (e.g., postherpetic neuralgia, nerve compression, or injury, neuroma)
- Trauma (e.g., female genital cutting, obstetrical)
- Iatrogenic (e.g., postoperative, chemotherapy, radiation)
- Hormonal deficiencies (e.g., genitourinary syndrome of menopause [vulvovaginal atrophy], lactational amenorrhea)

B. Vulvodynia—vulvar pain of at least 3 months' duration, without clear identifiable cause, which may have potential associated factors. The following are the descriptors:
- Localized (e.g., vestibulodynia, clitorodynia) or generalized or mixed (localized and generalized)
- Provoked (e.g., insertional, contact) or spontaneous or mixed (provoked and spontaneous)
- Onset (primary or secondary)
- Temporal pattern (intermittent, persistent, constant, immediate, delayed)

[a]Women may have both a specific disorder (e.g., lichen sclerosus) and vulvodynia.

[Reprinted from Bornstein J, Goldstein AT, Stockdale CK, Bergeron S, Pukall C, Zolnoun D, Coady D; consensus vulvar pain terminology committee of the International Society for the Study of Vulvovaginal Disease (ISSVD).; International Society for the Study of Women's Sexual Health (ISSWSH).; International Pelvic Pain Society (IPPS). 2015 ISSVD, ISSWSH, and IPPS Consensus Terminology and Classification of Persistent Vulvar Pain and Vulvodynia. J Sex Med.2016;13(4): 607–12. With permission from Elsevier].

that acknowledges the complexity of the clinical presentation and pathophysiology involved in vulvar pain and vulvodynia, and incorporates new information derived from evidence-based studies conducted since the last terminology.

The 2015 terminology of vulvar pain reflects key developments in understanding vulvar disorders and chronic pain over the recent years. The main difference between the 2015 terminology and the 2003 terminology is the addition of "potential associated factors" [1]. The inclusion of the associated factors emphasizes that treatment should be chosen according to the characteristics of the individual case and the possible associated factors, rather than as a "one-size-fits-all" approach (see Table 20-4).

Epidemiology of Dyspareunia/Coital Pain and Associated Comorbidities

Vulvodynia is not a rare condition: many studies now suggest that up to 15% of gynecologic clinic populations have the disorder at any given time [19]. Up to 14-million women are affected with vulvodynia at some point during their lifetimes, and the condition accounts for 10-million doctor visits annually. Results from research on the epidemiology (the study of the distribution and causes) of vulvodynia have helped to clarify the magnitude of the problem. Its frequency is underestimated partially because not recognized by doctors (some physicians dismiss this problem as psychological and relatively unimportant), and also because many affected women are reluctant to discuss their symptoms, which are perceived as unusual and possibly "all in the head."

Dyspareunia is the word currently more used in the epidemiological research when pain as intercourse is considered. Prevalence of dyspareunia is 14% in Europe (Figure 20-1) with data collected from a mail survey (Women's International Sexuality and Health Survey [WISHeS] Study) of 2467 women aged 20–70 years from Germany, UK, France and Italy and USA, where coital pain is reported by 21% of women aged 18–55 years of age (Figure 20-2).

Other researches indicate a prevalence of 16%: as indicated by a 2001 study of women in the Boston area, chronic burning, knifelike pain, or pain on contact that lasted at least 3 months or longer in the lower genital tract occurred frequently. These symptoms were reported by White, African-American, and Hispanic women of all ages, and nearly 40% of these women chose not to seek treatment. Of the women who sought treatment, 60% saw three or more doctors. These researchers estimate that up to 16% of women will experience symptoms consistent with vulvodynia in their lifetimes. The incidence of symptom onset was highest between the ages of 18 and 25 and lowest after age 35. Compared to controls, women with vulvar pain were seven times more likely to report difficulty and pain with their first tampon use. Almost 40% never sought medical care; 60% of those who sought medical care reported visiting more than three providers to receive a diagnosis and 40% remained undiagnosed after three medical consults. Although the reproductive age was the most affected, it was found that almost 4% of women between the ages of 45 and 54, and another 4% aged 55 to 64 years, reported burning or knifelike vulvar pain or pain on contact; in 50% of cases, pain limited sexual intercourse [22]. Lifelong mild vaginismus contributing to lifelong dyspareunia may occur in 10–15% of women.

Compared to controls, women with vulvodynia were significantly more likely to report chronic medical conditions, including bladder pain syndrome/interstitial cystitis (BPS/IC), fibromyalgia and irritable bowel syndrome. It was estimated that among women with urologist diagnosed IC, more than half (51.4%) were diagnosed with vulvodynia. This strong link may be related to a common etiology for these two conditions. The vulva and bladder are both derived from the embryonic urogenital sinus and share common sacral nerve innervation pathways. Conditions that affect the bladder may therefore lead to symptoms in the vulva, and vice versa [23]. Between 12 and 68% of patients diagnosed with BPS/IC report vulvodynia symptoms [24].

Current available epidemiological data do not differentiate between introital and deep dyspareunia, nor in terms of leading etiology.

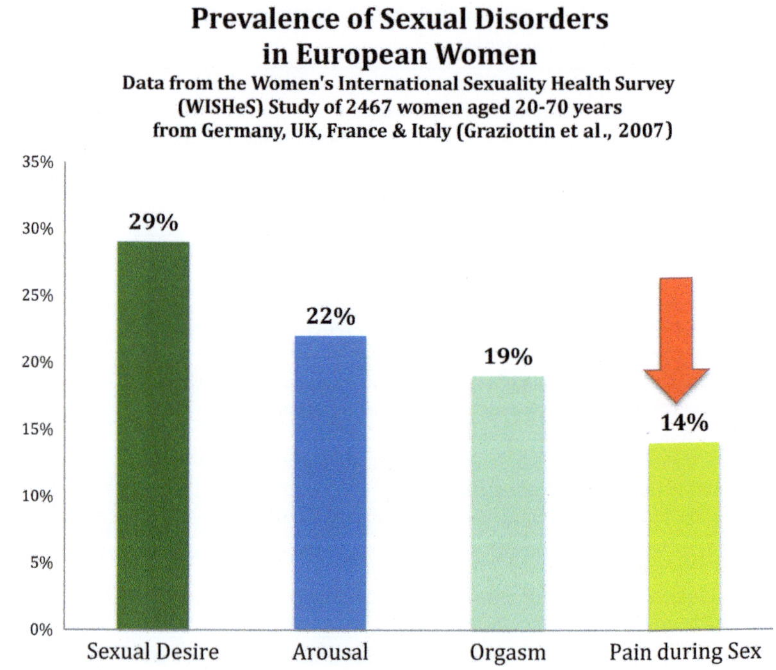

FIGURE 20-1. Prevalence of sexual disorders in European women [Based on data from Ref. 20].

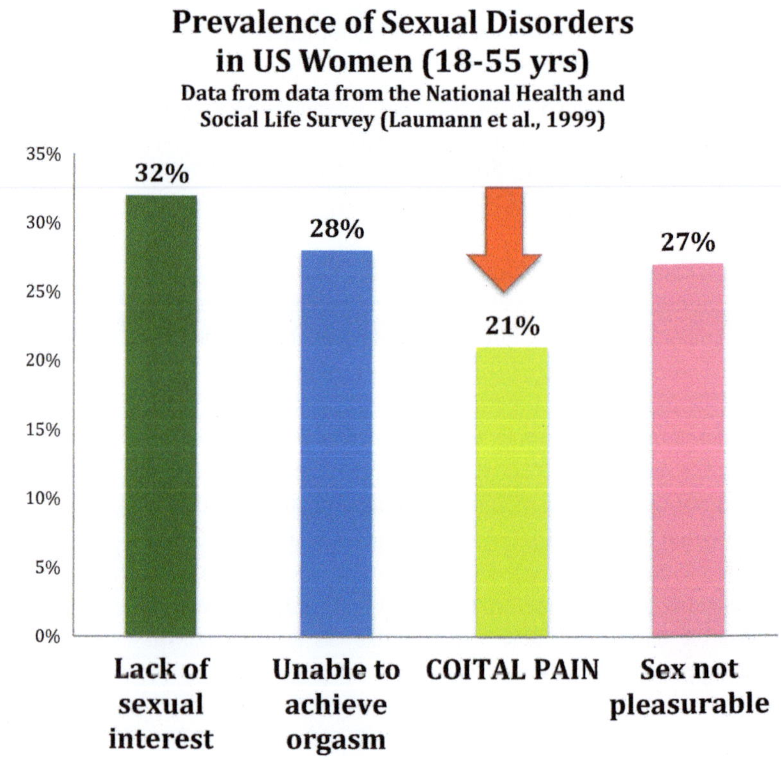

FIGURE 20-2. Prevalence of sexual disorders in US women [Based on data from Ref. 21].

Pathophysiology

Meaning of Pain

Coital pain has the same meaning of pain in every other tissue and/or organ. Yet this meaning is dismissed, forgotten, marginalized, because of the intimate nature of sexual pain and the potential for many emotional interferences. This is a major mistake in terms of diagnostic accuracy, prognostic value and, more important, for the whole health and quality of life of the woman and of the couple.

Key Point

What is then the **meaning of pain**? **Danger**! Which danger? **Tissue damage, loss of physical integrity, impaired function(s), disease and, potentially, death,** in general terms. Just think of pain associated, e.g., to a myocardial infarction or to a dissecting aneurysm of the aorta. The meaning of pain is the same, in any tissue and organ. Coital pain is no exception. Coital pain is therefore the sexual tip of the iceberg of an underlying inflammatory condition in the genitals and in the pelvis [16].

Biological Correlates of Pain

The prominent and more frequent **biological correlate of pain** is **inflammation**. This term, from the Latin word *inflammare*, means "to set on fire," to activate a biochemical fire, a real tissue war. Among other, it is the common denominator of cardiovascular diseases, neurodegenerative diseases and cancer. A real "secret killer," as inflammation may gradually destroy the basic organ and tissue survival mechanisms up to the death of the individual (e.g., when a massive myocardial infarction is in play). In case of GPPPD, inflammation is histologically documented at genital, vestibular and vaginal sites, and in other organs (bladder, colon, pelvis, ...) when an important comorbidity is reported.

Mast cells, defined as the powerful director of the inflammatory orchestra, are the single biological agents that bridge inflammation to pain. The mast cell can be activated by a spectrum of very heterogeneous stimuli: infections, estrogens fluctuations, which trigger flares of pain during periods, chemical and physical *noxae*, menstrual blood when released in the tissues (outside the uterus) as it happens in endometriosis, the mechanical trauma of intercourse in case of vaginal dryness, introital pain, hyperactive pelvic floor with vaginismus, just to mention a few leading etiologies [6, 25].

Vulvodynia can trigger dyspareunia, and a painful intercourse may worsen or precipitate vulvar pain, and concur to maintain it. A lifelong hyperactive pelvic floor ("myogenic hyperactivity," associated or not with phobia of penetration) anatomically reduces the entrance of the vagina. This predisposes the introital vestibular mucosa to microabrasions mechanically provoked by any attempt of intercourse. The contributing factor is an inadequate genital arousal, due to the reflex inhibition pain has on vaginal lubrication and vulvar congestion and/or fear of pain, either lifelong or acquired. The mechanical mucosal damage immediately activates the mast cell response: when the intercourse's attempts are recurrent, and/or the coital damage persistent, and/or if concomitant factors such as a Candida vaginitis further contribute to the inflammatory state, three key consequences are in play [16]:

1. the **mast cell is hyperactivated**, with hyperproduction of inflammatory molecules and neurotrophins such as the Nerve Growth Factor (NGF), which induces:
2. the **proliferation of pain nerve fibers**, responsible for the introital hyperalgesia, and allodynia, and induces or worsen:
3. the **hyperactivity of the pelvic floor**.

This vicious circle may move on the other way round: beginning with recurrent/chronic inflammation of the introital mucosa, caused by infections (from Candida, Herpes, Gardnerella), by physical damages (laser therapy or diatermocoagulation), by chemical irritation (from soaps, perfumes, douche gel, or other substances), allergies, iatrogenic insults (epiotomyrraphy, or any other perineal surgery such as the removal of a Bartholin's cysts), lifestyles, such as too tight blue-jeans, or neurogenic stimuli, that induce the hyperactivation of mast cell, the defensive contraction of the elevator ani and the proliferation of pain nerve fibers, NGF induced [16]. It results frequently in the progression of vulvodynia from provoked (by any genital or sexual stimulus or gynecologic examination) to unprovoked, from localized to generalized, with progressive comorbidity with bladder symptoms, and from dyspareunia to acquired loss of desire, arousal difficulties (mental and genital), orgasmic difficulties up to a progressive avoidance of intercourse, with important consequences on the quality of physical and emotional intimacy and the couple relationship [26].

Impact of Vulvodynia on Physical and Psychosexual Health

Vulvodynia is a prevalent and highly distressing disorder in women, with major health, psychosexual, interpersonal and social consequences.

Health related issues: besides being a serious medical problem per se, vulvodynia may trigger a spreading pain process becoming a real "red alert" in the pelvis. As a chronic inflammatory process, vulvar pain may secondarily involve/extend to other pelvic organs: the most frequent comorbidity is with bladder symptoms (post-coital cystitis, burning bladder syndrome). Other significant associations include endometriosis, chronic pelvic pain, irritable bowel syndrome, fibromyalgia, chronic fatigue syndrome, coccygodynia, headache, and depression.

Preliminary evidence suggests that the pathophysiology of comorbidity recognizes:

1. **a chronic inflammatory process** involving **different pelvic organs**. The common denominator seems to be the hyperactivity of the mast cell, the director of the inflammatory process, which produces and releases different molecules, responsible for the local inflammatory process, for the activation of the pain system and for the defensive contraction of muscles in the painful area. The mast cell is a travelling cell, patrolling all the body and specifically the boundaries such as the colonic mucosa, the bladder mucosa and the vestibular area: this may help to understand comorbidities among organs and system located in different sites (Table 20-5).

Table 20-5. Vulvodynia and comorbidities

– 50% of persons with irritable bowel syndrome had interstitial cystitis
– 38% of patients with interstitial cystitis had irritable bowel syndrome
– 26% of those with interstitial cystitis had vulvodynia

[Modified from Graziottin A, Murina F. Epidemiology of Vulvar Pain and its Sexual Comorbidities. In: Graziottin A, Murina F (eds). Vulvodynia Tips and tricks. Milan, Italy: Springer-Verlag; 2011: 1–5. With permission from Springer Verlag].

2. **the involvement of nerves innervating organs in close proximity** (e.g., the pudendal nerve): the term of **cross-talk** has been used to express this process of "sharing pain."

Practical tip: every time a woman complains of painful intercourse, always actively investigate if she suffers as well of: postcoital cystitis (24–72 h after intercourse), bladder pain syndrome/interstitial cystitis, vestibular/vaginal burning pain after intercourse, IBS, chronic pelvic pain, fibromyalgia, headache.

Psychosexual issues: having pain in a "secret" area of the body, the difficulty to disclose about it, and/or being medically labeled as "inventing pain" feeling of being "the only one," may worsen the intimate suffering of the woman. As unwanted pain is the strongest reflex inhibitor of desire, of mental and physical arousal, vulvodynia is associated with a progressive inhibition of the sexual response: with low desire, vaginal dryness, orgasmic (coital) difficulties and increasing dissatisfaction or frank frustration with sexual intimacy. Chronic pain, of whatever type, destroys the vital energy, leaving the affected woman weak, fatigued, anergic, moody, fearful, distressed, depressed, pessimistic up to a frank catastrophism, the shadow of whom she was when pain had not yet devastated her life.

Interpersonal and social issues:

1. **in the couple**: having a partner who complains of chronic genital pain is a challenge even for the most loving companion for a number of reasons:
   (a) it chronically limits any sexual intimacy up to a complete avoidance of any intimate behavior;
   (b) it monopolizes the conversation and the life content around the vulvar pain and related symptoms;
   (c) it irritates, and causes anger, aggressiveness, verbal and physical abuses, when the physician tell the partner that "she has nothing, pain is all in her head," or that "she is inventing pain"; or that she is "just trying to avoid intercourse";
   (d) it has increasing costs: countable (for visits, exams, loss of working days) and uncountable (for the waste of life, the dark days, the depression, the loss of happiness within the relationship);
2. **in the family**: when mom is ill, all children feel that something is wrong; they are deprived of attention, tenderness, cures with increasing impact with increasing severity of the disease;
3. **at work**: women with vulvodynia, and more generally with GPPPD, report increasing loss of working days, increasing difficulties in concentrating or even to stay seated at their desk for hours; many have to ask for the part time or leave their job and feel forced in an undesired "housewifing" [27].

Neuroinflammation, due to the flooding of the brain by the cytokines produced by the mast cells and by the microglia, is the biological trigger of depression and of the sickness behavior typical of GPPPD [6, 26, 28].

Involvement of Central Nervous System

Chronic pain is associated with changes in the central nervous system (CNS), which may maintain the perception of pain in the absence of acute injury. Recent evidence from human studies has significantly expanded the understanding of pain perception and has demonstrated that a complex series of spinal, midbrain, and cortical structures are involved in pain perception [16].

Pain transmission from the periphery to the higher brain centers via the spinal cord is not a simple, passive process involving exclusive pathways. The relationship between a stimulus causing pain, and the way it is perceived by an individual, is dramatically affected by circuitry within the spinal cord and the brain. The sensation of pain is modulated as it is transmitted upwards from the periphery to the cortex. It is modulated at a segmental level and by descending control from higher centers, with the main neurotransmitters involved being serotonin, noradrenaline, and endogenous opioids [25].

The peripheral nociceptors are simple bare-endings nerve fibers and they are widespread in the superficial layers of the skin. Nociceptors are classified Aδ, which are small diameter, lightly myelinated, and C-fibers, which are not myelinated. The nociceptors neurons pass in the peripheral nerves and enter the spinal cord at the dermatomal level ascribed by their insertion. Innervation to the vulva is via the pudendal nerve, which originates from the S2-4 nerve roots and the ileoinguinal and genitofemoral nerves, arising from L1-2. The two latter nerves are predominantly sensory, but the pudendal nerve contains motor, sensory, and sympathetic fibers, which supply the complex autonomic reflexes of the pelvic organs. The vagina itself is relatively insensitive to pain, while the vulva and particularly the vulvar vestibule have an high level of free nerve endings.

Spinal cord. Following spinal cord integration of afferent inputs there are neurons (second-order neurons) that transmit the information to the higher centers via ascending pathways. The classical ascending pathway ascribed to pain is the spinothalamic one; other pathways relevant in pain modulation include the spinomesencephalic, spinoreticular, and dorsal column pathways.

Cerebral cortex. Cortical pain perception can be roughly divided into a lateral, somatosensory system involved in discrimination of pain location and intensity, and a medial system which mediates the anticipatory, fearful, affective quality of pain through limbic structures. In broad terms, pain has elements that are sensory and localizing with other elements that are involved with memory, cognition, and affect.

Descending pathways. Some of spinothalamic fibers project to the periaqueductal grey (PAG) and hypothalamus and then to the dorsal horn of the spinal cord. The PAG is one area of the brain that is rich in opioid receptors and thus involved with the endogenous opioid system. The descending pathways are, therefore, inhibitory at the dorsal horn reducing ascending nociceptive inputs.

Neuropathic pain is defined as pain initiated or caused by a primary lesion or dysfunction in the nervous system. Neuropathic pain results from damage to the nervous system anywhere along the neuraxis: peripheral nervous system, spinal or supraspinal nervous system, or brain. Clinically, neuropathic pain is expressed by two abnormal sensory processes: **hyperalgesia** and/or **allodynia**. Hyperalgesia is defined as an increased response to a stimulus that is normally painful, while allodynia as pain due to a stimulus that is not normally painful.

Vulvodynia patients exhibit these two basilar elements: hyperalgesia and/or allodynia.

Peripheral change after nerve damage. Free nerve endings injury induces structural and functional changes in both injured and uninjured parts of the nerve. These changes increase ectopic and spontaneous firing after nerve damage, furthermore "cross-talk" from neighboring nerves can augment this effect. Regeneration of axon terminals after nerve damage may enhance cross-talk, although the degree of sprouting does not correlate with the severity of pain behaviors. Hyperalgesia and allodynia are the symptomatic expression of these phenomena. Inflammation has been suggested to be pivotal to the development of peripheral sensitization. Nerve grow factor (NGF) appear to be a key molecule in the orchestration of peripheral inflammation. NGF is released from many cells after tissue injury and has several pro-inflammatory roles. Indeed, NGF has a significant action on the expression of other inflammation mediators (interleukin-1ß, tumor necrosis factor, etc.) and it is also capable of direct and indirect sensitization of nociceptors. Inflammation-driven release of cytokine from immune cells provokes hyperalgesia through stimulation and production of other pro-inflammatory agents.

Mast cells are the main source of inflammatory mediators. These peripheral cell types are located in the dermis, adjacent to blood vessels, nerve endings and glandular ducts, and have a cytoplasm filled with spherical granules. Mast cells' granules contain many factors implicated in neurogenic inflammation like *NGF, tumor necrosis factor (TNF), protease, and cytokines* [6].

Physical, chemical and mechanical stimuli activate local mast cells causing degranulation and secretion of mediators which have been found to sensitize and induce the proliferation of C-afferent nerve fibers.

These nerve fibers release inflammation mediators, including NGF, which increase the proliferation and degranulation of mast cells, causing hyperesthesia, and enhance the inflammatory response. Mast cells show particularly complexity regard the inflammation and their density in inflamed tissue changes over time. In tissue where there is an acute inflammatory response, the concentration of mast cells is high. As the inflammation becomes more chronic the number of mast cells decreases and there is a parallel increase in neuronal proliferation. At this stage of the inflammatory process neuropathic symptoms became prominent, but mast cell reactivation can occur at any time with a symptoms accentuation or promoting an acceleration of the neurogenic inflammation processes [26].

Central mechanism. The dorsal horn is now known to play a key role in the modulation of pain and development of chronic pain states. Pain is only perceived if this electrical activity reaches the brain and, hence, any modulation of alteration within the dorsal horn can have profound effect on pain sensation. Lamina IV and V of the dorsal horn contain peculiar neurons called wide dynamic range (WDR). Repetitive stimulation by C-fibers causes some WDR cells in the dorsal horn to augment their response. Thus, for a given input stimulus, the output is enhanced; this process is referred to as "wind up." Wind up is a part of a process termed "central sensitization." Cortical functioning has both localizing, emotional and memory component. Descending modulatory control is bidirectional in nature. These descending control system link the brain cortex to the dorsal horn, acting either directly on primary afferents or indirectly via inhibitory and excitatory interneurones.

The phenomena described above lead to the central sensitization, pivotal aspect of neuropathic pain. Central sensitization involves an increase in the receptive fields of a nociceptor, an increase in the magnitude and duration of response to a noxious stimulus. And a reduction in the threshold required to stimulate nociceptors [29].

A vestibular proliferation of C-afferent receptors (ten folds increase in the density of nerve endings) and a significant number of activated mast cells (assessed by measuring the mast cell degranulation levels) has been reported in vestibulodynia patients.

Biopsies from the area around the ductal openings of the Bartholin's glands, the most sensitive vestibular area in most vestibulodynia patients, showed significantly more intraepithelial free nerve endings than in healthy control subjects.

It is possible that the epithelium of the vulvar vestibule expresses an abnormal response to trigger inflammatory events such as infection, trauma and repeated exposure to an irritant or allergen, with a subsequent increase in number of activated mast cells. Their activation is associated with discharge of various mediators from the granules, such as NGF, tryptase, and bradykinin. The various mediators that are secreted by the mast cells are known to sensitize C-nerve fibers and induce their proliferation.

Neurogenic inflammation is the most appropriate definition of this series of events.

Recent lines of evidence highlight a potential genetic predisposition to chronic inflammation among vestibulodynia afflicted women. These genetic polymorphism leads to a reduced capacity to terminate and to an exaggerated inflammatory response.

The findings of multiple case–control studies of women with provoked vestibulodynia suggest that they experience more frequent vaginal infections.

A history of recurrent candidiasis infections is one of the most consistently reported findings associated with the onset of vestibolodynia. A reduced capacity to control *Candida albicans* action due to a polymorphism in the gene coding for mannose-binding lectin, an innate immune system antimicrobial protein, has been reported and this polymorphism has also been associated with vestibulodynia.

It was also demonstrated that women with vulvodynia more frequently react to patch tests for *Candida albicans*, and it was postulated that exposure to *Candida albicans* at low concentrations may involve neurotransmitters that have been shown to influence contact hypersensitivity and are present in abundance in the vulvar vestibule. In vulvodynia patients there is not an **active inflammation**, rather we can find a **neurogenic inflammation**, where the prolonged or severe infectious, thermal, or chemical irritation caused excessive local responses (mast cell activation) [16].

The name "vulvar vestibulitis," in our opinion, should be reconsidered given the histological evidence of tissue inflammation, with significant increase of:

1. number of mast cells;
2. number of degranulated mast cells;
3. number of mast cells in close proximity to pain nerve fibers.

The wording "provoked vestibulodynia" is pertinent as it describes the pain evoked by the examining finger, probes, or intercourse. However, the substantial inflammatory nature of the disorder must not be dismissed.

The morphological findings of nerve endings proliferation was not demonstrated for generalized vulvodynia, but new elements have been identified also in this subtype of disease where we have a scarcity of research on the pathophysiology.

As with patients with neuropathic pain, women with generalized vulvodynia exhibit hyperalgesia and/or allodynia that we can consider the functional corresponding of neural hyperplasia.

A recent study of ours indicated that the current perception threshold (CPT) values were lower in women affected by vulvodynia than those in controls, suggesting hypersensitivity [16].

The CPT measures provide objective and quantitative determinations of the sensory nerve conduction and nerve functional integrity; it uses an electrical stimulus selective for the large and small myelinated and unmyelinated fibers that are involved in the transmission of painless and painful sensation.

Each of the three major sensory fiber types has a characteristic neurophysiological profile, sensory function, sensation evoked by electrical stimulation, and conduction block susceptibility.

Because findings of enhanced pain perception are typical of neuropathic pain syndromes, our results add strength to a neuropathic hypothesis for pain also in generalized vulvodynia.

Always it is difficult to find a trigger inflammatory events in generalized vulvodynia.

Women with generalized vulvodynia experience symptoms anywhere within the distribution of the pudendal nerve.

The pudendal nerve is an extrapelvic nerve; it quickly exits the pelvis, wrapps around ischial rectal fossa, enters the pudendal canal, and provides innervation to the external genitalia, the urethral sphincter, the anal sphincter, and the external genitalia.

The branch that innervates the vulva and vestibule is very superficial, while the branch that innervates the clitoris is deeper. Thus, there is the possibility of repeated micro-trauma to the vulvar branch, like during bicycling and horseback riding, which could lead to neurogenic inflammation. Particularly, some authors have demonstrated that vestibulodynia patients perceive light and moderate touch to the vulvar vestibule more intensely than control women do. The increase in perception was reflected in more significantly activated neural areas than in control women. In addition, it has been showed that vestibulodynia in young women is associated with increased gray matter density in pain modulatory and stress-related brain regions.

It was speculated that increased gray matter density could be caused by microglial proliferation, maybe due to excess excitatory neural activity.

Phenomenology/Diagnostic Criteria

The diagnosis of this pathological condition, namely GPPPD, is prominently clinical based on:

1. an extremely careful *listening to* the symptoms and their narrative in the patient' own "reading" of the sexual penetration problem(s)
2. *questioning with an investigative mind on* predisposing, precipitating, and perpetuating factors, while activating the mental file « what is the pathophysiologic correlate of those factors? »
3. the *medical visit* of vulva, vagina and degree of elevator ani contraction, with a sexual medicine perspective, integrating listening, questioning and physical examination finding in a meaningful pathophysiologic reading of the current sexual complaint. This is the basis for a well-tailored, individualized treatment.

Moreover, in the clinical setting, patients affected with (years of) sexual pain definitely prefer a comprehensive, focused, and empathic dialog with the health care provider specifically trained in sexual medicine with a solid experience in diagnosing and curing sexual pain disorders instead of filling up many questionnaires (Graziottin, unpublished data).

Until the publication of fifth edition of the *Diagnostic and Statistical Manual of Mental Disorders* (DSM-5; American Psychiatric Association, 2013) dyspareunia and vaginismus were typically classified as distinct sexual pain disorders. This new classification unifies vaginismus and dyspareunia into one category called "**genito-pelvic pain/penetration disorder**" due to the clinical difficulties to distinguishing these condition. This disorder is defined as **marked difficulty** with at least one of the following:

(a) **vaginal intercourse/penetration pain**
(b) **genito-pelvic pain**
(c) **fear of vaginal intercourse/penetration/pain or**
(d) **heightened pelvic floor muscle tension during attempted penetration** (American Psychiatric Association, 2013) as seen in Table 20-6.

The new GPPPD definition is inspired by the desire to avoid overlapping between dyspareunia and vaginismus, and conditions such as the genito-pelvic pain, that are leading biological contributor to introital dyspareunia. However it does not simplify the clinical diagnosis and may even be perceived as more complicated and "obscure" by the vast majority of clinical practitioner and family physicians.

In the clinical setting, "painful intercourse" is the wording more easy to be discussed with patients and physicians not trained in sexual medicine. The specific characteristics may then be perfectly described both with the old and the new classification system, if the basic criteria of the diagnosis (listening, questioning, examining) are carefully respected.

Table 20-6. DSM-5 Diagnostic Criteria for Genito-Pelvic Pain/Penetration Disorder 302.76 (F52.6)

A. Persistent or recurrent difficulties with one (or more) of the following:
   1. Vaginal penetration during intercourse.
   2. Marked vulvovaginal or pelvic pain during vaginal intercourse or penetration attempts.
   3. Marked fear or anxiety about vulvovaginal or pelvic pain in anticipation of, during, or as a result of vaginal penetration.
   4. Marked tensing or tightening of the pelvic floor muscles during attempted vaginal penetration.

B. The symptoms in Criterion A have persisted for a minimum duration of approximately 6 months.

C. The symptoms in Criterion A cause clinically significant distress in the individual.

D. The sexual dysfunction is not better explained by a nonsexual mental disorder or as a consequence of a severe relationship distress (e.g., partner violence) or other significant stressors and is not attributable to the effects of a substance/medication or another medical condition.

Specify whether:
Lifelong: The disturbance has been present since the individual became sexually active.
Acquired: The disturbance began after a period of relatively normal sexual function.
Specify current severity:
Mild: Evidence of mild distress over the symptoms in Criterion A.
Moderate: Evidence of moderate distress over the symptoms in Criterion A.
Severe: Evidence of severe or extreme distress over the symptoms in Criterion A.

Patients and partners find extremely empowering their healing hope, and comforting, to be explained the "biomechanics" of pain, with the aid of a mirror during clinical examination, focusing on the hyperactive pelvic floor or other vulvar/vaginal lesions or conditions contributing to sexual pain, such as retracting episiotomy/rraphy, retracting scars of Bartolin's gland removal, too tightened colporraphy, vaginal and/or vulvar atrophy etc.

This is helpful in educating the patient—and the caring partner—to "see" the retracted centrum tendineum of the perineum, or the pain-contributing condition/lesion, while combining the visual aspect of the genitalia with the feeling of contraction and burning worsening and then relaxation, of stretching and massage of the muscle.

Educating the patient to listen to "body feelings" elicited by different level of contraction, relaxation, and stretch of the pelvic floor is difficult but it is really "the" turning point of the therapeutic process of curing sexual pain disorders.

Filling-up questionnaires is certainly essential from the research point of view. It is useful to quantify some "elusive" aspect of the sexual response for a better monitoring of the diagnosis and treatment but cannot surrogate the accurate end experienced clinical approach.

In other words, patients and couples affected with sexual pain disorders, or GPPPD, can be successfully and completely cured without filling one single questionnaire. While they can fill up tens of questionnaires but cannot be cured without a competent clinical approach, the most neglected area in GPPPD.

Researchers and students who like to refine their knowledge on *best practice or evidence-based approach to diagnosis* including diagnostic tests, instruments, or rating scales are referred to NIH PROMIS MEASURES (PROMIS references Sexual measures: https://www.assessmentcenter.net/documents/Sexual%20Function%20Manual.pdf General introduction: http://www.healthmeasures.net/explore-measurement-systems/promis/intro-to-promis).

This document describes resources for measuring sexual function and satisfaction using the PROMIS© system.

Section 1 of the PROMIS © manual presents a brief, comprehensive measure of sexual function for men and women, known as the PROMIS Sexual Function and Satisfaction Measures Brief Profile. For many users, this short measure (8 items for males, 10 items for females) will suffice.

The PROMIS Sexual Function and Satisfaction Measures Brief Profile (PSxFBP) provides scores on seven different subdomains of sexual function: Interest in Sexual Activity, Vaginal Discomfort (women only), Lubrication (women only), Erectile Function (men only), Orgasm, and Global Satisfaction with Sex Life (see below for subdomain definitions).

Clinicians may use the female questionnaire for the woman complaining of GPPPD, while the male questions may be used to explore the he/partner sexuality (In case of a she/partner, the female questionnaires should be used for both partner).

Section 2 of the PROMIS © manual is intended for users who might want to create a more customized assessment of sexual function. Parts of the second section require the reader to have greater sophistication in measurement methodology.

Clinical Diagnosis

When Sex Hurts: Key Questions

To ease the learning process, clinical cases will be presented focusing on real-life dialogs.

"When did you first experience pain at intercourse? What happened in the weeks/months before? Did you experience pain from the very beginning or your sexual life or later on, after months/year of normal joyful sex? What in your opinion is the leading cause of it? Do you have it with every partner and in every circumstance or not?"

This is just the beginning of a structured interview the physician should have in mind [16].

In summary, when the health care provider aims at understanding the etiology of dyspareunia, he/she should first ask **three basic questions**:

- where does it hurt?
- when does it hurt?
- what are the associated symptoms?

These are three basic questions every physician asks routinely when a patient report pain anywhere in the body. Coital pain is no exception. Yet physicians seem to forget this medical approach when coital pain is reported and shift to the psychogenic reading of pain.

Key Point

The biological etiology of sexual pain should be evaluated carefully in the first line of the medical approach to coital pain.

Where Does It Hurt

According to the pelvic site, he or she should first distinguish between:

Pain in the vagina

1. **introital/midvaginal pain** (introital dyspareunia).
2. **deep vaginal pain** (deep dyspareunia).

Each type of pain typically involves different sets of contributing factors (Figures 20-3 and 20-4). A woman complaining of sexual pain will usually describe her pain in very different ways when it is a pain at the introitus (vaginal opening) as compared to deep pain. Pain at the introitus will create difficulties with vaginal penetration, while deep pain usually becomes worse during the thrusting phase of intercourse.

Pain at the urethra-trigonal level

Women may report that pain is more excruciating at the urethral level, during and after intercourse, when **painful bladder syndrome is comorbid** and/or when the woman complains of **frequency, urgency and burning at micturition after the intercourse.**

Careful evaluation of the tonus of the levator ani and the presence of pathogenic biofilm in the bladder wall is mandatory.

Pain at anal level

Women who enjoy anal intercourse may find distressing having pain because of hemorrhoids, ragads, or postpartum lesions or painful outcomes of physical or sexual abuse. This is an underreported, underdiagnosed, and undertreated subset of genito-pelvic pain/penetration disorders.

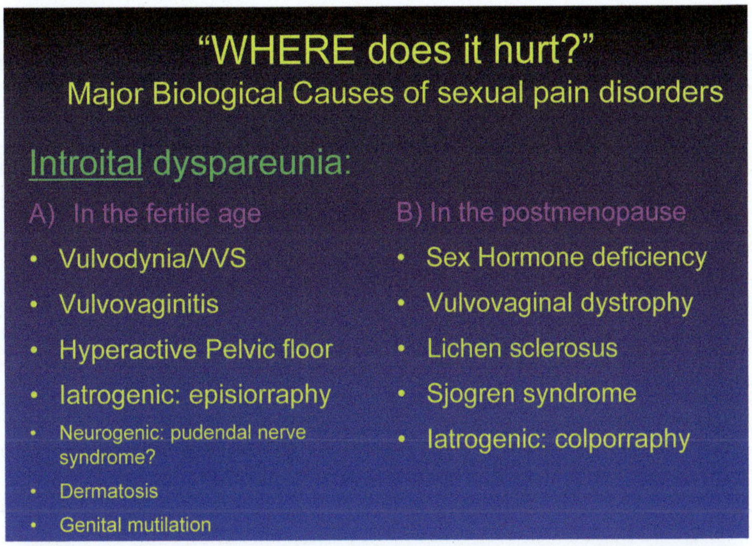

FIGURE 20-3. Major biological causes of sexual pain disorders: introital dyspareunia [Courtesy of Alessandra Graziottin].

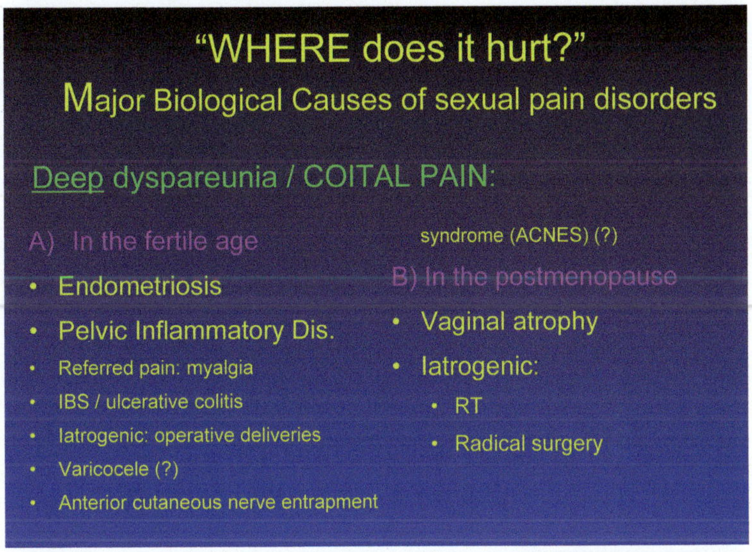

FIGURE 20-4. Major biological causes of sexual pain disorders: deep dyspareunia/coital pain [Courtesy of Alessandra Graziottin].

Clitoral Pain

Women may complain of clitoral pain during sexual intercourse/penetration when the corpus cavernosus congestion typical of genital arousal may elicit/worsen clitoral pain during thrusting or at the orgasm.

Pain deep in the pelvis

Worsening during periods is frequently reported. Comorbidity with endometriosis, pelvic inflammatory diseases, and/or chronic pelvic pain is frequently reported.

The clinical evaluation of dyspareunia consists of taking a thorough clinical history and performing a physical examination. Whenever sexual pain disorders are being diagnosed, the following subtypes should be specified [1]:

- lifelong versus acquired, focusing on time-related characteristics;
- generalized versus situational, according to the context, physical or relational, where it is reported to be experienced;
- organic, psychogenic, mixed, or unknown, focusing on the etiology;
- highly distressing, moderately distressing, or non-distressing, according to how intensely the woman experiences her coital pain.

Clinical Cases of Painful Intercourse from Women's Wording to the Clinical Diagnosis

Case histories may help students and learning physicians to focus on the real complaint and associated comorbidities, sexual and urogenital, with their impact on the real life of patients. They will illustrate how sexual pain can affect a woman's life and how an early diagnosis can definitely change the woman's and couple's sexual experience for the better. All names in the following case stories have been changed.

Readers should focus what should be listened to, selected as critical info from the narrative of the problem, and evaluated to get the proper diagnosis and a well tailored effective treatment [16].

Case 1

"I had pain from the very first intercourse. I hoped it would have gone better over time. I tried many times, but pain became more and more excruciating. I had tears every time we tried. When I tried to make love, I felt that my vagiht and dry. I cannot get aroused anymore, because I'm afraid of pain. Even my sexual desire has gone away. My family physician prescribed the contraceptive pill for me, suggesting that perhaps I was afraid of getting pregnant and did not relax. The pain didn't change. It's three years now that we do nothing. We have lost any type of intimacy, for fear that he gets aroused and we try again to have sex. I feel guilty for disappointing him and being unable to do what is so easy and funny for the majority of women. Now I'm here because we would love to have a child."

Laura, 33 years of age

Clinical Evaluation

Laura' wording suggests a lifelong vaginismus, with acquired loss of desire, and significant distress. When asked, Laura reports that:

(a) since her first periods, she could not use tampons during menstruation, because she could not insert them: "I felt I had a wall there";
(b) since she was a girl, she was afraid of feeling pain at intercourse, in spite of longing for a closer intimacy with her boyfriend;
(c) she was not abused or harassed;
(d) she received a strict catholic education, where sex was considered not appropriate for a girl until marriage.

These observations suggest that she could have a lifelong vaginismus, severe enough to prevent intercourse, and a hyperactive pelvic floor. Attempts of penetration may have caused microabrasions of the mucosa at the entrance of the vagina leading to vulvar vestibulitis/provoked vestibulodynia, sufficient to predispose her to introital dyspareunia.

Clinical Examination

Her body language indicated a systemic anxiety and fear of being examined. She could not relax in spite of her physician's reassuring manner. Exquisite pain was elicited at 5 and 7 o'clock (when viewing the vaginal opening as a clock face with the anus at 6 o'clock), between the hymen remnants and the introitus vagina (the opening of the vagina). Tender points were elicited where the muscle levator ani inserts at the spine.

Diagnosis

Lifelong vaginismus and dyspareunia, comorbid with vulvar vestibulitis and a tightened, myalgic pelvic floor. Lifelong vaginismus could be the predisposing factor to dyspareunia (both vaginismus and vulvar vestibulitis will be described below). Acquired genital arousal disorder and acquired loss of sexual desire were the comorbid female sexual disorders (FSD). Currently the diagnosis would be: Genito-Pelvic Pain/Penetration Disorder, comorbid with other FSD.

Comment

Comorbidity between different FSDs and between FSD and medical conditions is frequent in women. A careful clinical history is essential to identify predisposing, precipitating, and maintaining/perpetuating factors, which may be biological, psychosexual and/or relational. In this case, the natural history of the current complaint had vaginismus as a likely predisposing factor, while intercourse was the precipitating factor. Maintaining factors were biological (vulvar vestibulitis) and psychosexual (systemic fear and anxiety about the pain). Acquired desire and arousal disorders increased the vulnerability of the introital mucosa to the mechanical trauma, due to the lack of lubrication in response to sexual stimulation.

Cases 2 and 3

"I had a satisfying sexual life since my first intercourse, at age 16. I do not want to catch diseases, so I had always used condoms as a protection against sexually transmitted infections (STI) and as contraceptive. I never had STI. My last gynecological examination was performed three years ago, with a normal record and normal pap-smear. Now I have a worsening acute pain during intercourse at deep penetration. Pain got worse in the last two years. Yes, periods were progressively more painful since my adolescence. They are now so debilitating, that I have to take two days off work to stay home because of my "cramping" *periods."*

Maria, 25 years.

"My periods are a curse: every month I have two days of pain, I cannot go to school, meet my friends, do anything. I'm just lying in bed ingurgitating painkillers until pain goes down a bit. Last year I had my first intercourse. I had little pain at the entrance of the vagina and a horrible pain deep in the vagina. My gynaecologist says that I have endometriosis, located in the vaginal wall between the vagina and the rectum, and that endometriosis invade the "utero-sacral" ligaments that connect the uterus to the sacrum. This is why intercourse is so painful. He says I should be operated but I'm very afraid."

Rebecca, 21 years.

Clinical Evaluation

Maria's and Rebecca's wording suggests endometriosis. Two leading suggestive symptoms are the invalidating and worsening pain during periods and pain deep in the vagina, suggesting endometriosis of the uterosacral ligaments and/or in the Douglas pouch, in the posterior fornix or the rectovaginal septum.

Clinical Examination

Maria has a specific tenderness at the location of the uterosacral ligaments, with acutely elicited pain when these ligaments are palpated. An ovarian cyst of apricot size is present on the right side. The blood sample of the specific marker CA-125 is elevated (56 mU/ml). The ultrasound confirms an ovarian cyst of 5.2 cm in diameter, on the right, suggestive of endometriosis. MR confirms these findings. Rebecca report an acute pain, a stabbing pain, at the gynecological examination, when the uterosacral ligament in investigated. She has the very same pain when she has intercourse and when she underwent vaginal ecographic evaluation.

Diagnosis

Acquired deep dyspareunia, due to pelvic endometriosis.

Comment

The incapacitating dysmenorrhea is a key symptom of endometriosis. Unfortunately it is often neglected or ignored until more serious conditions develop, such as ovarian endometrioma, deep dyspareunia, and/or infertility. Besides endometriosis, which is the most frequent etiology of deep dyspareunia, pelvic inflammatory disease should be considered as the second leading cause of deep dyspareunia, particularly in promiscuous women who do not consistently use condom.

Case 4

"I had my first intercourse when I was 16. Little pain the first time, then sex was fun and love. Last year, at 27, I had recurrent bronchitis and had two strong antibiotic treatments. Two weeks later I had a very painful vaginitis from Candida, that never went away completely. Sex became more and more painful at the entrance of the vagina. Even worse, this burning pain at the entrance of the vagina may last up to two–three days or more. Yes, since that antibiotic treatment, even my bowel habits have changed. I have alternating days of diarrhea and constipation. Could this contribute to my symptoms?"

Victoria, 27 years

Clinical Evaluation

Victoria's wording suggests that Candida vaginitis has been triggered by two strong antibiotic courses, with major consequences on the intestinal and vaginal microbiota. Recurrent vaginal Candida is the precipitating cause of vulvar vestibulitis/provoked dyspareunia. Irritable bowel syndrome (IBS) is often comorbid after repeated antibiotic courses.

Clinical Examination

At inspection, the genital region appears inflamed. The vulva is red, with white leakage suggesting a Candida vaginitis; the centrum tendineum of the perineum is retracted and the pelvic floor is tightened. When the woman is requested to breath in with abdominal breathing and then push, she pulls instead. This suggests an "inverted command" of the pelvic floor and it is an indication to electromyographic biofeed-back to help the woman to improve her awareness about the pelvic floor muscles relaxation while having an analgesic effect too on the introital pain. At examination, the swab test elicit an acute burning pain at 5 and 7, when looking at the vaginal entrance as a clock–face. At the insertion of the levator ani at the ischiatic spine, mid vagina left and right, tender points are appreciated suggesting levator ani myalgia and suggesting the need of biofeedback relaxation training. The remaining gynecological examination is within the normal range. The colon appears tense (*corda colica*) and inflamed, suggesting a likely comorbidity with irritable bowel syndrome (IBS), with diarrhea alternated to constipation, often comorbid with VVS/VP, after antibiotic courses.

Diagnosis

Candida vulvovaginitis, vulvar vestibulitis/provoked vestibulodynia, levator ani myalgia, comorbid with IBS.

Comment

In rats, three episode of vaginal candida are sufficient to trigger vulvar vestibulitis/PV. The levator ani hyperactivity can be provoked by the increasing inflammation and pain. IBS can be comorbid with VVS/PV in 30–50% of cases (the "evil twins"). Treatment should consider normalizing the bowel inflammation as well, in synergy with a competent gastroenterologist.

Case 5

"I could not imagine that having a baby would have killed my sexual life. Sex was good until I got pregnant. Then I started to fear that having intercourse would have damaged the child or the pregnancy course. I avoided any more penetration. The delivery was a nightmare. There were complications. The physician made me a big cut on the genitals (episiotomy) and then jumped on my belly to push the child out (Kristeller's maneuver). I had a terrible pain: I felt I was broken into pieces. The cutting was low to heal, very painful. When we tried to have intercourse after three months, pain was horrible, like having a knife pushing inside. I shouted so loud that he lost his erection. I cried all my tears. I have no more desire as I'm afraid of pain. Yes, I'm still without periods. My husband is very nervous and aggressive now. He was supportive at the beginning but now he says that after two years without sex he cannot think of spending his life in such a way. He says that If a do not find a solution he will get divorce."

Louise, 35 years

Clinical Evaluation

Louise' wording suggests postpartum dyspareunia, comorbid with low desire and genital arousal difficulties.

Clinical Examination

Her episiotomy scar was tense, retracted and painful. The vaginal pH was 6, suggesting vaginal dryness caused by the lack of estrogens, due to the continued breastfeeding, and a substantial change of the vaginal microbiota. This could be a concomitant etiological factor.

Diagnosis

Acquired dyspareunia, acquired genital arousal disorder, and acquired loss of sexual desire causing severe distress and interpersonal difficulties.

Comment

The postpartum period is a difficult transitional phase for the woman and the couple. Besides making the adjustment to meeting their infant's needs, the couple has to face a major reassessment of the erotic intimacy. The most frequent complaint is the vaginal dryness, which correlates with a genital arousal disorder. Comorbidity with low desire is common, while dyspareunia is more frequent when episiotomy/episiorraphy has been performed with a poor scarring outcome. What is the persisting problem? The **lack of professional recognition**, i.e., the medical neglect of sexual pain after delivery as Glazener stigmatized in her paper about genital sexual pain/dyspareunia in 1997 [30]. This neglect about women's and couples sex life after delivery is still the leading cause of persisting pain even 18 month after delivery in 23% of women [31]. Variables include operative deliveries, macrosomic baby, poor surgical outcomes, persisting breastfeeding with vaginal dryness, and lack of genital arousal [32].

Case 6

"Julia is a 60-year-old woman. She has been very happily married for thirty-four years and has three children. She is also the proud grandmother of two girls. She had no specific complaints at menopause, besides moderate hot flashes, so she decided not to use hormone therapy. She has developed progressive vaginal dryness. In the last year intercourse has become frankly painful."

"I love my husband and I do not want to make him feel rejected. He feels that if I'm dry I have no more desire for him. Well, yes, I do not have the drive I was used to, but I still enjoy our intimacy were it not for that pain that is becoming worse and worse. By the way, I often suffer from vaginitis with the same germ, Escherichia coli."

Julia, 60 years

Clinical Evaluation

Julia wording suggests a specific menopause-triggered biological problem: vaginal dryness, predisposing to introital dyspareunia, in the context of a good couple relationship and a serene family life.

Clinical Examination

External genitalia present with vulvar dystrophy, involution of the labia, white hair. The vaginal pH is 7.0, which suggests vaginal atrophy because of the persistent lack of estrogens.

Diagnosis

Acquired genital arousal disorder with acquired dyspareunia and personal distress. Comorbidity with recurrent vaginitis from saprophytic pathogens (*Escherichia coli*).

Comment

Vaginal dryness is the second most frequent sexual complaint during the postmenopausal years, after loss of desire. Comorbidity with recurrent vaginitis and cystitis is frequent. Comorbidity between genital arousal disorder and dyspareunia is also frequent, when the atrophic vaginitis is complicated by vulvar dystrophy, which contributes to introital dyspareunia. Unfortunately, vaginal dryness is underreported, underdiagnosed and undertreated in the majority of postmenopausal women. An easy to be treated problem may therefore turn into a major cause of loss of sexual intimacy and sexual avoidance even between loving partners.

Conclusions

Genito-pelvic/pain penetration disorder is a comprehensive wording to include all the pain symptoms women may experience before, during, and after intercourse.

Vulvar pain is leading contributor to GPPPD. It is a common disorder, which still remains unaddressed for years in the majority of affected women. It was wrongly considered as "psychogenic," but vulvodynia is a disorder with solid biological etiologies, that are in the domain of a medical diagnosis. It can be multifactorial: the diagnosis requires a careful listening to the woman's symptoms, an accurate reading of vulvodynia's pathophysiology, a competent physical examination focused on detecting all the clinical signs, and an attention to the frequent comorbidities (medical and sexual) that vulvar pain can be associated with—bladder symptoms (postcoital cystitis, painful bladder syndrome), endometriosis, irritable bowel syndrome, fibromyalgia, headache; and sexual comorbidities, with coital pain (dyspareunia) being the leading symptom, with its cohort of secondary loss of desire, vaginal dryness, orgasmic difficulties, and sexual dissatisfaction that can deeply affect the couple relationship [16].

The challenge for every physician is to diagnose all the predisposing, precipitating, and perpetuating factors contributing to GPPPD, to give to every affected woman and couple a timely comprehensive diagnosis and a competent help.

References

1. Bornstein J, Goldstein AT, Stockdale CK, et al. 2015 ISSVD, ISSWSH and IPPS consensus terminology and classification of persistent vulvar pain and vulvodynia. Obstet Gynecol. 2016;127:745–51.
2. Graziottin A, Gambini D, Bertolasi L. Genital and sexual pain in women. In: Vodusek D, Boller F, editors. Neurology of sexual and bladder disorders (Handbook of clinical neurology, Vol 130, 3rd Series). Amsterdam: Elsevier; 2015. p. 395–412.
3. Graziottin A, Rovei V. Sexual pain disorders. In: Owens AF, Tepper MS, editors. Sexual health. Westport, CT; London, UK: Praeger; 2007. p. 287–313.
4. Graziottin A. Sexual pain disorders: dyspareunia and vaginismus. In: Porst H, Buvat J, editors. ISSM (International Society of Sexual Medicine) standard committee book, standard practice in sexual medicine. Oxford: Blackwell; 2006. p. 342–50.
5. Graziottin A. Female sexual dysfunction: assessment In: Bø K, Berghmans B, Mørkved S, Van Kampen M, editors. Evidence-based physical therapy for the pelvic floor-bridging science and clinical practice. 2nd ed. Oxford: Elsevier; 2015. p. 243–57.
6. Graziottin A. Mast cells and their role in sexual pain disorders In: Goldstein A, Pukall C, Goldstein I, editors. Female sexual pain disorders: evaluation and management. Chichester; Hoboken: Blackwell Publishing; 2009. p. 176–9.
7. Graziottin A. Recurrent cystitis after intercourse: why the gynaecologist has a say. In: Studd J, Seang LT, Chervenak FA, editors. Current progress in obstetrics and gynaecology, vol. 2. Mumbai: Suketu P. Kothari-Tree Life Media; 2014. p. 319–6.
8. Graziottin A, Serafini A. HPV infection in women: psychosexual impact of genital warts and intraepithelial lesions. In: Takac I, editor. Recent advances in cervical cancer. Kerala: Transworld Research Network; 2012. p. 69–85.
9. Graziottin A. Iatrogenic and post-traumatic female sexual disorders. In: Porst H, Buvat J, editors. ISSM (International Society of Sexual Medicine) standard committee book, standard practice in sexual medicine. Oxford: Blackwell; 2006. p. 351–61.
10. Graziottin A. Psychogenic causes of chronic pelvic pain and impact of CPP on psychological status. In: Vercellini P, editor. Chronic pelvic pain. Oxford: Blackwell Publishing; 2011. p. 29–39.
11. Lukasiewicz ME, Graziottin A. Women' sexuality after gynecologic cancers. In: Studd J, Seang LT, Chervenak FA, editors. Current progress in obstetrics and gynaecology, Vol. 3. 2nd ed. Mumbai: Kothari Medical; 2015. p. 95–116.
12. Graziottin A, Zanello PP. Pathogenic biofilms: their role in recurrent cystitis and vaginitis (with focus on D-mannose as a new prophylactic strategy). In: Studd J, Seang LT, Chervenak FA, editors. Current progress in obstetrics and gynaecology, Vol. 3. 2nd ed. Mumbai: Kothari Medical; 2015. p. 218–38.
13. Graziottin A. Lukasiewicz M. Psychosexual issues and quality of life after oncologic pelvic surgery, with focus on cervical cancer. In: Carbone A, Palleschi G, Pastore AL, Messas A, editors. Functional urologic surgery in neurogenic and oncologic diseases. Berlin: Springer Verlag; 2016. p. 113–32 (in press).
14. Graziottin A, Lukasiewicz M. Female sexual dysfunction and premature menopause In: Lipshultz L, Pastuszak A, Perelman M, Giraldi AM, Buster J, editors. Sexual health in the couple: management of sexual dysfunction in men and women. Berlin: Springer (in press)
15. Vincenti E, Graziottin A. Sexual pain disorders: management by anesthetic blocks. In: Goldstein I, Meston C, Davis S, Traish A, editors. Women's sexual function and dysfunction: study diagnosis and treatment. London: Taylor and Francis; 2006. p. 524–8.
16. Graziottin A, Murina F. Vulvodynia tips and tricks. Italia: Springer-Verlag; 2011.
17. Goldstein AT, Pukall CF. Provoked vestibulodynia. In: Goldstein AT, Pukall CF, Goldstein I, editors. Female sexual pain disorders: evaluation and management. Oxford (UK): Wiley-Blackwell; 2009. p. 43–8.
18. Andrews JC. Vulvodynia interventions—systematic review and evidence grading. Obstet Gynecol Surv. 2011;66:299–315.
19. Harlow BL, Stewart EG. A population-based assessment of chronic unexplained vulvar pain: have we underestimated the prevalence of vulvodynia? J Am Med Womens Assoc. 2003 Spring;58(2):82–8.
20. Graziottin A. Prevalence and evaluation of sexual health problems—HSDD in Europe. J Sex Med. 2007 Mar;4(Suppl 3):211–9.
21. Laumann EO, Paik A, Rosen RC. Sexual dysfunction in the United States: Prevalence and predictors. JAMA. 1999;281(6):537–44.
22. Arnold LD, Bachmann GA, Rosen R, Rhoads GG. Assessment of vulvodynia symptoms in a sample of US women: a prevalence survey with a nested case control study. Am J Obstet Gynecol. 2007;196(2):128.e1–6.
23. Gunter J. Is there an association between vulvodynia and interstitial cystitis? Obstet Gynecol. 2000;95:S4.
24. Kennedy CM, Nygaard IE, Bradley CS, Galask RP. Bladder and bowel symptoms among women with vulvar disease: are they universal? J Reprod Med. 2007 Dec;52(12):1073–8.

25. Bornstein J, Goldschmid N, Sabo E. Hyperinnervation and mast cell activation may be used as histopathologic diagnostic criteria for vulvar vestibulitis. Gynecol Obstet Invest. 2004;58(3):171–8.
26. Graziottin A, Skaper SD, Fusco M. Mast cells in cronich inflammation, pelvic pain and depression in women. Gynecol Endocrinol. 2014;30(7):472–7.
27. Brotto LA, Basson R, Gehring D. Psychological profi les among women with vulvar vestibulitis syndrome: a chart review. J Psychosom Obstet Gynaecol. 2003;24(3):195–203.
28. Graziottin A, Skaper S, Fusco M. Inflammation and chronic pelvic pain: a biological trigger for depression in women? J Depression Anxiety. 2013;3:142–50.
29. Abraham SN, St John AL. Mast cell-orchestrated immunity to pathogens. Nat Rev Immunol. 2010;10(6):440–52.
30. Glazener CM. Sexual function after childbirth: women's experiences, persistent morbidity and lack of professional recognition. Br J Obstet Gynaecol. 1997 Mar;104(3):330–5.
31. McDonald EA, Gartland D, Small R, Brown SJ. Dyspareunia and childbirth: a prospective cohort study. BJOG. 2015 Apr;122(5):672–9.
32. Hauck YL, Lewis L, Nathan EA, White C, Doherty DA. Risk factors for severe perineal trauma during vaginal childbirth: a Western Australian retrospective cohort study. Women Birth. 2015 Mar;28(1):16–20.

21 Treatment of Genito-Pelvic Pain/Penetration Disorder

Andrea Rapkin, Salome Masghati, and Tamara Grisales

Sexual pain disorders are classified as genito-pelvic pain/penetration disorder (GPPPD) in the Diagnostic and Statistical Manual of Mental Disorders 5th edition [1]. By definition, GPPPD consists of persistent or recurring difficulties within one or more of four of the following often interrelated symptom dimensions: (1) Difficulty having vaginal intercourse or penetration, (2) Genito-pelvic pain, (3) Fear of pain or vaginal penetration, (4) Tension of pelvic floor muscles. Symptoms must not be explained by another "non-sexual" mental disorder or serious relationship dysfunction and should cause significant distress for a minimum of 6 months [1]. Difficult vaginal penetration ranges from situations involving sexual contact (intercourse or other vaginal penetration) to difficulty placing tampons or undergoing a gynecologic examination. Genito-pelvic pain is characterized by pain during vaginal penetration. The location of the pain can be superficial (vulvovaginal) and/or deep (vaginal canal or pelvic); provoked (by genital contact) and/or spontaneous. Marked fear or anxiety about vulvovaginal or pelvic pain either in anticipation of, during, or as a result of vaginal penetration can result from myriad physical, psychosocial, cultural, and religious factors [2]. Pronounced tensing or involuntary tightening of the pelvic floor muscles during attempted vaginal penetration can follow experiences of pain, fear, or anxiety or develop without obvious reason. This chapter reviews evidence based therapeutic interventions and expert opinion for the management of female sexual pain disorders. Treatment of vulvodynia, vaginismus, and other specific disorders causing superficial vulvovaginal pain or deep/pelvic pain with sexual activity is addressed.

Vulvodynia

In 2015, the International Society for the Study of Vulvovaginal Disease (ISSVD), the International Society for the Study of Women's Health Sexual Health (ISSWSH) and the International Pelvic Pain Society (IPPS) revised the terminology and classification of persistent vulvar pain and vulvodynia [3]. In the 2015 nomenclature, pain is categorized as vulvar pain caused by a specific disorder or as vulvodynia. Vulvodynia is defined as vulvar pain for a minimum of 3 months without a clearly identifiable cause. Specific disorders causing vulvar pain include infectious, inflammatory, neoplastic, neurologic, traumatic, iatrogenic (e.g., chemotherapy, radiation, surgery) or hormonal deficiency. Factors that are associated with vulvodynia and potentially affect management are now included in the Appendix of the classification system. These currently include comorbid pain or psychiatric disorders, genetic predisposition to pain or inflammation, sex steroid hormone deficiency, inflammation, pelvic musculoskeletal abnormalities, relevant neurological changes, and psychosocial issues. Further descriptors for vulvodynia in the classification system germane to treatment include pain localization, triggers and timing of onset. "Localized" refers to pain of the vulvar vestibule (vestibulodynia) or clitoris (clitorodynia); "generalized" refers to pain over entire vulva, and "mixed" refers to pain that is both localized and generalized. Pain trigger refers to pain that is "provoked" (pain stimulated only by genital contact) or "spontaneous" (pain occurs without contact), or "both". Timing of onset includes "primary" (pain occurring from the first genital penetration attempt) or "secondary" (pain onset after a period of painless genital contact).

In this section, treatment options for vestibulodynia and generalized vulvodynia when associated with associated pain with sexual contact are discussed. The preponderance of literature addresses provoked vestibulodynia. The diagnosis of vulvodynia can only be made after ruling out specific causes of persistent vulvar pain (see Specific Causes of Vulvar Pain and Superficial Dyspareunia).

Vestibulodynia

Vestibulodynia, either solely upon contact (provoked) (PVD) or provoked and spontaneous is the most common cause of introital pain with penetration, affecting up to 8% of

W.W. IsHak (ed.), *The Textbook of Clinical Sexual Medicine*, DOI 10.1007/978-3-319-52539-6_21

reproductive aged women [4]. By definition, the diagnosis of PVD is based on findings of allodynia (pain with normally non painful stimuli) and varying degrees of erythema of the vestibule, in the absence of a specific disorder. Vulvar pain in areas of the vulva outside the vestibule or clitoris in the absence of neurological, dermatological, neoplastic, musculoskeletal, or other specific findings is called generalized vulvodynia. Generalized vulvodynia often co exists with vestibulodynia and is managed similarly, with the exception of surgical excision.

The pathophysiology of vestibulodynia, similar to other unexplained chronic pain disorders, is complex and likely multifactorial. Histological investigations of many but not all studies of vestibular tissue demonstrate proliferation of nociceptive nerve fibers, increased inflammatory infiltrate dominated by mast cells, and increased neuroinflammatory neurokines, cytokines, chemokines, and prostanoids [5]. Biopsy of the vestibule of an individual patient is not useful for guiding diagnosis or management. There is evidence for peripheral sensitization based on hypersensitivity of the vestibule to tactile, thermal, and chemical stimuli. Hypersensitivity to pressure is also found in tissues other body regions consistent with the presence of central sensitization. Pelvic floor muscle over activity and tenderness is found in most but not all women. Psychological and relationship factors in affected women include depression, anxiety, and lower sexual desire, arousal, orgasm, and overall lower sexual and relationship satisfaction [5].

History and Examination

Comprehensive medical, pain, psychological, and sexual history is indicated [6, 7] (Figure 21-1). After general physical exam, the vulva is closely inspected for dermatitis, dermatoses, infection, lesions, scars, atrophy, and other abnormal anatomic changes. Neurological exam of the relevant dermatomes of the lower abdomen and external vulva (T12 –S 5) for light touch and pinprick can help to rule out neuralgia. Cotton swab test of the vestibule at 12, 2, 5, 6, 7, and 10 o'clock should be performed. Vestibular pain during cotton swab application for 1 s to a depth of 1/3 of the cotton tip is pathognomonic of provoked vestibulodynia. Pain can be rated by the patient on a numeric rating scale (NRS) 0–10 and recorded to compare findings over time. Pelvic floor muscles are evaluated with a single lubricated digit for tone, function and pain (NRS 0–10) [8]. Saline and KOH prep for examination of the vaginal secretions under the microscope can rule out yeast or bacterial infection and highlight estrogen status. Bimanual pelvic exam is then performed and again a single digit can be placed in the vagina to prevent excessive pain with the traditional two finger bimanual exam. Imaging and other studies to diagnose comorbid pelvic and other pain conditions may be indicated based on history and examination. Anxiety, depression, coping skills, sexual functioning, history of trauma, and relationship factors must be discussed. Validated questionnaires can be used [7].

Treatment of Vulvodynia

State-of-the-art research is attempting to define clinically relevant subgroups or phenotypes can that predict the success of specific treatments for vulvodynia. However in practice, a multidisciplinary approach is recommended, with therapy based on presenting symptoms, side effect profile of recommended treatments, cost, and patient preference (Figure 21-1). Predisposing or associated factors that contribute to, magnify or maintaining pain (mood, relationship or sexual concerns, hormonal deficiency, etc.) must be addressed.

Treatment approaches can be divided into distinct categories: surgical, pharmacological (oral, topical, injection), psychological (cognitive-behavioral, psychotherapy, mindfulness based relaxation therapy), physical (manipulative, myofascial physical therapy (PT), EMG biofeedback, dilators, and complementary/alternative such as acupuncture or hypnotherapy [6, 9–13]. The majority of studies are small, single site, and retrospective, uncontrolled or case series. Some methodologically stronger randomized trials (active control or placebo control) have emerged. There are few trials of multimodal therapy [14–16]. Treatment should begin with vulvar care, i.e., eliminating pads allergens fabric softeners, soaps and other potentially irritating chemicals. Initial management will depend on findings but usually includes physical therapy, relaxation therapy, and topical medications outlined below. Oral medication and injections may follow and surgery may be considered if other approaches fail.

Vestibulectomy

Surgical removal of the painful vulvar vestibular tissue is the most widely investigated approach for dyspareunia in women with vestibulodynia, though controlled trials are lacking. The overall success rates are high (85–90%) but success refers to improvement of at least 50% and need not include painless intercourse. Surgery has risks, side effects, and some less than optimal outcomes [17]. Surgical intervention for vestibulodynia has been described with either laser ablation or excisional vestibulectomy. Laser ablation is no longer recommended. There are only a few studies of laser, either CO_2 or flash lamp-excited dye laser and none are more successful than excisional surgery, while laser seems to increase scarring and prolong healing [18]. The first known surgical treatment of vestibulodynia (formerly called vulvar vestibulitis syndrome) was described by Woodruff in 1981 [19].

The original Woodruff procedure involved removal of semicircular segment of perineal skin, mucosa of the posterior vestibule, and the posterior hymnal ring, extending to Hart's line (the junction between vestibule and perineal skin just above the anal orifice). Different surgical techniques and

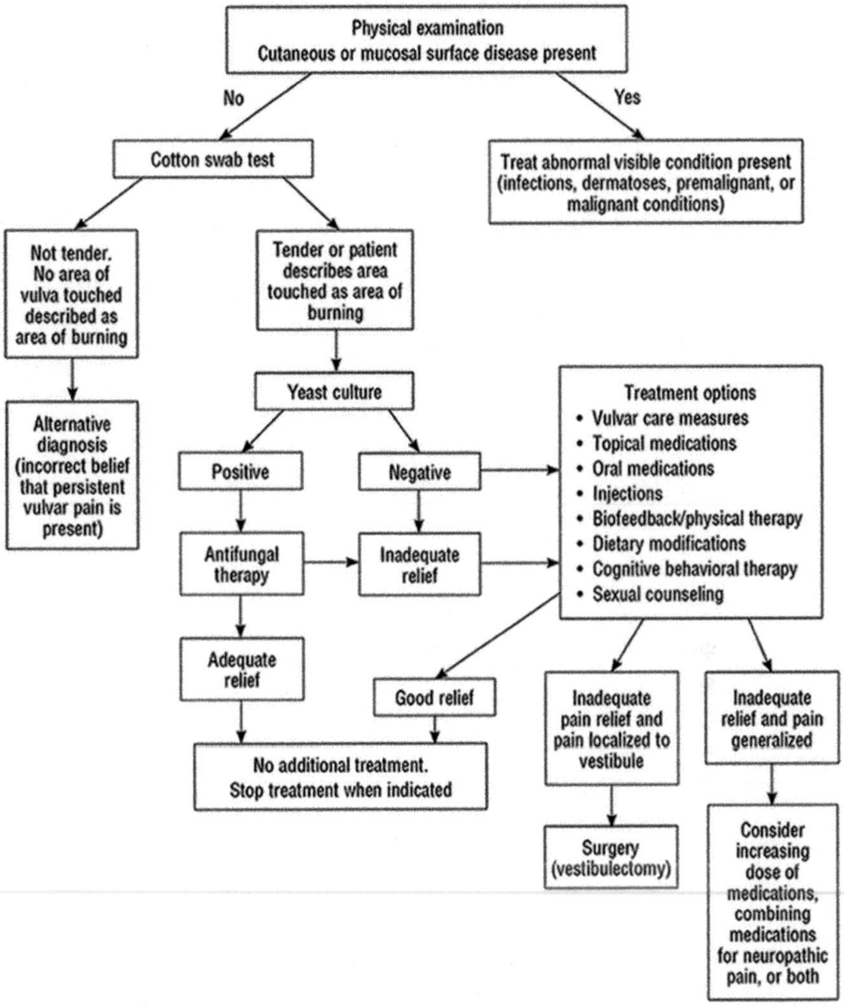

FIGURE 21-1. Persistent vulvar pain treatment algorithm [Adapted from Haefner HK, Collins ME, Davis GD, Edwards L, Foster DC, Hartmann ED, et al. The vulvodynia guideline. J Low Genit Tract Dis. 2005;9:40–51. With permission from Wolters Kluwer Health].

modifications have since been described such as limited posterior vestibulectomy, modified vestibulectomy, simplified vestibulectomy, and vestibuloplasty. Studies have failed to predict which subgroups of patients (primary vs secondary, provoked or spontaneous or both) would best respond to surgery. Most do not include long-term follow-up. There are no randomized studies comparing operative techniques [10]. Despite these caveats, the majority of studies have shown success rates between 50% and 90% for provoked pain in women with vestibulodynia [2, 20]. In less than 5% pain can become more severe after surgery [10]. In an extensive review of 17 studies, the authors concluded approximately 80% reported significant relief of pain with penetration [18].

A large randomized, prospective study [21] compared vestibulectomy, biofeedback and cognitive-behavioral treatment at 6 month and 2.5 years follow-up. Reduced pain and improvement of sexual functioning resulted from all three treatments and improvement was maintained 2.5 years after treatment. Higher pretreatment pain and presence of psychosocial complaints were negatively correlated with treatment outcome. Patients with negative attitude towards sex were less fitting candidates for vestibulectomy as they had poorer outcome compared with the other treatment groups. At 6 months follow-up, all treatment groups were associated with significant reduction in pain, while vestibulectomy resulted in almost twice the degree of pain reduction than the two other treatment groups. It is noteworthy that at 2.5 years self-reported pain during intercourse was similar in the cognitive-behavioral treatment and vestibulectomy groups. CBT has the advantage of being noninvasive and cost-effective. While the long-term benefits of vestibulectomy supports the theory of augmented peripheral nociception, the salutary effects of CBT underline the role of central neurological and psychological factors [22]. Postoperative use of dilators and sex therapy has been associated with improved outcome of vestibulectomy [23].

In a multimodal design combining various modalities, 502 women with vestibulodynia were given oral tricyclic antidepressants or gabapentin and a low-oxalate diet with calcium supplementation followed by biofeedback. Participants then had the option of surgical treatment with either vestibulectomy or vestibulectomy plus excision of the Bartholin's glands. Participants were followed up for a minimum of 12 months. Ninety eight (20%) women had tolerable pain or low pain during intercourse with conservative treatment alone. 80% chose surgery; postoperatively, 97% of women subjected to vestibulectomy with Bartholin's gland removal and 95% of those undergoing vestibulectomy alone reported pain free intercourse [16].

On the basis of over 15 studies, vestibulectomy seems to be a very effective treatment option, but excellent results can be obtained with other noninvasive modalities. Opinion leaders recommend surgery as the last resort. Surgical risks include hematoma formation, infection, delayed healing, obstruction of the Bartholin's glands, and increased pain a small percentage. Adjuvant treatment (cognitive/behavioral therapy, sexual counseling, physical therapy) is often required to manage other problems that contribute to a less than optimal outcome such as anxiety, depression, fear, relationship or sexual dysfunction, comorbid pain conditions, and pelvic floor dysfunction.

Obviously if pain is not localized to the vestibule, vestibulectomy is not indicated. Generalized vulvodynia is managed with nonsurgical modalities as outlined below.

Pharmacological Treatment

Medical options include topical application or injections of local anesthetics or injections of botulinum toxin A, oral neuropathic pain medications such as anticonvulsants or antidepressants (tricyclic antidepressants—TCAs and serotonin norepinephrine re-uptake inhibitors—SNRIs). In controlled trials, the placebo response rate is as high as 50%. Finally, up to 20% of women experience spontaneous improvement [24].

Tricyclic antidepressants modulate pain in the central nervous system at the level of the dorsal horn of the spinal cord and brain [25]. TCAs are an excellent medication for generalized vulvodynia and may be effective for localized provoked although the only RCT failed to find differences compared with placebo. Uncontrolled and active control trials support use of TCAs. A randomized, prospective trial utilizing multimodal therapy by compared CBT, physical, and sex therapy to low-dose oral amitriptyline (10–20 mg daily) with or without topical triamcinolone [26]. Women ($n = 43$) with localized and generalized pain, provoked or unprovoked, were included. There was significant improvement in pain and functioning in both groups but no significant differences between the treatment groups were demonstrated. The one randomized, double blind, controlled trial of TCAs evaluated desipramine and topical lidocaine, as monotherapy or in combination compared with placebo. All groups had with similar response rates (defined as at least 50% pain reduction) ranging from 24% to 43%. Topical lidocaine alone produced the least improvement but the desipramine treatment arms had the highest dropout rates due to anticholinergic and noradrenergic side effects of dry mouth, tachycardia, hot flashes, and dizziness [25]. Uncontrolled studies have shown more than 50% reduction in pain with tricyclic antidepressants, in particular amitriptyline [27].

Topical medications are frequently used for vestibulodynia. Topical amitriptyline avoids systemic side effects such as drowsiness. In a non-controlled prospective study of women with vestibulodynia, topical amitriptyline 2% cream yielded a 56% response rate with 10% pain free and 30% reporting a moderate degree of improvement [28]. Overall, there is insufficient evidence to support the benefits of TCAs in the treatment of vulvodynia [29], but only one RCT has been performed and in clinical practice many women seem to benefit. Clearly further trials are warranted.

Gabapentin inhibits excitatory neurotransmitter glutamate and potentiates inhibitory GABAergic transmission. Oral gabapentin has proven effective in post-herpetic neuralgia, diabetic neuropathy, and fibromyalgia. A multisite study of oral gabapentin for vulvodynia is in progress but in clinical practice anticonvulsants are useful for generalized vulvodynia and for spontaneous pain in women with localized vulvar pain. Topical gabapentin largely avoids systemic side effects such as sedation, dizziness, constipation [30]. A retrospective study of 51 patients with both localized and generalized vulvodynia who received low dose (2%) and high dose (6%) topical gabapentin found 80% of women were responders (at least 50% improvement in pain scores). The treatment was well tolerated with 14% discontinuing for local irritation and urinary complaints [30].

Lidocaine, a sodium channel blocker, inhibits transmission of C-fibers and continuous exposure is suggested to impede irritable nociceptors, and thus its role substantial role in neuropathic pain management. Topical lidocaine 5% is the most commonly prescribed medication for vestibulodynia, used twice per day to the vestibule and before any sexual activity [31]. In a randomized non-blinded trial, lidocaine 5% ointment was compared with pelvic floor EMG. No differences were found between these two active interventions [32]. An uncontrolled study also showed promise with aver 50% reduction pain in 61 women with dyspareunia who applied topical 5% lidocaine ointment nightly to the vestibule. At 6 months follow-up, 77% reported ongoing use [33]·5% lidocaine ointment for treatment of is a reasonable initial treatment alone or as adjunctive therapy with CBT and/or PT in women with vulvodynia.

Injections with lidocaine and methyl prednisone aim to decrease the local inflammatory reaction and take advantage of the sodium channel blocking effects of lidocaine. After one case study demonstrated complete relief of persistent vulvar vestibular pain with submucosal infiltration of betamethasone and lidocaine in the vestibular area [34], a prospective, non-randomized study of 22 patients utilized the same treatment. 32% experienced complete response and 36% experienced significant improvement, but 32% failed to respond despite multiple injections [35]. It should be noted that topical corticosteroid creams are not effective. In another non controlled trial, multilevel local anesthetic nerve blockade (caudal block, pudendal block, vulvar infiltration) using ropivacaine and bupivacaine in 26 patients with generalized vulvodynia showed 57% average improvement [36]. The same protocol was used in patients with vestibulodynia with similar improvement in both pain and sexual functioning [37].

Botulinum toxin A reduces muscle hypertonicity and has antinociceptive effects in studies of neuropathic pain. Two small RCTS found significant improvement in both dyspareunia, but response was similar in the Botulinum toxin A and the saline injection groups [38]. Another small study noted the placebo group reported a significantly larger reduction in sexual distress than the Botulinum toxin group [39]. Reported side effects are rare but include hematoma and bleeding, toxin reactions and loss of pelvic sphincter control. Botulinum toxin should be considered as a second-line treatment for vestibulodynia. It is also recommended for pelvic floor hypertonus and in women with vulvodynia if physical therapy and CBT are unsuccessful [40].

Cromolyn sodium blocks mast cell degranulation and inhibits the release of inflammatory mediators. It has been reported to prevent hypersensitivity to seminal fluid when applied topically [41]. The effectiveness of topical cromolyn cream did not exceed that of placebo in a double-blinded RCT for vestibulodynia, although symptoms of burning and dyspareunia improved in both groups [42].

Capsaicin is an agonist of vanilloid receptors, located on the peripheral terminals of sensitive nociceptors. It has been recommended for treatment of post-herpetic neuralgia or peripheral neuropathy and was therefore investigated for vestibulodynia. Application of capsaicin to the skin causes irritation and pain, but used long term results in degeneration of C (pain) nerve fibers and desensitization [43]. In a prospective uncontrolled trial, 33 women were treated with topical capsaicin 0.05%, with 19 patients reporting improvement in dyspareunia [43]. The second study evaluating capsaicin in dyspareunia was a chart review of 42 women with vulvodynia. Post treatment, 95% of the patients was having vaginal intercourse compared with 62% prior to treatment. Given the retrospective nature of the study, the researchers could not evaluate which participants used additional therapies [44]. Currently topical capsaicin is not currently recommended due to the burning sensation after application; however, other substance P antagonists lacking this side effect are under evaluation.

Hormonal Treatment

Some but not all studies have associated oral contraceptives (OCPs), particularly long term intake prior to the age of 18 with increased risk for vestibulodynia [45–47]. OCPs inhibit luteinizing hormone and therefore decrease ovarian estradiol and testosterone production. Oral intake of estrogens and progestins also increases hepatic production of sex hormone binding globulin which further lowers circulating free testosterone. Lack of testosterone has been shown to impact vestibular morphology, lubrication as well as libido [48]. Vestibular glands which produce protective mucin are also rich in androgen receptors. The lower endogenous estrogen and bioavailable testosterone have been suggested to thin the vestibule, predisposing to inflammation and development of neuropathic pain [49].

Application of topical estradiol 0.03% and testosterone 0.1% twice per day may be effective in patients who suffer from vestibulodynia while taking oral contraceptives (OCPs). However it is preferable to discontinue hormonal contracepetives that suppress ovarian steroids. Levonorgestrel or copper IUD can be used. In a retrospective study, participants who had developed vestibular pain while using OCPs were asked to discontinue all oral hormones and to apply the above compounded estradiol-testosterone cream twice daily. After 6 months, significant improvement in vestibular pain scores were noted [48]. Topical estrogen (± testosterone) is the first choice when vestibular pain is associated with hypoestrogenic disorders such the climacteric, menopause, puerperium, lactation, hypothalamic amenorrhea, or systemic hormonal contraceptives [50].

Physical Therapy (PT) and Biofeedback

Women with vestibulodynia demonstrate increased pelvic floor muscle hypertonus, muscular instability, poor muscle control, decreased strength, and restriction of the vaginal opening [51, 52]. Chronic vulvar pain can also trigger chronic pelvic floor tightening as part of the normal pain response [53]. Pelvic floor hypertonic dysfunction can activate viscerosomatic reflexes and visceral afferent neurons causing muscle over activity and a vaginismus type response [12]. Muscle trigger points can cause referred, localized or radiating pain and can present as sensations of vulvar burning, itching, and tingling [54]. Physical therapy techniques for management include internal and external tissue mobilization and myofascial trigger point release, joint manipulation, biofeedback, electrical stimulation, use of dilators [55]. PT improves pain threshold and dyspareunia, as well as overall sexual pain, pain catastrophizing, and pain related anxiety [56–58]. In a retrospective study, physical therapy yielded a 52% success rate with a significantly decreased pain, increased intercourse frequency, levels of sexual desire and arousal [59]. Biofeedback with surface electromyography (EMG) to treat pelvic floor hypertonicity was also found to be an effective tool for pelvic floor myalgia and dysfunction in patients with vestibulodynia. 52% of participant were pain free at 6 months follow-up [60] with treatment gains maintained 3–5 years post treatment [61]. In another uncontrolled study, EMG biofeedback alleviated introital tenderness by up to 50% and allowed up to 90% of study participants to have intercourse without discomfort [62].

Transcutaneous Electrical Nerve Stimulation (TENS)

Beneficial effects of TENS were demonstrated in a randomized placebo-controlled trial of 40 women with vestibulodynia. After 20 sessions, the TENS treatment arm showed significant improvement of pain and sexual function compared with placebo [63].

Psychological Interventions

Psychological factors play a significant role in development, maintenance and management of vulvodynia. Pain is both a physical and emotional experience. These factors should be addressed prior to and during treatment [64]. Psychological interventions target emotions, cognitions, and dysfunctional couple interactions that impact sexual functioning and genital pain. Vulvar pain can have a tremendous impact on the patient's body image, sexual self-esteem, and sexual functioning in their intimate relationship [65]. Women with vulvodynia often report a sense of shame, isolation and blame themselves for their disease. There is a sense of loss and unfairness associated with anger, powerlessness, or depression. Anxiety, fear, and lower levels of pain self-efficacy are associated with more sexual impairment in women with vestibulodynia [64, 66]. Women with history of depression or anxiety are four times more likely to be diagnosed with vulvodynia [5]. Vulvodynia sufferers are almost three times more likely to report severe physical or sexual abuse and continued fear of abuse [5].

Hypnotherapy

In addition to personal history of mood disorders or sexual, physical, and emotional trauma, the quality of patient's relationship with their partner plays an important role. Women with vulvodynia report more problematic relationships [12, 67]. Vestibulodynia is also associated with psychological and sexual consequences for sexual partners. In couples with provoked vestibulodynia, the partner's perceptions and behaviors influence both the partner's and the patient's coping mechanisms and sexual outcomes. A perception of injustice can negatively impact the intimate relationship [68, 69]. Relationship factors such as partner catastrophizing and solicitousness also influence pain and sexual outcomes [70].

Cognitive Behavioral Therapy (CBT)

CBT is the most studied psychological intervention for vulvodynia. Individual and group CBT are validated, noninvasive options for treatment. CBT stresses self-management, relaxation, coping mechanisms [71]. The goal of CBT is to help women understand how thoughts and emotions impact behaviors and to modify these factors by redirecting negative thought pathways leading to behavioral changes. CBT reduces anxiety by giving patients more control over their pain sexual interactions [21]. CBT has been shown to significantly decrease catastrophizing scores and improve sexual functioning [72]. Compared with supportive psychotherapy, CBT showed a greater improvement in pain severity on exam, overall sexual functioning, and greater global treatment satisfaction. Participants in both psychological treatment groups reported significant improvements in pain severity with sex, sexual and emotional functioning, and decreased anxiety and depression.

Acceptance-based psychological treatment approaches are of great value for couples where one partner suffers from genito-pelvic pain and who report perceived injustice [68]. Couples who underwent CBT together experienced better sexual function, and less anxiety and depression for both partners after 12 sessions [73].

A comprehensive treatment approach for provoked vestibulodynia combined pelvic floor exercises, desensitization techniques (vaginal acupressure, masturbation, tampon use) and CBT. The 10 week therapy period included education about genital anatomy, relationship problems, sexual disorders, and practical exercises. Patients were instructed to perform daily self-examination with touch and massage using a hand mirror. Tampon use was encouraged. Once the home work was successfully executed, exercises with the partner were included. Sexual interest, sexual pleasure and frequency of masturbation were all increased and sexual pain was decreased at 6 month follow-up [74].

Two studies showed equivalent outcomes between CBT and vestibulectomy for patients with vestibulodynia [31, 75]. Surgical and psychosocial modalities can be complementary; addressing factors such as fear of sex and poor body image can improve surgical outcome [21]. The literature highlights the impact of psychosocial factors and role for psychosocial interventions in women with chronic vulvar pain [71].

Mindfulness Based Stress Reduction (MBSR) Therapy

Mindfulness is the practice of relaxed wakefulness, defined as nonjudgmental moment awareness, and is an ancient eastern practice with roots in Buddhist meditation [76]. Many pain programs now blend CBT and mindfulness treatments [77]. In a recent study, 85 patients with vulvodynia who were treated with MBSR demonstrated significant improvements in pain, sexual distress, and depressive symptoms [78].

Hypnotherapy has shown promising results in the treatment of vulvar vestibulitis in a small pilot study of eight women with vestibulodynia who underwent six hypnotherapy sessions. Dyspareunia, pain associated with gynecologic exams, sexual satisfaction, and overall sexual function were improved [79].

Addressing Relationship Factors in the Treatment of Vulvodynia

The partner's response to pain reinforces and perpetuates the pain experience. Several studies have shown that partner response to women's pain is affects pain intensity, sexual function, and sexual satisfaction [80]. The dynamics of a couple's relationship and their implications for emotional and physical aspects of the patient's condition have to be taken into consideration when treating patients with vestibulodynia [81]. Lower ambivalence in communication is associated with better outcomes of sexual and relationship satisfaction in couples with vestibulodnia [82]. Patients with vestibulodynia who perceived their partners to have negative perceptions of their pain condition reported higher levels of pain during intercourse [83, 84]. Relationships where partners were sympathetic, encouraged coping mechanisms and demonstrated less negative attitude such as anger were associated with lower pain intensity, less catastrophizing and increased sexual and relationship satisfaction [85]. Patient's self-reports of high levels of relationship satisfaction and sexual intimacy had a protective impact on the sexual well-being in the context of pain [86]. Patients also had lower pain scores during intercourse when the partner's pain acceptance was higher [87, 88].

Studies highlight the importance of including the partner in the psychological/behavioral treatment. One randomized clinical trial still in progress will examine the efficacy of cognitive behavioral couples therapy compared to topical lidocaine [89]. This study is based on a successful pilot study of cognitive-behavioral couple therapy for couples coping with provoked vestibulodynia. Significant improvement in pain and sexual outcome for both women and partners, as well as pain related cognitions, anxiety, and depression symptoms for both partners was noted [73].

Acupuncture

A small ($n = 36$) randomized study examined acupuncture in women with vulvodynia compared with a wait-list control group. Vulvar pain significantly decreased in patients who underwent acupuncture whereas sexual functioning was not improved [90].

Multimodal Approaches

Multidisciplinary approaches which integrate psychological, medical, and physical therapy treatments are difficult to study in a controlled fashion but reflect the current recommended standard of care for women with vulvodynia [91]. A retrospective questionnaire survey evaluated the long-term outcome of a multimodal approach to provoked vestibulodynia. Over 81% reported pain reduction and had resumed intercourse [92]. A qualitative retrospective study using semi-structured interviews demonstrated enhanced knowledge, improved mood and psychological well-being, and an increased sense of empowerment in patients who had been offered CBT, pelvic PT, and sexual education in addition to medical therapy [12]. A large study of 132 women with provoked vestibulodynia enrolled in a 10-week program incorporating pelvic floor PT, psychological skill training, and medical management resulted in significant improvement in dyspareunia, arousal, desire, and orgasmic function [93]. Given the multifaceted nature of vulvodynia, treatments targeting pain as well as associated psychological, sexual, and relational consequences have more impact than interventions aiming at reducing pain alone.

Vaginismus

Vaginismus is a highly prevalent condition that can overlap with provoked vestibulodynia [94]. Vaginismus was described in 1547 by Trotula of Salerno as a condition of "tightening of the vulva so that even a women who has been seduced may appear a virgin" [94]. In 1862, Sims first used the term "vaginismus" which he described as "involuntary spasmodic closure of the mouth of the vagina" [94]. The DSM 5 classification identifies vaginismus as a vaginal penetration disorder of any form, making the use of tampons, fingers, vaginal dilators, gynecological examinations, and intercourse painful or impossible [95]. The prevalence of vaginismus in the population is difficult to assess since such studies would require gynecological examinations that patients prefer to avoid. Furthermore, studies have shown that only a third of sufferers with sexual problems consult health professionals, with barriers being negative past experiences, poor self-perceived health, embarrassment and shame [96]. In the USA, prevalence rates have been reported between 5 and 17% [97]. The severity of the condition is influenced by the amount of vaginal spasm and the degree of fear and anxiety. Patients can have a visceral reaction to examination with palpitations sweating, hyperventilation, shaking, screaming, and a feeling of becoming unconscious [98].

Vaginismus and vestibulodynia overlap and can pose a challenge to differentiate the two diagnoses based solely on exam. Fear and vaginal muscle tension were greater in the vaginismus group as compared the dyspareunia/PVD and control group. Genital pain however did not differ significantly between vaginismus patients and patients with dyspareunia [94].

Treatment of Vaginismus

Desensitization

The use of dilators, also called vaginal trainers (VTs), of gradually increasing sizes is one of the most commonly recommended treatments for vaginismus, despite lack of systematic research [99]. A Cochrane uncontrolled trial concluded systematic desensitization with insertion training is effective for vaginismus if the outcome is measured by the ability to have intercourse [97] VTs may help overcome the physical aspects of vaginismus, as well as the fear of penetration [95]. However, simply asking women to buy a dilator set without providing support and counseling on their use is a setup for failure. Patients require instructions on how to use the dilators, how to overcome the anxiety associated with the use, the importance of progression to larger sizes and how to transition to intercourse, and education on sexual positions that allow relaxation of the pelvic floor. Dilators come in various sizes and materials (plastic, silicone, glass). Some patients find it helpful to use vibrators to relax during the dilation process. With adequate use, patients are potentially able to sleep with a dilator at night and progress with morning dilation to the next size up [95]. Psychological, sexual and behavioral therapy in conjunction with VTs leads to the best outcome. However, it should be acknowledged that successful penetration alone is not enough to guarantee a couple's satisfaction and pleasurable feeling [100].

Dilator therapy consisting of vaginal penetration exercises by patient, in the presence of a female therapist or patient's partner led to improvement of sexual distress, coital fear and pain and 89% of participants who had the intervention were able to have intercourse [101]. Interestingly, 11% of the patients assigned to the 3 month wait list group were also able to have intercourse, highlighting the small chance of spontaneous resolution of symptoms in motivated couples who recognize the nature of the problem.

Pharmacological Interventions

Anxiolytic medication, such as diazepam or antidepressants such as amitriptyline, alone has not shown to resolve vaginismus symptoms, but in conjunction with psychotherapy they can be used for patients with high levels of anxiety [102].

Botulinum toxin decreases overactive muscle tone of the pelvic floor [103]. Small non controlled studies are supportive. Botulinum toxin A was injected into puborectalis muscles of 24 patients with vaginismus refractory to other treatments and 23 of the patients showed no vaginismus symptoms on the post-injection visit 1 week later with effects lasting up to 12 months [104]. In another study, 39 patients who underwent injections into the levator ani under EMG guidance had improvement in pain, sexual function and vaginal spasms and 63% completely recovered from vaginismus [105].

Psychological Interventions

CBT in group format offers the opportunity to practice pain and sexual coping strategies which can help reduce pelvic muscle contraction [106]. CBT can also include be used in conjunction with physical therapy techniques such as vaginal dilation and sensate focus. Sensate focus consists of non-penetrative, touching exercises that aim to increase the participant's awareness of their senses [9]. There are a few studies looking specifically at the success of CBT in patients with vaginismus. In a 2010 study, 44 patients completed questionnaires regarding ability to have intercourse, sexual pain and enjoyment of intercourse after 14 sessions of CBT with follow-up several months later (mean of 39 months). A large proportion of the women (61%) were able to have pain-free intercourse [107].

Gradual exposure to intercourse using CBT can decrease fear of penetration and avoidance behavior [108]. In a wait list controlled trial, 81 patients were randomly assigned to a 3 month CBT group and 36 to a waiting list group. CBT was more successful as defined by coitus frequency, decrease in fear, and changes in avoidance behavior [108]. Graded exposure exercises with dilators or fingers, as directed by the therapist, with homework assignments (alone or with partner) was effective for 31 out of 35 patients in the active group who were able to have sexual intercourse compared to 4 out of 35 in the waiting list control group [101].

Including the Partner in Treatment

Treating the couple and not just the affected woman is recommended. Partners of women with vaginismus can develop sexual dysfunction secondarily to their partner's complaint. 5–45% of men have reported erection disorders or premature ejaculation [109, 110]. Of 56 couples were treated with CBT, 80% were able to have penetrative sex, with most prognostic indicator of positive treatment outcome being mild and moderate as opposed to severe vaginismus [110]. An interesting approach allowing participants to use surrogate partners for penetration exercises compared 16 using surrogates to 16 patients treated with their own partner. Treatment involved dilators, tampons or finger insertion followed by sensate focus exercises with the partner or surrogate. The patients using surrogates had 100% success rate with intercourse vs 69% in the established couples [111]. The high success rate depicted in this trial highlights the importance of a cooperative, nonjudgmental partner in the process of treating vaginismus.

Specific Causes of Vulvar Pain and Superficial Dyspareunia

Women presenting with vulvar pain and entry dyspareunia should be evaluated to exclude a specific etiology before a diagnosis of vulvodynia is given [3]. Burning and aching in the Sacral 2–4 nerve dermatomal distribution can also be caused by dermatoses, dermatitis, infections, referred visceral pain from the bladder or the rectum, or levator ani syndrome.

Neuralgia/Neuropathy

The International Association for the Study of Pain (IASP) definition of neuropathic pain is pain caused by a lesion or a disease of the somatosensory nervous system. Pudendal neuralgia due to injury or entrapment is one of the most common causes of neuropathic vulvar, perineal, and/or buttocks pain. Other nerves including the genitofemoral nerve, ilioinguinal nerve, inferior cluneal nerve (branch of posterior femoral cutaneous nerve, and the obturator nerve also innervate the genital region).

Pudendal Neuropathy

Pudendal neuralgia or neuropathy is related to direct injury or entrapment associated with ligamentous and muscular inflammation and fibrosis. Pudendal neuropathy can be caused by various types of injury: distortion of bony pelvis due a fall on coccyx or other trauma to spine or pelvis, heavy lifting, traction on lower limbs, traction on nerves due to straining with constipation, prolonged sitting, repetitive workouts, biking, childbirth with large baby or prolonged second stage, pelvic sidewall hematoma, and vaginal prolapse or other pelvic surgery. In the case of idiopathic entrapment of the pudendal nerve between the sacrospinous and sacrotuberous ligaments, the pain typically increases with sitting and diminishes or resolves in the supine position. More severe pudendal nerve involvement can produce numbness and tingling but lack of sensation is more typical of a severe pudendal nerve injury or other neurological disorder as opposed to entrapment.

Diagnosis of Pudendal Neuropathy/Neuralgia

The diagnosis of pudendal neuropathy is clinical; there is no diagnostic imaging, laboratory, or electrophysiological tests. The pudendal nerve motor latency test measures the time between the stimulation of the pudendal nerve at the ischial spine to the contractile response of the external anal sphincter. However unless a nerve is severely injured, the motor function of the nerve is unaffected.

The Nantes criteria for pudendal neuralgia related to entrapment include essential, complementary, and exclusion criteria [112]. Essential criteria: (1) pain in the territory of the pudendal nerve (anal-rectal, vulvo-vaginal, and distal urethral tissues) (2) pain mostly while sitting which may become continuous over time, (3) pain does not wake the patient at night, (4) pain without sensory deficit, and (5) relief by diagnostic pudendal nerve block. Complementary diagnostic criteria include burning, shooting, stabbing pain and numbness, allodynia or hyperalgesia in the pudendal nerve territory, rectal or vaginal foreign body sensation, worsening of the pain during the day, predominately unilateral pain, pain triggered by defecation, and exquisite tenderness on palpation of the ischial spine. Exclusion criteria include exclusively coccygeal, gluteal, pubic, or hypogastric pain, itching, exclusively paroxysmal pain and imaging abnormalities that account for the pain. Associated signs that do not exclude the diagnosis include buttock pain on sitting, referred sciatic pain, pain referred to the medial aspect of the thigh, suprapubic pain, urinary frequency, or pain on a full bladder. Although sexual intercourse is not generally painful, postcoital pain is typical.

Gluteal pain is not dependent on the pudendal nerve, and isolated buttock pain cannot be considered to be due to pudendal neuralgia, but perineal pain and buttocks pain can be due to compression or concomitant lesion of the posterior femoral cutaneous or inferior gluteal nerve. Buttocks pain can be due to spasms in the deep gluteal muscles, obturator internus and piriformis. Referred sciatic pain due to compression of the posterior femoral cutaneous nerve or sciatic trunk, with or without piriformis or obturator internus syndrome may be confused with pudendal neuralgia. If the pain is referred to the urethra and medial thigh only, one should consider obturator internus muscle spasm as an etiology.

Management of Pudendal Neuropathy

Pharmacological Management

The initial step in diagnosis and management of pudendal neuropathy is to perform a neural blockade, using local anesthetic ± corticosteroid. If the pain is relieved immediately after the block and then pain improvement outlasts the duration of the local anesthesia, the blocks can be repeated without the steroids every 2 weeks to 1 month to downgrade the pain signaling. The blocks can be imaging guided using CT or ultrasound to improve accuracy. There are no controlled studies of the outcomes of treating pudendal neuralgia with local anesthetic blocks. Some recommend Botulinum toxin A injection as well.

Medical therapy for pudendal neuralgia is similar to treatment of other neuropathies but controlled trials are lacking. Tricyclic antidepressants, such as nortriptyline, desipramine or amitriptyline, beginning with 10 mg at night and increasing to 50–150 mg are useful. Amitriptyline has the most antihistaminergic and anticholinergic side effects and is most sedating, therefore useful for urinary frequency or difficulty sleeping. Desipramine is the least sedating and can lead to anxiety or irritability. All the TCAs increase constipation and prolong QT interval, therefore they should not be using elderly patients without consulting with primary care physician. Selective serotonin and norepinephrine reuptake inhibitors have also been used to treat pudendal neuropathy, duloxetine 30–60 mg, one to two times per day, or venlafaxine 37.5 mg once or twice per day, up to 225 mg. Anticonvulsants, such as gabapentin, in doses of 300 mg at night up to 600–900 mg three times daily, pregabalin 75 mg per day up to 300 mg twice daily, topiramate 50–100 mg twice daily are in the armamentarium. Topical lidocaine 5% or other compounded preparations of the above medications can be used off label. Muscle relaxants orally or vaginally may be helpful.

Physical Therapy

PT is an important part of treatment and pelvic floor disorders often accompany pudendal nerve pain. All the muscles between ribs and knees should be examined; myofascial trigger points (hyperirritable spots within a taut band of muscle or fascia) should be treated. Common trigger points are located in the rectus abdominis, obturator internus, piriformis, gluteal muscles, quadratus lumborum abductus; these will respond to manual therapy, dry needling or trigger point injections. Connective tissue restrictions and muscle hypertonicity in pelvic floor must be addressed. PT consists of exercise for the pelvic girdle and pelvic floor; soft tissue mobilization/myofascial release of the pelvic girdle, pelvic floor and associated structures; joint mobilization/manipulation; bowel/bladder retraining. It is important to treat trigger points, teach self-care: muscle strengthening and stretching, and trigger point release can include injections of local anesthetics or Botulinum toxin A.

Neuromodulation and Surgery

Case reports of pudendal neuromodulation for the treatment of chronic refractory pelvic and perineal pain are supportive [113]. Initially one should recommend PT for compressed nerves and pelvic muscle dysfunction. If medical management for 6 months has failed and gastrointestinal, genitourinary, gynecological and musculoskeletal diagnoses have been ruled out (Negative CT or MRI, ±laparoscopy) then pulsed radio frequency ablation or surgery are the last resort.

Pudendal nerve decompression surgery is quite an involved surgery is not routinely performed by gynecologists or neurosurgeons; finding an experienced surgeon may be geographically challenging. Indications for surgery include diagnosis of pudendal neuropathy by Nantes criteria and failed conservative management. The surgical procedure entails freeing the nerve from compressed position from the sacrospinous and sacrutuberous ligaments or by obturator fascia in Alcock's canal. There are transgluteal trans-ischial rectal fascia approaches. In small uncontrolled trials, 2/3 of the patients improved, with good relief in 20%, some relief in up to 60% of patients. Unfortunately, in 30%, pain may be unchanged or worsened. One randomized controlled trial of surgical decompression exists; Eligible patients had positive temporary response to local anesthetic nerve block at the ischial spine and Alcock's canal. After 3 months 50% of the surgery group ($n = 16$) reported improvement in pain versus 6.2% of the control group ($n = 16$). At 12 months, 71.4% of the surgery group was improved, compared to 13% of the control group, and after 4 years, 8 remained improved; no complications were encountered [114]. Women who have better response to conservative measures are more likely to have improvement with surgery. Unfortunately, only the operative finding of nerve entrapment and postoperative relief can completely confirm the diagnosis.

Vulvar Dermatoses

Lichen Sclereous

Vulvar/introital pain with sexual activity can also result from chronic inflammatory autoimmune conditions lichen sclerosus (LS) or lichen planus (LP). LS is a chronic inflammatory autoimmune disorder which may be associated with LP, pernicious anemia, alopecia areata, and autoimmune thyroid disease. The disease affects 1 in 70 women and the average age of onset is 51 years. Women with LS are more likely than unaffected women to have dyspareunia, decreased orgasm, and decreased coital frequency. Standard medical therapy to treat LS results in improved of sexual functioning but does not completely normalize.

Typical symptoms include itching, vulvar pain/burning and dyspareunia. Biopsy is useful for diagnosis and imperative if cancer is suspected, but diagnosis of LS can also be made clinically. Signs and symptoms are localized to areas of skin changes. Skin changes consist of white epithelium, thickened plaques, and fissures between the labia minora and majora, anterior commissure, posterior fourchette, and scarring of clitoral prepuce often causing phimosis. Scarring of introiotus, perineum and perirectal area (vagina is rarely involved) narrow the vaginal caliber and can tear with intercourse.

Treatment of Lichen Sclereosus

The treatment of lichen sclerosus begins with ultra-potent steroid ointments such as clobetasol 0.05% twice a day for 1 month and then tailoring the medication over 3 months the used once or twice a week as needed with exams every 4–6 months. Another approach after obtaining remission is to use the lowest potency of corticoid steroid ointment on a daily basis that prevents recurrent symptoms. Daily application may be preferable to as needed higher potency approach as women may not be aware of LS exacerbation until they have significant scarring or cancer. For those that do not respond, tacrolimus ointment, a macrolide immunosuppressant, can be used in a similar regiment. A slight increased risk of squamous cell carcinoma with tacrolimus used for lichen sclerosis has been reported [115].

A review of 7 RCTs, with a total of 249 participants, covering 6 treatments found clobetasol propionate 0.05% was effective for genital lichen sclerosus and mometasone furaote 0.05% showed somewhat less improvement, especially for investigator-rated change in degree of phimosis. Trials found no significant differences in reported adverse drug reactions between the corticosteroid and placebo groups. The data from four trials found no significant benefit for topical testosterone, dihydrotestosterone, and progesterone. One trial found no differences between pimecrolimus and clobetasol propionate in relieving symptoms pruritus (itching) and burning/pain but pimecrolimus was less effective than clobetasol propionate with regard to the investigator rated changes. There were no significant differences in reported adverse drug reactions between the pimecrolimus and placebo groups [116].

To maintain the integrity of the vestibule, topical estradiol and testosterone are helpful, applied once or twice daily. For those who have not been sexually active and who have minor degrees of narrowing dilators can be effective. Treatment is successful in over 80% of individuals, and surgery is needed for less than 0.5% of women [117].

The main cause of dyspareunia is intractable scarring with narrowing of the introitus to the point of midline fusion at times with urethral outlet obstruction, buried clitoris can lead to decrease sensation or retention pseudocysts and introital stenosis can lead to dyspareunia. These findings are indications for surgery. Surgical approaches, including release of adhesions with laser or cautery, perineoplasty. Ultra-potent topical steroids 2 weeks before and then resumed with healing and vaginal dilators are crucial [118, 119].

Lichen Planus (LP)

LP affects 1–2% of the population. Symptoms include pain, burning, dyspareunia, and postciotal bleeding. LP affects the vestibule and inner labia minora and majora, vagina, and mouth. Signs include erosions in 74%, redness in approximately 65%, scarring and lacy changes with white overlying red epithelium in 63%, and in 56% vestibule and vagina are involved. Abnormal vaginal discharge consists of yellow non odorous discharge; under the microscope reveals multiple white blood cells and immature vaginal epithelial cells. If there is a question as to whether there is estrogen deficiency and atrophy is suspected, treat with estrogen first, and biopsy for definitive diagnosis.

Treatment of Lichen Planus

Ultra- and mid-potent corticoid steroids ointments for vulva are recommended. The vagina can be treated with clobetasol or mometasone furaote cream, hydrocortisone suppositories, or tacrolimus. Some patients may require prophylaxis for candida infection with weekly fluconazole. Dilators and physical therapy are also needed. Some patients require systemic therapy which is generally in concert with dermatology [120].

Vulvar Granuloma Fissuratum

The etiology of vulvar granuloma fissuratum may be atrophy, such as with menopause or estrogen suppression related to hormonal contraceptives, lichen planus or lichen sclerosus, vulvar intraepithelial neoplasia, hypertonic pelvic floor muscles or a poorly healed episiotomy. Vulvar granuloma fissuratum is a granuloma -like lesion of the posterior fourchette. Causes pain with intercourse and postciotal bleeding. Severe cutting pain of posterior fourchette is typical [121]. The diagnosis is made on visual examination with findings of a thin friable erythematous posterior fourchette and biopsy may reveal granulomatous tissue. Wet mount with saline prep and KOH are performed to rule out infectious etiologies. Pelvic floor muscle evaluation must be performed. Targeted treatments include hormonal or topical corticoid steroids, depending on the etiology, dilators, physical therapy, sexual therapy, and if not successful, surgery. Surgery consists of perineoplasty and vaginal advancement flap [121].

Vulvovaginal Atrophy

Vulvovaginal atrophy or thinning is a common cause of dyspareunia occurring in the setting of prolonged estrogen deficiency, typically with menopause. Atrophic changes can affect reproductive aged women with low endogenous estrogen and/or androgen levels due to idiopathic central amenorrhea, prolonged postpartum amenorrhea due to lactation, and hormonal contraceptives., such as low dose combined hormonal oral contraceptives, progestogen implants or injections.

Symptoms include poor lubrication, pain on contact in the region of the vestibule and the vagina, dryness, burning, irritation, urinary urgency, and in more severe cases, pain with urination and recurrent urinary tract infections. Deficiency of estrogen leads to anatomic changes in the external genitalia, including the labia, majora and minora, the clitoris, the vestibule, the vagina, the urethra, and bladder [122]. Androgen deficiency can contribute. Estrogen promotes maturation of the vaginal epithelium, increases vaginal blood flow, and improves the integrity and elasticity of the tissue, quality and quantity of vaginal secretions. The mature estrogenized vaginal cells contain glycogen, the substrate for lactobacilli. The lactobacilli ferment the glycogen restoring the acid pH of 4.5 and reducing colonization with enterobacteria, and subsequently, atrophic vaginitis [123].

Treatment of Atrophy

Successful management of vulvo vaginal atrophy can take up to 18 months for restoration of elasticity for those who have not maintained coitus and who have a narrow introits, although improvement dryness, burning and itching can be expected after 2–3 months of estrogen. Treatment must continue as long as the estrogen deficient state persists.

Nonhormonal approaches are first line for managing urogenital atrophy [124]. Hormonal therapies consist of topical or systemic estrogen or selective estrogen receptor modulators.

Systemic estrogen therapy is not necessary, although the topical and systemic estrogen can be used concurrently. Topical therapies are equally effective and consist of "bio-identical" 17 beta estradiol rings, vaginal tablets or creams. Conjugated equine estrogen cream is a more potent formulation such that lower doses are recommended to prevent endometrial stimulation. If higher doses are needed, concurrent progestogen therapy for 10 days every 3 months or endometrial monitoring with ultrasound may be needed [125]. The 17 beta estradiol preparations in standard doses do not yield systemic estrogen levels outside the menopausal range and have not been shown to cause endometrial proliferation, even with long-term use. When the vaginal epithelium is still thin, absorption is higher; however, after atrophy has been corrected absorption is nil. The estrogen vaginal rings contain 17 beta estradiol and are replaced every 3 months. The estradiol vaginal tablets contain 10 mcg of estradiol and after 14 days of continuous dosing are then used twice a week. The estradiol cream 0.01% is used in a dose of 1 to 2 mg nightly for 14 days then two to three times per week.

In practice, for those with persistent vestibular pain, a ring or tablets with estradiol vaginally can be combined with an estrogen cream for the vestibule, sometimes compounded with 0.1% testosterone for nighty application. Those who do not respond after resolution of atrophy should be evaluated for vestibulodynia.

Women with a history of estrogen-dependent breast cancer who are unresponsive to nonhormonal remedies can consider vaginal estrogen as above according to a recent opinion from the American College of Obstetrics and Gynecology [126]; however, this decision should be made in coordination with oncologist. The data do not reveal increased risk for women undergoing treatment of breast cancer currently or those with a prior history of breast cancer [126].

For those women who cannot tolerate a vaginal estrogen preparation, a selective estrogen receptor modulator called ospemifene can be considered. It approved by the US Food and Drug Administration and is effective and well tolerated; however, hot flashes have been reported in up to 7% of patients in the dose of 60 mg per day. Endometrial hyperplasia occurs in less than 1% of women. The drug is contraindicated in women with a history of deep vein thrombosis, pulmonary embolism and retinal vein thrombosis. The effect on the breast is not known [127]. Vaginal dehydroepiandrosterone (DHEA) has been subjected to open label studies only. The 6.5 mg suppository is compounded and used intervaginally 3.27 times per week. DHEA significantly improved dyspareunia, dryness and irritation without endometrial hyperplasia [128].

Nonhormonal therapies include vegetable oil based lubricants, such as coconut oil or olive oil, silicon based lubricants, vaginal moisturizing agents such as polycarbophil polymers that attach to the vaginal tissues and retain water [122]. Lidocaine 4% aqueous can be applied to the vestibule 3–4 min before contact [129].

Vaginal laser has been shown to improve glycogen storage and epithelial thickening and therefore vaginal dryness, burning, itching, and dyspareunia; however, only two small studies have been published and large or long-term controlled trials are lacking. There is no evidence that laser therapy improves symptoms for women with vestibulodynia [130].

Deep Dyspareunia

Most women suffering from chronic lower abdominal/pelvic pain disorders (CPP) experience deep dyspareunia. Pain with intercourse can originate from reproductive organs or from other pelvic structures with shared innervations including the bladder, large intestine, pelvic and abdominal wall musculature and nerves. Women with CPP typically have multiple pain diagnoses and more than one "pain generator" can contribute to dyspareunia [131]. Endometriosis, the most common gynecological disorder associated with deep dyspareunia, often coexists with bladder pain syndrome/interstitial cystitis (BPS/IC), pelvic floor myalgia, and vulvodynia. These "idiopathic" pain disorders are associated with disturbed sleep, abnormalities of autonomic functioning, psychological distress, widespread myofascial pain, and amplification of pain signals in the central nervous system [132, 133]. Psychological contributors such as trauma (emotional, physical, or sexual), decreased resilience in the face of stress, anxiety, and depression intensify the pain experience.

Of women with CPP who are subjected to diagnostic laparoscopy, approximately a third have no visible pathology, a third have endometriosis implants which may not be the cause of their pain, and the remainder evidence other findings that generally do not cause pain including adhesions, stigmata of past pelvic inflammatory disease (hydro salpinges), leiomyomata, congested pelvic vessels or small ovarian cysts.

Endometriosis

Endometriosis is defined as the presence of endometrial glands and stroma outside of the endometrial cavity. Definitive diagnosis of endometriosis can only be made at the time of surgery (laparoscopy or laparotomy) therefore the true prevalence is not known but is estimated to affect 10% of women without symptoms and up to 50% of women with CPP or infertility. Genetic, inflammatory, hormonal, and immunological factors influence the development of the disease.

The size and location of the endometriosis implants and the amount of anatomic distortion due to inflammation and adhesions do not correlate with the presence or degree of pain. Prostaglandins, cytokines, and de novo innervation of lesions play a role in pain. Neurogenesis and deeply infiltrating endometriosis in the cul-de-sac often cause deep dyspareunia. Allodynia (pain with a usually painless stimulus) and hyperalgesia (increased pain with a painful stimulus) are found on neuromuscular assessment in women with endometriosis [133, 134] Brain imaging studies reveal altered connectivity in areas related to pain processing [134].Women with endometriosis and dyspareunia who have other pelvic pain generators, comorbid idiopathic pain conditions, anxiety, depression, catastrophizing, or abdominal wall and pelvic floor hyperalgesia and trigger points are likely to have augmented processing of pain signals in the central nervous system (CNS) [135] and require multidisciplinary therapy to address all pain generators, stress, coping skills, and mood.

Common symptoms of endometriosis include severe menstrual and premenstrual pain, CPP, deep dyspareunia, dyschezia (pain with bowel movements), abnormal uterine bleeding, and subfertility.

The pelvic exam can be normal. Signs of significant disease include focal tenderness, retro-verted (tipped) uterus fixed to the rectum, nodules in the cul de sac behind the uterus or the uterosacral ligaments, and ovarian endometriosis cysts (endometriomata). Ultrasound and pelvic MRI are helpful but can be negative.

There is no optimal therapy for endometriosis related pain and disease can recur within 1–5 years after treatment. Endometriosis is a chronic disease. Although it may regress without continued therapy, hormonal contraceptives or progestogens are recommended after achieving symptom control. The disease atrophies with menopause.

Pharmacological Treatment of Endometriosis

First line treatment of women with suspected endometriosis or adenomyosis should be initiated after clinical evaluation. Surgery is reserved for women who are currently attempting fertility, have an adnexal mass, or have failed medical management. Medical management is recommended by expert consensus on the basis of low cost, high response rate and low risk profile. Endometriosis is an estrogen-dependent disease state; and the mainstay of hormonal therapy focuses on suppressing ovarian functioning, thereby lowering estrogen levels to those within a therapeutic window.

Medical treatment consists of "first line" therapy: low dose hormonal contraceptives (cyclically or continuously), continuous progestogens (oral, depo injection, removable implant, intrauterine device) and "second line": gonadotrophin releasing hormone agonists that create a temporary medical menopause [136].

Combined estrogen-progestin regimens suppress ovulation, thin the endometrium, promote decidualization and lead to atrophy of endometriotic implants. These regimens are effective taken cyclically (21/7 or 24/4 on/off regimens) or in an extended regimen of continuous active pills. If a patient does not respond to a cyclic regimen, a continuous regimen may be effective. A 4- to 6-month trial of therapy is recommended before switching to another treatment modality. Side effects can include nausea, bloating, irregular bleeding, headache, moodiness and breast tenderness. When given continuously, for the first 6 months breakthrough bleeding or spotting is common. Rare adverse events include venous thromboembolism (VTE), myocardial infarction, and stroke. Absolute contraindications to estrogen containing contraceptives are history of VTE, stroke, estrogen dependent tumor, liver disease, pregnancy, undiagnosed abnormal uterine bleeding, hypertriglyceridemia, migraine with aura, and smoking (>15 cig/day) in a women over 35. Relative contraindications include poorly controlled hypertension, migraine headaches without aura. With anticonvulsant intake, there may be decreased efficacy of either the OC or the anticonvulsant, as both are metabolized by the same P450 system liver enzymes.

Progestogens suppress the hypothalamic pituitary axis and consequently estrogen levels and they decidualize and atrophy in situ and ectopic endometrium. Progestogens effectively treat endometriosis in clinical trials with over 80% obtaining partial or complete relief of pain [137]. Norethindrone 2.5–5 mg daily or dienogest 2 mg daily can be used.

GnRH agonists are effective for treatment of pain due to endometriosis [138]. GnRH agonists down regulate GnRH receptors with a resultant suppression of ovarian functioning simulating menopause. Side effects include vasomotor symptoms, mood changes, headaches, insomnia, myalgia, arthralgia, urogenital atrophy, and bone loss. Due to these concerns, GnRH agonists are approved for a 6-month course but can be probably administered safely for 2 years when low dose add-back estrogen and progestin or progestin-only therapy is administered for bone protection. Norethindrone acetate 5 mg is recommended as first line for add-back therapy as it has been shown to preserve bone density levels while still providing effective relief from vasomotor side effects without interfering with efficacy. Low dose of estrogen can also be added (0.5 mg of estradiol daily).

Danazol, an androgen analog, has been shown to be effective in treating the painful symptoms of endometriosis and in reducing the size of endometriotic implants, but is rarely used today due to side effects such as weight gain, muscle cramps, decreased breast size, acne, hirsutism, oily skin, hot flashes, mood changes, depression, increased liver enzymes, all of which can be treated by lowering the dose. Unlike GnRH agonists, add-back therapy is not useful for minimizing side effects.

Aromatase inhibitors (AI) regulate local formation of estrogen within endometriotic lesions by inhibiting the overstimulated aromatase enzyme as well as by decreasing estrogen production in the ovary, brain, and periphery. AIs may be effective in women with refractory endometriosis pain. Because AIs stimulate FSH release, they can cause multifollicular cyst development, they require ovarian suppression by another hormonal agent such as an OC, progestin, or GnRH agonist. They can also cause bone loss with prolonged use [139].

Surgery

During laparoscopic surgery, implants are fulgurated or excised and anatomy is restored. Lesions are often not completely removed due to depth or extent or location on the ureter or bowel. Pain recurrence and reoperation rates are up to 50–60% within 5 years. Reoperation rates have been found to be lower after hysterectomy than laparoscopy indicating that removal of the uterus may contribute to the therapeutic effect of the surgery. Removal of both ovaries and the uterus resulted in the lowest rate of reoperation at 7 years (8.3%) compared with hysterectomy alone (23%). When the ovaries are preserved, it is important to prevent ovulation to decrease the incidence of pain recurrence. When the ovaries are removed, low dose estrogen/progestagen hormone replacement therapy (HRT) can be given to prevent bone loss and vasomotor side effects [140]. There is a low likelihood of symptom recurrence with HRT in women who had all endometriosis resected. Progestin may decrease the small risk of cancer in endometrial implants stimulated by unopposed estrogen.

The only well-designed, randomized clinical trials of surgical intervention for endometriosis have been limited by brief follow-up, small numbers and loss to follow-up, although many observational and retrospective studies have demonstrated favorable results. Surgical and medical therapies improve sexual functioning, general health, quality of life, emotional wellbeing. Recent studies confirm dyspareunia, sexual functioning, quality of life, and mood improved significantly after surgical excision of endometriosis [141–143].

Adenomyosis

A uterine form of endometriosis called adenomyosis is characterized by endometrial glands penetrating into the myometrium (muscle wall of the uterus). Adenomyosis can also cause deep dyspareunia, dysmenorrhea, and menorrhagia, but rarely does it cause chronic daily intermenstrual pain. Medical treatment for endometriosis is generally effective for adenomyosis and hysterectomy is curative.

Pelvic Congestion Syndrome

Pelvic vein varicosities and congested pelvic organs has been associated with dyspareunia. Factors other than venous congestion likely contribute to pain, as most women with pelvic varicosities have no pain. Diagnosis is via pelvic MRI venogram. Treatment consists of ovarian hormone suppression which decreases blood flow to the pelvic organs. Outcome is improved if cognitive behavioral therapy is added confirming the need for multimodal therapy in most cases of CPP. A few non controlled studies suggest embolization of involved veins may be helpful but long term or controlled studies are lacking. Hysterectomy and oophorectomy can be beneficial for women who have completed childbearing, but are rarely indicated.

Genitourinary Pelvic Pain

Genitourinary pelvic pain is a common cause of deep dyspareunia. Pain that localizes to the bladder or urethra can be difficult to diagnose and treat due to the interplay of the urinary tract with the vulva, vagina, pelvic floor, and the network of nerves supplying this area.

Comprehensive physical examination and evaluation for infection, urolithiasis, dermatitis, vaginitis both infectious and noninfectious, neurogenic and muscular etiologies is key for these patients. Often, referral is made when there are persistent symptoms despite treatment for cystitis or vaginitis, or when symptoms are present despite negative basic workup of cystitis or vaginitis. Bladder base tenderness is present in 34% of women with pelvic pain, compared with 3% without pelvic pain (OR 16.3) [144] and is specifically associated with deep dyspareunia, pelvic floor muscle tenderness, and abdominal wall trigger point. A thorough evaluation of all bladder complaints in patients with pelvic pain and dyspareunia is important, and may facilitate diagnosis in certain cases. When the diagnosis is not straightforward, this assessment is optimally performed by a specialist with expertise in both urology and gynecology systems or in a multidisciplinary fashion.

Recurrent Urinary Tract Infections (UTIs)

UTIs can result in an acute and post-infectious inflammation of the bladder. UTIs should be treated based on urine culture. Particularly in patients with persistent symptoms, antibiotic choice should be determined by a culture with sensitivity. Recurrent UTIs can be managed with long-term antibiotics or antiseptics for the urine. Two randomized controlled trials have demonstrated reduction of recurrent UTIs in postmenopausal women using local vaginal estrogen. Acidification of urine has also been shown to decrease the risk of recurrent UTIs. Several small studies suggest reduction in recurrent UTIs with cranberry extract and vitamin C supplementation. However, caution must be used as acidification of the urine can increase symptoms in noninfectious painful bladder syndromes or interstitial cystitis.

Trauma

Trauma from vaginal or pelvic surgery, accidental trauma, and radiation can contribute to pain that localizes to the bladder or urethra. Patients with a history of pelvic or vaginal trauma benefit from consultation with a urogynecologists.

Bladder Pain Syndrome/Interstitial Cystitis

Bladder Pain Syndrome/Interstitial Cystitis (BPS/IC) is associated with pelvic pain and dyspareunia. Several studies have demonstrated a strong association between IC/BPS and deep dyspareunia, sexually related distress, and a decline in desire and orgasm frequency [145]. It is estimated that 85% of chronic pelvic pain cases originate with bladder pain [146].

According to the International Continence Society, BPS is defined as chronic (>6 months) pelvic pain, pressure, or discomfort perceived to be related to the urinary bladder accompanied by at least one other urinary symptom such as persistent urge to void or frequency [147]. The prevalence of sexual function among women with BPS/IC has been reported as high as 87% [148]. BPS/IC specific sexual dysfunction has also been significantly associated with more severe BPS/IC symptoms, younger age, and worse depression. BPS/IC is commonly associated with other comorbid conditions such as vulvodynia and IBS. Studies have demonstrated 38% of patients with interstitial cystitis had irritable bowel syndrome and 26 percent of those with interstitial cystitis had vulvodynia [149]. Each of these diagnoses independently carry negative implications for sexual activity. Patients diagnosed with multiple concomitant pain syndromes are at higher risk of suffering from dyspareunia.

A multidisciplinary approach with the involvement of a specialist has been demonstrated to result in more satisfactory treatment strategy for these patients [150]. Management should ideally aim to treat all painful areas and comorbid conditions simultaneously.

First line treatment of BPS/IC involves behavioral modifications including dietary changes, fluid management, and bladder training. The AUA considers these interventions first line therapies and recommends they be offered to all patients with BPS/IC. They have minimal risk of adverse effects. Identification of dietary triggers and avoidance of irritants should be recommended to all patients with bladder discomfort. Common triggers include caffeine, tea, citrus, artificial sweeteners, alcohol, carbonated drinks, and spices. Though restrictive bladder diets are recommended by some experts, there is insufficient quality data supporting significant symptoms improvement [151]. Physical therapy has been shown to improve pain and dyspareunia in women with IC who are found to have pelvic floor spasm or tenderness on exam [152].

Medical Management

Most oral medications are considered second line therapy by the AUA Guidelines [153].

Tricyclic antidepressants are used to manage several chronic pain syndromes. Amitriptyline is most commonly used for BPS/IC. Though data from two RCTs showed conflicting results, both suggest that amitriptyline at doses higher than 50 mg daily is associated with marked reduction of symptoms [154, 155]. Adverse effects include typical anticholergic effects such as dry mouth, constipation, and urinary retention as well as drowsiness and cardiac arrhythmia.

Antihistamines have also been used as treatment of BPS/IC based on the theory that the development of IC may be due to a hypersensitivity reaction involving increased mast cell activity and histamine release. Hydroxyzine is most commonly used, though no studies definitely support its efficacy for improvement of bladder pain and drowsiness is common. Cimetidine has also been tried with conflicting evidence, though the only RCT ($n = 36$) demonstrated improvement over placebo [156–158].

Elmiron: Pentosan polysulfate sodium (PPS) is believed to improve symptoms of interstitial cystitis by providing a protective coating to the damaged bladder wall.

Pentosan polysulfate sodium (PPS) is considered second line treatment for BPS/IC, and can be used orally or intravesically [153]. Despite its use, studies regarding its efficacy for improvement of bladder symptoms and pain have been inconclusive [159], though it seems that those that do respond to PPS also report improvement in sexual function. In well-designed, randomized, controlled trials in patients with moderate or severe IC, pentosan polysulfate was more effective than placebo, with greater proportions of pentosan polysulfate recipients (28 and 32%) than placebo recipients (13% and 16%) [160].

In another prospective study, pentosan polysulfate 300 mg daily resulted a greater than 30% reduction in pain and bladder symptoms in 44% of patients. Those who achieved greater than 30% improvement in symptoms also reported a significant improvement in sexual function [161]. Common side effects include hair loss, and gastrointestinal complaints.

Bladder instillations: Intravesical therapy is based on clinical experience. It may be used as rescue therapy for acute bladder pain. There is no standard combination or concentration used. Potential adverse reactions may include urinary tract infection, urethral irritation, and bladder pain. Intravesical instillations of lidocaine, heparin, or dimethyl sulfoxide (DSMO) are considered second line therapies for interstitial cystitis by the American Urological Association [153]. The most common intravesical instillation is a solution of heparin, lidocaine, and bicarbonate. This solution has been shown to improve symptoms in a percentage of patients with BPS/IC. In one study evaluating patients with IC and dyspareunia, among patients with tenderness localizing to the bladder on exam, 85% achieved resolution of dyspareunia with a series of heparin/lidocaine/bicarbonate instillations at 3 week follow-up [162]. Only 29% of those without bladder base tenderness reported resolution of dyspareunia suggesting that the presence of bladder base tenderness may predict response to treatment.

Intravesical DSMO has been shown in two small RCTs to reduce bladder symptoms in patients with IC. However, it is more commonly associated with acute symptom exacerbation prior to improvement. The intravesical use of hyaluronic acid and chondroitin sulfate remain experimental. Though several small trials report improvement of symptoms with hyaluronic acid, it is currently not approved by the FDA in the USA for treatment if IC.

Cystoscopy and hydrodistention: Though cystoscopy is not required for diagnosis or management of BPS/IC, cystoscopic evaluation with hydrodistention and fulguration of Hunner's ulcers when present is considered third line treatment for IC by the AUA. Hydrodistention involves filling the bladder to a pressure of 60–80 cm H20 for a duration of 5–10 min while under anesthesia. In a retrospective study of 84 patients with IC, those undergoing cystoscopy with hydrodistention were more likely to experience improvement in overall pain, vaginal pain, and dyspareunia than those undergoing cystoscopy alone [163]. Though it can provide therapeutic relief in some patients, it may worsen symptoms in others and response has proven difficult to predict. Hydrodistention may allow visualization of some of the cystoscopic findings suggestive of IC such as glomerulations or Hunner's ulcers. Despite this, cystoscopy is not required for a diagnosis of IC and evidence regarding its utility is sparse.

Onabutilinum Toxin A: Intravesical botox has been approved by the FDA for treatment of overactive bladder and is considered a fourth line treatment option for IC by the AUA [154]. Recent studies suggest that botox modulates pain by altering muscle function of detrusor, decreasing release of noxious neurotransmitters, and reducing inflammation [164]. Botox results in muscle paralysis and relief of pain may be in part to relaxation of pelvic floor muscle spasm or repeated detrusor spasms. Botox has also been demonstrated in animal studies to decrease nerve growth factor (NGF) in bladder tissue [165, 166] and to block release of noxious neurotransmitters such as glutamate and substance P from neurons [167–172]. Recent studies suggest a possible CNS effect of botox, that may result in a cascade of cellular level changes which could reverse some of the changes resulting from central sensitization [134, 164, 167, 169–172]. Botox may also reduce chronic inflammation in BPS/IC patients by decreasing abnormal cytokine release in the bladder.

Clinical studies on botox used in BPS/IC have demonstrated overall improvement in subjective bladder pain scores and urinary frequency. Two randomized controlled trials comparing intravesical botox to normal saline injections have demonstrated a statistically significant improvement in pain on mean visual analog scores (VAS), urinary frequency, and bladder capacity after botox injection compared to placebo at 2–3 month follow-up [173, 174]. Several other small studies support this conclusion though there remains some controversy regarding the optimal dose and site of injection. There is little data specifically evaluating improvement in sexual function after intravesical botox injection for IC. One small study demonstrated an improvement sexual function in women with multiple sclerosis who received intravesical botox.

Neuromodulation

Sacral neuromodulation is also considered a fourth line management strategy for patients with IC [153]. Though a well-established treatment option for urinary frequency and overactive bladder, the studies assessing pain related outcomes including dyspareunia are conflicting and poor quality [175, 176].

Management of bladder-related pain and associated dyspareunia is complex, and often requires involvement of a specialist. Treatment of the potential sources of pain localizing to the bladder such as infection, postoperative scarring, radiation changes, and BPS/IC is key. As with most chronic pain syndromes, behavioral modifications, lifestyle changes, and optimization of psychosocial support and coping mechanisms remain first line strategies for BPS/IC. There are several systemic and local medications as well as surgical procedures that are available to address the specific sources of discomfort in BPS/IC. Among the etiologies of bladder pain, BPS/IC is the most difficult to treat. Multimodal management as described above, often with a multidisciplinary team, is recommended to optimize treatment.

Gastrointestinal (GI) Pain

GI sources of dyspareunia can include irritable bowel syndrome (IBS), functional abdominal pain syndrome (FAPS), celiac disease, neoplasm, and inflammatory bowel disease. IBS is the most common GI cause of CPP. Symptoms include pain at times of alteration in form or frequency of bowel movements, increased pain before and improved pain after a BM, and pain with stress and eating. Dyspareunia was reported by 16.4% of females with IBS. Sexual dysfunction is associated with GI symptom severity, but not with the severity of psychological symptoms [177]. Treatment includes bulking agents, dietary changes such as adding fiber, avoiding lactose or gluten, and FODMAP diet to decrease fermentable carbohydrates. Antispasmotics, antidepressants, and laxatives (for constipation-predominant IBS) or antidiarrheal agents (for diarrhea predominant IBS) may be indicated. Stress reduction, MBSR and CBT can be helpful.

Neurological and Myofascial Pain

Pain of neuromuscular origin is an often unrecognized cause of dyspareunia and the prevalence is unknown. Low back pain, abdominal wall and pelvic floor pain usually increase with sexual activity, bladder or bowel filling and evacuation, and stress.

Abdominal wall and pelvic floor trigger points and nerve entrapments are not uncommon causes of deep dyspareunia. In one study of 177 women with CPP, 74% had dermatomal hypersensitivity and trigger point-like pain in abdominal wall (83%), vagina (71%), and/or sacrum (25%) that reproduced their pain [178]. Successful long term reduction of pain in 100% of women with only abdominal wall points and 84% of women overall with injection of local anesthetic into fat pad above fascia and 63% required two or fewer visits.

Myalgia

Trigger points and myalgia of the abdominal wall, and pelvic floor muscles cause CPP and deep dyspareunia, and also vulvodynia [179, 180]. It is recommended to assess the pelvic floor for myalgia, dysfunction, trigger points [8]. Treatment of pelvic floor myalgia, dysfunction, and trigger points is primarily through physical therapy. Muscle relaxants show insufficient evidence (cyclobenzaprine or tizanidine (alpha-2 adrenergic agonist)). Sedatives and hypnotics (clonazepam, alprazolam, and diazepam) can be effective for myofascial pain [181].

Entrapped or Compressed Nerves

Entrapped nerves in the abdominal wall (iliohypogastric and ilioinguinal) or pelvic floor (pudendal nerve) are unrecognized sources of pain and dyspareunia. The nerves may become entrapped after surgery or physical trauma, pregnancy and delivery, repetitive strain, or occupational injury. Detailed history and exam can make the diagnosis. Symptoms of ilioinguinal or Iliohypogastric neuralgia are burning, aching pain over nerve distribution, referred to hip, labia, anterior thigh, increased pain with exercise, forced stretch of affected part, bending, lifting, valsalva (chronic cough), prolonged sitting, pannus, or tight clothes. To make the diagnosis one should look for scars, and examine for pinprick hyper or hyperalgesia in L1, L2 dermatomal territory. Ask patient to localize areas of worst tenderness with one finger. Perform Carnett's test as follows: mark areas of pain with pen. Palpate the area with one finger and ask for a numeric pain score 0–10. Ask patient to raise both extended legs or perform abdominal crunch (sit-up), re-palpate marked area during the abdominal tensing. Persistent or increased pain constitutes a positive Carnett's test. Diagnostic nerve block can be performed with injection of 5–10 cc of 0.25% bupivacaine between the internal and external oblique muscles.

In addition to avoiding neve injury at the time of abdominal surgery, early recognition with removal of offending fascial suture within 1 month of surgery can be curative. Treatment of neuralgia starts with avoiding perpetuating activities (lifting, hyperflexion or hyperextension of thigh, tight clothes, and prolonged sitting) and decreasing stress. Injection therapy is very helpful. Weekly or every other week injections of local anesthetic 5–10 cc 0.25% bupivacaine in the form of a nerve block. As long as improvement continues, blocks can be repeated. Criteria found to be good predictors of successful treatment of abdominal wall pain include localized pain or tenderness under 2.5 cm and positive Carnett's test. In a study of 84 female CPP patients who fulfilled these criteria with mean pain duration 23 mos., 36 were reinjected with 1–27 injections (4.3 average procedures). Long-term relief in the 70–80% range were noted but those with scars needed more injections Similar response rates are reported in the literature [182]. Topical local anesthetic creams and patches are also helpful for pain flares as are medications for neuropathic pain such as anticonvulsants and antidepressants.

References

1. American Psychiatric Association. Diagnostic and statistical manuel of mental disorders (5th ed., Text Rev). Washington: American Psychiatric Association; 2013.
2. Bergeron S, Corsini-Munt S, Aerts L, Rancourt K, Rosen N. Female sexual pain disorders: a review of the literature on etiology and treatment. Curr Sex Health Rep. 2015;7(3):159–69.
3. Bornstein J, Goldstein AT, Stockdale CK, Bergeron S, Pukall C, Zolnoun D, Coady D. Consensus vulvar pain terminology committee of the International Society for the Study of Vulvovaginal Disease (ISSVD), the International Society for the Study of Women's Sexual Health (ISSWSH), and the International Pelvic Pain Society (IPPS). Obstet Gynecol. 2016;127(4):745–51. doi:10.1097/AOG.0000000000001359.
4. Harlow BL, Kunitz CG, Nguyen RH, Rydell SA, Turner RM, MacLehose RF. Prevalence of symptoms consistent with a diagnosis of vulvodynia: population-based estimates from 2 geographic regions. Am J Obstet Gynecol. 2014;210(1):40.
5. Pukall CF, Goldstein AT, Bergeron S, Foster D, Stein A, Kellogg-Spadt S, Bachmann G. Vulvodynia: definition, prevalence, impact, and pathophysiological factors. J Sex Med. 2016;13(3):291–304. doi:10.1016/j.jsxm.2015.12.021.
6. American College of Obstetricians and Gynecologists Committee Opinion. Persistent vulvar pain. Number 673, September 2016;128:78–84.
7. Lamvu G, Nguyen RH, Burrows LJ, Rapkin A, Witzeman K, Marvel RP, Hutchins D, Witkin SS, Veasley C, Fillingim R, Zolnoun D. The evidence-based vulvodynia assessment project. A national registry for the study of vulvodynia. The evidence-based vulvodynia assessment project. A national registry for the study of vulvodynia. J Reprod Med. 2015;60(5–6):223–35.
8. Sarton J. Assessment of the pelvic floor muscles in women with sexual pain. J Sex Med. 2010;7:3526–9.
9. Al-Abbadey M, Liossi C, Curran N, Schoth DE, Graham CA. Treatment of female sexual pain disorders: a systematic

review. J Sex Marital Ther. 2016;42(2):99–142. doi:10.1080/0092623X.2015.1053023.. Epub 2015 Jun 2.
10. Goldstein AT, Pukall CF, Brown C, Bergeron S, Stein A, Kellogg-Spadt S. Vulvodynia: assessment and treatment. J Sex Med. 2016;13(4):572–90. doi:10.1016/j.jsxm.2016.01.020.. Epub 2016 Mar 25.
11. Landry T, Bergeron S, Dupuis MJ, Desrochers G. The treatment of provoked vestibulodynia: a critical review. Clin J Pain. 2008;24(2):155–71. doi:10.1097/AJP.0b013e31815aac4d.
12. Sadownik LA. Etiology, diagnosis, and clinical management of vulvodynia. Int J Womens Health. 2014;6:437–49.
13. Yong PJ, Sadownik L, Brotto LA. Concurrent deep-superficial dyspareunia: prevalence, associations, and outcomes in a multidisciplinary vulvodynia program. J Sex Med. 2015;12(1):219–27.
14. De Andres J, Sanchis-Lopez N, Asensio-Samper JM, Fabregat-Cid G, Villanueva-Perez VL, Monsalve Dolz V, Minguez A. Vulvodynia—an evidence-based literature review and proposed treatment algorithm. Pain Pract. 2016;16(2):204–36. doi:10.1111/papr.12274.. Epub 2015 Jan 12.
15. Goetsch MF. Surgery combined with muscle therapy for dyspareunia from vulvar vestibulitis: an observational study. J Reprod Med. 2007;52(7):597–603.
16. Baggish MS, Miklos JR. Vulvar pain syndrome: a review. Obstet Gynecol Surv. 1995;50(8):618–27.
17. Andrews JC. Vulvodynia interventions—systematic review and evidence grading. Obstet Gynecol Surv. 2011;66(5):299–315.
18. Tommola P, Unkila-Kallio L, Paavonen J. Surgical treatment of vulvar vestibulitis: a review. Acta Obstet Gynecol Scand. 2010;89(11):1385–95. doi:10.3109/00016349.2010.512071.
19. Woodruff JD, Genadry R, Poliakoff S. Treatment of dyspareunia and vaginal outlet distortions by perineoplasty. Obstet Gynecol. 1981;57(6):750–4.
20. Bohm-Starke N, Rylander E. Surgery for localized, provoked vestibulodynia: a long-term follow-up study. J Reprod Med. 2008;53(2):83–9.
21. Bergeron S, Binik Y, Khalifé S, Pagidas K, Glazer H. A randomized comparison of group cognitive–behavioral therapy, surface electromyographic biofeedback, and vestibulectomy in the treatment of dyspareunia resulting from vulvar vestibulitis. Pain. 2001;91(3):297–306. doi:10.1016/S0304-3959(00)00449-8.
22. Tommola P, Unkila-Kallio L, Paavonen J. Long-term well-being after surgical or conservative treatment of severe vulvar vestibulitis. Acta Obstet Gynecol Scand. 2012;91(9):1086–93. doi:10.1111/j.1600-0412.2012.01466.x.. Epub 2012 Jul 2.
23. Nunns D, Mandal D, Byrne M, McLelland J, Rani R, Cullimore J, Bansal D, Brackenbury F, Kirtschig G, Wier M. British Society for the Study of Vulval Disease (BSSVD) guideline group. guidelines for the management of vulvodynia. Br J Dermatol. 2010;162(6):1180–5. doi:10.1111/j.1365-2133.2010.09684.x.. Epub 2010 Mar 16.
24. Reed BD, Haefner HK, Sen A, Gorenflo DW. Vulvodynia incidence and remission rates among adult women: a 2-year follow-up study. Obstet Gynecol. 2008;112(2 Pt 1):231–7. doi:10.1097/AOG.0b013e318180965b.
25. Foster DC, Kotok MB, Huang LS, Watts A, Oakes D, Howard FM, Poleshuck EL, Stodgell CJ, Dworkin RH. Oral desipramine and topical lidocaine for vulvodynia: a randomized controlled trial. Obstet Gynecol. 2010;116(3):583–93. doi:10.1097/AOG.0b013e3181e9e0ab.
26. Brown CS, Wan J, Bachmann G, Rosen R. Self-management, amitriptyline, and amitripyline plus triamcinolone in the management of vulvodynia. J Womens Health (Larchmt). 2009;18(2):163–9. doi:10.1089/jwh.2007.0676.
27. Reed BD, Caron AM, Gorenflo DW, Haefner HK. Treatment of vulvodynia with tricyclic antidepressants: efficacy and associated factors. J Low Genit Tract Dis. 2006;10(4):245–51.
28. Pagano R, Wong S. Use of amitriptyline cream in the management of entry dyspareunia due to provoked vestibulodynia. J Low Genit Tract Dis. 2012;16(4):394–7. doi:10.1097/LGT.0b013e3182449bd6.
29. Leo RJ, Dewani S. A systematic review of the utility of antidepressant pharmacotherapy in the treatment of vulvodynia pain. J Sex Med. 2013;10(10):2497–505. doi:10.1111/j.1743-6109.2012.02915.x.. Epub 2012 Sep 13.
30. Boardman LA, Cooper AS, Blais LR, Raker CA. Topical gabapentin in the treatment of localized and generalized vulvodynia. Obstet Gynecol. 2008;112(3):579–85. doi:10.1097/AOG.0b013e3181827c77.
31. Bergeron S, Khalifé S, Glazer H, Binik Y. Surgical and behavioral treatments for vestibulodynia: two-and-one-half-year follow-up and predictors of outcome. Obstet Gynecol. 2008;111(1):159–66. doi:10.1097/01.AOG.0000295864.76032.a7.
32. Danielsson I, Torstensson T, Brodda-Jansen G, Bohm-Starke N. EMG biofeedback versus topical lidocaine gel: a randomized study for the treatment of women with vulvar vestibulitis. Acta Obstet Gynecol Scand. 2006;85(11):1360–7.
33. Zolnoun DA, Hartmann KE, Steege JF. Overnight 5% lidocaine ointment for treatment of vulvar vestibulitis. Obstet Gynecol. 2003;102(1):84–7.
34. Segal D, Tifheret H, Lazer S. Submucous infiltration of betamethasone and lidocaine in the treatment of vulvar vestibulitis. Eur J Obstet Gynecol Reprod Biol. 2003 Mar 26;107(1):105–6.
35. Murina F, Tassan P, Roberti P, Bianco V. Treatment of vulvar vestibulitis with submucous infiltrations of methylprednisolone and lidocaine. An alternative approach. J Reprod Med. 2001;46(8):713–6.
36. McDonald JS, Rapkin AJ. Multilevel local anesthetic nerve blockade for the treatment of generalized vulvodynia: a pilot study. J Sex Med. 2012;9(11):2919–26. doi:10.1111/j.1743-6109.2012.02909.x.. Epub 2012 Aug 27.
37. Rapkin AJ, McDonald JS, Morgan M. Multilevel local anesthetic nerve blockade for the treatment of vulvar vestibulitis syndrome. Am J Obstet Gynecol. 2008;198(1):41.e1–5 .Epub 2007 Oct 22
38. Abbott J. The use of botulinum toxin in the pelvic floor for women with chronic pelvic pain-a new answer to old problems? J Minim Invasive Gynecol. 2009;16(2):130–5. doi:10.1016/j.jmig.2008.11.006.. Epub 2009 Jan 22. Review.
39. Petersen CD, Giraldi A, Lundvall L, Kristensen E. Botulinum toxin type A-a novel treatment for provoked vestibulodynia? Results from a randomized, placebo controlled, double blinded study. J Sex Med. 2009;6(9):2523–37. doi:10.1111/j.1743-6109.2009.01378.x.. Epub 2009 Jul 10.
40. Abbott JA, Jarvis SK, Lyons SD, Thomson A, Vancaille TG. Botulinum toxin type A for chronic pain and pelvic floor spasm in women: a randomized controlled trial. Obstet Gynecol. 2006;108(4):915–23.
41. Bosso JV, Aiken MJ, Simon RA. Successful prevention of local and cutaneous hypersensitivity reactions to seminal fluid with intravaginal cromolyn. Allergy Proc. 1991;12(2):113–6.
42. Nyirjesy P, Sobel JD, Weitz MV, Leaman DJ, Small MJ, Gelone SP. Cromolyn cream for recalcitrant idiopathic vulvar vestibulitis: results of a placebo controlled study. Sex Transm Infect. 2001;77(1):53–7.
43. Murina F, Radici G, Bianco V. Capsaicin and the treatment of vulvar vestibulitis syndrome: a valuable alternative? MedGenMed. 2004;6(4):48.
44. Steinberg AC, Oyama IA, Rejba AE, Kellogg-Spadt S, Whitmore KE. Capsaicin for the treatment of vulvar vestibulitis. Am J Obstet Gynecol. 2005;192(5):1549–53.
45. Bouchard C, Brisson J, Fortier M, Morin C, Blanchette C. Use of oral contraceptive pills and vulvar vestibulitis: a case-control study. Am J Epidemiol. 2002;156(3):254–61.
46. Edgardh K, Abdelnoor M. Vulvar vestibulitis and risk factors: a population-based case-control study in Oslo. Acta Derm Venereol. 2007;87(4):350–4.

47. Lee M, Morgan M, Rapkin A. Clitoral and vulvar vestibular sensation in women taking 20 mcg ethinyl estradiol combined oral contraceptives: a preliminary study. J Sex Med. 2011;8(1):213–8. doi:10.1111/j.1743-6109.2010.02074.x.. Epub 2010 Oct 18.
48. Burrows LJ, Goldstein AT. The treatment of vestibulodynia with topical estradiol and testosterone. Sex Med. 2013;1(1):30–3. doi:10.1002/sm2.4.
49. Goldstein A, Burrows L, Goldstein I. Can oral contraceptives cause vestibulodynia? J Sex Med. 2010;7(4 Pt 1):1585–7.
50. Simonelli C, Eleuteri S, Petruccelli F, Rossi R. Female sexual pain disorders: dyspareunia and vaginismus. Curr Opin Psychiatry. 2014;27(6):406–12.
51. Reissing ED, Brown C, Lord MJ, Binik YM, Khalifé S. Pelvic floor muscle functioning in women with vulvar vestibulitis syndrome. J Psychosom Obstet Gynaecol. 2005;26(2):107–13.
52. Bortolami A, Vanti C, Banchelli F, Guccione AA, Pillastrini P. Relationship between female pelvic floor dysfunction and sexual dysfunction: an observational study. J Sex Med. 2015;12(5):1233–41. doi:10.1111/jsm.12882.. Epub 2015 Apr 8.
53. Albrecht KB. "How-To" guide to pelvic floor muscle dysfunction. Clin Obstet Gynecol. 2015;58(3):546–50. doi:10.1097/GRF.0000000000000135.
54. Hong CZ, Simons DG. Pathophysiologic and electrophysiologic mechanisms of myofascial trigger points. Arch Phys Med Rehabil. 1998;79(7):863–72.
55. Haefner HK, Collins ME, Davis GD, Edwards L, Foster DC, Hartmann ED, Kaufman RH, Lynch PJ, Margesson LJ, Moyal-Barracco M, Piper CK, Reed BD, Stewart EG, Wilkinson EJ. The vulvodynia guideline. J Low Genit Tract Dis. 2005;9(1):40–51.
56. Goldfinger C, Pukall CF, Gentilcore-Saulnier E, McLean L, Chamberlain S. A prospective study of pelvic floor physical therapy: pain and psychosexual outcomes in provoked vestibulodynia. J Sex Med. 2009;6(7):1955–68.
57. Goldfinger C, Pukall CF, Thibault-Gagnon S, McLean L, Chamberlain S. Effectiveness of cognitive-behavioral therapy and physical therapy for provoked vestibulodynia: a randomized pilot study. J Sex Med. 2016;13(1):88–94.
58. Gentilcore-Saulnier E, McLean L, Goldfinger C, Pukall CF, Chamberlain S. Pelvic floor muscle assessment outcomes in women with and without provoked vestibulodynia and the impact of a physical therapy program. J Sex Med. 2010;7(2 Pt 2).
59. Bergeron S, Brown C, Lord MJ, Oala M, Binik YM, Khalifé S. Physical therapy for vulvar vestibulitis syndrome: a retrospective study. J Sex Marital Ther. 2002;28(3):183–92.
60. Glazer HI, Rodke G, Swencionis C, Hertz R, Young AW. Treatment of vulvar vestibulitis syndrome with electromyographic biofeedback of pelvic floor musculature. J Reprod Med. 1995;40(4):283–90.
61. Glazer HI. Dysesthetic vulvodynia. Long-term follow-up after treatment with surface electromyography-assisted pelvic floor muscle rehabilitation. J Reprod Med. 2000;45(10):798–802.
62. McKay E, Kaufman RH, Doctor U, Berkova Z, Glazer H, Redko V. Treating vulvar vestibulitis with electromyographic biofeedback of pelvic floor musculature. J Reprod Med. 2001;46(4):337–42.
63. Murina F, Bianco V, Radici G, Felice R, Di Martino M, Nicolini U. Transcutaneous electrical nerve stimulation to treat vestibulodynia: a randomised controlled trial. BJOG. 2008;115(9):1165–70. doi:10.1111/j.1471-0528.2008.01803.x.
64. Desrochers G, Bergeron S, Khalifé S, Dupuis MJ, Jodoin M. Fear avoidance and self-efficacy in relation to pain and sexual impairment in women with provoked vestibulodynia. Clin J Pain. 2009;25(6):520–7. doi:10.1097/AJP.0b013e31819976e3.
65. Maillé DL, Bergeron S, Lambert B. Body image in women with primary and secondary provoked vestibulodynia: a controlled study. J Sex Med. 2015;12(2):505–15. doi:10.1111/jsm.12765.. Epub 2014 Nov 13.
66. Desrochers G, Bergeron S, Landry T, Jodoin M. Do psychosexual factors play a role in the etiology of provoked vestibulodynia? A critical review. J Sex Marital Ther. 2008;34(3):198–226. doi:10.1080/00926230701866083.
67. Smith KB, Pukall CF. A systematic review of relationship adjustment and sexual satisfaction among women with provoked vestibulodynia. J Sex Res. 2011;48(2–3):166–91. doi:10.1080/00224499.2011.555016.
68. Pâquet M, Bois K, Rosen NO, Mayrand MH, Charbonneau-Lefebvre V, Bergeron S. Why us? perceived injustice is associated with more sexual and psychological distress in couples coping with genito-pelvic pain. J Sex Med. 2016;13(1):79–87. doi:10.1016/j.jsxm.2015.11.007.
69. Jackson B, Kubzansky L, Wright R, Rosalind J. Linking perceived unfairness to physical health: the perceived unfairness model. Rev Gen Psychol. 2006;10(1):21–40. doi:10.1037/1089-2680.10.1.21.
70. Rosenbaum TY, Barnard E, Wilhite M. Psychosexual aspects of vulvar disease. Clin Obstet Gynecol. 2015;58(3):551–5. doi:10.1097/GRF.0000000000000136.
71. Masheb RM, Kerns RD, Lozano C, Minkin MJ, Richman S. A randomized clinical trial for women with vulvodynia: cognitive-behavioral therapy vs. supportive psychotherapy. Pain. 2009;141(1–2):31–40. doi:10.1016/j.pain.2008.09.031.. Epub 2008 Nov 20.
72. Desrochers G, Bergeron S, Khalifé S, Dupuis MJ, Jodoin M. Provoked vestibulodynia: psychological predictors of topical and cognitive-behavioral treatment outcome. Behav Res Ther. 2010;48(2):106–15. doi:10.1016/j.brat.2009.09.014.. Epub 2009 Oct 7.
73. Corsini-Munt S, Bergeron S, Rosen NO, Mayrand MH, Delisle I. Feasibility and preliminary effectiveness of a novel cognitive-behavioral couple therapy for provoked vestibulodynia: a pilot study. J Sex Med. 2014;11(10):2515–27.
74. Lindström S, Kvist LJ. Treatment of provoked vulvodynia in a Swedish cohort using desensitization exercises and cognitive behavioral therapy. BMC Womens Health. 2015;15:108. doi:10.1186/s12905-015-0265-3.
75. Weijmar Schultz WC, Gianotten WL, van der Meijden WI, van de Wiel HB, Blindeman L, Chadha S, Drogendijk AC. Behavioral approach with or without surgical intervention to the vulvar vestibulitis syndrome: a prospective randomized and non-randomized study. J Psychosom Obstet Gynaecol. 1996;17(3):143–8.
76. Bishop S, Lau M, Shapiro S, Carlson L, Anderson N, Carmody J, Segal Z, Abbey S, Specca M, Velging D, Devins G. Mindfulness: a proposed operational definition. Clin Psychol. 2004;11(3):230–41. doi:10.1093/clipsy.bph077.
77. Brotto LA, Basson R. Group mindfulness-based therapy significantly improves sexual desire in women. Behav Res Ther. 2014;57:43–54. doi:10.1016/j.brat.2014.04.001.. Epub 2014 Apr 18.
78. Brotto L, Basson R, Smith K, Driscoll M, Sadownik L. Mindfulness-based Group therapy for women with provoked vestibulodynia. Mindfulness. 2015;6(3):417–32.
79. Pukall C, Kandyba K, Amsel R, Khalifé S, Binik Y. Effectiveness of hypnosis for the treatment of vulvar vestibulitis syndrome: a preliminary investigation. J Sex Med. 2007;4(2):417–25.
80. Rosen NO, Bergeron S, Leclerc B, Lambert B, Steben M. Woman and partner-perceived partner responses predict pain and sexual satisfaction in provoked vestibulodynia (PVD) couples. J Sex Med. 2010,7(11):3715–24. doi:10.1111/j.1743-6109.2010.01957.x.
81. Sheppard C, Hallam-Jones R, Wylie K. Why have you both come? Emotional, relationship, sexual and social issues raised by heterosexual couples seeking sexual therapy (in women referred to a

sexual difficulties clinic with a history of vulval pain). Sex Relat Ther. 2008;23(3):217–26. doi:10.1080/14681990802227974.

82. Awada N, Bergeron S, Steben M, Hainault VA, McDuff P. To say or not to say: dyadic ambivalence over emotional expression and its associations with pain, sexuality, and distress in couples coping with provoked vestibulodynia. J Sex Med. 2014;11(5):1271–82. doi:10.1111/jsm.12463.. Epub 2014 Feb 19.
83. Desrosiers M, Bergeron S, Meana M, Leclerc B, Binik YM, Khalifé S. Psychosexual characteristics of vestibulodynia couples: partner solicitousness and hostility are associated with pain. J Sex Med. 2008;5(2):418–27 .Epub 2007 Dec 17
84. Lemieux AJ, Bergeron S, Steben M, Lambert B. Do romantic partners' responses to entry dyspareunia affect women's experience of pain? The roles of catastrophizing and self-efficacy. J Sex Med. 2013;10(9):2274–84. doi:10.1111/jsm.12252.. Epub 2013 Jun 27.
85. Rosen NO, Bergeron S, Glowacka M, Delisle I, Baxter ML. Harmful or helpful: perceived solicitous and facilitative partner responses are differentially associated with pain and sexual satisfaction in women with provoked vestibulodynia. J Sex Med. 2012;9(9):2351–60. doi:10.1111/j.1743-6109.2012.02851.x.. Epub 2012 Jul 19.
86. Bois K, Bergeron S, Rosen NO, McDuff P, Grégoire C. Sexual and relationship intimacy among women with provoked vestibulodynia and their partners: associations with sexual satisfaction, sexual function, and pain self-efficacy. J Sex Med. 2013;10(8):2024–35. doi:10.1111/jsm.12210.. Epub 2013 Jun 26.
87. Boerner KE, Rosen NO. Acceptance of vulvovaginal pain in women with provoked vestibulodynia and their partners: associations with pain, psychological, and sexual adjustment. J Sex Med. 2015;12(6):1450–62. doi:10.1111/jsm.12889.. Epub 2015 Apr 13.
88. Rosen NO, Bergeron S, Sadikaj G, Delisle I. Daily associations among male partner responses, pain during intercourse, and anxiety in women with vulvodynia and their partners. J Pain. 2015;16(12):1312–20. doi:10.1016/j.jpain.2015.09.003.. Epub 2015 Sep 25.
89. Corsini-Munt S, Bergeron S, Rosen NO, Steben M, Mayrand MH, Delisle I, McDuff P, Aerts L, Santerre-Baillargeon M. A comparison of cognitive-behavioral couple therapy and lidocaine in the treatment of provoked vestibulodynia: study protocol for a randomized clinical trial. Trials. 2014;15:506.
90. Schlaeger JM, Xu N, Mejta CL, Park CG, Wilkie DJ. Acupuncture for the treatment of vulvodynia: a randomized wait-list controlled pilot study. J Sex Med. 2015;12(4):1019–27. doi:10.1111/jsm.12830.. Epub 2015 Jan 30.
91. Backman H, Widenbrant M, Bohm-Starke N, Dahlof LG. Combined physical and psychosexual therapy for provoked vestibulodynia-an evaluation of a multidisciplinary treatment model. J Sex Res. 2008;45(4):378–85. doi:10.1080/00224490802398365.
92. Spoelstra SK, Dijkstra JR, van Driel MF, Weijmar Schultz WC. Long-term results of an individualized, multifaceted, and multidisciplinary therapeutic approach to provoked vestibulodynia. J Sex Med. 2011;8(2):489–96. doi:10.1111/j.1743-6109.2010.01941.x.
93. Brotto LA, Yong P, Smith KB, Sadownik LA. Impact of a multidisciplinary vulvodynia program on sexual functioning and dyspareunia. J Sex Med. 2015;12(1):238–47. doi:10.1111/jsm.12718.. Epub 2014 Oct 30.
94. Lahaie MA, Amsel R, Khalifé S, Boyer S, Faaborg-Andersen M, Binik YM. Can fear, pain, and muscle tension discriminate vaginismus from dyspareunia/provoked vestibulodynia? Implications for the new DSM-5 diagnosis of genito-pelvic pain/penetration disorder. Arch Sex Behav. 2015;44(6):1537–50. doi:10.1007/s10508-014-0430-z.. Epub 2014 Nov 15.
95. Pacik PT. Understanding and treating vaginismus: a multimodal approach. Int Urogynecol J. 2014;25(12):1613–20. doi:10.1007/s00192-014-2421-y.. Epub 2014 Jun 4.
96. Shifren JL, Johannes CB, Monz BU, Russo PA, Bennett L, Rosen R. Help-seeking behavior of women with self-reported distressing sexual problems. J Womens Health (Larchmt). 2009;18(4):461–8. doi:10.1089/jwh.2008.1133.
97. Melnik T, Hawton K, McGuire H. Interventions for vaginismus. Cochrane Database Syst Rev. 2012;12:CD001760. doi:10.1002/14651858.CD001760.pub2.
98. Pacik PT. Vaginismus: review of current concepts and treatment using botox injections, bupivacaine injections, and progressive dilation with the patient under anesthesia. Aesthetic Plast Surg. 2011;35(6):1160–4. doi:10.1007/s00266-011-9737-5.. Epub 2011 May 10. Review.
99. Macey K, Gregory A, Nunns D, das Nair R. Women's experiences of using vaginal trainers (dilators) to treat vaginal penetration difficulties diagnosed as vaginismus: a qualitative interview study. BMC Womens Health. 2015;20(15):49. doi:10.1186/s12905-015-0201-6.
100. Schnyder U, Schnyder-Lüthi C, Ballinari P, Blaser A. Therapy for vaginismus: in vivo versus in vitro desensitization. Can J Psychiatry. 1998;43(9):941–4.
101. ter Kuile MM, Melles RJ, Tuijnman-Raasveld CC, de Groot HE, van Lankveld JJ. Therapist-aided exposure for women with lifelong vaginismus: mediators of treatment outcome: a randomized waiting list control trial. J Sex Med. 2015;12(8):1807–19. doi:10.1111/jsm.12935.. Epub 2015 Aug 6.
102. Lahaie MA, Boyer SC, Amsel R, Khalifé S, Binik YM. Vaginismus: a review of the literature on the classification/diagnosis, etiology and treatment. Womens Health (Lond). 2010;6(5):705–19. doi:10.2217/whe.10.46.
103. Ferreira JR, Souza RP. Botulinum toxin for vaginismus treatment. Pharmacology. 2012;89(5–6):256–9.
104. Ghazizadeh S, Nikzad M. Botulinum toxin in the treatment of refractory vaginismus. Obstet Gynecol. 2004;104(5 Pt 1):922.
105. Bertolasi L, Frasson E, Cappelletti JY, Vicentini S, Bordignon M, Graziottin A. Botulinum neurotoxin type A injections for vaginismus secondary to vulvar vestibulitis syndrome. Obstet Gynecol. 2009;114(5):1008–16. doi:10.1097/AOG.0b013e3181bb0dbb.
106. ter Kuile MM, Weijenborg PT. A cognitive-behavioral group program for women with vulvar vestibulitis syndrome (VVS): factors associated with treatment success. J Sex Marital Ther. 2006;32(3):199–213.
107. Engman M, Wijma K, Wijma B. Long-term coital behaviour in women treated with cognitive behaviour therapy for superficial coital pain and vaginismus. Cogn Behav Ther. 2010;39(3):193–202. doi:10.1080/16506070903571014.
108. ter Kuile MM, van Lankveld JJ, de Groot E, Melles R, Neffs J, Zandbergen M. Cognitive-behavioral therapy for women with lifelong vaginismus: process and prognostic factors. Behav Res Ther. 2007;45(2):359–73.
109. Akhavan-Taghavi MH, Asghari-Moghaddam MA, Froutan SK, Jadid-Milani M. Vaginismus in Iran: a single center report of 7 years experience. Nephrourol Mon. 2015;7(6):e30077. doi:10.5812/numonthly.30077.. eCollection 2015.
110. Munasinghe T, Goonaratna C, de Silva P. Couple characteristics and outcome of therapy in vaginismus. Ceylon Med J. 2004; 49(2):54–7.
111. Ben-Zion I, Rothschild S, Chudakov M, Aloni R. Surrogate versus couple therapy in vaginismus. J Sex Med. 2007;4(3):728–33.
112. Labat JJ, Riant T, Robert R, Amarenco G, Lefaucheur JP, Rigaud J. Diagnostic criteria for pudendal neuralgia by pudendal nerve entrapment (Nantes criteria). Neurourol Urodyn. 2008;27(4):306–10.
113. Carmel M, Lebel M, Tu le M. Pudendal nerve neuromodulation with neurophysiology guidance: a potential treatment option for refractory chronic pelvi-perineal pain. Int Urogynecol J. 2010;21(5):613–6. doi:10.1007/s00192-009-1054-z.. Epub 2009 Dec 12.
114. Robert R, Labat JJ, Bensignor M, Glemain P, Deschamps C, Raoul S, Hamel O. Decompression and transposition of the

pudendal nerve in pudendal neuralgia: a randomized controlled trial and long-term evaluation. Eur Urol. 2005;47(3):403–8.
115. Lee A, Bradford J, Fischer G. Long-term management of adult vulvar lichen sclerosus: a prospective cohort study of 507 women. JAMA Dermatol. 2015;151(10):1061–7. doi:10.1001/jamadermatol.2015.0643.
116. Chi CC, Kirtschig G, Baldo M, Brackenbury F, Lewis F, Wojnarowska F. Topical interventions for genital lichen sclerosus. Cochrane Database Syst Rev. 2011;7(12):CD008240. doi:10.1002/14651858.CD008240.pub2.
117. Burrows LJ, Creasey A, Goldstein AT. The treatment of vulvar lichen sclerosus and female sexual dysfunction. J Sex Mad. 2011;8(1):219–22.
118. Goldstein AT, Burrows LJ. Surgical treatment of clitoral phimosis caused by lichen sclerosus. Am J Obstet Gynecol. 2007;196(2):126.e1–4.
119. Gurumurthy M, Morah N, Gioffre G, Cruickshank ME. The surgical management of complications of vulval lichen sclerosus. Eur J Obstet Gynecol Reprod Biol. 2012;162(1):79–82.
120. Bradford J, Fischer G. Management of vulvovaginal lichen planus: a new approach. J Low Genit Tract Dis. 2013;17(1):28–32.
121. Goldstein A. Perineoplasty and vaginal advancement flap for vulvar granuloma fissuratum. J Sex Med. 2011;8(11):2984–7.
122. Palacios S, Castelo-Branco C, Currie H, Mijatovic V, Nappi RE, Simon J, Rees M. Update on management of genitourinary syndrome of menopause: a practical guide. Maturitas. 2015;82(3):308–13. doi:10.1016/j.maturitas.2015.07.020.. Epub 2015 Jul 26.
123. Palma F, Volpe A, Villa P, Cagnacci A, Writing group of AGATA study. Vaginal of women in postmenopause. Results from a multicentric observational study: The AGATA study atrophy. Maturitas. 2016;83:40–4.
124. North American Menopause Society. Management of symptomatic vulvovaginal atrophy: 2013 position statement of The American Menopause Society. Menopause. 2013;20(9):888–902.
125. Suckling J, Lethaby A, Kennedy R. Local oestrogen for vaginal atrophy in postmenopausal women. Cochrane Database Syst Rev. 2006;4:CD001500.
126. American College of Obstetricians and Gynecologists Committee Opinion. The Use of Vaginal Estrogen in Women With a History of Estrogen-Dependent Breast Cancer Number 659, March 2016 p. 618–9.
127. Simon JA, Lin VH, Radovich C, Bachmann GA, Ospemifene Study Group. One-year long-term safety extension study of ospemifene for the treatment of vulvar and vaginal atrophy in postmenopausal women with a uterus. Menopause. 2013;20(4):418–27. doi:10.1097/gme.0b013e31826d36ba.
128. Portman DJ, Labrie F, Archer DF, Bouchard C, Cusan L, Girard G, Ayotte N, Koltun W, Blouin F, Young D, Wade A, Martel C, Dubé R, Other participating members of VVA Prasterone Group. Lack of effect of intravaginal dehydroepiandrosterone (DHEA, prasterone) on the endometrium in postmenopausal women. Menopause. 2015;22(12):1289–95.
129. Goetsch MF, Lim JY, Caughey AB. A practical solution for dyspareunia in breast cancer survivors: a randomized controlled trial. J Clin Oncol. 2015;33(30):3394–400.
130. Perino A, Calligaro A, Forlani F, Tiberio C, Cucinella G, Svelato A, Saitta S, Calagna G. Vulvo-vaginal atrophy: a new treatment modality using thermo-ablative fractional CO2 laser. Maturitas. 2015;80(3):296–301.
131. Zondervan KT, Yudkin PL, Vessey MP, Jenkinson CP, Dawes MG, Barlow DH, Kennedy SH. Chronic pelvic pain in the community – symptoms, investigations, and diagnoses. Am J Obstet Gynecol. 2001;184(6):1149–55.
132. Diatchenko L, Nackley AG, Slade GD, Fillingim RB, Maixner W. Idiopathic pain disorders – pathways of vulnerability. Pain. 2006;123(3):226–30.
133. Stratton P, Khachikyan I, Sinaii N, Ortiz R, Shah J. Association of chronic pelvic pain and endometriosis with signs of sensitization and myofascial pain. Obstet Gynecol. 2015;125(3):719–28.
134. As-Sanie S, Kim J, Schmidt-Wilcke T, Sundgren PC, Clauw DJ, Napadow V, Harris RE. Functional connectivity is associated with altered brain chemistry in women with endometriosis-associated chronic pelvic pain. J Pain. 2016;17(1):1–13. doi:10.1016/j.jpain.2015.09.008.. Epub 2015 Oct 9.
135. Brawn J, Morotti M, Zondervan KT, Becker CM, Vincent K. Central changes associated with chronic pelvic pain and endometriosis. Hum Reprod Update. 2014;20(5):737–47.
136. Kavoussi SK, Lim CS, Skinner BD, Lebovic DI, As-Sanie S. New paradigms in the diagnosis and management of endometriosis. Curr Opin Obstet Gynecol. 2016;28(4):267–76.
137. Prentice A, Deary AJ, Bland E. Progestagens and anti-progestagens for pain associated with endometriosis. Cochrane Database Syst Rev. 2000;CD002122.
138. Brown J, Pan A, Hart RJ. Gonadotrophin-releasing hormone analogues for pain associated with endometriosis. Cochrane Database Syst Rev. 2010;8(12):CD008475.
139. Ferrero S, Gillott DJ, Venturini PL, Remorgida V. Use of aromatase inhibitors to treat endometriosis-related pain symptoms: a systematic review. Reprod Biol Endocrinol. 2011;9:89. doi:10.1186/1477-7827-9-89.
140. Muzii L, Di Tucci C, Achilli C, Di Donato V, Musella A, Palaia I, Panici PB. Continuous versus cyclic oral contraceptives after laparoscopic excision of ovarian endometriomas: a systematic review and metaanalysis. Am J Obstet Gynecol. 2016;214(2):203–11.
141. Deguara CS, Pepas L, Davis C. Does minimally invasive surgery for endometriosis improve pelvic symptoms and quality of life? Curr Opin Obstet Gynecol. 2012;24(4):241–4.
142. Fritzer N, Hudelist G. Love is a pain? Quality of sex life after surgical resection of endometriosis: a review. Eur J Obstet Gynecol Reprod Biol. 2016. pii: S0301-2115(16)30187-7.
143. Lukic A, Di Properzio M, De Carlo S, Nobili F, Schimberni M, Bianchi P, Prestigiacomo C, Moscarini M, Caserta D. Quality of sex life in endometriosis patients with deep dyspareunia before and after laparoscopic treatment. Arch Gynecol Obstet. 2016;293(3):583–90. doi:10.1007/s00404-015-3832-9.. Epub 2015 Aug 6.
144. Nourmoussavi M, Bodmer-Roy S, Mayji N, Williams C, ALlaire C, Yong PJ. Bladder base tenderness in etiology of deep dyspareunia. J Sex Med. 2014;12:3078–84.
145. Peters KM, Killinger KA, Carrico DJ, Ibrahim IA, Diokno AC, Grasiottin A. Sexual function and sexual distress in women with interstitial cystitis a case control study. Urology. 2007;70(3):543–7.
146. Mathias SD, Kuppermann M, Liberman RF, et al. Chronic pelvic pain: prevalence, health-related quality of life, and economic correlates. Obstet Gynecol. 1996;87:321Y327.
147. Doggweiler R, Whitmore KE, Meijlink JM, Drake MJ, Frawley H, Nordling J, Hanno P, Fraser MO, Homma Y, Garrido G, Gomes MJ, Elneil S, van de Merwe JP, Lin AT, Tomoe H. A standard for terminology in chronic pelvic pain syndromes: a report from the chronic pelvic pain working group of the international continence society. NeurourolUrodyn. 2016. doi:10.1002/nau.23072.. [Epub ahead of print].
148. Bogart LM, Suttorp MJ, Elliott MN, Clemens JQ, Berry SH. Prevalence and correlates of sexual dysfunction among women with bladder pain sydrome/interstitial cystitis. Female Urology. 2011;77(3):576–80.
149. Graziottin A. Sexual pain disorders: dyspareunia and vaginismus. Oxford: Blackwell; 2006. p. P342 35.International Society of Sexual Medicine. Chapter 25
150. Gardella B, Porru D, Ferdeghini F, Martinotti Gabellotti E, Nappi RE, Rovereto B, Spinillo A. Insight into urogynecologic features of women with interstitial cystitis/painful bladder syndrome. Eur

Urol. 2008;54(5):1145–51. doi:10.1016/j.eururo.2008.01.079.. Epub 2008 Feb 6.
151. www.ichelp.org/TreatmentAndSelfHelp/ICAandDiet.html. Accessed 24 Jan 2012.
152. Fitzgerald MP, Anderson RU, Potts J, Payne CK, Peters KM, Clemens JQ, Kotarinos R, Fraser L, Cosby A, Fortman C, Neville C, Badillo S, Odabachian L, Sanfield A, O'Dougherty B, Halle-Podell R, Cen L, Chuai S, Landis JR, Mickelberg K, Barrell T, Kusek JW, Nyberg LM, Urological Pelvic Pain Collaborative Research Network. Randomized multicenter feasibility trial of myofascial physical therapy for the treatment of urological chronic pelvic pain syndromes. J Urol. 2013;189(1 Suppl):S75–85. doi:10.1016/j.juro.2012.11.018.
153. Hanno PM, Burks DA, Clemens JQ, et al. AUA guideline for the diagnosis and treatment of interstitial cystitis/bladder pain syndrome. J Urol. 2011;185:2162.
154. Foster Jr HE, Hanno PM, Nickel JC, et al. Effect of amitriptyline on symptoms in treatment naïve patients with interstitial cystitis/painful bladder syndrome. J Urol. 2010;183:1853.
155. van Ophoven A, Pokupic S, Heinecke A, Hertle L. A prospective, randomized, placebo controlled, double-blind study of amitriptyline for the treatment of interstitial cystitis. J Urol. 2004;172:533.
156. Thilagarajah R, Witherow RO, Walker MM. Oral cimetidine gives effective symptoms relief in painful bladder disease: a prospective, randomized double blind placebo controlled trial. BJU Int. 2001;87:207.
157. Seshadri P, Emerson L, Morales A. Cimetidine in the treatment of interstitial cystitis. Urology. 1994;44:614.
158. Dasgupta P, Sharma SD, Womack C, et al. Cimetidine in painful bladder syndrome: a histopathological study. BJU Int. 2001;88:183.
159. Nickel JC, Herschorn S, Whitmore KE, Forrest JB, Hu P, Friedman AJ, Baseman AS. Pentosan polysulfate sodium for treatment of interstitial cystitis/bladder pain syndrome: insights from a randomized, double-blind, placebo controlled study. J Urol. 2015;193(3):857–62. doi:10.1016/j.juro.2014.09.036.. Epub 2014 Sep 20.
160. Anderson VR, Perry CM. Pentosan polysulfate: a review of its use in the relief of bladder pain or discomfort in interstitial cystitis. Drugs. 2006;66(6):821–35.
161. Nickel JC, Parsons CL, Forrest J, Kaufman D, Evans R, Chen A, Wan G, Xiao X. Improvement in sexual functioning in patients with interstitial cystitis/painful bladder syndrome. J Sex Med. 2008;5(2):394–9 .Epub 2007 Dec 14
162. Welk BK, Teichman JM. Dyspareunia response in patients with interstitial cystitis treated withintravesical lidocaine, bicarbonate, and heparin. Urology. 2008;71(1):67–70. doi:10.1016/j.urology.2007.09.067.
163. Ottem DP, Teichman JM. What is the value of cystoscopy with hydrodistension for interstitial cystitis? Urology. 2005;66(3):494–9.
164. Jhang JF, Kuo HC. Novel treatment of chronic bladder pain syndrome and other pelvic pain disorders by Onabotulinumtoxin A injection. Toxins. 2015;7:2232–50.
165. Giannantoni A, Conte A, Farfariello V, Proietti S, Vianello A, Nardicchi V, Santoni G, Amantini C. Onabotulinumtoxin-A intradetrusorial injections modulate bladder expression of NGF, TrkA, p75 and TRPV1 in patients with detrusor overactivity. Pharmacol Res. 2013;68(1):118–24. doi:10.1016/j.phrs.2012.11.009.. Epub 2012 Dec 13.
166. Conte A, Giannantoni A, Proietti S, Giovannozzi S, Fabbrini G, Rossi A, Porena M, Berardelli A. Botulinum toxin A modulates afferent fibers in neurogenic detrusor overactivity. Eur J Neurol. 2012;19(5):725–32. doi:10.1111/j.1468-1331.2011.03618.x.. Epub 2011 Dec 28.
167. Kaya S, Hermans L, Willems T, Roussel N, Meeus M. Central sensitization in urogynecological chronic pelvic pain: A systematic literature review. Pain Physician. 2013;16:291–308.
168. Aoki KR. Evidence for antinociceptive activity of botulinum toxin type A in pain management. Headache. 2003;43(Suppl 1):S9–15.
169. Foran PG, Mohammed N, Lisk GO, Nagwaney S, Lawrence GW, Johnson E, Smith L, Aoki KR, Dolly JO. Evaluation of the therapeutic usefulness of botulinum neurotoxin B, C1, E, and F compared with the long lasting type A. Basis for distinct durations of inhibition of exocytosis in central neurons. J Biol Chem. 2003;278(2):1363–71 .Epub 2002 Oct 14
170. Durham PL, Cady R, Cady R. Regulation of calcitonin gene-related peptide secretion from trigeminal nerve cells by botulinum toxin type A: implications for migraine therapy. Headache. 2004;44(1):35–42 .discussion 42-3
171. Khera M, Somogyi GT, Kiss S, Boone TB, Smith CP. Botulinum toxin A inhibits ATP release from bladder urothelium after chronic spinal cord injury. Neurochem Int. 2004;45(7):987–93.
172. Nijs J, van Houdenhove B, Oostendorp RA. Recognition of central sensitization in patients with musculoskeletal pain: application of pain neurophysiology in manual therapy practice. Man Ther. 2010;15(2):135–41. doi:10.1016/j.math.2009.12.001.. Epub 2009 Dec 24.
173. Kuo HC, Chancellor MB. Comparison of intravesical botulinum toxin type A injections plus hydrodistention with hydrodistention alone for the treatment of refractory interstitial cystitis/painful bladder syndrome. BJU Int. 2009;104(5):657–61. doi:10.1111/j.1464-410X.2009.08495.x.. Epub 2009 Mar 30.
174. Kuo HC, Jiang YH, Tsai YC, Kuo YC. Intravesical botulinum toxin-A injection reduce bladder pain of interstital cystitis/bladder pain syndrome refractory to conventional treatment—A prospective, multicenter, randomized, double blind, placebo-controlled clinical trial. NeurourolUrodyn. 2016;35(5):609–14. doi:10.1002/nau.22760.. Epub 2015 Apr 24.
175. Marcelissen T, Jacobs R, van Kerrebroeck P, de Wachter S. Sacral neuromodulation as a treatment for chronic pelvic pain review article. J Urol. 2011;186(2):387–93.
176. Lombardi G, Finazzi Agrò E, Del Popolo G. Sacral neuromodulation and female sexuality. Int Urogynecol J. 2015;26(12):1751–7. doi:10.1007/s00192-015-2708-7.. Epub 2015 Apr 16.
177. Fass R, Fullerton S, Naliboff B, Hirsh T. Mayer EA sexual dysfunction in patients with irritable bowel syndrome and non-ulcer dyspepsia. Digestion. 1998;59(1):79–85.
178. Slocumb J. Neurological factors in chronic pelvic pain: trigger points and the abdominal pelvic pain syndrome. Am J Obstet Gynecol. 1984;149(5):536–43.
179. Tu FF, Holt J, Gonzales J, Fitzgerald CM. Physical theapy evaluation of patients with chronic pelvic pain: a controlled study. Am J Obstet Gynecol. 2008;198(3):272–7.
180. Mui J, Allaire C, Williams C, Yong PJ. Abdominal wall pain in women with chronic pelvic pain. J Obstet Gynaecol Can. 2016;38(2):154–9.
181. Annaswamy TM, De Luigi AJ, O'Neill BJ, Keole N, Berbrayer D. Emerging concepts in the treatment of myofascial pain: a review of medications, modalities, and needle-based interventions. PMR. 2011;3(10):940–61. doi:10.1016/j.pmrj.2011.06.013.
182. Nazareno J, Ponich T, Gregor J. Long-term follow-up of trigger point injections for abdominal wall pain. Can J Gastroenterol. 2005;19(9):561–5.

22 Evaluation and Treatment of Sexual Disorders Due to Medical Conditions

Alexander Joseph Steiner and Waguih William IsHak

Introduction

The Diagnostic and Statistical Manual of Mental Disorders (DSM), Fourth Edition, Text Revision reported that sexual dysfunction is diagnosed when problems secondary to the disorder result in marked distress or interpersonal problems [1]. In addition, the DSM-IV-TR considered sexual dysfunction to be the result of either psychological and physiological causes or a combination of both psychological and physiological factors [1]. With the introduction of the Fifth Edition of the DSM (DSM 5), new criteria were established that prohibited a sexual disorder to be considered a psychiatric diagnosis, if the disorders presumed etiology was a medical condition (or several concurrent medical conditions) [2]. While the requirement of biological foundations influence sexual responsiveness, a plethora of psychiatric disorders can also influence an individual's sexual function. Emotional functioning, psychiatric distress, and a variety of psychosocial issues have been identified to directly affect sexual responsiveness. Yet it is common practice for a physician to encounter a clinical context, in which a precise understanding of the specific cause of a sexual problem remains unidentified. Thus, the clinician bears the responsibility of ensuring due diligence to determine and recognize the constellation of factors that may impact a patients reported sexual dysfunction.

The American Psychiatric Association provided a new nosology for sexual disorders with the introduction of the DSM-5 [2]. Notably, a sexual dysfunction diagnosis requires the treating clinician to rule out a multitude of problems that could be better explained by a nonsexual psychiatric disorder (e.g., major depressive disorder, posttraumatic stress disorder, generalized anxiety disorder), by the direct and indirect effects of a specific substance (e.g., medication or drug), by a medical condition (e.g., diabetes mellitus), or by profound interpersonal and psychosocial stress [2]. In the event that sexual dysfunction is most probably explained by another psychiatric condition, then the other mental disorder diagnosis should be made in place of the sexual dysfunction disorder. If however, the sexual disorder is attributed to a medical condition, then an individual cannot be diagnosed with a psychiatric illness. In particular, Sexual Dysfunction due to a General Medical Condition is no longer a DSM diagnosis and clinicians will need to assess and treat medical conditions with their sexual consequences without separate psychiatric diagnostic labels.

One complicating issue worth noting is the likely scenario in which the exact etiological relationship between a concurrent medical disorder and a sexual disorder cannot be established, which is a commonly encountered problem facing treating physicians. This in turn, makes the diagnosis of a sexual disorder dependent on the clinicians understanding of how a host of medical conditions can influence sexual function and responsiveness. Furthermore, clinical judgment plays a critical role in ensuring that the cultural and religious context of each patient is considered when assessing and treating sexual disorders, as well as how a patient's cultural and religious morals, values, beliefs, customs, and practice influence sexual function and responsiveness. Another important concern, when addressing patients' sexual dysfunction is the awareness that aging is often associated with a normative decrease in sexual responsiveness. Taken together, a clinicians approach to the initial evaluations of patients' sexual disorders can be a complex and often rigorous process that requires a respect for the multitude of factors that can result in sexual dysfunction.

Notably, the current state of affairs pertaining to sexual education in medical schools in the United States of America is rather complex. Research suggest that while the importance of sexuality to patients is acknowledged, there is continued concern relating to both the quantity and quality of education on sexual medicine in North American medical schools [3]. It follows that we hope this chapter can assist medical students understanding of both the clinical rationale and medical necessity to provide patients with evidence-based and theory grounded treatments for sexual disorders. For the purpose of this chapter, we focus on sexual disorders

W.W. IsHak (ed.), *The Textbook of Clinical Sexual Medicine*, DOI 10.1007/978-3-319-52539-6_22

that are due to medical conditions. The inherent outline of this chapter assumes that the suspected etiology or presumed cause of a given sexual disorder is the result of a particular medical diagnosis, or as is often the case, a collection of medical conditions. The primary objective of this chapter is to cover the evaluation and treatment of common sexual disorders including genito-pelvic pain/penetration disorder, erectile disorder, delayed ejaculation, premature ejaculation, male hypoactive sexual desire disorder, female orgasmic disorder, and female sexual interest/arousal disorder, all of which are outlines in the DSM-5 [2].

These sexual disorders can be further classified as belonging to one of the following: disorders of desire, arousal, orgasm, or sexual pain. All information will focus on the most common medical and physiological conditions, which can potentially lead to any of the four previously mentioned and distinct types of sexual disorders [4]. In addition to covering the plethora of medical conditions known to affect sexual responsiveness, we begin by covering epidemiology, etiology, pathophysiology, and diagnostic criteria for the various disorders. We then provide an overview of common evidence-based practice and best approaches to the diagnosis of sexual disorders due to medical conditions. This section includes a review of diagnostic tests that may be useful in the treatment of sexual disorders. Finally, we conclude by highlighting key findings from studies focused on the treatment of sexual disorders by reviewing evidence-based approaches to treatment, including biological treatments (i.e., medications, devices), psychosocial treatments, and prognosis of sexual disorders.

Epidemiology

While there are increasing interests for clinical services of sexual dysfunction, and growing concern for the potential impact such dysfunction can have on interpersonal relationships and quality of life, there continues to be a dearth of epidemiologic data [5, 6]. Epidemiological data is further complicated by the varying methodological approaches and research designs in population based studies. Furthermore, prior studies have failed to separate sexual disorders into two distinct groups based upon either a psychiatric etiology or a medical etiology, which ultimately makes it difficulty to have a reliable estimate of varying sexual disorders to date.

Incidence and Prevalence

It is often difficult for researchers to accurately estimate or predict the prevalence rates of sexual disorders. One complicating factor is the sensitive nature of seeking professional care for sexual dysfunction. Nevertheless, several population-based studies have reported general estimates on the prevalence rates of sexual disorders. As is often the case, there are a variety of risk factors and modifying demographic variables that place certain cohorts at increased risk for sexual dysfunction. For example, data from the National Health and Social Life Survey, which was a large probability sample of sexual behavior for adults living in the USA found that sexual dysfunction is more prevalent for women (43%) compared to men (31%), and is associated with a variety of demographic factors including age and education [7]. One robust finding is that as men age, they are more than three times as likely to experience erectile problems and to report low sexual desire compared to younger men [7]. In addition, non-married women are approximately 1.5 times more likely to have climax problems compared to women, with non-married men reporting significantly higher rates of sexual dysfunction as well compared to their married peers [7]. Interestingly, high educational attainment has been reported to be negatively associated with the experiencing of sexual dysfunction for both sexes, as women and men with lower educational attainment report less pleasurable sexual experience [7].

There are some interesting, yet variable, associations between race and ethnicity and sexual problems. African American women tend to have greater rates of low sexual desire and report experiencing less pleasure compared with Caucasian women, while Caucasian women are more likely to have sexual pain than African American women, and Hispanic women consistently report lower rates of sexual problems [7]. Ethnic and racial differences for men are not as well documented, as findings are often mixed.

Delayed ejaculation is the least common male sexual complaint [2], with less than 1% of men complaining of problems with reaching ejaculation lasting more than a 6-month period [8]. With that said, while the prevalence of delayed ejaculation is relatively constant until approximately age 50, when the incidence rates start to increase significantly [2]. In addition, research suggest that men in their eighties are twice as likely as men younger than 59 to report difficulty with ejaculating [9]. Relatedly, prevalence rates of male hypoactive sexual desire disorder are variable, with nearly 6% of younger men (between 16 and 24 years old) and 41% of older men (between 66 and 74 years old) report problems of sexual desire [10].

Premature (early) ejaculation prevalence rate estimates have substantial variability depending on the operational definitions of the disorder. Research suggests that over 20% to 30% of men between the ages of 18 and 70 have concern about rapid ejaculation [11]. In another study, of 1491 adults living in the USA, early ejaculation (26.2%) and erectile difficulties (22.5%) were the most common male sexual problems [12].

Regarding erectile disorder, incidence rates for erectile dysfunction remain scarce. Yet a study of Caucasian males in the USA reported an incidence of 26 cases per 1000 man-years

[13]. The exact prevalence for erectile disorder secondary to a medical condition, presents as a difficult estimate to gather as the nature of erectile disorder is often complicated by several psychological and emotional factors. However, literature indicates that both the prevalence and incidence rates of erection problems are related to aging, particularly after 50 years of age [13]. Various community studies have reported that the prevalence rate of erectile dysfunction ranges from 7% to as high as 52% [13]. Roughly 13–21% of men between the age of 40 and 80 complain of occasional problems with erections [2]. Only 2% of men younger than ages 40–50 complain of frequent problems with erections, while up to 40%–50% of men older than 60–70 years of age have been reported to have significant problems with erections [14]. Another disorder isolated to males is Peyronie's disease, which is often referred to as penile curvature. Peyronie's disease afflicts 3% of the male population and can lead to incomplete erection and erectile dysfunction; this condition typically occurs between 45 and 60 years of age. While the average age for contracting Peyronie's disease is 50, it can also occur in men as young as 18.

A substantial amount of males living with diabetes suffer from erectile dysfunction, which often manifesting as a precursor sign of diabetes. Statistics by the Erectile Dysfunction institute reported that males with diabetes were two to five times more likely to develop erectile dysfunction compared to men without the disease. Other research has found that erectile dysfunction is strongly correlated with aging, from 65 in ages 20 to 24 years old to 52% in men between the ages of 55 and 59 years old [15]. In addition, men who have diabetes develop impotence approximately 10–15 years earlier than men without diabetes and more than 50% of men develop diabetic impotence within 10 years of getting diabetes. Around 50 to 60% of diabetic men over age 50 have erectile problems and around 50 to 70% of diabetic men will experience some degree of erectile difficulties through the course of their illness. In addition, men with type-1 diabetes often experience erectile dysfunction at an earlier age, as they typically have the disease for a longer period of time, and men with type 2 diabetes are more likely to experience problems later in life.

One national US survey conducted in 1999 and published in *JAMA* found that 15% of women report recurrent pain during intercourse [7]. While vaginusmus is considered an outdated term, previous estimates suggested that one out of every 100 women may suffer from vaginismus. This condition occurs when there is an involuntary muscle constriction of the outer third of the vagina that interferes with penile insertion and intercourse. There is evidence that this response occurs during routine gynecological examinations, during which time involuntary vaginal constriction prevents the introduction of the speculum into the vagina [16]. Notably, literature suggests that complaints related to genito-pelvic pain may peak in early adulthood or during perimenopausal and postmenopausal phases of life [2].

Approximately 10–42% of woman may experience female orgasmic disorder, yet there are a number of demographic factors that have been implicated in affecting the prevalence rates of this disorder (e.g., duration, severity of symptoms, culture, age) [17]. Nevertheless, rates of distress in women can vary dependent upon a number of factors including whether or not women manifest low interest or if lubrication insufficiency of dyspareunia are present, with the later group reporting greater distress [18]. Other researchers caution that variation in how symptoms are assessed can influence prevalence rates of female orgasmic disorder across studies [8]. One large study reported that a lack of sexual interest (33.2%) and lubrication difficulties (21.5%) were the two most common problems reported by women out of all types of sexual dysfunction [12].

Prevalence rates of the psychiatric diagnosis of female sexual interest/arousal disorder are reportedly unknown [2]. However, a variety of factors including duration of symptoms, age, presence of distress, and cultural factors can influence the aforementioned prevalence rates [17, 19, 20]. For example, literature indicates that older women may be more likely to report lower levels of distress about low sexual desire compared to younger women, with the acknowledgement that sexual desire may decrease with age for a variety of reasons [21].

Etiology

The exact manner or cause of a specific sexual disorder or condition can have myriad explanations. One further complicating factor is the reality that for many patients, there may be competing etiological considerations, as an individual can have several medical conditions that impact sexual response and function [22]. In general, medical conditions affecting sexual function can be further divided into distinct categories or classes. Other conditions that can affect sexual function are advanced age, chronic diseases in general, malnutrition as well as medication side effects, nicotine, drug and alcohol use and abuse. Table 22-1 provides a general overview of both direct and indirect causes of sexual dysfunction, as well as the mechanisms for a variety of factors with specific examples.

Urinary track symptoms have been identified to impact arousal and pain disorders for women and erectile dysfunction for men [7]. In addition, pelvic problems including endometriosis (the presence of uterine tissue outside of the uterus), cystitis (bladder infection), or vaginitis (inflammation of vaginal tissue which leads to vaginal dryness and decreased arousal) can all lead to arousal disorder in women. Treating the underlying cause responsible for the arousal

TABLE 22-1. Factors involved in sexual dysfunction associated with chronic disease and cancer

Type	Mechanisms	Examples
Direct	Change in sexual desire from disease	Typically reduced, e.g., from high prolactin and anemia of chronic renal failure [1]. May be increased, e.g., from some brain disorders [2]
	Disruption of genital response from disease	ED from multiple sclerosis [3], hypertension [4], orgasmic disorder from multiple sclerosis [5]
	Disruption of genital response from surgery	Radical prostatectomy and ED [6], radical hysterectomy and reduced genital congestion/reduced lubrication [7], orgasmic disorder after radical vulvectomy [8]
	Disruption of genital response from radiation	ED from vascular (and also likely nerve) damage after radiotherapy for prostate cancer [9]; vaginal stenosis and friability from radiation for pelvic cancer [10]
	Dyspareunia and disruption of sexual desire and response from chemotherapy	Sudden ovarian failure after chemotherapy for breast cancer [11]; testicular failure after intensive chemotherapy for hematopoietic transplantation [12]
	Disruption of sexual desire and response from antiandrogen treatment	GnRH therapy for prostate cancer [13]
	Disruption of genital response from aromatase inhibitors	Loss of sexual genital sensitivity, and exacerbation of vaginal atrophy from aromatase inhibition post breast cancer [14]
	Disruption of sexual desire and response from pain	Pain from any chronic condition is a potent sexual distraction
	Disruption of sexual desire and response from nonhormonal medications	Narcotics can depress desire through gonadotropin suppression [15]; selective serotonin reuptake inhibitors reduce desire and response [16]
Indirect	Reduction of self-image	Reduced by disfiguring surgeries, stomas, incontinence, altered appearance (e.g., drooling and altered faces of Parkinson's, altered skin color and muscle wasting of renal failure)
	Depressed mood	Depression and mood lability commonly accompany chronic illness; depression major determinant of sexual function in women with renal failure [17] or multiple sclerosis [18]; strong link between ED and subsequent depression [19]
	Impaired mobility	Reduced ability to caress, hug, and hold a partner; to sexually self-stimulate, to stimulate a partner, to move into positions for intercourse, to pelvically thrust in spinal cord injury, Parkinson's, brain injury, postamputation
	Reduced energy	Fatigue may take its toll on sexuality especially desire, e.g., from renal failure or chemotherapy
	Partnership difficulties	Difficulties finding a partner, dysfunction in the partner who assumes a care giver role, institutionalization, fear of becoming a burden to a partner, lack of independence. Relationship discord from stressors of living with medicalized lives (e.g., three times weekly hemodialysis)
	Sense of loss of sexuality from imposed infertility	From surgery removing gonads or uterus, from chemotherapy or radiotherapy causing gonadal failure
	Fear of sex worsening medical condition	Avoiding sex fearing a further stroke

ED Erectile dysfunction. [Reprinted from Basson R, Rees P, Wang R, Montejo AL, Incrocci L. Sexual Function in Chronic Illness. J Sex Med. 2010;7:374–388. with permission from Elsevier].

disorder through surgical intervention (i.e., endometriosis), or the use of antibiotics for the treatment of urinary tract infections, have proven to be effective interventions to alleviate symptoms of arousal disorder in women. A variety of surgical procedures, including hysterectomy and mastectomy, have the potential to influence a woman's sense of femininity and in turn affect both sexual desire and arousal. In addition, there are natural biological processes that impact hormonal fluctuations and changes, including pregnancy and menopause, which can in turn diminish sexual arousal. In men, endocrine disorders like hyperprolactinemia can substantially affect sexual desire and erectile function [23, 24].

One of the more difficult challenges clinicians face when treating erectile disorder is ruling out problems that are most likely attributable to medical factors. In addition to a plethora of psychological factors, male erectile disorder can have several physiological etiologies. Acquired erectile disorder has been associated with biological factors including diabetes and cardiovascular diseases. Therefore, it is important for clinicians to distinguish erectile disorder as a mental disorder, where psychological factors may cause erectile dysfunction, or if erectile dysfunction is the result of another medical condition. In addition, there are modifiable risk factors for acquired erectile disorder such as tobacco smoking history, sedentary lifestyle, and diabetes that should be considered [25]. A compilation of data from the National Cancer Institute, the American Diabetes Association, the Bureau of Health Statistics, and the American Cancer Society have found that for all of the erectile dysfunction cases caused by physical or medical factors, 40% is due to vascular disease,

30% is a result of diabetes, 11% is secondary to medications, drug abuse, and hormone deficiency, 10% is a result of neurological disorders, and 9% of all physical cases of ED is due to pelvic surgery and trauma. More recent literature has suggested that hyperthyroidism may also be associated with an increased risk of erectile dysfunction [24]. In sum, these numbers suggest that for the majority of cases of male erectile dysfunction, there is a vasculogenic origin; in particular, endothelial dysfunction appears to be the primary culprit for erectile dysfunction. Some data suggest that around 75–80% of men with heart failure in different stages can suffer from sexual dysfunction, a relationship that is independent of the etiology of the heart disease [26, 27].

The treatment of medical conditions poses a threat to the development of sexual disorders. In particular, gastrointestinal, cytotoxic, hormonal agents, and cardiovascular medications have been reported to be related to sexual dysfunction [2]. In addition, approximately 30% of surgical interventions of the female genitalia have been documented to result in temporary pain during sexual intercourse [16]. Conversely, pain during intercourse in males is an area that remains understudied. Typically, pain during intercourse in males is associated with Peyronie's disease where sclerotic plaques invade the sheath, which covers the penis. Pelvic pain syndrome (prostatodynia) has also been associated with painful erection, ejaculation, and pain during intercourse in males. The exact cause of prostatodynia remains unknown, yet some physicians consider local trauma to the penis and external genitalia or vigorous sexual activity as potential risks for developing pelvic pain syndrome.

There are a variety of medical conditions that can influence female orgasmic disorder including multiple sclerosis, pelvic nerve damage from radical hysterectomy or spinal cord injury [2]. In the presence of vulvovaginal atrophy, with symptoms including vaginal pain, itching, or dryness, women are significantly more likely to have difficulty with orgasm compared to women without this disorder [28]. Conversely, other research suggests that the relationship between vulvovaginal atrophy, dryness, pain, and estrogen remains as a poorly understood phenomenon [29]. The findings on the relationship between menopause and its effect on a woman's ability to achieve orgasm are mixed, with data suggesting there is no consistent relationship between the two [30]. A more recent review article suggests that there may be a genetic contribution to female orgasmic disorder [31].

In the case of female sexual interest/arousal disorder, vaginal dryness in older women is related to age and menopausal status, which indirectly can lead to the onset of this disorder if not properly treated [11, 32]. One review article suggests that there is a strong genetic influence in female sexual interest/arousal disorder [31]. Arthritis, diabetes mellitus, endothelial disease, thyroid dysfunction, urinary incontinence, inflammatory or irritable bowel disease (e.g., Crohn's disease, ulcerative colitis), and neurological disorders have all been identified to affect sexual interest and arousal in women [2, 33–35].

One research study suggests that premature (early) ejaculation may have a moderate genetic contribution in patients with lifelong symptoms of the disorder [36]. More recent research suggests that premature (early) ejaculation is potentially associated with the dopamine transporter gene polymorphism [37]. Likewise, the serotonin transporter gene polymorphism may also play a role in premature (early) ejaculation [38]. Clearly more research is needed to further elucidate the contributing factors of premature ejaculation.

Pathophysiology

There are a variety of medical factors that can compromise the pathophysiology of optimal sexual function. One's inability to ejaculate can be the result of an interruption of the nerve supply to the genitals, which is often observed following traumatic surgical injury to the lumbar sympathetic ganglia, abdominoperitoneal surgery, or a lumber sympatectomy [39]. Other physiological causes of a male's inability to ejaculate can be related to other surgical procedures including prostatectomy or any type of genitourinary interventions. As ejaculation is controlled by the autonomic nervous system involving the hypogastric (sympathetic) and pudendal (parasympathetic) nerves, there are several neurodegenerative diseases (e.g., multiple sclerosis, diabetic neuropathy, alcoholic neuropathy) that can result in an inability to ejaculate [40]. In addition, there is age-related loss of fast-conducting peripheral sensory nerves as well as decreased steroid secretion associated with aging that are possible physiological factors which may increase delayed ejaculation in men over 50 years of age [40]. Furthermore, neurological disorders that involve the lumbosacral spine or pain and paresthesia stemming from the external genitalia can affect a man's ability to orgasm (i.e., pelvic pain syndrome).

Premature ejaculation in men is thought to rarely have a physical cause. Rather premature ejaculation can be the result of psychological factors. Nevertheless, neurological disorders, prostatitis (inflammation of the prostate), or urethritis (inflammation of the urethra), are all plausible causes of premature ejaculation. It follows that once a physician has identified the etiology of a patients premature ejaculation, treating the underlying cause can alleviate this specific sexual disorder. Research indicates that there are a variety of cases in which premature (early) ejaculation is reversible. In particular, several medical conditions (e.g., prostatitis, hyperthyroidism), when treated, can lead to ejaculatory latencies at baseline [41].

If there is a medical condition that compromises a man's ability to have adequate blood pressure to carry blood to the penis, or if there are any "leaks" in the penile venous system caused by a medical condition, then erectile dysfunction can occur. In addition, for a male to sustain an erection, adequate levels of testosterone are required. In relation, the process of clitoral swelling and vaginal lubrication directly relies upon adequate blood flow to the vaginal area. In the event that a medical condition impedes this process, a woman's ability to become aroused during sexual activity is compromised [42]. Accordingly, physicians must take a thorough medical and sexual history, conduct physical examination of the organ systems, and request laboratory examinations in order to determine whether or not a medical condition is responsible for a sexual disorder pertaining to arousal. At the same time, the physician must also factor in psychological and cultural considerations that may be contributing to low sexual arousal.

There are a variety of surgical and gynecological interventions like hysterectomy, ileostomy and mastectomy that can significantly affect body image and lead to women feeling less feminine and sexual. Furthermore, decreased blood flow to the pelvic region following surgery involving the pelvic floor, abdomen, bladder, and genitals, or medical conditions like diabetes or atherosclerosis, can directly and indirectly impair sexual desire. Relatedly, sexual desire and interest disorders in both genders are related to altered hormonal levels. Specifically, decreased sex drive and absence of sexual fantasies have been observed to be the result of decreased estrogen, with the mechanism for estrogen's effect on sex drive thought to be indirect, by enhancing mood, vasomotor symptoms, and genital atrophy. Conversely, other studies have demonstrated that progesterone (another female hormone) might negatively impact sexual desire by affecting mood and the availability of androgens (sex hormones). Androgens are presumed to influence sexual function in both genders through their effects on sexual motivation and desire. Low testosterone levels have been correlated with sexual infrequency and reduced libido as well. Hypogonadism is another medical condition identified to influence sexual desire in men [2]. Lastly, excess of prolactin, a hormone in adults that regulates the behavioral aspects of reproduction and infant care, can lead to diminished libido in both males and females [16, 24].

Genito-pelvic pain/penetration disorder can have a variety of pathophysiological causes. Of note, as pelvic floor symptoms are implicated in this disorder, the probability of a comorbid medical disorder that impacts the pelvic floor or reproductive organs is quite high, with interstitial cystitis, constipation, vaginal infection, endometriosis, and irritable bowel disorder being common differentials to consider [2]. In general, pain during intercourse has the potential to significantly affect an individual's ability to experience pleasure during sex, and in several instances can result in anxiety and depression, which may in turn deter and discourage the person from sexual activity. Pain during sexual intercourse can have several causes. When viral or vaginal fungal infections are present in women, pain is often reported during sexual activity. If there is a fibroid growth in the female reproductive tract, pain may be located in the uterus. The presence of infections of the ovaries or prior surgeries can also leave scar tissue, which can also lead to pain. In addition, there are a significant amount of gynecological medical conditions that have shown to be responsible for pain before, during, or after intercourse. Cystitis, which is inflammation of the bladder, can lead to painful sex, and women should try to urinate immediately after intercourse to avoid urinary tract infections. Vaginitis is a condition that refers to the inflammation of vaginal tissue and its causes may be due to irritants or bacteria. Women who experience this condition secondary to pelvic inflammatory disease usually complain of painful intercourse and treatment of the underlying cause is necessary to eradicate pain. Urethritis is inflammation of the urethra due to urinary tract infection, which can result in painful sex. Like cystitis, treatment (e.g., antibiotics) of underlying cause should alleviate any pain. Genital Herpes can cause herpetic lesions, which may lead to discomfort and pain during intercourse. Genital warts caused by the human papilloma virus can make sexual activity painful depending on the location. In the case of endometriosis, there is abnormal uterine tissue growth in distinct parts of the body (ovaries are the most common site). Endometriosis can lead to abnormal bleeding, inflammation, scarring, pain, fatigue, and infertility. The pain can usually manifest when the uterus contracts during orgasm. Cystocele is a condition that occurs when the bladder bulges or herniates into a woman's vagina, which leads to painful intercourse. Uterine prolapse occurs when the uterus falls or "slides" from its normal position into the vaginal canal; the resulting shift in position may lead to painful intercourse. Lastly, rectal disease (i.e., cancer) often leads to complications such as pain that occurs due to the close proximity of the rectum (posterior) to the vagina.

Endothelial Dysfunction

In regards to male erectile disorder, endothelial dysfunction continues to gain increasing notoriety as a primary etiological consideration as to the pathogenesis of atherosclerosis [43]. Atherosclerosis has been identified as the most common cause of vasculogenic erectile dysfunction, particularly in older men. As such, it is frequently considered another manifestation of vascular disease. Hence, the risk factors for the development of endothelial dysfunction leading to coronary artery disease, for example, are similar to the risk factor leading to vasculogenic erectile dysfunction. Men who have underlying diseases leading to vascular abnormalities, including diabetes, have dysfunctional neurogenic and endothelium-dependent penile smooth muscle relaxation that result in erectile dysfunction. At the cellular level, impairment of the L-arginine NO pathway at a number of sites is plausible. As the precise mechanisms have not been clearly defined, endothelial damage can either decrease basal release of NO, or may lead to increased breakdown. Furthermore, eNOS activity may be attenuated by accumulation of NOS inhibitors. In addition to endothelial alterations, vascular smooth muscle cells appear to have a blunted response to nitric oxide. Endothelial function is also possibly related to microalbuminuria, which seems to influence endothelium-dependent and independent vasodilation. Men who have type 2 diabetes mellitus have documented impairment in vasodilation in response to both endothelium-dependent and -independent agonists and increased generation of reactive oxygen species that damage endothelial cells either directly or indirectly via effects on lipid peroxidation and by scavenging nitric oxide to produce peroxynitrite (which is a potent oxidant). There are a variety of other mechanisms that can lead to endothelial dysfunction, including decreased release of acetylcholine by cholinergic nerves, peripheral and autonomic neuropathy, and sparse penile noradrenergic nervous innervation [44]. Endothelial dysfunction has been identified as a possible risk factor for sexual dysfunction in woman as well [33].

Hypertension

One of the hallmark traits of primary hypertension is the increased peripheral sympathetic activity, increased vasoconstrictor tone, and decreased endothelium-dependent vasodilation. Certain cases of hypertension-associated endothelial dysfunction are possibly related to eNOS gene variations. Additional changes in the cyclooxygenase pathway may play a major role, as increases in cyclooxygenase activity can lead to increases in reactive oxygen species, with further disruption of normal endothelial activity. Notably, it is important to emphasize that dysfunctional endothelium-dependent vasodilation is not merely a cause of hypertension. Rather, dysfunctional endothelium-dependent vasodilation is present in multiple disease states and the degree of endothelial dysfunction is not related to blood pressure values. On the other hand, hypertension plays an etiologic role in the development of male sexual dysfunction beyond its correlation with endothelial dysfunction. Lastly, structural alterations with vascular and corporal remodeling occur that reduce vasodilatory capacity.

Dyslipidemia

Hypercholesterolemia has a strong relationship to endothelial dysfunction and oxidized low-density lipoprotein is a key mediator. For cases of familial hypercholesterolemia, endothelial dysfunction can be seen prior to clinical arterial disease. This effect has even been seen in the setting of angiographically normal coronary arteries, and reduced endothelium-derived NO bioavailability has been seen in the setting of hypercholesterolemia. Not only is endothelial dysfunction related to LDL concentration, but it is also related to LDL size, with smaller particles being associated with the aforementioned dysfunction. Yet what remains to be examined are the effects of hypertriglyceridemia, which are less clear.

Obesity

Obese patients have disrupted endothelial function as seen in both resistance and conductance arteries, independent of other vascular comorbidities. A possible mechanism is the relationship between obesity and a chronic inflammatory state. Specifically, elevated levels of the circulating intercellular adhesion molecules-1 (ICAM-1), vascular adhesion molecule (VCAM-1), E and P selectins, tumor necrosis factor alpha (TNFa) and interleukin 6 (IL-6) have been reported in obese men and women. Importantly, these specific cytokines have been demonstrated to influence endothelial function and are key contributors in the early atherogenic process. In addition, this inflammatory process contributes to and can result in oxidative stress, which leads to free radical formation and thereby secondarily decreasing NO bioavailability. Furthermore, other factors including oxygen radicals can further contribute to endothelial dysfunction in obesity. Thus, it comes as no surprise that obesity, in particular abdominal obesity, is not only linked to endothelial dysfunction but also to erectile dysfunction in men [43]. Obese women with endothelial dysfunction are also at risk for compromised sexual functioning [33, 45].

Men with erectile dysfunction have been documented to impair endothelial-dependent and independent vasodilation beyond what is explained by vascular risk factors [43]. One study compared brachial artery flow-mediated dilation (FMD) and nitroglycerine-mediated dilation (NMD) in three sets of patients: those with presumed vasculogenic ED and cardiac risk factors, those with similar risk factors but no ED, and a control population without cardiac risk factors or ED [46]. This study demonstrated that brachial artery FMD and NMD were significantly reduced in patients with ED compared to healthy controls. The patients without ED but who had similar risk factors had decreased FMD, but not NMD compared with healthy controls, which suggests impairment in endothelial-independent vasodilation. Other research groups have discovered that patients with erectile dysfunction have impaired FMD and NMD compared with healthy controls [47].

Cardiovascular Diseases in General

There is a significantly high prevalence rate of erectile dysfunction in men who have underlying cardiovascular diseases. Men with chronic cardiovascular diseases commonly experience decreased libido and decreased frequency of sexual activity, as well as erectile dysfunction. In addition, there are a number of medical risk factors common to the development of coronary artery disease, heart failure, and erectile dysfunction including diabetes mellitus, hypertension, smoking, and dyslipidemia. Many patients with coronary atherosclerosis (arteries diseased by cholesterol plaque buildup) have great likelihoods of having diseased arteries outside of the heart. In the case that the arteries supplying blood to the penis are sufficiently diseased, adequate achievement or maintenance of an erection is frequently prevented, often termed "penile angina." Moreover, potential changes in the pudendal arteries in the penis, stenoses of the common iliac, the hypogastric artery, which supplies the inguinal region with blood in men with peripheral atherosclerosis can lead to erectile dysfunction. For women, high blood pressure and heart disease are also systemic conditions that may be responsible for diminishing sexual arousal. Sexual frigidity and dissatisfaction leading to sexual dysfunction, at least for a prolonged period of time, has also been reported in women after myocardial infarction [48, 49]. Endocrine diseases like hypothyroidism, diabetes, and hyperprolactinemia can also affect a woman's ability to achieve an orgasm [16].

Diabetes

As previously mentioned, in order for a man to achieve an erection, he must have healthy nerves and blood vessels. For males, diabetes often causes hardening and narrowing of the blood vessels that supply the erectile tissue of the penis, which then directly hampers the process of achieving an erection. Diabetes may also damage the nerves that innervate erectile tissue and the penis can also be less firm during an erection.

Prostate Cancer

Males with a medical history significant for prostate cancer, or who have received surgical and medical intervention for the treatment of prostate cancer, can develop erectile dysfunction. In the presence of a cancerous prostate, nerve impulses are impeded as well as blood flow to the penis, which subsequently leads to erectile dysfunction. In fact, erectile difficulties can indeed be one of the first signs of prostate cancer. Other distinct treatments for eradicating prostatic cancer can result in erectile dysfunction. For example, a radical prostatectomy that completely removes the prostate runs the risk of destroying nervous tissue that surrounds the prostate, which aids the male's ability to achieve an erection. While surgeons strive to preserve the nerve bundles surrounding the prostate, surgical intervention frequently runs the risk of damaging and severing nerve bundles, which can compromise their integrity and function. Radiation therapy may also result in erectile dysfunction by directly damaging arteries that carry blood to the penis or lead to the formation of scar tissue (fibrosis) near the prostate, which then affects blood flow to the penile tissue. Erectile dysfunction that stems from radiation therapy usually does not develop as rapidly as a radical prostatectomy, and is often not apparent for years.

Neurologic and Spinal Cord Disorders

When a patient sustains a spinal cord injury, it can impede or reduce nerve impulses from the brain to the penis and erectile dysfunction may range from partial to complete. In addition, pelvic injuries also result in harm to nerves that innervate the penis and lead to erectile dysfunction. A collection of studies has shed light on the possibility that frequent bicycling may lead to erectile difficulties, as it is hypothesized that the bicycle seat compresses the path of blood to the penis. Multiple sclerosis is another neurological disorder, where cells of the body's immune system attack the outer insulating the nerve sheath of axons, thereby causing the production of scar tissue in random spots through out the central nervous system. Consequentially, the fibrotic tissue formed can then interfere and affect the propagation of nerve impulses to the penis thereby causing erectile dysfunction. Further concern is warranted in cases of a suspected neurodegenerative process or movement disorder. In particular, there are a wide range of neurodegenerative disorders (e.g., Alzheimer's disease, frontotemporal dementia, amyotrophic lateral sclerosis) and movement disorders (e.g., Dementia with Lewy Bodies, multiple systems atrophy, corticobasal degeneration, progressive supranuclear palsy, Huntington's disease), also known as "Parkinson's plus" disorders, that may result in compromised autonomic function, pain, sensory-motor disruption, or sleep disturbance [50]. In addition, the presence of sexual dysfunction may be secondary by medication regimens used in the management of neurodegenerative diseases and movement disorders. Table 22-2 provides a general overview of the epidemiology of sexual disorders or dysfunction related to neurological dysfunction and offers treatment recommendations for each etiology.

TABLE 22-2. Epidemiology of sexual dysfunctions in neurological disorders with comments re treatment

	Prevalence of sexual difficulty	Comments with regard to etiology	Comments with regard to treatment	LOE
Head injury	36–54% for severer levels of TBI compared with 15% of healthy controls [20]. Mostly erectile/ejaculatory dysfunction in men, reduced lubrication/dyspareunia in women. Pituitary injury prevalence unclear	Depression more important than severity of TBI in both sexes [21]. Medications (especially mood altering) account for up to one-quarter of cases of ejaculatory failure [22]. Screen for pituitary damage at 3 and 12 months	Treat spasticity with baclofen, tizanidine, botox, sclerosing agents	4
			Treat hypersexuality with CBT, SSRIs, clobazam, antiandrogens, dopamine antagonists, and some atypical antipsychotics [3]	4
			Replace testosterone according to TES [23]	4
Spinal cord injury	Orgasm is achieved by less than half of subjects of either gender. About 50% of men are able to ejaculate when incomplete cord lesions are included. As few as 4% of men with complete, high lesions achieve ejaculation even though reflex erections remain intact [24]	Chronic pain in relation to cord injury occurs in as many as one-third of cases, at least in men, to potentially interact with depression and the autonomic aspects of sexual dysfunction [24]	Sildenafil for ED [25]	2
			PGE1 for ED [3	4
			Tadalafil for EjD [26]	1
			Vardenafil for EjD [27]	1
			Midodrine to supplement PVS for EjD [28]	4
			Sildenafil for reduced lubrication [29]	2
			Treat spasticity with baclofen, etc.	4
Multiple sclerosis (MS)	Of men who are still ambulant, 60% have ED and 40–50% have ejaculatory/orgasmic dysfunction with reduced desire [30]. In ambulant, newly diagnosed women (mean time since first symptom of MS, 2.7 years), sexual dysfunctions according to FSFI scores were present in 34.9% of sample compared with 21.3% healthy controls [5]	Eventually well over half of either sex are affected, predominantly by ED in 75% of men and by loss of genital sensation in up to 62% of women [3]	Sildenafil for ED [31]	1
			PGE1 for ED [32]	3
			Sildenafil for reduced vaginal lubrication [33]	2
			Treat spasticity with Baclofen, etc.	4
Stroke	An internally controlled study of 75 men and 25 women showed a dissatisfaction rate of 58.6% of men compared with 21.3% before the stroke and in 44% of the women compared with 20% prior to the stroke [34]	With depression as one of the exclusion criteria, sexual desire poststroke in patients aged 40–80 years was still decreased or absent compared with prestroke in 61.9% of men ($n = 63$) and 52.5% of women ($n = 40$) having mild or no neurological disability after 6 months [35] ED has better prognosis in men <65 years [36]	Sildenafil for ED [3]	4
			Treat spasticity with Baclofen, etc.	4
			Treat hypersexuality as for head injury	4
Parkinsonism	Both men and women [37, 38] with PD report sexual dissatisfaction more commonly than controls—the major determinants being age, severity of disease, and depression	Caregiver partners (especially women partners) show an important degree of sexual dysfunction in several studies [39]	Sildenafil [40] or apomorphine [41] for ED	2
			PGE1 for ED [3]	4
			Deep brain stimulation to subthalamic nucleus for ED [42]	4
			Treat hypersexuality by d/c dopamine agonists, add quetiapine if necessary [3, 43]	3/4
Epilepsy	Hyposexuality follows but does not predate the onset of epilepsy [3] and is more common in TLE. Men with localization-related epilepsy taking no AEDs have abnormally low sexual function [44]. Women with epilepsy have higher rates of disinterest and orgasmic dysfunction compared with controls [45]	Epilepsy has biological as well as psychological effects upon sexual well-being. AEDs may increase SHBG and lower t-levels (phenobarbitone, phenytoin, and carbamazepine) or reduce SHBG (valproic acid). Lamotrigine seems sexually neutral.	Choose AEDs that are neutral to P450 enzyme system and therefore do not alter SHBG [46]	4
			In men, replace t [47]	3

AED = antiepileptic drug; *CBT* = cognitive behavioral therapy; *ED* = erectile dysfunction; *EJD* = ejaculatory disorder; *FSFI* = Female Sexual Function Index; *LOE* = level of evidence; *PD* = Parkinson's disease; *PGE* = prostaglandin E1; *PVS* = penile vibrostimulation; *SHBG* = sex hormone binding globulin; *SSRI* = selective serotonin reuptake inhibitor; *t* = testosterone; *TBI* = traumatic brain injury; *TES* = The Endocrine Society (American); *TLE* = temporal lobe epilepsy.

[Reprinted from Basson R, Rees P, Wang R, Montejo AL, Incrocci L. Sexual Function in Chronic Illness. J Sex Med 2010;7:374–388, with permission from Elsevier].

Peyronie's Disease

Peyronie's disease is characterized by the presence of hardened and calcified tissue (plaque) in the *tunica albuginea* of the penis. This sheath encompasses the spongy tissue of the penis. Peyronie's disease has three main symptoms: lumps present in the penis, pain, and curvature of the penis during erection. While not all causes of Peyronie's disease are known, physicians agree that sudden trauma to the penis or vigorous sexual activity can lead to this condition. Peyronie's disease itself can lead to psychological or physical erectile dysfunction [51].

Diagnostic Criteria

Sexual dysfunctions as a whole are a variety of rather heterogeneous disorders that are characterized by a clinically significant disturbance in an individual's ability to respond sexually or experience sexual pleasure [2]. There are several of cases where a patient may have multiple sexual disorders due to a medical condition, as a variety of medical conditions often lead to sexual dysfunction and responsiveness across the sexual disorders. As has already been discussed, with the introduction of the DSM-5, a sexual dysfunction diagnosis requires the treating clinician to rule out a multitude of problems that could be better explained by a nonsexual psychiatric disorder, by the direct and indirect effects of a specific substance, by a medical condition, or by profound interpersonal and psychosocial stress [2]. Accordingly, when sexual dysfunction is better explained by a medical condition, then an individual cannot receive a psychiatric diagnosis as outlined in DSM-5. With that said, there are a variety of medical conditions that would cause or result in sexual disorders as characterized in the DSM-5.

For example, in the cases of sexual disorders pertaining to desire or sexual interest (e.g., female sexual interest/arousal disorder, male hypoactive sexual desire disorder), there are a variety of chronic illnesses and medical conditions known to affect these disorders [22]. In the event that chronic illnesses deplete a patient's energy or compel the patient to adapt and make life long adjustments, depression and anxiety can follow, which in turn can affect sexual drive. According to Sadock, sexual arousal disorders surround the focus, intensity, and duration of sexual activity in which individuals engage [16]. In the event that sexual stimulation is inadequate in focus, intensity, or duration, the diagnosis of an arousal disorder in men or women should not be made. In short, two factors that can influence sexual arousal in females are insufficient vaginal lubrication and clitoral swelling, while a man may be unable to attain or maintain an adequate erection, both of which can be heavily influenced by comorbid medical conditions.

The DSM-5 diagnostic criteria for female orgasmic disorder requires the presence of either (a) marked delay in, marked infrequency of, or absence of orgasm, or (b) markedly reduced intensity of orgasmic sensation on almost all or all (~75%–100%) of occasions of sexual activity. In the majority of cases, this condition is the result of sexual inexperience in either one or both partners, often stemming from a lack of adequate clitoral or vaginal stimulation. However, a multitude of psychological factors, chronic physical conditions, or medications can result in symptoms consistent with female orgasmic disorder. For all intensive purposes, the treating physician must determine the cause of this particular sexual disorder. If a medical etiology is identified, treating that condition may restore orgasmic sensation.

In the case of genito-pelvic pain/penetration disorder, DSM-5 requires persistent or recurrent difficulties with one or more of the following: (a) vaginal penetration during intercourse (b) marked vulvovaginal or pelvic pain during vaginal intercourse or penetration attempts, (c) marked fear or anxiety about vulvovaginal or pelvic pain in anticipation of, during, or as a result of vaginal penetration, (d) marked tensing or tightening of the pelvic floor muscles during attempted vaginal penetration [2]. However, in the event that sexual dysfunction is better explained by another medical condition, the psychiatric diagnosis cannot be made. Furthermore, with the introduction of the DSM-5, there was a transition from the former edition (DSM-IV-TR), which was a linear approach to diagnosing female sexual dysfunction, to a more multidimensional conceptualization of sexual disorders in women [20]. It follows that physicians are required to conduct a thorough evaluation of possible medical conditions that can lead to these symptoms, as many of these medical conditions are readily treated and can result in a reversal of symptomatology. Figure 22-1 provides a decision tree and flowchart for clinicians to adequately establish a diagnosis of sexual dysfunction in females.

Best Practice and Evidence-Based Approach to Diagnosis

Often the best treatment for any disorder is a thorough review of the medical history of each patient, to ensure all etiological differentials are considered. Accordingly, the clinician is responsible for completing a comprehensive review of a patient's sexual history, in addition to conducting both physical examination and laboratory examinations as deemed necessary for treatment. Table 22-3 highlights important steps to evaluate and properly treat sexual dysfunction that is related to chronic medical illness or psychiatric and social factors.

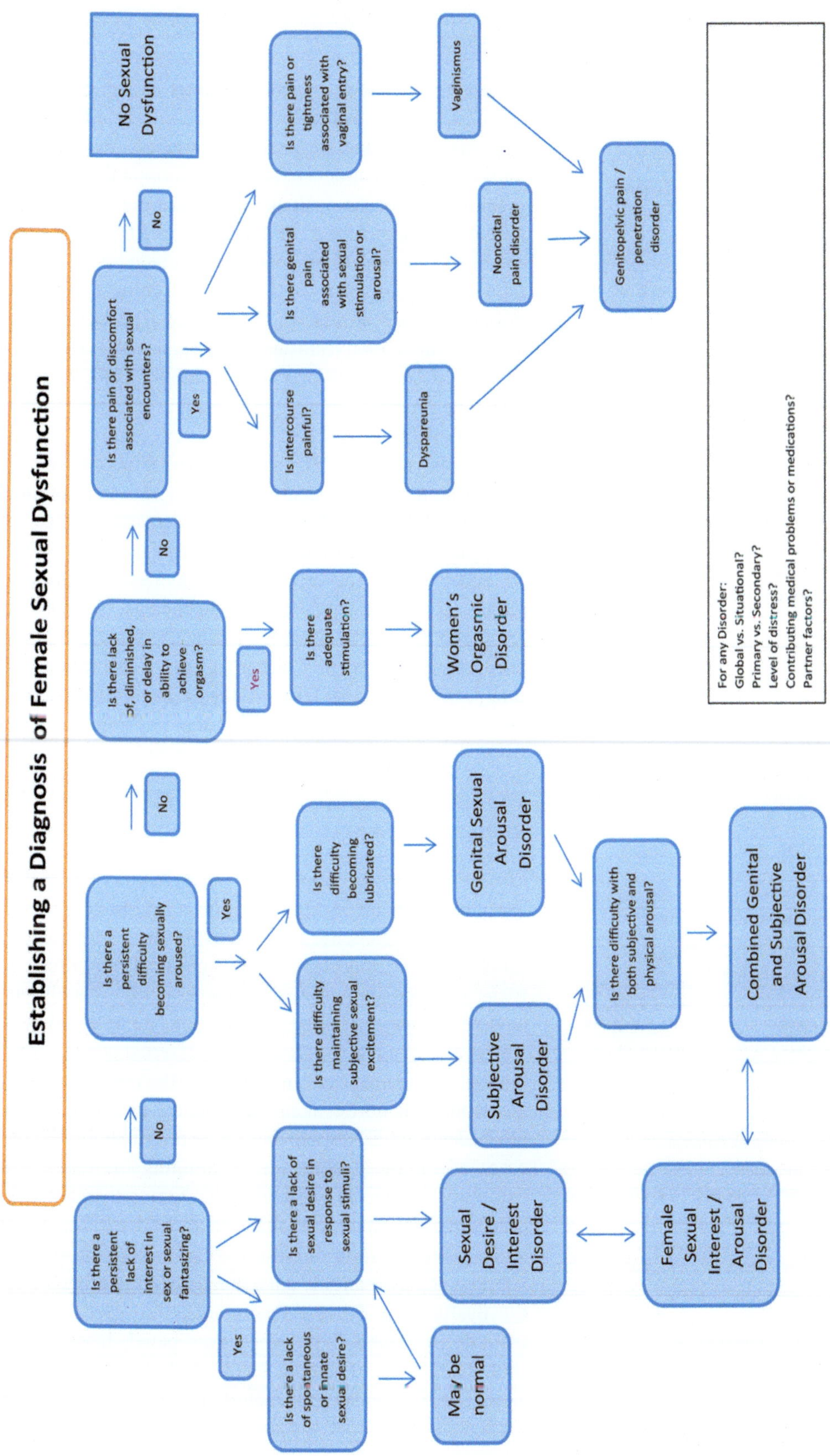

FIGURE 22-1. Establishing a diagnosis of female sexual dysfunction [Reprinted from Latif E. & Diamond MP. Arriving at the diagnosis of female sexual dysfunction. Fertil Steril. 2013;100:898–904. with permission from Elsevier].

TABLE 22-3. Assessment of sexual dysfunction associated with chronic illness

- Review past medical and psychiatric history
- Review current medical status: consider respiratory, cardiac, mobility, and continence requirements for sexual activity including intercourse, self-stimulation, and orgasm
- Review current medications
- List the sexual dysfunctions, their duration, and whether the dysfunction is also present with self-stimulation or with other partners
- Clarify relationship status and quality
- Review the environment for sex: home/institution/"medicalization," e.g., hemodialysis machines, respirators, lack of independence in daily living
- Review any chronic pain
- Assess consequences of illness on sexual self image (concerns with regard to attractiveness, physical appearance)
- Review dysfunctions in detail:
  - Clarify motivations for sex including "desire/drive" and desire to satisfy partner; identify reasons for avoiding sex
  - For ED check erections on waking from sleep
  - Clarify subjective arousal/excitement, pleasure
  - Review variety and usefulness of sexual stimuli
  - Assess couple's sexual communication
  - Consider the importance of distracting thoughts or negative emotions during sex
  - Determine if wanted orgasms are possible, very delayed, nonintense, painful
  - Identify ejaculation difficulties—delayed, too early, painful, absent
  - Review if intercourse is possible
  - Assess female dyspareunia: introital, deeper, how constant, exacerbation from partner's ejaculation fluid, postcoital burning, postcoital dysuria
  - Asses male dyspareunia: immediate, delayed, any physical changes
- Clarify sexual response pre illness: any dysfunction, how rewarding, how important was sex, any desire discrepancy, paraphilia
- Review impact of medications on desire and response
- Review treatment of sexual dysfunction to date
- Complete a full physical exam including genital exam: usually necessary because of the medical condition, particularly important for neurological illness and when there is ED, dyspareunia, or pain with arousal
- Complete psychological exam exploring mood, anxiety, insomnia, and life stressors
- Laboratory investigations—as necessary especially when needed to monitor anemia, high prolactin, hypogonadism, thyroid disorders. Estrogen levels usually assessed by the history and the genital/pelvic examination
- Specialized testing of genital blood flow, e.g., Doppler studies of cavernosal flow for ED—rarely indicated as results do not alter treatment options

ED = erectile dysfunction.

[Reprinted from Basson R, Rees P, Wang R, Montejo AL, Incrocci L. Sexual Function in Chronic Illness. J Sex Med 2010;7:374–388. with permission from Elsevier].

Diagnostic Tests

General

Complete metabolic panels, complete blood count, lipid profiles, urine analysis, thyroid function tests, kidney function tests, liver function tests, and hormonal levels are standard in sexual disorders evaluation. Hormonal levels are an essential part of the evaluation although normal ranges are still debated and depend on laboratory methods and lack of established norms. Hormonal levels include luteinizing hormone (LH) normal = 5–15 mIU/mL, follicle-stimulating hormone (FSH) (normal = 5–15 mIU/mL), prolactin (normal <15 mIU/mL), total testosterone (normal = 300–1000 ng/dL in adult males and 30–120 ng/dL in adult females), free testosterone (normal using the equilibrium ultrafiltration method = 5.00–21.00 ng/dL in adult males and 0.3–0.85 ng/dL in adult females). Serum for testosterone measurement should be drawn between 8 and 10:00 am, and not during the early follicular phase in premenopausal women. Sex hormone-binding globulin (SHBG) is the specific plasma transport protein for sex steroid hormones (dihydrotestosterone, testosterone, and estradiol) in humans. Normal values are 0.6–3.5 mg/L in adult men and 2.5–5.4 mg/L in adult non-pregnant women. Caution needs to be exercised in interpreting hormonal level results as they are affected by a number of factors including medical or physiological conditions, diet, and stress.

Specific Disorders

For erectile dysfunction, there are a number of available diagnostic test and best-practice procedures to determine the cause of and pathophysiological explanations for such dysfunction. It is important for the physical examination to focus on secondary sexual characteristics, in addition to completing an abdominal examination, pulse examination, S2–S4 neurological assessment, and external genitalia examination. Abdominal examinations have the potential to reveal an abdominal aortic aneurysm, which previous statistics have identified as responsible for approximately 1% of all cases of erectile dysfunction. Examining the major lower extremity pulses, in particular the femoral and popliteal pulses, are important to evaluate as they are markers for systemic atherosclerotic disease. Further evaluation of S2–S4 neural pathways can rule out a diagnosis of neurogenic erectile dysfunction. Per the recommendation of the National Institute of Health (NIH) consensus panel, laboratory test should include hematological and metabolic laboratory analyses. These panel screens should also include a measure of serum glucose in order to rule out diabetes mellitus. Additional assessment of both thyroid and liver function can provide valuable insight in ruling out any abnormalities of these two organ systems. It goes without saying that hormonal assessment is of absolute importance. Total and free testosterone levels as well as LH and prolactin levels should also be measures when determining the cause of erectile dysfunction. In addition to traditional laboratory tests, there is a number of other tests that investigators have identified to aid the physician in determining the cause of a male's erectile dysfunction including the following: vascular testing such as duplex ultrasound and dynamic infusion cavernosometry, nocturnal penile tumescence and rigidity analysis, and somatosensory evoked potentials and pudendal electromyelography. While some consider these test to be rather controversial, these specific tests are solely reserved for patients who have a high chance of being cured including young males with arteriogenic ED secondary to trauma or males with crural leaks. Nocturnal penile tumescence testing and erectile turgidity measurements during sleep may aid to differentiate organic and psychogenic etiologies for erectile problems, with the assumption that any erections during REM sleep would indicate a more psychological etiology [52]. In addition, both Doppler ultrasonography and intravascular injection of vasoactive agents, in addition to invasive diagnostic test like dynamic infusion caversnosography, are other validated tests that can measure vascular integrity [2]. In cases where there is concern for peripheral neuropathy, pudendal nerve conduction studies that measure somatosensory evoked potentials are other available tools in the evaluation of erectile dysfunction [2].

In the event that a woman presents with a disorder of arousal, a physician must rule out or determine if the influence of a medical condition is impacting sexual arousal. Several physiologic diagnostic tests are useful in aiding physicians to measure blood flow and engorgement. During a vaginal photoplethysmography, an acrylic tampon-shaped instrument is inserted in the vagina in order to measure blood flow and temperature. Vaginal pH testing is often utilized by probing to detect bacteria that may lead to vaginal tissue inflammation. In general, the normally acidic pH of the vagina is protective against disease causing pathogens and it is important to examine pH levels to ensure adequate homeostasis. Diminished vaginal secretions and hormone levels are commonly seen in perimenopausal and postmenopausal women, which can also make the vaginal pH more but can be readily detected through this process. A biothesiometer is another important instrument that can examine the sensitivity of the labia and clitoris to pressure and temperature. Comprehensive laboratory test and utilization of these measures/instruments will help ensure that the required biomechanical function, which promote arousal are intact.

When clinicians encounter female orgasmic disorder in a clinical context, a woman's self-report is always the diagnostic marker. However, during female orgasm, there are a variety of physiological changes that can be readily measured including brain activation, hormone levels, and pelvic floor musculature, yet research indicates that there is a significant amount of variability among these physiological markers across women as a group [2, 53]. There are currently no validated physiological measures to assess the varying symptom constellations present in genito-pelvic pain/penetration disorder [2].

With premature (early) ejaculation, the identification of what region of interest in the brain may enhance our understanding of this disorder. Interestingly, measures of regional cerebral blood flow during ejaculation using positron emission tomography scans have revealed that there is primary activation in the mesocephalic transition zone, which includes the ventral tegmental area [2]. Other diagnostic markers for premature (early) ejaculation include measuring ejaculatory latency in research settings by sexual partners using a timing device to record latency. Naturally, there are some ecological concerns to this method, as this does not replicate real-life sexual situations [2].

Best Practice and Evidence-Based Approach to Treatment

As the fields of science and medicine continue to progress, new diagnostic tools, biological agents, surgical techniques, and psychosocial interventions are becoming increasingly and readily available. In the sections that follow, emphasis is placed on evidence-based approaches to the treatment of sexual disorders secondary to medical conditions. A comprehensive biopsychosocial plan takes into account interventions that address all the factors involved in predisposing, precipitating or perpetuating the sexual dysfunction. It is essential to treat endocrinal abnormalities such as hypothyroidism, correct hormonal deficiencies such as low testosterone, and manage physically limiting disorders such as arthritis. Because the dysfunction could be caused by the actual treatment for the medical condition in question, identifying and replacing (or discontinuing) agents responsible for sexual disorders is the definitive treatment in many situations where sexual functioning could be ameliorated. Despite treating the medical cause of sexual dysfunction, sexual dysfunction might necessitate to provide biological treatments such as oral medications (phosphodiestrase-5 inhibitors, non PDE-5 agents, antidepressants, hormones), injections, pellets, implants, and devices, as well as psychosocial treatments such as individual psychotherapy, couple therapy, and sex therapy. Figure 22-2 depicts the steps for assessing and treating sexual dysfunction proposed by the International Consultation on Sexual Medicine.

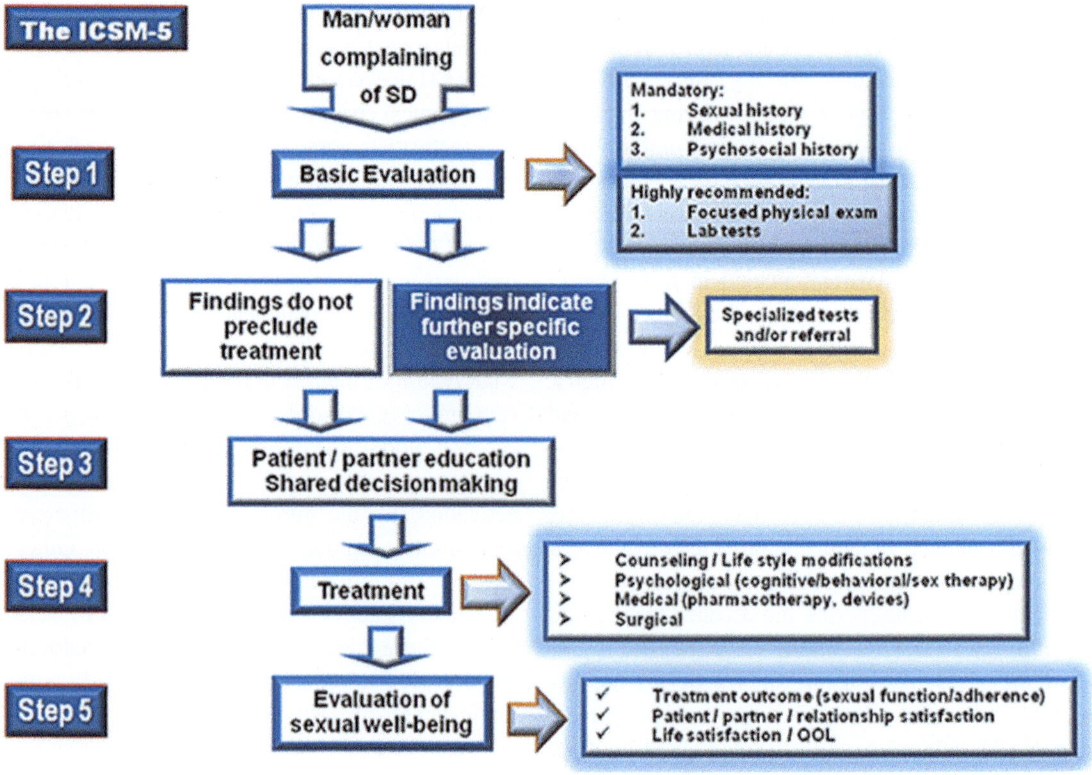

FIGURE 22-2. The steps of the International Consultation on Sexual Medicine (ICSM-5). *SD* = sexual dysfunction; *QoL* = quality of life [Reprinted from Montorsi F, Adaikan G, Becher E, et al. Summary of the Recommendations on Sexual Dysfunctions in Men. J Sex Med. 2010;7:3572–3588. with permission from Elsevier].

Biological Treatments

There has been significant progress in our understanding of the role pharmacotherapy can play in treating sexual dysfunction, particularly in female populations [54]. Likewise, pharmacological intervention is an important and often substantially beneficial to male patients with sexual dysfunction. For example, in the event that male erectile dysfunction is present, improving blood flow regionally, either through means of drugs like phosphodiesterase-5 inhibitors (PDE-5Is) or through interventional or surgical techniques, can result in improvement of sexual dysfunction in some cases [55]. The use of PDE-5Is, specifically sildenafil (Viagra), has been implicated in the treatment of all causes of erectile dysfunction, especially diabetes. Viagra stimulates blood flow to the penis and along with the other PDE-5 inhibitors (vardenafil and tadalfil) is often the first line of treatment of impotence [55]. Viagra does however fail in about 30– 40% percent of male patients who use it. Given that diabetes can potentially damage peripheral vascular system, Viagra or any other of the PDE-5 inhibitors may not be an appropriate treatment option. Figure 22-3 provides an illustration of the pathophysiological pathways and mechanics of PDE-5 inhibitors in regulating the penile corpus cavernous smooth muscle relaxation.

For diabetic male patients who do not benefit from PDE-5 inhibitor therapy, other treatments including as penile implants, vacuum devices, drug injections, and urethral suppositories have repeatedly been shown to be successful in treating erectile dysfunction. Implants have also been used for decades and have shown to be quite effective in treating erectile dysfunction. Implants have been modified over a long period and since their advent, nearly 300,000 males have had the procedure for treating their erectile problems. Other drugs including alprostadil, papavarine, and phentolamine are used in injection therapy, and these medications aim to relax penile muscle tissue, which then promotes blood flow to the penis. Vacuum erection devices also draw blood into the penis, and an elastic band is then placed around the base of the penis in order to preserve the erection. Other topical medications, including creams rubbed on the skin of the penis, and pellets (containing the medication alprostadil), are placed in the tip of the urethra, and have shown promising outcomes in treating erectile dysfunction. Vascular surgery has also proven to be an effective intervention for improving blood flow to the penis and correcting leaking veins which prevent the male from having an erection [56].

In general, testosterone supplementation as a treatment for sexual dysfunction is presumed to have a positive benefit.

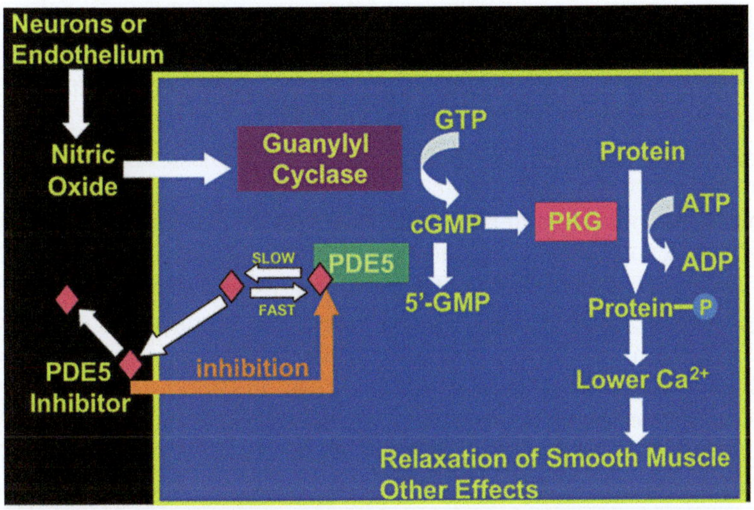

FIGURE 22-3. Regulation of penile corpus cavernosum smooth muscle relaxation and effect of phosphodiesterase type 5 inhibitors. *GTP* = guanosine triphosphate; *cGMP* = cyclic guanosine monophosphate; *PKG* = protein kinase G; *ATP* = adenosine triphosphate; *ADP* = adenosine diphosphate; *PDE5* = phosphodiesterase type 5 [Reprinted from Montorsi F, Adaikan G, Becher E, et al. Summary of the Recommendations on Sexual Dysfunctions in Men. J Sex Med. 2010;7:3572–3588. with permission from Elsevier].

One recent meta-analysis reported that testosterone supplementation had a positive effect in hypogonadal subjects, but that the role of testosterone supplementation in men who are not clearly hypogonadal remains unknown [57]. Furthermore, low testosterone levels in men have been associated with increase mortality, while testosterone treatment is associated with decreased mortality in men [58]. In the event that a male has prostate cancer, hormone therapy is used to decrease the level of androgens, in particular testosterone. Sildenafil, intracavernous injection therapy, and penile implants are also used with some success in the treatment of patients who have received treatment for prostate cancer.

Endocrine disorders present frequently when treating patients with sexual disorders due to medical conditions. In women with diabetes, diligent blood sugar control continues to be effective in alleviating symptoms of poor clitoral swelling and vaginal lubrication. In addition, restoring thyroid hormone levels to baseline can be helpful in restoring arousal in female patients with hypothyroidism. In cases of low sexual desire or interest, hormone replacement therapy can also restore hormone levels affected by age, hormone dysfunction, or surgery to normal levels thereby restoring sexual desire and function [59, 60]. Another study found that a testosterone transdermal patch showed effectiveness in the treatment of sexual desire in surgically menopausal women [61]. A more recent study demonstrated that long-term intranasal oxytocin in premenopausal and postmenopausal woman improved sexual function [62]. As the excess of the hormone prolactin can lead to diminished libido in both males and females, there are a variety of biological treatment options. A first step treatment approach is to target the underlying cause of hyperprolactinemia (high blood prolactin levels) with medication or through surgical intervention (i.e., removal of a pituitary gland tumor), which has been shown to restore sexual drive. Other pharmacological options include anti-prolactin dopamine agonists, including bromocriptine and cabergoline, which have also been shown to be effective in restoring sexual functioning though the normalization of prolactin levels.

When a patient presents with premature ejaculation, low doses of selective serotonin reuptake inhibitors may be successfully utilized to treat males with this disorder; these findings have been demonstrated regardless of the underlying physical etiology. One recent systematic review and meta-analysis paper found that dapoxetine significantly improves intravaginal ejaculation latency time but that the treatment effect size is modest [63]. The clinical efficacy, of other biological treatments including PDE5is, TAs, and tramadol remain unclear given the large amount of heterogeneity in the methodology of randomized clinical trials [63]. In cases of Peyronie's disease, there are a variety of available treatment options that are quite successful in alleviating erectile difficulties secondary to Peyronie's disease. These include sildenafil, penile implants, vacuum devices, injection therapy, and urethral suppositories, all of which have been used to treat erectile dysfunction due to this condition. In addition, penile implants have been very useful in treating erectile dysfunction in patients with Peyronie's disease.

There are no definitive treatments available for alleviating the pain associated with prostatodynia in men. Yet some male patients have reported benefited from monthly prostatic massage from their urologists, sitz baths, herbal medications (i.e., Graminex), and acupuncture. In women who experience marked tensing or tightening of the pelvic floor muscles during attempted vaginal penetration, local injections of the botulinum toxin (aka Botox) has been documented to be a safe and effective way of resolving these symptoms when other treatment responses have been unsuccessful. One study tested a cohort of 24 women who received treatments of Botox to alleviate symptoms, and found that 18 of the 23 patients (one patient dropped out) were able to have intercourse following the first injection, while four patients reported some pain with intercourse, and one reported being cured following a second series of injections; interestingly, none of the patients experienced a return of symptoms [64]. Other common medical conditions known to cause pain during sexual intercourse but that are treatable are numerous. Treatment of genital warts caused by the human papilloma virus is through ablative surgery or cryotherapy. The preventable way to minimize the risk of cystitis is for women to urinate immediately after intercourse to avoid urinary tract infections.

While vaginismus is a relatively outdates term, it is primarily believed to stem from psychological factors. Several treatment modalities have been established and are currently being studied in order to treat and cure this condition. Approximately 10% of women with vaginismus are not treated by standard treatments such as lubricants, anesthetic creams, antianxiety medications, or Kegel exercises. A conventional treatment of females with vaginismus consists mainly of teaching the patient muscle relaxation techniques by having the patient alternate between contracting and relaxing the pelvic muscles. Some females with this condition can achieve vaginal dilatation by using dilators with increasing diameter or commercial tampons; such instruments are placed in the vagina twice daily for a period of 15 min. Once the diameter of the dilator matches the size of the partner's penis, penetration with the penis can commence. Vaginitis, urethritis, and cystitis can be treated with a variety of remedies (e.g., antibiotics). Treatments for endometriosis include hormone therapy, pain medications, pregnancy, and surgical interventions. Women with this disease should also try to position themselves on top during intercourse to control the amount of penile penetration. Surgical intervention is usually needed to correct cystocele.

The countless biological treatments discussed above are not meant to be an all-encompassing list. We encourage the reader to reference the following review, meta-analytic, and original research articles for a more comprehensive understanding of biological treatment options for sexual dysfunction [22, 24, 51, 55, 57, 60, 63].

Psychosocial Treatments

In the event that physicians encounter patients with sexual dysfunction, it is important to provide support and query as to how you can best be of service in helping restore optimal sexual function. In fact, one recent and large national survey study reported that less than 25% of men and women with a sexual problem had sought help for their sexual problem, or multiple problems, from a health professional [12]. This raises concern for two reasons. First, there may be stigma, embarrassment, or fear of judgment that may hinder an individual's willingness to seek treatment for sexual dysfunction. Secondly, the findings from this study not only suggest that there may be a variety of barriers to patients' willingness to seeking treatment but also infer that a strong majority of patients with sexual dysfunction remain untreated.

One concern that continues to persist in the field of psychosocial treatments and interventions in both women and men with sexual dysfunctions is the relatively poor quality of methodological rigor and design across studies. An inherent problem that arises from poor research design and rigor is that researchers attempts to conduct systematic reviews and meta-analysis across studies are compromised. Nevertheless, there are numerous psychosocial treatment interventions that have been validated for a number of sexual disorders, with the majority of treatment modalities being either a concept derived from Masters and Johnson or traditional cognitive-behavioral therapy interventions [65–67].

Notably, one meta-analytic study reported that the use of pharmacological agents (i.e., PDE5-Is) in combination with psychological intervention to treat erectile dysfunction has better outcomes than either treatment alone [55]. Among men with diabetes, adequate blood glucose control is vital for preventing/treating their erectile disorder. When diabetes is well controlled, there is diminished risk of the development of any secondary complications including erectile dysfunction. In addition, optimal blood pressure control and discontinuing of tobacco products and alcohol may help diabetic patients in preventing sexual dysfunction. Continued assessment of serum lipids is important in the treatment, as men with erectile disorder 40 years old and older has been identified to predict future risk of coronary artery disease [68].

In the aftermath of myocardial infarction, a substantial proportion of men are at risk of developing a fear that a subsequent cardiac event could be triggered by a variety of phenomena (e.g., stress, anxiety) or others events that are combined with an increase of endogenous catecholamines, such as sexual activity. This often leads to the finding that nearly one third of men will cease all sexual activity initially after myocardial infarction, while another proportion may not resume prior sexual activity out of fear that an infarction or even sudden cardiac death will subsequently occur. Conversely, less than 1% of all heart attacks occur during sexual activity, and the actual rate of sudden death during sexual activity is quite low (around 0.3% of all cases of sudden cardiac death). Therefore, it is important for physicians to provide education as to the nature and risk of sexual activity in men who have had a myocardial infarction.

Women's rates of orgasm are consistently higher during masturbation than during sexual activity with a partner [69]. This aforementioned finding is an important point to consider when structuring psychosocial interventions as it may be important to query as to whether or not a patient is able to reach orgasm during masturbation, which would be more suggestive of a psychological process. Relatedly, a substantial amount of women who have genito-pelvic pain/penetration disorder are at risk of interpersonal romantic relationship problems and there is evidence to suggest that women with this disorder report that their sense or feelings of femininity are diminished in the context of this disorder [70]. Another research study using a mouse model found that even after vaginal infections resolve and there is no residual physical finding, pain may continue to persist [71]. Clearly, the implications of such findings may be clinically relevant to psychosocial treatments and interventions.

It is relatively well documented that being overweight or obese is as a major risk factor for sexual dysfunction in men and women [43, 45]. Visceral fat in particular has been identified as a stronger predictor of cardiovascular and metabolic disease risk than the amount of overall body fat alone [72]. As such, weight loss may be an important treatment goal in obese or overweight patients who are experiencing sexual dysfunction. In addition to improvements in quality of life, weight loss can also improve sexual function. In particular, severely obese women who received a multidisciplinary intervention for weight loss had significant improvements in a variety of indices for sexual functioning (e.g., arousal, lubrication, satisfaction) with the suspected mechanisms being improvements in endothelial function and insulin resistance [33]. Accordingly, this may be an important topic of focus in psychosocial treatment and interventions.

In addition to traditional behavioral techniques or cognitive-behavioral therapy interventions, there are a number of new and promising interventions that have been identified to improve sexual functioning. One systematic review paper reported that behavioral techniques have proven to be effective in men with premature ejaculation [65]. Another recent study identified that mindfulness-based group therapy significantly improved sexual arousal, sexual desire, sexual satisfaction, and lubrication in a group of women who received immediate treatment compared to a delayed treatment group [73]. In relation, the robust treatment efficacy of mindfulness-based cognitive behavioral interventions to improve sexual function has been reported in other cohorts, including women treated for gynecological cancer or women with provoked vestibulodynia or dyspareunia [74, 75]. Likewise, one randomized controlled trial demonstrated that a 12-week yoga exercise program significantly improved arousal and lubrication in a cohort of women with metabolic syndrome compared to a wait-listed control group [76]. In sum, new validated interventions with excellent treatment efficacy continue to emerge for a variety of sexual disorders.

Nonetheless, there is a dearth of literature for a number of specific sexual disorders. For example, the availability of validated randomized clinical trials of psychological treatments for hypoactive sexual desire disorder remains an understudied area [77]. Other research suggest that while there is a lack of systemic study of a variety female sexual dysfunction disorders, orgasmic disorder and sexual pain (e.g., vaginismus, dyspaurenia) are the most studied disorders for treatment and tend to have better outcomes than other disorders [67].

Certain cohorts of men or women living with a medical illness require exceptionally tailored and individualized psychosocial treatment interventions to address sexual dysfunction. There are a variety of reasons that explain this rational or line of thinking, as variability in the subtle nuances of differing medical conditions and diseases all present with myriad physiological, neurological, psychological, social, and existential components that often make the experience of living with a particular disorder rather unique. For example, individuals living with cancer or those who have received surgical treatments that effect sexual function are particularly in need of customized psychosocial interventions, the essence of which is beyond the scope of this chapter. However, one review article suggests that for men with prostate cancer, sexual functioning can improve as a result of psychosocial interventions [78]. As a heterogeneous group, women with either a current diagnosis of cancer or those who have previously been diagnosed with cancer and then subsequently treated, are also reported to benefit from a variety of psychosocial interventions [79, 80].

Another example of a population that requires highly specialized treatment is for individuals living with systemic lupus erythematous. Specifically, one recent study reported that patients' illness perceptions were more important predictors of sexual functioning than either socio-demographic or medical characteristics, and that psychosocial interventions that target illness perception modification and coping style may provide the most benefit to increasing sexual functioning [81]. Likewise, patients living with an inflammatory bowel disease, often present with a variety of psychological factors affecting sexual functioning. As sexual dysfunction is a broad term, psychosocial interventions should incorporate psychological, disease-related, surgical, and medical considerations into the focus of treatment for these patients [34].

While we have discussed a variety of psychosocial treatments for sexual dysfunction related to medical conditions, our coverage is not meant to be all-inclusive. The reader is encouraged to reference a number of studies and review papers, which go into more detail and discussion for specific treatment recommendations for sexual dysfunction with varying medical populations [22, 45, 55, 65, 78, 80]. In addition, it is of critical importance to emphasize that while sexual dysfunction may be a result of a particular medical condition (or several comorbid medical conditions in unison), there are a variety of psychological, interpersonal, and sociocultural factors that play a substantial role in optimal sexual functioning for both men and women, and a variety of validated psychotherapy interventions [51, 66, 67, 77, 80, 82–85]. Notably, there is evidence of distinct psychosocial factors that have been identified to affect sexual dysfunction between males and females. In men, medical factors and the presence of psychological factors (i.e., performance anxiety) have been reported to be two of the most likely factors to be associated with sexual dysfunction, while for women, relationship factors are more strongly related to sexual dysfunction [83]. In regards to successful treatment outcomes, relationship satisfaction pretreatment of cognitive behavioral therapy may be one of the strongest predictors of improved sexual functioning for women, and that while low relationship satisfaction prior to treatment can still result in improved sexual functioning, it may not be enough to alleviate sexual distress [84]. In trans persons, patients who were more satisfied with hormonal replacement therapy had significantly lower rates of hypoactive sexual desire disorder [85]. Lastly, one study reported that hypoactive sexual desire disorder was more prevalent in trans women compared to trans men, and the majority of trans women reported decreased sexual desire after sex reassignment therapy, while the opposite was observed in trans men [85].

Prognosis

While studies have reported that men who were able to achieve firm erections prior to surgery were less likely to develop ED, nearly 50% through 80% of men who undergo a radical prostatectomy become impotent. In cases where the surgeon was able to spare part or all of the nerves, trauma from the procedure still can cause some difficulty with erectile function through the first year following the operation. Hormone therapy utilized in the treatment of prostate cancer has shown to lead to ED as early as 2–4 weeks following the initiation of treatment and is usually accompanied with a loss of sex drive. Again, prognosis can have a variable course across patient populations, given the substantial amount of variability within and between distinct cohorts. With that said, we recommend that clinicians have an open and honest conversation with patients where the benefits and risk associated with treatment are discussed, as well as the potential complications related to medication side effects, pharmacological intervention, or surgical procedures.

Conclusion

Sexual disorders that stem from medical conditions often result in substantial psychological toll on an individual, affecting one's sense of general well-being and quality of life. Sexual dysfunction covered in this chapter can be caused by both psychological and physical or medical factors and conditions. The aim of this chapter is to introduce the most common general medical conditions that can potentially lead to any of the major sexual disorders. We further discuss epidemiology, etiology, pathophysiology, diagnostic criteria, and best evidence-based practice and approaches to the diagnosis of sexual disorders due to medical conditions, and review diagnostic tests often used by physicians to aid in diagnosis and monitoring of treatment outcomes for sexual disorders. We further provide current information on the treatment of sexual disorders using evidence-based approaches including biological treatments (e.g., medications, devices) and psychosocial treatments. Notably, in any given clinical context, the appropriate diagnosis and treatment of the underlying cause for sexual dysfunction will increase the likelihood that a physician is able to restore normal sexual functioning and subsequently restore well-being and promote an enjoyable life for each patient.

References

1. American Psychiatric Association. Diagnostic and statistical manual of mental disorders. 4th Ed., Text Revision. Washington, DC: American Psychiatric Association; 2000.
2. American Psychiatric Association. Diagnostic and statistical manual of mental disorders (DSM-5). Washington, DC: American Psychiatric Association; 2013.
3. Shindel AW, Parish SJ. Sexuality education in North American medical schools: current status and future directions. J Sex Med. 2013;10(1):3–17.
4. Golombok S, Rust J, Pickard C. Sexual problems encountered in general practice. Br J Sex Med. 1984;11:171–5.
5. Fugl-Meyer AR, Lodnert G, Branholm IB, Fugl-Meyer KS. On life satisfaction in male erectile dysfunction. Int J Impot Res. 1997;9(3):141–8.
6. Morokoff PJ, Gillilland R. Stress, sexual functioning, and marital satisfaction. J Sex Res. 1993;30(1):43–53.
7. Laumann EO, Paik A, Rosen RC. Sexual dysfunction in the United States: prevalence and predictors. JAMA. 1999;281(6):537–44.
8. Mercer CH, Fenton KA, Johnson AM, Wellings K, Macdowall W, McManus S, et al. Sexual function problems and help seeking behaviour in Britain: national probability sample survey. BMJ. 2003;327(7412):426–7.
9. Bacon CG, Mittleman MA, Kawachi I, Giovannucci E, Glasser DB, Rimm EB. Sexual function in men older than 50 years of age: results from the health professionals follow-up study. Ann Intern Med. 2003;139(3):161–8.
10. Fugl-Meyer A, Sjogren F-MK. Sexual disabilities, problems and satisfaction in 18-74 year old Swedes. Scand J Sexol. 1999;2:79.
11. Laumann EO, Nicolosi A, Glasser DB, Paik A, Gingell C, Moreira E, et al. Sexual problems among women and men aged 40-80 y: prevalence and correlates identified in the global study of sexual attitudes and behaviors. Int J Impot Res. 2005;17(1):39–57.
12. Laumann EO, Glasser DB, Neves RC, Moreira Jr ED. A population-based survey of sexual activity, sexual problems and associated help-seeking behavior patterns in mature adults in the United States of America. Int J Impot Res. 2009;21(3):171–8.
13. Lewis RW. Epidemiology of erectile dysfunction. Urol Clin North Am. 2001;28(2):209–16 .vii

14. Prins J, Blanker MH, Bohnen AM, Thomas S, Bosch JL. Prevalence of erectile dysfunction: a systematic review of population-based studies. Int J Impot Res. 2002;14(6):422–32.
15. McCulloch DK, Campbell IW, Wu FC, Prescott RJ, Clarke BF. The prevalence of diabetic impotence. Diabetologia. 1980;18(4):279–83.
16. Sadock V. Normal human sexuality and sexual and gender identity disorders. In: Kaplan & Sadock's comprehensive textbook of psychiatry. Baltimore: Lippincott Williams & Wilkins; 2000. p. 1577–607.
17. Graham CA. The DSM diagnostic criteria for female orgasmic disorder. Arch Sex Behav. 2010;39(2):256–70.
18. Oberg K, Fugl-Meyer AR, Fugl-Meyer KS. On categorization and quantification of women's sexual dysfunctions: an epidemiological approach. Int J Impot Res. 2004;16(3):261–9.
19. Brotto LA. The DSM diagnostic criteria for hypoactive sexual desire disorder in women. Arch Sex Behav. 2010;39(2):221–39.
20. Latif EZ, Diamond MP. Arriving at the diagnosis of female sexual dysfunction. Fertil Steril. 2013;100(4):898–904.
21. Bancroft J, Loftus J, Long JS. Distress about sex: a national survey of women in heterosexual relationships. Arch Sex Behav. 2003;32(3):193–208.
22. Basson R, Rees P, Wang R, Montejo AL, Incrocci L. Sexual function in chronic illness. J Sex Med. 2010;7:374–88.
23. Brotto LA. The DSM diagnostic criteria for hypoactive sexual desire disorder in men. J Sex Med. 2010;7(6):2015–30.
24. Maggi M, Buvat J, Corona G, Guay A, Torres LO. Hormonal causes of male sexual dysfunctions and their management (hyperprolactinemia, thyroid disorders, GH disorders, and DHEA). J Sex Med. 2013;10(3):661–77.
25. Beutel ME, Weidner W, Brahler E. Epidemiology of sexual dysfunction in the male population. Andrologia. 2006;38(4):115–21.
26. Schwarz ER, Rastogi S, Kapur V, Sulemanjee N, Rodriguez JJ. Erectile dysfunction in heart failure patients. J Am Coll Cardiol. 2006;48(6):1111–9.
27. Schwarz ER, Rodriguez J. Sex and the heart. Int J Impot Res. 2005;17(Suppl 1):S4–6.
28. Levine KB, Williams RE, Hartmann KE. Vulvovaginal atrophy is strongly associated with female sexual dysfunction among sexually active postmenopausal women. Menopause. 2008;15(4 Pt 1):661–6.
29. Kao A, Binik YM, Amsel R, Funaro D, Leroux N, Khalife S. Biopsychosocial predictors of postmenopausal dyspareunia: the role of steroid hormones, vulvovaginal atrophy, cognitive-emotional factors, and dyadic adjustment. J Sex Med. 2012;9(8):2066–76.
30. Avis NE, Stellato R, Crawford S, Johannes C, Longcope C. Is there an association between menopause status and sexual functioning? Menopause. 2000;7(5):297–309.
31. Burri AV, Cherkas LM, Spector TD. The genetics and epidemiology of female sexual dysfunction: a review. J Sex Med. 2009;6(3):646–57.
32. Richters J, Grulich AE, de Visser RO, Smith AM, Rissel CE. Sex in Australia: sexual difficulties in a representative sample of adults. Aust N Z J Public Health. 2003;27(2):164–70.
33. Aversa A, Bruzziches R, Francomano D, Greco EA, Violi F, Lenzi A, et al. Weight loss by multidisciplinary intervention improves endothelial and sexual function in obese fertile women. J Sex Med. 2013;10(4):1024–33.
34. Ghazi LJ, Patil SA, Cross RK. Sexual dysfunction in inflammatory bowel disease. Inflamm Bowel Dis. 2015;21(4):939–47.
35. Shifren JL, Monz BU, Russo PA, Segreti A, Johannes CB. Sexual problems and distress in United States women: prevalence and correlates. Obstet Gynecol. 2008;112(5):970–8.
36. Jern P, Santtila P, Witting K, Alanko K, Harlaar N, Johansson A, et al. Premature and delayed ejaculation: genetic and environmental effects in a population-based sample of Finnish twins. J Sex Med. 2007;4(6):1739–49.
37. Santtila P, Jern P, Westberg L, Walum H, Pedersen CT, Eriksson E, et al. The dopamine transporter gene (DAT1) polymorphism is associated with premature ejaculation. J Sex Med. 2010;7(4 Pt 1):1538–46.
38. Waldinger MD. Toward evidence-based genetic research on lifelong premature ejaculation: a critical evaluation of methodology. Korean J Urol. 2011;52(1):1–8.
39. McMahon CG, Abdo C, Incrocci L, Perelman M, Rowland D, Waldinger M, et al. Disorders of orgasm and ejaculation in men. J Sex Med. 2004;1(1):58–65.
40. Richardson D, Goldmeier D. Recommendations for the management of retarded ejaculation: BASHH special interest group for sexual dysfunction. Int J STD AIDS. 2006;17(1):7–13.
41. Rowland D, McMahon CG, Abdo C, Chen J, Jannini E, Waldinger MD, et al. Disorders of orgasm and ejaculation in men. J Sex Med. 2010;7(4 Pt 2):1668–86.
42. Basson R. The complexities of female sexual arousal disorder: potential role of pharmacotherapy. World J Urol. 2002;20(2):119–26.
43. Esposito K, Giugliano D. Obesity, the metabolic syndrome, and sexual dysfunction. Int J Impot Res. 2005;17(5):391–8.
44. Rodriguez JJ, Al Dashti R, Schwarz ER. Linking erectile dysfunction and coronary artery disease. Int J Impot Res. 2005;17(Suppl 1):S12–8.
45. Kolotkin RL, Zunker C, Ostbye T. Sexual functioning and obesity: a review. Obesity (Silver Spring). 2012;20(12):2325–33.
46. Yavuzgil O, Altay B, Zoghi M, Gurgun C, Kayikcioglu M, Kultursay H. Endothelial function in patients with vasculogenic erectile dysfunction. Int J Cardiol. 2005;103(1):19–26.
47. Kaiser DR, Billups K, Mason C, Wetterling R, Lundberg JL, Bank AJ. Impaired brachial artery endothelium-dependent and -independent vasodilation in men with erectile dysfunction and no other clinical cardiovascular disease. J Am Coll Cardiol. 2004;43(2):179–84.
48. Abramov LA. Sexual life and sexual frigidity among women devel oping acute myocardial infarction. Psychosom Med. 1976;38(6):418–25.
49. Vacanti LJ, Caramelli B. Age and psychologic disorders. Variables associated to post-infarction sexual dysfunction. Arq Bras Cardiol. 2005;85(2):110–4.
50. Bronner G, Aharon-Peretz J, Hassin-Baer S. Sexuality in patients with Parkinson's disease, Alzheimer's disease, and other dementias. Handb Clin Neurol. 2015;130:297–323.
51. Montorsi F, Adaikan G, Becher E, Giuliano F, Khoury S, Lue TF, et al. Summary of the recommendations on sexual dysfunctions in men. J Sex Med. 2010;7(11):3572–88.
52. Wylie K. Erectile dysfunction. Adv Psychosom Med. 2008;29:33–49.
53. Meston CM, Levin RJ, Sipski ML, Hull EM, Heiman JR. Women's orgasm. Annu Rev Sex Res. 2004;15:173–257.
54. Nappi RE, Cucinella L. Advances in pharmacotherapy for treating female sexual dysfunction. Expert Opin Pharmacother. 2015;16(6):875–87.
55. Schmidt HM, Munder T, Gerger H, Fruhauf S, Barth J. Combination of psychological intervention and phosphodiesterase-5 inhibitors for erectile dysfunction: a narrative review and meta-analysis. J Sex Med. 2014;11(6):1376–91.
56. Montague DK, Jarow JP, Broderick GA, Dmochowski RR, Heaton JP, Lue TF, et al. Chapter 1: The management of erectile dysfunction: an AUA update. J Urol. 2005;174(1):230–9.
57. Corona G, Isidori AM, Buvat J, Aversa A, Rastrelli G, Hackett G, et al. Testosterone supplementation and sexual function: a meta-analysis study. J Sex Med. 2014;11(6):1577–92.
58. Shores MM, Smith NL, Forsberg CW, Anawalt BD, Matsumoto AM. Testosterone treatment and mortality in men with low testosterone levels. J Clin Endocrinol Metab. 2012;97(6):2050–8.
59. Bachmann GA, Leiblum SR. The impact of hormones on menopausal sexuality: a literature review. Menopause. 2004;11(1):120–30.

60. Belkin ZR, Krapf JM, Goldstein AT. Drugs in early clinical development for the treatment of female sexual dysfunction. Expert Opin Investig Drugs. 2015;24(2):159–67.
61. Braunstein GD, Sundwall DA, Katz M, Shifren JL, Buster JE, Simon JA, et al. Safety and efficacy of a testosterone patch for the treatment of hypoactive sexual desire disorder in surgically menopausal women: a randomized, placebo-controlled trial. Arch Intern Med. 2005;165(14):1582–9.
62. Muin DA, Wolzt M, Marculescu R, Sheikh Rezaei S, Salama M, Fuchs C, et al. Effect of long-term intranasal oxytocin on sexual dysfunction in premenopausal and postmenopausal women: a randomized trial. Fertil Steril. 2015;104(3):715–23.e4.
63. Castiglione F, Albersen M, Hedlund P, Gratzke C, Salonia A, Giuliano F. Current pharmacological management of premature ejaculation: a systematic review and meta-analysis. Eur Urol. 2016;69(5):904–16.
64. Ghazizadeh S, Nikzad M. Botulinum toxin in the treatment of refractory vaginismus. Obstet Gynecol. 2004;104(5 Pt 1):922–5.
65. Berner M, Günzler C. Efficacy of psychosocial interventions in men and women with sexual dysfunctions—a systematic review of controlled clinical trials: part 1-the efficacy of psychosocial interventions for male sexual dysfunction. J Sex Med. 2012;9(12):3089–107.
66. Frühauf S, Gerger H, Schmidt HM, Munder T, Barth J. Efficacy of psychological interventions for sexual dysfunction: a systematic review and meta-analysis. Arch Sex Behav. 2013;42(6):915–33.
67. Pereira VM, Arias-Carrion O, Machado S, Nardi AE, Silva AC. Sex therapy for female sexual dysfunction. Int Arch Med. 2013; 6(1):37.
68. Inman BA, Sauver JL, Jacobson DJ, McGree ME, Nehra A, Lieber MM, et al. A population-based, longitudinal study of erectile dysfunction and future coronary artery disease. Mayo Clin Proc. 2009;84(2):108–13.
69. Laumann EO. The social organization of sexuality: sexual practices in the United States: University of Chicago Press; 1994.
70. Binik YM, Bergeron S, Khalifé S. Dyspareunia and vaginismus: so-called sexual pain. Principles and practice of sex therapy. 2007New York: Guilford. p. 124–56.
71. Farmer MA, Taylor AM, Bailey AL, Tuttle AH, MacIntyre LC, Milagrosa ZE, et al. Repeated vulvovaginal fungal infections cause persistent pain in a mouse model of vulvodynia. Sci Transl Med. 2011;3(101):101ra91.
72. Lamarche B. Abdominal obesity and its metabolic complications: implications for the risk of ischaemic heart disease. Coron Artery Dis. 1998;9(8):473–81.
73. Brotto LA, Basson R. Group mindfulness-based therapy significantly improves sexual desire in women. Behav Res Ther. 2014;57:43–54.
74. Brotto LA, Erskine Y, Carey M, Ehlen T, Finlayson S, Heywood M, et al. A brief mindfulness-based cognitive behavioral intervention improves sexual functioning versus wait-list control in women treated for gynecologic cancer. Gynecol Oncol. 2012;125(2):320–5.
75. Brotto LA, Basson R, Smith KB, Driscoll M, Sadownik L. Mindfulness-based group therapy for women with provoked vestibulodynia. Mindfulness. 2015;6:417–32.
76. Kim HN, Ryu J, Kim KS, Song SW. Effects of yoga on sexual function in women with metabolic syndrome: a randomized controlled trial. J Sex Med. 2013;10(11):2741–51.
77. Pyke RE, Clayton AH. Psychological treatment trials for hypoactive sexual desire disorder: a sexual medicine critique and perspective. J Sex Med. 2015;12(12):2451–8.
78. Chisholm KE, McCabe MP, Wootten AC, Abbott JA. Review: psychosocial interventions addressing sexual or relationship functioning in men with prostate cancer. J Sex Med. 2012;9(5):1246–60.
79. Falk SJ, Dizon DS. Sexual dysfunction in women with cancer. Fertil Steril. 2013;100(4):916–21.
80. Rosenberg SM, Tamimi RM, Gelber S, Ruddy KJ, Bober SL, Kereakoglow S, et al. Treatment-related amenorrhea and sexual functioning in young breast cancer survivors. Cancer. 2014; 120(15):2264–71.
81. Daleboudt GM, Broadbent E, McQueen F, Kaptein AA. The impact of illness perceptions on sexual functioning in patients with systemic lupus erythematosus. J Psychosom Res. 2013;74(3):260–4.
82. Brotto L, Atallah S, Johnson-Agbakwu C, Rosenbaum T, Abdo C, Byers ES, et al. Psychological and interpersonal dimensions of sexual function and dysfunction. J Sex Med. 2016;13(4):538–71.
83. McCabe MP, Connaughton C. Psychosocial factors associated with male sexual difficulties. J Sex Res. 2014;51(1):31–42.
84. Stephenson KR, Rellini AH, Meston CM. Relationship satisfaction as a predictor of treatment response during cognitive behavioral sex therapy. Arch Sex Behav. 2013;42(1):143–52.
85. Wierckx K, Elaut E, Van Hoorde B, Heylens G, De Cuypere G, Monstrey S, et al. Sexual desire in trans persons: associations with sex reassignment treatment. J Sex Med. 2014;11(1):107–18.

23 Evaluation and Treatment of Substance/Medication-Induced Sexual Dysfunction

Richard Balon

Sexual dysfunction associated with medications or substances of abuse is a fairly frequent phenomenon. The frequency (or prevalence) varies based on the type of medication or abused substance. In general, sexual dysfunction may be associated/reported with any medication—however, the frequency of sexual dysfunction associated with different groups (and even within these groups) of medications and substances varies significantly. Medications and substances of abuse may impact sexual functioning in its entirety or may impact a particular phase of sexual functioning. Some medications and substances may have more impact on sexual desire, some more arousal, and some on orgasm. A disturbance of one phase of sexual functioning could, of course, impact other aspects of sexual functioning—a man having erectile difficulties may subsequently be unable to ejaculate.

Reports of sexual dysfunction (SD) with some medications (e.g., tricyclic antidepressants—TCA) began to appear during the 1960s and 1970s. SD associated with these medications did not receive as much attention as other side effects during those times. This was probably because other side effects were perceived as more serious, and there was enthusiasm about the availability of new, effective treatments for depression and other mental disorders which allowed considering some side effects as a "necessary evil." However, with the arrival of newer antidepressants in the late 1980s and 1990s, the reporting of SD associated with antidepressants, namely selective serotonin reuptake inhibitors (SSRIs), increased. As Balon [1] wrote, "The reasons for the increased reporting are not entirely clear, although the trend is very likely multifactorial. Possible reasons include a much wider, more liberal use of the newer antidepressants for other conditions; pharmacotherapy of less severe depression that was previously more likely to be treated with psychotherapy; a more sophisticated approach to evaluation of side effects; a greater emphasis on patients' quality of life; and even marketing competition among pharmaceutical companies. It is also possible that patients taking SSRIs simply experience more sexual dysfunction than patients taking tricyclic antidepressants [2] and other antidepressants." The observation of SD associated with antidepressants probably served as an impetus to examine sexual functioning during treatment with other medications. Subsequently, the increased attention paid to substance abuse and quality of life led to realization that substances of abuse may also cause SD.

Sexual dysfunction associated with medications or substances of abuse could present as a complicated clinical conundrum, especially with certain medications. Take the example of a patient reporting SD during treatment of depression. Her/his SD may be (a) part of depressive symptomatology, (b) side effect of antidepressant medication, (c) due to concomitant medical illness (e.g., diabetes, hypertension), (d) side effect of medication used for her/his physical illness (e.g., antihypertensive), (e) consequence of substance use (e.g., opioids, marijuana), (f) primary sexual dysfunction, (g) associated with relationship difficulties, and (h)—combination of some or all these factors (see Table 23-1).

Epidemiology (Incidence/Prevalence)

The incidence and prevalence of SD associated with medications and substances of abuse differ significantly depending on the specific medication, group of medications and substances of abuse. There are also gender differences in estimates of prevalence of SD associated with medications and illicit substances. SD associated with medications if frequently underreported. It is well known that patients, especially in earlier clinical studies, underreport or do not report SD spontaneously. Several studies demonstrated differences between spontaneous reporting of SD and reports of SD when patients were actively asked by investigators—the frequency yielded during active questioning by investigators was always higher. The difference between spontaneous and actively obtained frequency of SD probably explains the

W.W. IsHak (ed.), *The Textbook of Clinical Sexual Medicine*, DOI 10.1007/978-3-319-52539-6_23

TABLE 23-1. Types of sexual dysfunction associated with selected groups of medications and effects of substances of abuse

Medications/substances of abuse	Sexual dysfunction(s)
Antipsychotics (significantly less frequent with most atypical antipsychotics)	Decreased libido (probably most frequent) Erectile dysfunction Delayed ejaculation/orgasm Priapism (rare) Retrograde ejaculation (thiothixene) Painful ejaculation Amenorrhea Galactorrhea
Antidepressants	Changes in libido (mostly decreased) Erectile dysfunction (mostly TCSs) Changes in lubrication Delayed ejaculation/orgasm (SSRIs, clomipramine) Anorgasmia (SSRIs, clomipramine) Priapism (trazodone and others) Clitoral engorgement Painful ejaculation (TCAs) Penile or vaginal anesthesia (rare)
Anxiolytics (infrequent)	Decreased libido Delayed or inhibited ejaculation Sexual disinhibition (?)
Antacids (mainly H2 antagonists)	Decreased libido Erectile dysfunction Gynecomastia
Anticonvulsants	Decreased libido Ejaculatory dysfunction Anorgasmia/ejaculatory failure Less satisfying orgasm Loss of sensation of orgasm Unpleasant feeling upon touching genitalia erogenous zones
Cardiovascular medications (mostly antihypertensives)	Decreased or absent libido Erectile dysfunction (most frequent) Decreased vaginal lubrication Delayed ejaculation/orgasm Anorgasmia Retrograde ejaculation Priapism
Substances of abuse	
Alcohol	Impotence with chronic use Acute intake: may increase desire, however interferes with erection, vaginal lubrication, and orgasm
Amphetamines	Acute intake: reduced sexual inhibition, increased satisfaction Chronic intake: erectile dysfunction, delayed ejaculation/orgasm
Cannabis	Chronic use may lead to decreased libido Acute use: Increased sexual pleasure, satisfaction, orgasm quality
Cocaine	Acute use: increased libido, rarely priapism Chronic use: impotence, anorgasmia, hyperprolactinemia

(continued)

TABLE 23-1. (continued)

Medications/substances of abuse	Sexual dysfunction(s)
Ecstasy	Increased desire, satisfaction; erectile failure, prolonged orgasm, priapism (?)
Opioids (including methadone and buprenorphine; buprenorphine seems to have less SD than methadone)	Decreased libido, ejaculatory failure, anorgasmia, premature ejaculation upon withdrawal Acute heroin administration may induce intense sexual pleasure similar to orgasmic feeling
Tobacco	Erectile dysfunction

originally low incidence of SD associated with fluoxetine mentioned in *Physician's Desk Reference* [3]—1.9%—and much higher frequencies in later studies (e.g., 52.9% [4]).

Various articles summarized the evidence of SD associated with antidepressants. Serretti and Chiesa [5] in their meta-analysis reported significantly higher rate of total and specific treatment-emergent SD and specific phases of dysfunction compared with placebo for the following drugs in decreasing order of impact; sertraline, venlafaxine, citalopram, paroxetine, fluoxetine, imipramine, phenelzine, duloxetine, escitalopram, and fluvoxamine; while no significant difference compared to placebo was found for agomelatine, amineptine, bupropion, moclobemide, mirtazapine, and nefazodone. The frequency of SD in their analysis ranged from 25.8 to 80.3%. The widespread differences in reporting SD with antidepressants and the fact that most studies lacked using a validated sexual functioning rating scale and a baseline evaluation of SD or a placebo control or both, lead Montgomery, Baldwin and Riley [6] to the conclusion that the existing literature confirms sexual dysfunction as a possible adverse event of all antidepressants. They also pointed out the occurrence of sexual dysfunction in various mental disorders (e.g., mood disorders, anxiety disorders, schizophrenia) which also varies significantly and may impact the reporting of SD associated with treatments for these disorders. However, the evidence is not sufficiently robust to support most claims for differences in the incidence of SD between existing antidepressant therapies, especially since most studies reporting SD with antidepressants were not comparative. The DSM-5 ([7], p. 449) concluded that approximately 25–80% of individuals taking monoamine oxidase inhibitors (MAOIs), TCAs, SSRIs, and combined serotonergic-adrenergic antidepressants (SNRIs) report sexual side effects.

It is probably prudent to expect SD in 40–50% of patients treated with antidepressants, if carefully evaluated.

Approximately 50% of patients taking antipsychotics will experience SD, including problems with sexual desire (mostly), erection, lubrication, ejaculation, orgasm, priapism, retrograde ejaculation [7, 8]. There are probably individual differences among various antipsychotics and it seems that the prevalence of SD with second generation (atypical) antipsychotics may be lower than that with the first generation (typical) antipsychotics. However, as with antidepressants, there are no good comparative studies and many studies are marred by methodological issues such as lack of baseline evaluation, and lack of validated rating tools. The evidence of SD associated with other psychotropic drugs such as anxiolytics and mood stabilizers is scarce and not providing data to estimate prevalence. It seems that buspirone may be associated with less SD than other medications used to treat anxiety disorders.

The exact prevalence and incidence of SD associated with non-psychotropic medications such as cardiovascular, gastrointestinal, hormonal, and cytotoxic agents are unknown [7, 8]. Some of these medications seem to have a high incidence of specific SD (e.g., erectile dysfunction associated with cimetidine is estimated to be 40–60%). Estimating the prevalence of SD associated with some of these medications may be difficult due to intrinsic patient and medication factors. Examples include some antihypertensives and some anticancer drugs. Hypertension is a well-known risk factor for erectile dysfunction (vascular damage) and thus untangling what part of SD is due to vascular disease and what part is duc to medication may be difficult. Similarly, cancer is associated with psychological problems which may lead to SD, and cytotoxic medications may cause general fatigue and damage to nerves and gonads—thus, it may be again difficult to determine what part of SD is due to a direct medication effect, indirect effect (fatigue) or the illness itself. The situation in estimating SD associated with medications used in obstetrics and gynecology, namely hormones, is similar.

There are many reports on SD associated with illicit drugs [7–9]. However, the estimates of incidence and prevalence are rare or nonexistent. In addition to previously mentioned methodological problems, the estimates of prevalence of SD associated with illicit drugs is complicated by the fact that some of these drugs may acutely help with sexual functioning, but later lead to deterioration of it (e.g., alcohol may decrease anxiety; cocaine may increase libido, cannabis may increase sexual pleasure and satisfaction and enhance orgasm).

In several studies the majority of subjects abusing opioids reported SD and the prevalence of SD in those abusing heroin is estimated to be 60–80% [7, 9]. Tobacco smoking is also associated with SD—increased incidence of erectile dysfunction in over 50% smokers has been reported in some studies [10] and in a meta-analysis by Tengs and Osgood [11], 40% of impotent men were current smokers compared with 28% of men in the general population. Tobacco smoking increases the risk of sexual dysfunction. As with other substances and medications, it is difficult to estimate the share of tobacco smoking in SD, as tobacco smoking is associated with poor overall general health and other risks of SD such as cardiovascular disease.

Etiology

The etiology of SD associated with medications or substances of abuse is clearly related to a specific substance and its impact on various neurotransmitters/receptors and hormones regulating sexual functioning. The regulation of sexual behavior and sexual response is complex and not fully understood. It involves the central nervous system (CNS), peripheral nerves and endocrine glands. Various neurotransmitters that are influenced by psychotropic medications play also an important role in mediating the sexual response. The serotonergic system generally inhibits sexual functioning (e.g., [8, 12])—by actually inhibiting all three major phases of the sexual response cycle, desire, arousal, and orgasm. However, the involvement of the serotonergic system is more complex, as some serotonergic receptors inhibit sexual functioning while others (e.g., 5-HT_{1A}) stimulate it. It is well known that serotonergic antidepressants are associated with SD, most significantly with delayed orgasm and anorgasmia. However, there are differences among serotonergic antidepressants in their impact, e.g., on ejaculation. For instance, paroxetine delays ejaculation significantly more than sertraline or citalopram [13, 14]. Presumably, strongly serotonergic medication may influence sexual functioning at the CNS (e.g., amygdala, hippocampus) and peripheral level. Dopamine, another neurotransmitter influenced by various medications, plays an important role in regulating sexual desire and arousal (e.g., 12). Dopamine (motor neurotransmitter of the reward system) activates nucleus accumbens and some hypothalamic regions that are important for sexual motivation and desire [12]. Thus medications blocking the dopamine receptors, such as antipsychotics, impact sexual functioning, namely desire and arousal. However, dopamine also regulates the secretion of prolactin from the pituitary gland—D_2 receptor blockage by antipsychotics increases the secretion of prolactin. Prolactin decreases sexual desire and the decreases levels of some sex hormones, such as estrogen and testosterone. On the other hand, prolactin seems to provide the body with sexual gratification after sex. Thus, psychotropic medications blocking the dopamine receptors (especially D_2 receptor) may profoundly impact sexual functioning. As noted before, sexual functioning may be also impacted by mental illness treated with a particular medication (e.g., antidepressant), that may contribute to SD. Further factor complicating the determination of a relationship between the substance and SD include possible multiple diseases, their treatments, marital discord, alcohol abuse and general life stress [8]. Another complicating issue may be the delayed onset of action of the substance implicated in SD (e.g., carbamazepine- and estrogen-induced increases in serum hormone binding globulin, thus decreasing the availability of free testosterone—[8]).

The etiology of SD associated with medications used to treat various physical illnesses is again tied to the specific mechanism of a particular medication. For instance, the erectile dysfunction associated with some beta-blockers, especially the nonselective ones, is due to their direct effect on penile vascular smooth muscle cells causing vasoconstriction from the unopposed alpha-adrenergic stimulation, leading to decreased perfusion in the corpora cavernosa [15]. In addition, some beta blockers (e.g., atenolol, propranolol, pindolol) have been reported to decrease the levels of testosterone and follicle stimulating hormone [15]. The underlying cardiovascular illness may again play an additional role in SD in this case. Quite frequent sexual side effects of cimetidine, an H_2 blocker, have been attributed to its antiandrogenic and estrogenic (increase of estradiol) properties [8, 16], ganglionic blockage, and an effect on central histaminic function [8].

As noted, the etiology of SD associated with substances of abuse again depends on the specific substance. Sexual dysfunction associated with chronic use of stimulants (cocaine) is related to the dopaminergic system. Alcohol related SD seems to be related to alcohol-induced hepatic catabolism of testosterone and its transformation to estradiol, and also possibly to the phytoestrogen content of alcoholic beverages [9]. SD associated with cannabis use is probably related to the disinhibition provided by delta-9-tetrahydrocannabinol [9]. SD associated with tobacco use could be explained by the strong vasoconstrictive effect of nicotine, its effect on the penile endothelium and its increase of sympathetic nervous tone [17]. Finally, SD associated with opioid use is probably related to the inhibition of the hypothalamic–pituitary–gonadal axis and increase in prolactin levels [9]. Sexual functioning during abuse of illicit substances is probably also impacted by poor physical health due to substance abuse (e.g., liver disease).

Pathophysiology

The physiology/regulation of human sexual response is quite complex. It involves CNS structures (e.g., amygdala, thalamus, paragigantocellularis nucleus), spinal cord and peripheral nerves (e.g., inferior mesenteric plexus, superior hypogastric plexus, pelvic plexus), endocrine glands (gonads, pituitary gland, and "peripheral" other endocrine organs, e.g., neuropathy due to diabetes), blood vessels, and smooth muscles.

Each phase of the sexual cycle is regulated by a complex interplay of biological, psychological, and environmental factors. For instance, the core of the excitatory system involved in sexual desire appears to be formed by the brain dopamine systems (incertohypothalamic and mesolimbic) that link the hypothalamus and the limbic system [18]. This system also includes melanocortins, oxytocin, and norepinephrine [18]. Brain opioid, endocannabinoid, and serotonin systems are activated during periods of sexual inhibition and blunt the ability of excitatory systems to be activated [18]. Thus, as Pfaus wrote [18], drugs (medications and drugs of abuse) that stimulate the activation of hypothalamic dopamine or that blunt endocannabinoid or serotonin release and/or postsynaptic binding may be effective in stimulating sexual desire. On the other hand, substances that inhibit or block dopamine or stimulate serotonin or endocannabinoid release seem to decrease or suppress desire. In addition, plasma testosterone is necessary for desire or interest in both men and women [12], as it influences specific brain regions sensitive to internal and external cues. Testosterone release is directly inhibited by, among others, prolactin. Substances that reduce dopamine or thyroid dysfunction may thus indirectly decrease testosterone availability.

Dopamine receptor activation may also be associated with penile erection, which also involves the inhibition of alpha-adrenergic influences and beta-adrenergic stimulation plus the release of a noncholinergic vasodilator substance and possibly vasoactive peptide [19]. Substances inhibiting the dopamine pathways or substances with alpha-adrenergic stimulation properties may impair erection centrally (the alpha-adrenergic influence could impair erection also on the peripheral level, e.g., in the regulation of vasoconstriction of peripheral vessels). Arousal regulation in both men and women involves the autonomic nervous system (e.g., acetylcholine is involved in parasympathetic activation which leads to vasodilatation in the penis, clitoris and vaginal wall). There are also intracellular mechanisms involved in medicating erection, e.g., cyclic guanosine monophosphate (c-GMP) and adenosine monophosphate (AMP). As explained e.g., by McVary [20] and many others, increased concentration of nitric oxide (NO) in smooth muscles (e.g., by nonadrenergic noncholinergic fibers; release is connected to sexual desire) leads to relaxation of cavernous sinusoids of penis through a complex way. The increase of NO leads to activation of guanylate cyclase which produces cGMP, and to a decrease in intracellular calcium through a pathway mediated by cGMP and that leads to muscle relaxation (cAMP may also decrease the intracellular calcium). Relaxation of smooth muscles leads to increased blood flow into corpora cavernosa. Substances that affect the cGMP pathway (e.g., drugs blocking phosphodiesterase-5 which metabolizes cGMP) or the cAMP pathway (alprostadil), or both pathways (papaverine) thus prolong muscle relaxation and inflow of blood into corpora cavernosa. Phosphodiesterase-5 inhibitors are medications used to treat erectile dysfunction through this complex mechanism. However, impairment of these pathways via various substances or due to physical illnesses (e.g., cardiovascular—endothelial damage) may lead to SD. It is hypothesized that similar mechanisms are involved in women [8]. Many of the same neurotransmitters involved in the regulation of erection have been identified in clitoris and/or vaginal wall [8].

Ejaculation involves the sympathetic nervous system (alpha-adrenergic fibers) [19]. The activation of this system leads to contraction of the smooth muscles in the epididymis, vas deferens and seminal vesicles, thus propelling the ejaculate to the posterior urethra [12]. Then spasms of the surrounding muscles lead to propulsion of the ejaculate from the urethra. Activation of dopamine or 5-HT_{1A} receptors promotes ejaculation. Serotonergic stimulation appears to inhibit the ejaculatory reflex. Opioids (endogenous and exogenous) inhibit ejaculation. Norepinephrine (primary messenger in the sympathetic nervous system) and prolactin also influence ejaculation. Finally, oxytocin seems also involved in regulating ejaculation/orgasm., especially the pleasant sensations experienced during orgasm and the affiliative feelings. All nerves and neurotransmitter/hormone systems could be impacted by medications or substances of abuse at various stages. The detailed physiology of female orgasm (beyond spasms of orgasmic platform, uterus, and anal sphincter) is less well understood and involves the coordination of sympathetic, parasympathetic, and somatic efferent system innervating the genital organs [21]. The reflexive cascade of contractions may be modulated by serotonin and dopamine; however, other neurotransmitters, hormones, and other substances are involved, too.

Clayton and colleagues [12] summarized the possible genetic/pharmacogenetic predisposition to SD associated with SSRIs. There are studies (e.g., [22]) reporting a higher incidence of SD associated with paroxetine in poor metabolizers of cytochrome CYP450 2D6. The role of genetics SD associated with medications or substances of abuse is not clear. Clayton and colleagues [12] noted that there is a lot of ongoing research into the pharmacogenetics affecting liver metabolism, the blood–brain barrier, serotonin receptor subunits, neurotropic factors, and glutamate receptor subunits.

Intact sexual functioning also depends on overall physical health, namely of the cardiovascular and endocrine systems. Medications and substances of abuse could negatively impact these systems.

The physiology of sexual functioning is clearly quite complicated and not fully understood. The pathophysiology of SD is even less well understood. The mechanisms of drug-induced sexual side effects include antiandrogenic, anticholinergic, antiestrogenic, alpha-adrenergic, beta-adrenergic, dopaminergic, and serotonergic effects; and the suppression of gonadotropin release and inhibition of NO synthase [8]. It is obvious that medications and substances of abuse can impact the regulation and physiology of human sexual response at numerous points.

Phenomenology and Diagnostic Criteria

The phenomenology of SD associated with medications and substances of abuse is basically the same as the phenomenology of sexual dysfunction in general. Medications and substances of abuse can be associated with an impairment of a particular phase of the sexual response cycle (decreased desire, impaired arousal, impaired—delayed or suppressed orgasm/ejaculation), or with an overall suppression/impairment of all phases of the sexual response cycle. Some less-known sexual side effects, such as retrograde or painful ejaculations, ejaculatory anhedonia and genital anesthesia may occur with some psychotropic medications (antipsychotics, tricyclic antidepressants).

The DSM-5 [7] diagnostic criteria of substance/medication-induced sexual dysfunction are outlined in Table 23-2.

The DSM-5 ([7], p. 446) notes that the diagnosis of substance/medication-induced SD should be made instead of a diagnosis of substance intoxication or substance withdrawal only when the symptoms in Criterion A predominate in the clinical picture and are sufficiently severe to warrant clinical attention.

The DSM-5 [7] also delineates the following *Specifiers* regarding the onset and severity of sexual dysfunction:

With regard to the onset:

With onset during intoxication: If the criteria are met for intoxication with the substance and symptoms develop during intoxication.

With onset during withdrawal: If the criteria are met for withdrawal from the substance and the symptoms develop during, or shortly after, withdrawal.

With onset after medication use: Symptoms may appear either at initiation of medication or after a modification or change in use.

Table 23-2. DSM-5 Diagnostic Criteria for Substance/Medication-Induced Sexual Dysfunction

A clinically significant disturbance in sexual function is predominant in clinical picture
B. There is evidence from the history, physical examination, or laboratory findings of both (1) and (2):
1. The symptoms in Criterion A developed during or soon after substance intoxication or withdrawal or after exposure to medication.
2. The involved substance/medication is capable of producing the symptoms in Criterion A.
C. The disturbance is not better explained by a sexual dysfunction that is not substance/medication-induced. Such evidence of an independent sexual dysfunction could include the following: The symptoms precede the onset of the substance/medication use; the symptoms persist for a substantial period of time (e.g., about 1 month) after the cessation of acute withdrawal or severe intoxication; or there is other evidence suggesting the existence of an independent non-substance/medication-induced sexual dysfunction (e.g., a history of recurrent non-substance/medication-related episodes)
D. The disturbance does not occur exclusively during the course of a delirium
E. The disturbance causes clinically significant distress in the individual

[Reprinted with permission from the Diagnostic and Statistical Manual of Mental Disorders, Fifth Edition, (Copyright 2013). American Psychiatric Association].

With regard to severity:

Mild: Occurs on 25–50% of occasions of sexual activity.

Moderate: Occurs on 50–75% of occasions of sexual activity.

Severe: Occurs on 75% or more of occasions of sexual activity.

Of note: The DSM-5 [7] also presents a complicated way of coding substance/medication-induced sexual dysfunction related to use and severity of use of a specific substance. The name of the substance/medication-induced sexual dysfunction should begin with the specific substance, e.g., alcohol or fluoxetine. The coding of medication-induced sexual dysfunction or of substances that do not fit into any of the classes should use the code (DSM or ICD) for "other substance." If the specific substance is not known but judged to be an etiological factor, the category of "unknown substance" should be used. The diagnosis should be followed by specifiers. The coding seems to be a bit cumbersome from a clinical point of view, but may be useful in future surveillance studies.

In contrast to other sexual dysfunctions, the DSM-5 criteria for substance/medication-induced SD do not specify the duration of this SD. However, the DSM-5 [7] text mentions that the onset of antidepressant-associated SD may occur as early as 8 days after the medication is first taken. It also mentions that about 30% of patients with mild to moderate orgasm delay may experience spontaneous remission within 6 months. SD associated with medications and substances of abuse may increase with age [7]. The question whether the SD persists after the discontinuation of medication/substance of abuse in some individuals remains unresolved. Rare cases of SD associated with SSRIs persisting for 4–24 months after SSRIs discontinuation have been reported [23].

Best Approach to Diagnosis (Including Possible Diagnostic Tests, or Rating Instruments)

The cornerstone of the best approach to the diagnosis is a thorough clinical interview and questioning. The interview should help to differentiate between SD and sexual complaint. Sexual complaints are almost universal, frequently related to relationship problems or life stress, are transient and inconsistent in symptomatology, and frequently remit spontaneously.

Questioning should be rather specific, with a focus on the character of SD (decreased libido, arousal impairment, orgasm delay or absence), intensity, persistence, and especially the onset of SD and time relationship to the start of a particular medication or taking of a substance of abuse. Baseline evaluation (= prior to starting the medication) of sexual functioning is of utmost importance. It is difficult to rely on the patient's *retrospective* interpretation of the relationship/time between the onset of SD and the start of a particular medication. Frequently, the underlying illness treated with a particular medication is also associated with SD (e.g., depression, schizophrenia, diabetes, cardiovascular disease) and it may be difficult to decipher the relationship between the illness, medication, and SD without having the baseline evaluation of SD. Similarly, relationship problems may be a complicating factor. Thus an astute clinician should evaluate sexual functioning at the initial clinical interview, at the start of prescribing any medication and, actually, regularly at follow-up visits. Balon [1] outlined the elements of an evaluation of sexual functioning during baseline evaluation of patients with depression that is applicable to the evaluation of sexual functioning prior to starting any medication. The elements include: (a) pretreatment and, if possible, premorbid sexual functioning; (b) comorbid psychiatric disorders and substance use (including tobacco and alcohol), (c) physical illnesses; (d) all concurrent medications (including over-the-counter ones); (e) sexual functioning during the recent episode of illness (depression, anxiety, etc.) but before initiation of treatment; (f) potential interpersonal context of the SD (marital conflict etc.).

Both the clinician and the patient should be comfortable with discussing sexual functioning and SD [24]. Questions should be asked in a serious manner, and should progress from open-ended ones with gradual narrowing the focus and following the cues [24]. Vague general questions, such as "How is your sex life?" are not advisable and are frequently met with similarly vague answers, such as "OK." The clinician should not assume anything. At times, it may be very useful to interview the patient's partner.

There is *no valid and reliable diagnostic instrument* in the area of human sexuality/SD. The Structured Clinical Interviews for various versions of DSM have not included the diagnostic interview for sexual dysfunctions. However, there are many instruments to measure various phases and aspects of sexual functioning and its impairment [24–26]. Some of them are useful for measuring changes of sexual functioning/side effects during medication administration and have been used in a number of clinical trials—see Table 23-3.

At times, general psychopathology scales items (e.g., Hamilton Depression Rating Scale (HDRS)—[27]) of sexual functioning, or general side effects scales items for sexual functioning have been used for the evaluation of SD during treatment with various medications [28]. No valid and/or reliable scales for measuring SD associated with substances of abuse exist.

There are no diagnostic laboratory tests of SD. However, some laboratory tests may help to elucidate the etiology of SD. Prolactin level could be useful in patients treated with antipsychotics who report SD or galactorrhea. Free testosterone level may be useful in patients reporting low sexual

TABLE 23-3. Selected instruments to measure sexual dysfunction associated with medications

Instrument	Modality	Number of items	Administration time	Domains
Arizona Sexual Experience Scale (ASEX) [29]	SR	5	Less than 5 min	Drive, arousal, erection, vaginal lubrication orgasm, satisfaction
Changes in Sexual Functioning Questionnaire (CSFQ) [30]	CI and SR	35 (female) 36 (male)	Less than 20 min	Desire interest, desire frequency, pleasure arousal, orgasm, total score
Modified Rush Sexual Inventory (MRSI) [31]	SR	24 (female) 31 (male)	Unknown	Desire, satisfaction functioning, behavior sensitivity, pain
Psychotropic Related Sexual Dysfunction Questionnaire (PRSexDQ orSALSEX) [32]	SR	7	5 min	Desire, arousal ejaculation/orgasm degree of tolerability of any change in functioning
Sex Effects Scale (SexFx) [33]	SR/CR	13	5–10 min	Desire, arousal, orgasm, global satisfaction
Derogatis Interview for Sexual Functioning (DISF/DISF-SR) [34]	CR (semi-structured)	26	15 min	Sexual cognition/fantasy, arousal, sexual behavior/experience, orgasm, sexual drive/ relationship
International Index of Erectile Function (IIEF) [35]	SR (males only)	15	10 min	Erectile function, orgasm function, sexual desire, intercourse satisfaction, overall satisfaction

CR clinician rated; *CI* clinical interview; *SR* self-report.

desire—possibly to help rule out hypogonadism. Thyroid stimulating hormone could be ordered to rule out hypothyroidism. Finally, fasting glucose and glycosylated hemoglobin A_{1C} may be obtained in older men reporting erectile problems on medication, as one of the first signs of diabetes may be erectile dysfunction. Urine drug screen for substances of abuse may be useful in some patients to provide a starting point for the connection of SD and substance abuse.

Best Practice for Management

The best practice starts with addressing sexual functioning during the initial evaluation. Good sexual functioning is important for patients in general and even during illnesses (e.g., in depression) in which many clinicians assume sexual functioning is of no importance to patients. The discussion should address sexual functioning, the patient's expectations, fantasies and reality (age, lifestyle, partner, etc.), healthy lifestyle, and possibility of SD during the suggested treatment. As a matter of standard practice, patients should be encouraged to lead a healthy lifestyle, including avoiding substances of abuse including tobacco, maintain a healthy weight and a weight loss, healthy diet (Mediterranean diet may improve sexual functioning—e.g., [36]), exercise [37, 38], and adherence to proper treatment of physical illnesses (e.g., diabetes). A healthy lifestyle may help patients not only with possible improvement of sexual functioning but also with overall physical and mental health, a sense of well-being, and enhancement of self-image. The discussion of physical illness, the possibility of associated SD and approaches to SD may help to dispel some patients' fears and myths. For instance, a male patient with cardiovascular disease (especially after myocardial infarction) may be counseled about his sexual activity [8]—suggesting to resume sex as soon as he desires, avoiding sex after meals (wait 3 h) or after alcohol consumption, avoiding sex in extreme temperatures, avoiding sex when tired, fatigued, avoiding sex during periods of extreme stress. Patients should report unusual symptoms during or after sexual activity to their physician (e.g., marked fatigue, prolonged palpitations). Patients may be also assured that myocardial infarction during sexual activity is very rare.

The possibility of SD associated with medications should be openly discussed with the patient prior to starting the medication. Patients may be asking about the chance of sexual dysfunction with a particular medication, other options of treatment, and what could be done if SD occurs with their treatment. Free, open communication and good doctor–patient relationship is always helpful in managing this clinical situation.

As part of good management practice, the physician should always consider starting the patient on a medication with a lower probability of associated SD, especially in sexually active patients. For example, one may choose bupropion, mirtazapine, or nefazodone (still available, in generic form) as an initial treatment of depression in patients concerned about possible SD associated with medication. The situation will be, of course, different in a patient who has been treated with multiple medications and none of these three drugs worked or could not be considered for other reasons (e.g., seizure disorder or eating disorder in case of bupropion).

Good management practice also includes active monitoring of sexual functioning during treatment. A number of studies (e.g., [39, 40]) demonstrated large differences between reporting in response to direct questioning vs. spontaneous reporting of SD in clinical trials (58% vs. 14% (39) and 41% vs. 6% [40]).

The outlined good management strategies also apply to SD associated with substance abuse. However, the first step in the management of substance abuse-associated SD should be an attempt to educate the patient and discontinue the offending substance.

Management Strategies

Over the last 2 decades a number of reviews and chapters [1, 8, 12, 41–51] outlined various management strategies for psychotropic medications-associated SD (see Table 23-4). These references [1, 8, 12, 41–51] also provide summaries of evidence for each strategy and the reader is encouraged to look for references there, as a review of all evidence is beyond the scope of this chapter.

It should be noted that most of these strategies were originally developed for antidepressant-associated SD and some of them may not be applicable to SD associated with other medications (see below). Systematic reviews (e.g., [46, 49, 51]) also point out that that the currently available evidence for efficacy of these strategies is rather limited, with a small number of trials published (some strategies are based on case reports or on one study). For instance, the latest Cochrane Database Review [51] concluded that "For men with antidepressant-induced erectile dysfunction, the addition of sildenafil or tadalafil appears to be an effective strategy. For women with antidepressant-induced sexual dysfunction the addition of bupropion at higher doses appears to be the most promising approach studied so far." Similarly, a Cochrane Database Review on antipsychotic-associated SD [49] concluded that there are no good studies available and that "Sildenafil may be a useful option in the treatment of antipsychotic-induced sexual dysfunction in men with schizophrenia, but this conclusion is based only on one small short trial. Switching to olanzapine may improve sexual functioning in men and women, but the trial assessing this was a small, open label trial."

TABLE 23-4. Management strategies for sexual dysfunctions associated with psychotropic medications

1.	Selecting a medication with a low incidence of sexual dysfunction, especially in sexually active patients and in patients on psychotropic medication for the first time
2.	Encouraging lifestyle changes or adjustments (diet, exercise, no substances of abuse)
3.	Waiting for spontaneous remission of sexual dysfunction or patient's accommodation to it
4.	Reduction of medication to the lowest effective dose
5.	Scheduling sexual activity around dosing of medication (e.g., before the once a day nighttime dose)
6.	Switching to another medication from the same class with a lower frequency of SD
7.	Using drug holidays
8.	Using "antidotes" or other medications (e.g., phosphodiesterase-5 inhibitors) to counteract SD
9.	Using psychotherapy (CBT?), sex therapy
10.	Exercise—general and before sexual activity, also Kegel exercise (?)
11.	Use of mechanical intervention (vacuum pump, vibrators, EROS-CTD* [52]?)

• *EROS-CTD* EROS Clitoral Therapy Device (FDA approved for SD in women) [Based on data from Refs. [41–51].

? = Unclear whether to use, sugegsted by some authors

Thus, management of SD associated with various medications remains more a clinical art than science, combining the weak evidence from the literature with clinical skills and improvisation based on the clinical picture, medication profile, and the patient's interest and willingness. The two most frequently used strategies for already developed SD associated with antidepressants are switching to an antidepressant with a lower frequency of SD and using "antidotes" or other medications to alleviate SD.

Maintaining a healthy lifestyle and exercise makes sense for any case of sexual dysfunction and thus should be suggested to all patients with SD as a general measure (especially as suggested by studies by Lorenz and Meston [37, 38] that exercise helped immediately prior to sexual activity in women with SD associated with antidepressants). Patients should be recommended to abstain from substances of abuse, to lose weight, and possibly start a Mediterranean diet. Cognitive-behavioral (CBT) and sex therapies have been more frequently suggested as one of the management strategies for SD associated with medications. While there is evidence in the literature that CBT and sex therapy help in various sexual dysfunctions, including sexual pain, there is no literature available to support the efficacy of these two therapy modalities in SD associated with medications. Intuitively, their use makes sense, though.

Management Strategies Application Within Specific Classes/Groups of Medications

Antidepressants

Selecting antidepressant with a low frequency of SD: Several antidepressants (bupropion, mirtazapine, moclobemide, nefazodone, and vortioxetine) have been reported to have very low incidence of associated SD and thus may be a good first choice in a sexually active patient.

Waiting for spontaneous remission or accommodation of SD (as noted, up to 30% of patients with mild to moderate orgasm delay may experience spontaneous remission of SD within 6 months –[7]): This strategy is used infrequently. Achieving a remission may take a long time. This strategy may be acceptable only to patients with a low frequency of sexual activity. There are reports of spontaneous remission of SD with phenelzine and sertraline. On the other hand, this strategy is usually not helpful in TCA-associated anorgasmia. Implementing this strategy requires a good doctor–patient relationship, as adherence to the medication will become an issue.

Reduction to a minimal effective dose of antidepressant: This strategy seems to make sense, as SD with antidepressants is dose-dependent [53]. However, implementation may be complicated. It is known that antidepressant doses should be kept the same even during remission. It may be difficult to balance between the minimal therapeutic versus subtherapeutic doses. This strategy has been touted for erectile dysfunction associated with antidepressants. It has been working with SD associated with some SSRIs.

Scheduling sexual activity around dosing of medication (e.g., *before the once a day nighttime dose)*: This strategy has been occasionally suggested for antidepressants with a shorter half-life (e.g., paroxetine, sertraline). While it again seems to make some sense, it has not been really tested.

Switching to another medication from the same class with a lower frequency of SD: There are several reports on successfully switching patients with SD associated with SSRIs to bupropion and also to mirtazapine, nefazodone, and vortioxetine [54]. Presumably, switching to other antidepressants with relatively low incidence of associated SD, such as moclobemide and vilazodone, may also help. Switching to bupropion would probably be the most preferable. However, one has to remember that the antidepressant effect may not be the same as with the previous antidepressant. This strategy could also be considered when antidepressants are used in other indications than depression, e.g., in anxiety disorders. In such a case, one may consider switching to buspirone or benzodiazepines.

Using drug holidays: This strategy was tested in one small, open label, 4-week study. Three SSRIs (fluoxetine, paroxetine, sertraline) were stopped on Thursday and resumed on Sunday noon. Sexual activity was recommended just before the antidepressants were restarted. The strategy was effective for patients on paroxetine and sertraline, but not for patients on fluoxetine (probably because of the substantially longer half-life of fluoxetine). Nevertheless, most experts [1, 8, 12] do not recommend this strategy, as it may encourage nonadherence, withdrawal symptoms may occur during the period after stopping medication (not tested in the original study), and the long-term effects of this approach are unknown. Some case reports also suggested partial drug holiday—decreasing the dosage of antidepressant for a few days with sexual activity at the end of the period of lower dose.

Using "antidotes" or other medications (e.g., *phosphodiesterase-5 inhibitors) to counteract SD*:

A number of various "antidotes" and other medications have been reported to counteract SD associated with antidepressants (see Table 23-5)

Table 23-5. Antidotes and other medications and preparations used for management of SD associated with antidepressants

Amantadine	Mirtazapine
Adenosyl methionine	Mianserin[a]
Bethanechol	Nefazodone
Bromocriptine	Neostigmine
Bupropion	Pemoline[b]
Buspirone	Rosa damascene oil
Cyproheptadine	Sildenafil
Dextroamphetamine	Tadalafil
Gingko biloba	Testosterone
Granisetron	Trazodone
Loratidine	Vardenafil [55]
Maca root	Yohimbine
Methylphenidate	

[a]Not available in the USA.
[b]Withdrawn from the US market.

Most of these "antidotes" have not been properly tested and the evidence of their efficacy is based on case reports. Several open label studies or case series demonstrated efficacy of some antidotes such as buspirone, bupropion, and yohimbine [8]. The evidence from case reports or open label studies may be problematic. Gingko biloba can serve as example—one open label study [56] reported that it may be helpful in SSRIs associated SD, while another open label study [57] and two blinded studies [58, 59] did not confirm these findings. Some double-blind studies may not provide definite evidence either: in one double-blind placebo-controlled study Michoulon and colleagues [60] did not find differences between amantadine, buspirone and placebo in the management of SD associated with fluoxetine. However, the doses of both antidotes—amantadine 100 mg/day, buspirone 20–30 mg/day—were clearly lower than reported in case reports. Other studies (e.g., [61]) found sildenafil to be effective in women reporting SSRI associated SD. This finding is interesting in view of the fact that sildenafil trials in sexual dysfunction were stopped by the sildenafil maker seemingly for lack of efficacy. As there may be a subgroup of women responding to sildenafil, it still seems advisable to try sildenafil in women reporting SD with antidepressants. It would be interesting to see whether the newly approved medication for female hypoactive sexual desire disorder—flibanserin—could and would be used in SSRI associated SD (this may have to be taken with caution as flibanserin is a failed SSRI).

All these findings prompted Rudkin and colleagues [51] to reach the previously mentioned conclusion that the current evidence supports only the use of sildenafil in erectile dysfunction associated with antidepressants and bupropion in women reporting SSRI-associated SD. This should not, however, totally discourage creativity in management of SD associated with antidepressants or stop clinicians using various antidotes. Their use should be based on the entire clinical picture.

Use of mechanical intervention (vacuum pump, vibrators, EROS-CTD: There is no evidence for usefulness of these devices in SD associated with antidepressants, though some suggested their use. EROS-CTD is actually one of the two FDA-approved treatments for sexual dysfunction. It is basically a mechanical pump applied over the clitoris.

Interestingly, one study demonstrated efficacy of acupuncture in sexual dysfunction secondary to antidepressants [62].

Antipsychotics

Selecting a medication with a low frequency of sexual dysfunction, especially in sexually active patients and patients on psychotropic medication for the first time: Among the typical antipsychotics, loxapine and molindone were reported to have lower frequency of associated SD. However, the production of molindone was discontinued. The frequency of SD associated with atypical antipsychotics (with the exception of risperidone, which is really not atypical) is usually low, though the reports have been inconsistent. One may consider starting patients on olanzapine, quetiapine and particularly on aripiprazole among atypical antipsychotics. However, some of the atypical antipsychotics may be also more prone to raise prolactin, which may contribute to SD.

Waiting for spontaneous remission of sexual dysfunction or patient's accommodation to it: There are no reports on usefulness of this strategy. There is some evidence of alleviation of SD with antidepressants over the time.

Reduction of medication to a minimal effective dose: Again, there are no reports on the usefulness of this strategy. As with antidepressants, it may be difficult to balance between the minimal effective dose and subtherapeutic dose. This should be reserved for patients who are adherent to treatment and have good social support.

Scheduling sexual activity around dosing of medication (e.g., *before the once a day nighttime dose)*: There are no reports on this strategy. This strategy could not be applied to long-acting antipsychotics associated SD.

Switching to another medication from the same class with a lower frequency of SD: The best choice to switch within the typical antipsychotics would be to switch to loxapine. It seems than switching to olanzapine or quetiapine may be useful within the group of atypical antipsychotics (or even switching from a typical to an atypical antipsychotic). However, the best antipsychotic to switch to seems to be aripiprazole. In one small open study [63], switching to aripiprazole from several other antipsychotics led to improvements of desire, erection, ejaculation, and overall sexual satisfaction. Prolactin levels and menstrual dysfunction were reduced. It seems that switching to aripiprazole may be the best option within this strategy. The decision about switching could be also based on a specific SD associated with a particular antipsychotic (erectile failure?—less alpha-adrenergic blockade; low libido—consider atypical antipsychotics).

Using drug holidays: This strategy is not advisable for patients on antipsychotics medications.

Using "antidotes" or other medications (e.g., *phosphodiesterase-5 inhibitors) to counteract SD*:

Several "antidotes" have been suggested for antipsychotics-associated SD [8, 12]. These include bromocriptine (especially for low libido), cabergoline (again, especially for low libido) [64], imipramine (for anorgasmia with thioridazine), bethanechol, neostigmine, aripiprazole [63], and sildenafil (especially for erectile dysfunction—[65]). One should be careful with dopaminergic medications such as bromocriptine and cabergoline as they may worsen psychotic symptomatology.

Mood Stabilizers

No good data exist on management of SD associated with mood stabilizers. Waiting for spontaneous remission might be an option. Reduction of mood stabilizer dose is probably not the best idea. Switching to another mood stabilizer such as lamotrigine (low incidence of SD) or valproic acid (not in women of childbearing potential, though—[66]), or even to an atypical antipsychotic may be an option. Antidotes, such as bupropion and phosphodiesterase inhibitors could also be considered.

Antianxiety Medications

The frequency of SD associated with antianxiety medication (unless SSRIs are used for treatment of anxiety and related disorders) is usually low. There are no solid reports of management strategies beyond case reports. Suggested strategies [8] include reduction of dose (SD seems to be more frequent with higher doses of benzodiazepines), switching to another benzodiazepine or buspirone in case of benzodiazepine-associated SD, or considering a trial of sildenafil.

Cardiovascular Medications

Again, very little is known about the management of SD associated with cardiovascular medications. The guidelines for managing SD with antihypertensives are not very clear [67]. However, the main recommendation seems to be either switching to antihypertensives with a better safety profile (e.g., calcium channel blockers or angiotensin-converting enzyme inhibitors, or captopril which has been reported to have a lower incidence of associated SD) or intervention with phosphodiesterase-5 inhibitors. One may also consider reducing the dose after years of effective treatment, or scheduling sexual activity around the dose of antihypertensive [8].

Other Medications

As noted before, medications used to treat some gastrointestinal diseases (e.g., H_2 antagonist antacids) are frequently associated with SD. However, there are no data on the management of this group of side effects. Similarly, there is no clear guidance on the management of SD associated with medications used to treat cancer. Due to possible disfigurement, loss of some sexual organs, including ovaries and testes, the management of SD associated with chemotherapy may be quite a complicated issue requiring more substantial involvement of psychological intervention, hormones and various "antidotes" or other medications used to counteract SD such as phoshodiesterase-5 inhibitors or intracavernosal injections (e.g., alprostadil) [8]. Dyspareunia due to chemotherapy may be relieved by vaginal lubricants or estrogen vaginal creams or rings. Hormone replacement has to be considered against unknown risks of hormonal use. Vibrators, vacuum pumps, and EROS-CTD use could be also considered.

Substances of Abuse

There are no management strategies for substance abuse associated SD. Discontinuation of the offending substance should be the primary goal and strategy. Substance abuse patients should be properly counseled about the deleterious effects of substances of abuse on sexual functioning.

Prognosis

There is no solid information about the prognosis of substance/medication-associated SD. As noted, medication-associated SD may improve or remit over time in some cases [7, 8]. On the other hand, as reported, SD associated with some antidepressants does not remit even after medication discontinuation [23]. The success rate of various management strategies is unknown as there are no good studies to evaluate these strategies available. The prognosis is probably dependent on multiple factors including demographic, clinical, medication, and physiological ones.

References

1. Balon R. SSRI-associated sexual dysfunction. Am J Psychiatry. 2006;163:1504–9.
2. Steffens DC, Krishnan KRR, Helms MJ. Are SSRIs better than TCA? Comparison of SSRIs and TCAs: a meta-analysis. Depress Anxiety. 1997;6:10–8.
3. *Physicians' Desk Reference*. 56 ed. Montvale, NJ: Medical Economics Company; 2002.
4. Gelenberg AJ, Dunner DL, Rothschild AJ, Pedersen R, Dorries KM, Ninan PT. Sexual functioning in patients with recurrent major depressive disorder enrolled in the PREVENT study. J Nerv Ment Dis. 2013;201:266–73.
5. Serretti A, Chiesa A. Treatment-emergent sexual dysfunction related to antidepressants: a meta-analysis. J Clin Psychopharmacol. 2009;29:259–66.
6. Montgomery SA, Baldwin DS, Riley A. Antidepressant medications: a review of the evidence for drug-induced sexual dysfunction. J Affect Disord. 2002;69:109–40.
7. American Psychiatric Association. Diagnostic and statistical manual of mental disorders. 5th ed. Arlington, VA: American Psychiatric Association; 2013.
8. Segraves RT, Balon R. Sexual pharmacology: fast facts. New York: WW Norton & Comp; 2003.
9. Palha AP, Esteves M: Drugs of abuse and sexual functioning. In: Balon R, editor. Sexual dysfunction. The brain-body connection. Basel, Switzerland: Karger AG; 2008, p. 131–49.
10. Hatzimouratidis K. Epidemiology of male sexual dysfunction. Am J Mens Health. 2007;1:103–25.
11. Tengs TO, Osgood ND. The link between smoking and impotence: two decades of evidence. Prev Med. 2001;32:447–52.
12. Clayton AH, Alkiis AR, Parikh NB, Votta JG. Sexual dysfunction due to psychotropic medication. In: Mago R,editor. Adverse effects of psychotropic treatments. Psychiatr Clin North Am 2016; 39: 427–463
13. Waldinger MD, Zwinderman AH, Olivier B. Antidepressants and ejaculation: a double-blind, randomized, placebo-controlled, fixed-dose study with paroxetine, sertraline and nefazodone. J Clin Psychopharmacol. 2001;21:293–7.
14. Waldinger MD, Zwinderman AH, Olivier B. SSRIs and ejaculation: a double-blind, randomized, fixed-dose study with paroxetine and citalopram. J Clin Psychopharmacol. 2001;21:556–60.
15. Chrysant S. Antihypertensive therapy causes erectile dysfunction. Curr Opin Cardiol. 2015;30:383–90.
16. Galbraith RA, Michnovicz JJ. The effects of cimetidine on the oxidative metabolism of estradiol. N Engl J Med. 1989;321:269–74.
17. Biebel MG, Burnett AL, Sadeghi-Nejad H. Male sexual function and smoking. Sex Med Rev. 2016;4:366–75.
18. Pfaus JG. Pathways of sexual desire. J Sex Med. 2009;6:1506–33.
19. Segraves RT. Effects of psychotropic drugs on human erection and ejaculation. Arch Gen Psychiatry. 1989;46:275–84.
20. McVary KT. Erectile dysfunction. N Engl J Med. 2007;357:2472–81.
21. Giraldi A, Marson L, Nappi R, Pfaus J, Traish AM, Vardi Y, Goldstein I. Physiology of female sexual function: animal models. J Sex Med. 2004;1:237–53.
22. Zourkova A, Ceskova E, Hadasova E, Ravcukova B. Links among paroxetine-induced sexual dysfunctions, gender, and CYP2D6 activity. J Sex Marital Ther. 2007;33:343–55.
23. Csoka AB, Bahrick A, Mehtonen OP. Persistent sexual dysfunction after discontinuation of selective serotonin reuptake inhibitors. J Sex Med. 2008;5:227–33.
24. Derogatis LR, Balon R. Clinical evaluation of sexual dysfunctions. In: Balon R, Segraves RT, editors. Clinical manual of sexual disorders. Arlington, VA: American Psychiatric Publishing, Inc.; 2009. p. 23–57.
25. Rizvi SJ, Yeung NW, Kennedy SH. Instruments to measure sexual dysfunction in community and psychiatric populations. J Psychosom Res. 2011;70Z:99–109.
26. Derogatis LR. Measures of sexual dysfunction and disorders. In: Rush AJ Jr, First MB, Blacker D, editors. Handbook of psychiatric measures. 2nd ed. Arlington, VA: American Psychiatric Publishing, Inc.; 2008. p. 601–20.
27. Hamilton M. A rating scale for depression. J Neurol Neurosurg Psychiatry. 1960;23:56–62.
28. Lingjaerde O, Ahlfors UG, Bech P, Dencker SJ, Elgen K. The UKU side effects rating scale. A new comprehensive rating scale for psychotropic drugs and a cross-sectional study of side effects in neuroleptic-treated patients. Acta Psychiatr Scand Suppl. 1987;334:1–100.
29. McGahuey CA, Gelenberg AJ, Laukes CA, Moreno FA, Delgado PL, McKnight KM, Manber R. The arizona sexual experience scale (ASEX): reliability and validity. J Sex Marital Ther. 2000;26:25–40.

30. Clayton AH, McGarvey EL, Clavet GJ. The changes in sexual functioning questionnaire (CSFQ): development, reliability, and validity. Psychopharmacol Bull. 1997;33:747–53.
31. Rao D, Zajecka J, Skubiak T. The modified rush sexual inventory: preliminary psychometric findings. Psychiatry Res. 2005;137:175–81.
32. Montejo AL, Ricco-Villademoros F. Psychometric properties of the psychotropic-related sexual dysfunction questionnaire (PRSexDQ-SALSEX) in patients with schizophrenia and other psychotic disorders. J Sex Marital Ther. 2008;34:227–39.
33. Kennedy SH, Rizvi SJ, Fulton K, Ellis J, Quilty LC, Ravindran L. The sex effects scale: pilot validation in a healthy population. Psychopharmacol Bull. 2010;43:15–25.
34. Derogatis LR. The derogatis interview for sexual functioning (DISF/DISF-SR): and introductory report. J Sex Marital Ther. 1997;23:291–304.
35. Rosen RC, Riley A, Wagner G, Osterloh IH, Kirpatrick J, Mishra A. The international index of erectile function (IIEF): a multidimensional scale for assessment of erectile dysfunction. Urology. 1997;49:822–30.
36. Guigliano F, Maiorino MI, Bellastella G, Autorino R, De Sio M, Guigliano D, Esposito K. Adherence to mediterranean diet and erectile dysfunction in men with type 2 diabetes. J Sex Med. 2010;7:1911–7.
37. Lorenz TA, Meston CM. Exercise improves sexual function in women taking antidepressants: results from a randomized crossover trial. Depress Anxiety. 2014;31:188–95.
38. Lorenz TA, Meston CM. Acute exrcise improves physical sexual arousal in women taking antidepressants. Ann Behav Med. 2012;43:352–61.
39. Montejo-Gonzales AL, Llorca G, Izquierdo JA, Ledesma A, Bousono M, Calcedo A, Carrasco JL, Ciudad J, Daniel E, De la Gandara J, Derecho J, Franco M, Gomez MJ, Macias JA, Martin T, Sanchez JM, Sanchez D, Vicens E. SSRI-induced sexual dysfunction: fluoxetine, paroxetine, sertraline, and fluvoxamine in a prospective, multicenter, and descriptive clinical study of 344 patients. J Sex Marital Ther. 1997;23:176–94.
40. Landen M, Hogberg P, Thase ME. Incidence of sexual side effects in refractory depression during treatment with citalopram or paroxetine. J Clin Psychiatry. 2005;66:100–6.
41. Harvey KV, Balon R. Clinical implications of antidepressant drug effects on sexual function. Ann Clin Psychiatry. 1995;7:189–201.
42. Clayton DO, Shen WW. Psychotropic induced sexual function disorders: diagnosis, incidence and management. Drug Saf. 1998;19:299–312.
43. Rosen RC, Lane RM, Menza M. Effects of SSRIs on sexual function: a critical review. J Clin Psychopharmacol. 1999;19:67–85.
44. Baldwin DS. Depression and sexual function. Br Med Bull. 2001;57:81–99.
45. Taylor MJ, Rudkin L, Hawton K. Strategies for managing antidepressant-induced sexual dysfunction: systematic review of randomized controlled trials. J Affect Disord. 2005;88:241–54.
46. Taylor MJ. Strategies for managing antidepressant-induced sexual dysfunction: a review. Curr Psychiatry Rep. 2006;8:431–6.
47. Labbate LA. Psychotropics and sexual dysfunction: the evidence and treatment. In: Balon R, editor. Sexual dysfunction. The brain-body connection. Basel, Switzerland: Karger AG; 2008, p. 107–30.
48. Balon R. Medications and sexual function and dysfunction. In: Balon R, Segraves RT, editors. Clinical manual of sexual disorders. Arlington, VA: American Psychiatric Publishing, Inc.; 2009. p. 95–115.
49. Schmidt HM, Hagen M, Kriston L, Soares-Weiser K, Maayan N, Berner MM. Management of sexual dysfunction due to antipsychotic drug therapy. Cochrane Database Syst Rev. 2012, Nov 14;11:CD003546.
50. Nunes LV, Moreira HC, Razzouk D, Nunes SO, Mari Jde J. Strategies for the treatment of antipsychotic-induced sexual dysfunction and/or hyperprolactinemia among patient of the schizophrenia spectrum: a review. J Sex Marital Ther. 2012;38:281–301.
51. Taylor MJ, Rudkin L, Bullermor-Day P, Lubin J, Chukwujekwu C, Hawton K. Strategies for managing sexual dysfunction induced by antidepressant medication. Cochrane Database Syst Rev. 2013;5:CD003382.
52. Billups KL, Berman L, Berman J, Metz ME, Glennon ME, Goldstein I. A new non-pharmacological vacuum therapy for female sexual dysfunction. J Sex Marital Ther. 2001;27:435–41.
53. Benazzi F, Mazzali M. Fluoxetine-induced sexual dysfunction: a dose-dependent effect? Pharmacopsychiatry. 1994;27:246.
54. Jacobsen PL, Mahableshwarkar AR, Chen Y, Chrones L, Clayton AH. Effect of vortioxetine vs. escitalopram on sexual functioning in adults with well-treated major depressive disorder experiencing SSRI-induced sexual dysfunction. J Sex Med. 2015;12:2036–48.
55. Berigan T. Antidepressant-induced sexual dysfunction treated with vardenafil. Can J Psychiatry. 2004;49:643.
56. Cohen AJ, Bartlik B. Gingko biloba for antidepressant-induced sexual dysfunction. J Sex Marital Ther. 1998;24:139–43.
57. Ashton AK, Ahrens K, Gupta S, Masand PS. Antidepressant-induced sexual dysfunction and Gingko biloba. Am J Psychiatry. 2000;157:836–7.
58. Kang BJ, Lee SJ, Kim MD, Cho MJ. A placebo-controlled, double-blind trial of Gingko biloba for antidepressant-induced sexual dysfunction. Hum Psychopharmacol. 2002;17:279–84.
59. Wheatley D. Triple-blind, placebo-controlled trial of Gingko biloba in sexual dysfunction due to antidepressant drugs. Hum Psychopharmacol. 2004;19:545–8.
60. Michelson D, Bancroft J, Targum S, Kim Y, Tepner R. Female sexual dysfunction associated with antidepressant administration: a randomized, placebo-controlled study of pharmacological intervention. Am J Psychiatry. 2000;157:239–43.
61. Nurnberg HG, Hensley PL, Heiman JR, Croft HA, Debattista C, Paine S. Sildenafil treatment of women with antidepressant-associated sexual dysfunction: a randomized controlled trial. JAMA. 2008;300:395–404.
62. Khamba B, Aucoin M, Lytle M, Vermani M, Maldonado A, Iorio C, Cameron C, Tsirgielis D, D'Ambrosio C, Anand L, Katzman MA. Efficacy of acupuncture treatment of sexual dysfunction secondary to antidepressants. J Altern Complement Med. 2013;19:862–9.
63. Mir A, Shivakumar K, Williamson RJ, McAllister V, O'Kkeane V, Aitchinson KJ. Change in sexual dysfunction with aripiprazole: a switching or add-on study. J Psychopharmacol. 2008;22:244–53.
64. Kalkavoura CS, Michopoulos I, Arvanitakis P, Theodoropoulou P, Dimopoulou K, Tzebelikos E, Lykouras L. Effects of cabergoline on hyperprolactinemia, psychopathology, and sexual functioning in schizophrenic patients. Exp Clin Psychopharmacol. 2013;21:332–241.
65. Gopalakrishnan R, Jacob KS, Kuruvilla A, Vasantharaj B, John JK. Sildenafil in the treatment of antipsychotic-induced erectile dysfunction: a randomized, double-blind, placebo-controlled, flexible-dose, two-way crossover trial. Am J Psychiatry. 2006;163:494–9.
66. Balon R, Riba M. Should women of childbearing potential be prescribed valproate? A call to action. J Clin Psychiatry. 2016;77:525–6.
67. Al Khaja KA, Sequeira RP, Alkhaja AK, Damanhori AH. Antihypertensive drugs and male sexual dysfunction: a review of adult hypertension guideline recommendations. J Cardiovasc Pharmacol Ther. 2016;21:233–44.

24 Evaluation and Treatment of Hypersexual and Other Sexual Dysfunctions

Waguih William IsHak

Introduction

Hypersexual disorder is a diagnostic label given to a variety of behaviors revolving around recurrent and intense sexual fantasies, sexual urges, and sexual behavior that cause significant distress or interfere with social and occupational functioning. Manifestations of this behavior include excessive engagement in sexual intercourse, masturbation, pornography, and online or computer-based sexual activities [1]. Kafka proposed this new category with specific diagnostic criteria; however, it was not included in the DSM-5 [2]. Such sexual behaviors are also seen in the context of manic and hypomanic episodes in bipolar disorder, cyclothymia, and schizoaffective disorder, as well as neurological conditions such as traumatic brain injury, Kluver-Bucy syndrome, partial complex seizures, frontal lobe lesions, and sexual disinhibition in dementia and delirium [3]. Illicit drugs such as poppers and methamphetamine, alcohol, and prescription medications such as dopamine agonists used in Parkinson's disease have also been associated with similar behaviors [4]. Hypersexual disorder could be considered to be a type of addiction, compulsion, or an impulse control disorder [5, 6]. The overlap with increased sexual desire and the behaviors of increased sexual activity [7] raised the possibility of labeling it as hyperactive sexual desire disorder [8].

Epidemiology

Depending on how hypersexual behaviors are defined [9], the prevalence is reported to be between 3 and 6% in the general population [10]. Kinsey et al. defined hypersexual behavior as having seven or more orgasms per week and found in their survey that 7.6% of men met that definition for at least five consecutive years [11]. Kafka recommended defining hypersexual disorder as daily orgasms for 6 months [12]. Overall, about 5–10% of males [13] and 6.8% of females meet the criteria [9].

Phenomenology/Diagnostic Criteria

The phenomenology of hypersexual disorder is better understood along a number of models describing what drives the sexual behaviors [1]. Gold and Heffner in 1998 highlighted three models used to describe hypersexual disorder [6]:

The Addiction Model

This model considers sex similar to substances of use, in terms of patients spending excessive time looking for sex, engaging in sex, or recovering from its effects and experiencing tolerance and withdrawal with impairment of functioning, as well as medical, legal, and financial consequences [14]. This model showed that patients have experienced successful outcomes following 12-step self-help groups based on the principles of Alcoholics Anonymous such as Sex Addicts Anonymous and Sexaholics Anonymous, as well as following cognitive behavioral therapy, as shown by Carnes in 2002 [15].

The Compulsive Model

This model emphasizes that the behavior reflects sexual thoughts, images, or impulses that are experienced as obsessions that increase tension/anxiety leading to compulsions in the form of repetitive engagement in sex to decrease tension/anxiety [16]. Favorable outcomes with clomipramine and SSRIs approved for obsessive-compulsive disorder (OCD) lend credence to this model. However, OCD medications' mechanism of action in hypersexual disorder is not fully determined because significant reduction in sexual desire is also a side effect of the same medicines.

W.W. IsHak (ed.), *The Textbook of Clinical Sexual Medicine*, DOI 10.1007/978-3-319-52539-6_24

The Impulse Control Disorder Model

In this model, hypersexuality is seen similar to pathological gambling where an impulse is experienced with high intensity leading to repeated sexual activity followed by significant remorse [17]. High rates of comorbidity of impulse control disorders (ICD) and hypersexual disorder give support for this model especially that patients frequently respond to the same SSRIs used for ICD.

DSM-5 Diagnostic Criteria (Proposed, Not Approved)

The DSM-5 proposed specific diagnostic criteria for hypersexual disorder [18]; however, the category was not approved, and the criteria were not included in the DSM-5. The full criteria are depicted in Table 24-1. The proposed criteria highlighted age 18 as a minimum, 6 months of recurrent and intense sexual fantasies, sexual urges, and sexual behavior in association with at least four out of five criteria including excessive time, in response to dysphoric mood states, stressful life events, unsuccessful efforts to control or reduce, and disregard the risk to self or others. Additional criteria include clinically significant personal distress or impairment in functioning, and that it is not due to substances, medical conditions, or manic episodes. The proposed specifiers included masturbation, pornography, sexual behavior with consenting adults, cybersex, telephone sex, and strip clubs [18].

TABLE 24-1. DSM-5 Proposed Criteria for Hypersexual Disorder

A. Over a period of at least 6 months, recurrent and intense sexual fantasies, sexual urges, and sexual behavior in association with four or more of the following five criteria:
1. Excessive time is consumed by sexual fantasies and urges and by planning for and engaging in sexual behavior
2. Repetitively engaging in these sexual fantasies, urges, and behavior in response to dysphoric mood states (e.g., anxiety, depression, boredom, and irritability)
3. Repetitively engaging in sexual fantasies, urges, and behavior in response to stressful life events
4. Repetitive but unsuccessful efforts to control or significantly reduce these sexual fantasies, urges, and behavior
5. Repetitively engaging in sexual behavior while disregarding the risk for physical or emotional harm to self or others
B. There is clinically significant personal distress or impairment in social, occupational, or other important areas of functioning associated with the frequency and intensity of these sexual fantasies, urges, and behavior
C. These sexual fantasies, urges, and behavior are not due to direct physiological effects of exogenous substances (e.g., drugs of abuse or medications), a co-occurring general medical condition, or to manic episodes
D. The person is at least 18 years of age
Specify if masturbation, pornography, sexual behavior with consenting adults, cybersex, telephone sex, and strip clubs

[Reprinted from Reid RC, Carpenter BN, Hook JN, Garos S, Manning JC, Gilliland R, Cooper EB, McKittrick H, Davtian M, Fong T. Report of findings in a DSM-5 field trial for hypersexual disorder. J Sex Med. 2012;9(11):2868–77. with permission from Elsevier].

Subtypes of Hypersexual Disorder

Using the criteria proposed by Kafka for the DSM-5 [18], Kaplan and Krueger described in the details the subtypes of hypersexual disorders [19].

1. Masturbation: The rates of excessive masturbation within hypersexual disorder range from 50 to 75% according to a number of studies [20–22].
2. Pornography: Research studies show that 50–60% of patients with hypersexual disorder are dependent on pornography [20, 23].
3. Sexual behavior with consenting adults: This behavior involved significant promiscuity, which ranges from 24 to 84% in men. Reid et al., in 2009, showed that 7% of a treatment-seeking male sample solicited sex workers regularly, 12% had unprotected multiple anonymous sex, and 21% had extramarital affairs [23].
4. Cybersex: This behavior is defined as having online sexual conversations in chat rooms or text-messaging applications ("sexting"). Despite its provision of privacy and health protection sounding involvement, it is very clear that hypersexual behaviors encompassing excessive use, time spent, and associated dysfunctional behaviors are leading to significant impairments of social, occupational, and relationship functioning [24]. The exact prevalence of these behaviors is still understudy.
5. Telephone sex: Studies from the late 1990s showed that about 37% of males struggling with hypersexual behaviors had excessive telephone sex [20]. However, in light of technological advancement of the Internet, telephone sex seems to be on the decline.
6. Strip clubs: Many patients who are suffering from hypersexual behaviors report frequent dependence on strip clubs and their associated financial cost, excessive alcohol use, shame, and guilt. However, there is very little research in this area.

Best Practice and Evidence-Based Approach to Evaluation

The evaluation of hypersexual disorder includes three crucial components:

(a) A thorough medical evaluation to rule out any potential medical, endocrinal/hormonal, and neurological causes of the behaviors.
(b) A thorough evaluation of the effects of any substances (prescribed, over the counter, dietary supplements, herbs, or street drugs).
(c) The impact on functioning. The negative impact of hypersexual disorder on functioning was described by Reid et al. [18] using data from the field trials of the DSM-5 proposed criteria, as depicted in Table 24-2.

It is also important to utilize measurement instruments during the evaluation and treatment of hypersexual disorders. The literature reports at least 22 questionnaires to measure hypersexual behavior [25, 26]. Table 24-3 displays the three most utilized rating scales.

Best Practice and Evidence-Based Approaches to Treatment

The field still has yet to define and approve clinical and/or research diagnostic criteria that could pave the road for empirical research and establish solid evidence for specific interventions. For the time being, a biopsychosocial approach will need to be followed in order to help patients with hypersexual disorder reduce/eliminate the effects of biological and psychosocial factors that might have predisposed, precipitated, or perpetuated the symptoms. This approach should encompass biological interventions to address the effects of medical contributing factors and the effects of substances, as well as psychosocial interventions to address not only the effects of psychiatric disorders and traumas/losses but also the results of the behaviors which commonly worsen patients' suffering. Guilt and shame about hypersexual behaviors coupled with loss of control/ability to stop, despite commitments to abstinence, not uncommonly lead to hopelessness and helplessness with or without full-blown depressive symptoms. The behaviors themselves end up by providing transient mood elevations and respite from self-deprecation and facing one's reality of mounting social, occupational, and financial complications.

TABLE 24-2. Consequences associated among patients with hypersexual disorder

Has happened several times, %	Has happened once or twice, %	Hypersexual behavior consequences scale (sample items from the HBCS)
1.6	15.7	Caused job loss
16.5	22.8	Ended a romantic relationship
5.5	22.0	Contracted a sexually transmitted infection
0.8	16.5	Caused legal problems
29.1	23.6	Experienced unwanted financial losses
67.7	22.0	Emotionally hurt a loved one
66.9	11.0	Interfered with ability to experience healthy sex
73.2	20.5	Negatively affected mental health

Missing data reduced this sample from $n = 138$ to $n = 127$.
[Reprinted from Reid RC, Carpenter BN, Hook JN, Garos S, Manning JC, Gilliland R, Cooper EB, McKittrick H, Davtian M, Fong T. Report of findings in a DSM-5 field trial for hypersexual disorder, J Sex Med. 2012; 9(11):2868–77. with permission from Elsevier].

Biological Interventions

To start, it is important to address any medical contributing factors such as traumatic brain injury, hormonal issues, and neurological problems, as well as the effects of substances such as stimulants and dopaminergic agents. Psychiatric issues such as manic episodes will need to be addressed accordingly. The most frequently used medications for hypersexual disorder include:

1. Selective serotonin reuptake inhibitors (SSRIs): The most commonly used SSRIs for this disorders are fluoxetine 60–80 mg per day, paroxetine 40–60 mg per day, and fluvoxamine 100–200 mg per day [4].
2. Tricyclic antidepressants (TCAs): Serotonergic TCAs such as clomipramine are used at doses ranging from 150–300 mg per day.
3. Opioid antagonists: Naltrexone has been used successfully to treat hypersexual behaviors occurring alone or comorbid with neurological disorders, in the range of 50–150 mg per day [30].
4. Antiandrogens: Medroxyprogesterone 300–500 mg IM injection weekly has been used in severe hypersexual behaviors especially in conjunction with paraphilias or

TABLE 24-3. Rating scales for hypersexual disorder

Rating scale, author (Reference)	Description/items	Psychometric properties	Sample item
The sexual compulsivity scale [27]	Ten items rated on a four-point Likert scale from 1="Not at all like me" to 4="Very much like me"	Internal consistency Cronbach's $\alpha = 0.84$. Test-retest reliability = 0.73	"I feel that sexual thoughts and feelings are stronger than I am"
Hypersexual behavior inventory [28]	19 items using a five-point Likert scale to obtain a total score and measure three factors: control, coping, and consequences	Internal consistency Cronbach's α: total score = 0.90, control = 0.78 coping = 0.86, and consequences = 0.78	"My sexual behavior controls my life"
The hypersexual disorder screening inventory [29]	7 items scored from 0 = "Never true" to 4 = "Almost always true". The items are divided to 2 sections: Recurrent and intense sexual fantasies, urges and behaviors; Distress and impairment During the last 6 months	Internal consistency Cronbach's α: = 0.88	"I have tried to reduce or control the frequency of sexual fantasies, urges, and behavior but I have not been very successful"

treatment-refractory head injury associated with hypersexuality [31]. Cyproterone at 100–300 mg po daily in divided doses or 300–600 mg IM injection weekly has also been used but more commonly in sexual offenders [32].
5. Luteinizing hormone-releasing hormone agonists: Leuprolide (or leuprorelin) 7.5 mg monthly IM injection has been used in this disorder [33].
6. Gonadotropin-releasing hormone (GnRH) agonists: Triptorelin 3.75 mg was found to decrease secretion of gonadotropins (FSH and LH) by the pituitary gland leading to a decrease in hypersexual behaviors [34].
7. Other medications: Lithium and other mood stabilizers are used to treat manic symptoms that might be contributing to hypersexual behaviors.

Psychosocial Interventions

Hypersexual patients are often dealing with depressive and anxiety symptoms and a vicious cycle of shame and guilt. Therefore, psychotherapy is one of the essential interventions in hypersexual disorder.

1. Behavioral therapy: Shift stimulus control, feedback, and self-monitoring are examples of behavioral techniques used to reduce hypersexual behaviors especially in patients with traumatic brain injury [35].
2. Cognitive behavioral therapy (CBT): Techniques used to decrease hypersexual behaviors include cognitive restructuring, covert sensitization, and victim empathy therapy. CBT has been shown to be the best non-pharmacological treatment of hypersexual behaviors [36].
3. Group psychotherapy: As opposed to 12-step programs, motivating patients to participate in hypersexual support groups has been shown to be difficult [37]. Studies of group psychotherapy in hypersexual disorder are still lacking.
4. Self-help 12-step groups: There are many variations of 12-step programs including Sex Addicts Anonymous, Sexaholics Anonymous, Sex and Love Addicts Anonymous, Sexual Compulsives Anonymous, and S-Anon for family members. Although clinical trials about the effectiveness of 12-step programs are still needed, patients and families report major improvements [38].
5. Couples Therapy: Involving the couple in the treatment of hypersexual behaviors has been found helpful [39], especially when sex therapy was added later in the course [40].

Prognosis

The prognosis of hypersexual disorder is guarded and is highly dependent on adherence to treatment interventions especially psychotherapy and 12-step programs as well as compliance with medications interventions.

Other Sexual Dysfunctions

The DSM-5 lists two categories where symptoms of sexual dysfunction cause significant distress but do not meet the full diagnostic criteria. "Other specified sexual dysfunction" is used when the clinicians names the dysfunction, e.g., sexual aversion, whereas "other unspecified sexual dysfunction" is reserved for dysfunction where the clinician chooses not to specify the reason [41].

References

1. IsHak WW. The guidebook of sexual medicine. Beverly Hills, CA: A&W Publishing; 2008.
2. Kafka MP. Hypersexual disorder: a proposed diagnosis for DSM-V. Arch Sex Behav. 2010;39(2):377–400.
3. Sadock VA, IsHak WW, Rodack V. Hypersexuality: addiction or compulsion? presented at the annual meeting of the American Psychiatric Association. San Diego; May 1997.
4. Turner D, Schöttle D, Bradford J, Briken P. Assessment methods and management of hypersexuality and paraphilic disorders. Curr Opin Psychiatry. 2014;27(6):413–22.
5. Parsons JT, Rendina HJ, Ventuneac A, Moody RL, Grov C. Hypersexual, sexually compulsive, or just highly sexually active? Investigating three distinct groups of gay and bisexual men and their profiles of HIV-related sexual risk. AIDS Behav. 2016; 20(2):262–72.
6. Gold SN, Heffner CL. Sexual addiction: many conceptions, minimal data. Clin Psychol Rev. 1998;18(3):367–81.
7. Winters J, Christoff K, Gorzalka B. Dysregulated sexuality and high sexual desire: distinct constructs? Arch Sex Behav. 2010;39:1029–43.
8. Leiblum SR, Rosen RC. Sexual desire disorders. New York: Guilford; 1988.
9. Langstrom N, Hanson RK. High rates of sexual behavior in the general population: correlates and predictors. Arch Sex Behav. 2006;35:37–52.
10. Black DW. The epidemiology and phenomenology of compulsive sexual behavior. CNS Spectr. 2000;5:26–72.
11. Kinsey AC, Pomeroy WB, Martin CE. Sexual behavior in the human male. Philadelphia: W.B. Saunders Company; 1948.
12. Kafka MP. Hypersexual desire in males: an operational definition and clinical implications for males with paraphilias and paraphilia-related disorders. Arch Sex Behav. 1997;26:505–26.
13. Atwood JD, Gagnon J. Masturbatory behavior in college youth. J Sex Education Ther. 1987;13:35–42.
14. Carnes PJ. Out of the shadows: understanding sexual addiction. Center City, MN: Hazelden Information & Edu; 1983.
15. Carnes PJ, Adams KM. Clinical management of sex addiction. New York: Brunner-Routledge; 2002.
16. Quadland MC. Compulsive sexual behavior: definition of a problem and an approach to treatment. J Sex Marital Ther. 1985;11(2):121–32.
17. Barth RJ, Kinder BN. The mislabeling of sexual impulsivity. J Sex Marital Ther. 1987;13(1):15–23.
18. Reid RC, Carpenter BN, Hook JN, Garos S, Manning JC, Gilliland R, et al. Report of findings in a DSM-5 field trial for hypersexual disorder. J Sex Med. 2012;9(11):2868–77.
19. Kaplan MS, Krueger RB. Diagnosis, assessment, and treatment of hypersexuality. J Sex Res. 2010;47(2):181–98.
20. Kafka MP, Hennen J. The paraphilia-related disorders: an empirical investigation of nonparaphilic hypersexuality disorders in outpatient males. J Sex Marital Ther. 1999;25(4):305–19.

21. Raymond NC, Coleman E, Miner MH. Psychiatric comorbidity and compulsive/impulsive traits in compulsive sexual behavior. Compr Psychiatry. 2003;44(5):370–80.
22. Wines D. Exploring the applicability of criteria for substance dependence to sexual addiction. Sex Addict Compulsivity. 1997;4:195–220.
23. Reid RC, Carpenter BN, Lloyd TQ. Assessing psychological symptom patterns of patients seeking help for hypersexual behavior. Sex Relation Ther. 2009;24:47–63.
24. Daneback K, Ross MW, Mansson SA. Characteristics and behaviors of sexual compulsives who use the Internet for sexual purposes. Sex Addict Compulsivity. 2006;13:53–67.
25. Womack SD, Hook JN, Ramos M, et al. Measuring hypersexual behavior. Sex Addict Compulsivity. 2013;20:65–78.
26. Karila L, Wéry A, Weinstein A, Cottencin O, Petit A, Reynaud M, Billieux J. Sexual addiction or hypersexual disorder: different terms for the same problem? A review of the literature. Curr Pharm Des. 2014;20(25):4012–20.
27. Kalichman SC, Adair V, Rompa D, Multhauf K, Johnson J, Kelly J. Sexual sensation-seeking: scale development and predicting AIDS-risk behavior among homosexually active men. J Pers Assess. 1994;62(3):385–97.
28. Reid RC, Garos S, Carpenter BN. Reliability, validity, and psychometric development of the Hypersexual Behavior Inventory in an outpatient sample of men. J Sex Addict Compulsivity. 2011;18(1):30–51.
29. Parsons JT, Rendina HJ, Ventuneac A, Cook KF, Grov C, Mustanski B. A psychometric investigation of the hypersexual disorder screening inventory among highly sexually active gay and bisexual men: an item response theory analysis. J Sex Med. 2013;10(12):3088–101.
30. Piquet-Pessôa M, Fontenelle LF. Opioid antagonists in broadly defined behavioral addictions: a narrative review. Expert Opin Pharmacother. 2016;17(6):835–44.
31. Hebebrand K, Hebebrand J, Remschmidt H. Pharmacological agents for treatment of paraphilias and hypersexual disorders. Fortschr Neurol Psychiatr. 2002;70(9):462–75.
32. Khan O, Ferriter M, Huband N, Powney MJ, Dennis JA, Duggan C. Pharmacological interventions for those who have sexually offended or are at risk of offending. Cochrane Database Syst Rev. 2015;2:CD007989.
33. Guay DR. Drug treatment of paraphilic and nonparaphilic sexual disorders. Clin Ther. 2009;31(1):1–31.
34. Safarinejad MR. Treatment of nonparaphilic hypersexuality in men with a long-acting analog of gonadotropin-releasing hormone. J Sex Med. 2009;6:1151–64.
35. Zencius A, Wesolowski MD, Burke WH, Hough S. Managing hypersexual disorders in brain-injured clients. Brain Inj. 1990;4(2):175–81.
36. Krueger RB, Kaplan MS. Behavioral and psychopharmacological treatment of the paraphilic and hypersexual disorders. J Psychiatr Pract. 2002;8(1):21–32.
37. Tierens E, Vansintejan J, Vandevoorde J, Devroey D. Diagnosis and treatment of participants of support groups for hypersexual disorder. Arch Ital Urol Androl. 2014;86(3):175–82.
38. Carnes P. Sexual addiction and compulsion: recognition, treatment, and recovery. CNS Spectr. 2000;5(10):63–72.
39. Bird MH. Sexual addiction and marriage and family therapy: facilitating individual and relationship healing through couple therapy. J Marital Fam Ther. 2006;32:297–311.
40. Schneider JP. Sexual problems in married couples recovering from sexual addiction and coaddiction. Am J Prevent Psychiatr Neurol. 1990;2(3):33–8.
41. American Psychiatric Association. Diagnostic and statistical manual of mental disorders: DSM-5. Washington, D.C: American Psychiatric Press; 2013.

Part III
Special Topics In Sexual Medicine

25
Myths About Sexual Health

Irene María López García and Nicolás Mendoza Ladrón de Guevara

Introduction and Objectives

Sexual health can be defined as a state of physical, emotional, mental and social well-being that is related to sexuality and not merely the absence of disease, dysfunction or infirmity. The sexual health of individuals requires them to have a positive and respectful attitude towards sexuality and sexual relations and the possibility of having sexual experiences that are pleasurable, safe and free of coercion, discrimination and violence. Therefore, sexual health is not exclusive to the prevention of sexually transmitted diseases; it also entails a broader approach that is related to the full development of a person's welfare, health, education and love [1].

Achieving sexual health requires the sexual rights of individuals to be recognized and guaranteed. In this sense, in 1997, the XIII World Congress of Sexology of Valencia (Spain) proposed an initial declaration of sexual rights that was reviewed and approved in 1999 by the General Assembly of the World Association for Sexology (WAS, a body linked to the WHO). In March 2014, the WAS made the most recent revision to this declaration of sexual rights that has been issued to date [2].

Among the cited sexual rights are "the right to comprehensive sexual education" and "the right to information based on scientific knowledge", which imply that sexual information should be generated through free and ethical scientific research and appropriately disseminated at all social levels. However, sexology remains a neglected educational discipline in the general population, in particular among physicians, and it is therefore possible that misinformation leads to the proliferation of myths and misconceptions about sexuality.

Based on the above considerations, the main objective of this chapter is to understand what these myths or misconceptions are and how ingrained they are in our population. We then present some answers and recommendations about sexual health.

Material and Methods

Opinion Poll on "Myths in Medical Sexology"

The construction and evaluation of our survey of the opinions of students and professors in the Faculty of Medicine of Granada were based on Likert scale.

A scale is a set of items or statements that have been selected to constitute a valid, reliable and accurate set of criteria for measuring social phenomena. In this case, the measured phenomenon was the degree of belief in and opinions on various issues related to sexual health. The Likert scale uses ordinal levels. This is a type of scale in which the subject being interviewed is offered a number of selected statements and asked to qualify their degree of agreement/disagreement with each statement. These statements reflect positive or negative attitudes towards a construct, and these attitudes are scored to as favourable and unfavourable, respectively. For each statement, the degree of agreement/disagreement is assessed using a score of 0–4.

The Likert scale is known as a combined scale because the score for each unit of analysis (in our case, survey respondents) is obtained by determining the sum of the responses to a particular item or statement. The main advantage of this type of scale is that all respondents share the same order of statements and that the degree of agreement/disagreement is very easily understood by the respondent.

The survey was administered to students and teachers in the degree of Medicine on paper, completed anonymously and collected in a closed box that was locked with a key and then opened when all the volunteers had returned the survey.

Statistical Method

To analyse the degree of credibility of each myth group (teachers and students or men and women), both the average score for each question in each group and the average of the

W.W. IsHak (ed.), *The Textbook of Clinical Sexual Medicine*, DOI 10.1007/978-3-319-52539-6_25

sum of all questions were calculated. The mean difference was also computed to identify differences in the credibility of the groups.

To analyse the differences in beliefs between groups, a nonparametric statistical method, the Mann-Whitney test of two unpaired samples, was applied to compare two independent samples. This test, which is based on the sum of ranges, was applied to test the following assumptions:

H0: The data distribution is identical in both groups.

H1: The data distribution is more biased to the right in group X than in group Y, that is, there is a greater probability that $X > Y$ than $X < Y$.

We considered all possible combinations of groups using two levels to ensure that the maximum number of conclusions could be extracted from the available data.

Questions and Doubts of the Population Concerning Sexual Health

According to the multitude of entries concerning problems related to sexual life that we detected in our search on the subject, questions regarding sex are very significant across both male and female Internet users. Additionally, we observed in the media that doubts arise about sexuality without taboos. Of the most prevalent myths, we chose the 14 that were in our opinion the most interesting to draft responses to myths about sexology as supported by the latest and best evidence available (Table 25-1).

TABLE 25-1. Myths about sex

1.	"There is a relationship between sex education and sexual ability"
2.	"Sexual desire and sexual potency decrease markedly after the age of 45 years"
3.	"By nature, women have less sexual desire than men and take longer to reach orgasm"
4.	"Penis size influences women's pleasure during sex"
5.	"There are different types of orgasms in women"
6.	"Removing the uterus and ovaries causes women to lose their sexual appetite and prevents them from feeling sexual enjoyment"
7.	"Sexual intercourse should be avoided during pregnancy"
8.	"There are no frigid women, but inexperienced men"
9.	"Race plays a role in enjoying greater sexual impulses and power"
10.	"Ejaculation is synonymous with orgasm; when a man ejaculates, intercourse ends"
11.	"Premature ejaculation only occurs in young men"
12.	"A solution to premature ejaculation is to have unpleasant thoughts and/or thoughts unrelated to intercourse"
13.	"It is deviant to have sexual fantasies about someone else during sex"
14.	"Male or female masturbation is a sign that something is wrong sexually with the couple"

Answers to Myths

1. "There is an association between sex education and sexual ability".

Sexuality, sexual behaviour and sexual relationships are important and necessary for the development of every individual. However, in our society, explicit sexuality issues are taboo and not openly discussed, and they are therefore rarely treated appropriately in the family, and this affects women and men from an early age. However, if we provide appropriate education and information, we will be better able to develop this important personal characteristic and enjoy adult sexuality in a more healthy and satisfying way.

Issues related to sexual health are relevant to all people because they have personal and social significance. However, these issues are particularly emphasized during a vital stage of change, i.e. during adolescence. In this stage, there are profound changes in one's manner of thinking, emotional ties and relationships with others. These changes are influenced by multiple biological, psychological, interpersonal and sociocultural factors. In adolescence, the sex organs mature, and the person becomes capable of reproducing. This process coincides with an increase in testosterone that resulted in increased sexual interest.

Psychologically, adolescence is characterized by self-centredness. Adolescents feel invincible, believe that their own experiences are unique, question everything that was previously set in stone and sometimes come to view sex as a symbol of freedom. Girls usually become sexually mature earlier than boys, are concerned about the size of their breasts and their ability to attract partners and hope to fall in love with someone or something greater. In contrast, boys are concerned about the size of their penis and other sexual characteristics and crave their first sexual intercourse.

Among the interpersonal factors that influence adolescence are family, friends and romantic partners. Adolescent sexuality depends largely on the type of family an individual grows up with and parental attitudes. Sexuality is affected by a lack of communication with the parents because parents often shy away from talking about sex. Even when they do, they usually focus on the preventive aspects of sex education, which do not always capture the interest of the adolescent.

The freedom of the adolescent from his or her nuclear family and the great importance of being "equal" during this vital stage result in friendships becoming an important source of information on sexuality.

Sociocultural factors have a major influence on differences in sexual behaviours between boys and girls. Educational materials, the school environment and the messages released by the media are largely responsible for this influence.

According to a recent study in Spain, seven out of ten teenagers are afraid to talk about sexuality and cite lectures in school, friendships and the Internet as their most common sources for sexual health information. A higher percentage of girls considered talks in schools to be the most useful source of information about sexuality. The second most useful source was friendships, which was cited more often by girls. Finally, the third most valued source of information was the Internet, which was used more by boys [3].

Sex education is one of the best investments society can make to promote sexual health in the population because it teaches and transforms individual's knowledge, attitudes and values regarding sexuality in all its manifestations. In addition, a sexually healthy society must ensure that its entire population has access to sex education throughout people's lifetime. Sex education should be initiated early in life, be adapted to the age of the audience and degree of development of each person and promote a positive attitude towards sexuality.

Sex education in children and adolescents should involve the participation of families, schools, health services and the community in general. The healthy development of adolescents requires them to acquire a mature and responsible sexual identity. Responsible sexual behaviour is an incredibly important public health problem and should include delaying sexual intercourse, choosing respectful and supportive partners and using condoms and effective contraceptive methods.

Comprehensive sex education programmes provide children and young people with the information, skills and values they need to be responsible for their own sexual health and wellness. In these programmes, information is provided regarding contraception and the benefits of delaying first intercourse, which has been shown to have positive effects on sexual behaviour. Accordingly, good sex education programmes are aimed at sending the message to young people that they should wait until they are ready to have sex [4].

In contrast, educational models based on sexual abstinence have been demonstrated to lack effectiveness. They do not produce changes in sexual behaviour over the long term.

In developed countries, adolescents are becoming sexually active at increasingly younger ages, at an average age of 16 years old [5]. According to statistics, 30% of girls aged 15–17 years have had sex, and this figure increases to 70% among girls aged 17–19 years. In boys, the respective figures are 31% and 64% [6]. Early sex among adolescents seems to be associated with different family circumstances, such as limited parental control, a lack of parental availability, an uncaring family atmosphere, pressure and the attitudes of other people towards the teen.

However, there is no evidence showing that sexual education delays first sexual experience. In a study on comprehensive sex education programmes, two-thirds of the programmes were found to have a positive effect on sexual behaviour in that they delayed the onset of sex, reduced the number of sexual partners and increased the use of condoms or other contraceptives. None of the programmes delayed first sexual experience. In addition, while some of them reduced the frequency of sexual intercourse, none encouraged the young people who received the programmes to have sex more frequently than other young people [7].

Good sex education not only prevents diseases and infections but also contributes to the integral development of individuals, teaching them respect and non-discrimination. Sex education includes the ability to make autonomous decisions about one's sexual life within the context of personal and social ethics and the ability to control and enjoy our bodies.

As previously mentioned, sex education should promote the integral development of adolescents [8] by achieving the following:

- Helping them to assess their body and appropriately express their sexuality, love and intimacy.
- Teaching them to maintain a proper and respectful relationship with people of both genders and to avoid being emotionally exploited, which is very important for preventing abuse and violence.
- Raising awareness of the need to respect other's value systems and improving the understanding that sex should be something that is consensual, pleasurable and nonexploitative.
- Enhancing critical communication with family members, friends and partners and promoting the development of a critical view of the information that is received.
- Promoting their sense of responsibility for their own choices and behaviours and improving their ability to select reasoned decisions.

Sex education is another key objective in combating the main risks of irresponsible sexual behaviour, including sexually transmitted infections and unwanted pregnancies.

- Sexually transmitted infections (STIs) are very common in adolescence. In the USA, 24% of adolescents between 14 and 19 years of age were carriers of at least one of the following STIs: human papilloma virus (HPV), which is the most common, *Chlamydia trachomatis*, *Trichomonas vaginalis*, the herpes simplex type 2 virus and *Neisseria gonorrhoeae* [9].
- In the span of a few months, many teenagers become infected. Repeated acquisition of STIs is also considered a risk factor for the later development of HIV. In the USA, in 1 year, 80% of the reported HIV cases occurred in the population aged 20–24 years [7].
- In 2014, in Spain, 3568 new cases of syphilis, 4562 new cases of gonorrhoea and 66,967 cumulative cases of

HIV were recorded in men, while 17,076 were reported in women.

- Another important sexual health issue is unwanted pregnancy. In the USA, 80% of teenage pregnancies are unwanted pregnancies. This has a profound influence on the lives of the affected teens because half of them will never finish a secondary education. In 2013, a total of 108,690 abortions were reported in Spain, and of these, 12% were performed in women under 20 years old [10].

Drawing on the conclusions of different authors, we found that effective and quality sex education programmes should include the following characteristics. They should:

- Provide comprehensive sex education for all children and young people that address a wide range of topics, including contraception.
- Be implemented by trained educators, including competent and committed teachers.
- Involve a training programme that is appropriate to each age because young people are till maturing. It is preferable to start before a young person has had his or her first sexual experience.
- Provide accurate and objective information.
- Target the social factors that affect sexual behaviour and promote fundamental values including a consent and mutual respect, the right to information, safety, health and equality and a responsibility for oneself and others.
- Use participatory learning methods in small groups to develop skills and not only to acquire knowledge.
- Require the participation of parents and caregivers.

In short, it has been shown that sex education delays the onset of sexual relationships between young people, reduces the number of sexual partners, improves condom use when they do become sexually active and does not increase the frequency of intercourse. Therefore, teaching young people about sexuality and contraception does not lead to early sexual activity. The objective of sex education is to provide children and young people with the information, skills and values they need to take responsibility for their own sexual health and to engage in pleasurable and safe sex. A good sex education results in every person initiating relationships when they feel ready without being carried away by the tips for success they may receive from other people or the frequent myths that surround sexuality. In addition, a quality sex education reduces risky sexual behaviour, which is the most effective and inexpensive way by which we can aim at ending or at least alleviating two major problems in our society: sexually transmitted infections and unwanted pregnancies.

2. "Sexual desire and sexual potency decrease markedly after the age of 45 years".

In our culture, different myths are related to the sexual health of older adults, and these can be summarized in three following points: the elderly are not sexually desirable, older people have no sexual desire and the elderly are not sexually capable. While it is true that sexual response deteriorates with age, it is also true that this circumstance does not prevent elderly individuals from enjoying a healthy sex life.

The physical, psychological and sociocultural changes that occur in middle-aged people may favour sexual intercourse, but it is more common for them to harm or even completely interrupt sexual activity. Sexuality at this age is conditioned by previous sexual experiences and is often affected by health problems and the treatment of these problems with medications. Age and disease most often affect sexual desire in women (hypoactive sexual desire disorder), and erection most often affects men (erectile dysfunction) [11].

Sexual desire is very complex and depends on physical, psychological, social and cultural factors. In men, the sexual response has a linear progression and usually begins with desire. However, in women, the sexual response is cyclical, and desire does not usually initiate a sexual response. All physical factors influence the emotions and experiences of women.

In general, spontaneous sexual desire decreases with age in women. Thus, when with a well-established partner, what motivates a woman to seek sexual activity is the desire for emotional closeness and intimacy with her partner. In addition, women often experience excitement before desire. Therefore, when in a long-term relationship, it is common for some women to begin sexual intercourse without desire and to obtain excitement after sexual relations have been initiated [12].

Factors Determining Sexual Desire

Age should not be considered a factor that is responsible for impaired sexual function. In the elderly, certain factors affect sexual desire and sexual potency in men and women more significantly. Of the factors that may affect female and male sexual desire, we include the following [11]:

- Hormonal factors

Sexual activity is influenced by blood levels of specific hormones. Testosterone stimulates sexual desire, but in individuals between 30 and 40 years old, decreased serum testosterone levels are observed. In addition, peak testosterone secretion occurs during only half of the ovarian cycle and does not occur in postmenopausal women. A lack of desire is more common in middle-aged women (45–64 years old) and increases following menopause [13].

Additionally, a progressive decrease in testosterone levels has been associated with decreased sexual activity and power and reduced levels of sexual desire in men. However, hormonal factors do not fully explain the changes that are observed in sexuality with increasing age.

Oestrogens negatively affect desire in men, but in women, they help to maintain trophism and vaginal lubrication. In postmenopausal women, decreased oestrogen levels lead to atrophy and decreased vaginal lubrication. These changes can lead to less pleasurable or painful intercourse in women (dyspareunia), which could adversely affect their motivation and sexual desire.

- Physical factors

Organic diseases can affect desire, though they rarely fully prevent sexual activity. However, genitourinary diseases that require surgical treatment or are cancer based have a greater impact on people's sexual health.

At this age, a frequent consumption of drugs may be responsible for decreased desire, including antihypertensives, antidepressants, opioid analgesics, and drugs used for the treatment of benign prostatic hyperplasia.

- Psychological and relationship factors

Different psychological problems can lead to decreased sexual desire. These include depressive syndrome or anxiety disorders, especially in men. During menopause, changes in mood or sleep disturbances can influence desire in women. Additionally, decreased self-esteem or changes in body images that occur as a result of a disease or its treatment may lead to a deterioration in sexual health.

Relationship problems with partners can lead to decreased libido, especially in women. A bad relationship in and of itself can cause sexual health problems.

Certain stressful life situations, especially the death of a partner, can lead to a permanent abandonment of sexual activity.

- Cultural factors

In our society, the belief that people do not have sex after a certain age is pervasive. This can unconsciously lead older adults to consider it to be normal to not have sexual relationships, motivation or desire. This myth is negated by studies showing that over 80% of people over 60 years of age continue having sex.

The cultural perception of sexuality in young people as a fiery and intense activity and attempts to enforce the social standards of youth and power could influence the sexual activity of the elderly. They leave no opportunity for a more leisurely and intimate sexuality, which could be the ideal type of sexuality for this population.

Factors Determining Sexual Potency

Men's sexual power can be negatively affected by a variety of factors that influence penile erection, including the following:

- A progressive reduction in testosterone levels is responsible for a decrease in male sexual potency, a decrease in nocturnal erections, a decreased duration and stability of erections and an increase in the refractory period after an orgasm that reaches hours or days. Erectile dysfunction affects almost 50% of men between 60 and 70 years old in Spain, and at approximately 70 years old, men may have testosterone levels that are similar to those observed in hypogonadism.
- At any age, toxic habits, such as the use of alcohol, tobacco and other drugs, can decrease sexual potency and increase the risk of erectile dysfunction in men. However, the main habits that affect erection are a sedentary lifestyle and an unbalanced diet.
- Some health problems that are common in older and middle-aged people may be associated with erectile dysfunction. These include the presence of cardiovascular risk factors (e.g. hypertension, sedentary lifestyle, atherosclerosis and high cholesterol), metabolic diseases (e.g. diabetes), chronic renal failure and psychological problems, among other conditions.

On the other hand, the physical factors and physiological changes that occur with ageing do not determine the sexual activity of older people because there are other factors that determine this behaviour, including the following:

- Previous sexual history: The level of sexual activity of each person during earlier life stages is very important to sexual activity in the second part of his or her life.
- The interest and existence of a partner in addition to the health of this partner have special importance in these stages of life. Older people discontinue sexual activities more as a result of a lack of available partners than a lack of interest.
- Physical and psychological health: Health problems can hinder sexual activity. If necessary and to avoid complications related to health problems, changing the usual recommended positions to perform sexual activity using a side or rear position may be advised. The use of a support pillow might also be advised.

Treatment of Sexual Problems During Menopause/Andropause

Treatments for sexual health problems should be adapted to the needs of each patient and must entail a multidisciplinary approach that involves the couple themselves in addition to their physicians, sex therapists, psychiatrists and physiotherapists. Currently, the following different treatment modalities are available that can resolve or alleviate the sexual problems that may arise with age:

- **Couples therapy** should be the first step because it resolves 65% of sexual problems and involves none of the risks associated with more aggressive treatments. It is particularly effective for solving problems related to stress and for enhancing intimacy between partners.
- **Changes in lifestyle** can prevent a sedentary lifestyle, excessive fatigue, obesity and stress or increase the quantity and quality of time spent with one's family. The following changes can be effective: making "appointments" to create time and intimacy with a partner, reducing stress through yoga, participating in support groups, broadening one's sexual repertoire, using lubricants and sexual devices or caring for and improving one's image to increase self-esteem and desire.
- **Drug treatment** is used when previous therapies have failed and can differ according to the sex of the patient:
  - In postmenopausal women with impaired sexual health, the best alternative is treatment with *tibolone*, which addresses sexual desire and improves the symptoms of menopause, such as hot flashes or mood swings.
  - Treatment with oestrogen cream is the most suitable option for women with vaginal atrophy but no other symptoms of menopause.
  - In men, erectile dysfunction can be treated with phosphodiesterase type 5 inhibitors such as *sildenafil*, *vardenafil* or *tadalafil*. These are fairly safe drugs but should not be used if the patient is taking nitrates because of the risk of hypotension.
  - In men with androgen deficiency, the complementary use of testosterone patches or intramuscular testosterone appears to improve sexual responses and mood and to maintain virile characteristics, muscle and bone mass and sexual health.
  - If drug therapy fails, there are alternative therapies that may improve erectile function, such as the use of elastic, a constrictor ring or vacuum systems, the injection of prostaglandin E1 into the corpora cavernosa of the penis or even a prosthetic penis.

In conclusion, even though sex may be constrained by the physical, psychological and social changes that accompany age, this should not disrupt sexual activity. Maturity can be an opportunity for a more intimate or relaxed type of sex. The acceptance of physical changes and a history of good sexual experiences can positively influence the maintenance of sexual health as the years pass. At any age, especially in long-term relationships, a good relationship is the most important factor that influences desire and sexual health. Pharmacological treatments should be reserved for cases in which couples therapy or changing lifestyles have not been effective at improving sexual health.

3. "By nature, women have less sexual desire than men and take longer to reach an orgasm".

Sexual desire is a complex condition that depends on physical, psychological, social and cultural factors and has a different meaning for women and for men. The factors that can affect sexual desire include the following:

- **Physical and hormonal factors**

The serum levels of certain hormones, including testosterone, oestrogen, oxytocin, beta endorphins and prolactin, influence sexual activity. Testosterone is a hormone that stimulates sexual desire in both men and women, but from 30 to 40 years of age, testosterone levels decrease in the blood. Women of childbearing age have a peak secretion of testosterone and androstenedione for half of the ovarian cycle that coincides with ovulation that has been associated with an increase in spontaneous desire. Oestrogens help to maintain trophism and vaginal lubrication. Hence, they indirectly enable pleasurable sex. In postmenopausal women, a decrease in oestrogen levels results in atrophy and decreased vaginal lubrication. These changes may be responsible for less pleasurable or painful intercourse in women (dyspareunia), which could adversely affect their motivation and sexual desire [11].

The existence of organic disease can decrease sexual desire, although it rarely fully prevents sexual activity. However, neurological diseases have a greater significance and can reduce the motivation for sex. The use of certain medications, including antihypertensives, antidepressants, opioid analgesics, anti-androgens and oral contraceptives, may also be responsible for decreased desire [14].

- **Psychological factors**

Different psychological problems, including depression and anxiety, can lead to a decreased sex drive. Psychological disorders that are specifically related to sexual behaviour, such as sexual aversion disorder or hypoactive sexual desire disorder, can also have this effect [11].

Hypoactive sexual desire disorder is characterized by a deficiency or absence of sexual fantasies or the desire for sexual activity, which can cause marked distress in women and difficulties in their relationships with their partner [15].

Additionally, decreased self-esteem and body image changes can occur as a result of certain diseases, and the side effects of some treatments for these conditions can deteriorate sexual health in women [11].

- **Social and cultural factors**

Relationship problems with partners can lead to a decrease in libido, especially in women. A good relationship is fundamental because a stable and harmonious relationship promotes the prompt and satisfactory resolution of any sexual conflicts that may arise. Conversely, a bad relationship itself can cause problems in a couple's sexual life [16]. Additionally, drugs can affect sexual experiences and lead to risky sexual behaviour and social conflicts within the couple [11].

Continued stressful situations facilitate the production of prolactin, and increased in serum prolactin levels decrease sexual desire [17].

In our society, models of education that do not encourage the acceptance of sexuality can have negative effects on sexual desire. Additionally, the false belief that older women do not have sex can unconsciously cause a loss of motivation and desire [11].

The sexual response of men progresses linearly and usually begins with desire. This desire can be triggered by sexual thoughts and fantasies or the urgency to experience sexual satisfaction. However, the female sexual response resembles that of males only occasionally, in particular at the beginning of romantic relationships, after which, women require more stimulation. In general, spontaneous sexual desire decreases with women's increasing age [11].

According to Rosemary Basson, the progression of the sexual response in women is cyclical, and the phases of the female sexual response (desire, excitement, plateau, orgasm and resolution) do not necessarily follow this order but can overlap with each other or progress in an order that can vary according to the situation. Therefore, desire does not usually mark the start of the female sexual response. This entire cycle can be influenced by emotional intimacy, sexual stimulation and the woman's satisfaction with the relationship [18].

The human sexual response to exciting stimuli involves a cycle of motivation that is based on incentives and that comprises the physiological changes and subjective experiences of the individual. Psychological and biological factors influence the processing of sexual stimuli in the brain, causing it to allow or not allow the activation of the next phase of sexual response. The results obtained during both sexual and non-sexual intercourse influence an individual's future motivation to seek intimacy [14].

In conclusion, more so than desire, increasing emotional closeness and commitment to the couple are more frequent motivators for women to initiate a sexual relationship. Once initiated, continuous stimulation can cause an increase in sexual arousal, which can then lead to desire [19]. The fact that sex can be initiated without desire is normal and in no way should be considered a disorder of female sexuality.

Treatment for women who experience problems with sexual desire depends on their phase in reproductive life. Different treatment recommendations can be made, including the following:

- Treating disorders that are responsible for the lack of desire, whether they are natural or psychiatric causes.
- Introducing changes in or decreasing the doses of drug treatments that can influence the lack of desire.
- Introducing changes in lifestyle.
- Initiating sex and couples therapy.
- Initiating drug therapy in some cases.

Drug therapy may be useful in postmenopausal women who are experiencing problems with sexual desire and in premenopausal women with hypoactive sexual desire disorder. In **postmenopausal women**, the use of a drug (*tibolone*) with an effect similar to oestrogen and testosterone has been shown to resolve problems with desire and to improve symptoms [20]. It is also beneficial for treating vaginal atrophy when administered as an oestrogen cream. In women with surgical menopause, treatment with testosterone patches has been shown to improve sexual desire and orgasms [11].

Moreover, in seeking a "female Viagra", different drugs that increase sexual desire in women have been tested or are being tested, including *flibanserin* (initially investigated as an antidepressant drug and approved in the USA only for the **treatment of hypoactive sexual desire in premenopausal women**), *ORL101* (a synthesized melatonin that increases sexual desire for 2 h that is in the research phase) and *Lybrido* (an experimental drug that acts on the brain to increase dopamine secretion and inhibit serotonin, thereby enhancing relaxation and activating sexual desire).

As in the case with desire, the **female orgasm** is a complex process that has biological, psychological and social components. The female orgasm is accompanied by intermittent muscle contractions of the genital and pelvic floor. In addition, involuntary contractions of other muscles (e.g. the sphincter or carpopedal spasms), increases in blood pressure, respiration and heart rate and the sudden release of nervous tension occur. According to some authors, women who reach orgasms more easily have an assertive attitude with their partner (showing understanding but not submitting to their partner's will) and have more sexual fantasies, less anxiety and a more androgynous role and are less submissive, less shy and more demanding. However, the female orgasm is more influenced by qualitative aspects such as **affectivity** than quantitative aspects or the duration of sexual activity. Therefore, to achieve satisfaction in a relationship, individuals are encouraged to view a sexual relationship as a relationship that is based on situations involving emotional intimacy and not one that is focused exclusively on coital activity [12].

The female orgasm may be affected by different disorders, including the following:

- **Physical causes**, such as neurological conditions (e.g. paraplegia and multiple sclerosis), vascular conditions (e.g. myocardial infarction or hypertension), endocrinology-related conditions (e.g. diabetes and thyroid disorders), serious illnesses and the consequences of treatments for them (e.g. breast cancer) or drugs (e.g. antidepressants, anxiolytics, barbiturates and beta blockers).
- **Psychological causes**, such as anxiety about execution (before sexual performance), negative feelings about sex, depressive disorders and traumatic experiences.
- **Cultural factors**, such as girls' education that does not favour the acceptance of sexuality, genitals and pleasure.

In women with orgasmic function disorders, different therapeutic measures can be adopted, such as:

- Treatment for physical or psychological disorders.
- Introducing changes to or decreasing the dose of drug treatments that may have negative influences.
- Reassurances to decrease anxiety.
- Encouragement of communication between the woman and her partner.
- Providing a report to refute false myths.
- Training the pubococcygeus muscles.

Anorgasmia is a sexual function disorder that can affect women. Today, the term "preorgasmia", which assumes that all women are capable of reaching orgasms but must learn to how to do so, is preferred.

In short, the answers to the myth that "by nature, women have less desire and take longer to reach an orgasm" are that no studies support this claim and that sexual desire has a different meaning to women and men. The sexual response of women varies depending on the situation, and unlike men, in women, desire is often not the first stage of a sexual response. This is normal and should not be considered a sexual disorder because in women, motivation may be more important than desire. In women, the most common motivation for starting a sexual encounter is increasing emotional closeness and commitment to the couple. Similar to desire, women's orgasms depend on multiple biological, psychological and social factors. However, the female orgasm is more influenced by qualitative aspects, such as affectivity.

4. "Penis size influences women's pleasure during sex".

The erect penis is a symbol of masculinity. In many cultures, it has become a symbol of different qualities, such as strength, courage, endurance, intelligence, knowledge, dominance over other men, possession of women or love and being loved. During puberty, significant growth of the penis occurs as a result of the actions of testosterone [21].

Men place more importance on penis size than women [22]. A study found that men are especially concerned about their height, their weight and the size of their penis [23]. Several factors can influence the perception that a man has of his penis. These can include self-assessment of one's body image and the influence of the media. Two types of disorders have been described in which there is an unrealistic perception that a penis is abnormal: small penis anxiety (also *small penis syndrome*) and body dysmorphic disorder, or BDD [24].

Penis size is determined by measuring various parameters, such as the flaccid length, stretched flaccid length, erect length, flaccid girth and erect girth. A variety of studies have been performed to analyse penis size. In an analysis of previous works, the following average values were found: 9–10 cm flaccid length, 12–13 cm stretched length, 14–16 cm erect length, 9–10 cm flaccid girth and 12–13 cm erection circumference. Typically, a flaccid penis is shorter than the same penis when erect by 6.5 cm. A few racial differences were also observed [21]. However, in a recent study of men over 17 years of age who were of different races and at different ages, the following average values were found: flaccid length, 9.16 cm; stretched length, 13.24 cm; erect length, 13.12 cm; flaccid circumference, 9.31 cm; and erect circumference, 11.66 cm [25].

When a penis is less than 7.5 cm in length while erect or 4 cm while in a flaccid state, it is considered a micropenis. Only 2.28% of the male population has an abnormally small penis [26].

Some studies have resulted in hypotheses concerning the relationships between penis size, physical characteristics and age. However, significant relationships have not been found between penis size and weight, body mass index, the length of the fingers, foot size, the size of the testicles or age. On the contrary, there was a relationship between height and the length of the penis when stretched or erect [27]. These findings refute various myths that continue to persist in our society.

The female orgasm is an intense feeling of pleasure that is achieved by stimulating erogenous zones and is influenced by biological, psychological and social components [7]. The work of Masters and Johnson established that women can reach orgasm using different forms of stimulation (e.g. clitoral, vaginal penetration, erotic dreams and fantasies) but that a single physiological response is common to all of them. In the vagina, the area of greatest sensitivity is the bottom of the front wall. This area is known as the G-spot (*Grafënberg spot*). If we consider the contributions of recent publications, penis size does not have an influence on the sexual pleasure of women. The satisfaction of a woman is based on orgasms and resolutions, and orgasms are always produced by a women's erectile organ, which is effectively stimulated by sexual intercourse, masturbation or simply using a finger. Sexual arousal affects the female erectile organ, resulting in clitoral erection, congestion and the thickening of the labia minora and spongy body of the female urethra. Because these erectile bodies are the triggers for orgasms, they could be considered the *female penis*. Consequently, whether it is vaginal stimulation or stimulation of the G-spot should not matter when attempting to achieve an orgasm [20].

However, other studies have focused on orgasms that are obtained by vaginal penetration without clitoral stimulation. It appears that women who are able to obtain orgasms mainly by vaginal stimulation are taught to understand that it is important to focus their attention on vaginal sensations during intercourse. Additionally, long penises are preferable for achieving orgasms using this method because they have a greater capacity for causing sexual arousal by stimulating the deep areas of the vagina [28, 29]. These women attribute more importance to sex with vaginal penetration, which presents a challenge to relationships without intercourse [30]. However, these data have been discussed because the alleged vaginal orgasms may actually be caused by the stimulation of the erectile bodies that surround the vaginal entrance [31].

Therefore, although the clitoris is the centre of the orgasmic response in women, sexual arousal is not produced exclusively by clitoral stimulation because a woman's sexual enjoyment involves a balance between physical and emotional factors that should be enhanced [32].

In conclusion, this myth is deeply ingrained in the population, yet it has no medical basis because the most sensitive area of the vagina is the first 2 cm of its entrance, suggesting that penises as small as 6 cm in length can reach these erogenous zones. Even simple friction caused by a wider penis should be able to stimulate these areas without requiring deep penetration.

5. "There are different types of orgasms in women".

The female orgasm is a complex process that has biological, psychological and social components. From a point of view of experiencing pleasure, an orgasm is the culmination of a sexual response that is achieved as a result of the stimulation of erogenous zones. In women, this is characterized by intermittent and rhythmic contractions of the muscles of the pelvic floor and the outermost portion of the vagina (the "orgasmic platform" described by Masters and Johnson) in addition to anal and sometimes uterine contractions [12].

The myth regarding the distinction between vaginal and clitoral orgasms began in studies performed by Sigmund Freud, who considered clitoral orgasms to be a phenomenon of immature women and believed that the response of a mature woman was a vaginal orgasm without clitoral stimulation. Thus, removing the sexuality of the clitoris was a requirement for the development of femininity. In contrast, Alfred Kinsey was one of the first researchers to criticize Freud's ideas about sexuality and the female orgasm. In 1953, he discovered that most women could not have vaginal orgasms, and he thus considered the clitoris to be the main centre of the female sexual response [33]. However, the method used in that study was later questioned [34].

In 1967, research by Masters and Johnson resolved the old psychoanalytic idea of a vaginal orgasm occurring before a clitoral orgasm. Their studies on female sexual responses led them to defend the existence of a single orgasm with different origins. They determined that clitoral structures surround and extend along and inside the vagina that most women can only have clitoral orgasms and that all orgasms involve the same stages of physical response. Based on these findings, they argued that clitoral stimulation was the basis of both types of orgasm, whether it results from either the direct or indirect stimulation of the nerve fibres through penetration (Masters and Johnson). Therefore, they determined that the routes would differ according to the type of orgasm (e.g. clitoral, penetration, erotic dreams and fantasies) but that the physiological response would be common to all of them. Hence, although one might think that there are several types of orgasm, there is actually only one type (clitoral), and what varies is the mechanism of stimulation and input.

In the 1980s, discussions concerning the G-spot (*Grafënberg spot*) arose, and this caused the controversy over the existence of different types of orgasms to re-emerge. Some authors argued for a distinction between vulvar and uterine orgasms, the latter being caused by the stimulation of the G-spot. In fact, there was not a particular point but a particularly sensitive area that was located in the anterior and inferior wall of the vagina [35].

According to other authors, the G-spot consists of a shaft located inside the vagina that coordinates the operation of the structure formed by the clitoris, urethra and vaginal wall and the associated network of nerves, muscles and glands (the clitoral-urethral-vaginal complex) [27, 36]. Stimulating this area would trigger an orgasmic response in women. There appears to be anatomical and physiological evidence supporting the existence of the G-spot or the clitoral-urethral-female orgasm [31].

Sexual thoughts and fantasies are present during sexual activity and differ between women and men. Studies that utilize imaging techniques to explore the brain mechanisms that are involved in orgasms seem to confirm that there are differences in the processing of sexual stimuli between women and men. However, the levels of the hormone oxytocin in the blood increase during all sexual activity in both women and men, and they reach maximum values during orgasm [37].

The assumption that women may experience only the clitoral, external orgasm is not based on the best available scientific evidence [38]. In some researches, women have greater orgasm during deeper penile-vaginal intercourse without concurrent clitoral masturbation and even they prefer longer penis [30]. However, according to Puppo V and

Puppo V and Puppo G, G-spot/vaginal/clitoral orgasm, vaginally activated orgasmand clitorally activated orgasm, are incorrect terms; the correct term is "female orgasm"[31].

Multi-orgasms involve achieving several orgasms during the same sexual response. Currently, no clear hypotheses are available to explain the mechanisms that produce this phenomenon. Orgasms are followed by a refractory period during which further stimulation produces no excitation. It is therefore difficult to cause a sexual response during this time. Women often do not present a refractory period except after intense orgasms, and they may therefore be able to quickly experience an additional or multiple orgasms. It is thought that this period is related to the release of the hormone prolactin [39, 40].

Consequently, the answer to this myth is that in women, there is only one type of orgasm physiologically, but it can be reached through different pathways, such as clitoral stimulation, penetration, erotic dreams, sexual fantasies or a mixture thereof. Although there are differences in how orgasms are perceived, the mechanisms involved in their production are similar in all cases. In women, the ability to achieve several orgasms (multi-orgasms) during the same sexual response has been observed.

6. "Removing the uterus and ovaries causes women to lose their sexual appetite and prevents them from feeling sexual enjoyment".

The uterus has historically been considered a regulator and controller of important physiological functions in addition to a sexual organ and a source of energy, vitality and maintenance of youthfulness and attractiveness in women. It is therefore not surprising that some women may feel that their sex life could be affected by the removal of the organ [41].

Female sexual responses are complex because they are influenced by physical and emotional factors and women's sexual experiences. Unlike what occurs in men, desire is not usually the beginning of the female sexual response. The female orgasm is also a complex process that is characterized by intermittent and rhythmic muscle contractions of the pelvic floor and the outermost portion of the vagina, anus and sometimes the uterus, which results in a more pleasurable feeling [42].

Women in stable relationships may be more concerned about emotional intimacy with their partners, and although in some cases, the frequency of sexual intercourse can be related to a better sex life; female sexual functions are more a matter of quality than quantity. Thus, the sexual well-being of women should not be defined as the mere absence of sexual dysfunction.

The operation that is used to surgically remove the uterus is called a hysterectomy. Hysterectomies may be limited to the uterus body (subtotal hysterectomy) or the body and the uterus neck (total hysterectomy), or they may also include the fallopian tubes, ovaries and surrounding lymph nodes (radical hysterectomy). The application of one or another of these surgical techniques depends on the type of pathology to be treated, whether it is benign or malignant and, if necessary, the degree of tumour extension.

A hysterectomy may be necessary to treat tumours of the neck or body of the uterus or advanced endometriosis or prolapse, among other conditions. These conditions may be responsible for pelvic pain, painful intercourse (dyspareunia) or vaginal bleeding unrelated to menstruation, all of which can negatively influence the sexual health of women. Therefore, removing the uterus may improve the sexual relations of women who are affected by these problems.

When a subtotal or total hysterectomy is performed, it may affect the ligaments, blood vessels and nerves that are involved in sexual function. Moreover, following a total hysterectomy, the shortening of the dome of the vagina could be responsible for dyspareunia. However, there are currently conservative surgical techniques that can preserve the nerves that innervate the pelvic organs [43].

A hysterectomy does not adversely affect sexual health. Most women who have only their uterus removed will have equal or better sexual function after the surgery than before, probably because their symptoms and previous problems are relieved. In this sense, some authors claim that after a subtotal or total hysterectomy, women experience a decrease in abdominal pain and increased desire, excitability and the frequency of intercourse. However, in women whose previous sexual experiences were not good, their sexual health is often worse after surgery [44].

In addition to hysterectomies, the removal of the ovaries may be necessary for the treatment of some benign, premalignant or malignant diseases of the internal genitalia [45]. In postmenopausal women, the removal of the ovaries causes no symptoms or major changes to their sexual health, but in premenopausal woman, it causes surgical menopause, with sudden and intense hormonal changes and subsequent consequences, mainly climacteric syndrome (hot flashes, sweating, psychological problems, insomnia, etc.) and impaired sexual function [46]. In this sense, women with surgical menopause show an increased risk of developing hypoactive sexual desire disorder [28] and more emotional involvement than premenopausal women who experience natural menopause [13]. Additionally, a lower frequency of sexual intercourse, difficulty in lubrication, reduced sexual satisfaction, dyspareunia and difficulty achieving orgasm [47] has been observed in women with surgical menopause.

The bilateral removal of the ovaries in premenopausal women causes a significant decrease in the levels of oestrogen and testosterone in the blood [46], which may explain some of the changes observed in these patients. Lower levels of oestrogen cause atrophy and decreased vaginal lubrication, which can cause less pleasurable or even painful sex in women, and this could negatively influence their sexual motivations and desire. The hypothesis in which a decline in blood testosterone causes hypoactive sexual desire disorder and sexual dysfunction in women with surgical menopause has not been supported [48]. In all hysterectomy cases, it is recommended that women practice sexual self-stimulation 2 weeks after surgery because it allows them to experience pleasure without the pressure that can be exerted when in a relationship [12].

Some problems related to surgical menopause can be treated by oestrogen hormone therapy, which mitigates hot flashes and vaginal dryness and reduces dyspareunia, but it is less clear what effect this therapy may have on improving sexual function [47]. Testosterone replacement therapy patches seem to improve sexual desire and the frequency of intercourse and orgasms. In our experience, the use of tibolone has proved more effective in improving the sexual health of these women [11].

Moreover, psycho-educational therapy has been proposed to help women with surgical menopause to manage their sexual health problems. Short educational sessions on sexual health, body awareness and relaxation techniques seem to have a positive effect [49]. Preoperative knowledge of the possible side effects decreased sexual distress after surgery [50].

In conclusion, removing the uterus does not adversely affect the sexual health of women. In most cases, the relief of symptoms and previous problems leads equal to or better sexual performance than they experienced before the surgery. In postmenopausal woman, removing the ovaries does not cause major changes. However, in premenopausal woman, it induces surgical menopause, which leads to sudden hormonal changes and impaired sexual functions and can be treated with hormone therapy and psycho-educational methods.

7. "Sexual intercourse should be avoided during pregnancy".

Pregnancy should be understood as a physiological state that is considered within normal limits. A pregnant woman does not have to significantly vary her behaviour or abandon activities for which she is qualified solely because she is pregnant. However, basic precautions should be taken. We must therefore abandon the false beliefs that "a pregnant woman is a sick woman" or "sexual activity during pregnancy may harm the foetus".

To support this response, we provide the following arguments.

During pregnancy, women experience changes that may affect their sex life. These changes are due to:

- **Biological factors** that are the result of the hormonal and structural changes that characterize pregnancy. Some of these can be positive, such as vasocongestion in the vagina, which increases lubrication and could favour orgasms. Some women experience uterine contractions after orgasms due to the production of oxytocin, but this normal phenomenon does not cause alterations in the foetus.
- **Emotional factors**. The sexual activity of women is strongly influenced by emotional aspects, in which false beliefs, a fear of harm coming to the foetus and inadequate medical advice come into play.

During pregnancy, sexual activity is often decreased, but after pregnancy, an increase in physical sexual contact is often not experienced. It is essential that the couple maintain a positive attitude and that they observe the changes that occur in the woman while adapting their sexual activity to retain a satisfactory level. The relationship must be a source of support for the pregnant women, and the couple should consider communication to be a fundamental component of the relationship because many women have feelings of guilt due to the decreased sexual desire they experience and because their partner may feel unsatisfied.

Most pregnant women experience increased sexual desire during the second trimester of pregnancy, when they perceive that the risk of abortion has decreased. In contrast, there is usually a significant decrease in sexual activity at the end of pregnancy due to hormonal changes, the women's level of discomfort and a fear of causing harm to the child [51].

Sexual activity during pregnancy has **positive aspects**. As previously mentioned, sexual activity during pregnancy carries psychological and marital benefits, but it is also positive for the course of pregnancy, as has been shown by some studies. It has been found, for example, that vaginal penetration during week 39 of gestation is positive for childbirth because semen contains substances (prostaglandins) that help the maturation of the cervix. In addition, tactile stimulation of the nipples stimulates the release of oxytocin, which causes uterine contractions and helps induce labour in term pregnancies (between 37 and 42 weeks of gestation) but does not favour the occurrence of premature birth (before 37 weeks). Sexual intercourse during pregnancy reduces the number of cases in which it is medically necessary to induce labour [52].

It has been hypothesized that oral sex may decrease the risk of preeclampsia (a type of hypertension in pregnancy that can be severe) as a result of immune tolerance to the semen of the father [53].

The Influence of Sexual Activity on Some Complications of Pregnancy

One factor that influences the reduction of sex during pregnancy is the mistaken belief that damage can be inflicted on the foetus during sexual activity.

It is not possible to cause direct harm to the foetus during penetration because it is surrounded by the amniotic sac and protected by the closed cervix. In addition, the angle of the vagina and the penis during penetration does not allow the penis to have direct contact with the bottom of the vagina and cervix. However, face-to-face intercourse with the man above the woman is discouraged, and couples are encouraged to seek other positions that better accommodate the woman's anatomy. The side-to-side position has been proposed as the most desirable, manageable and enjoyable position for women [54].

One way the foetus could be harmed is by the occurrence of complications. Only some of the possible complications of pregnancy require taking precautions during sexual activity, including the following:

- In women with a high risk of abortion in the first trimester of pregnancy, sexual activity is discouraged as part of commonly prescribed rest. However, this does not justify the requirement that woman without a risk of abortion should maintain sexual abstinence during the first trimester of pregnancy [51].
- When vaginal bleeding occurs before delivery as a result of placenta previa or any other cause, sexual abstinence is recommended.
- In women at high risk of preterm delivery, sexual abstinence is recommended because there is some evidence supporting this practice. Abstinence is advised as an easy measure to prevent potential complications. In women at low risk of preterm delivery, it is not necessary to take these precautions except in women with frequent sexual activity who suffer from genital tract colonization of certain microorganisms (e.g. *Trichomonas vaginalis* and *Mycoplasma hominis*). Sexual activity does not increase the risk of preterm labour in women who have no symptoms/evidence of infection [51].
- An increased risk of premature membrane rupture (amniotic sac) was identified only in asymptomatic women with small breaks.

However, no evidence has indicated that sexual activity during pregnancy increases the risk of complications such as pelvic inflammatory disease or preeclampsia or that it increases the risk of having twins [51].

In conclusion, sex is safe throughout pregnancy, especially in low-risk pregnancies. In the absence of complications, the only precaution is to adopt a safe and comfortable position for the woman. Sex is only discouraged in the event of pregnancy complications, such as a high risk of abortion during the first trimester, a diagnosis of placenta previa or a high risk of preterm delivery.

8. "There are no frigid women, but inexperienced men".

In the past, men were concerned with only their own sexual satisfaction. In fact, some elderly men still boast of having been *very quick* in their youth, possibly referring to premature ejaculation. However, social changes occurred during the second half of the twentieth century, and new knowledge has become available about sexuality and effective contraception that have enabled human reproduction to be separated from the search for pleasurable sex. In addition, some reports about female sexuality have been of great importance, such as the *Kinsey Report*, which allowed the sexual demands of women to be made public.

The facts show that women increasingly need to be sexually satisfied, but in the context of a macho social environment, men assume responsibility for female pleasure. In the realm of sex, men's success came to be defined by their power and their latency time to ejaculation, which allowed women to achieve multiple orgasms. Thus, if we add sexual stress to the life stress that exists in our society, we should not be surprised that some men suffer from performance anxiety, a disorder that occurs as a result of fear of inadequate sexual performance or "not measuring up" in which the couple remains sexually unsatisfied. This can significantly affect erections and the ejaculatory response. It is likely that high levels of anxiety cause erection problems, whereas more moderate anxiety is responsible for premature ejaculation [17].

The female orgasm depends less on quantitative aspects (e.g. the duration of sexual activity) and more on qualitative aspects (e.g. affectivity). It is therefore wise to seek accurate information about sexual health and to discredit social and sexual stereotypes to prevent relationships from becoming stressful rather than pleasant for intimacy with one's partner, which should be the real goal of any sexual relationship [12].

Education and attitudes can help people to achieve this goal. The following tips should be useful for disproving this false myth:

- As a couple, analyse issues such as responsibility and roles in sexual intercourse to learn to understand that each person is responsible for his or her own orgasmic response.
- Improve the couple's level of knowledge of female and male sexual responses and prevent coital activity from being the focus of all sexual activities.
- Explore new perspectives of sexuality to show that it can be based on situations involving emotional intimacy and consider that sexual relationships do not need to end with ejaculation.

In conclusion, this false belief is based on two recent social phenomena: women claimed their need for sexual gratification and men have assumed the responsibility for women's sexual pleasure because of a chauvinistic social environment. The acceptance of this social role by men may cause performance anxiety in some individuals, leading to disorders in sexual functions and thereby adversely affecting the individual's health and that of their sexual partners. Therefore, with regard for sexual stereotypes, it is advisable to avoid them and to advance one's knowledge so that he or she can enjoy pleasant moments of intimacy with one's partner.

9. "Race plays a role in enjoying greater sexual impulses and power".

In the information provided in the answers to some of the other myths, we indicated that multiple factors could influence sexual desire, potency or orgasm in both women and men. These factors can be biological (e.g. testosterone, oestrogen, medications, cardiovascular disease, diabetes, neurologic disorders, cancer and their treatments), psychological (e.g. anxiety and depression), social (e.g. drug use, one's relationship with their partner or continued stress) or cultural (e.g. type of education or sexual myths that are deeply rooted in society). However, we have not identified any studies that indicate that certain racial groups have greater impulses or sexual potency. On the contrary, differences in attitudes and sexual behaviour are probably due to social, cultural or religious factors.

Some data that may help to dismantle this false myth are:

- In some studies, the association between race or ethnicity and the frequency of sexual problems were studied, and higher frequencies of certain sexual problems were observed in blacks. The black population seemed to experience more frequent sexual problems, while Hispanics were less likely to suffer from them [55].
- Black women have higher rates of low sexual desire and unpleasant relationships than white women, who are more likely to have problems with vaginal lubrication during sexual intercourse. In contrast, Hispanic women have lower rates of sexual problems. However, other studies have reported that black women with disorders have a lower frequency of sexual desire [56].
- A recent study of young US women compared differences in attitudes towards sexuality between black and white women. Black women generally had less positive attitudes towards juvenile sex outside of marriage, contraception and motherhood and fewer expectations of sexual desire. The factors responsible for these differences were not racial but were religious, social and family related and included lower educational levels and lower socioeconomic status among black women [48].
- In men, racial differences appear to be more limited, but black men have reported having less pleasant relationships. It has been argued that being black is a risk factor for erectile dysfunction [57]. In some military studies performed on black populations, higher rates of erectile dysfunction and other sexual problems were reported [58, 59]. However, the increased frequency of erectile dysfunction that was observed in black men was not motivated by race itself but by other highly prevalent factors that present risks to the African American population (e.g. obesity, diabetes, physical inactivity and lower socioeconomic status) [59, 60]. Genitourinary diseases are also more common in people of colour [61].

In conclusion, there are no data supporting the notion that certain races have better sexual health. A person in good general health, whether they are male or female, black or white or European or American, has an excellent chance of enjoying a good sex drive. Greater or lesser sexual power is not determined by the colour of one's skin but is related to a number of both complex biological, psychological, social and /or spiritual variables. It is expected that a person in optimal health will have a good sex drive, regardless of their race or ethnicity. If, on the other hand, the person is in poor health, he or she could experience poor sexual performance.

10. "Ejaculation is synonymous with orgasm; when a man ejaculates, intercourse ends".

Sexual responses are influenced by testosterone levels in the blood and facilitated by dopamine-mediated activities in the anterior hypothalamus of the brain [62]. Male sexual responses generally have a linear progression, as described in the models proposed by Masters and Johnson and Helen S. Kaplan, and consists of several interactive consecutive phases: desire, arousal, plateau, orgasm and resolution [63, 64]. Next, we present the most relevant information for each of these characteristic phases.

Sexual desire is triggered by sexual thoughts and fantasies and the urge to experience sexual satisfaction. Hormonally, prolactin decreases sexual desire, whereas testosterone enhances sexual interest.

In the **excitement phase**, there is an increase in the heart rate, muscle tension and vascular congestion in the genitals, during which penile erection and the secretion of a fluid that lubricates the urethra occurs. This phase can last from a few minutes to several hours and coincides with an increase in the blood hormone vasopressin. The excitement phase is influenced by several factors, including age, the situation or novelty of the couple and the frequency of sexual activity.

In the **plateau phase**, the above changes become more intense, the sphincter of the bladder closes so that the semen and urine do not mix, and rhythmic contractions of muscles in the penis begin.

In men, the **orgasm phase** is usually achieved with the ejaculation of semen, though this is not always the case. During the orgasm phase, serum levels of the hormone oxytocin reach maximum levels [65].

In the **resolution phase**, a general sense of well-being occurs, vital signs and muscle tone return to normal levels, and pelvic vascular congestion is reduced.

Finally, a **refractory period** takes place in which it is difficult to reach a new orgasm. This phase can last from a few minutes to several days, although a partial or complete penile erection can often be maintained. The refractory period increases as men age. Increased levels of the hormone prolactin have been detected in the blood during this stage [66].

Orgasm and ejaculation are two different physiological processes that are sometimes difficult to distinguish [67]. Ejaculation is a complex physiological process involving neuronal, neurochemical and hormonal control. In the ejaculatory reflex, sensory receptors in the genitals, nerve pathways, sensory areas of the brain and motor centres of the brain and spinal cord interact with the muscles and organs of the genital area. This reflex is the result of complex interactions between neurons in the central nervous system (CNS, the brain and spinal cord) that use characteristic neurotransmitters, particularly serotonin and dopamine, and the less available neurotransmitters acetylcholine, norepinephrine, oxytocin, GABA and nitric oxide [68].

Antegrade (outward) ejaculation consists of two phases: emission and expulsion. Serotonin inhibits seminal emission and expulsion, while dopamine promotes both. In the emission phase, semen (a sperm mixture containing prostatic fluid and seminal fluid) is prepared for subsequent expulsion. This process involves a sympathetic reflex contraction in which the epididymis, vas deferens, seminal vesicles and prostate facilitate the movement of the components of semen into the prostatic urethra. During this phase, the relaxation of the prostatic urethra is accompanied by a sense of inevitable ejaculation but allows some degree of voluntary control. The expulsion phase is the precise moment when the semen is expelled out of the body. Expulsion is a parasympathetic reflex during which the prostatic urethra is dilated as a result of the accumulation of semen and the triggering of rhythmic contractions of the muscles in the penis and the pelvic floor, which cause the expulsion of the prepared semen. The extent of voluntary control during this phase is either very limited or non-existent, and controlling it requires one to control the progression of sexual arousal [69].

In contrast, an orgasm is a transient feeling of intense pleasure that is accompanied by an altered state of consciousness [67]. Orgasm is a process that develops at the level of the cortex in the brain and is both a cognitive and emotional experience. In men, orgasms are the result of the brain processing a series of sensory stimuli that are caused by the physical changes that accompany ejaculation, such as the initial increase and subsequent release of pressure in the prostatic urethra, the stimulation of the opening of the ejaculatory ducts, the contraction of accessory sex organs and bulbourethral-glands and the perception of muscle contractions in addition to with the expulsion of the semen [69].

Currently, some authors defend the existence of **non-genital orgasms**. In men, orgasmic sensations may occur as a result of the stimulation of certain non-genital body areas, such as the neck, earlobes, armpits, inner thighs, toes, hands, mouth, anus (with or without penetration) and prostate. These orgasms or orgasmic sensations have particular characteristics that are based on the different patterns of innervation of each body area and the region of the brain that processes the information [70].

Orgasms generated in the brain by electrical stimulation of the frontal cortex have also been described. Additionally, epileptic patients describe feelings that are similar to an orgasm before they experience a seizure (orgasmic aura) [71]. It is unclear whether wet dreams during sleep originate in the brain. Furthermore, the effects of some drugs produce experiences that are similar to orgasms.

In the male sexual response, increased arousal reaches a threshold that triggers the ejaculatory reflex. **Ejaculatory latency** is defined as the time it takes a man to ejaculate after vaginal penetration occurs. The latency time (based on the amount of stimulation that the penis receives) thus varies between individuals and even within the same individual, depending on the situation. In general, ejaculatory latency allows for the sexual satisfaction of the partner. Otherwise, premature ejaculation can result in dissatisfaction. In these cases, much of the dissatisfaction is because of a lack of knowledge about the female sexual response and the fact that the sexual relationship is focused almost exclusively on intercourse. The education received by men in our society favours the inhibition of their emotional needs. Hence, many men may try to satisfy their emotional needs through coital sex because situations involving emotional intimacy can cause feelings of shame, insecurity and/or fear.

It is therefore important to consider that intercourse is not the only alternative to emotional intimacy and to explore new perspectives on sexual relationships with partners that are based on situations of emotional intimacy while taking into account that intercourse does not end with ejaculation. The time spent on foreplay and the development of fantasies allows the couple to relax and enjoy physical contact without focusing exclusively on a genital response, and this allows men to reduce their excitability and to thereby maintain better control over their ejaculation [72].

In short, the answer to this myth is that ejaculation and orgasm are two different concepts. Ejaculation is a complex reflexive action that involves neurochemical and hormonal control mechanisms and that consists of two phases: the preparation of semen and its expulsion. However, an orgasm is a transient feeling of intense pleasure that involves the brain, which processes the sensory stimuli that accompany the expulsion of semen. Therefore, the relationship does not end with ejaculation, although some men feel that the goal of every intimate relationship is to reach orgasm through intercourse. Because the real purpose of a relationship should be for the couple to share an intimate and enjoyable time, it does not necessarily require ejaculation.

11. "Premature ejaculation only occurs in young men".

The frequency of premature ejaculation in the male population varies greatly in different studies, probably as a result of the different methods that are used to obtain data. The results indicate that premature ejaculation could affect approximately 15–30% of adult males. Some authors consider problems with premature ejaculation to be the most common problem in male sexual health, although in many cases go undiagnosed or untreated [73, 74].

In adult males, premature ejaculation occurs in all age groups. Theoretically, younger men tend to ejaculate more quickly than older men, perhaps because of the novelty of sex, and controlling ejaculation seems to be associated with sexual experience. However, this should not lead to the assumption that premature ejaculation affects only young men.

Different studies have investigated the prevalence of premature ejaculation in different ages and provided conflicting results. In a study of men aged 18–59 years old, no significant differences were found the age of affected individuals [55]. One study reported that the frequency of premature ejaculation became lower with advanced age [74], whereas some authors have noted that older men have a shorter ejaculatory latency (the time from vaginal penetration to ejaculation) than younger men, and consequently, older age was associated with a tendency towards faster ejaculation [75].

Premature ejaculation is more common in men with a low level of academic training and in those who have infrequent sex. Some authors have found it to be more common in black men [76].

The causes of premature ejaculation are not well understood, but different hypotheses involving biological and psychological theories have been proposed, most of which have not been supported. The validation of some of these theories is used to justify current treatments for premature ejaculation that involve SSRIs and cognitive behavioural therapies.

One hypothesis suggests that there is a genetic predisposition to inheriting **intravaginal ejaculatory latency time** (IELT). Ejaculation is regulated by various neurotransmitters, one of which is serotonin. Serotonin is involved in the ejaculation reflex and acts by inhibiting the expulsion of semen. One study demonstrated that there is a relationship between different forms of the gene for the serotonin transporter protein and IELT, and some genotypes are associated with shorter IELT [77]. These results could explain the presence of primary premature ejaculation (lifelong) and the high frequency of this dysfunction in some families [68].

Acquired premature ejaculation can result from sexual performance anxiety, psychological or relationship problems, inflammation of the prostate, erection problems, hyperthyroidism or the use of some drugs and drug detoxification processes.

One theory that seeks to explain secondary premature ejaculation suggests that a high level of performance anxiety and excessive concern over possible failure could distract the male and reduce his ability to control and recognize the sensations that precede an impending ejaculation, which would facilitate the expulsion of semen [68].

In conclusion, premature ejaculation can occur in adult males at any age. However, in the studies conducted to date, its frequency in different age group is not well defined, with some studies finding no significant differences between age groups and other studies identifying a lower frequency of premature ejaculation in older age groups.

12. "A solution to premature ejaculation is to have unpleasant thoughts and/or thoughts unrelated to intercourse".

Premature ejaculation is a disorder that has been studied for over 100 years. Hence, the concept and definition of this sexual dysfunction has changed over time and should be periodically updated [78]. In this regard, the International Society of Sexual Medicine (ISSM) convened a group of experts in 2013 to establish a set of recommendations for diagnosing and treating premature ejaculation [79].

Current definitions include three key aspects related to a diagnosis of premature ejaculation (PE) [54]:

- A short ejaculatory latency (the time from vaginal penetration to ejaculation)
- A perceived lack of control or an inability to delay ejaculation
- Distress and interpersonal difficulties in the individual and/or a couple-related disorder

The Diagnostic and Statistical Manual of Mental Disorders (5th Edition, DSM 5) defines premature ejaculation as "a persistent or recurrent pattern of ejaculation produced during sexual activity with a partner that happens approximately the minute after vaginal penetration and before the person wishes" [80].

The definition proposed by the ISSM in 2013 includes the three characteristics mentioned above and defines premature ejaculation as "a male sexual dysfunction characterized by ejaculation that always or nearly always occurs prior to or within the first minute of vaginal penetration, present from the first sexual or in consecutive experiences, a frustrating change in ejaculatory latency, an inability to delay ejaculation in all or nearly all vaginal penetrations, with negative personal consequences, such as distress, worry, frustration and/or avoidance of sexual intimacy" [79].

According to this definition, there are two main types of premature ejaculation: primary PE (lifelong), which begins with early sexual experiences, and acquired PE (has an onset after a period of normal ejaculatory function). However, it is limited to heterosexual men who are performing vaginal intercourse because few available studies have explored premature ejaculation in homosexual men or men performing other forms of sexual expression [68].

Men who have sporadic ejaculation problems often think that their partner is not satisfied, which increases their anxiety and creates low self-esteem, thus reinforcing the problem. This can cause difficulties with erection or avoidance of sexual intercourse. Thus, the couple and the relationship may be affected by the man's reaction. In these cases, the goal should be the satisfaction of the couple and not ejaculatory control because focusing on the first of these may lead to anxiety levels being reduced to the extent that control over ejaculation could occur on its own.

If the goal is to decrease anxiety and to control arousal, men should be aware of their level of excitement so that they can reduce it, if necessary. Therefore, strategies that promote "thinking about something else" are not recommended. According to some authors, distraction is a self-help mechanism that is used in 80% of men with premature ejaculation, even though this could cause problems with erection. Conversely, it may be advisable to reduce physical sexual arousal using pelvic movements, more relaxed penetration positions and breathing more slowly using the diaphragm (abdominal breathing) [72].

The perception of the time it takes to ejaculate in a sexual relationship is subjective and differs for each man. Men with **premature ejaculation, whether subjective or variable** (false or occasional, respectively), may have unrealistic expectations of treatment outcomes that are based on incorrect perceptions of normal sexual functions. In these cases, psycho-educational interventions can be used without drugs [68].

Treating premature ejaculation can involve the use of pharmacological agents, either daily or as needed, as the sole treatment for delaying ejaculation or a combination of drug therapy and psychosexual counselling as part of an integrated programme of treatment to delay ejaculation and reduce the anxiety associated with the disorder.

Pharmacotherapy

Daily drug treatment is performed using SSRI antidepressants (selective serotonin reuptake inhibitors) such as *paroxetine*, *sertraline*, *fluoxetine*, *citalopram* and *clomipramine* (a tricyclic antidepressant). At the doses used to treat premature ejaculation, these drugs are effective, safe and well tolerated. The delay in ejaculation begins 5–10 days after a patient starts treatment, but its effect is not achieved until 2 or 3 weeks after initiation. Adverse effects are rare, include mild nausea, diarrhoea, fatigue, yawning and perspiration, and usually disappear within 2 or 3 weeks. It is also important to not abruptly stop treatment [81].

Drug treatment that is administered as needed, for example, before initiating sexual intercourse, is performed using another SSRI, *dapoxetine*, which was developed specifically to treat male sexual dysfunction. This medication should be taken 1–3 h before initiating a scheduled sexual relationship and plays an important role in ejaculatory control, the sexual satisfaction of the patient and his partner, reduced personal distress and improvement in the couple and the relationship. Side effects, such as headache, dizziness, nausea and diarrhoea, are rare and depend on the dose (30 or 60 mg) [82].

Treatment with a local anaesthetic cream, gel or aerosol that is a desensitizing topical agent is based on the theory that men with premature ejaculation may have a high sensitivity to the stimulation of their penis. Local anaesthetics are moderately effective in delaying ejaculation, but they may decrease the sensitivity of the penis and cause a lack of orgasm in women if a condom is not used [83].

Behavioural Psychotherapy

Sexual psychotherapy techniques are based on the theory that premature ejaculation occurs because a man does not pay enough attention to his level of sexual arousal prior to orgasm. Although the success of some methods is relatively positive in the short term, there is no conclusive evidence regarding the long-term results of these methods [68].

- The *stop-start* manoeuvre of Semans consists of self-stimulation that is aimed at identifying the sensations that precede ejaculation, stopping motion and then repeating the manoeuvre. After a period of training, the man is joined by his partner, and when the couple has become familiar with the procedure, they are instructed to practice vaginal penetration in succession, asking the man to stop when pre-ejaculatory sensations are perceived.
- The Masters and Johnson model involves a systematic desensitization technique that consists of sensate focusing. The couple exchanges caresses without performing intercourse. The focus on the senses is intended to allow the patient to focus on his own feelings and not the feelings of the couple. This reduces anxiety and increases comfort with erotic situations.
- Once the phase prior to coitus has been reached, the compression technique can be used. This involves pressing the tip of the penis when the sensation prior to ejaculation is

perceived and asking the couple to apply the pressure to reduce arousal and erection.

In conclusion, the answer to this myth is that distracting thoughts during intercourse are not a solution for premature ejaculation. Pharmacological treatments (primarily *dapoxetine*) and behavioural psychological therapies (when there is performance anxiety) are currently available that have been shown to be successful treatment options for these individuals. However, when the problem is only occasional, it is advisable to discuss it with the couple to try to control anxiety and thus ejaculation.

13. "It is deviant to have sexual fantasies about someone else during sex".

Sexual fantasies are thoughts with sexual content that are positively experienced by most individuals. They comprise mental representations of erotic desires that can occur spontaneously or voluntarily or be caused by other thoughts and perceptions of our senses.

Sexual fantasies are important because they seem to be associated with **better sexual functioning** [37]: they increase desire, enhance arousal in both women and men and increase sexual satisfaction. In addition, **most people fantasize during sex**, during masturbation or when daydreaming [84].

Based on their content, four types of sexual fantasies can be distinguished [85]:

- Intimate: those that place importance on feelings and relate to commitment to a limited number of sexual partners.
- Exploratory: those that relate to sexual variety, promiscuity and group sex.
- Impersonal: those that place little value on feelings and relate to fetishes, such as clothes or erotic films.
- Sadomasochistic: those that focus on causing or suffering from pain during sexual arousal and therefore on dominant or submissive attitudes.

The most common sexual thoughts are very similar in both sexes. However, there are differences between the sexual fantasies of men and women. These differences are likely the result of social factors, such as gender roles, rather than a consequence of biological sex [86].

Men's fantasies have very varied subjects, are often explicit, involve visual and domination fantasies and include more sexual activities that involve a group. Women's fantasies are more submissive. Women usually imagine a smaller variety of sexual activities and include intimate and romantic fantasies and fewer sexual partner issues [37].

Thus, the five most common fantasies between women and men are, in order of occurrence [87]:

- Sexual activity with a partner: both women and men
- Sexual activity with another couple: both women and men
- Sexual activity with two or more women: more frequent in men
- Sexual activity with a stranger: more frequent in women
- Sexual activity with a co-worker: both men and women

Sexual thoughts can be perceived both positively and/or negatively. Positive sexual thoughts are acceptable, pleasant and enjoyable for the person experiencing them, while negative sexual thoughts are unacceptable and unpleasant, and the person experiencing them does not want to perform these actions. The most common negative thoughts are sadomasochistic and have been implicated with neurotic and obsessive personality traits.

Attitude towards fantasies are also important because having a favourable attitude towards sexual fantasies and perceiving them as something positive increases desire and the frequency of masturbation and sexual satisfaction. In contrast, negative thoughts are related to low desire and arousal and lower satisfaction [37].

Another positive aspect of erotic fantasies is their possible use in sex therapy during the process of rehabilitation in people with sexual dysfunctions because the development of sexual fantasies can reduce anxiety and increase desire, thereby improving sexual health [12].

In conclusion, having sexual fantasies is a good way to promote sexual health in both healthy people and people with sexual dysfunctions. A good tool to facilitate this could be erotic literature.

14. "Male or female masturbation is a sign that something is wrong sexually with the couple".

Masturbation is completely natural. It is a private act that can be practiced alone or with a partner, and it does not cause physical or mental problems, as implied by some sexual myths. Only in the event of feelings of fear or guilt could problems with sexual health occur.

Masturbation is usually preceded by erotic fantasies and is probably influenced by testosterone levels [12]. These events coincide with **increased testosterone**, as reflected in:

- **Fantasies** and erotic dreams
- The physical excitement of others

- Lubrication and spontaneous genital swelling
- The **need to masturbate** or to find a partner

According to some studies, 81% of adolescents have masturbated. Males masturbate more often, although 10% of them experience feelings of guilt. Boys experience masturbation more positively than girls, who have more negative attitudes and reserve pleasure for a relationship [88].

Nevertheless, masturbation has a number of benefits, such as:

- Encouraging self-awareness of the body and helping to increase the safety and quality of future sex.
- Relieving sexual tension and helping individuals relax.
- Maintaining interest in sexual activity and energy.
- In girls, it helps to reduce the discomfort that may accompany menstruation.

Adolescents and adult men can grow to understand their sexual responses using masturbation and thereby learn to control their ejaculation using techniques such as the stop-start manoeuvre and the compression technique [31]. Therefore, those who masturbate slowly while fantasizing have better ejaculatory responses than those who compulsively masturbate to relieve tension [12].

In women, stimulating the vagina using masturbation at an early age seems to improve the ability to achieve orgasms through vaginal penetration in adulthood [29].

In short, masturbation is a **sexual practice that is as valid as any other** that plays an important role in the establishment of self-knowledge and personal sexual preferences. Masturbation, including sexual fantasies, is not only acceptable in all its forms but can also be used to treat certain sexual dysfunctions because it can help to improve self-knowledge and the development of sexuality. Based on these findings, masturbation and sexual fantasies are recommended for all persons who wish to practice them, either alone or with a partner.

References

1. World Health Organization. Defining sexual health: report of a technical consultation on sexual health, 28–31 January 2002. Geneva: WHO; 2006.
2. World Association for Sexual Health (WAS). Declaration for sexual rights. March 2014. http://www.worldsexology.org.
3. Liga Española de la Educación, Ministerio de Sanidad, Servicios Sociales e Igualdad. Relaciones afectivas y sexualidad en la adolescencia. Madrid; 2013.
4. Sex Education Forum. Sex educational supplement. March 2016. http://www.sexeducationforum.org.uk.
5. Guttmacher Institute. Review of key findings of "Emerging answers 2007". Report on Sex Education Programs. Guttmacher Institute; 2007.
6. Lorrie Gavin L, MacKay AP, Brown K, Harrier S, Ventura SJ, Kann L, et al. Sexual and reproductive health of persons aged 10-24 years, United States, 2002-2007. MMWR Surveill Summ. 2009;58(6):1–58.
7. Kirby D. Emerging answers 2007: research findings on programs to reduce teen pregnancy and sexually transmitted diseases. Washington DC: The National Campaign to Prevent Teen and Unplanned Pregnancy; 2007.
8. Sexuality Information and Education Council of the United States. The guidelines for comprehensive sexuality education: grades K-12. 3rd ed. National Guidelines Task Force; 2004. Kth= Kindergarten 12th It´s a National Guidelines (USA)
9. Forhan SE, Gottlieb SL, Sternberg MR, Xu F, Datta SD, McQuillan GM, et al. Prevalence of sexually transmitted infections among female adolescents aged 14 to 19 in the United States. Pediatrics. 2009;124:1505–12.
10. Ministerio de Sanidad, servicios sociales e igualdad. Interrupciones voluntarias de embarazo. 2014. http://www.msssi.gob.es/profesionales/saludPublica/prevPromocion/embarazo.
11. Sánchez-Borrego R, Molero F, Castaño R, Castelo-Branco C, Honrado M, Jurado AR, et al. Spanish consensus on sexual health in men and women over 50. Maturitas. 2014;78:138–45.
12. Cabello SF. Manual de sexología y terapia sexual. Madrid: Editorial Síntesis; 2010.
13. Dennerstein L, Koochaki P, Barton I, Graziottin A. Hypoactive sexual desire disorder in menopausal women: a survey of Western European women. J Sex Med. 2006;3(2):212–22.
14. Basson R. Human sexual response. Handb Clin Neurol. 2015;130:11–8.
15. Warnock JJ. Female hypoactive sexual desire disorder: epidemiology, diagnosis and treatment. CNS Drugs. 2002;16(11):745–53.
16. Leiblum SR, Koochaki PE, Rodenberg CA, Barton IP, Rosen RC. Hypoactive sexual desire disorder in postmenopausal women: US results from the Women's International Study of Health and Sexuality (WISHeS). Menopause. 2006;13(1):46–56.
17. Cabello SF. Aspectos psicosociales del manejo de la disfunción eréctil. Hábitos tóxicos y estilo de vida. La pareja en la disfunción eréctil. Psicoterapia y terapia de pareja. Arch Esp Urol. 2010;63(8):693–702.
18. Basson R, Brotto LA, Laan E, Redmond G, Utian WH. Assessment and management of women's sexual dysfunctions: problematic desire and arousal. J Sex Med. 2005;2(3):291–300.
19. Kingsberg SA. Hypoactive sexual desire disorder: understanding the impact on midlife women. Female Patient. 2011;36:1–4.
20. Mendoza N, Abad P, Barón F, Cancelo MJ, Llaneza P, Manubens M, et al. Spanish menopause society position statement: use of tibolone in postmenopausal women. Menopause. 2013;20(7):754–60.
21. Wylie KR, Eardley I. Penile size and the "small penis syndrome". BJU Int. 2007;99:1449–55.
22. Lever J, Frederick DA, Peplau LA. Does size matter? Men's and women's views on penis size across the lifespan. Psychol Men Masc. 2006;7:129–43.
23. Tiggemann M, Martins Y, Churchett L. Beyond muscles: unexplored parts of men's body image. J Health Psychol. 2008;13:1163–72.
24. Veale D, Miles S, Read J, Troglia A, Wylie K, Muir G. Sexual functioning and behavior of men with body dysmorphic disorder concerning penis size compared with men anxious about penis size and with controls: a cohort study. Sex Med. 2015;3:147–55.
25. Veale D, Miles S, Bramley S, Muir G, Hodsoll J. Am I normal? A systematic review and construction of nomograms for flaccid and erect penis length and circumference in up to 15.521 men. BJU Int. 2015;115:978–86.
26. Wessells H, Lue TF, McAninch JW. Penile length in the flaccid and erect states: guidelines for penile augmentation. J Urol. 1996;156:995–7.

27. Lenck LC, Vanneuville G, Monnet JP, Harmand Y. Urethral sphincter (G point). Anatomo-clinical correlations. Rev Fr Gynecol Obstet. 1992;87(2):65–9.
28. Brody S, Weiss P. Vaginal orgasm is associated with vaginal (not clitoral) sex education, focusing mental attention on vaginal sensations, intercourse duration, and a preference for a longer penis. J Sex Med. 2010;7(8):2774–81.
29. Brody S, Klapilova K, Krejčová L. More frequent vaginal orgasm is associated with experiencing greater excitement from deep vaginal stimulation. J Sex Med. 2013;10(7):1730–6.
30. Costa RM, Miller GF, Brody S. Women who prefer longer penises are more likely to have vaginal orgasms (but not clitoral orgasms): implications for an evolutionary theory of vaginal orgasm. J Sex Med. 2012;9(12):3079–88.
31. Puppo V, Puppo G. Anatomy of sex: revision of the new anatomical terms used for the clitoris and the female orgasm by sexologists. Clin Anat. 2015;28(3):293–304.
32. Pauls RN. Anatomy of the clitoris and the female sexual response. Clin Anat. 2015;28(3):376–84.
33. Kinsey AC, Pomeroy WB, Martin CE, Gebhard P. Sexual behaviour in the human female. Philadelphia: WB Saunders Co; 1953.
34. Wyatt GE, Peters SD, Guthrie D. Kinsey revisited, part I: comparisons of the sexual socialization and sexual behavior of white women over 33 years. Arch Sex Behav. 1988;17(3):201–39.
35. Perry JD, Whipple B. Multiple components of the female orgasm. In: Graver B, editor. Circunvaginal musculature and sexual function. New York: Karger; 1982.
36. Puppo V, Gruenwald I. Does the G-spot exist? A review of the current literature. Int Urogynecol J. 2012;23(12):1665–9.
37. Moyano Muñoz MN. Fantasías sexuales: análisis de factores determinantes y de su influencia en la salud sexual [Tesis Doctoral]. Granada: Editorial Universidad de Granada; 2014.
38. Jannini EA, Rubio-Casillas A, Whipple B, Buisson O, Komisaruk BR, Brody S. Female orgasm(s): one, two, several. J Sex Med. 2012;9(4):956–65.
39. Darling CA, Davidson Sr JK, Jennings DA. The female sexual response revisited: understanding the multiorgasmic experience in women. Arch Sex Behav. 1991;20(6):527–40.
40. Levin RJ. Recreation and procreation: a critical view of sex in the human female. Clin Anat. 2015;28(3):339–54.
41. Thakar R. Is the uterus a sexual organ? Sexual function following hysterectomy. Sex Med Rev. 2015;3:264–78.
42. Mas M. Fisiología de la respuesta sexual femenina: actualización. Rev Int Androl. 2007;5(1):11–21.
43. Watson T. Vaginal cuff closure with abdominal hysterectomy. A new approach. J Reprod Med. 1994;39:903–7.
44. Flory N, Bissonnette F, Amsel RT, Binik YM. The psychosocial outcomes of total and subtotal hysterectomy: a randomized controlled trial. J Sex Med. 2006;3:483–91.
45. ACOG. ACOG, practice bulletin no. 89. elective and risk-reducing salpingo-oophorectomy. Obstet Gynecol. 2008;111:231–41.
46. Finch A, Metcalfe KA, Chiang JK, Elit L, McLaughlin J, Springate C, et al. The impact of prophylactic salpingo-oophorectomy on menopausal symptoms and sexual function in women who carry a BRCA mutation. Gynecol Oncol. 2011;121:163–8.
47. Tucker PE, Bulsara MK, Salfinger SG, Jit-Sun Tan J, Green H, Cohen PA. Prevalence of sexual dysfunction after risk-reducing salpingo-oophorectomy. Gynecol Oncol. 2016;140:95–100.
48. Barber JS, Yarger JE, Gatny HH. Black-white differences in attitudes related to pregnancy among young women. Demography. 2015;52:751–86.
49. Bober SL, Recklitis CJ, Bakan J, Garber JE, Patenaude AF. Addressing sexual dysfunction after risk-reducing salpingo-oophorectomy: effects of a brief, psychosexual intervention. J Sex Med. 2015;12:189–97.
50. Brotto LA, Branco N, Dunkley C, McCullum M, McAlpine JN. Risk-reducing bilateral salpingo-oophorectomy and sexual health: a qualitative study. J Obstet Gynaecol Can. 2012;34(2):172–8.
51. Chan C, Farine D. Sex in pregnancy. CMAJ. 2011;183(7):815–8.
52. Tan PC, Andi A, Azmi N, Noraihan MN. Effect of coitus at term on length of gestation, induction of labor, and mode of delivery. Obstet Gynecol. 2006;108(1):134–40.
53. Koelman CA, Coumans AB, Nijman HV, Doxiadis II, Dekker GA, Claas FH. Correlation between oral sex and a low incidence of preeclampsia: a role for soluble HLA in seminal fluid? J Reprod Immunol. 2000;46(2):155–66.
54. McMahon CG, Althof SE, Waldinger MD, Porst H, Dean J, Sharlip I, et al. An evidence-based definition of lifelong premature ejaculation: report of the International Society for Sexual Medicine (ISSM) ad hoc committee for the definition of premature ejaculation. J Sex Med. 2008;5:1590–606.
55. Laumann EO, Paik A, Rosen RC. Sexual dysfunction in the United States: prevalence and predictors. JAMA. 1999;281(6):537–44.
56. West SL, D'Aloisio AA, Agans RP, Kalsbeek WD, Borisov NN, Thorp JM. Prevalence of low sexual desire and hypoactive sexual desire disorder in a nationally representative sample of US women. Arch Intern Med. 2008;168(13):1441–9.
57. Kupelian V, Link CL, Rosen RC, McKinlay JB. Socioeconomic status, not race/ethnicity, contributes to variation in the prevalence of erectile dysfunction: results from the Boston Area Community Health (BACH) Survey. J Sex Med. 2008;5(6):1325–33.
58. Armed Forces Health Surveillance Center (AFHSC). Erectile dysfunction among male active component service members, U.S. Armed Forces, 2004-2013. Med Surveill Mon Rep. 2014; 21(9):13–6.
59. Hosain GM, Latini DM, Kauth MR, Goltz HH, Helmer DA. Racial differences in sexual dysfunction among postdeployed Iraq and Afghanistan veterans. Am J Mens Health. 2013;7(5):374–81.
60. Simon RM, Howard L, Zapata D, Frank J, Freedland SJ, Vidal AC. The association of exercise with both erectile and sexual function in black and white men. J Sex Med. 2015;12:1202–10.
61. Laumann EO, West S, Glasser D, Carson C, Rosen R, Kang J-H. Prevalence and correlates of erectile dysfunction by race and ethnicity among men aged 40 or older in the United States: from the Male Attitudes Regarding Sexual Health survey. J Sex Med. 2007;4:57–65.
62. Clement P, Giuliano F. Physiology and pharmacology of ejaculation. Basic Clin Pharmacol Toxicol. 2016;119 Suppl 3:18-25.
63. Masters WH, Johnson VE. The human female: anatomy of sexual response. Minn Med. 1960;43:31–6.
64. Kaplan HS. The new sex therapy. New York: Brunner/Mazel; 1974.
65. Carmichael MS, Humbert R, Dixen J, Palmisano G, Greenleaf W, Davidson JM. Plasma oxytocin increases in the human sexual response. J Clin Endocrinol Metab. 1987;64:27–31.
66. Puppo V, Puppo G. Comprehensive review of the anatomy and physiology of male ejaculation: premature ejaculation is not a disease. Clin Anat. 2016;29(1):111–9.
67. Alwaal A, Breyer BN, Lue TF. Normal male sexual function: emphasis on orgasm an ejaculation. Fertil Steril. 2015;104(5):1051–60.
68. McMahon CG. Management of ejaculatory dysfunction. Intern Med J. 2014;44:124–31.
69. Rowland D, McMahon CG, Abdo C, Chen J, Jannini E, Waldinger MD, Ahn TY. Disorders of orgasm and ejaculation in men. J Sex Med. 2010;7:1668–86.
70. Komisaruk BR, Whipple B. Love as sensory stimulation: physiological consequences of its deprivation and expression. Psychoneuroendocrinology. 1998;23(8):927–44.
71. Heath RG. Pleasure and brain activity in man. Deep and surface electroencephalograms during orgasm. J Nerv Ment Dis. 1972;154(1):3–18.

72. Fernández S-BM. Terapia sexual de las disfunciones eyaculatorias y orgásmicas: alternativas e innovaciones. Rev Int Androl. 2007; 5(3):297–307.
73. Lindau ST, Schumm LP, Laumann EO, Levinson W, O'Muircheartaigh CA, Waite LJ. A study of sexuality and health among older adults in the United States. N Engl J Med. 2007;357(8):762–74.
74. Nicolosi A, Laumann EO, Glasser DB, Moreira Jr ED, Paik A, Gingell C. Sexual behavior and sexual dysfunctions after age 40: the global study of sexual attitudes and behaviors. Urology. 2004;64(5):991–7.
75. Waldinger MD, Quinn P, Dilleen M, Mundayat R, Schweitzer DH, Boolell M. A multinational population survey of intravaginal ejaculation latency time. J Sex Med. 2005;2(4):492–7.
76. Laumann EO, Nicolosi A, Glasser DB, Paik A, Gingell C, Moreira E, Wang T. Sexual problems among women and men aged 40–80 years: prevalence and correlates identified in the Global Study of Sexual Attitudes and Behaviors. Int J Impot Res. 2005;17:39–57.
77. Janssen PKC, Bakker SC, Rethelyi J, Zwinderman AH, Touw DJ, Olivier B, et al. Serotonin transporter promoter region (5-HTTLPR) polymorphism is associated with the intravaginal ejaculation latency time in Dutch men with lifelong premature ejaculation. J Sex Med. 2009;6:276–84.
78. Serefoglu EC, Saitz TR, Trost L, Hellstrom WJ. Premature ejaculation: do we have effective therapy? Transl Androl Urol. 2013;2(1):45–53.
79. Althof SE, McMahon CG, Waldinger MD, Serefoglu EC, Shindel AW, Adaikan PG, et al. An update of the International Society of Sexual Medicine's guidelines for the diagnosis and treatment of premature ejaculation (PE). Sex Med. 2014;2:60–90.
80. American Psychiatric Association. Diagnostic and statistical manual of mental disorders. 3rd ed. Arlington, VA: Asociación Americana de Psiquiatría; 2013.
81. Waldinger MD, Zwinderman AH, Schweitzer DH, Olivier B. Relevance of methodological design for the interpretation of efficacy of drug treatment of premature ejaculation: a systematic review and meta-analysis. Int J Impot Res. 2004;16: 369–81.
82. McMahon CG. Current and emerging treatments for premature ejaculation. Sex Med Rev. 2015;3:183–202.
83. Morales A, Barada J, Wyllie MG. A review of the status of topical treatments for premature ejaculation. BJU Int. 2007;100:493–501.
84. Zamboni BD, Crawford I. Using masturbation in sex therapy: relationships between masturbation, sexual desire, and sexual fantasy. J Psychol Human Sex. 2002;14:123–41.
85. Wilson GD. The secrets of sexual fantasy. London: Dent; 1978.
86. Eagly AH, Wood W. Feminism and the evolution of sex differences and similarities. Sex Roles. 2011;64:758–67.
87. Kahr B. Sexo y fantasías: la investigación más completa y reveladora sobre nuestro mundo sexual interior. Madrid: Ediciones Martínez Roca; 2010.
88. Heras D, Lara F. La sexualidad en los primeros años de la adolescencia: una investigación con chicos y chicas de 2 y 3 de ESO. Sexología Integral. 2009;6(1):20–5.

26 Sex and Pharmacological Sexual Enhancement

Thomas Parisi, Robert N. Pechnick, and Waguih William IsHak

Introduction

Sexual dysfunctions are the primary focus of sexual medicine practice using treatments such as couple therapy, individual psychotherapy, sex therapy, and pharmacological agents. However, an important paradigm shift is needed involving enhancement of sexual function in all the phases of the sexual response cycle from desire to arousal to orgasm. Sexual enhancement interventions range from dietary [1] to improving technique [2] to pharmacological interventions.

As the experience of sexual behavior enlists the interplay between the peripheral and the central nervous systems, the direction of drug development in this field could possibly benefit from treatments that employ both central and peripheral mechanisms [3]. The pharmacological agents are listed in the chapter alphabetically; however, Table 26-1 shows classification of agents by sex according to stage of the sexual response cycle.

Alprostadil

Synopsis

Alprostadil is a synthetic prostaglandin E1 that was discovered to improve sexual dysfunction. It was the first medication approved by the FDA for erectile dysfunction (ED) in 1995, and it is the only approved medication by intracavernosal injection. It is also approved as an intraurethral suppository for ED. However, topical alprostadil has been developed and approved in Europe and Canada for ED (Vitaros®) and for phase III clinical trials for female sexual interest/arousal disorder (Femprox®).

Clinical Studies

Alprostadil acts on prostaglandin E receptors leading to an increase in cAMP through membrane-bound adenylyl cyclase as well as a decrease in noradrenaline through alpha-adrenergic receptors. Studies showed the safety and efficacy of intra-cavernosal alprostadil doses from 1 to 40 μg [4]. Intraurethral application using the Medicated Urethral System for Erection (MUSE) has not gained traction partly because of side effects such as local pain/burning as well the significant difference between its effects compared to intra-cavernosal administration where complete penile rigidity has been achieved in only 10% of patients on MUSE (1000 micro-gm) compared to 43% of patients on intra-cavernosal alprostadil (20 μg) [5]. For sexual enhancement, the more exciting topical route is gaining more attention especially because it is combined with a cutaneous permeation enhancer. Phase II and Phase III trials show rapid onset from 10 to 12 min and erections lasting >60 min, with satisfactory erection rates ranging from 74% to 83% at dose of 300 μg every 4–7 days [6]. Although large placebo-controlled trials led to topical alprostadil's approval in Europe and Canada [7], it is still considered less effective than oral PDE5 inhibitors or alprostadil injection in ED. Nevertheless, the convenience of its administration places it as a combination agent or in mild cases.

Side Effects

Serious Side Effects

Fainting and dizziness have been rarely reported (0.5%) and erections >4 h (0.4%) [6].

Common Side Effects

Topical preparations are associated with burning sensation and erythema in 12.2%, pain/tenderness in 4.4%, and 2.1% of the female partners of male using alprostadil complained about vaginal burning or itching sensation [6].

Dosing (Off Label According to Research Studies)

Topical alprostadil: 200–300 μg every 4–7 days.

W.W. IsHak (ed.), *The Textbook of Clinical Sexual Medicine*, DOI 10.1007/978-3-319-52539-6_26

Table 26-1. Classification of pharmacological agents by sex and stage of sexual response cycle

Stage of the sexual response cycle	Women	Men
Desire	Bupropion	Bupropion
	Flibanserin	Ropinirole
	Melanocortin	Testosterone
Arousal		Alprostadil
	Apomorphine	Apomorphine
	Buspirone	Bupropion
	Sildenafil	Melanocortin
		PDE5 inhibitors
		Yohimbine
Orgasm	Bupropion	Bupropion
		Dapoxetine
		PDE5 inhibitors
		Yohimbine

Apomorphine

Synopsis

Apomorphine is a dopamine receptor agonist with its effects being mediated by interacting with dopamine D1 and D2 receptors [8]. It also increases growth hormone-releasing hormone, growth hormone, and somatomedin C secretions [9]. By virtue of its central activity, apomorphine is thus able to activate a neuronal cascade, with effects reaching the periphery via natural signal amplification [10]. Classically prescribed as an anti-Parkinson's agent, apomorphine has been explored for the use both in the treatment of male erectile disorder (ED) as well as in the treatment of female hypoactive sexual desire disorder (HSDD).

Clinical Studies

Apomorphine has been found in a small (n = 24) study to produce subjective and objective changes in the sexual arousal phase of women with orgasmic sexual dysfunction. A clitoral hemodynamic measure, known as peak systolic velocity, was found to improve post-stimulus from 72.5% with placebo to 139.14% with apomorphine. Moreover, arousal and lubrication were subjectively found to improve with administration of apomorphine [11]. In a placebo-controlled study of 62 premenopausal women with HSDD, six women benefited from as-needed apomorphine (2–3 mg). With daily 3 mg administration, the effects on arousal and desire were better than with 2 mg. Enjoyment, orgasm, and satisfaction also improved during treatment with daily apomorphine [12]. The effect of treatment with apomorphine in premenopausal women with HSDD merits more investigation.

Apomorphine was studied in 5000 men who participated in phase II/III clinical trials assessing the safety and efficacy of apomorphine. The 3 mg dose has similar efficacy to the 4 mg dose, but with less adverse effects. A positive outcome was defined primarily as attempts resulting in erections firm enough for intercourse, as well as by percentage of attempts resulting in intercourse, and by improvement in erection. From a baseline of 24.4% of erections firm enough for intercourse, apomorphine treatment resulted in 49.4% success. Erections were found to occur between 18 and 19 min after dosing [13]. Another study of 849 men—11.5% with mild, 23.8% with moderate, and 48.1% with severe ED—examined a dose-optimized regimen of sublingual apomorphine. Erections firm enough for intercourse increased from a baseline of 13.1 to 39.4% with apomorphine. Attempts resulting in intercourse rose from a baseline of 12.7 to 38.3% with treatment. Average time to erection was 23 min, while average duration of erection was 13 min [14]. Another study comparing the 3 mg and 4 mg dosing found that a median time to erection was 18.8 min, with efficacy not being greatly impacted by dosing [15]. A double-blind, placebo-controlled multicenter trial over 8 weeks with 569 subjects showed that between 48 and 53% of men, compared to 35% with placebo, reported erections firm enough for intercourse and between 45 and 51% of men, compared with 33% with placebo, reported attempts resulting in intercourse [16].

A European study of 507 patients with varying etiologies and severities of ED, but all with pharmacologically treated comorbidities, such as hypertension, coronary artery disease, diabetes, or benign prostatic hypertrophy, examined safety and tolerability of a forced-dose escalation of 4 mg. Adverse effects were not found to limit treatment [17].

Of note, inhaled apomorphine showed faster onset of action, as a significant number of patients achieved an erection of long enough duration for successful intercourse, within 10 min of dosing [18].

Side Effects

Nausea is a common dose-related effect, but has been found to decrease with treatment duration [16]. Other common ones include sweating, dizziness, and drowsiness [19].

Serious Reactions

Hallucinations, sudden sleep episodes, orthostatic hypotension, syncope, myocardial infarction, cardiac arrest, priapism, abuse potential, and neuroleptic malignant syndrome-like symptoms if abrupt discontinuation

Common Reactions

Yawning, somnolence, dyskinesia, nausea/vomiting, falling, injection site reaction, dizziness, orthostatic hypotension, rhinorrhea, chest pain/pressure, hallucinations, peripheral edema, confusion, arthralgia, insomnia, headache, depression, UTI, anxiety, CHF, back/limb pain, Parkinson's disease exacerbation, pneumonia, diaphoresis, dyspnea, fatigue/weakness, ecchymosis, constipation, diarrhea, and compulsive behavior [20]

Contraindications

The concomitant use of nitrates (any form) either regularly or intermittently and concomitant use with a guanylate cyclase stimulator (e.g., riociguat)

Dosing (Off Label According to Research Studies)

Start with 2 mg subcutaneously and then increase as needed to 4 mg [16].

Inhaled for faster onset of action [18], 0.5 or 0.8 mg [21]. (Inhalational form is not available in the US.)

Avanafil

Synopsis

Avanafil is the newest among the oral phosphodiesterase-5 (PDE5) inhibitors prescribed for the treatment of ED. PDE5 inhibitors' mechanism of action is depicted in Figure 26-1. It offers enhanced selectivity, faster action of onset, and a lower side effect profile relative to its other drugs in this class [22]. It is a competitive antagonist of cyclic guanosine monophosphate and has a high degree of selectivity for PDE5 compared to other PDE subtypes [23]. Avanafil is rapidly absorbed and has a short time to peak response [24]. It has a plasma half-life comparable to that of sildenafil and vardenafil [25]. Table 26-2 shows the onset of action and duration of action for each of the FDA-approved PDE5 inhibitors. Avanafil's selectivity for PDE5 over PDE1, PDE6, and PDE1 causes it to produce fewer musculoskeletal, hemodynamic, and vision-related effects compared to less-selective PDE5 inhibitors [26]. Avanafil is effective for patients seeking on-demand treatment of ED [27].

Table 26-2. Onset and duratin of action for PDE5 inhibitors for treatment of ED

PDE5 inhibitor	Trade name	Onset of action (h)	Duration of action (h)
Avanafil	Strendra®	0.25–0.5	4–6
Sildenafil	Viagra®	0.5–4	4–6
Tadalafil	Cialis®	1–4	4–36
Vardenafil	Levitra®	0.25–4	4–8

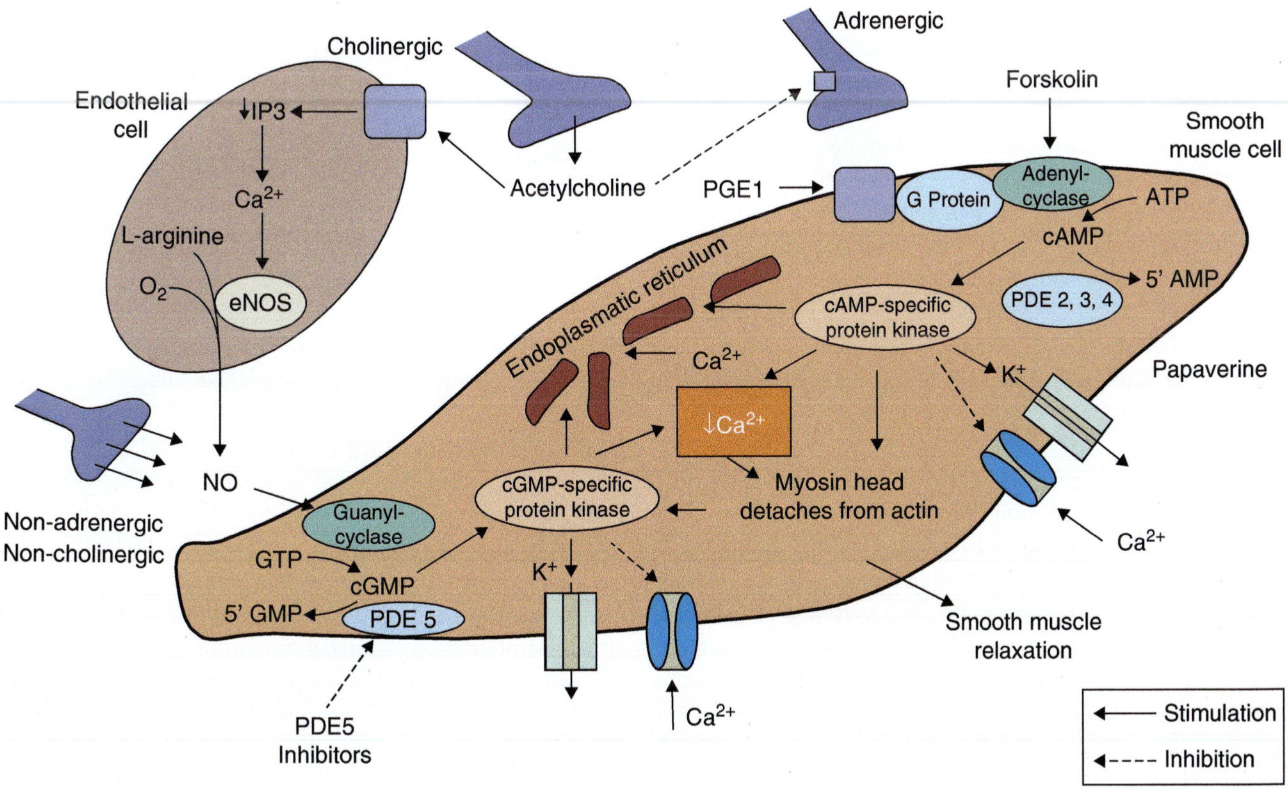

Figure 26-1. Regulation of penile corpus cavernosum smooth muscle relaxation and effect of PDE5 inhibitors. *ATP* adenosine triphosphate, *cAMP* cyclic adenosine monophosphate, *cGMP* cyclic guanosine monophosphate, *eNOS* endothelial nitric oxide synthase, *GTP* guanosine-5′-triphosphate, *IP3* inositol trisphosphate, *NO* nitric oxide, *PDE* phosphodiesterase, *PGE1* prostaglandin E1 [Reprinted from Hatzimouratidis K, Salonia A, Adaikan G, Buvat J, Carrier S, El-Meliegy A, McCullough A, Torres LO, and Khera M. Pharmacotherapy for Erectile Dysfunction: Recommendations From the Fourth International Consultation for Sexual Medicine (ICSM 2015). J Sex Med 2016;13(4):465-88 with permission from Elsevier].

Clinical Studies

Avanafil's rapid onset of action was demonstrated in a randomized, double-blind, placebo-controlled trial by a 64–71% success rate at successful intercourse within 15 min of dosing in 300 sexual attempts compared with 27% in placebo-treated subjects. Moreover, 59–83% of the sexual attempts of the 80 subjects occurred at more than 6 h after dosing compared to 25% on placebo, indicating continuing effect of avanafil [28]. In a multicenter, randomized, placebo-controlled, double-blind trial, 200 subjects with ED showed significantly improved erectile function on avanafil compared to placebo, and after 12 weeks, the proportions of patients achieving normal Erectile Function Domain (EDF) scores were 39.4% and 45.6% on avanafil 100 mg and 200 mg, respectively, compared to 16.7% in the placebo group [29]. One study even demonstrated that treatment with avanafil could be efficacious in as little as 10 min after dosing. The proportion of successful sexual attempts within 15 min, defined by achievement of erection sufficient for vaginal penetration, as well as by successful completion was shown to improve by 25.9% in the 100 mg group and by 29.1% in the 200 mg group with on-demand avanafil therapy [30].

The fast onset of action of avanafil has made it an attractive option among the PDE5 inhibitors in addition to vardenafil. Using visual sexual stimulation, avanafil showed a peak response of 20–40 min after dosing with tumescence and rigidity standing superior to that associated with placebo. In comparison, sildenafil exhibited peak responses in the 60–80 min and 100–120 min ranges [27].

Avanafil also has been shown to be effective in ED patients with medical comorbidities. For example, the treatment of ED in men with diabetes mellitus (most with type II) was explored in a 12-week study of 390 men. Not only was avanafil (100 mg and 200 mg) found safe and effective as early as 15 min after dosing, but also the study revealed that successful intercourse could be initiated more than 6 h after dosing [31].

Avanafil has been investigated in more difficult-to-treat patient populations. A study to investigate the efficacy and safety of avanafil 100 mg and 200 mg in the treatment of ED after nerve-sparing radical prostatectomy was undertaken with 298 subjects. 16.1% of the men were age 65 years or older, and 71.5% had severe ED. Among the features measured were erectile function and successful vaginal insertion. At 12 weeks, patients on avanafil had 36.4% of sexual attempts that were successful at 15 min (or less), versus 4.5% for placebo [32].

To evaluate the long-term efficacy and tolerability of avanafil, a 52-week extension trial of two 12-week trials with 686 patients measured the percentage of sexual attempts ending in successful vaginal penetration and intercourse, as well as erectile function. Success rates improved from 44 to 83% in vaginal penetration and from 13 to 68% in intercourse after avanafil (100 mg and 200 mg). Moreover, 65% of patients who did not respond to 100 mg of avanafil did respond when the dose was increased to 200 mg [33].

Side Effects

Serious Reactions

Hypersensitivity reaction, priapism, sudden hearing loss, vision loss, and non-arteritic anterior ischemic optic neuropathy

Common Reactions

Headache, flushing, nasal congestion, nasopharyngitis, and back pain [34]

Contraindications

The concomitant use with serotonin 5-HT [3] receptor antagonists including antiemetics

Dosing

50–200 mg PO 15–30 min before sexual activity

Start: 100 mg PO 15 min before sexual activity; max: 200 mg/dose up to one dose/24 h [35]

Bupropion

Synopsis

Bupropion is an antidepressant in the aminoketone family. It is a weak, dopaminergic reuptake inhibitor [36], and its metabolite, hydroxybupropion [37], is a norepinephrine reuptake inhibitor. It also acts as a noncompetitive antagonist at nicotinic acetylcholine receptors, specifically blocking $\alpha3\beta2$ and $\alpha4\beta2$ and weakly blocking $\alpha7$ nicotinic acetylcholine receptors [38]. Bupropion is used to treat depression, attention deficit hyperactivity disorder, and for smoking cessation. It is marketed under the following brand names: Wellbutrin®/SR/XL/Aplenzin®/Forfivo™/Zyban®/Budeprion®.

The antidepressant activity of bupropion has been demonstrated in double-blind, placebo-, and drug-controlled studies, with a number of significant advantages over other antidepressants: less weight gain [39], less cardiovascular effects [40], and less cardiotoxicity in cases of overdose [41]. Compared to SSRIs, bupropion has been found not only to have a lower negative impact on sexual function across desire, arousal, and orgasm domains but also to enhance sexual function in both depressed and nondepressed women and men [42, 43]. Among the first placebo-controlled clinical trials demonstrating an improvement in the psychological components of sexual dysfunction (inhibited sexual desire, inhibited sexual arousal, and/or inhibited orgasm), 63% of male and female patients treated for 12 weeks by bupropion exhibited greater improvements in libido and on the global assessment of sexual functioning. Moreover, a trend toward increased sexual activity was observed [44].

Studies comparing sertraline to bupropion showed that while the two agents proved similar over time across rating scales for depression, sertraline was more associated with sexual dysfunction in men and women compared to bupropion [45]. Similar studies comparing the effects between fluoxetine and bupropion sustained-release (bupropion SR) found that significantly more men and women experienced less sexual dysfunction with bupropion than with fluoxetine [46] and sertraline [47]. Before the DSM-V merged both HSDD and female sexual arousal disorder (FSAD) into female sexual interest/arousal disorder, bupropion studies were performed using the DSM-IV criteria for HSDD and FSAD [48, 49]. One 4-week study assessing the effect of bupropion sustained-release (SR) in nondepressed women with HSDD showed that sexual desire and sexual function overall increased in 29% of subjects [50]. Another study examining the effect of bupropion on premenopausal women found it to increase sexual arousal, as well as orgasm completion and sexual satisfaction over a 112-day trial [51]. Sexual thoughts/desire scores more than doubled in patients with regular menstrual cycles suffering from HSDD who were treated for 12 weeks by bupropion [52].

Along with primary sexual dysfunction, bupropion SR has been investigated as an adjunctive agent to reverse selective serotonin reuptake inhibitor (SSRI)-induced sexual dysfunction in menstruating women. Although improvements in scores for desire, arousal, lubrication, orgasm, and satisfaction were significantly higher in a bupropion SR for SSRI-induced female sexual dysfunction, the desire domain increased most after treatment [53, 54]. It also seems that higher doses are most efficacious for treatment with bupropion SR of SSRI-induced sexual dysfunction [55]. Two studies comparing the effects of escitalopram and bupropion extended-release (bupropion XL) on sexual functioning and depression showed a significantly decreased percentage of orgasm dysfunction and decreased "worsened sexual functioning" in women treated with bupropion XL compared to escitalopram [56]. In a 43-person study, desire and frequency of sex increased most significantly after treatment of men with SSRI-induced sexual dysfunction after bupropion SR was added [54].

The use of bupropion in the treatment of delayed ejaculation has been investigated, with mixed outcomes. Although 70% of men and women reported improvement in libido, arousal, and orgasmic function during bupropion treatment of ejaculation/orgasmic delays [57], bupropion 150 mg daily showed limited benefit as an agent in the treatment of lifelong delayed ejaculation [58].

Side Effects

Serious Reactions

Cardiac arrhythmias, seizures, angle closure glaucoma, mania, and suicidal thoughts

Common Reactions

Nausea, constipation, dry mouth, headache, insomnia, nervousness, tachycardia, and dermatologic reactions (rare delayed urticarial)

Contraindications

Seizure disorders, eating disorders, abruptly discontinuing alcohol, benzodiazepines, barbiturates, or antiepileptic drugs [38]

Dosing (for Sexual Dysfunction)

75–450 mg PO per day (BID or TID).

Bupropion regular-release: 75 mg and 100 mg tablets.

Bupropion SR/Zyban: 100 mg, 150 mg, and 200 mg tablets.

Bupropion XL: 150 mg and 300 mg tablets.

Aplenzin: 174 mg, 348 mg, and 522 mg extended-release tablets.

Usual dosage: start with 100 mg SR BID and then increase after 3–7 days to 150 mg SR BID or 300 mg XL daily.

Buspirone

Synopsis

Buspirone is FDA approved for the management of anxiety disorders. Its mechanism of action suggests activity in a wide variety of neuronal systems [59]. It is a presynaptic and postsynaptic partial agonist selectively at the 5-hydroxytryptamine-1A (5-HT1A) receptor, lending to its antianxiety and antidepression properties [60]. Among anxiolytics, it is an azaspirodecanedione and does not interact with gamma-aminobutyric (GABA) receptors [61]. It is used for longer-term treatment of anxiety, because compared to the benzodiazepine-type anxiolytics, it is not associated with dependence, and there are no additive effects when taken with ethanol or benzodiazepines [62].

Clinical Studies

An HSDD study in women posited that although testosterone increases sensitivity to sexual cues, it might increase sexual inhibitory mechanisms in women predisposed to sexual inhibition by 5-HT1A-mediated mechanisms in the prefrontal cortex. The study found that a single dose of buspirone in combination with testosterone enhanced sexual responsiveness in women with high sexual inhibition with HSDD [63]. The same combination of testosterone and buspirone also worked for the treatment of low desire in women with SSRI-induced sexual dysfunction [64]. Moreover, buspirone alone was shown to be effective in the reversal of SSRI-induced sexual dysfunction [65].

Side Effects

Serious Reactions

Serotonin syndrome, akathisia, extrapyramidal symptoms, tardive dyskinesia, dystonia, hostility, and depression (source: Epocrates) [62]

Common Reactions

Nausea, dizziness, drowsiness, headache, nervousness, fatigue, insomnia, xerostomia, impaired concentration, hostility, confusion, depression, blurred vision, diarrhea, abdominal pain, numbness, and weakness [66]

Dosing

Available in 5, 7.5, 10, 15, and 30 mg in divided doses

For treatment of anxiety/sexual dysfunction: 20–30 mg/day PO divided BID-TID

Clomiphene and Enclomiphene

Synopsis

Clomiphene citrate is a nonsteroidal, ovulatory stimulant indicated for female infertility. It binds to estrogen receptors in the hypothalamus and pituitary where it has both estrogenic and antiestrogenic effects, leading to increases in GnRH, LH, and FSH release [67]. Increasing LH levels in men leads to a rise in testosterone levels, justifying its use for treating males with low testosterone. With fewer side effects than clomiphene, enclomiphene citrate—the trans-stereoisomer of clomiphene citrate—is becoming an alternative to testosterone replacement therapy.

Clinical Studies

For the past three decades, multiple studies showed that clomiphene citrate consistently increases serum testosterone levels in men. For instance, a study of 25 mg daily of clomiphene citrate increased testosterone levels and the testosterone/estradiol ratio in men with hypogonadism [68]. Enclomiphene citrate 25 mg daily increased levels of total testosterone in men within 2 weeks into the normal range, and the effects persisted for at least 1 week of treatment discontinuation [69].

Side Effects

Serious Reactions

Pancreatitis, visual function loss, and psychotic disorder

Common Reactions in Men

Hot flushes occurred in 10% of patients on clomiphene citrate, whereas less than 5% experienced nausea, vomiting, headaches, and visual disturbances

Contraindications

Liver disease, intracranial lesions, uncontrolled thyroid, or adrenal dysfunction

Dosing

Clomiphene citrate in men: 25–50 mg daily and then increase to 50 mg PO BID

Enclomiphene citrate in men: 12.5–25 mg daily

Dapoxetine

Synopsis

Dapoxetine, a potent SSRI that is similar to fluoxetine in structure, was specifically developed for premature ejaculation (PE). Despite its approval in Europe, the Middle East, and Mexico, it has not yet been approved in the United States [70]. Dapoxetine has a rapid onset and is administered 1–3 h before intercourse or on a daily basis [71].

Clinical Studies

Dapoxetine has been evaluated using randomized, double-blind, placebo-controlled studies. Five industry sponsored of 6081 men showed that the geometric mean average stopwatch-measured intravaginal ejaculatory latency time (IELT) increased from 0.8 min at baseline to 2 min on dapoxetine 30 mg and 2.3 min on dapoxetine 60 mg versus 1.3 min on placebo (p for both comparisons <0.001) [72].

Side Effects

Serious Side Effects

Dapoxetine is contraindicated in case of liver impairment.

Common Side Effects

Common adverse effects were higher in frequency at the 60 mg dose and included nausea, dizziness, and headache [73].

Dosing (Off Label According to Research Studies)

Start with 30 mg 1–3 h before intercourse or daily and could be increased to 60 mg.

Flibanserin

Synopsis

Flibanserin is a novel multifunctional serotonin agonist and antagonist. Its mechanism of action is as a 5-HT1A agonist and secondarily a 5-HT2A antagonist. Additional action includes weaker antagonism at 5-HT2C and 5-HT2B and partial agonist activity at D4-dopamine receptors [74]. A centrally acting agent, it preferentially activates mesolimbic, dopaminergic, and hypothalamic structures involved in response to sexual stimuli [75]. Flibanserin is used to treat premenopausal women with acquired HSSD [76]. Thus, flibanserin offers a new direction in the treatment of HSDD [77].

Clinical Studies

Flibanserin increases the number of reported satisfying sexual events and general sexual function and decreases sexual distress. In terms of experiencing meaningful benefits, women taking flibanserin (37.6%) reported to have benefited compared to placebo (28.0%) [78]. Flibanserin clinical trials are named after a series of flowers.

In 2010 the DAISY study initiated a series of 24-week studies on the effects of flibanserin on premenopausal women with HSDD. This study sets out to assess efficacy and tolerability of flibanserin, revealing a direct relationship between optimal dosing (100 mg at bedtime) of flibanserin and improvements in satisfying sexual events, sexual desire, sexual function, and sexual distress. Still, improvements in female sexual distress and female sexual function were reported with all dosage (25 mg twice daily and 50 mg twice daily) regimens [79]. The VIOLET study aimed to evaluate efficacy and safety of flibanserin. It revealed at 50 mg and 100 mg once daily at bedtime that flibanserin was well tolerated and associated with similar results to the DAISY study [80]. This helped establish the safety of optimal dosing of flibanserin.

The 24-week trial standard was extended to one of 52 weeks in the SUNFLOWER study. Women participating in this trial were not only premenopausal as in the other studies, but they had already completed a trial of flibanserin or placebo. By study end, 42% of those with active HSDD showed improvement of sexual distress to remission level, and the percentage of those in remission rose from 83 to 90% [81].

The 24-week BEGONIA trial sets out to assess the efficacy and safety of flibanserin in premenopausal women with HSDD. This randomized, placebo-controlled trial was geared toward optimal dosing of 100 mg at night. A significant number of women reported reductions in distress associated with sexual dysfunction, as well as reductions in distress associated with low sexual desire [82]. The SNOWDROP trial reaffirmed that flibanserin, compared with placebo, is associated with improvement in sexual desire, increased number of satisfying sexual events, and reduced distress secondary to low sexual desire [78]. Prior to the August 2015 FDA approval of flibanserin for women experiencing HSDD, there had been two prior failed FDA reviews, mainly due to concerns for flibanserin's efficacy and the product's risk/benefit profile [83]. A systematic review and meta-analysis of randomized clinical trials assessing the safety of flibanserin for the treatment of HSDD in women revealed that treatment with flibanserin, on average, resulted in only one-half additional satisfying sexual event per month while statistically and clinically significantly increasing the risk of dizziness, somnolence, nausea, and fatigue [84]. To limit risk, it is encouraged that flibanserin be taken at bedtime, and the concomitant use of alcohol with flibanserin should be discouraged [83].

Side Effects

Serious Side Effects

Hypotension/syncope, accidental injury, appendicitis, and central nervous system (CNS) depression [85]

Common Side Effects

Somnolence, dizziness, and fatigue [79, 82] with adverse events leading to discontinuation in 9.6% of women receiving flibanserin vs. 3.7% on placebo. Nausea and headaches have also been reported [78].

Contraindications

Concomitant ethanol use, hepatic impairment, and concomitant use of moderate or strong CYP3A4 inhibitors

Dosing

For the treatment of HSDD, acquire 100 mg PO QHS; for premenopausal female patient, discontinue after 8 weeks if no improvement is noted [86].

Melanocortin

Synopsis

Melanocortins constitute a group of peptide hormones, which include adrenocorticotropic hormone and melanocyte-stimulating hormones, and are derived from the proopiomelanocortin, which is made in the pituitary gland. By binding to one of five melanocortin receptors, melanocortins influence a variety of functions, including pigmentation, inflammation, energy homeostasis, and sexual function [87, 88]. Melanocortins play a role in the central pathways involved in mediating arousal and orgasm in females, as well as in erection in males [89]. Successful efficacy in preclinical treatment studies of ED using centrally acting melanocortin receptor agonists was limited by side effects such as nausea, severe enough to warrant discontinuation [90]. The melanocortin agonist available on the market is called Melanotan II, available in subcutaneously injectable form.

Clinical Studies

A study to investigate the effect of a selective melanocortin analog known as bremelanotide on 18 premenopausal women diagnosed with female sexual arousal disorder revealed that even upon exposure to sexually explicit visual stimuli, it improved subjective sexual desire and more positive feelings of genital arousal. This change occurred within 24 h of treatment with nasal bremelanotide [91]. Another study of 80 married, premenopausal women, average age 31, showed that intranasal bremelanotide was associated with improvements in arousal, as well as with significant gains in intercourse satisfaction [92].

The use of a nonselective melanocortin analog, known as Melanotan II, was investigated on 20 men with psychogenic and organic ED. Without sexual stimulation, Melanotan II led to penile erection in 17 out of 20 men. Moreover, participants reported 68% increased sexual desire, as opposed to 19% in placebo [93]. The melanocortin 4 receptor, specifically, has been found to be of interest, as its agonists in both oral and in sublingual form have been shown to be safe and effective at 200 mg in the treatment of ED up to a similar efficacy level as that exhibited by sildenafil [94], as well as in those who fail sildenafil therapy [95]. Likewise with another study of healthy patients and of patients who had failed sildenafil therapy, in doses of 0.3–10 mg, a cyclic heptapeptide melanocortin analog offered statistically significant erection improvement in patients who had not responded to phosphodiesterase 5 (PDE5) inhibitor therapy [96].

Side Effects

Nausea, stretching, yawning, spontaneous penile erection, and increased pigmentation [97]

Dosing

Healthy patients: 1.0 mg SC

Erectile dysfunction: 4 or 6 mg SC [96] or up to 200 mg PO or up to 200 mg sublingual [95]

Oxytocin

Synopsis

Oxytocin (OT) is a neuropeptide made of nine amino acids naturally produced by the paraventricular and supraoptic nuclei of the hypothalamus and then stored in the posterior pituitary where it could be released to the bloodstream or is secreted from the paraventricular nuclei projections into brain structures such as the amygdala, hypothalamus, and hippocampus and nucleus accumbens [98]. OT is responsible for contractility and social bonding. Synthetic OT has been prescribed to induce labor (IV form) and mild ejection (intranasal form) and experimentally to improve social skills in autism [99] and schizophrenia [100].

Clinical Studies

Using a continuous blood sampling technique and anal electromyography, Carmichael et al. reported in 1994 a positive correlation between oxytocin levels and the intensity, but not duration, of orgasmic contractions in males and females [101]. IsHak et al. in 2008 used intranasal oxytocin successfully in treatment refractory anorgasmia [102]. Oxytocin is administered intranasally during intercourse (due to its half-life of 2–3 min), at the point when ejaculation is sought. For multiorgasmic women, the amount of oxytocin level increase was positively correlated with subjective reports of orgasm intensity [103]. A number of case reports have documented the role of oxytocin in producing remarkable improvement in sexual function [104] and improving orgasmic difficulties [105]. In a 2013 review of oxytocin, Wudarczyk et al. proposed the use of oxytocin for enhancement of romantic/sexual relationships [106].

Side Effects

Serious Side Effects (Reported in Pregnant Women)

More intense or more frequent contractions, postpartum hemorrhage, and ruptured uterus

Common Side Effects

Loss of appetite, nausea, vomiting, cramping, stomach pain, and runny nose [107]

Contraindications (Reported for Pregnant Women)

Placenta previa, vasa previa, and cord prolapse

Dosing

Off-label use for delayed orgasm: 24 IU intranasally [108]

Ropinirole

Synopsis

Dopamine agonists—ropinirole originally novel—were first used in patients diagnosed with moderate to advanced Parkinson's disease (PD), as they allowed for reduction in dosing and hence decreased adverse motor response reactions to levodopa [109, 110]. Ropinirole is a potent and selective D2-dopaminergic agonist [111, 112]. In contrast to pramipexole, a D2-agonist ergot ropinirole is a non-ergoline [113], centrally acting agent, which was also employed to alleviate restless legs syndrome [114]. It also came to be explored as an agent to combat sexual dysfunction, a common side effect of antidepressants [115]. Ropinirole has a half-life of about 6 h and has approximately 50% bioavailability, with low plasma protein binding [116]. Although not classically offered for the treatment of sexual dysfunction, ropinirole merits attention as a dopaminergic agent with potential for the treatment of sexual dysfunction.

Clinical Studies

Dopaminergic agents have gained attention in the treatment of antidepressant-induced sexual dysfunction. An early report of 13 patients, 10 of whom were men, indicated that over 4 weeks of daily treatment, 54% of patients reported improvement in sexual function, suggesting that ropinirole may be part of the arsenal in the strategy against antidepressant-induced sexual dysfunction [115].

A case report of a 45-year-old man with 20 years of PD, medicated with a high dose of ropinirole, indicates that this patient displayed hypersexuality and exhibitionism. The account urges caution as to sexual impulses and reduced control of behavior in the face of dopaminergic agents [117]. Moreover, pathological hypersexuality is documented to have developed in 13 patients with PD, with hypersexuality exhibited in 14 out of 15 cases beginning within 8 months after onset of treatment with ropinirole [118].

An analysis of 1580 adverse drug events from the United States and 21 other countries suggesting impulse control disorders (pathological gambling, hypersexuality, and compulsive shopping) revealed that 710 cases had involved in them patients taking dopaminergic agents, with 188 of these patients on ropinirole [119]. Further, a screening interview of 272 patients with idiopathic PD revealed that, in fact, 4% of them suffered from an impulse control disorder [120, 121]. Further exploration into the use of dopaminergic agents for the treatment of sexual dysfunction is warranted.

Dosing

Start at 0.25 mg PO daily and titrate up to 2–4 mg PO daily over 4 weeks, as tolerated [115].

Side Effects

Serious Reactions

Sudden sleep episodes, orthostatic hypotension, bradycardia, syncope, mental status alterations, hallucinations, dyskinesia, melanoma risk, fibrotic complications, hypersensitivity reaction, and NMS-like symptoms if abruptly discontinued.

Common Reactions

Nausea, somnolence, abdominal pain, dizziness, orthostatic hypotension, headache, asthenia, dyskinesia, paresthesia, vomiting, hallucinations, dyspepsia, edema, vision changes, constipation, anxiety, diaphoresis, pharyngitis, xerostomia, diarrhea, hypertension, anorexia, chest pain, rebound/augmentation in treatment of restless leg syndrome, and compulsive behaviors [122]

Sildenafil

Synopsis

Sildenafil is the first in its class of vasoactive drugs developed for the oral treatment of ED. It is a peripherally acting agent that inhibits cyclic guanosine monophosphate (cGMP)-specific PDE5 from the corpus cavernosa. PDE5 is the chief PDE type in the corpus cavernosum and plays a key role in penile erection [123]. Erection is dependent on NO and on its second messenger, cGMP [124]. Sildenafil potentiates the NO-stimulated cGMP signal that mediates relaxation of penile cavernosal smooth muscle during sexual stimulation [125]. Sildenafil has also been shown to successfully treat female sexual arousal disorder in hormonally replete women without contributing psychosocial stressors [126, 127], likely clarified by NO-mediated relaxation of clitoral and vaginal smooth muscle [128]. PDE5 contains two N-terminal domains (GAF A and GAF B) and is activated upon cGMP binding to the GAF A domain. Moreover, activated PDE5 demonstrates higher sensitivity toward sildenafil than does nonactivated PDE5. In fact, PDE5 is activated directly upon cGMP binding to the GAF A domain, without the need for PDE5 phosphorylation [129]. Sildenafil also has direct muscle relaxant potential, likely inhibiting Ca^{2+} influx through both receptor-mediated and voltage-dependent Ca^{2+} channels [130]. PDE6 is also inactivated by sildenafil, explanatory for adverse visual disorders [131]. Cyclic adenosine monophosphate (cAMP)-dependent signaling mechanisms also interplay with cGMP-dependent signaling mechanisms in human cavernous arteries [132]. By nature of being a PDE5 inhibitor, sildenafil may have an effect on adrenal steroidogenesis, as its administration has been shown to be associated with an increase in testosterone levels, likely secondary to a direct effect on the testis [133]. Employed classically for the treatment of ED, sildenafil affects the domains of desire and of orgasm less so than it does arousal [134], with a duration of approximately 4 h [135]. Table 26-2 shows the onset of action and duration of action for each of the FDA-approved PDE5 inhibitors.

Clinical Studies

A direct relationship between sildenafil dosing and efficacy is documented. The first published large-scale clinical trial for sildenafil included a 24-week-dose-response study of 532 men and a 12-week, flexible dose-escalation study of 329 men, followed by a 32-week, open-label extension study of 225 of the 329 men. The dose-response study showed a direct relationship between dosage and erectile function (achieving and maintaining erection); a 100% increase in the number of men achieving erections was observed for men receiving 100 mg of sildenafil. During the final 4 weeks of the dose-escalation study, there was a 69% success rate at sexual intercourse, compared to 22% for those receiving placebo. There was a staggering near 400% increase in attempts at sexual intercourse for these men [136]. Men with ED treated with 100 mg compared to 50 mg sildenafil have also been shown to attain greater gains in erectile function and, even within the first 2 weeks of treatment, have experienced completely hard and rigid erections [137]. The dose-response relationship was poignantly evinced in a study of 54 men with refractory ED, who had failed treatment with 100 mg sildenafil, with 37%, 46.3%, and 68% of these patients experiencing improved erections using 100 mg, 150 mg, and 200 mg sildenafil, respectively [138].

Relative safety was shown in a 1998 data analysis of 2722 sildenafil patients and 1552 placebo patients, who collectively had undergone double-blind, placebo-controlled, and ten open-label extension studies of sildenafil. Adverse effects, such as headache, flushing, and dyspepsia, were transient, mild, or moderate. Discontinuation secondary to side effects nearly matched that of placebo [139]. Successful ongoing improvement of ED has been shown to be dependent upon continued treatment with sildenafil [140].

Different types of ED have been successfully treated with sildenafil therapy. One double-blind, placebo-controlled study of 329 patients suffering from ED of organic, psychogenic, or mixed etiology revealed that 74% of patients receiving sildenafil versus 16% for placebo had improved erections and that 65% of patients receiving sildenafil versus 20% for placebo reported successful attempts at sexual intercourse [141]. A study of 514 men with a mean age of 56 years, with 32% diagnosed with organic ED, 25% with psychogenic ED, and 43% with mixed ED, showed between 67 and 86% relative to placebo improved erections, helping to establish sildenafil as well tolerated and efficacious among ED of various etiologies [142]. Likewise, with age matching to healthy subjects across broad-spectrum ED etiologies, one study demonstrated that sildenafil is associated with near normalization of ED [143].

Sleep-related erectile activity, especially tip rigidity, was shown to be enhanced in 77% of the 30 patients tested, 23 of whom experienced ED due to established medical or biological "organic" reasons [144]. Another study of organic impotence demonstrated that sildenafil improves nocturnal penile activity (rigidity and tumescence) in organic ED. Moreover, ED due to psychogenic etiology in the same study was shown to benefit rigidity, as opposed to tumescence [145]. Even men without ED, who in fact were potent, demonstrated improved nocturnal erections with sildenafil [146]. Refractory time was cut from 10.8±0.9 min to 2.6±0.7 min in a study of 20 healthy men in stable relationships with proven fertility [147].

Investigation of the treatment of ED in men with diabetes is important because diabetes is a common comorbidity in ED. A randomized, double-blind, placebo-controlled, flexible dose-escalation clinical trial over 7 months of 268 men with a diagnosis of diabetes (mean = 12 years) and with a diagnosis of ED (mean = 5.6 years), showed improved erections in 56% of patients receiving sildenafil versus 10% on placebo. The proportion of men with a minimum of one successful attempt at sexual intercourse was 61%, compared to 22% for the placebo group [148]. This study, as well as another to investigate sildenafil's efficacy in diabetes mellitus, hypertension, history of pelvic surgery, and ischemic heart disease, helped establish sildenafil as an effective treatment of ED in men with these common comorbidities [149]. Men with moderately severe congestive heart failure also exhibited good tolerance, improved erectile function, and relief of depressive symptoms with low-dose (50 mg) sildenafil [150].

Sildenafil has gained notice as a well-tolerated and efficacious pharmacological treatment of ED in men with spinal cord injuries. One analysis of a two-part pilot study to assess the efficacy of sildenafil in the treatment of ED was conducted on patients with spinal cord injury. Results revealed that 65% of patients receiving sildenafil versus 8% for placebo had erections of at least 60% rigidity. Moreover, 67% of these men wanted to continue treatment with sildenafil. None of the subjects discontinued due to adverse effects [151]. Another study of spinal cord injury patients showed similar results to the pilot study; [152] while another study elucidated that the efficacy of sildenafil depends on sparing of sacral (S2–S4) or thoracolumbar (T10–L2) spinal segments, which help mediate psychogenic erections in males with spinal cord injuries [153].

The studies of ED and comorbidities using sildenafil treatment called for the need to study its effects on medication treatment. In a study of 1685 men with at least 6 months of ED, who were taking antihypertensive medication, sildenafil was found not to have clinically significant effects on blood pressure and heart rate in the acute, short-term treatment of ED [154]. One study of men with ED and taking two or more antihypertensive medications likewise revealed similar efficacy and tolerability [155].

Psychiatric symptoms are commonly encountered in ED, especially depressive symptoms. "Positive affect" was a change of particular note in one of the early sildenafil studies [156]. Another study showed that Hamilton depression scale scores were lower in 76% of patients treated by sildenafil, while 14% of patients did not exhibit a significant decrease in depressive symptoms. Improvement of ED was shown to reduce depressive symptoms and improve quality of life in mild to moderate depressive disorder [157]. Ten post-traumatic stress disorder (PTSD) patients with ED taking antidepressants demonstrated significant improvements in all sexual domains (particularly arousal), following treatment with sildenafil 50 mg daily as needed [158].

About 81% of patients with antidepressant-associated ED who did not respond to treatment responded fully to open-label sildenafil [159]. As antipsychotic use is associated with ED and remains a common reason for poor compliance, sildenafil has been studied in patients with ED on antipsychotics. While one study showed that ED decreased significantly after treatment with sildenafil of ED in patients with schizophrenia on risperidone [160], another study revealed an odds ratio with sildenafil of 4.07 for adequate erections [161].

As the first approved agent, sildenafil is often compared to other agents. A pilot study of 10,750 ED patients was conducted prior to the release of vardenafil and tadalafil, comparing sildenafil, apomorphine, yohimbine, and alprostadil. The results showed that 81% were satisfied with the treatment outcome with all the interventions; however, 85% reported particularly satisfaction with sildenafil's onset of action, duration of action, efficacy, and tolerability [162].

Additional effects were detected with sildenafil. Ejaculatory latency secondary to treatment by serotonin reuptake inhibitors was decreased in nine out of ten men in remission from MDD by treatment with 150–200 mg sildenafil [163]. Conversely, sildenafil was found more efficacious relative to paroxetine and the squeeze method in the treatment of premature ejaculation [164]. Adding sildenafil to a fluoxetine regimen also significantly improved rates of premature ejaculation when compared to fluoxetine by itself [165]. Similarly, adding sildenafil to talk therapy in the treatment of ED proved more efficacious than the former alone [166].

Side Effects

Serious Reactions

Myocardial infarction, stroke, sudden death, ventricular arrhythmias, severe hypotension, cerebrovascular hemorrhage, pulmonary hemorrhage, subarachnoid hemorrhage, retinal hemorrhage, non-arteritic anterior ischemic optic neuropathy, vision loss, intraocular pressure increase, hearing loss, hypersensitivity reaction, dyspnea, ataxia, shock, anemia, leukopenia, priapism, and seizures

Common Reactions

Headache, flushing, dyspepsia, nasal congestion, UTI, visual disturbance, diarrhea, dizziness, rash, and photosensitivity [167]

Dosing

Erectile dysfunction: 50 mg PO ×1; start 0.5–4 h prior to intercourse; maximum 100 mg/dose up to 1 dose/day; consider starting at 25 mg PO × 1 in patients above 65 years old [168].

Range of onset to erection 12–30 min, mean time 27 min, duration of action at least 4 h [169].

Remains clinically active 12 h after administration in patients with ED at 100 mg [170, 171].

No significant loss of efficacy occurs when sildenafil is taken shortly before or with a meal [172].

Tadalafil

Synopsis

Tadalafil is among the PDE5 inhibitors class of vasoactive drugs developed for the oral treatment of ED. Erection is dependent on nitric oxide and on its second messenger, cGMP [124]. The long-acting active inhibition by tadalafil of PDE5 lends to increased cGMP and hence smooth muscle relaxation in the penis for up to 36 h [135, 173], with the longest plasma presence among the PDE5 inhibitors [174]. It is also the only PDE5 inhibitor whose pharmacokinetic profile is not affected by fatty food [175]. Table 26-2 shows the onset of action and duration of action for each of the FDA-approved PDE5 inhibitors. Tadalafil exhibits peripheral action by inhibiting cGMP-specific PDE5 from the corpus cavernosum [123]. PDE6 is not inhibited by tadalafil, explaining its nearly nonexistent visual side effect profile [131]. Tadalafil is unique among the PDE inhibitors in that it also inhibits PDE11, an effect that does not have any known clinical implications [176]. Another set of distinctions it holds among PDE5 inhibitors is that it lacks significant effect on noradrenaline [130].

Clinical Studies

By virtue of a longer half-life, tadalafil conceivably offers a specific advantage over sildenafil, as patients might less closely link dosing with planning of sexual intercourse. In a multicenter study of 207 men, it was found that 82.8% of those treated with tadalafil experienced improved erections, versus 19.6% taking placebo. Of note, the higher rate of successful intercourse attempts occurred between 4 and 36 h after dosing [177]. The length of time that tadalafil works has proven favorable and gained significant patient satisfaction [178]. Sexual partner satisfaction has mirrored that of patients in the treatment of ED by tadalafil [179, 180].

The versatility in dosing of tadalafil is also noteworthy. One large ($n = 4262$), multicenter study looking at male preference for on-demand tadalafil treatment versus three times weekly tadalafil treatment found that although 57.8% of men preferred the on-demand regimen of tadalafil 20 mg, a considerable 42.2% of men preferred the three times weekly treatment [181], especially that tadalafil proved efficacious up to 36 h. Moreover, men of different age groups demonstrated significantly changed sexual behavior on the three-time weekly dosing [182]. These men engaged in having sex distributed over a wider period of time, having sex beyond the 4-h window, and having sex during the morning and the evening hours [183]. In fact, in one study of 367 PDE5 inhibitor-naïve men with ED, 71% preferred tadalafil and 29% chose sildenafil as their preference [184].

As ED is increasingly common with advancing age, a study of 188 men with a mean age of 71.6 years without depression and without diabetes mellitus demonstrated 81% improved erections and 56% successful completion of sexual encounters up to 36 h after tadalafil 20 mg dosing. Moreover, only 5% of patients discontinued treatment due to adverse effects [185]. Long-term treatment with tadalafil 5 mg once daily has also been shown to be well tolerated and effective in a 472-patient study [186]. Moreover, 46.3% of patients in one trial continued to show normal erectile function after 4 weeks of no treatment, following a period of 1 year of tadalafil therapy [187].

In order to understand the effect of tadalafil over time on men with ED with medical comorbidities and their medication treatment, a multicenter, open-label study of 1173 men with ED who were taking concomitant medications for such conditions as diabetes (30.5%) and hypertension (29.5%) was conducted. The study demonstrated the overall safety and tolerability for tadalafil at doses of 5, 10, or 20 mg taken once daily for 18–24 months [188]. A larger study ($n = 1911$) showed adequate tolerance and efficacy for tadalafil 20 mg for men with ED who had comorbid diabetes mellitus, cardiovascular disease including hypertension and hyperlipidemia, and depression and with men with two or more comorbidities [189]. Moreover, men with ED secondary to traumatic spinal cord injury showed improved erectile function and good tolerance to treatment with tadalafil [190]. One study revealed that patients with ED due to treatment by SSRIs, who were treated with tadalafil 20 mg, demonstrated significantly improved sexual function [191]. The effect of tadalafil versus fluoxetine versus the combination of tadalafil and fluoxetine versus placebo on PE was investigated, with results indicating statistically significant increase in intravaginal ejaculatory latency time by 49.57±25.87 to 336.13±224.77 s [192].

The treatment of ED is typically ongoing and success depends on compliance. In five double-blind, placebo-controlled 12-week studies, 308 men were randomized to placebo, 321 to tadalafil 10 mg, and 258 to tadalafil 20 mg. Dose-dependent success was demonstrated [193]. Tadalafil has shown efficacy within 3 days at 2.5 mg and 5 mg once-daily dosing [194]. Dose-dependent success, beyond first-time success, has been demonstrated by improved erections in 79% of tadalafil 20 mg patients, 67% of tadalafil 10 mg patients, and 22% of placebo patients. Successful completion of sexual intercourse was achieved in 62% of tadalafil 20 mg patients, 50% of tadalafil 10 mg patients, and 31% of placebo patients [195].

As ED presents in various severities, a study of 443 men—47% with mild, 30% with moderate, and 23% with severe ED—was undertaken. Erectile function improved to normal in 64% of patients treated with tadalafil, as opposed to 16% in the placebo group [196]. Tadalafil 20 mg has also proven as efficacious in Hispanic and in African-American groups as in the Caucasian reference group [197]. Similarly, tadalafil has been shown to be effective in Egyptian and Turkish men with ED [198] and as effective and well tolerated for the treatment of ED in East Asian, Southeast Asian [199], and Japanese men [200].

One study investigated the effect of tadalafil on ED by examining 1112 men (age range 22–82, mean age = 59), suffering with mild to severe ED of various etiologies. They were randomized to placebo or tadalafil in five randomized, double-blind trials of 12-week duration. Tadalafil exhibited significant improvements in erectile function from baseline, intercourse attempts, and successful completion. Moreover, the tadalafil group showed 81% improved erections at endpoint, compared with 35% in the control group [201].

Another study looked at the effect of tadalafil at 24 and 36 h after dosing. It stratified patients by baseline severity of ED and then randomized within the severity group to tadalafil 20 mg or placebo. Patients were asked to attempt sexual intercourse at approximately these time marks, with success being defined as completion to ejaculation. Not only was tadalafil well tolerated by patients at both time points, but also the 36-h group exhibited 59.2% success relative to placebo, whereas the 24-h group showed 52.9% success [202].

Side Effects

Serious Reactions

Angina, MI, stroke, severe hypotension, hypertension, syncope, tachycardia, priapism, vision loss, hearing loss, nonarteritic anterior ischemic optic neuropathy, Stevens-Johnson syndrome, and exfoliative dermatitis

Common Reactions

Headache, dyspepsia, back pain, myalgia, nasal congestion, flushing, limb pain, and diarrhea [203]

Dosing

Erectile dysfunction: [PRN dosing regimen] 5–20 mg PO × 1 prior to sexual activity; start at 10 mg PO × 1 and adjust based on individual response; maximum 20 mg/dose, 1 dose/24 h; 10 mg/dose, 1 dose/72 h if strong CYP3A4 inhibitor use; effects may last for 36 h [204].

Testosterone

Synopsis

Testosterone is generally considered the chief male sex hormone, playing a pivotal role in the development of male reproductive tissues, such as the testes and the prostate, as well as in formation of secondary sex characteristics, such as growth and pattern of body hair, muscle mass, and bone mass. Despite the inverse relationship between testosterone levels and time, the decline in testosterone levels in men that comes with age is not mutually exclusive with acquisition of erectile dysfunction (ED) [205] nor is the relationship between age and ED firm and fixed. Nonetheless, sexual function is revived in severely hypogonadal men who receive androgen replacement therapy [206, 207]. It has been demonstrated that testosterone treatment in men with lower levels increases the number of nocturnal erections, the frequency of sexual thoughts, and the rate of successful intercourse and improves erectile function and overall sexual satisfaction scores. The effects of testosterone on eugonadal men, however, are not significant [208]. Although much attention has been paid to the treatment of ED, testosterone therapy has also been explored for women for the treatment of HSDD symptoms related to menopause and of decreased sexual desire secondary to medication. Testosterone plays a vital role for both sexes in the treatment of sexual dysfunction.

Clinical Studies

The use of testosterone therapy for the treatment of HSDD after oophorectomy in menopausal women was explored in a 24-week, randomized, double-blind, placebo-controlled trial of 87 people. Transdermal testosterone therapy was shown to improve sexual desire, as well as other domains of sexual function. The testosterone-treated group showed a significantly greater change from baseline in sexual desire, compared with placebo. Arousal, orgasm, sexual concerns, responsiveness, and self-image also significantly improved with testosterone therapy [209]. A larger study of 132 surgically postmenopausal women with HSDD looked at the effect of testosterone treatment on frequency of sexual activity and sexual desire. The study showed that 52% of the women who received testosterone therapy reported a "meaningful treatment benefit" or desire progressing from "seldom" to "sometimes," compared with 31% who received placebo [210].

The use of estrogen as hormonal treatment for the symptoms of menopause is common. The addition of testosterone to this regimen has been explored. A 52-week trial in which 814 women with HSDD were assigned testosterone or placebo showed benefits with testosterone treatment. These postmenopausal women had not received estrogen therapy prior to treatment with testosterone. The effects of testosterone without estrogen on sexual function, specifically satisfying sexual episodes, were modest, though significant [211].

A 3-month assessment of the effect of testosterone cream on 36 women who had undergone hysterectomy and were taking transdermal estrogen revealed that testosterone cream significantly improved sexual desire and frequency of sex [212]. Testosterone undecanoate added twice weekly to an already in-place hormonal regimen was also noted to improve sexual function among postmenopausal women, more so than the estrogen treatment alone [213].

A study to assess naturally occurring menopause in 277 women with HSDD both with and without conventional hormone therapy to treat the menopause revealed that a transdermal testosterone patch over 6 months was associated with significant improvements in sexual desire versus placebo [214].

The effect of testosterone treatment on antidepressant-induced female sexual dysfunction, focusing on the facet of emergent loss of libido, was not published until 2014. What was discovered was that transdermal testosterone therapy resulted in a significant increase in the number of satisfying sexual events, compared to placebo in women with SSRI-/serotonin-norepinephrine reuptake inhibitor (SNRI)-emergent loss of libido, suggesting that transdermal testosterone therapy might be a smart option for SSRI-/SNRI-emergent loss of libido in patients who need to remain on antidepressant therapy [215].

The use of testosterone injection in hypogonadal men for the treatment of low sexual desire has been long-standing. It is common for ED to be comorbid with low testosterone levels [216]. Studies of men without hypogonadism have been found, though to a much lesser extent, and merit investigation. An early double-blind crossover comparison of testosterone and placebo injection in two groups of men with normal testosterone levels—ten with loss of sexual interest and ten with erectile failure—suggested a "significant increase in sexual interest" in the former group. These results pointed to the notion that testosterone influences sexual interest, even in men with normal levels [217].

As comorbid depression and antidepressant side effects typically include sexual dysfunction, a test involving men with major depressive disorder (MDD) who were taking an SSRI and exhibited low or low-normal testosterone level was conducted. Ejaculatory ability was improved by testosterone. In this 6-week, double-blind, placebo-controlled trial of testosterone gel versus placebo in 100 men, it was found that the subgroup of men with the higher baseline testosterone levels showed nearly the same improvement in ejaculatory ability than those with the lower baseline testosterone levels. This implies that the improved ejaculatory ability was unlikely to be secondary to correction of hypogonadism [218].

Side Effects

Serious Reactions

Application site reactions, venous thromboembolism, MI risk, stroke risk, CHF exacerbation, generalized edema, BPH, polycythemia, oligospermia, priapism, prostate cancer, sleep apnea, and hematuria

Common Reactions

Application site reactions, back pain, prostate hypertrophy, headache, allergic contact dermatitis, depression, gynecomastia, hyperlipidemia, edema, hematocrit elevation, PSA elevation, rigors, diarrhea, fatigue, polyuria, dysuria, prostatitis, rash, acne, libido changes, and confusion [219]

Dosing

Surgically menopausal women with HSDD: 300 microgram/day transdermal [209] or 10 mg topical daily (2 cm AndroFeme cream) [212]

Menopausal women with HSDD on daily oral estrogen: oral testosterone decanoate 40 mg twice weekly added to daily oral estrogen [213]

Menopausal women with HSDD: 300 micrograms patch daily [211]

Female sexual dysfunction secondary to SSRI/SNRI therapy: testosterone 300 microgram patch daily [215]

Parenteral injections (testosterone enanthate or testosterone cypionate): every 2–3 weeks; oral, scrotal patch: 5 mg daily (Testoderm); nonscrotal patch: 5 mg daily (Androderm); or skin gel (Androgel) [205]

Tibolone

Synopsis

Tibolone as an agent is a synthetic steroid [220], an analog of the progestin norethynodrel. It has tissue-specific effects on receptors and enzymes involved in the synthesis and metabolism of endogenous estrogen, progesterone, and androgen. It is transformed via intestinal bioconversion into metabolites that have tissue-specific agonistic and/or antagonistic estrogenic and progestogenic/androgenic properties. Tibolone—marketed as Livial and Tibofem, except in the United States, where it was rejected in 2006 by the FDA [221]—has been used as an agent for the treatment of symptomatic menopause [222, 223]. Tibolone stands apart, however, from traditional hormone replacement therapy in climacteric in that it is tissue-specific, associated with low breast tissue proliferation among estrogen therapy alone or combined with progestogens, and is also associated with less vaginal bleeding [224, 225]. Nevertheless, tibolone has also been found to increase breast cancer recurrence [226]. Tibolone also increases free estradiol and testosterone levels, thereby reducing climacteric vasomotor symptoms, as well as alleviating atrophic vaginitis, vaginal dryness, and dyspareunia [227]. It has also been employed in the reduction of hot flashes and sweating, as well as in the improvement of mood and libido [228].

Clinical Studies

Hormone replacement is often used to alleviate symptoms of menopause, which can include decreased sex drive. As tibolone acts as both an estrogen agonist and as a progesterone agonist, its use in postmenopausal women is suggested as an alternative treatment for postmenopausal women with decreased sex drive. A 3-month study of 38 postmenopausal women to examine its impact on sexual function and on climacteric symptoms was conducted. Vaginal blood flow during erotic stimulation by fantasy and film was measured, and sexual responses recorded. Vaginal blood flow was shown to significantly increase with the use of tibolone during fantasy periods, but not during visual film erotic stimulation, suggesting a preferential pathway of female sexual response. Not only did increased vaginal blood flow correspond to fantasy periods but also tibolone was associated with significant increases in sexual desire, as well as frequency of arousability and of sexual fantasies [229].

The relationship between sexual satisfaction and its relation to quality of life is important in the exploration of menopause. As hormone replacement therapy is frequently employed to address the decrease in sexual desire often associated with menopause, a 3-month study of 48 postmenopausal women showed that tibolone had more effect on sexuality than did continuous combined hormone therapy alone. Specifically, tibolone was associated with perceived improvement of sexual performance, including general sexual satisfaction, sexual interest, sexual fantasies, sexual arousal, and orgasm [230].

A 6-month study of 80 postmenopausal women, randomized to either tibolone or to continuous combined conjugated equine estrogens and medroxyprogesterone acetate, revealed significantly higher scores in the tibolone group, when assessing for sexual desire, sexual excitement, intercourse frequency, and vaginal dryness [231]. A study of 140 postmenopausal women comparing tibolone to conventional hormonal therapy likewise showed a significant improvement with tibolone treatment in the sexual domain desire, arousal, and orgasm, whereas conventional hormone therapy was not shown to improve the sexual sub-score of a climacteric questionnaire [232].

The effect of tibolone on sexual functioning was examined in postmenopausal women on hormone replacement therapy and showed that different components of libido, as well as satisfaction with sexual life, were significantly improved in women with tibolone added to their regimen. Effects were attributed to an increase in genital blood flow, as well as to the estrogenic/andronergic mechanism of tibolone [233].

The physiology of tibolone therapy is of interest in understanding its positive effects on the treatment of sexual dysfunction. A study of 50 postmenopausal women under hormone therapy, who reported sexual dysfunction (specifically low libido and arousal disorders), revealed that clitoral circulation in postmenopausal women with sexual dysfunction under hormone therapy treated with tibolone is significantly increased, relative to women not receiving treatment with tibolone [234].

Side Effects

Although it has been in Europe and the rest of the world for about 20 years, tibolone was rejected by the FDA in 2006, probably due to reports of liver injury. For instance, a subacute, drug-induced liver damage in a 54-year-old woman being treated for urinary incontinence and climacteric symptoms normalized after nearly 2 months of discontinuation of tibolone and flavoxate treatment [235]. Tibolone also has been found to increase the risk of stroke in older women with osteoporosis [236].

Adverse Reactions

Increased bone mineral density and increased breast cancer recurrence in women with normal bone mineral density [226]

Common Reactions

Headache, dizziness, nausea, abdominal pain, swollen feet and itching, and slight bleeding or spotting initially [237]

Dosing

Tibolone is usually prescribed at 2.5 mg PO daily in postmenopausal women with climacteric symptoms, but 1.25 mg PO daily has been shown to induce more prompt improvement of sexual function than the higher dose [238].

Vardenafil

Synopsis

Vardenafil is an oral PDE5 inhibitor agent prescribed for the treatment of ED, although it is biochemically more potent and selective than sildenafil [173]. PDE5 is the chief PDE type in the corpus cavernosum and plays a key role in penile erection [123]. In the presence of erectile stimulus, vardenafil potentiates the intracellular actions cGMP [239]. It is hepatically metabolized and has a half-life of 4–6 h [240]. Vardenafil used to have the fastest onset of action in its class [175], until avanafil was approved. Table 26-2 shows the onset of action and duration of action for each of the FDA-approved PDE5 inhibitors. It offers greatest gains with regard to the rate of achieved erection [241] while having high first-dose success rates [242]. It has been shown to be efficacious in the treatment of severe ED, as well as in some patients who are refractory to sildenafil treatment [176]. It also stands out in its class as the only one with a cardiac conduction precaution [243]. One study showed that among the PDE5 inhibitors used for treatment of ED, vardenafil was preferred by younger men, as well as by newlyweds [244]. Its potency in part is explained by it having the highest inhibitory activity of PDE5. An oral dispersible tablet form is attractive not only for its rapid onset and superior bioavailability but also for its ability to be consumed without water [245, 246].

Clinical Studies

A 6-month, multicenter, placebo-controlled, fixed-dose study of men with erectile dysfunction has shown vardenafil to improve erectile function and maintenance of erections, as well as to increase success rates for penetrations [247]. A study of 580 men with erectile dysfunction demonstrated similar gains, as well as advances in orgasmic function, intercourse satisfaction, and overall satisfaction over 12 weeks [248]. One powerful study involved 566 men with ED who, over 24 months of on-demand treatment with vardenafil, showed successful penetration in 92–94% of attempts and erections that maintained in 87–89% [249], supporting long-term efficacy and reliability of vardenafil in men with ED. Likewise in another large study, 600 vardenafil-naïve patients showed 87% success at first attempt of penetration and 74% of erection maintenance [250].

Due to its rapid onset, vardenafil was found in two studies over 12–26 weeks to improve success rates of attempted intercourse as early as 15 min or less and through 4–8 h after dosing in ability to penetrate and as early as 15 min or less and through 8–12 h after dosing in maintenance of erection [251]. An at-home study of 732 men with ED showed that within the first four doses, 50% of men on vardenafil 10 mg and 53% of men on vardenafil 20 mg achieved erection within 25 min of dosing [252]. Vardenafil improved successful intercourse rates compared with placebo in Japanese diabetes mellitus patients from as early as 15 min after dosing [253]. Moreover, like tadalafil, vardenafil's ability to provide efficacy for up to 8 h post-dose offers couples more flexibility in their sexual life [254], making it a strong choice in the treatment of ED.

The study of vardenafil in the treatment of ED in men with comorbidities has shown dosage-related success. Dose-dependent improvements in erection in men with ED who had diabetes have been shown [255, 256], suggesting that higher doses of vardenafil should be employed in populations that are more challenging to treat. Moreover, vardenafil is well tolerated in diabetic men with ED regardless of the level of glycemic control [257]. First-dose vardenafil in the treatment of ED among men not only with diabetes but also with dyslipidemia and hypertension has been shown to lead to a consistently high rate of penetration and maintenance of erection [258]. Men with spinal cord injuries experienced improved erectile function with vardenafil, especially at higher 20 mg dosing, relative to 10 mg [259].

Vardenafil therapy for ED has also been studied in depressed patients. In a study of 280 men with ED and mild depression, vardenafil was found highly efficacious in improving erectile function [260]. Vardenafil therapy has also found a place in the management of PE. In a study designed to assess which of sertraline or vardenafil had a better effect on PE in men with ED, 67% reported improved ejaculation latency times with vardenafil, compared to 40% in the sertraline group [261]. A study of men with lifelong PE was undertaken to assess the effect of vardenafil. Significant improvements in ejaculatory latency times were observed with vardenafil with 189.5 s, compared with 62.7 s on placebo [262]. Interestingly, one study examining the effects on semen characteristics demonstrated that vardenafil did not have adverse effects on sperm concentration, compared with sildenafil and placebo [263]. Moreover, sperm motility was shown to significantly increase in a group of 205 infertile males [264].

Side Effects

Serious Reactions

Anaphylaxis, angina, myocardial ischemia/infarction, hypertension, hypotension, syncope, tachycardia, QT prolongation, priapism, glaucoma, non-arteritic anterior ischemic optic neuropathy, vision loss, and hearing loss

Common Reactions

Headache, flushing, rhinitis, dyspepsia, sinusitis, flu syndrome, dizziness, nausea, CK elevated, abnormal LFTs, back pain, arthralgia/myalgia, and photosensitivity [265]

Dosing

ED: 10 mg PO × 1; start 1 h prior to intercourse; maximum 20 mg/dose up to 1 dose/day; start 5 mg PO × 1 in patients age 65 and older [266].

Regarding the time of dosing, moderate-fat meal consumption has no clinically relevant effect on vardenafil pharmacokinetics [267], setting it apart in its class with regard to planning around meals.

Yohimbine

Synopsis

Yohimbine is an indole alkaloid from the bark of the *Pausinystalia* yohimbe tree, the *Rauwolfia* root, and the *Aspidosperma quebracho* tree. Although it was employed in the United States as a treatment for ED prior to the release of sildenafil, it has been utilized as part of traditional medicinal treatment for ED in West Africa, where for centuries it has been considered an aphrodisiac [268]. Yohimbine is a centrally acting alpha(2A)-adrenoceptor competitive antagonist that overall increases sympathetic outflow [269]. By binding alpha(2A)-adrenoceptors in the cavernosa, yohimbine prevents the contractility of smooth muscle [268], helping to facilitate erection. It exhibits a multifaceted effect, lending to increases in dopamine and in noradrenaline and a decrease in serotonin. More specifically, yohimbine displays high affinity at alpha(2A)-, alpha(2B)-, and alpha(2C)-adrenoceptors; significant affinity for 5-HT(1A), 5-HT(1B), 5-HT(1D), and dopamine 2-receptors; and weak affinity for dopamine 3-receptors. It wields antagonist actions at alpha(2A)-adrenoceptors, 5-HT(1B), 5-HT(1D), and dopamine 2-receptors, but partial agonist actions at 5-HT(1A) sites. It enhances striatal dopamine turnover, suppresses striatal 5-HT turnover, decreases activity of serotonergic neurons in the raphe nuclei, and increases hippocampal noradrenaline turnover [270]. It has monoamine oxidase activity and may also interact with vasoactive intestinal peptidergic receptors. It could be over-the-counter today as a sexual enhancement product.

Clinical Studies

An early study investigating the use of yohimbine enrolled 48 subjects with psychogenic ED participated in a 10-week placebo-controlled, double-blind, partial crossover trial of yohimbine for the restoration of erectile function. Overall, 46% of participants who received yohimbine had a positive response, suggesting that yohimbine could be employed for the treatment of psychogenic ED and that it was as effective as sex and marital counseling for restoring satisfactory sexual function [271].

Yohimbine was investigated as an agent in the treatment of decreased sexual desire, specifically secondary to antidepressant treatment. Non-geriatric patients with new-onset sexual dysfunction secondary to treatment with fluoxetine participated in this open trial. A remarkable eight out of nine patients reported improved sexual function with yohimbine. Putting the side effect profile aside (five patients discontinued due to adverse effects), the use of yohimbine as treatment for fluoxetine-induced sexual dysfunction now deserved more attention [272].

The use of yohimbine with trazodone, a serotonergic agent, as treatment for pure psychogenic ED was also established in a study of 63 patients. Erectile function, ejaculation, interest in sex, and sexual thoughts were examined at the end of two 8-week courses, as well as at 3- and 6-month follow-ups. Results were promising, with 71% reporting improved sexual function at 8 weeks, 58% reporting improved sexual function at 3 months, and 56% reporting improved sexual function at 6 months [273].

To help identify whether yohimbine was useful in the treatment of male sexual dysfunction for organic versus non-organic causes, a double-blind placebo-controlled study of 31 patients demonstrated that yohimbine was not superior to placebo in organic patients but that nonorganic patients exhibited significant improvements in sexual function. Moreover, nocturnal penile tumescence and rigidity were not improved by yohimbine, helping to further establish it as an appropriate option in the treatment of psychogenic male sexual dysfunction [274]. Sexual desire, arousal, and ejaculatory response evoked by visual sexual stimulation were assessed in one study. Interestingly, sexual arousal and erectile response increased during masturbation, but not during intercourse. Nonetheless, with nocturnal penile tumescence again showing no improvement secondary to treatment by yohimbine, development would focus on the treatment of psychogenic erectile problems [275]. The efficacy of yohimbine in the treatment of nonorganic erectile dysfunction in 86 patients over 8 weeks in a similar study showed a 71% versus a 45% response rate in yohimbine versus placebo, respectively. This improvement represented changes in sexual desire, sexual satisfaction, frequency of sexual contacts, and quality of erection during sexual contact/intercourse. Objective measurement was determined via polysomnography in a sleep laboratory [276].

Appropriate for the treatment of common causes of non-organic sexual dysfunction, another investigation into yohimbine therapy for SSRI-induced sexual side effects in patients treated for obsessive compulsive disorder, trichotillomania, anxiety, or affective disorders revealed that five out of six patients treated with yohimbine experienced improved sexual functioning [277]. A larger study of the therapeutic effect of yohimbine on ED in a mixed group of men, some with diabetes and vascular pathological conditions, showed that within 2–3 weeks yohimbine helped 34% of participants reported either partial or full restoration of full and sustained erections [278]. One study of the treatment with yohimbine of orgasmic dysfunction of varying etiology found that 16 out of 29 men were able to ejaculate either during masturbation or during sexual intercourse [279].

Side Effects

Serious Reactions

Hypertension: Alpha 2-adrenoceptor antagonists such as yohimbine are known to cause an increased blood pressure [280]. Yohimbine increased the risk for impulsivity secondary to noradrenergic stimulation [281] and respiratory depression

Common reactions: urinary retention, hyperglycemia, tachycardia, irritability, tremor, diaphoresis, nausea, vomiting, dizziness, headache, flushing, nervousness, and blood pressure elevation [282]

Dosing

For the treatment of ED: 10 mg PO TID × 8 weeks [276]

Note: to be decreased if adverse reactions occur to ½ tab PO TID and then increased back to 1 tab PO TID [283]

Conclusion

Improving and enhancing sexual function pharmacologically include approved and off-label medications. The pharmacological interventions highlighted above have scientific basis for their use in sexual enhancement; however, large randomized controlled trials remain needed to establish their value in subthreshold diagnosis and transient dysfunction and to examine more closely placebo response and side effect profile.

More research is also needed to identify new and existing pharmacological agents that have novel mechanisms of action in sexual enhancement.

References

1. Aldemir M, Okulu E, Neselioglu S, Erel O, Kayigil O. Pistachio diet improves erectile function parameters and serum lipid profiles in patients with erectile dysfunction. Int J Impot Res. 2011;23(1):32–8.
2. Vatsyavana, Burton RF, Muhammed U. The kama sutra. New York: Diadem Books; 1984.
3. Farmer M, Yoon H, Goldstein I. Future targets for female sexual dysfunction. J Sex Med. 2016;13(8):1147–65.
4. Porst H, Buvat J, Meuleman E, et al. Intracavernous Alprostadil Alfadex—an effective and well tolerated treatment for erectile dysfunction. Results of a long-term European study. Int J Impot Res. 1998;10:225–31.
5. Porst H. Transurethral alprostadil with MUSE (medicated urethral system for erection) vs intracavernous alprostadil—a comparative study in 103 patients with erectile dysfunction. Int J Impot Res. 1997;9:187–92.
6. Moncada I, Cuzin B. Clinical efficacy and safety of Vitaros(c)/Virirec(c) (Alprostadil cream) for the treatment of erectile dysfunction. Urologia. 2015;82:84–92.
7. Padma-Nathan H, Yeager JL. An integrated analysis of alprostadil topical cream for the treatment of erectile dysfunction in 1732 patients. Urology. 2006;68(2):386–91.
8. Schechter MD, Greer NL. Evidence that the stimulus properties of apomorphine are mediated by both D1 and D2 receptor activation. Life Sci. 1987;40(25):2461–71.
9. Brambilla F, Bellodi L, Perna G, Anrancio C, Bertani A. Dopamine function in obsessive-compulsive disorder: growth hormone response to apomorphine stimulation. Biol Psychiatry. 1997;42(10):889–97.
10. Rampin O. Mode of action of a new oral treatment for erectile dysfunction: apomorphine SL. BJU Int. 2001;88(Suppl 3):22–4.
11. Bechara A, Bertolino MV, Casabé A, Fredotovich N. A double-blind randomized placebo control study comparing the objective and subjective changes in female sexual response using sublingual apomorphine. J Sex Med. 2004;1(2):209–14.
12. Caruso S, Agnello C, Intelisano G, Farina M, Di Mari L, Cianci A. Placebo-controlled study on efficacy and safety of daily apomorphine SL intake in premenopausal women affected by hypoactive sexual desire disorder and sexual arousal disorder. Urology. 2004;63(5):955–9.
13. Altwein JE, Keuler FU. Oral treatment of erectile dysfunction with apomorphine SL. Urol Int. 2001;67(4):257–63.
14. Mulhall JP, Bukofzer S, Edmonds AL, George M, Apomorphine SL Study Group. An open-label, uncontrolled dose-optimization study of sublingual apomorphine in erectile dysfunction. Clin Ther. 2001;23(8):1260–71.
15. Dula E, Bukofzer S, Perdok R, George M. Apomorphine SL Study Group. Double-blind, crossover comparison of 3 mg apomorphine SL with placebo and with 4 mg apomorphine SL in male erectile dysfunction. Eur Urol. 2001;39(5):558–3; discussion 564.
16. Dula E, Keating W, Siami PH, Edmonds A, O'neil J, Buttler S. Efficacy and safety of fixed-dose and dose-optimization regimens of sublingual apomorphine versus placebo in men with erectile dysfunction. The Apomorphine Study Group. Urology. 2000;56(1):130–5.
17. Von Keitz AT, Ströberg P, Bukofzer S, Mallard N, Hibberd M. A European multicentre study to evaluate the tolerability of apomorphine sublingual administered in a forced dose-escalation regimen in patients with erectile dysfunction. BJU Int. 2002;89(4):409–15.
18. Riley A, Main M, Morgan F. Inhalation device allows novel administration of apomorphine in men with erectile dysfunction-efficacy and safety findings. J Sex Med. 2010;7(4 Pt 1):1508–17.
19. Heaton JP, Dean J, Sleep DJ. Sequential administration enhances the effect of apomorphine SL in men with erectile dysfunction. Int J Impot Res. 2002;14(1):61–4.
20. Athenahealth, Inc. [Internet]. San Mateo (CA): Epocatres, Inc. https://online.epocrates.com/drugs/366605/Apokyn/Adverse-Reactions. Accessed 15 Aug 2016.
21. Grosset KA, Malek N, Morgan F, Grosset DG. Phase IIa randomized double-blind, placebo-controlled study of inhaled apomorphine as acute challenge for rescuing 'off' periods in patients with established Parkinson's disease. Eur J Neurol. 2013;20(11):1445–50.
22. Limin M, Johnsen N, Hellstrom WJ. Avanafil, a new rapid-onset phosphodiesterase 5 inhibitor for the treatment of erectile dysfunction. Expert Opin Investig Drugs. 2010;19(11):1427–37.
23. Kyle JA, Brown DA, Hill JK. Avanafil for erectile dysfunction. Ann Pharmacother. 2013;47(10):1312–20.
24. Egui-Rojo MA, Moncada-Iribarren I, Carballido-Rodriguez J, Martinez-Salamanca JI. Avanafil for the treatment of erectile dysfunction. An updated review. Arch Esp Urol. 2014;67(10):839–47.
25. Kedia GT, Uckert S, Assadi-Pour F, Kuczyk MA, Albrecht K. Avanafil for the treatment of erectile dysfunction: initial data and clinical key properties. Ther Adv Urol. 2013;5(1):35–41.
26. Wang R, Burnett AL, Heller WH, Omori K, Kotera J, Kikkawa K, et al. Selectivity of avanafil, a PDE5 inhibitor for the treatment of erectile dysfunction: implications for clinical safety and improved tolerability. J Sex Med. 2012;9(8):2122–9.
27. Hellstrom WJ, Freier MT, Serefoglu EC, Lewis RW, DiDonato K, Peterson CA. A phase II, single-blind, randomized, crossover evaluation of the safety and efficacy of avanafil using visual sexual stimulation in patients with mild to moderate erectile dysfunction. BJU Int. 2013;111(1):137–47.
28. Goldstein I, McCullough AR, Jones LA, Hellstrom WJ, Bowden CH, Didonato K, et al. A randomized, double-blind, placebo-controlled evaluation of the safety and efficacy of avanafil in subjects with erectile dysfunction. J Sex Med. 2012;9(4):1122–33.
29. Zhao C, Kim SW, Yang DY, Kim JJ, Park NC, Lee SW, et al. Efficacy and safety of avanafil for treating erectile dysfunction: results of a multicentre, randomized, double-blind, placebo-controlled trial. BJU Int. 2012;110(11):1801–6.
30. Hellstrom WJ, Kaminetsky J, Belkoff LH, Goldstein I, Tursi JP, Uy J, et al. Efficacy of Avanafil 15 minutes after dosing in men with erectile dysfunction: a randomized, double-blind, Placebo Controlled Study. J Urol. 2015;194(2):485–92.
31. Goldstein I, Jones LA, Belkoff LH, Karlin GS, Bowden CH, Peterson CA, et al. Avanafil for the treatment of erectile dysfunction: a multicenter, randomized, double-blind study in men with diabetes mellitus. Mayo Clin Proc. 2012;87(9):843–52.
32. Mulhall JP, Burnett AL, Wang R, McVary KT, Moul JW, Bowden CH, et al. A phase 3, placebo controlled study of the safety and efficacy of avanafil for the treatment of erectile dysfunction after nerve sparing radical prostatectomy. J Urol. 2013;189(6):2229–36.
33. Belkoff LH, McCullough A, Goldstein I, Jones L, Bowden CH, DiDonato K, et al. An open-label, long-term evaluation of the safety, efficacy and tolerability of avanafil in male patients with mild to severe erectile dysfunction. Int J Clin Pract. 2013;67(4):333–41.
34. Athenahealth, Inc. [Internet]. San Mateo (CA): Epocatres, Inc. https://online.epocrates.com/drugs/685705/Stendra/Adverse-Reactions. Accessed 15 Aug 2016.
35. Athenahealth, Inc. [Internet]. San Mateo (CA): Epocatres, Inc. https://online.epocrates.com/drugs/685701/Stendra/Adult-Dosing. Accessed 15 Aug 2016.

36. Ferris RM, Maxwell RA, Cooper BR, Soroke FE. Neurochemical and neuropharmacological investigations into the mechanisms of action of bupropion. HCl–a new atypical antidepressant agent. Adv Biochem Psychopharmacol. 1982;31:277–86.
37. Ascher JA, Cole JO, Colin JN, Feighner JP, Ferris RM, Fibiger HC, et al. Bupropion: a review of its mechanism of antidepressant activity. J Clin Psychiatry. 1995;56(9):395–401.
38. Rappa L. Condensed psychopharmacology 2016: a pocket reference for psychiatry and psychiatric medications. Fort Lauderdale: RXPSYCH LLC; 2015.
39. Preskorn SH, Othmer SC. Evaluation of bupropion hydrochloride: the first of a new class of atypical antidepressants. Pharmacotherapy. 1984;4(1):20–34.
40. Remick RA, Campos PE, Misri S, Miles JE, Van Wyck Fleet J. A comparison of the safety and efficacy of bupropion HCL and amitriptyline hcl in depressed patients. Prog Neuropsychopharmacol Biol Psychiatry. 1982;6(4–6):523–7.
41. Wenger TL, Cohn JB, Bustrack J. Comparison of the effects of bupropion and amitriptyline on cardiac conduction in depressed patients. J Clin Psychiatry. 1983;44(5 Pt 2):174–5.
42. Pereira VM, Arias-Carrión O, Machado S, Nardi AE, Silva AC. Bupropion in the depression-related sexual dysfunction: a systematic review. CNS Neurol Disord Drug Targets. 2014;13(6):1079–88.
43. Kennedy SH, Fulton KA, Bagby RM, Greene AL, Cohen NL, Rafi-Tari S. Sexual function during bupropion or paroxetine treatment of major depressive disorder. Can J Psychiatry. 2006;51(4):234–42.
44. Crenshaw TL, Goldberg JP, Stern WC. Pharmacological modification of psychosexual dysfunction. J Sex Marital Ther. 1987;13(4):239–52.
45. Croft H, Settle Jr E, Houser T, Batey SR, Donahue RM, Ascher JA. A placebo-controlled comparison of the antidepressant efficacy and effects on sexual functioning of sustained release bupropion and sertraline. Clin Ther. 1999;21(4):643–58.
46. Coleman CC, King BR, Bolden-Watson C, Book MJ, Segraves RT, Richard N, et al. A placebo-controlled comparison of the effects on sexual functioning of bupropion sustained release and fluoxetine. Clin Ther. 2001;23(7):1040–58.
47. Segraves RT, Kavousi R, Hughes AR, Batey SR, Johnston JA, Donahue R, et al. Evaluation of sexual functioning in depressed outpatients: a double-blind comparison of sustained-release bupropion and sertraline treatment. J Clin Psychopharmacol. 2000;20(2):122–8.
48. Lodise NM. Hypoactive sexual desire disorder in women: treatment options beyond testosterone and approaches to communicating with patients on sexual health. Pharmacotherapy. 2013;33(4):411–21.
49. American Psychiatric Association (APA). Diagnostic and statistical manual of mental disorders. 4th ed., text revision. Washington, DC: American Psychiatric Publishing Inc.; 2000.
50. Segraves RT, Croft H, Kavoussi R, Ascher JA, Batey SR, Foster VJ, et al. Bupropion sustained release (SR) for the treatment of hypoactive sexual desire disorder (HSDD) in non-depressed women. J Sex Marital Ther. 2001;27(3):303–16.
51. Segraves RT, Clayton A, Croft H, Wolf A, Warnock J. Bupropion sustained release for the treatment of hypoactive sexual desire disorder in premenopausal women. J Clin Psychopharmacol. 2004;24(3):339–42.
52. Safarinejad MR, Hosseini SY, Asgari MA, Dadkhah F, Taghva A. A randomized, double-blind, placebo-controlled study of the efficacy and safety of bupropion for treating hypoactive sexual desire disorder in ovulating women. BJU Int. 2010;106(6):832–9.
53. Safarinejad MR. Reversal of SSRI-induced female sexual dysfunction by adjunctive bupropion in menstruating women: a double-blind, placebo-controlled and randomized study. J Pscyhopharmacol. 2011;25(3):370–8.
54. Clayton AH, Warnock JK, Kornstein SG, Pinkerton R, Sheldon-Keller A, McGarvey EL. A placebo-controlled trial of bupropion SR as an antidote for selective serotonin reuptake inhibitor-induced sexual dysfunction. J Clin Psychiatry. 2004;65(1):62–7.
55. Taylor MJ, Rudkin L, Bullemor-Day P, Lubin J, Chukwujekwu C, Hawton K. Strategies for managing sexual dysfunction induced by antidepressant medication. Cochrane Database Syst Rev 2013;(5):CD003382.
56. Clayton AH, Croft HA, Horrigan JP, Wightman DS, Krishen A, Richard NE, et al. Bupropion extended release compared with escitalopram: effects on sexual functioning and antidepressant efficacy in 2 randomized, double-blind, placebo-controlled studies. J Clin Psychiatry. 2006;67(5):736–46.
57. Modell JG, May RS, Katholi CR. Effect of bupropion-SR on orgasmic dysfunction in nondepressed subjects: a pilot study. J Sex Marital Ther. 2000;26(3):231–40.
58. Abdel-Hamid IA, Saleh e-S. Primary lifelong delayed ejaculation: characteristics and response to bupropion. J Sex Med. 2011;8(6):1772–9.
59. Riblet LA, Eison AS, Eison MS, Newton RE, Taylor DP, Temple Jr DL. Buspirone: an anxioselective alternative for the management of anxiety disorders. Prog Neuropsychopharmacol Biol Psychiatry. 1983;7(4–6):663–8.
60. Robinson DS, Alms DR, Shrotriya RC, Messina M, Wickramaratne P. Serotonergic anxiolytics and treatment of depression. Psychopathology. 1989;22(Suppl 1):27–36.
61. Goldberg HL. Benzodiazepine and nonbenzodiazepine anxiolytics. Psychopathology. 1984;17(Suppl 1):45–55.
62. Feighner JP, Boyer WF. Serotonin-1A anxiolytics: an overview. Psychopathology. 1989;22(Suppl 1):21–6.
63. Van Rooij K, Poels S, Bloemers J, Goldstein I, Gerritsen J, van Ham D, et al. Toward personalized sexual medicine (part 3): testosterone combined with a Serotonin1A receptor agonist increases sexual satisfaction in women with HSDD and FSAD, and dysfunctional activation for sexual inhibitory mechanisms. J Sex Med. 2013;10(3):824–37.
64. Van Rooij K, Poels S, Worst P, Bloemers J, Koppeschaar H, Goldstein A, et al. Efficacy of testosterone combined with a PDE5 inhibitor and testosterone combined with a serotonin (1A) receptor agonist in women with SSRI-induced sexual dysfunction. A preliminary study. Eur J Pharmacol. 2015;753:246–51.
65. Landén M, Eriksson E, Agren H, Fahlén T. Effect of buspirone on sexual dysfunction in depressed patients treated with selective serotonin reuptake inhibitors. J Clin Psychopharmacol. 1999;19(3):268–71.
66. Athenahealth, Inc. [Internet]. San Mateo (CA): Epocatres, Inc. https://online.epocrates.com/drugs/46305/buspirone/Adverse-Reactions. Accessed 15 Aug 2016.
67. Dean JD, McMahon CG, Guay AT, Morgentaler A, Althof SE, Becher EF, Bivalacqua TJ, Burnett AL, Buvat J, El Meliegy A, Hellstrom WJ, Jannini EA, Maggi M, McCullough A, Torres LO, Zitzmann M. The international society for sexual medicine's process of care for the assessment and management of testosterone deficiency in adult men. J Sex Med. 2015;12(8):1660–86.
68. Shabsigh A, Kang Y, Shabsign R, Gonzalez M, Liberson G, Fisch H, Goluboff E. Clomiphene citrate effects on testosterone/estrogen ratio in male hypogonadism. J Sex Med. 2005;2(5):716–21.
69. Wiehle R, Cunningham GR, Pitteloud N, Wike J, Hsu K, Fontenot GK, Rosner M, Dwyer A, Podolski J. Testosterone restoration by enclomiphene citrate in men with secondary hypogonadism: pharmacodynamics and pharmacokinetics. BJU Int. 2013;112:1188–200.
70. Buvat J, Tesfaye F, Rothman M, Rivas DA, Giuliano F. Dapoxetine for the treatment of premature ejaculation: results from a randomized, double-blind, placebo-controlled phase 3 trial in 22 countries. Eur Urol. 2009;55(4):957–67.

71. McMahon CG, Althof SE, Kaufman JM, Buvat J, Levine SB, Aquilina JW, Tesfaye F, Rothman M, Rivas DA, Porst H. Efficacy and safety of dapoxetine for the treatment of premature ejaculation: integrated analysis of results from five phase 3 trials. J Sex Med. 2011;8(2):524–39.
72. McMahon CG. Dapoxetine: a new option in the medical management of premature ejaculation. Ther Adv Urol. 2012;4(5):233–51.
73. McMahon CG, Giuliano F, Dean J, Hellstrom WJ, Bull S, Tesfaye F, Sharma O, Rivas DA, Aquilina JW. Efficacy and safety of dapoxetine in men with premature ejaculation and concomitant erectile dysfunction treated with a phosphodiesterase type 5 inhibitor: randomized, placebo-controlled, phase III study. J Sex Med. 2013;10(9):2312–25.
74. Stahl SM, Sommer B, Allers KA. Multifunctional pharmacology of flibanserin: possible mechanism of therapeutic action in hypoactive sexual desire disorder. J Sex Med. 2011;8(1):15–27.
75. Gelez H, Clement P, Compagnie S, Gorny D, Laurin M, Allers K, et al. Brain neuronal activation induced by flibanserin treatment in female rats. Psychopharmacology (Berl). 2013;230(4):639–52.
76. Food and Drug Administration [Internet]. Silver Spring: FDA; cc2015 [updated 2015 August]. Accessdata; [about 1 screen]. http://www.accessdata.fda.gov/drugsatfda_docs/label/2015/022526lbl.pdf. Accessed 2 Aug 2016.
77. Holloway V, Wylie K. Sex drive and sexual desire. Curr Opin Psychiatry. 2015;28(6):424–9.
78. Simon JA, Kingsberg SA, Shumel B, Hanes V, Garcia Jr M, Sand M. Efficacy and safety of flibanserin in postmenopausal women with hypoactive sexual desire disorder: results of the SNOWDROP trial. Menopause. 2014;21(6):633–40.
79. Thorp J, Simon J, Dattani D, Taylor L, Kimura T, Garcia Jr M, et al. DAISY trial investigators: treatment of hypoactive sexual desire disorder in premenopausal women: efficacy of flibanserin in the DAISY study. J Sex Med. 2012;9(3):793–804.
80. Derogatis LR, Komer L, Katz M, Moreau M, Kimura T, Garcia Jr M, et al. Treatment of hypoactive sexual desire disorder in premenopausal women: efficacy of flibanserin in the VIOLET study. J Sex Med. 2012;9(4):1074–85.
81. Jayne C, Simon JA, Taylor LV, Kimura T, Lesko LM, SUNFLOWER study investigators. Open-label extension study of flibanserin in women with hypoactive sexual desire disorder. J Sex Med. 2012;9(12):3180–8.
82. Katz M, DeRogatis LR, Ackerman R, Hedges P, Lesko L, Garcia Jr M, et al. Efficacy of flibanserin in women with hypoactive sexual desire disorder: results from the BEGONIA trial. J Sex Med. 2013;10(7):1807–15.
83. Baksh SN, Gellad WF, Alexander GC. Maximizing the post-approval safety of flibanserin: a role for regulators, clinicians, and patients. Drug Saf. 2016;39(5):375–80.
84. Jaspers L, Feys F, Bramer WM, Franco OH, Leusink P, Laan ET. Efficacy and safety of flibanserin for the treatment of hypoactive sexual desire disorder in women: a systematic review and meta-analysis. JAMA Intern Med. 2016;176(4):453–62.
85. Robinson K, Cutler JB, Carris NW. First pharmacological therapy for hypoactive sexual desire disorder in premenopausal women: flibanserin. Ann Pharmacother. 2016;50(2):125–32.
86. Athenahealth, Inc. [Internet]. San Mateo (CA): Epocatres, Inc. https://online.epocrates.com/drugs/730801/Addyi/Adult-Dosing. Accessed 15 Aug 2016.
87. Gantz I, Fong TM. The melanocortin system. Am J Physiol Endocrinol Metab. 2003;284(3):E468–74.
88. Yang YK, Harmon CM. Recent developments in our understanding of melanocortin system in the regulation of food intake. Obes Rev. 2003;4(4):239–48.
89. Ückert S, Bannowsky A, Albrecht K, Kuczyk MA. Melanocortin receptor agonists in the treatment of male and female sexual dysfunction: results from basic research and clinical studies. Expert Opin Investig Drugs. 2014;23(11):1477–83.
90. Porst H. The future of erectile dysfunction (ED). Arch Esp Urol. 2010;63(8):740–7.
91. Diamond LE, Earle DC, Heiman JR, Rosen RC, Perelman MA, Harning R. An effect on the subjective sexual response in premenopausal women with sexual arousal disorder by bremelanotide (PT-141), a melanocortin receptor agonist. J Sex Med. 2006;3(4):628–38.
92. Safarinejad MR. Evaluation of the safety and efficacy of bremelanotide, a melanocortin receptor agonist, in female subjects with arousal disorder: a double-blind placebo-controlled, fixed dose, randomized study. J Sex Med. 2008;5(4):887–97.
93. Wessells H, Levine N, Hadley ME, Dorr R, Hruby V. Melanocortin receptor agonists, penile erection, and sexual motivation: human studies with Melanotan II. Int J Impot Res. 2000;12(Suppl 4):S74–9.
94. Lansdell MI, Hepworth D, Calabrese A, Brown AD, Blagg J, Burring DJ, et al. Discovery of a selective small-molecule melanocortin-4 receptor agonist with efficacy in a pilot study of sexual dysfunction in humans. J Med Chem. 2010;53(8):3183–97.
95. Safarinejad MR, Hosseini SY. Salvage of sildenafil failures with bremelanotide: a randomized, double-blind, placebo-controlled study. J Urol. 2008;179(3):1066–71.
96. Rosen RC, Diamond LE, Earle DC, Shadiack AM, Molinoff PB. Evaluation of the safety, pharmacokinetics and pharmacodynamics effects of subcutaneously administered PT-141, a melanocortin receptor agonist, in healthy male subjects and in patients with an inadequate response to Viagra. Int J Impot Res. 2004;16(2):135–42.
97. Dorr RT, Lines R, Levine N, Brooks C, Xiang L, Hruby VJ, et al. Evaluation of melanotan-II, a superpotent cyclic melanotropic peptide in a pilot phase-I clinical study. Life Sci. 1996;58(20):1777–84.
98. IsHak WW, Kahloon M, Fakhry H. Oxytocin role in enhancing well-being: a literature review. J Affect Disord. 2011;130(1–2):1–9.
99. Ooi YP, Weng SJ, Kossowsky J, Gerger H, Sung M. Oxytocin and autism spectrum disorders: a systematic review and meta-analysis of randomized controlled trials. Pharmacopsychiatry. 2016. [Epub ahead of print] PubMed.
100. Oya K, Matsuda Y, Matsunaga S, Kishi T, Iwata N. Efficacy and safety of oxytocin augmentation therapy for schizophrenia: an updated systematic review and meta-analysis of randomized, placebo-controlled trials. Eur Arch Psychiatry Clin Neurosci. 2016;266(5):439–50.
101. Carmichael MS, Warburton VL, Dixen J, Davidson JM. Relationships among cardiovascular, muscular, and oxytocin responses during human sexual activity. Arch Sex Behav. 1994;23:59–77.
102. IsHak WW, Berman DS, Peters A. Male anorgasmia treated with oxytocin. J Sex Med. 2008;5(4):1022–4.
103. IsHak WW. The guidebook of sexual medicine. Beverly Hills, CA: A&W Publishing; 2008.
104. MacDonald K, Feifel D. Dramatic improvement in sexual function induced by intranasal oxytocin. J Sex Med. 2012;9(5):1407–10.
105. Macdonald K, Macdonald TM. The peptide that binds: a systematic review of oxytocin and its prosocial effects in humans. Harv Rev Psychiatry. 2010;18(1):1–21.
106. Wudarczyk OA, Earp BD, Guastella A, Savulescu J. Could intranasal oxytocin be used to enhance relationships? Research imperatives, clinical policy, and ethical considerations. Curr Opin Psychiatry. 2013;26(5):474–84.
107. Farina Z, Fawcus S. Oxytocin–ensuring appropriate use and balancing efficacy with safety. S Afr Med J. 2015;105(4):271–4.
108. Daughters K, Manstead AS, Hubble K, Rees A, Thapar A, van Goozen SH. Salivary oxytocin concentrations in males following intranasal administration of oxytocin: a double-blind, cross-over study. PLoS One. 2015;10(12):e0145104.
109. Rabey JM. Second generation of dopamine agonists: pros and cons. J Neural Transm Suppl. 1995;45:213–24.

110. Montastruc JL, Rascol O, Sendard JM. Treatment of Parkinson's disease should begin with a dopamine agonist. Mov Disord. 1999;14(5):725–30.
111. de Mey C, Enterling D, Meineke I, Brendel E. Effects of the novel D2-dopaminergic agonist ropinirol on supine resting and stimulated circulatory and neuroendocrine variables in healthy volunteers. Arzneimittelforschung. 1990;40(1):7–13.
112. Eden RJ, Costall B, Domeney AM, Gerrard PA, Harvey CA, Kelly ME, et al. Preclinical pharmacology of ropinirole (SK&F 101468-A) a novel dopamine D2 agonist. Pharmacol Biochem Behav. 1991;38(1):147–54.
113. Rascol O. Dopamine agonists: what is the place of the newer compounds in the treatment of Parkinson's disease? J Neural Transm Suppl. 1999;55:33–45.
114. Ondo W. Ropinirole for restless legs syndrome. Mov Disord. 1999;14(1):138–40.
115. Worthington 3rd JJ, Simon NM, Korbly NB, Perlis RH, Pollack MH, Anxiety Disorders Research Program. Ropinirole for antidepressant-induced sexual dysfunction. Int Clin Psychopharmacol. 2002;17(6):307–10.
116. Kaye CM, Nicholls B. Clinical pharmacokinetics of ropinrole. Clin Pharmacokinet. 2000;39(4):243–54.
117. Berger C, Mehrhoff FW, Beier KM, Meinck HM. Sexual delinquency and Parkinson's disease. Nervenarzt. 2003;74(4):370–5.
118. Klos KJ, Bower JH, Josephs KA, Matsumoto JY, Ahlskog JE. Pathological hypersexuality predominantly linked to adjuvant dopamine agonist therapy in Parkinson's disease and multiple system atrophy. Parkinsonism Relat Disord. 2005;11(6):381–6.
119. Moore TJ, Glenmullen J, Mattison DR. Reports of pathological gambling, hypersexuality, and compulsive shopping associated with dopamine receptor agonist drugs. JAMA Intern Med. 2014;174(12):1930–3.
120. Weintraub D, Siderowf AD, Potenza MN, Goveas J, Morales KH, Duda JE, et al. Association of dopamine agonist use with impulse control disorders in Parkinson disease. Arch Neurol. 2006;63(7):969–73.
121. Driver-Dunckley ED, Noble BN, Hentz JG, Evidente VG, Caviness JN, Parish J, et al. Gambling and increased sexual desire with dopaminergic medications in restless legs syndrome. Clin Neuropharmacol. 2007;30(5):249–55.
122. Athenahealth, Inc. [Internet]. San Mateo (CA): Epocatres, Inc. https://online.epocrates.com/drugs/117405/ropinirole/Adverse-Reactions. Accessed 15 Aug 2016.
123. Carrier S. Pharmacology of phosphodiesterase 5 inhibitors. Can J Urol. 2003;10(Suppl 1):12–6.
124. Boolell M, Allen MJ, Ballard SA, Gepi-Attee S, Muirhead GJ, Naylor AM, et al. Sildenafil: an orally active type 5 cyclic GMP-specific phosphodiesterase inhibitor for the treatment of penile erectile dysfunction. Int J Impot Res. 1996;8(2):47–52.
125. Ballard SA, Gingell CJ, Tang K, Turner LA, Price ME, Naylor AM. Effects of sildenafil on the relaxation of human corpus cavernosum tissue in vitro and on the activities of cyclic nucleotide phosphodiesterase isoenzymes. J Urol. 1998;159(6):2164–71.
126. Berman JR, Berman LA, Toler SM, Gill J, Haughie S, Sildenafil Study Group. Safety and efficacy of sildenafil citrate for the treatment of female sexual arousal disorder: a double-blind, placebo controlled study. J Urol. 2003;170(6 Pt 1):2333–8.
127. Caruso S, Intelisano G, Lupo L, Agnello C. Premenopausal women affected by sexual arousal disorder treated with sildenafil: a double-blind, cross-over, placebo-controlled study. BJOG. 2001;108(6):623–8.
128. IsHak WW. The guidebook of sexual medicine. Beverly Hills: A&W Publishing Group; 2008.
129. Rybalkin SD, Rybalkina IG, Shimizu-Albergine M, Tang XB, Beavo J. PDE5 is converted to an activated state upon cGMP binding to the GAF A domain. EMBO J. 2003;22(3):469–78.
130. Lau LC, Adaikan PG. Mechanisms of direct relaxant effect of sildenafil, tadalafil and vardenafil on corpus cavernosum. Eur J Pharmacol. 2006;541(3):184–90.
131. Huang YY, Li Z, Cai YH, Feng LJ, Wu Y, Li X, et al. The molecular basis for the selectivity of tadalafil toward phosphodiesterase 5 and 6: a modeling study. J Chem Inf Model. 2013;53(11):3044–53.
132. Waldkirch E, Uckert S, Yildrim H, Sohn M, Jonas U, Stief CG, et al. Cyclic AMP-specific and cyclic GMP-specific phosphodiesterase isoenzymes in human cavernous arteries—immunohistochemical distribution and functional significance. World J Urol. 2005;23(6):405–10.
133. Spitzer M, Bhasin S, Travison TG, Davda MN, Stroh H, Basaria S. Sildenafil increases serum testosterone levels by a direct action on the testis. Andrology. 2013;1(6):913–8.
134. Rosas SE, Wasserstein A, Kobrin S, Feldman HI. Preliminary observations of sildenafil treatment for erectile dysfunction in dialysis patients. Am J Kidney Dis. 2001;37(1):134–7.
135. Seftel AD. Phosphodiesterase type 5 inhibitor differentiation based on selectivity, pharmacokinetic, and efficacy profiles. Clin Cardiol. 2004;27(4 Suppl 1):I14–9.
136. Goldstein I, Lue TF, Padma-Nathan H, Rosen RC, Steers WD, Wicker PA. Oral sildenafil in the treatment of erectile dysfunction. Sildenafil Study Group. N Engl J Med. 1998;338(20):1397–404.
137. Kirby M, Creanga DL, Stecher VJ. Erectile dysfunction hardness and tolerability in men treated with sildenafil 100 mg vs 50 mg for erectile dysfunction. Int J Clin Pract. 2013;67(10):1034–9.
138. McMahon CG. High dose sildenafil citrate as salvage therapy for erectile dysfunction. Int J Impot Res. 2002;14(6):533–8.
139. Morales A, Gingell C, Collins M, Wicker PA, Osterloh IH. Clinical safety of oral sildenafil citrate (VIAGRA) in the treatment of erectile dysfunction. Int J Impot Res. 1998;10(2):69–73.
140. Christiansen E, Guirguis WR, Cox D, Osterloh IH, Sildenafil Multicentre Study Group. Long-term efficacy and safety of oral Viagra (sildenafil citrate) in men with erectile dysfunction and the effect of randomized treatment withdrawal. Int J Impot Res. 2000;12(3):177–82.
141. Padma-Nathan H, Steers WD, Wicker PA. Efficacy and safety of oral sildenafil in the treatment of erectile dysfunction: a double-blind, placebo-controlled study of 329 patients. Sildenafil Study Group. Int J Clin Pract. 1998;52(6):375–9.
142. Montorsi F, McDermott TE, Morgan R, Olsson A, Schulz A, Kirkeby HJ, et al. Efficacy and safety of fixed-dose oral sildenafil in the treatment of erectile dysfunction of various etiologies. Urology. 1999;53(5):1011–8.
143. Dinsmore WW, Hodges M, Hargreaves C, Osterloh IH, Smith MD, Rosen RC. Sildenafil citrate (Viagra) in erectile dysfunction: near normalization in men with broad spectrum erectile dysfunction compared with age-matched healthy control subjects. Urology. 1999;53(5):1072.
144. Montorsi F, Maga T, Strambi LF, Salonia A, Barbieri L, Scattoni V, et al. Sildenafil taken at bedtime significantly increases nocturnal erections: results of a placebo-controlled study. Urology. 2000;56(6):906–11.
145. Terradas C, Levalle O, Nagelberg A, Mormandi E. Sildenafil improves nocturnal penile erections in organic impotence. Int J Impot Res. 2001;13(2):125–9.
146. Yaman O, Tokath Z, Inal T, Anafarta K. Effect of sildenafil on nocturnal erections of potent men. Int J Impot Res. 2003;15(2):117–21.
147. Aversa A, Mazzilli F, Rossi T, Delfino M, Isidori AM, Fabbri A. Effects of sildenafil (Viagra) administration on seminal parameters and post-ejaculatory refractory time in normal males. Hum Reprod. 2000;15(1):131–4.
148. Rendell MS, Rajfer J, Wicker PA, Smith MD. Sildenafil for treatment of erectile dysfunction in men with diabetes: a randomized controlled trial. Sildenafil Diabetes Study Group. JAMA. 1999;281(5):421–6.

149. Meuleman E, Cuzin B, Opsomer RJ, Hartmann U, Bailey MJ, Maytom MC, et al. A dose-escalation study to assess the efficacy and safety of sildenafil citrate in men with erectile dysfunction. BJU Int. 2001;87(1):75–81.
150. Webster LJ, Michelakis ED, Davis T, Archer SL. Use of sildenafil for safe improvement of erectile function and quality of life in men with New York Heart Association classes II and III congestive heart failure: a prospective, placebo-controlled, double-blind crossover trial. Arch Intern Med. 2004;164(5):514–20.
151. Maytom MC, Derry FA, Dinsmore WW, Glass CA, Smith MD, Orr M, et al. A two-part study of sildenafil (VIAGRA) in men with erectile dysfunction caused by spinal cord injury. Spinal Cord. 1999;37(2):110–6.
152. Giuliano F, Hultling C, El Masry WS, Smith MD, Osterloh IH, Orr M, et al. Randomized trial of sildenafil for the treatment of erectile dysfunction in spinal cord injury. Sildenafil Study Group. Ann Neurol. 1999;46(1):15–21.
153. Schmid DM, Schurch B, Hauri D. Sildenafil in the treatment of sexual dysfunction in spinal cord-injured male patients. Eur Urol. 2000;38(2):184–93.
154. Zusman RM, Prisant LM, Brown MJ. Effect of sildenafil citrate on blood pressure and heart rate in men with erectile dysfunction taking concomitant antihypertensive medication. Sildenafil Study Group. J Hypertens. 2000;18(12):1865–9.
155. Pickering TG, Shepherd AM, Puddey I, Glasser DB, Orazem J, Sherman N, et al. Sildenafil citrate for erectile dysfunction in men receiving multiple antihypertensive agents: a randomized controlled trial. Am J Hypertens. 2004;17(12 Pt 1):1135–42.
156. Müller MJ, Benkert O. Lower self-reported depression in patients with erectile dysfunction after treatment with sildenafil. J Affect Disord. 2001;66(2–3):255–61.
157. Seidman SN, Roose SP, Menza MA, Shabsigh R, Rosen RC. Treatment of erectile dysfunction in men with depressive symptoms: results of a placebo-controlled trial with sildenafil citrate. Am J Psychiatry. 2001;158(10):1623–30.
158. Reznik I, Zemishlany Z, Kotler M, Spivak B, Weizman A, Mester R. Sildenafil citrate for the sexual dysfunction. Psychother Psychosom. 2002;71(3):173–6.
159. Nurnberg HG, Fava M, Gelenberg AJ, Hensley PL, Paine S. Open-label sildenafil treatment of partial and non-responders to double-blind treatment in men with antidepressant-associated sexual dysfunction. Int J Impot Res. 2007;19(2):167–75.
160. Aviv A, Shelef A, Weizman A. An open-label trial of sildenafil addition in risperidone-treated male schizophrenia patients with erectile dysfunction. J Clin Psychiatry. 2004;65(1):97–103.
161. Gopalakrishnan R, Jacob KS, Kuruvilla A, Vasantharaj B, John JK. Sildenafil in the treatment of antipsychotic-induced erectile dysfunction: a randomized, double-blind, placebo-controlled, flexible-dose, two-way crossover trial. Am J Psychiatry. 2006;163(3):494–9.
162. Jünemann KP, Cassens S, Lippert H, Burkart M. Quality assurance in the urologist's practice. Erectile dysfunction as an example of a multicenter approach to documenting treatment results. Urologe A. 2005;44(7):785–93.
163. Seidman SN, Pesce VC, Roose SP. High-dose sildenafil citrate for selective serotonin reuptake inhibitor-associated ejaculatory delay: open clinical trial. J Clin Psychiatry. 2003;64(6):721–5.
164. Wang WF, Wang Y, Minhas S, Ralph DJ. Can sildenafil treat primary ejaculation? A prospective clinical study. Int J Urol. 2007;14(4):331–5.
165. Hosseini MM, Yarmohammadi H. Effect of fluoxetine alone and in combination with sildenafil in patients with premature ejaculation. Urol Int. 2007;79(1):28–32.
166. Abdo CH, Afif-Abdo J, Otani F, Machado AC. Sexual satisfaction among patients with erectile dysfunction treated with counseling, sildenafil, or both. J Sex Med. 2008;5(7):1720–6.
167. Athenahealth, Inc. [Internet]. San Mateo (CA): Epocatres, Inc. https://online.epocrates.com/drugs/138805/Viagra/Adverse-Reactions. Accessed 15 Aug 2016.
168. Athenahealth, Inc. [Internet]. San Mateo (CA): Epocatres, Inc. https://online.epocrates.com/drugs/138801/Viagra/Adult-Dosing. Accessed 15 Aug 2016.
169. Eardley I, Ellis P, Boolell M, Wulff M. Onset and duration of action of sildenafil for the treatment of erectile dysfunction. Br J Clin Pharmacol. 2002;53(Suppl 1):61S–5S.
170. Moncada I, Jara J, Subirá D, Castaño I, Hernández C. Efficacy of sildenafil citrate at 12 hours after dosing: re-exploring the therapeutic window. Eur Urol. 2004;46(3):357–60.
171. Gingell C, Sultana SR, Wulff MB, Gepi-Attee S. Duration of action of sildenafil citrate in men with erectile dysfunction. J Sex Med. 2004;1(2):179–84.
172. Zinner N. Do food and dose timing affect the efficacy of sildenafil? A randomized placebo-controleld study. J Sex Med. 2007;4(1):137–44.
173. Rosen RC, McKenna KE. PDE5 inhibition and sexual response: pharmacological mechanisms and clinical outcomes. Annu Rev Sex Res. 2002;13:36–88.
174. Abdel-Aziz AA, Asiri YA, El-Azab AS, Al-Omar MA, Kunieda T. Tadalafil. Profiles Drug Subst Excip Relat Methodol. 2011;36:287–329.
175. Wright PJ. Comparison of phosphodiesterase type 5 (PDE5) inhibitors. Int J Clin Pract. 2006;60(8):967–75.
176. Carson CC. PDE5 inhibitors: are there differences? Can J Urol. 2006;13(Suppl 1):34–9.
177. Seftel AD, Wilson SK, Knapp PM, Shin J, Wang WC, Ahuja S. The efficacy and safety of tadalafil in United States and Puerto Rican men with erectile dysfunction. J Urol. 2004;172(2):652–7.
178. Carson C, Shabsigh R, Segal S, Murphy A, Fredlung P, Kuepfer C, et al. Efficacy, safety, and treatment satisfaction of tadalafil versus placebo in patients with erectile dysfunction evaluated at tertiary-care academic centers. Urology. 2005;65(2):353–9.
179. Althof SE, Eid JF, Talley DR, Brock GB, Dunn ME, Tomlin ME, et al. Through the eyes of women: the partner's perspective on tadalafil. Urology. 2006;68(3):631–5.
180. Rubio-Aurioles E, Kim ED, Rosen RC, Porst H, Burns P, Zeigler H, et al. Impact on erectile dysfunction and sexual quality of life of couples: a double-blind, randomized, placebo-controlled trial of tadalafil taken once daily. J Sex Med. 2009;6(5):1314–23.
181. Mirone V, Costa P, Damber JE, Holmes S, Moncada I, Van Ahlen H, et al. An evaluation of an alternative dosing regimen with tadalafil, 3 times/week, for men with erectile dysfunction: SURE study in 14 European countries. Eur Urol. 2005;47(6):846–54.
182. Wespes E, Moncada I, Schmitt H, Jungwirth A, Chan M, Varanese L. The influence of age on treatment outcomes in men with erectile dysfunction treated with two regimens of tadalafil: results of the SURE study. BJU Int. 2007;99(1):121–6.
183. Moncada I, Damber JE, Mirone V, Wespes E, Casariego J, Chan M, et al. Sexual intercourse attempt patterns with two dosing regimens of tadalafil in men with erectile dysfunction: results from the SURE study in 14 European countries. J Sex Med. 2005;2(5):668–74.
184. Eardley I, Mirone V, Montorsi F, Ralph D, Kell P, Warner MR, et al. An open-label, multicentre, randomized, crossover study comparing sildenafil citrate and tadalafil for treating erectile dysfunction in men naïve to phosphodiesterase 5 inhibitor therapy. BJU Int. 2005;96(9):1323–32.
185. Sharlip ID, Shumaker BP, Hakim LS, Goldfischer E, Natanegara F, Wong DG. Tadalafil is efficacious and well tolerated in the treatment of erectile dysfunction (ED) in men over 65 years of age: results from Multiple Observations in Men with ED in National Tadalafil Study in the United States. J Sex Med. 2008;5(3):716–25.

186. Porst H, Rajfer J, Casabé A, Feldman R, Ralph D, Vieiralves LF, et al. Long-term safety and efficacy of tadalafil 5 mg dosed once daily in men with erectile dysfunction. J Sex Med. 2008;5(9):2160–9.
187. Porst H, Glina S, Ralph D, Zeigler H, Wong DG, Woodward B. Durability of response following cessation of tadalafil taken once daily as treatment for erectile dysfunction. J Sex Med. 2010;7(10):3487–94.
188. Montorsi F, Verheyden B, Meuleman E, Jünemann KP, Moncada I, Valiquette L, et al. Long-term safety and tolerability of tadalafil in the treatment of erectile dysfunction. Eur Urol. 2004;45(3):339–44.
189. Goldstein I, Kim E, Steers WD, Pryor JL, Wilde DW, Natanegara F, et al. Efficacy and safety of tadalafil in men with erectile dysfunction with a high prevalence of comorbid conditions: results from MOMENTUS: multiple observations in men with erectile dysfunction in National Tadalafil Study in the US. J Sex Med. 2007;4(1):166–75.
190. Giuliano F, Sanchez-Ramos A, Löchner-Ernst D, Del Popolo G, Cruz N, Leriche A, et al. Efficacy and safety of tadalafil in men with erectile dysfunction following spinal cord injury. Arch Neurol. 2007;64(11):1584–92.
191. Evliyaoglu Y, Yelsel K, Kobaner M, Alma E, Saygili M. Efficacy and tolerability of tadalafil for treatment of erectile dysfunction in men taking serotonin reuptake inhibitors. Urology. 2011;77(5):1137–41.
192. Mattos RM, Marmo Lucon A, Srougi M. Tadalafil and fluoxetine in premature ejaculation: prospective, randomized, double-blind, placebo-controlled study. Urol Int. 2008;80(2):162–5.
193. Schulman CC, Shen W, Stothard DR, Schmitt H. Integrated analysis examining first-dose success, success by dose, and maintenance of success among men taking tadalafil for erectile dysfunction. Urology. 2004;64(4):783–8.
194. Seftel A, Goldfischer E, Kim ED, Dula E, Zeigler H, Burns P. Onset of efficacy of tadalafil once daily in men with erectile dysfunction: a randomized, double-blind, placebo-controlled trial. J Urol. 2011;185(1):243–8.
195. Carrier S, Brock GB, Pommerville PJ, Shin J, Anglin G, Whitaker S, et al. J Sex Med. 2005;2(5):685–98.
196. Skoumal R, Chen J, Kula K, Breza J, Calomfirescu N, Basson BR, et al. Efficacy and treatment satisfaction with on-demand tadalafil (Cialis) in men with erectile dysfunction. Eur Urol. 2004;46(3):362–9.
197. Morgentaler A, Barada J, Niederberger C, Donatucci C, Garcia CS, Natanegara F, et al. Efficacy and safety of tadalafil across ethnic groups and various risk factors in men with erectile dysfunction: use of a novel noninferiority study design. J Sex Med. 2006;3(3):492–503.
198. Saylan M, Khalaf I, Kadioglu A, Shoair KZ, Beheiry A, Wang WC, et al. Efficacy of tadalafil in Egyptian and Turkish men with erectile dysfunction. Int J Clin Pract. 2006;60(7):812–9.
199. Yip WC, Chiang HS, Mendoza JB, Tan HM, Li MK, Wang WC, et al. Efficacy and safety of on demand tadalafil in the treatment of East and Southeast Asian men with erectile dysfunction: a randomized double-blind, parallel, placebo-controlled clinical study. Asian J Androl. 2006;8(6):685–92.
200. Nagao K, Kimoto Y, Marumo K, Tsujimura A, Vail GM, Watts S, et al. Efficacy and safety of tadalafil 5, 10, and 20 mg in Japanese men with erectile dysfunction: results of a multicenter, randomized, double-blind, placebo-controlled study. Urology. 2006;68(4):845–51.
201. Brock GB, McMahon CG, Chen KK, Costigan T, Shen W, Watkins V, et al. Efficacy and safety of tadalafil for the treatment of erectile dysfunction: results of integrated analyses. J Urol. 2002;168(4 Pt 1):1332–6.
202. Porst H, Padma-Nathan H, Giuliano F, Anglin G, Varanese L, Rosen R. Efficacy of tadalafil for the treatment of erectile dysfunction at 24 and 36 hours after dosing: a randomized control trial. Urology. 2003;62(1):121–5.
203. Athenahealth, Inc. [Internet]. San Mateo (CA): Epocatres, Inc. https://online.epocrates.com/drugs/355905/Cialis/Adverse-Reactions. Accessed 15 Aug 2016.
204. Athenahealth, Inc. [Internet]. San Mateo (CA): Epocatres, Inc. https://online.epocrates.com/drugs/355901/Cialis/Adult-Dosing. Accessed 15 Aug 2016.
205. Rajfer J. Relationship between testosterone and erectile dysfunction. Rev Urol. 2000;2(2):122–8.
206. Davidson JM, Camargo CA, Smith ER. Effects of androgen on sexual behavior in hypogonadal men. J Clin Endocrinol Metab. 1979;48:935–41.
207. Morales A, Johnston B, Heaton JP, Lundie M. Testosterone supplementation for hypogonadal impotence: assessment of biochemical measures and therapeutic outcomes. J Urol. 1997;157:849–54.
208. Isidori AM, Giannetta E, Gianfrilli D, Greco EA, Bonifacio V, Aversa A, et al. Effects of testosterone on sexual function in men: results of a meta-analysis. Clin Endocrinol (Oxf). 2005;63(4):381–94.
209. Davis SR, van der Mooren MJ, van Lunsen RH, Lopes P, Ribot C, Rees M, et al. Efficacy and safety of a testosterone patch for the treatment of hypoactive sexual desire disorder in surgically menopausal women: a randomized, placebo-controlled trial. Menopause. 2006;13(3):387–96.
210. Kingsberg S, Shifren J, Wekselman K, Rodenberg C, Koochki P, Derogatis L. Evaluation of the clinical relevance of benefits associated with transdermal testosterone treatment in postmenopausal women with hypoactive sexual desire disorder. J Sex Med. 2007;4(4 Pt 1):1001–8.
211. Davis SR, Moreau M, Kroll R, Bouchard C, Panay N, Gass M, et al. Testosterone for low libido in postmenopausal women not taking estrogen. N Engl J Med. 2008;359(19):2005–17.
212. El-Hage G, Eden JA, Manga RZ. A double-blind, randomized, placebo-controlled trial of the effect of testosterone cream on the sexual motivation of menopausal hysterectomized women with hypoactive sexual desire disorder. Climacteric. 2007;10(4):335–43.
213. Tungmunsakulchai R, Chaikittisilpa S, Snabboon T, Panyakhamlerd K, Jaisamrarn U. Effectiveness of a low dose testosterone undecanoate to improve sexual function in postmenopausal women. BMC Womens Health. 2015;15:113.
214. Panay N, Al-Azzawi F, Bouchard C, Davis SR, Eden J, Lodhi I, et al. Testosterone treatment of HSDD in naturally menopausal women: the ADORE study. Climacteric. 2010;13(2):121–31.
215. Fooladi E, Bell RJ, Jane F, Robinson PJ, Kulkarni J, Davis SR. Testosterone improves antidepressant-emergent loss of libido in women: findings from a randomized, double-blind, placebo-controlled trial. J Sex Med. 2014;11(3):831–9.
216. Spitzer M, Basaria S, Travison TG, Davda MN, Paley A, Cohen B, et al. Effect of testosterone replacement on response to sildenafil citrate in men with erectile dysfunction: a parallel, randomized trial. Ann Intern Med. 2012;157(10):681–91.
217. O'Carroll R, Bancroft J. Testosterone therapy for low sexual interest and erectile dysfunction in men: a controlled study. Br J Psychiatry. 1984;145:146–51.
218. Amiaz R, Pope Jr HG, Mahne T, Kelly JF, Brennan BP, Kanayama G, et al. Testosterone gel replacement improves sexual dysfunction in depressed men taking serotonergic antidepressants: a randomized, placebo-controlled clinical trial. J Sex Marital Ther. 2011;37(4):243–54.
219. Athenahealth, Inc. [Internet]. San Mateo (CA): Epocatres, Inc. https://online.epocrates.com/drugs/2015/testosterone-transdermal. Accessed 15 Aug 2016.
220. Nastri CO, Lara LA, Ferriani RA, Rosa-E-Silva AC, Figueiredo JB, Martins WP. Hormone therapy for sexual function in perimenopausal

and postmenopausal women. Cochrane Database Syst Rev. 2013;6:CD009762.
221. Drugs.com [Internet] Tibolone Information from Drugs.com. https://www.drugs.com/nda/tibolone_060602.html. Accessed 30 Aug 2016.
222. Notelovitz M. Postmenopausal tibolone therapy: biologic principles and applied clinical practice. MedGenMed. 2007;9(1):2.
223. Palacios S, Tobar AC, Menendez C. Sexuality in the climacteric years. Maturitas. 2002;43(Suppl 1):S69–77.
224. Huang KE, Baber R, Asia Pacific Tibolone Concensus Group. Updated clinical recommendations for the use of tibolone in Asian women. Climacteric. 2010;13(4):317–27.
225. Pompei LM, Cunha EP, Steiner ML, Theodoro TR, Mader AM, Petri G. Effects of estradiol, progestogens, and of tibolone on breast proliferation and apoptosis. Climacteric. 2015;18(4):518–22.
226. Bundred NJ, Kenemans P, Yip CH, Beckman MW, Foidart JM, Sismondi P, et al. Tibolone increases bone mineral density but also relapse in breast cancer survivors: LIBERATE trial bone substudy. Breast Cancer Res. 2012;14(1):R13.
227. Davis SR. The effects of tibolone on mood and libido. Menopause. 2002;9(3):162–70.
228. Verheul HA, Kloosterboer HJ. Metabolism of exogenous sex steroids and effect on brain functions with a focus on tibolone. J Steroid Biochem Mol Bio. 2006;102(1–5):195–204.
229. Laan E, van Lunsen RH, Everaerd W. The effects of tibolone on vaginal blood flow, sexual desire and arousability in postmenopausal women. Climacteric. 2001;4(1):28–41.
230. Wu MH, Pan HA, Wang ST, Hsu CC, Chang FM, Huang KE. Quality of life and sexuality changes in postmenopausal women receiving tibolone therapy. Climacteric. 2001;4(4):314–9.
231. Uyguy D, Yesildaglar N, Erkaya S. Effect on sexual life—a comparison between tibolone and continuous combined conjugated equine estrogens and medroxyprogesterone acetate. Gynecol Endocrinol. 2005;20(4):209–12.
232. Ziaei S, Moghasemi M, Faghihzadeh S. Comparative effects of conventional hormone replacement therapy and tibolone on climacteric symptoms and sexual dysfunction in postmenopausal women. Climacteric. 2010;13(2):147–56.
233. Egarter C, Topcuoglu A, Vogl S, Sator M. Hormone replacement therapy with tibolone: effects on sexual functioning in postmenopausal women. Acta Obstet Gynecol Scand. 2002;81(7): 649–53.
234. Nappi RE, Ferdeghini F, Sampaolo P, Vaccaro P, De Leonardis C, Albani F, Salonia A, Polatti F. Maturitas. 2006;55(3):288–95.
235. Rigato I, Cravatari M, Avellini C, Ponte E, Crocé SL, Tiribelli C. Drug-induced acute cholestatic liver damage in a patient with mutation of UGT1A1. Nat Clin Pract Gastroenterol Hepatol. 2007;4(7):403–8.
236. Cummings SR, Ettinger B, Delmas PD, Kenemans P, Stathopoulos V, Verweij P. The effects of tibolone in older postmenopausal women. N Engl J Med. 2008;359(7):697–708.
237. Hammar M, Christau S, Nathorst-Böös J, Rud T, Garre K. A double-blind, randomized trial comparing the effects of tibolone and continuous combined hormone replacement therapy in postmenopausal women with menopausal symptoms. Br J Obstet Gynaecol. 1998;105(8):904–11.
238. Hudita D, Posea C, Ceausu I, Rusu M. Efficacy and safety of oral tibolone 1.25 or 2.5 mg/day vs. placebo in postmenopausal women. Eur Rev Med Pharmacol Sci. 2003;7(5):117–25.
239. Eardley I. Vardenafil: a new oral treatment for erectile dysfunction. Int J Clin Pract. 2004;58(8):801–6.
240. Crowe SM, Streetman DS. Vardenafil treatment for erectile dysfunction. Ann Pharmacother. 2004;38(1):77–85.
241. Kendirci M, Bivalacqua TJ, Hellstrom WJ. Vardenafil: a novel type 5 phosphodiesterase inhibitor for the treatment of erectile dysfunction. Expert Opin Pharmacother. 2004;5(4):923–32.
242. Morales AM, Mirone V, Dean J, Costa P. Vardenafil for the treatment of erectile dysfunction: an overview of the clinical evidence. Clin Interv Aging. 2009;4:463–72.
243. Campbell HE. Clinical monograph for drug formulary: erectile dysfunction agents. J Manag Care Pharm. 2005;11(2):151–71.
244. Zhang SX, Gao P. Experience of using three phosphodiesterase type 5 inhibitors in the same period for the treatment of erectile dysfunction. Zhonghua Nan Ke Xue. 2007;13(3):226–8.
245. Gamidov SI, Iremashvii VV, Popova Alu. Modernity in the treatment of erectile dysfunction: levitra (vardenafil) in the form of oral dispersible tablet. Urologiia. 2013;(3):102–4, 106.
246. Heinig R, Weimann B, Dietrich H, Böttcher MF. Pharmacokinetics of a new orodispersible tablet formulation of vardenafil: results of three clinical trials. Clin Drug Investig. 2011;31(1):27–41.
247. Hellstrom WJ, Gittelman M, Marlin G, Segerson T, Thibonnier M, Taylor T, et al. Sustained efficacy and tolerability of vardenafil, a highly potent selective phosphodiesterase type 5 inhibitor, in men with erectile dysfunction: results of a randomized, double-blind, 26-week placebo-controlled pivotal trial. Urology. 2003; 61(4 Suppl 1):8–14.
248. Porst H, Young JM, Schmidt AC, Buvat J, International Vardenafil Study Group. Efficacy and tolerability of vardenafil for treatment of erectile dysfunction in patients subgroups. Urology. 2003; 62(3):519–23.
249. Stief C, Porst H, Sáenz De Tejada I, Ulbrich E, Beneke M, Vardenafil Study Group. Sustained efficacy and tolerability with vardenafil over 2 years of treatment in men with erectile dysfunction. Int J Clin Pract. 2004;58(3):230–9.
250. Valiquette L, Young JM, Moncada I, Porst H, Vézina JG, Stancil BN, et al. Vardenafil Study Group. Sustained efficacy and safety of vardenafil for treatment of erectile dysfunction: a randomized, double-blind, placebo-controlled study. Mayo Clinic Proc. 2005;80(10):1291–7.
251. Valiquette L, Montorsi F, Hellstrom WJ, Giuliano F, Homering M, Taylor T, et al. Penetration and maintenance of erection with vardenafil: a time-from-dosing analysis. Can J Urol. 2005;12(3): 2687–98.
252. Montorsi F, Padma-Nathan H, Buvat J, Schwaibold H, Beneke M, Ulbrich E, et al. Earliest time to onset of action leading to successful intercourse with vardenafil determined in at-home setting: randomized, double-blind, placebo-controlled trial. J Sex Med. 2004;1(2):168–78.
253. Nagao K, Kobayashi H, Fujikawa K, Tachibana T, Iwamoto Y, Ishii N, et al. Vardenafil allows successful intercourse initiated rapidly after dosing in Japanese patients with diabetes mellitus and erectile dysfunction. J Sex Med. 2009;6(10):2851–7.
254. Porst H, Sharlip ID, Hatzichristou D, Rubio-Aurioles E, Gittelman M, Stancil BN, et al. Extended duration of efficacy of vardenafil when taken 8 hours before intercourse: a randomized, double-blind, placebo-controlled study. Eur Urol. 2006; 50(5):1086–94.
255. Goldstein I, Young JM, Fischer J, Bangerter K, Segerson T, Taylor T, et al. Vardenafil, a new phosphodiesterase type 5 inhibitor, in the treatment of erectile dysfunction in men with diabetes: a multicenter double-blind placebo-controlled fixed-dose study. Diabetes Care. 2003;26(3):777–83.
256. Ishii N, Nagao K, Fujikawa K, Tachibana T, Iwamoto Y, Kamidono S. Vardenafil 20-mg demonstrated superior efficacy to 10-mg in Japanese men with diabetes mellitus suffering from erectile dysfunction. Int J Urol. 2006;13(8):1066–72.
257. Ziegler D, Merfort F, van Ahlen H, Yassin A, Reblin T, Neureither M. Efficacy and safety of flexible-dose vardenafil in men with type 1 diabetes and erectile dysfunction. J Sex Med. 2006; 3(5):883–91.
258. Valiquette L, Montorsi F, Auerbach S, Vardenafil Study Group. First-dose success with vardenafil in men with erectile dysfunction

and associated comorbidities: RELY-I. Int J Clin Pract. 2006;60(11):1378–85.
259. Kimoto Y, Sakamoto S, Fujikawa K, Tachibana T, Yamamoto N, Otani T. Up-titration of vardenafil dose from 10 mg to 20 mg improved erectile function in men with spinal cord injury. Int J Urol. 2006;13(11):1428–33.
260. Rosen R, Shabsigh R, Berber M, Assalian P, Menza M, Rodriguez-Vela L, et al. Efficacy and tolderability of vardenafil in men with mild depression and erectile dysfunction: the depression-related improvement with vardenafil for erectile response study. Am J Psychiatry. 2006;163(1):79–87.
261. Suz XZ, Deng CH, Dai YP. A clinical study of sertraline and vardenafil in the treatment of premature ejaculation complicated by erectile dysfunction. Zhonghua Nan Ke Xue. 2007;13(7):610–2.
262. Gökce A, Demirtas A, Hallis F, Ekmekcioglu O. In vitro measurement of ejaculation latency time (ELT) and the effects of vardenafil on ELT on lifelong premature ejaculators: placebo-controlled, double-blind, cross-over laboratory setting. Int Urol Nephrol. 2010;42(4):881–7.
263. Jarvi K, Dula E, Drehobi M, Pryor J, Shapiro J, Seger M. Daily vardenafil for 6 months has no detrimental effects on semen characteristics or reproductive hormones in men with normal baseline levels. J Urol. 2008;179(3):1060–5.
264. Rago R, Salacone P, Caponecchia L, Marcucci I, Fiori C, Sebastianelli A. Effect of vardenafil on semen parameters in infertile men: a pilot study evaluating short-term treatment. J Endocrinol Invest. 2012;35(10):897–900.
265. Athenahealth, Inc. [Internet]. San Mateo (CA): Epocatres, Inc. https://online.epocrates.com/drugs/349605/Levitra/Adverse-Reactions. Accessed 4 Sep 2016.
266. Athenahealth, Inc. [Internet]. San Mateo (CA): Epocatres, Inc. [cited 2016 Aug 15]. Available from Athenahealth, Inc. [Internet]. San Mateo (CA): Epocatres, Inc. https://online.epocrates.com/drugs/349601/Levitra/Adult-Dosing. Accessed 4 Sep 2016.
267. Rajagopalan P, Mazzu A, Xia C, Dawkins R, Sundaresan P. Effect of high-fat breakfast and moderate-fat evening meal on the pharmacokinetics of vardenafil, an oral phosphodiesterase-5 inhibitor for the treatment of erectile dysfunction. J Clin Pharmacol. 2003;43(3):260–7.
268. Köhler TS, McVary KT, editors. Contemporary treatment of erectile dysfunction: a clinical guide. 2nd ed. New York: Humana Press; 2016.
269. Phillips MA, Szabadi E, Bradshaw CM. Comparison of the effects of clonidine and yohimbine on spontaneous pupillary functions in healthy human volunteers. Psychopharmacology (Berl). 2000;150(1):85–9.
270. Millan MJ, Newman-Tancredi A, Audinot V, Cussac D, Lejeune F, Nicolas JP, et al. Agonist and antagonist actions of yohimbine as compared to fluparoxan at alpha(2)-adrenergic receptors (AR)s, serotonin (5-HT)(1A), 5-HT(1B), 5-HT(1D) and dopamine D(2) and D(3) receptors. Significance for the modulation of frontocortical monoaminergic transmission and depressive states. Synapse. 2000;35(2):79–95.
271. Reid K, Surridge DH, Morales A, Condra M, Harris C, Owen J, et al. Double-blind trial of yohimbine in treatment of psychogenic impotence. Lancet. 1987;2(8556):421–3.
272. Jacobsen FM. Fluoxetine-induced sexual dysfunction and an open trial of yohimbine. J Clin Psychiatry. 1992;53(4):119–22.
273. Montorsi F, Strambi LF, Guazzoni G, Galli L, Barbieri L, Rigatti P, Pizzini G, Miani A. Effect of yohimbine-trazodone on psychogenic impotence: a randomized, double-blind, placebo-controlled study. Urology. 1994;44(5):732–6.
274. Mann K, Klingler T, Noe S, Röschke J, Müller S, Benkert O. Effects of yohimbine on sexual experiences and nocturnal penile tumescence and rigidity in erectile dysfunction. Arch Sex Behav. 1996;25(1):1–16.
275. Rowland DL, Kallan K, Slob AK. Yohimbine, erectile capacity, and sexual response in men. Arch Sex Behav. 1997;26(1):49–62.
276. Vogt HJ, Brandi P, Kockott G, Schmitz JR, Wiegand MH, Schadrack J, Gierend M. Double-blind, placebo-controlled safety and efficacy trial with yohimbine hydrochloride in the treatment of nonorganic erectile dysfunction. Int J Impot Res. 1997; 9(3):155–61.
277. Hollander E, McCarley A. Yohimbine treatment of sexual side effects induced by serotonin reuptake blockers. J Clin Psychiatry. 1992;53(6):207–9.
278. Susset JG, Tessier CD, Wincze J, Bansal S, Malhotra C, Schwacha MG. Effect of yohimbine hydrochloride on erectile impotence: a double-blind study. J Urol. 1989;141(6):1360–3.
279. Adeniyi AA, Brindley GS, Pryor JP, Ralph DJ. Yohimbine in the treatment of orgasmic dysfunction. Asian J Androl. 2007;9(3):403–7.
280. Haefeli WE. Individualising the evidence—single case randomized trial. Ther Umsch. 2006;63(12):777–81.
281. Swann AC, Lijffijt M, Lane SD, Cox B, Steinberg JL, Moeller FG. Norepinephrine and impulsivity: effects of acute yohimbine. Psychopharmacology (Berl). 2013;229(1):83–94.
282. Athenahealth, Inc. [Internet]. San Mateo (CA): Epocatres, Inc. https://online.epocrates.com/drugs/30505/yohimbine/Adverse-Reactions. Accessed 2 Sep 2016.
283. Athenahealth, Inc. [Internet]. San Mateo (CA): Epocatres, Inc. https://online.epocrates.com/drugs/30501/yohimbine/Adult-Dosing. Accessed 3 Sep 2016.

27 Sex and Natural Sexual Enhancement: Sexual Techniques, Aphrodisiac Foods, and Nutraceuticals

Waguih William IsHak, Steven Clevenger, Robert N. Pechnick, and Thomas Parisi

Introduction

Non-pharmacological methods for sexual enhancement have been reviewed and studied over the years [1]. In this section we describe a variety of sexual enhancement techniques that have been studied using research methods producing emerging or replicated evidence. Nevertheless, research on optimal sex has identified eight major components that constitute overarching concepts throughout all sexual enhancement techniques, dietary supplements, and herbs: being present, connected in sync, having deep sexual and erotic intimacy, having extraordinary communication, exploring interpersonal risk-taking and fun, and having authenticity, vulnerability, and transcendence [2].

Sexual Enhancement Techniques

Stimulation of the Grafenberg Spot or the G-Spot

The G-spot, first described by Grafenberg in the 1950s, is located on the anterior wall of the vagina, and when stimulated it enhances vaginal lubrication, orgasm, and sexual satisfaction (Figure 27-1).

The G-spot triggered a long drawn debate about its very existence. The anterior wall is linked a number of arousal structures, including the urethra, Halban's fascia in the vaginal-urethral septum, the internal clitoral structures, and the ligaments attached to the clitoris—called "the anterior wall erogenous complex" and was later was renamed the "clitorourethral complex" by excluding Halban's fascia.

Stimulation of the Anterior Fornix Erogenous (AFE) Zone or the A-Spot

The stimulation of the AFE zone, an area in the inner half of the anterior fornix of the vagina, leads to vaginal lubrication and facilitation of orgasm [3]. This technique probably end up by stimulating some of the structures described above in the G-spot.

Sex Positions and the Coital Alignment Technique (CAT)

Sex positions have been graphically described in the Kama Sutra among many other texts throughout the years. Research on sex positions has not yielded any preferential findings except for clinical trial evidence for the coital alignment technique (CAT) and the anecdotal evidence for the rear-entry position directly stimulating the anterior vaginal wall. CAT was introduced by Eichel, Eichel, and Kule in 1988, aimed at making contact with the clitoris during penile vaginal intercourse [4]. CAT includes a combination of the "riding high variation of the missionary" sexual position, and "genitally focused pressure–counterpressure stimulus" coordinated with sexual movement [4]. The goal is to execute a rocking movement of the penis up and down in the vagina (rather than thrusting in and out) so that the male's pubic bone and base of the penis are rubbing against the female's clitoris. CAT was shown to increase coital female orgasm frequency and simultaneous orgasms in addition to sexual satisfaction [4, 5]. Orgasm consistency training builds on the use of CAT and has shown improvements in the latter study [5].

Orgasm Synchronization (Simultaneous Orgasm)

Orgasm synchronization or simultaneous orgasm occurs when the couple manages to reach orgasm at the same time. Description of simultaneous orgasm appeared for the first time in 1926 in a book by the gynecologist Theodoor Van de Velde, who presented the idea as a requisite to normal and perfect coitus [6]. A 2006 French study of 1002 individuals (483 men and 519 women; age ≥35) showed that nearly 36% of the sample identified simultaneous orgasms and feelings

W.W. IsHak (ed.), *The Textbook of Clinical Sexual Medicine*, DOI 10.1007/978-3-319-52539-6_27

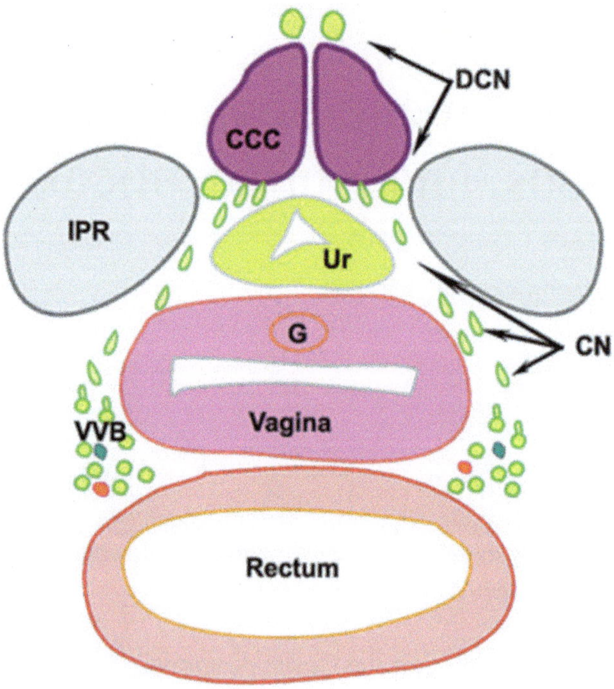

Figure 27-1. Schematic representation of the G-spot (G) in relation to perineal innervation at the level of the corporis cavernosum clitoridis (ccc). The cavernous nerves (CN) branch from the neurovascular bundle (NVB) and course between the ischiopubic ramus (IPR) and urethra (Ur). The dorsal clitoris nerve (DCN) originates from the pudendal nerve (not seen) [Reprinted from Kilchevsky A, Vardi Y, Lowenstein L, Gruenwald I. Is the female G-spot truly a distinct anatomic entity? J Sex Med. 2015; 9(3): 719–26 with permission from Elsevier].

of closeness as the most important accomplishments during sexual intercourse. Nearly 42% of men and 30% of women considered simultaneous orgasms as the most important accomplishment [7]. Simultaneous penile/vaginal orgasm was shown by Brody and Weiss, to be significantly associated with ratings of greater life, sexual, partnership, and mental health satisfaction [8].

New Functional-Sexological Treatment

The new functional-sexological treatment that could be used for sexual enhancement targets enjoyment of intercourse through prolongation and delaying ejaculation based on the premise that ejaculation cannot be controlled, whereas excitement leading to ejaculation can be controlled. The couple's knowledge of body cues and practice of controlling excessive sexual excitement can help prolong intercourse. Sexual excitement increases muscular tension, and speeds up thoracic breathing, and accelerates pelvic movement. In order to control the duration of intercourse this technique calls for voluntarily controlling of sexual excitement by reducing muscular tension, breathing slower and shifting to abdominal breathing, and slowing pelvic movement. Specific advice given by the creators of this technique include: "combine abdominal breathing with the pelvic movement; inhale when drawing the pelvis back, exhale when moving the pelvis forward", "spread legs apart, keep eyes opened", and "stop moving, relax every muscle, and breathe abdominally when approaching ejaculation" [9]. Research comparing this technique to behavioral therapy (squeeze and stop-and-start techniques; see below) and a wait-list control group, showed that it is as effective as behavioral therapy and is superior to the control group on measures of duration of intercourse, sexual satisfaction, and sexual functioning after treatment as well as at 3-month follow-up. In this study the mean duration of intercourse was extended from 42.5 s to 468 s (7 min, 48 s) on average after using the new functional-sexological treatment [9].

Start–Stop

The technique to prolong intercourse and prevent premature ejaculation was introduced in 1956 by Semans [10]. This behavioral exercise engages both partners and aims at applying stimulation to the penis and then stopping, and repeating the process in order to retrain the individual behaviorally to delay ejaculation [11].

Squeeze Technique

In the behavioral therapy squeeze technique, the coronal ridge of the penis is squeezed when the ejaculation feeling is approaching, thus inhibiting ejaculation, and repeating the process to retrain the individual to delay ejaculation [12].

Directed Masturbation

The nine-step masturbation technique described by LoPicclo and Lobitz still provides an initial, private individual way for women to work on improving orgasm [13].

Kegel Exercises

Kegel exercises constitute a method to strengthen pelvic floor muscles especially the pubococcygeus and have been linked to improvement in sexual functioning, especially orgasm facilitation in women and prolonging ejaculation time in men [14].

Sensate Focus

Since described by Masters and Johnson [12], the sensate focus exercises continue to represent an important intervention that couples could use with or without a sex therapist. Sensate One partner invites the other and performs pleasurable touching to the other for a minimum of 30 min and a maximum of 45 min, and then sometime during the week, the other partner will do the same. Sensate Focus I, involves pleasurable touching excluding the genitalia and the breasts before progressing to Sensate Focus II, which includes them [12].

Bibliotherapy

Bibliotherapy is the use of books or educational materials to improve or treat a variety of conditions. Bibliotherapy has been used successfully both to enhance orgasm as well as in the management of orgasmic problems in women. Research showed that bibliotherapy using the book "Becoming Orgasmic" led to significant increases in sexual arousability, sexual satisfaction and sexual repertoire in 17 women and their partners compared to controls [15]. Bibliotherapy has been also used successfully to improve premature ejaculation and prolong intercourse [16]. A study using the short text "The Practical Guide of Premature Ejaculation" compared to a control group ($n = 66$), showed significant improvements on all self-reported measures at 4–8 months ($n = 120$) and at 10–14 months ($n = 79$) after bibliotherapy [17].

Eros Clitoral Therapy Device (EROS-CTD)

The FDA approved in 2000 the clitoral vacuum device EROS-CTD, which is safe and effective method for treating female arousal disorder. A 2001 study shows that it was safe and effective in improving sensation, vaginal lubrication, ability to orgasm, and satisfaction in female arousal disorder ($n = 10$) as well as in women without the disorder ($n = 9$) [18].

Other Sexual Enhancement Techniques

Additional natural sexual enhancers include exercise, balanced nutrition, adequate sleep, stress reduction, and the use of erotic materials such as videos, clothing, and toys. Most importantly, the promotion of intimate and close emotional and sexual relationship could be a significant factor in natural sexual enhancement.

Sexual Enhancement Food Aphrodisiacs

Pomegranates

Pomegranates are a fruit known not only for their well-regarded taste but also their health benefits (Figure 27-2). In historical times the pomegranate was linked with fertility due to its abundance of seeds and it was used for many other medicinal purposes [19]. Pomegranate extract has been shown to benefit individuals suffering from a wide array of illnesses, including coronary artery disease, peripheral vascular disease, benign prostatic hypertrophy, and even infertility in men [20–22]. Atherosclerotic plaques can, over time, lead to reduced ability to deliver blood flow to areas of the body more distal to the heart, including the limbs in the case of peripheral arterial disease and the sex organs as in erectile dysfunction (ED). Pomegranate's ability to prevent arterial plaques occurs via several mechanisms. First, it blocks the expression of NF-kB, thus reducing inflammation that plays a key role in plaque development. Second, it lowers the activity of serum angiotensin-converting enzyme, reducing blood pressure that can lead to damaging of arterial intima. Third, it is a potent antioxidant due to high concentrations of tannins and flavonoids found in the peel that prevent peroxidation of lipids that lead to plaque development [20, 21].

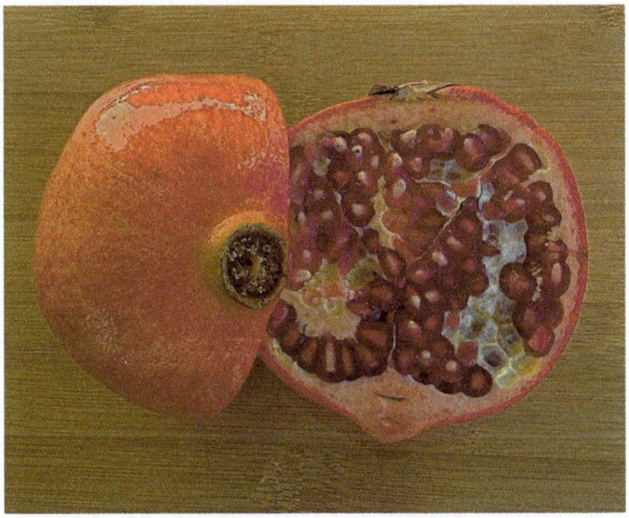

Figure 27-2. Pomegranates. Source: https://commons.wikimedia.org/wiki/File:89_-_IMG_20151128_144806.jpg.

Although it might not seem that these aspects of pomegranate make them a true aphrodisiac, cardiovascular health is essential in maintaining a healthy sexual drive, hormone production, and the ability to both attain and maintain erections in men. Indeed men and women who look after their cardiovascular health have much healthier sex lives into their older ages via improved ability and mood than those who neglect this aspect of their health [23]. Turk et al. noted in a rat study that groups of rats receiving medium and high doses of pomegranate nutrients had statistically significant increases in sperm concentration, and the high dose group had significant decreases in the production of abnormal sperm [19, 24].

Antioxidants

Like pomegranate, other foods that are reputed to have sexually enhancing properties likely act through improving cardiovascular health. Foods rich in antioxidants such as avocados, various nuts, olive oil, figs, arugula, and cherries are thought to enhance sexual desire and function [25–30].

Red wine has also been popularly associated with enhanced sexual desire. Recent research has revealed red wine to be rich in a potent antioxidant called resveratrol that like other antioxidants promoted cardiovascular health [31]. This potent health benefit in combination with the subjective increase in sexual desire experienced under the influence of alcohol likely contributes to the erotic reputation of red wine [32].

Omega-3 Fatty Acids

Similar to antioxidants, omega-3 fatty acids have strong anti-inflammatory effects that help reduce atherosclerotic plaques and improve cardiovascular health. Not surprisingly foods rich in omega-3 such as salmon and walnuts have been thought to promote sexual health [33–35].

Cinnamon and Coriander

Cinnamon and coriander are also known to have anti-inflammatory properties and along with cinnamon containing chai tea drinks might promote sexual health [36–38]. It is likely similar mechanisms of enhancing cardiovascular health lie behind these purported benefits.

Basil, Cardamom, and Garlic

Foods such as basil, cardamom, and garlic have been used for their aphrodisiac potential in various cultures. They also all have been documented to have blood pressure lowering effects. In a study by Tabassum and Ahmad, *Ocimum basilicum* (basil) caused a fall in mean arterial pressure (MAP), systolic, and diastolic blood pressure. The active ingredient in basal is thought to be eugenol [39]. Cardamon seed also has antihypertensive and antioxidant activity. In a study of 20, Stage 1 hypertensive individuals cardamom significantly lowered systolic, diastolic, and MAP [40].

Garlic is appreciated for many health benefits including its blood pressure lowering ingredient allicin (Figure 27-3). Allicin has been show to both increase blood flow in post-ischemic conditions and lower blood pressure in rat models [41, 42].

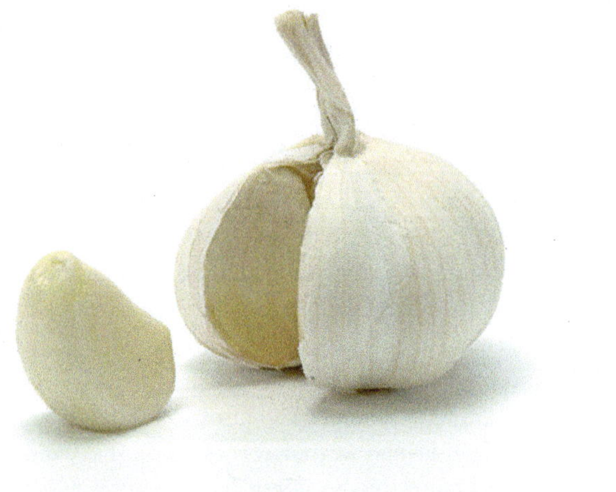

FIGURE 27-3. Garlic and garlic cloves. Source: https://commons.wikimedia.org/wiki/File:Opened_garlic_bulb_with_garlic_clove.jpg.

Watermelon

Watermelon has been reputed to have sexual enhancing properties due to its high content of L-citrulline (it is mostly in the rind, not the flesh) (Figure 27-4). L-citrulline is a precursor to L-arginine, the key source of nitrogenous substrate for the production of nitric oxide (NO) which in turn plays a central role in penile erection [43, 44].

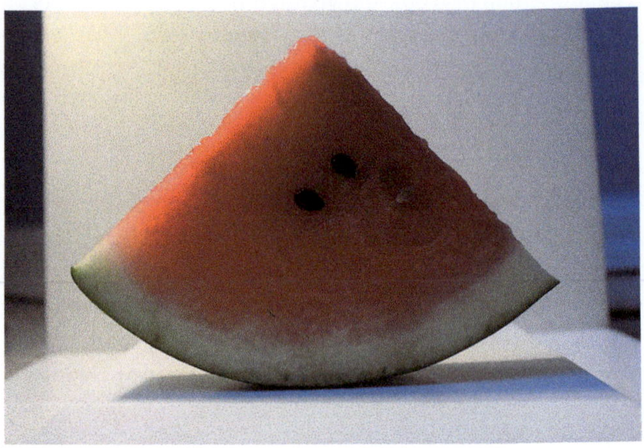

FIGURE 27-4. Watermelon slice. Source: https://commons.wikimedia.org/wiki/File:Watermelon_(2623545972).jpg.

Cormio et al. studied the effects of L-citrulline supplementation on erection strength in men and found that subjects on the supplement achieved a stronger erection. However, it was noted that the effect was not as great as PDE-5 inhibitors [45]. One additional health benefit of L-arginine is its ability to lower blood pressure [46].

Oysters, Okra, and Pumpkin Seeds

Foods rich in magnesium, such as oysters, okra, and pumpkin seeds, have been thought to enhance sexual drive and ability [47–49]. Several studies have attempted to shed light on this belief by evaluating the effects of magnesium on the production of testosterone. One study comparing Taekwondo athletes to a sedentary control group showed that supplementation with magnesium was associated with higher levels of free testosterone in both groups [50]. Maggio et al. studied the ability of magnesium supplements to increase free testosterone in older men who generally suffer from declining sex hormone production. The study found that magnesium levels were strongly and positively and independently associated with total testosterone levels. It was theorized that the possible mechanism behind this observation is that there is increased reactive oxygen species (ROS) production in magnesium deficiency, therefore low magnesium levels create a pro-inflammatory state [51]. Demirbag et al. found that testosterone production is strongly associated with the antioxidant capacity of hormone producing cells. Testosterone itself is thought to play a chief role in the libido of both men and women. Declines in libido in men have been associated with the decline in testosterone production that comes with age. Conversely, in women the decline in estrogen production with age leads to a higher relative level of testosterone and purported increase in libido [52, 53]. Thus, the positive association between testosterone and magnesium provides a plausible explanation for the potential aphrodisiac effects of magnesium rich foods.

Pine Nuts, Chickpeas and Cashews

Zinc containing foods, such as pine nuts, chickpeas, and cashews (Figure 27-5), are occasionally mentioned as a food with aphrodisiac potential in the popular literature. The scientific literature has found that zinc deficiency is associated with male hypogonadism [54]. In a rat study the aphrodisiac-like qualities of zinc were validated. Male rats given 5 mg/day of zinc supplements exhibited a significantly increased ejaculatory latency and increased penile thrusting. One possible explanation is that zinc supplementation increases serum testosterone levels in both unhealthy and healthy adult men. Jalalj et al. studied 100 males with end stage renal disease and found supplementation with zinc significantly increased serum testosterone levels.

Similarly, in a healthy population Prasad et al. found that serum testosterone increased significantly from 8.3 ± 6.3 to 16.0 ± 4.4 nmol/L with the administration of zinc [54, 55]. Given the central role of testosterone in both male and female libido, it is plausible that eating foods high in zinc could increase sex drive.

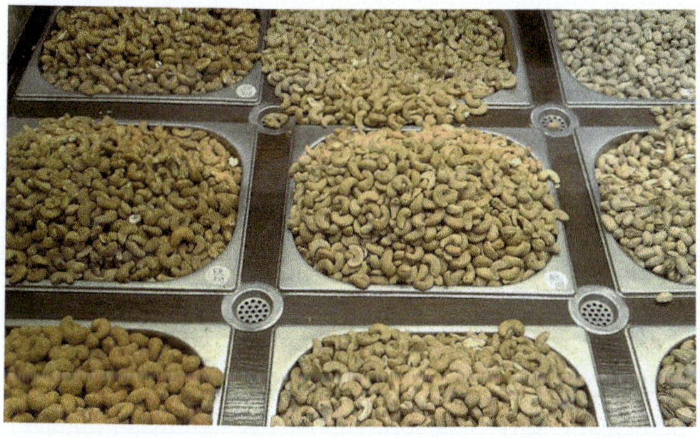

FIGURE 27-5. Cashew nuts. Source: https://commons.wikimedia.org/wiki/File:Jeddah_cashews_and_pistachios.jpg.

Celery

Celery is a vegetable that has been valued throughout history for its aphrodisiac qualities, with the Romans dedicating celery to Pluto. Celery is high not only in fiber but also hormones the androstenol and androsterone [56]. These two hormones are pheromones and are thought to play a role in human olfactory communication in regard to sexual attraction. In a study rating the subjective attractiveness of men it was found that women's rating on men in the areas of warmth, goodness, and masculinity were significantly and positively associated with androsterone levels measured in the male subject [57].

Chilies

Chilies and other spicy members of the genus *Capsicum* have long been believed to enhance sexual pleasure and function (Figure 27-6). The chemical responsible for the spicy flavor of these plants is capsaicin [58]. Capsaicin itself is used medicinally as a pain reliever. Capsaicin binds to a receptor called the vanilloid receptor subtype 1 (TRPV1), which modulates pain [59, 60].

Although beta endorphins act as analgesics and pleasure inducers there is little evidence that they enhance libido. To the contrary several rat studies have shown that increased B-endorphins suppressed mating behaviors [61, 62]. While capsaicin containing plants are medicinally valuable, there appears to be little evidence of their aphrodisiac value in humans.

Artichokes

Artichokes have been used since Roman times as a sexual stimulant. The mechanism of action seems to be related to

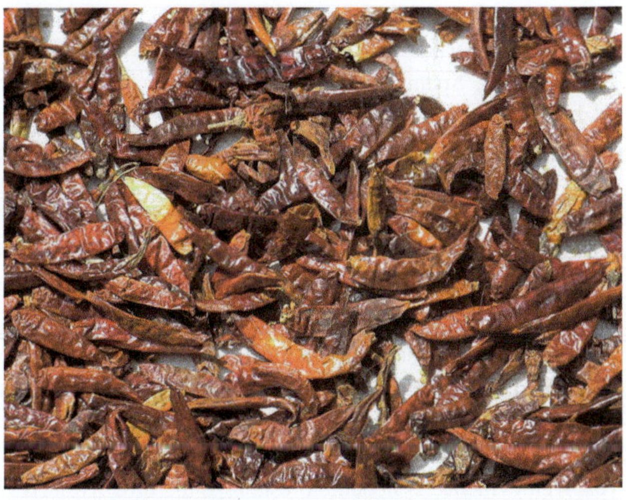

FIGURE 27-6. Chilies. Source: https://commons.wikimedia.org/wiki/File:Red_Chillies.JPG.

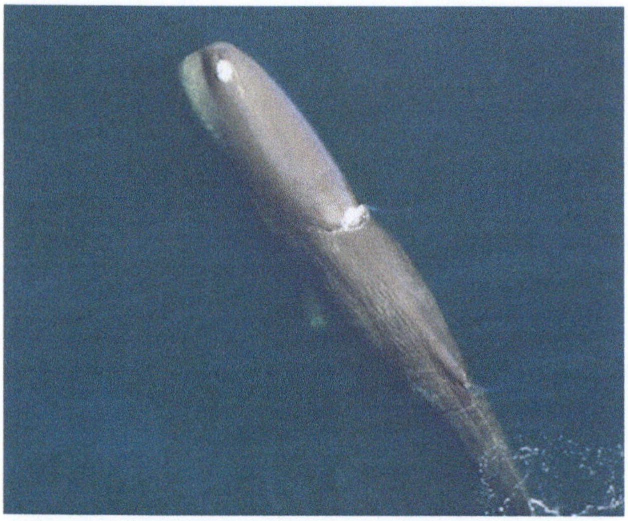

FIGURE 27-7. Sperm whale from above. Source: https://commons.wikimedia.org/wiki/File:Sperm_whale_from_above.jpg.

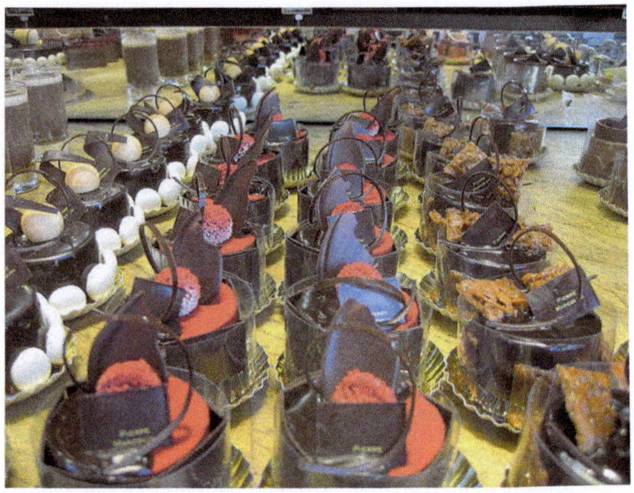

FIGURE 27-8. Chocolate. Source: https://commons.wikimedia.org/wiki/File:Chocolate_art.JPG.

improved endothelial function [63]. However, research studies still need to be performed to establish their exact effects on sexual functioning.

Ambergris (Ambrein, Ambra Grisea)

This natural product is found in the gut of the sperm whale (Figure 27-7) and is used in the Arab world as an aphrodisiac. Ambrein increases the concentration of several anterior pituitary hormones and serum testosterone as well as facilitation noradrenergic transmission and dopamine synthesis [64].

Arthropods

Arthropods such as lobster, Arizona bark scorpion, deathstalker, banana spider, Mediterranean black widow, Burmeister's triatoma, giant water bug, diving-beetle, Korean bug, diaclina, flannel moth, Spanish fly, migratory locust, red wood ant, and honeybee, were reviewed in 2012 by Pajovic and colleagues for their use as aphrodisiacs [65]. Although they have been used for this purpose for centuries, research is still needed to establish their effectiveness.

Bufo Toad

The skin and glands of the Bufo toad contain bufotenine, related to serotonin (as well as the "love stone" from the Caribbean and Chan su from China), which has been reported historically to improve sexual performance [64]. However, research evidence is needed to establish the effectiveness of this food element.

Pistachios

A 3-week uncontrolled trial of 17 patients with a 12-month diagnosis of ED involved taking took 100 g pistachio nuts daily for 3 weeks. All five domains of the International Index of Erectile Function (IIEF) as well as penile color Doppler ultrasound parameters significantly improved [66].

Asparagus

Asparagus has been reported for centuries to improve sexual performance. Through activating NO release, asparagus could potentially improve arousal and erection [67]. More studies would need to be performed to examine on the impact of asparagus on sexual functioning.

Chocolate

Chocolate has historically been thought to exert several effects on sexuality including acting as an aphrodisiac and enhancing sexual pleasure, especially in women [67] (Figure 27-8). Salonia et al. addressed this question in a study of 163 women that completed anonymous semi-structured interviews on their sexual function, sexual distress, and depression. The study found that women who consumed chocolate daily had a statistically significant higher score on sexual desire and total sexual function section the interview; however this difference was eliminated once adjusted for age [68].

One possible explanation for the effects of chocolate on human sexuality is its ability to have a significant impact on overall mood [69]. It is thought that the appeal of chocolate and its positive effect on mood are due its fat and sugar content along with its pleasant aroma [70–72]. At a biochemical level chocolate contains high levels of phenylethylamine, a compound that is detected at higher levels among people in love [72]. Additionally, chocolate has been associated with serotonin release that acts to produce arousal in women [67, 72]. Despite feasible mechanisms at a biochemical level there are no studies showing a significant association between chocolate consumption and libido.

Nutmeg

Nutmeg or *Myristica fragrans* is a dried kernel that is native to India and has historically been used as a medicine for stomach ailments and several other illnesses, and as a tonic, nerve stimulant, and aphrodisiac [73–76]. The aphrodisiac potential of nutmeg has been studied in animal models, though further testing is required in order to apply these results to humans and provide a plausible biological mechanism.

Saffron

Saffron or *Crocus sativus* is a plant from the Middle East and South Asia traditionally ascribed with medicinal value including aphrodisiac potential [77, 78]. In a study of male rats Hosseinzadeh et al. that found intraperitoneally injected crocin, a saffron extract constituent, produced increased frequency of mounting, intromission, and erection relative to controls [78]. To determine is these findings are applicable to humans Safarinejad et al. evaluated the ability of saffron to benefit patients suffering from ED in an open label, randomized crossover study [79]. Patients were given on demand sildenafil for 12 weeks followed by twice daily saffron for an additional 12 weeks. When compared to sildenafil, saffron did not exhibit satisfactory benefit in men with ED [79]. Saffron does show potential for enhancing sexual drive in mammals but no evidence to date indicates its usefulness in humans.

Caffeine

Caffeine is found in a variety of foods. Caffeine is a central nervous system stimulant, with peak plasma concentration occurring at 1–2 h, with an approximate half-life of 5 h. It is broadly consumed and often associated with withdrawal effects [80]. Approximately 80% of caffeine is metabolized to paraxanthine. Caffeine and paraxanthine are known increase diastolic blood pressure, plasma epinephrine levels, and free fatty acids [81]. It is anxiogenic, especially for those who consume it in large quantities. Caffeine has does not increase alertness in non- or low-consuming individuals, and with consistent consumption, tolerance develops to its anxiogenic effect [82]. A recent study investigated the effect of on-demand caffeine consumption in treating patients with PE [83]. The caffeine group, comprised of 40 healthy males, was treated with 100 mg of encapsulated caffeine 2 h prior to intercourse for 3 weeks, 2 h prior to each occurrence of sexual intercourse. There was a highly significant correlation between caffeine treatment and improvements in intravaginal ejaculation latency time, as well as index of sexual satisfaction [83].

Nutraceuticals: Dietary Supplements, Non-prescription/Over-the-Counter Products, Herbs, and Plants

This section on non-prescription products and the following section on herbal products review most sexual enhancement ingredients except for yohimbine, which is reviewed in the chapter on pharmaceutical sexual enhancers. Cui et al. identified the top-selling sexual enhancement ingredients in a recent 2015 review [84], as shown in Table 27-1.

TABLE 27-1. Top 20 most commonly identified ingredients based on product nutrition labels

Ingredient name	Number of products containing ingredient
Ginseng	13
Tribulus spp.	13
Zinc	13
Epimedium spp. (Horny goat weed)	11
Vitamin B6	10
Fenugreek	10
L-arginine	10
Vitamin B12	9
Maca	9
Vitamin B3 (also as niacin)	6
Saw Palmetto	6
Vitamin B9 (also as folate)	5
Dehydroepiandosterone (DHEA)	5
Vitamin E	5
Ginkgo biloba	5
Magnesium	5
Yohimbine	5
Vitamin B1 (also as thiamin)	4
Vitamin B2 (also as riboflavin)	4
Selenium	4

Reprinted from Cui T, Kovell RC, Brooks DC, Terlecki RP. A Urologist's Guide to Ingredients Found in Top-Selling Nutraceuticals for Men's Sexual Health. J Sex Med. 2015;12(11): 2105–17 with permission from Elsevier.

L-Arginine

L-arginine, an amino acid available over the counter, is the substrate for nitric oxide synthase (NOS) and is converted into NO [85]. This pathway affects the smooth muscle relaxation that is needed for sexual functioning [86]. NO relaxes blood vessel walls, thus improving circulation throughout the body, including in erectile tissue. L-arginine also increases elasticity of arteries, potentially decreasing blood pressure and improving the capacity of erectile tissue [87].

L-arginine appears to impact two desire and arousal stages of the sexual response cycle and has been explored as an intervention in both premenopausal and postmenopausal women. Two studies of a mixture that includes L-arginine suggested improvements in female sexual function, including desire, frequency of intercourse, and orgasm [88, 89]. Another study, assessed the effects on sexual function in healthy, postmenopausal women, this time using a mixture containing the dietary supplement pycnogenol and L-arginine, found that there were significant subjective improvements after 4 and 8 weeks in domains related to desire, arousal, lubrication, and orgasm [90]. L-arginine's effect on sexual function of healthy women of reproductive age with moderate sexual dysfunction was examined using a mixture containing pycnogenol and L-arginine, along with a management program of lifestyle, diet, exercise, and stress control. The results revealed significantly improved desire, arousal, lubrication, orgasm, satisfaction, and pain [91]. Some studies of L-arginine also have focused on its physiological impact. In one such study a mixture of oral L-arginine glutamate and yohimbine significantly increased vaginal pulse amplitude in response to an erotic film in postmenopausal women with female sexual arousal disorder [92].

In one study of 50 men with organic ED, of the 29 who took L-arginine, nine indicated subjective improvements in sexual function. Of note, all nine of these men had low levels of NO excretion or production [93]. L-arginine as an intervention for ED has been investigated primarily in combination with a variety of other agents. A combination of pycnogenol and L-arginine was tested in 40 men over 3 months. After 1 month of L-arginine treatment, there was no change in the percent of men who experienced normal erection, but after adding pycnogenol during the second month there was a significant improvement. After 3 months of treatment with the combination, successful erections were elicited in 92.5% of participants [94]. Another study of 50 men with moderate ED, treatment with a mixture including pycnogenol and L-arginine restored erectile function to normal over 1 month [95]. These results were replicated in the treatment of mild to moderate ED in Japanese men [96]. Prelox® Blue is an example of a commercially available product containing this combination of L-arginine and pycnogenol with the addition of L-taurine and aspartic acid. A combination of L-arginine and adenosine monophosphate one to 2 h prior to sexual intercourse showed gains in erectile function and in intercourse satisfaction [97]. Side effects of L-arginine include abdominal pain, bloating, diarrhea, gout, blood abnormalities, allergies, airway inflammation, asthma exacerbation, and hypotension. Doses for treatment of ED are about 5 g PO daily over 6 weeks [98]. For postmenopausal women with sexual arousal disorder, the dose is 6 g PO daily 1 h prior to intercourse [94].

L-Carnitine

L-carnitine acts as a vasodilator by activating prostaglandin synthesis [93]. Cavallini et al. compared androgen supplementation to L-carnitine (propionyl-L-carnitine 2 g/day plus acetyl-L-carnitine 2 g/day) and placebo for 6 months, and showed that L-carnitine was superior to androgen supplement in terms of nocturnal penile tumescence and IIEF [99].

Dehydroepiandrosterone (DHEA)

DHEA occurs naturally as a weak steroid hormone produced by the adrenal glands and by the brain. Its uses in the body are myriad, one herein significant being the improvement of sexual function. It leads to the production of androgens and estrogens, but its levels decline with age, more quickly in women than in men. DHEA is converted to androstenedione, testosterone, and dihydrotestosterone, and aromatized to estrogen. As DHEA, testosterone, and estrogen decrease over time, the employment of DHEA has not been limited to treatment of primary adrenal insufficiency, building the immune system, slowing the aging process, providing increased energy, improving memory and mood, and building bone and muscle strength [100]. Prasterone is a formulation of DHEA used, off label, to treat sexual dysfunction in postmenopausal women. It can be applied intravaginally as a cream [101]. Alternatively, low-dose DHEA therapy for sexual dysfunction in postmenopausal women is available in oral form [102]. DHEA also can be used orally in men for the ED off label.

DHEA was tested in 16 sexually functional postmenopausal women in whom sexual arousal was activated by erotic video. Subjective responses and physical sexual arousal increased significantly in the DHEA group versus the placebo group [103]. A time- and dose-dependent improvement in desire/interest, arousal, and orgasm was detected upon treatment with intravaginal DHEA in 216 postmenopausal women with moderate to severe symptoms of vaginal atrophy. Arousal/sensation improved by 68%, arousal/lubrication by 39%, orgasm by 75%, and dryness during intercourse by 57%, supporting the use of intravaginal DHEA in postmenopausal women with sexual dysfunction [101]. The treatment of dyspareunia, or pain with intercourse, was examined in one study of 114 postmenopausal women who were also treated with intravaginal DHEA. Intravaginal DHEA caused a rapid, efficient effect on dyspareunia [104]. The effect over 1 year of oral DHEA on sexual dysfunction in early post-menopausal women was also assessed. In 48 healthy post-menopausal women daily oral DHEA provided significant improvement in sexual function and in frequency of sexual intercourse [102]. One study significant for discerning DHEA treatment differences between sexes was undertaken. The premise was that outcome differences in dehydroepiandrosterone treatment in postmenopausal women and in men with HSDD were gender-based as a consequence of the peripheral conversion of DHEA to testosterone. Women, as opposed to, men had significant beneficial effect on arousal, suggesting that ongoing dosing with DHEA could be efficacious in the treatment of HSDD in women [105]. The Massachusetts Male Aging Study in 1994 reported an inverse correlation between DHEA and ED. A study to replace DHEA in men suffering from ED was therefore undertaken. Success was determined by the ability to maintain or achieve an erection sufficient for satisfactory sexual performance. Although the patient database was not large enough to perform meaningful statistical analysis, what was found was that DHEA treatment was associated with higher mean scores for the International Index of Erectile Function [106].

Side effects of DHEA include abdominal pain, acne, fatigue, alopecia, headache, hirsutism, hypertension, hypoglycemia, menstrual irregularities, nasal congestion, psychosis, voice changes [107]. DHEA is administered as a 10% vaginal cream to apply topically daily [108], and at 50–100 mg PO daily for ED [108, 109].

Zestra Oil

Zestra oil is an over the counter preparation that is applied to the clitoris and labia locally, and it leads to improved desire and arousal, and the effects are reported to start within 3–5 min and lasting up to 45 min [110, 111]. A 16-week randomized, placebo-controlled, double-blind study of 256 women, age 21–65, showed significant improvement in desire, arousal, and treatment satisfaction benefits. Zestra was well tolerated and the only significant safety finding was mild to moderate genital burning in 14.6% of patients [112].

SS Cream

SS cream contains extracts of plants and is used for the treatment of premature ejaculation. Placebo controlled studies showed that the mean ejaculatory latency time was nearly 11 min on the SS cream compared to nearly 2.5 min on placebo. Moreover, nearly 80% of SS cream patients had an ejaculatory latency time >2 min compared to 15% of placebo patients. Side effects of the SS cream included mild local burning and pain [113].

Ginkgo biloba

Ginkgo biloba leaves and extract are thought to stimulate NO production and on contribute to smooth muscle relaxation (Figure 27-9). Reports of improving sexual function led to more research to examine its effects. In a randomized placebo-controlled study, Meston et al. examined the effects of Ginkgo biloba 300 mg/day on women with sexual arousal disorder, compared to sex therapy or their combination, showing that Ginkgo biloba combined with sex therapy but not alone, increased sexual desire and contentment more than placebo with minimal side effects [114].

Vitamin B

Vitamin B for sexual enhancement includes B1, B3, B6, B9, and B12. B1 (Thiamine) was reported to improve erectile dysfunction during treatment of alcoholism [115]. B3 (Niacin) has been reported to improve sexual function in hyperlipidemia and diabetes mellitus [116]. B6 is involved in homocysteine regulation, which is implicated in NO synthesis, and B6 has been reported to improve erection scores when combined with PDE5 inhibitors in diabetics [117]. B9 (Folate) is also involved in homocysteine regulation and its deficiency affects energy level [118]. B12 deficiency is associated with fatigue and depression, and therefore B12 supplementation could improve mood, energy, and sexual functioning [118].

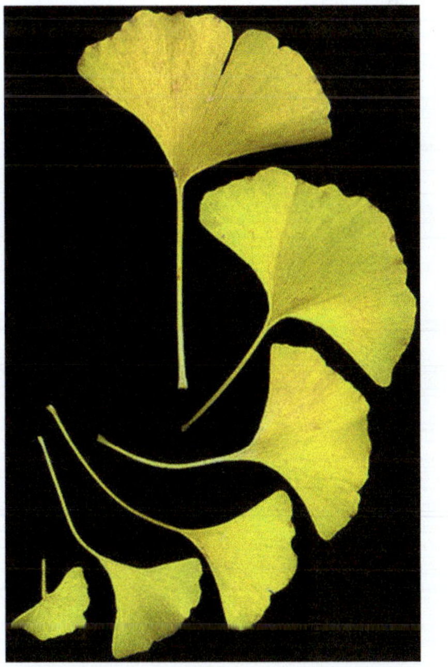

FIGURE 27-9. *Ginkgo biloba*. Source: https://commons.wikimedia.org/wiki/File:GinkgoLeaves.jpg.

Trace Elements (Zinc, Magnesium, Selenium)

Trace elements are important to maintain healthy metabolism and different body functions including sexual performance. Selenium daily intake for dose is 55 mcg. Zinc is very common element among men's sexual enhancement products with doses ranging from 1 to 30 mg with 11 mg being the daily recommend dose [84]. Zinc deficiency is associated with decreased testosterone [55]. Magnesium has a positive effect on the production of testosterone [50–53]. Selenium is frequently encountered in men's sexual health preparations [84], although no studies have linked its supplementation with sexual performance.

Ginseng

Ginseng is a plant of the *Panax* genus of the family Araliaceae used as a food and herbal remedy renowned for its health benefits, especially in East Asia and the Indian subcontinent (Figure 27-10). It has been explored as an agent to increase energy, decrease blood sugar, lower cholesterol levels, reduce stress, promote relaxation, improve psychomotor performance, and treat sexual dysfunction [119]. Ginseng promotes NO release and relaxation of the smooth muscle of the corpora cavernosa [120].

Two Korean studies tested the sexual enhancing properties of ginseng root. Compared to placebo, men who took 3000 mg of ginseng daily showed improved erection rigidity and ability to penetrate [121]. A placebo-controlled trial, the oral administration of Korean red ginseng extracts improved sexual arousal in menopausal women [122]. The use of a mixture contained ginseng, along with L-arginine, ginkgo, and damiana for 4 weeks of treatment showed improved satisfaction with their overall sex life in 73.5% of patients compared to 37.2% on placebo [89]. Perimenopausal women exhibited significant improvements in frequency of intercourse and satisfaction with sexual relationship in a placebo-controlled trial using the same mixture [90]. A double-blind crossover study of 45 with ED were treated with Korean red ginseng over 8 weeks showed significantly improved erections [123]. A subsequent study of 119 men with mild-to-moderate ED demonstrated improvement in all domains of sexual function when compared to placebo [124]. A 60 person study of patients with mild to moderate ED administered 1000 mg three times daily of ginseng and found that ratings for penetration and maintenance were significantly higher than those found in the placebo group [125].

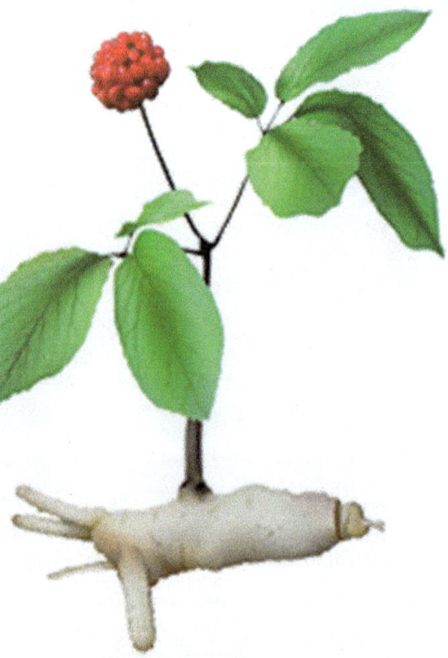

Figure 27-10. Ginseng plant and root. Source: https://commons.wikimedia.org/wiki/File:Ginseng_root.jpg.

Side effects of ginseng include: skin hypersensitivity reaction, amenorrhea, appetite decreased, cerebral arteritis, cholestatic hepatitis, diarrhea, edema, ejaculation delay (topical use), euphoria, excitability, ginseng abuse syndrome, headache, hypertension, hyperpyrexia, hypotension, insomnia, irritability, libido increase, local burning/irritation (topical use), mastalgia, arthralgia/myalgia, palpitations, pruritus, restlessness, rose spots, skin eruptions, Stevens-Johnson syndrome, tachycardia, vaginal bleeding, and vertigo [126]. Ginseng dosing is not well established and depends on the type of ginseng used. The usual treatment course lasts 3 weeks to 3 months. There is a 2-week ginseng-free period that is encouraged between treatment courses. Tea is prepared with 3 g root per 150 mL water [127].

Chlorophytum borivilianum

Chlorophytum borivilianum roots (vajikaran rasayana or safed musli) have been used in Ayurdedic medicine for its positive influence on sexual behavior [128]. In a comparative study comparing *C. borivalinum* to other traditional Indian herbs in a rat model, the group given *C. borivalinum* had the least hesitation time when initiating mating behavior in the presence of a female rat. Additionally the male rats had increased penile erection index which is a measure of NO activity [128]. The positive studies in rat models using *C. borivilianum* suggest that could be a source of promising research in regard to enhancing fertility and sexual drive in humans. Furthermore, there were no reports of serious side effects.

Monida whitei

Monida whitei is a sub-Saharan plant that has been used as an aphrodisiac since ancient times [129]. In an in vitro study it enhanced total and progressive motility human spermatozoa in a time-dependent manner [129]. One possible explanation is that *M. whitei* increases serum and intratesticular testosterone levels [130]. A later study by the same group showed that *M. whitei* extract had an anti-alpha adrenergic effect on penile smooth muscle, possibly enhancing erectile function [131]. Based on these findings *M. whitei* might have potential therapeutic benefits in males suffering low sperm counts and might help enhance erectile function. However, without human trials it is difficult to determine the safety and effectiveness of this herb.

Tribulus terrestris

Tribulus terrestris is a plant native to tropical and warm regions and used in both Indian and Chinese traditional medicine for sexual enhancement of men [132] (Figure 27-11). Other studies have shown that active ingredients *in T. terrestris*, improve sperm production in human and animal trials and increases levels of testosterone, LH, and DHEA [133–135] Some studies suggest that endothelium and nitric oxide-dependent mechanisms underlie its aphrodisiac and pro-erectile activities [136, 137]. In preclinical studies *Tribulus terrestris* increases intracavernosal pressure, suggesting that pro-erectile properties might be the result of increased androgen levels and subsequent release of NO from nerve endings that innervate the corpus cavernosum [138].

Given the proven pro-androgenic nature of *T. terrestris* it is understandable that it is used as an aphrodisiac. *Tribulus terrestris* has been found to be a useful agent in the treatment of HSDD in a study of 60 women. After 4 weeks of treatment with *Tribulus terrestris* significant improvements in desire, arousal, lubrication, satisfaction, and pain were found [139]. Another study based on hospital records of women of reproductive age with sexual dysfunction reported significant improvements in the Female Sexual Function Index scores [140].

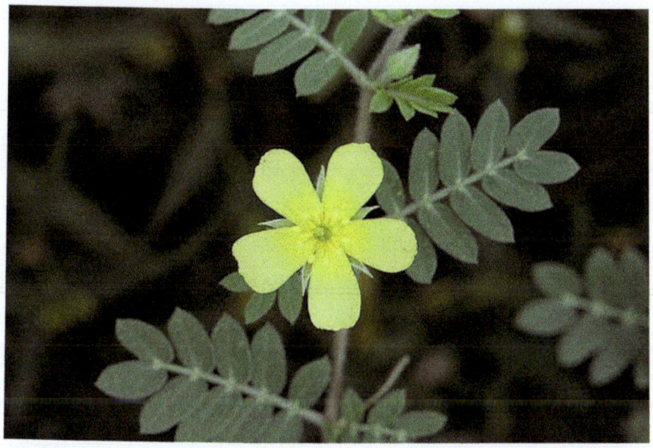

FIGURE 27-11. *Tribulus terrestris*. Source: https://commons.wikimedia.org/wiki/File:Tribulus_terrestris_3002.jpg.

A study of 60 women with sexual dysfunction secondary to menopause also showed that *Tribulus terrestris* was efficacious in the domains of vaginal lubrication during coitus and/or foreplay, sensation in the genitalia during sexual intercourse or other stimuli, sensation in the genital region, sexual intercourse and/or other sexual stimulation, and the ability to reach orgasm [141]. However, *Tribulus terrestris* was shown not to be more effective than placebo in improving symptoms of ED [142]. On the other hand, a compound containing *Tribulus terrestris* was investigated in comparison to tadalafil in the treatment of decreased libido and ED in elderly men, with results suggesting that libido was improved after 2 months, without the side effects attributed to tadalafil [143]. Despite the promise this herb presents it must be used with caution as it could induce nephrotoxicity, hepatotoxicity, and neurotoxicity on rare occasions [144, 145]. Priapism has been reported after consuming an herbal supplement comprised chiefly of *Tribulus terrestris* [146].

Trigonella foenum-graecum (Fenugreek)

Trigonella foenum-graecum or Fenugreek or "methi," is found in 10 of the top 30 selling GNC men's health supplements, and it contains sex hormones precursors such as steroidal saponins, e.g., diosgenin and was reported to have arginine [84]. A randomized double-blind, placebo-controlled study of 60 males without ED who received 600 mg or placebo daily for 6 week showed significant increases in self-report of sexual arousal and orgasm, improved quality of life, and no changes in testosterone and prolactin levels [147].

Horny Goat Weed or Yin Yang Huo (Epimedium, Icariin)

Horny goat weed (HGW, or Yin Yang Huo, Epimedium) is an herb from China and the Middle East has used for ED [148]. It was found in 11 of the top 30 GNC male sexual health products and thought to contain icariin, a PDE inhibitor [84]. Animal model studies showed its success in ED, though human studies are lacking [149].

Muira Puama (Potency Wood)

Muira Puama, a known as an aphrodisiac in South America extracted from a plant root and bark, improves sexual arousal through inhibition of GABA [150]. A formulation of Muira puama and Ginkgo biloba (Herbal vX) for 1 month was examined in 202 healthy women with low sex drive, in an uncontrolled trial. The self-reported measures showed statistically significantly improvement in 65% in desire, arousal, orgasm, and satisfaction with sex life, with good tolerability [151].

Korean Herbs

Korean herbs were reviewed in detail in 2015 by Shin and collaugues [152]. The unripe *Rubus coreanus* extract may help in ED cases that did not respond to sildenafil as shown in animal models to activate the corpus cavernosum NO-cGMP system [153]. *Schisandra chinensis* relaxes vascular tissue through an endothelium-dependent NO pathway and was shown to improve sildenafil citrate-induced relaxation [154]. *Artemisia capillaris* acts through the NO-cGMP and cAMP signaling pathways to relax penile vessels [155]. *Cuscuta chinensis* mechanism of action is thought to involve the NO-cGMP pathway and might be useful in sildenafil-unresponsive patients [156].

Essential Oils: Ylang-Ylang and Jasmine Oil

Essential oils have been reported to enhance sexual activity from early history. Ylang-ylang [157] and jasmine [158] oils have been frequently recommended for body or genital rubbing in women and men.

Phoenix dactylifera (Date Palm)

Phoenix dactylifera (date palm) is a sweet fruit cultivated in the Middle East [159] (Figure 27-12). The pollen of the date palm is reputed to be an aphrodisiac and has been used in traditional medicine [160]. Bahamanpour et al. tested the effects of date palm pollen on sperm parameters and reproductive system of male rats. They found increased sperm count, motility and improved sperm morphology.

Additionally there was an increase in the weight of the testis and epididymus [161]. Initial research in animal models appears to be promising for the application of date palm pollen to treating infertility and male libido issues.

Lepidium meyenii (Maca)

Lepidium meyenii is a plant that grows in the central Andes within a narrow altitude range between 4000 and 4500 m. Locals have used the root for its aphrodisiac and fertility enhancing abilities [160] (Figure 27-13). Several studies have evaluated the effects of Maca using animal models. Zheng et al. tested both mice and rats and found improved erectile function and increased mating frequency in the maca-treated groups compared to controls [162]. Bo Lin et al. observed similar results with oral administration of *L. meyenni* extract given to mice. In a double blind RCT study on human male subjects Gonzales et al. compared placebo to maca using subjective surveys on sexual desire. The study found improved sexual desire in men taking maca at 8 and 12 weeks [163]. In an additional study the same research group tested the ability of maca to affect serum reproductive hormones and found no significant increase after 12 weeks of administration when compared to the control group [164].

Although animal testing and subjective testing in humans seem to show an aphrodisiac-like effect, the lack of influence on reproductive hormones leaves open the question as to how it exerts its influence. As a supplement maca appears to be safe with no major reported side effects found in literature.

Kaempferia parviflora

Kaempferia parviflora is a plant native to Southeast Asia used to enhance male sexual function. The extracts do not affect on reproductive organ weight [160]. Alcohol extracts of the plant decreased ejaculatory latencies [160]. Chaturapanich et al. found an alcohol extract increased sexual performance, likely

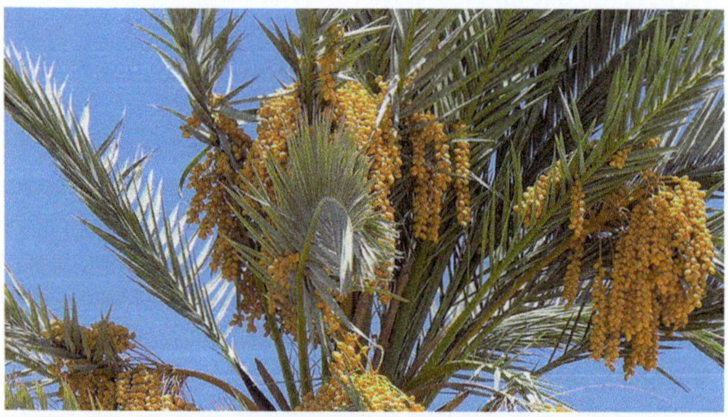

FIGURE 27-12. Date palms. https://commons.wikimedia.org/wiki/File:Dahab_Egypt_Phoenix_dactylifera.JPG.

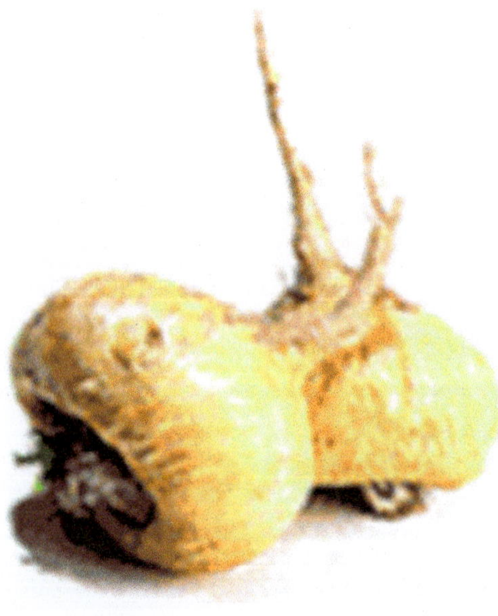

FIGURE 27-13. Maca roots. Source: https://commons.wikimedia.org/wiki/File:Maca.gif.

by increasing blood flow in the testis [165]. With little evidence to support the efficacy of this herb, more studies are needed to establish its use as an aphrodisiac.

Eurycoma longifolia (Tongkat Ali)

Eurycoma longifolia (Tongkat Ali) is a flowering plant native to Southeast Asia where it has gained a reputation among Malaysian men as an aphrodisiac due to its purported ability to increase virility and sexual prowess [160]. Animal studies showed that 9-hydroxycanthin-6-one, one of *Eurycoma longifolia*'s primary constituents induces penile erection and delays ejaculation, and a dose-dependent significant increase in penile reflex episodes [166]. A systematic review and meta-analysis of 342 articles identified analyzed data from 2 human studies with a total of 139 participants, and showed significantly improved scores on the International Index of Erectile Function (IIEF-5) only in subjects with lower baseline IIEF-5 [167].

Satureja khuzestanica Jamzad and *Satureja montana*

Satureja khuzestanica Jamzad is native to southern Iran thought to be an aphrodisiac [160] (Figure 27-14). Testing has been done on the *Satureja khuzestanica* essential oil (SKEO) in two different studies. Sulmaz et al. tested SKEO on rat fertility in male rats and found it improved potency, fecundity, and fertility index in male rats [168]. Rezvanfar et al. found that SKEO, when co-administered with cyclophosphamide, improved the negative side effects on the reproductive system that normally occurred with administration of cyclophosphamide. The likely mechanism is that SKEO has antioxidant and androgenic activities [169]. Upon histological examination of reproductive organs of rats receiving SKEO there was increased numbers of sperm and Leydig cells as well as sertoli cell hypertrophy [169].

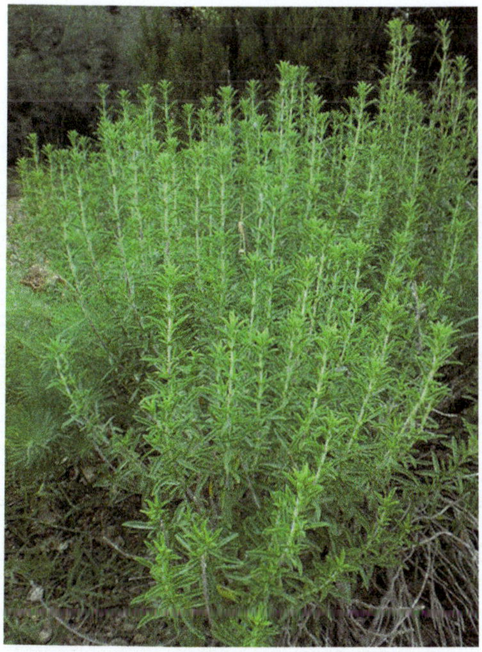

FIGURE 27-14. *Satureja montana*. Source: https://commons.wikimedia.org/wiki/File:Satureja_montana_1c.JPG.

Satureja montana has been used successfully in animal models for premature ejaculation [170]. In a recent controlled study of premature ejaculation in five urology clinics, patients were given an oral combination of Satureja montana, tryptophan, Tribulus terrestris, and Phyllanthus emblica extracts for 3 months, with significant improvements on ejaculation parameters (calculated as mean from that perceived by partner and that perceived by patient) [171].

Fadogia argestis

Fadogia argestis is a plant from Central Africa and the aqueous extracts of the stem contain saponins, alkaloids, anrthaquinones, and flavonoids [172]. The stems have been used as a traditional aphrodisiac in folk medicine [173]. Extract from this plant has been tested for its aphrodisiac potential in a study where the extract was administered orally to male rats and produced significant increases in mounting frequency and ejaculatory latency among other sexual parameters [172]. Research studies showed an increase in serum testosterone with *F. argestis* extract, with the potential toxic effects on the testicles at very high doses [174–176]. Evidence is limited in human trials, but positive findings in rodent models suggest that this herb's aphrodisiac potential should be further investigated.

Montanoa tomentosa

Montanoa tomentosa is a plant native to Mexico that has been used as an aqueous extract to treat reproductive impairments and also as a contraceptive early in pregnancy [177, 178]. In a study of its aphrodisiac potential in 2004, Carro-Juarez et al. administered *M. tomentosa* extract to male rats and found that is improved motivation, performance and drastically reduced ejaculatory latency [179]. In a later study, the effects of *M. tomentosa* on ejaculatory motor patterns in rats was tested. Two important findings were drawn from this study. First. *M. tomentosa* increased ejaculatory motor pattern expression, and second, this effect was neutralized by the administration of a selective oxytocin antagonist [180]. These findings suggest that *M. tomentosa* extract might act at the level of the spinal circuits that regulate ejaculatory function [181]. Although the active ingredient in this herb is still unknown, early studies suggest grandiflorenic acid might be responsible for the pro-ejaculatory effects observed in rat models [180, 181]. *M. tomentosa* extract appears to be safe for consumption, although women who are trying to become pregnant should avoid it due to its contraceptive effects on early pregnancy. More research still needs to be done on human subjects before its aphrodisiac potential can be confirmed.

Terminalia catappa

Terminalia catappa is a tropical tree native to tropical areas in Asia, Africa, and Australia [182]. The plant's seeds are considered an aphrodisiac in Ayurvedic medicine [183]. A study performed by Ratnasooriya evaluated the efficacy of seed extracts in male rats [184]. The study found that a dose of 1500 mg/kg produced improvements in sexual vigor of male rats. However, this relationship reversed at higher doses of 3000 mg/kg where all parameters of sexual behavior measured in the study other than mounting were temporarily diminished [185]. One concern revealed in this study is that higher doses of the seed produced moderate elevations of serum glutamic-oxaloacetic transaminase (SGOT) and glutamic-pyruvate transaminase (SGPT), indicating liver injury [184]. *T catappa* shows promise as a therapeutic herb for men; however, caution should be exercised to not exceed recommended doses so as to avoid potential liver damage and decrease in libido.

Casmiroa edulis

Casmiroa edulis is a widespread tropical plant with seeds that are valued for their aphrodisiac potential [160]. Ali et al. evaluated the aphrodisiac potential of *C. edulis* seed extract in male rats. The rats were given sildenafil or *C. edulis* extract, and whereas both groups exhibited statistically relevant increases in several mating parameters, sildenafil rat experienced greater enhancement than *C. edulis* rats. *C. edulis* is noted for its ability to produce hypotension much like sildenafil. Therefore, it is possible that both compounds function through a similar mechanism of action [186, 187]. Indeed, *C. edulis* was reported in Baisch et al. to exert its vasodilating effects via NO release [188]. Other than the expected side effects of hypotension, experimental animal studies have not found any concerning toxicity. *C. edulis* seed extract might very well offer an herbal alternative to sildenafil albeit slightly less effective.

Tunera diffusa

Tunera diffusa is a Mexican shrub that has historically been used by northern Mexican natives as a leaf decoction to treat muscle weakness, bladder inflammation, and as an aphrodisiac [189, 190] (Figure 27-15). Although there is little scientific evidence to support the claims that this plant is an aphrodisiac, several studies have showed some promise.

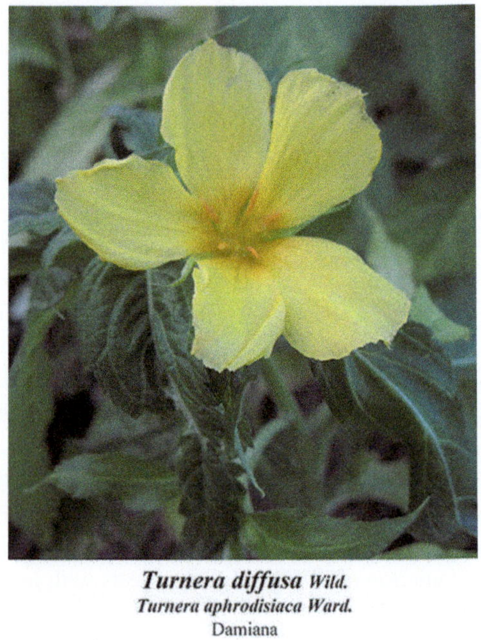

FIGURE 27-15. *Tunera diffusa* Damiana. Source: https://commons.wikimedia.org/wiki/File:Turnera_diffusa_damiana_1.jpg.

Arletti et al. studied "sexually sluggish" rats given *T. diffusa* extract and found that it improved the copulatory patterns [191]. Estrada-Reyes et al., evaluated *T. diffusa* extract in male rats exhibiting sexual exhaustion and subsequent sexual inhibition. Sexual exhaustion occurs after copulation with a single female leading to period of sexual inhibition where no further mating can occur until the male has recovered from the refractory period [192, 193]. They found that *T. diffusa* extract allowed male rats experiencing sexual exhaustion to copulate with an additional female rat sooner than would otherwise be possible via significantly reduction the post-ejaculatory interval [194]. A possible explanation for this finding is the high levels of flavonoids found in that have been found to exert biological activity in the central nervous system [194, 195]. Flavonoids and their derivatives enhance sexual behavior in male rodents and increase levels of NO in vascular tissue, a chief regulator of penile erection [196–198].

Mad Honey (*Rhododendron ponticum*, *Grayanotoxin*)

Grayanotoxin-containing honey is produced from the nectar of a plant called *Rhododendron ponticum*, which grows in Turkey, Nepal, Japan, and Brazil. Grayanotoxin activates the vagus nerve leading to improved sexual functioning. High doses have been associated with bradycardia, low blood pressure, cardiac events, A-V heart block, and loss of consciousness [199].

Other Herbal and Plant Products

Cinnamomum cassia (China) [200], aqueous extract of *Lecaniodiscus cupanioides* (Nigeria) [201], *Monsonia angustifolia* (South Africa) [202] are only a few examples of herbs showing emergent evidence in preclinical studies only in the recent years. Further research studies would need to be conducted to establish the evidence for the effectiveness of emerging agents.

Conclusion

Natural sexual enhancement is an important theme for the public and for the scientific community. Innovation of sexual enhancement techniques, aphrodisiacs, dietary supplements, and herbal preparations is in high demand. Randomized placebo-controlled clinical trials are warranted before such interventions could be recommended with confidence [199]. Evidence supporting the various interventions described in this chapter is still emerging. Rigorous study to examine the evidence for efficacy and safety remains highly needed.

References

1. Almås E, Landmark B. Non pharmacological treatment of sexual problems—a review of research literature 1970–2008. Sexologies. 2010;19(4):202–11.
2. Kleinplatz PJ, Menard D, Paquet M, Paradis N, Campbell M, Zuccarino D, et al. The components of optimal sexuality a portrait of "great sex". Can J Hum Sex. 2009;18(1):1–13.
3. Ann CC. A proposal for a radical new sex therapy technique for the management of vasocongestive and orgasmic dysfunction in women: the AFE Zone Stimulation Technique. Sex Marital Ther. 1997;12(4):357–70.
4. Eichel EW, Eichel JD, Kule S. The technique of coital alignment and its relation to female orgasmic response and simultaneous orgasm. J Sex Marital Ther. 1988;14(2):129–41.
5. Hurlbert DF, Apt C. The coital alignment technique and directed masturbation: a comparative study on female orgasm. J Sex Marital Ther. 1995;21(1):21–9.
6. van de Velde TH, Browne S, Rouben Mamoulian Collection (Library of Congress). Ideal marriage; its physiology and technique. New York: Covici-Friede; 1930.
7. Colson MH, Lemaire A, Pinton P, Hamidi K, Klein P. Sexual behaviors and mental perception, satisfaction and expectations of sex life in men and women in France. J Sex Med. 2006;3(1):121–31.
8. Brody S, Weiss P. Simultaneous penile-vaginal intercourse orgasm is associated with satisfaction (sexual, life, partnership, and mental health). J Sex Med. 2011;8(3):734–41.
9. de Carufel F, Trudel G. Effects of a new functional-sexological treatment for premature ejaculation. J Sex Marital Ther. 2006;32(2):97–114.
10. Semans JH. Premature ejaculation: a new approach. South Med J. 1956;49(4):353–8.
11. Masters WH, Johnson VE. Human sexual inadequacy. London: Churchill; 1970.
12. Masters WH, Johnson VE. Human sexual inadequacy. Boston: Little; 1970.
13. LoPiccolo J, Lobitz WC. The role of masturbation in the treatment of orgasmic dysfunction. Arch Sex Behav. 1972;2(2):163–71.
14. Kegel AH. Sexual functions of the pubococcygeus muscle. West J Surg Obstet Gynecol. 1952;60(10):521–4.
15. Trudel G, Laurin F. The effects of bibliotherapy on orgasmic dysfunction and couple interactions: an experimental study. Sex Marital Ther. 1988;3(2):223–8.
16. Trudel G, Proulx S. Treatment of premature ejaculation by bibliotherapy: an experimental study. Sex Marital Ther. 1987;2(2):163–7.
17. Kempeneers P, Andrianne R, Bauwens S, Georis I, Pairoux JF, Blairy S. Clinical outcomes of a new self-help booklet for premature ejaculation. J Sex Med. 2012;9(9):2417–28.
18. Wilson SK, Delk 2nd JR, Billups KL. Treating symptoms of female sexual arousal disorder with the Eros-clitoral therapy device. J Gend Specif Med. 2001;4(2):54–8.
19. Türk G, Ateşşahin A, Sönmez M, Yüce A, Çeribaşı AO. Lycopene protects against cyclosporine A-induced testicular toxicity in rats. Theriogenology. 2007;67:778–85.
20. Zhang Q, Radisavljevic ZM, Siroky MB, Azadzoi KM. Dietary antioxidants improve anteriogenic erectile dysfunction. Int J Androl. 2011;34(3):225–35.
21. Zarfeshany A, Asgary S, Javanmard SH. Potent health effects of pomegranate. Adv Biomed Res. 2014;3:100.
22. Trexler ET, Smith-Ryan AE, Melvin MN, Roelofs EJ, Wingfield HL. Effects of pomegranate extract on blood flow and running time to exhaustion. Appl Physiol Nutr Metab. 2014;39(9):1038–42.
23. Levine GN, Steinke EE, Bakaeen FG, Bozkurt B, Cheitlin MD, Conti JB, et al. Sexual activity and cardiovascular disease: a scientific statement from the American Heart Association. Circulation. 2012;125(8):1058–72.
24. Turk G, Sonmez M, Aydin M, Yuce A, Gur S, Yuksel M, et al. Effects of pomegranate juice consumption on sperm quality, spermatogenic cell density, antioxidant activity and testosterone level in male rats. Clin Nutr. 2008;27(2):289–96.
25. Mandalari G, Faulks RM, Rich GT, Lo Turco V, Picout DR, Lo Curto RB. Release of protein, lipid, and vitamin E from almond seeds during digestion. J Agric Food Chem. 2008;56(9):3409–16.
26. Azarenko O, Jordan MA, Wilson L. Erucin, the major isothiocyanate in arugula (Eruca sativa), inhibits proliferation of MCF7 tumor cells by suppressing microtubule dynamics. PLoS One. 2014;9(6):e100599.
27. Oliveras-López MJ, Molina JJ, Mir MV, Rey EF, Martín F, de la Serrana HL. Extra virgin olive oil (EVOO) consumption and antioxidant status in healthy institutionalized elderly humans. Arch Gerontol Geriatr. 2013;57(2):234–42.
28. Solomon A, Golubowicz S, Yablowicz Z, Grossman S, Bergman M, Gottlieb HE, et al. Antioxidant activities and anthocyanin content of fresh fruits of common fig (Ficus carica L.). J Agric Food Chem. 2006;54(20):7717–23.
29. Menghini L, Genovese S, Epifano F, Tirillini B, Ferrante C, Leporini L. Antiproliferative, protective and antioxidant effects of artichoke, dandelion, turmeric and rosemary extracts and their formulation. Int J Immunopathol Pharmacol. 2010;23(2):601–10.
30. McCune LM, Kubota C, Stendell-Hollis NR, Thomson CA. Cherries and health: a review. Crit Rev Food Sci Nutr. 2011;51(1):1–12.
31. Wu JM, Wang ZR, Hsieh TC, Bruder JL, Zou JG, Huang YZ. Mechanism of cardioprotection by resveratrol, a phenolic antioxidant present in red wine (review). Int J Mol Med. 2001;8(1):3–17.
32. Beckman LJ, Ackerman KT. Women, alcohol, and sexuality. Recent Dev Alcohol. 1995;12:267–85.
33. Lee JH, O'Keefe JH, Lavie CJ, Marchioli R, Harris WS. Omega-3 fatty acids for cardioprotection. Mayo Clin Proc. 2008;83(3):324–32.

34. Lane K, Derbyshire E, Li W, Brennan C. Bioavailability and potential uses of vegetarian sources of omega-3 fatty acids: a review of the literature. Crit Rev Food Sci Nutr. 2014;54(5):572–9.
35. Simopoulos AP. Omega-3 fatty acids in inflammation and autoimmune diseases. J Am Coll Nutr. 2002;21(6):495–505.
36. Mashhadi NS, Ghiasvand R, Askari G, Feizi A, Hariri M, Darvishi L, et al. Influence of ginger and cinnamon intake on inflammation and muscle soreness endued by exercise in Iranian female athletes. Int J Prev Med. 2013;4(Suppl 1):S11–5.
37. Reuter J, Huyke C, Casetti F, Theek C, Frank U, Augustin M, et al. Anti-inflammatory potential of a lipolotion containing coriander oil in the ultraviolet erythema test. J Dtsch Dermatol Ges. 2008;6(10):847–51.
38. Chao LK, Hua K-F, Hsu H-Y, Cheng S-S, Liu J-Y, Chang S-T. Study on the antiinflammatory activity of essential oil from leaves of Cinnamomum osmophloeum. J Agric Food Chem. 2005;53(18):7274–8.
39. Tabassum N, Ahmad F. Role of natural herbs in the treatment of hypertension. Pharmacogn Rev. 2011;5(9):30–40.
40. Verma SK, Jain V, Katewa SS. Blood pressure lowering, fibrinolysis enhancing and antioxidant activities of cardamom (Elettaria cardamomum). Indian J Biochem Biophys. 2009;46(6):503–6.
41. Batirel HF, Naka Y, Kayano K, Okada K, Vural K, Pinsky DJ, et al. Intravenous allicin improves pulmonary blood flow after ischemia-reperfusion injury in rats. J Cardiovasc Surg (Torino). 2002;43(2):175–9.
42. Elkayam A, Peleg E, Grossman E, Shabtay Z, Sharabi Y. Effects of allicin on cardiovascular risk factors in spontaneously hypertensive rats. Isr Med Assoc J. 2013;15(3):170–3.
43. Collins JK, Wu G, Perkins-Veazie P, Spears K, Claypool PL, Baker RA, et al. Watermelon consumption increases plasma arginine concentrations in adults. Nutrition. 2007;23(3):261–6.
44. Cartledge J, Minhas S, Eardley I. The role of nitric oxide in penile erection. Expert Opin Pharmacother. 2001;2(1):95–107.
45. Cormio L, De Siati M, Lorusso F, Selvaggio O, Mirabella L, Sanguedolce F, et al. Oral L-citrulline supplementation improves erection hardness in men with mild erectile dysfunction. Urology. 2011;77(1):119–22.
46. Dong JY, Qin LQ, Zhang Z, Zhao Y, Wang J, Arigoni F, et al. Effect of oral L-arginine supplementation on blood pressure: a meta-analysis of randomized, double-blind, placebo-controlled trials. Am Heart J. 2011;162(6):959–6.
47. Mathis CG. Aphrodisiacs: better sex or just bunk? [Internet]. 1999. WebMd.com. http://www.webmd.com/sex-relationships/features/want-better-sex? Accessed 1 Nov 2016.
48. Price CT, Langford JR, Liporace FA. Essential nutrients for bone health and a review of their availability in the average North American diet. Open Orthop J. 2012;6:143–9.
49. Glew RH, Glew RS, Chuang LT, Huang YS, Millson M, Constans D, et al. Amino acid, mineral and fatty acid content of pumpkin seeds (Cucurbita spp) and Cyperus esculentus nuts in the Republic of Niger. Plant Foods Hum Nutr. 2006;61(2):51–6.
50. Cinar V, Polat Y, Baltaci AK, Mogulkoc R. Effects of magnesium supplementation on testosterone levels of athletes and sedentary subjects at rest and after exhaustion. Biol Trace Elem Res. 2011;140:18–23.
51. Maggio M, De Vita F, Lauretani F, Nouvenne A, Meschi T, Dominguez LJ. The interplay between magnesium and testosterone in modulating physical function in men. Int J Endocrinol. 2011;2014:525249.
52. Scutti S. Male sex drive: is the mighty testosterone alone responsible for libido? [Internet]. 2013. MedicalDaily.com. http://www.medicaldaily.com/male-sex-drive-mighty-testosterone-alone-responsible-libido-246793. Accessed 10 Oct 2016.
53. Holt M. The health care blog [Internet]. San Francisco: Matthew Holt. 2003. http://www.thehealthcareblog.com/the_health_care_blog/. Accessed 13 Feb 2009.
54. Evaristo I, Batista D, Correia I, Correia P, Costa R. Chemical profiling of Portuguese Pinus pinea L. nuts. J Sci Food Agric. 2010;90(6):1041–9.
55. Prasad AS, Mantzoros CS, Beck FW, Hess JW, Brewer GJ. Zinc status and serum testosterone levels of healthy adults. Nutrition. 1996;12(5):344–8.
56. Asha MR, Hithamani G, Rashmi R, Basavaraj KH, Jagannath Rao KS, Sathyanarayana Rao TS. History, mystery and chemistry of eroticism: emphasis on sexual health and dysfunction. Indian J Psychiatry. 2009;51(2):141–9.
57. Maiworm RE, Langthaler WU. Influence of androstenol and androsterone on the evalulation of men of varying attractiveness levels. Chemical signals in vertebrates 6. 1st ed. New York: Springer Science+Business Media; 1992.
58. O'Neill J, Brock C, Olesen AE, Andresen T, Nilsson M, Dickenson AH. Unravelling the mystery of capsaicin: a tool to understand and treat pain. Pharmacol Rev. 2012;64(4):939–71.
59. Bach FW, Yaksh TL. Release of beta-endorphin immunoreactivity into ventriculo-cisternal perfusate by lumbar intrathecal capsaicin in the rat. Brain Res. 1995;701(1–2):192–200.
60. Lee YM, Kang SM, Chung JH. The role of TRPV1 channel in aged human skin. J Dermatol Sci. 2012;65:81–5.
61. Meyerson BJ. Neonatal beta-endorphin and sexual behavior. Acta Physiol Scand. 1982;115(1):159–60.
62. Wiesner JB, Moss RL. Behavioral specificity of beta-endorphin suppression of sexual behavior: differential receptor antagonism. Pharmacol Biochem Behav. 1986;24(5):1235–9.
63. Lupattelli G, Marchesi S, Lombardini R, Roscini AR, Trinca F, Gemelli F, Vaudo G, Mannarino E. Artichoke juice improves endothelial function in hyperlipemia. Life Sci. 2004;76(7):775–82.
64. Sandroni P. Aphrodisiacs past and present: a historical review. Clin Auton Res. 2001;11(5):303–7.
65. Pajovic B, Radosavljevic M, Radunovic M, Radojevic N, Bjelogrlic B. Arthropods and their products as aphrodisiacs—review of literature. Eur Rev Med Pharmacol Sci. 2012;16(4):539–47.
66. Aldemir M, Okulu E, Neşelioğlu S, Erel O, Kayıgil O. Pistachio diet improves erectile function parameters and serum lipid profiles in patients with erectile dysfunction. Int J Impot Res. 2011;23(1):32–8.
67. Thakur M, Thompson D, Connellan P, Deseo MA, Morris C, Dixit VK. Improvement of penile erection, sperm count and seminal fructose levels in vivo and nitric oxide release in vitro by ayurvedic herbs. Andrologia. 2011;43(4):273–7.
68. Salonia A, Fabbri F, Zanni G, Scavini M, Fatini GV, Briganti A. Original research—women's sexual health: chocolate and women's sexual health: an intriguing correlation. J Sex Med. 2006;3(6):476–82.
69. Benton D, Donohoe RT. The effects of nutrients on mood. Public Health Nutr. 1999;2:403–9.
70. Bruinsma K, Taren DL. Chocolate: food or drug? J Am Diet Assoc. 1999;99:1249–56.
71. Hetherington MM, Pirie LM, Nabb S. Stimulus satiation: effects of repeated exposure to foods on pleasantness and intake. Appetite. 2002;38:19–28.
72. Hetherington MM, Macdiarmid JI. Pleasure and excess: liking for and overconsumption of chocolate. Physiol Behav. 1995;57:27–35.
73. Bijlwan A, Kush L. The dietary aphrodisiacs. IJIRD. 2013;2(10):76–84.
74. Tajuddin SA, Shamshad A, Abdul L, Iqbal A. Aphrodisiac activity of 50% ethanolic extracts of Myristica fragrans Houtt. (nutmeg) and Syzygium aromaticum (L) Merr. and Perry (clove) in male mice: a comparative study. BMC Complement Altern Med. 2003;3:6.
75. Burkil IH. Dictionary of the economic products of the Malay Peninsula. London, England: 1Z Crown Agents; 1935. Vol. 2, p. 1554–6.

76. Ghani N. Khazeenatul Advia. Lucknow, India: Matba Munshi Nawal Kishore; 1921. Vol. 2, p. 241–2. Katrak 1985.
77. Khory RN, Katrak NN. Materia Medica of India and their therapeutics. Delhi: Neeraj Publishing House; 1985. p. 532–24.
78. Khazdair MR, Boskabady MH, Hosseini M, Rezaee R, Tsatsakis AM. The effects of Crocus sativus (saffron) and its constituents on nervous system: a review. Avicenna J Phytomed. 2015;5(5):376–91.
79. Hosseinzadeh H, Ziaee T, Sadeghi A. The effect of saffron, Crocus sativus stigma, extract and its constituents, safranal and crocin on sexual behaviors in normal male rats. Phytomedicine. 2008;15:491–5.
80. Safarinejad MR, Shafiei N, Safarinejad S. An open label, randomized, fixed-dose, crossover study comparing efficacy and safety of sildenafil citrate and saffron (Crocus sativus Linn.) for treating erectile dysfunction in men naïve to treatment. Int J Impot Res. 2010;22:240–50.
81. Bruce M, Scott N, Lader M, Marks V. The psychopharmacological and electrophysiological effects of single doses of caffeine in healthy human subjects. Br J Clin Pharmacol. 1986;22(1):81–7.
82. Benowitz NL, Jacob 3rd P, Mayan H, Denaro C. Sympathomimetic effects of paraxanthine and caffeine in humans. Clin Pharmacol Ther. 1995;58(6):684–91.
83. Rogers PJ, Hohoff C, Heatherley SV, Mullings EL, Maxfield PJ, Evershed RP, Deckert J, Nutt DJ. Association of the anxiogenic and alerting effects of caffeine with ADORA2A and ADORA1 polymorphisms and habitual level of caffeine consumption. Neuropsychopharmacology. 2010;35(9):1973–83.
84. Saadat SH, Ahmadi K, Panahi Y. The effect of on-demand caffeine consumption on treating patients with premature ejaculation: a double-blind randomized clinical trial. Curr Pharm Biotechnol. 2015;16(3):281–7.
85. Cui T, Kovell RC, Brooks DC, Terlecki RP. A urologist's guide to ingredients found in top-selling nutraceuticals for men's sexual health. J Sex Med. 2015;12(11):2105–17.
86. Schneider JY, Rothmann S, Schröder F, Langen J, Lücke T, Mariotti F, et al. Effects of chronic oral L-arginine administration on the L-arginine/NO pathway in patients with peripheral arterial occlusive disease or coronary artery disease: L-arginine prevents renal loss of nitrite, the major NO reservoir. Amino Acids. 2015;47(9):1961–74.
87. Monti LD, Galluccio E, Fontana B, Spadoni S, Comola M, Marrocco Trischitta MM. Metabolism. 2015;64(11):1582–91.
88. Schwedhelm E, Maas R, Freese R, Jung D, Lukacs Z, Jambrecina A, et al. Pharmacokinetic and pharmacodynamics properties of oral L-citrulline and L-arginine: impact on nitric oxide metabolism. Br J Clin Pharmacol. 2008;65(1):51–9.
89. Ito TY, Trant AS, Polan ML. A double-blind placebo-controlled study of ArginMax, a nutritional supplement for enhancement of female sexual function. J Sex Marital Ther. 2001;27(5):541–9.
90. Ito TY, Polan ML, Whipple B, Trant AS. The enhancement of female sexual function with ArginMax, a nutritional supplement, among women differing in menopausal status. J Sex Marital Ther. 2006;32(5):369–78.
91. Bottari A, Belcaro G, Ledda A, Cesarone MR, Vinciguerra G, Di Renzo A, et al. Lady Prelox® improves sexual function in post-menopausal women. Panminerva Med. 2012;4(1 Suppl 4):3–9.
92. Bottari A, Belcaro G, Ledda A, Luzzi R, Cesarone MR, Dugall M. Lady Prelox® improves sexual function in generally healthy women of reproductive age. Minerva Ginecol. 2013;65(4):435–44.
93. Meston CM, Worcel M. The effects of yohimbine plus L-arginine glutamate on sexual arousal in postmenopausal women with sexual arousal disorder. Arch Sex Behav. 2002;31(4):323–32.
94. Chen J, Wollman Y, Chernichovsky T, Iaina A, Sofer M, Matzkin H. Effect of oral administration of high-dose nitric oxide donor L-arginine in men with organic erectile dysfunction: results of a double-blind, randomized, placebo-controlled study. BJU Int. 1999;83(3):269–73.
95. Stanislavov R, Nikolova V. Treatment of erectile dysfunction with pycnogenol and L-arginine. J Sex Marital Ther. 2003;29(3): 207–13.
96. Stanislavov R, Rohdewald P. Improvement of erectile function by a combination of French maritime pine bark and roburins with aminoacids. Minerva Urol Nefrol. 2015;67(1):27–32.
97. Aoki H, Nagao J, Ueda T, Strong JM, Schonlau F, Yu-Jing S, et al. Clinical assessment of a supplement of Pycnogenol® and L-arginine in Japanese patients with mild to moderate erectile dysfunction. Phytother Res. 2012;26(2):204–7.
98. Neuzillet Y, Hupertan V, Cour F, Botto H, Libret T. A randomized, double-blind, crossover, placebo-controlled comparative clinical trial of arginine aspartate plus adenosine monophosphate for the intermittent treatment of male erectile dysfunction. Andrology. 2013;1(2):223–8.
99. Cavallini G, Caracciolo S, Vitali G, Modenini F, Biagiotti G. Carnitine versus androgen administration in the treatment of sexual dysfunction, depressed mood,and fatigue associated with male aging. Urology. 2004;63(4):641–6.
100. Gurnell EM, Hunt PJ, Curran SE, Conway CL, Pullenayegum EM, Huppert FA, et al. Long-term DHEA replacement in primary adrenal insufficiency: a randomized, controlled trial. J Clin Endocrinol Metab. 2008;93(2):400–9.
101. Labrie F, Archer D, Bouchard C, Fortier M, Cusan L, Gomez JL, et al. Effects of intravaginal dehydroepiandrosterone (Prasterone) on libido and sexual dysfunction in postmenopausal women. Menopause. 2009;16(5):923–31.
102. Genazzani AR, Stomati M, Valentino V, Pluchino N, Pot E, Casarosa E, et al. Effect of 1-year, low-dose DHEA therapy on climacteric symptoms and female sexuality. Climacteric. 2011;14(6):661–8.
103. Hackbert L, Heiman JR. Acute dehydroepiandrosterone (DHEA) effects on sexual arousal in postmenopausal women. J Womens Health Gend Based Med. 2002;11(2):155–62.
104. Labrie F, Archer DF, Bouchard C, Fortier M, Cusan L, Gomez JL, et al. Intravaginal dehydroepiandrosterone (prasterone), a highly efficient treatment of dyspareunia. Climacteric. 2011; 14(2):282–8.
105. Bloch M, Meiboom H, Zaig I, Schreiber S, Abramov L. The use of dehydroepiandrosterone in the treatment of hypoactive sexual desire disorder: a report of gender differences. Eur Neuropsychopharmacol. 2013;23(8):910–8.
106. Reiter WJ, Pycha A, Schatzi G, Pokorny A, Gruber DM, Huber JC, et al. Dehydroepiandrosterone in the treatment of erectile dysfunction: a prospective, double-blind, randomized, placebo-controlled study. Urology. 1999;53(3):590–4.
107. Athenahealth, Inc. [Internet]. San Mateo (CA): Epocatres, Inc. https://online.epocrates.com/drugs/alternativemedicines/284903/DHEA/Adverse-Reactions. Accessed 15 Aug 2016.
108. Athenahealth, Inc. [Internet]. San Mateo (CA): Epocatres, Inc. https://online.epocrates.com/u/1152850/DHEA/Reported+Doses. Accessed 3 Sep 2016.
109. Morales AJ, Haubrich RH, Hwang JY, Asakura H, Yen SS. The effect of six months treatment with a 100 mg daily dose of dehydroepiandrosterone (DHEA) on circulating sex steroids, body composition and muscle strength in age-advanced men and women. Clin Endocrinol (Oxf). 1998;49(4):421–32.
110. Ferguson DM, Hosmane B, Heiman JR. Randomized, placebo-controlled, double-blind, parallel design trial of the efficacy and safety of Zestra in women with mixed desire/interest/arousal/orgasm disorders. J Sex Marital Ther. 2010;36(1):66–86.
111. Bolour SY, Braunstein GD. Pharmacologic treatment options for hypoactive sexual desire disorder. Womens Health (Lond). 2005;1(2):263–77.

112. Ferguson DM, Steidle CP, Singh GS, Alexander JS, Weihmiller MK, Crosby MG. Randomized, placebo-controlled, double blind, crossover design trial of the efficacy and safety of Zestra for Women in women with and without female sexual arousal disorder. J Sex Marital Ther. 2003;29(Suppl 1):33–44.
113. Choi HK, Jung GW, Moon KH, Xin ZC, Choi YD, Lee WH, et al. Clinical study of SS-cream in patients with lifelong premature ejaculation. Urology. 2000;55:257–61.
114. Meston CM, Rellini AH, Telch MJ. Short- and long-term effects of Ginkgo biloba extract on sexual dysfunction in women. Arch Sex Behav. 2008;37(4):530–47.
115. Tjandra BS, Janknegt RA. Neurogenic impotence and lower urinary tract symptoms due to vitamin B1 deficiency in chronic alcoholism. J Urol. 1997;157:954–5.
116. Ng CF, Lee CP, Ho AL, Lee VW. Effect of niacin on erectile function in men suffering erectile dysfunction and dyslipidemia. J Sex Med. 2011;8:2883–93.
117. Hamidi Madani A, Asadolahzade A, Mokhtari G, Shahrokhi Damavand R, Farzan A, Esmaeili S. Assessment of the efficacy of combination therapy with folic acid and tadalafil for the management of erectile dysfunction in men with type 2 diabetes mellitus. J Sex Med. 2013;10:1146–50.
118. Stanger O, Fowler B, Piertzik K, et al. Homocysteine, folate and vitamin B12 in neuropsychiatric diseases: review and treatment recommendations. Expert Rev Neurother. 2009;9:1393–412.
119. Hartz AJ, Bentler S, Noyes R, Hoehns J, Logemann C, Sinift S, et al. Randomized controlled trial of Siberian ginseng for chronic fatigue. Psychol Med. 2004;34(1):51–61.
120. Kang YJ, Sohn JT, Chang KC. Relaxation of the canine corporal smooth muscle relaxation by ginsenoside saponin Rg3 is independent from eNOS activation. Life Sci. 2005;77(1):77–84.
121. Melnyk J, Marcone M. Aphrodisiacs from plant and animal sources—a review of current scientific literature. Food Res Int. 2011;44:840.
122. Oh KJ, Chae MJ, Lee HS, Hong HD, Park K. Effects of Korean red ginseng on sexual arousal in menopausal women: placebo-controlled, double-blind crossover clinical study. J Sex Med. 2010;7(4 Pt 1):1469–77.
123. Hong B, Ji YH, Hong JH, Nam KY, Ahn TY. A double-blind crossover study evaluating the efficacy of Korean red ginseng in patients with erectile dysfunction: a preliminary report. J Urol. 2002;168(5):2070–3.
124. Choi YD, Park CW, Jang J, Kim SH, Jeon HY, Kim WG, et al. Effects of Korean ginseng berry extract on sexual function in men with erectile dysfunction: a multicenter, placebo-controlled, double-blind clinical study. Int J Impot Res. 2013;25(2):45–50.
125. De Andrade E, De Mesquita AA, Claro Jde A, de Andrade PM, Ortiz V, Paranhos M, et al. Study of the efficacy of Korean red ginseng in the treatment of erectile dysfunction. Asian J Androl. 2007;9(2):241–4.
126. Athenahealth, Inc. [Internet]. San Mateo (CA): Epocatres, Inc. https://online.epocrates.com/drugs/alternative-medicines/293403/ginseng-Korean/Adverse-Reactions. Accessed 15 Aug 2016.
127. Athenahealth, Inc. [Internet]. San Mateo (CA): Epocatres, Inc. https://online.epocrates.com/drugs/alternative-medicines/293405/ginseng-Korean/Reported-Doses. Accessed 15 Aug 2016.
128. Thakur M, Chauhan NS, Bhargava S, Dixit VK. A comparative study on aphrodisiac activity of some ayurvedic herbs in male albino rats. Arch Sex Behav. 2009;38:1009–15.
129. Lampiao F, Krom D, du Plessis SS. The in vitro effects of Mondia whitei on human sperm motility parameters. Phytother Res. 2008;22:1272–3.
130. Watcho P, Fotsing D, Zelefack F, Nguelefack TB, Kamtchouing P, Tsamo E, et al. Effects of Mondia whitei extracts on the contractile responses of isolated rat vas deferens to potassium chloride and adrenaline. Indian J Pharmacol. 2006;38:33–7.
131. Watcho P, Fotsing D, Zelefack F, Nguelefack TB, Kamtchouing P, Tsamo E. Aphrodisiac effect of MH2 and MH6 isolated from Hexane extract of Mondia whitei in sexually inexperienced male rats. J Sex Med. 2006;5:382–452.
132. Gauthaman K, Adaikan PG, Prasad RN. Aphrodisiac properties of Tribulus terrestris extract (Protodioscin) in normal and castrated rats. Life Sci. 2002;71:1385–96.
133. Tomova M, Gjulemetova R, Zarkova S, Peeva S, Pangarova T, Simova M. Steroidal saponins fromTribulus terrestris L. with a stimulating action on the sexual functions. International conference of chemistry and biotechnology of bio-logically active natural products, Varna, Bulgaria. 1981 Sep 21–26;3:298–302.
134. Adimoelja A, Adaikan PG. Protodioscin from herbal plant Tribulus terrestris L. improves male sexual functions possibly via DHEA. Int J Impot Res. 1997;9(1):S64–74.
135. Gauthaman K, Adaikan PG, Prasad RN, Goh VH. Changes in hormonal parameters secondary to intravenous administration of Tribulus terrestris extract in primates. Int J Impot Res. 2000;2:6.
136. Neychev V, Mitev V. Pro-sexual and androgen enhancing effects of Tribulus terrestris L.: fact or fiction. J Ethnopharmacol. 2016;179:345–55.
137. Qureshi A, Naughton DP, Petroczi A. A systematic review on the herbal extract Tribulus terrestris and the roots of its putative aphrodisiac and performance enhancing effect. J Diet Suppl. 2014;11(1):64–79.
138. Gauthaman K, Ganesan AP, Prasad RN. Sexual effects of puncturevine (Tribulus terrestris) extract (protodioscin): an evaluation using a rat model. J Altern Complement Med. 2003;9(2):257–65.
139. Akhtari E, Raisi F, Keshavarz M, Hosseini H, Sohrabvand F, Bioos S, et al. Tribulus terrestris for treatment of sexual dysfunction in women: a randomized double-blind placebo-controlled study. Daru. 2014;22:40.
140. Gama CR, Lasmar R, Gama GF, Abreu CS, Nunes CP, Geller M, et al. Clinical assessment of Tribulus terrestris extract in the treatment of female sexual dysfunction. Clin Med Insights Womens Health. 2014;7:45–50.
141. Postigo S, Lima SM, Yamada SS, dos Reis BF, da Silva GM, Aoki T. Assessment of the effects of Tribulus Terrestris on sexual function of menopausal women. Rev Bras Ginecol Obstet. 2016;38(3):140–6.
142. Santos Jr CA, Reis LO, Destro-Saade R, Luiza-Reis A, Fregonesi A. Tribulus terrestris versus placebo in the treatment of erectile dysfunction: a prospective, randomized, double blind study. Actas Urol Esp. 2014;38(4):244–8.
143. Iacono F, Prezioso D, Illiano E, Romeo G, Ruffo A, Amato B. Sexual asthenia: tradamixina versus tadalafil 5 mg daily. BMC Surg. 2012;12(Suppl 1):S23.
144. Talasaz AH, Abbasi M-R, Abkhiz S, Dashti-Khavidaki S. Tribulus terrestris-induced severe nephrotoxicity in a young healthy male. Nephrol Dial Transplant. 2010;25(11):3792.
145. Ryan M, Lazar I, Nadasdy GM, Nadasdy T, Satoskar AA. Acute kidney injury and hyperbilirubinemia in a young male after ingestion of Tribulus terrestris. Clin Nephrol. 2015;83(3):177–83.
146. Campanelli M, De Thomasis R, Tenaglia RL. Priapism caused by 'Tribulus terrestris'. Int J Impot Res. 2016;28(1):39–40.
147. Steels E, Rao A, Vitetta L. Physiological aspects of male libido enhanced by standardized Trigonella foenum-graecum extract and mineral formulation. Phytother Res. 2011;25:1294–300.
148. Corazza O, Martinotti G, Santacroce R, Chillemi E, Di Giannantonio M, Schifano F, Cellek S. Sexual enhancement products for sale online: raising awareness of the psychoactive effects of yohimbine, maca, horny goat weed, and Ginkgo biloba. Biomed Res Int. 2014;2014:841798.
149. Shindel AW, Xin ZC, Lin G, Fandel TM, Huang YC, Banie L, Breyer BN, Garcia MM, Lin CS, Lue TF. Erectogenic and neurotrophic effects of icariin, a purified extract of horny goat weed

(Epimedium spp.) in vitro and in vivo. J Sex Med. 2010;7(4 Pt 1):1518–28.
150. Adimoelja A. Phytochemicals and the breakthrough of traditional herbs in the management of sexual dysfunctions. Int J Androl. 2000;23(Suppl 2):82–4.
151. Waynberg J, Brewer S. Effects of Herbal vX on libido and sexual activity in premenopausal and postmenopausal women. Adv Ther. 2000;17(5):255–62.
152. Shin YS, Zhao C, Zhang LT, Park JK. Current status and clinical studies of oriental herbs in sexual medicine in Korea. World J Mens Health. 2015;33(2):62–72.
153. Zhao C, Kim HK, Kim SZ, Chae HJ, Cui WS, Lee SW, et al. What is the role of unripe Rubus coreanus extract on penile erection? Phytother Res. 2011;25:1046–53.
154. Kim HK, Bak YO, Choi BR, Zhao C, Lee HJ, Kim CY, et al. The role of the lignan constituents in the effect of Schisandra chinensis fruit extract on penile erection. Phytother Res. 2011;25:1776–82.
155. Kim HK, Choi BR, Bak YO, Zhao C, Lee SW, Jeon JH, et al. The role of capillarisin from Artemisia capillaris on penile erection. Phytother Res. 2012;26:800–5.
156. Sun K, Zhao C, Chen XF, Kim HK, Choi BR, Huang YR, et al. Ex vivo relaxation effect of Cuscuta chinensis extract on rabbit corpus cavernosum. Asian J Androl. 2013;15:134–7.
157. Arun M, Satish S, Anima P. Phytopharmacological profile of Jasminum grandiflorum Linn. (Oleaceae). Chin J Integr Med. 2016;22(4):311–20.
158. Tan LT, Lee LH, Yin WF, Chan CK, Abdul Kadir H, Chan KG, Goh BH. Traditional uses, phytochemistry, and bioactivities of Cananga odorata (Ylang-Ylang). Evid Based Complement Alternat Med. 2015;2015:896314.
159. Morton J. Fruits of warm climates. Miami; 1987. p. 5–11.
160. Kotta S, Ansari SH, Ali J. Exploring scientifically proven herbal aphrodisiacs. Pharmacogn Rev. 2013;7(13):1–10.
161. Bahmanpour S, Talaei T, Vojdani Z, Panjehshahin MR, Poostpasand A, Zareei S. Effect of *Phoenix dactylifera* pollen on sperm parameters and reproductive system of adult male rats. Iran J Med Sci. 2006;31(4):208–12.
162. Zheng BL, He K, Kim CH, Rogers L, Shao Y, Huang ZY, et al. Effect of a lipidic extract from *Lepidium meyenii* on sexual behavior in mice and rats. Urology. 2000;55:598–602.
163. Gonzales GF, Córdova A, Vega K, Chung A, Villena A, Góñez C. Effect of *Lepidium meyenii* (Maca), a root with aphrodisiac and fertility-enhancing properties, on serum reproductive hormone levels in adult healthy men. J Endocrinol. 2003;176:163–8.
164. Gonzales GF, Córdova A, Vega K, Chung A, Villena A, Góñez C, et al. Effect of *Lepidium meyenii*(MACA) on sexual desire and its absent relationship with serum testosterone levels in adult healthy men. Andrologia. 2002;34:367–72.
165. Chaturapanich G, Chaiyakul S, Verawatnapakul V, Pholpramool C. Effects of *Kaempferia parviflora* extracts on reproductive parameters and spermatic blood flow in male rats. Reproduction. 2008;136:515–22.
166. Chiou WF, Wu TS. 9-hydroxycanthin-6-one induces penile erection and delays ejaculation. J Sex Med. 2012;9(4):1027–36.
167. Kotirum S, Ismail SB, Chaiyakunapruk N. Efficacy of Tongkat Ali (Eurycoma longifolia) on erectile function improvement: systematic review and meta-analysis of randomized controlled trials. Complement Ther Med. 2015;23(5):693–8.
168. Haeri S, Minaie B, Amin G, Nikfar S, Khorasani R, Esmaily H, et al. Effect of *Satureja khuzestanica*essential oil on male rat fertility. Fitoterapia. 2006;77:495–9.
169. Rezvanfar M, Sadrkhanlou R, Ahmadi A, Shojaei-Sadee H, Rezvanfar M, Mohammadirad A, et al. Protection of cyclophosphamide-induced toxicity in reproductive tract histology, sperm characteristics, and DNA damage by an herbal source; evidence for role of free-radical toxic stress. Hum Exp Toxicol. 2008;27:901–10.
170. Zavatti M, Zanoli P, Benelli A, Rivasi M, Baraldi C, Baraldi M. Experimental study on Satureja montana as a treatment for premature ejaculation. J Ethnopharmacol. 2011;133(2):629–33.
171. Sansalone S, Russo GI, Mondaini N, Cantiello F, Antonini G, Cai T. A combination of tryptophan, Satureja montana, Tribulus terrestris, Phyllanthus emblica extracts is able to improve sexual quality of life in patient with premature ejaculation. Arch Ital Urol Androl. 2016;88(3):171–6.
172. Yakubu MT, Akanji MA, Oladiji AT. Aphrodisiac potentials of the aqueous extract of Fadogia agrestis (Schweinf. Ex Hiern) stem in male albino rats. Asian J Androl. 2005;7(4):399–404.
173. Irvine FR. Woody plants of Ghana. London: Oxford University Press; 1961.
174. Yakubu MT, Akanji MA, Oladiji AT. Effects of oral administration of aqueous extract of *Fadogia agrestis* (Schweinf. Ex Hiern) stem on some testicular function indices of male rats. J Ethnopharmacol. 2008;115:288–92.
175. Breton S, Smith PTS, Lui B, Brown D. Acidification of the male reproductive tract by a proton pumping (H^+)-ATPase. Nat Med. 1996;2:470–2.
176. Butterworth PJ, Moss DW. The effect of urea on human kidney alkaline phosphatase. Biochem J. 1966;99:9–10.
177. Levine SD, Hahn DW, Cotter MI, Greenslade FC, Kanojia RM, Pasquale SA, et al. The Mexican plant zoapatle (*Montanoa tomentosa*) in reproductive medicine. Past, present and future. J Reprod Med. 1981;26:524–8.
178. Gallegos AJ. The zoapatle I. A traditional remedy from Mexico emerging to moder times. Contraception. 1983;27:211–25.
179. Carro-Juárez M, Cervantes E, Cervantes-Méndez M, Rodríguez-Manzo G. Aphrodisiac properties of *Montanoa tomentosa* aqueous crude extract in male rats. Pharmacol Biochem Behav. 2004;78:129–34.
180. Carro-Juarez M, Rodriguez-Manzo G. Evidence for the presence and functioning of the spinal patter generator for ejaculation in the neonatal male rat. Int J Impot Res. 2005;17:270–6.
181. Carro-Juárez M, Lobatón I, Benítez O, Espíritu A. Pro-ejaculatory effect of the aqueous crude extract of cihuapatli (*Montanoa tomentosa*) in spinal male rats. J Ethnopharmacol. 2006;106:111–6.
182. Oudhia P, Paull RE. West Indian almond Terminalia catappa L. Combretaceae. In: Janick J, Paull RE, editors. Encyclopedia of fruit and nuts. Wallingford, UK: CABI; 2008. p. 283–76.
183. Jayasinghe DM. Ayurveda pharmacopoeia. Colombo, Sri Lanka: Department of Ayurveda; 1997. p. 67–8.
184. Ratnasooriya WD, Dharmasiri MG. Effects of *Terminalia catappa* seeds on sexual behaviour and fertility of male rats. Asian J Androl. 2000;2:213–9.
185. Patel DK, Kumar R, Prasad SK, Hemalatha S. Pharmacologically screened aphrodisiac plant: a review of current scientific literature. Asian Pac J Trop Biomed. 2011;1:S131–8.
186. Ali ST, Rakkah NI. Probable neuro sexual mode of action of *Casimiroa edulis* seed extract versus correction of verses sildenafil citrate (Viagra (tm)) on mating behavior in normal male rats. Pak J Pharm Sci. 2008;21:1–6.
187. Goldstein I, Lue T, Padma-Nathan H, Rosen RC, Steers WD, Wicker PA. Oral sildenafil in the treatment of erectile dysfunction. N Engl J Med. 1998;338:1397–404.
188. Baisch AL, Urban H, Ruiz AN. Endotheliumdependent vasorelaxing activity of aqueous extract of lyophilized seeds of casimiroa edulis (AECe) on rat mesenteric arterial bed. J Ethnopharmacol. 2004;95(2–3):163–7.
189. Linares E, Bye R, Flores B. Plantas medicinales de mexico. Usos y remedies tradicionales. México: Instituto de Biología; 1999. p. 102.

190. Shultes RE, Hoffmann A. Plantas de los dioses. Origenes del uso de los alucinogenos. Mexico City: Fondo de Cultura Económica; 2000. p. 98.
191. Arletti R, Benelli A, Cavazzuti E, Scarpetta G, Bertolini A. Stimulating property of Turnera diffusa and Pfaffia paniculata extracts on the sexual-behavior of male rats. Psychopharmacology (Berl). 1999;143(1):15–9.
192. Beach FA, Jordan L. Sexual exhaustion and recovery in male rat. Q J Exp Psychol. 1956;8:121–33.
193. Fernandez-Guasti A, Rodriguez-Manzo G. Pharmacological and physiological aspects of sexual exhaustion in male rats. Scand J Psychol. 2003;44(3):257–63.
194. Estrada-Reyes R, Ortiz-López P, Gutiérrez-Ortíz J, Martínez-Mota L. *Turnera diffusa* Wild (Turneraceae) recovers sexual behavior in sexually exhausted males. J Ethnopharmacol. 2009;123:423–9.
195. Paladini AC, Marder M, Viola H, Wolfman C, Wasowski C, Medina JH. Flavonoids and the central nervous system: from forgotten factors to potent anxiolytic compounds. J Pharm Pharmacol. 1999;51(5):519–26.
196. Dhawan K, Sharma A. Restoration of chronic-Δ^9-THC-induced decline in sexuality in male rats by a novel benzoflavone moiety from *Passiflora incarnata* Linn. Br J Pharmacol. 2003;138(1):117–20.
197. Grassi D, Aggio A, Onori L, Croce G, Tiberti S, Ferri C, et al. Tea, flavonoids, and nitric oxide-mediated vascular reactivity. J Nutr. 2008;138(8):1554S–60S.
198. Toque HA, Teixeira CE, Lorenzetti R, Okuyama CE, Antunes E, De Nucci G, et al. Pharmacological characterization of a novel phosphodiesterase type 5 (PDE5) inhibitor lodenafil carbonate on human and rabbit corpus cavernosum. Eur J Pharmacol. 2008;591(1–3):189–95.
199. West E, Krychman M. Natural aphrodisiacs-a review of selected sexual enhancers. Sex Med Rev. 2015;3(4):279–88.
200. Goswami SK, Inamdar MN, Jamwal R, Dethe S. Effect of Cinnamomum cassia methanol extract and sildenafil on arginase and sexual function of young male Wistar rats. J Sex Med. 2014;11(6):1475–83.
201. Nurudeen QO, Ajiboye TO, Yakubu MT, Oweh OT, Nosarieme O. Aqueous root extract of Lecaniodiscus cupanioides restores nitric oxide/cyclic guanosine monophosphate pathway in sexually impaired male rats. J Ethnopharmacol. 2015;175:181–4.
202. Fouche G, Afolayan AJ, Wintola OA, Khorombi TE, Senabe J. Effect of the aqueous extract of the aerial parts of Monsonia angustifolia on the sexual behaviour of male Wistar rats. BMC Complement Altern Med. 2015;15:343.

28
Sex and Sexual Orientation

Maria Manuela Peixoto

Sexual Orientation

Sexual orientation can be defined as romantic, affective, and/or sexual attraction to same sex, opposite sex, or both. When a person is romantic, affective and/or sexually attracted to same sex they are usually named homosexual, when attracted to opposite sex they are usually classified as heterosexual, and when attracted to both sexes they are named bisexual. Sexual orientation can be addressed through self-identification, according to sexual behaviors or based on sexual fantasies. Commonly, a combination of these criteria was used to define sexual orientation.

Sexual orientation is clearly more complex than a dichotomy between heterosexuality and homosexuality, and can be metaphorically described as the colors of a rainbow [1]. Alfred Kinsey is a well-known sex researcher, who developed the Kinsey Sexual Orientation Scale. Kinsey interviewed more than 18,000 men and women from the USA and collected information about sexual behaviors. During this work, Kinsey and his team found out that individuals self-identified as heterosexuals, for instance, may have in their past had same-sex sexual activity. Therefore, Kinsey proposed a sexual orientation scale from "exclusively heterosexual" to "exclusively homosexual," with other options in between—"predominantly heterosexual, only incidentally homosexual," "predominantly heterosexual, but more than incidentally homosexual," "bisexual—equally heterosexual and homosexual," "predominantly homosexual, only incidentally heterosexual," "predominantly homosexual, but more than incidentally heterosexual."

Although same-sex behavior has been reported in different societies across time, sexual orientation concept is recent, being reported in medical discourse during the nineteenth century. The first reference to "homosexuality" backs to 1868 [2]. Nevertheless, the first studies conducted raised several empirical questions regarding sample collection and possible outcome generalization. Homosexual samples were collected in clinical contexts; therefore sample bias can be described, with individuals reporting more frequently higher levels of psychological symptoms. Additionally, when comparative studies were conducted, sample size of homosexual was significantly lower compared to heterosexual ones. Another concern was the definition of sexual orientation, where for some studies it was conceptualized based on sexual behaviors, for others based on self-identification, and for others defined by sexual attraction [2].

In 1973, it was proposed at an American Psychiatric Association meeting that homosexuality should no longer constitute a mental illness. Later, in 1974, the American Psychiatric Association members vote for the depathologization [2]. Consequently, the concept of homosexuality has been removed from the DSM-III, but it was replaced by "egodystonic homosexuality." The "egodystonic homosexuality" was only retrieved from DSM in 1988. Therefore, between 1973 and 1988, homosexuals who reported personal distress associated to their own sexual orientation were diagnosed with a mental disorder. This diagnosis promotes the discrimination against homosexuals during this decade.

Homosexuality gathers closer attention from social, media, and research fields, when compared to heterosexuality or bisexuality. When a HIV epidemic occurred in the USA, gay men were considered a risk group for HIV and sexually transmitted infections. Homosexuality was associated to a chronic illness with significant and negative impact on lifestyle. In order to overcome that prejudice, epidemiologists, especially those who work in the HIV field, since at least 1990, have started to apply the concept of "men who have sex with men". The acronyms MSM—"men who have sex with men," and later WSW—"women who have sex with women" [3]. It also allows conducting studies that transcend the social construction of sexual orientation. Nowadays, the acronyms MSM and WSW are widely spread in the sex research field.

W.W. IsHak (ed.), *The Textbook of Clinical Sexual Medicine*, DOI 10.1007/978-3-319-52539-6_28

Asexuality

According to Bogaert [4], asexuality is the absence of sexual attraction towards men and/or women, which can be addressed as the "*absence of a traditional sexual orientation*" ([4], p.279). Although asexuals did not experience sexual attraction, they can get involved in intimate relationships and experience romantic attraction [5]. In a study conducted by Bogaert [4], using a probability sample from the UK, the main findings suggested that only 1.05% of the population referred that they never felt sexual attraction to anyone. Interestingly, according to the author, the rate was similar to rates of same-sex attraction, which gathers much more attention from social, political, religious, or research disciplines. Nevertheless, in the past years, asexuality has received more attention from disciplines such as psychology and sexology [6].

Asexuality definition raises questions regarding clinical diagnose classifications, mainly associated to "personal distress." Asexuals do not experience sexual aversion; however, they often feel that something is wrong with them, revealing personal distress. Additionally, they also tend to classify less behaviors as sexual, when compared to non-asexuals, which is probably due to lack of associated pleasure experienced [7]. Although asexuality is commonly described as lack of sexual attraction, the definition can also include lack of sexual behavior or self-identification [5]. If self-identification is considered, asexuality can also be conceptualized as a sexual orientation.

Sexual Scripts and Heterosexual Bias

Activists and social media may be responsible for sexual orientation being a core theme nowadays. Several steps forward have been made regarding deconstruction of myths about sexual orientation and sexual minorities. Concerning sexuality and sexual functioning, sex researchers struggle with a major concern: heterosexual bias. Although research about sexuality among gays, lesbians, and bisexuals has increased across the years, the heterosexual script remains. The heterosexual script regulates how a sexual relationship/intercourse should happen; when the heterosexual script is used for a better understanding of sexuality among gays, lesbians, and bisexuals, specific information and details may be lost in the process, forming generalizations without empiric support.

Social interactions can be described and conceptualized according to individual beliefs regarding personal expectations [8]. Therefore, a script is learned through lifetime based in modeling behaviors. If we transfer the social scripts knowledge to sexuality field, there is a propensity for sexual scripts being taught from men to boys, and from women to girls, with men learning to perform perfectly in sexual context, and women learning to be sexually submissive [8]. Sexual scripts constitute universal rules about how we should sexually behave and how we expect others to sexually behave. Gender roles, sex roles, sexual expectations among others constitute sexual scripts [8, 9]. Culturally, individuals are raised in order to establish intimate and romantic relationships with someone from the opposite sex, and not with someone from the same sex. Likely, vaginal intercourse constitutes the major sexual behavior during sexual intercourse, while other sexual behaviors (e.g., oral sex, cuddling) are characterized as preliminary sexual behaviors [8, 9].

Homophobia and Internalized Homophobia

Homophobia can be defined by hostility and explicit prejudice against gays and lesbians. When the concept "homophobia" is used, we are describing a discriminatory attitude towards gay and lesbian, which implies serious political and social concerns. The concept "homophobia" may be considered inadequate for several reasons. First of all, the suffix "phobia," in psychology and psychiatry, refers to an irrational fear and a persistent avoidance. For that reason, the word "homonegativity" is preferred to "homophobia."

Internalized homophobia is defined by negative attitudes developed by homosexuals against themselves. It is considered a major vulnerability factor for health problems in gays and lesbians. Across life span, we are exposed to a heteronormative environment, and therefore some young gays, lesbians, and bisexuals develop feelings of internalized homophobia, characterized by negative attitudes towards their own sexuality. On the other hand, internalized homophobia promotes psychological distress, which impairs other life areas [2]. Internalized homophobia is conceptualized as a component of minority stress, by causing psychological distress associated to being part of a minority group, which is a target to discriminatory actions. Minority stress, is characterized by internalized homophobia, perceived stigma and experiencing discriminatory episodes. Nevertheless, internalized homophobia appears to be the core factor for experiencing psychological distress among sexual minority groups [2, 10, 11, 12]. Negative experiences associated to discriminatory attitudes promote psychological distress and poor psychological adjustment, which may lead to psychological and psychiatric disorders [12].

The American Psychological Association [13] established some guidelines regarding concepts in order to decrease the negative bias against gays, lesbians, and bisexuals. According to American Psychology Association, Division 44, the words "gay" and "lesbian" are preferable to "homosexual," because homosexuality has been considered a mental illness over decades, and therefore the word is still negatively associated to mental disorders. Additionally, "homosexual" can also be discriminatory for lesbian women once it recurrently used to refer to men, neglecting women [13].

Same-Sex Relationships

Research on same-sex couples is still considered sparse due to several reasons. A major explanation is the fact that same-sex marriage is still illegal in some countries or states in the USA. Therefore, when researchers aim to study same-sex relationships they have to clarify the inclusion criteria for describing a same-sex couple.

Despite of sexual orientation, in intimate and sexual relationships, men tend to appreciate physical appearance and body image, while women value contextual and intimate characteristics. Additionally, in romantic and intimate relationships, affectivity, shared interests, moral and social beliefs are often treasured in an intimate partner. The first longitudinal study with same-sex and opposite-sex couples in civil union was conducted by Balsam et al. [14]. The major finding suggested that same-sex couples reported better dyadic adjustment and less conflict situations when compared to opposite-sex couples. For lesbian couples, sex frequency activity was a major predictor of better and satisfactory relationship, while for gay couples, the length of the relationship was a significant predictor of satisfactory relationships, with longer civil unions being associated to a decrease in dyadic adjustment [14].

Non-monogamy is more common across same-sex relationships, particularly in gay couples. Nevertheless, non-monogamy can be established by mutual agreement and rules can be defined. According to Hoff et al. [15], the reasons why gay men establish rules for non-monogamous relationships are: building trust in their relationship, promote honesty and protect themselves in terms of sexual health. No significant differences have been found regarding relationship satisfaction between monogamous and non-monogamous couples.

Extra-dyadic relationships can occur in both same-sex and heterosexual relationships. Commonly, in heterosexual couples, extra-dyadic relationships occur in secrecy. An interesting characteristic of gay couples is that extra-dyadic relationships can occur with knowledge of both partners and with mutual agreement. Although not well empirically established, extra-dyadic relationships by mutual agreement may promote sexual and relationship satisfaction. When extra-dyadic relationships occur by mutual agreement, we no longer talk about infidelity.

Closed relationships may help prevent transmission of sexual infections, by decreasing sexual risk behavior. So gay couples may agree to allow a third person to be part of their sex lives. Along with the mutual agreement, protective sexual behaviors can be negotiated with all members at the same time.

Sex Roles in Gay and Bisexual Men Relationships

During penetrative sexual behavior, gay and bisexual men engage in sex roles labeled as insertive ("top"), receptive ("bottom"), or versatile. Gay and bisexual men who often engage in anal sex where they penetrate their partners usually label themselves as "top," gay and bisexual men who often engage in anal sex where they are penetrated by their partners usually label themselves as "bottom," and gay and bisexual men who engage in both types of anal sex are often labeled as "versatiles." Although these labels usually refer to anal sex, they can also be used to other sexual activities, such as oral sex or fisting [16]. Sex labels exist to describe and identify gay and bisexual men preferences during penetrative sexual behaviors. Nevertheless, social and cultural associations can be inferred. In some cases, the "top" gay or bisexual men may be considered as more dominant, comparatively to "bottom" gay or bisexual men, who are considered as submissive.

Gender roles and stereotypes associated to masculinity and feminity may have a role on sex labels and sexual behaviors among gay and bisexual men. According to Carballo-Diégouz et al. [17], versatile gay or bisexual men more likely engaged in a "top" sex role when they perceived their partners as less aggressive, with smaller penis, less taller and handsome, and with lighter skin. On the other hand, if they perceived their partners as more aggressive, more handsome, with darker skin, or with larger penis, which is considered as more masculine, they adopt a "bottom" sex role more often [17]. This findings support the idea that gender stereotypes, masculinity and feminity, play a major role in same-sex relationships, specially between two men. Sex roles in same-sex relationships may be dependent on gender representations, with "top" gay or bisexual men being considered more masculine and "bottom" gay or bisexual men being described as more feminine. The main characteristics associated to self-labeling are the physical appearance and penis size, with gay and bisexual men with smaller penis more often label themselves as "bottoms," because they believe they will not being able to satisfy their partners [16]. When looking for a partner, "top" gay or bisexual men often look for partners with more feminine characteristics, usually associated to "bottom" gay or bisexual men, while "bottom" gay or bisexual men usually look for partners with characteristics often associated to "bottom" gay or bisexual men [17, 18].

Sexual Difficulties

Sexual dysfunctions have been conceptualized by international classification systems according to a heterosexist perspective, which is based on classic models of sexual response (e.g., [18, 19]). Therefore, penile–vaginal penetration continues to play a major role in the definition of sexual difficulties. Nevertheless, along with sexual dysfunctions referred on international classification systems, complaints as "not having a steady sexual partner" or "sexual desire discrepancy" were often referred by gay men and lesbian women as the most frequent sexual problem experienced [20–23]. Therefore, self-perceived sexual difficulties can be distinct from the sexual dysfunctions referred by international classification systems, and should be addressed in clinical context.

Assessing Sexual Difficulties

Regarding measures for assessing both male and female sexual functioning, once again a heterosexist bias can be found. One of the most common self-reported measures for assessing male sexual difficulties is the International Index of Erectile Functioning (IIEF; [24]). The IIEF is a self-reported measure with 15 items assessing five domains: erectile function, orgasmic function, sexual desire, intercourse satisfaction, and overall satisfaction [24]. The IIEF [24] is a very reliable measure for both clinical and research context [25], however it has been developed according to a heterosexual perspective. Therefore, Coyne and her colleagues developed an adapted version of the IIEF for men who have sex with men (IIEF-MSM; [26]). The IIEF-MSM included the five domains assessed by the original IIEF [24], with modified questions, mainly adapted for both receptive and insertive anal intercourse. According to the study conducted by Coyne et al. [26], with a sample of 486 men who have sex with men, HIV-positive, Cronbach's alpha values were: 0.82 for erectile function; 0.83 for orgasmic function; 0.89 for sexual desire, 0.55 for intercourse satisfaction; and 0.42 for overall satisfaction. Despite of satisfaction questions, the other domains assessed by the IIEF-MSM revealed overall high internal consistency. Regarding satisfaction questions, the authors found out that the frequency of sexual intercourse attempts was not associated with the other items, which can be explained by the HIV status of the sample. Additionally, sexual satisfaction with a regular sexual partner was also unrelated to global sexual satisfaction, possibly due to types of sexual relationships maintained by the men in the sample [26]. The IIEF-MSM has been recently adapted, and research has shown good outcomes [26, 27]. However, anal sex pain is not assessed by the IIEF-MSM [28], and according to several studies it constitutes a major concern among men who have sex with men [29–32].

For women, the Female Sexual Functioning Index (FSFI; [33]) is the most frequent tool for assessing sexual functioning, constituted by 19 items evaluating sexual desire, orgasmic function, sexual arousal, lubrication, sexual satisfaction, and sexual pain. As a reliable measure for self-reported sexual difficulties in women, the FSFI [33] is widely used in both research and clinical context [33, 34]. However, the introduction to the measure states that sexual intercourse is defined as penile penetration of the vagina, which is inadequate for women who have sex with women [35]. Therefore, the psychometric properties of the FSFI were assessed in a sample of 350 lesbian women, with two major adaptations: the sexual intercourse definition was removed, and the period of time was modified from 4 weeks to 6 months. The decision was mainly based on previous studies that argue that lesbian couples engage less frequently in sexual activity [36, 37]. Findings from the study of the psychometric properties of the FSFI in a lesbian women sample showed good outcomes [35]. More specifically, the Cronbach's alpha values were: 0.84 for satisfaction; 0.89 for sexual desire; 0.93 for sexual arousal and orgasmic function; 0.95 for lubrication; 0.96 for sexual pain [35].

Despite of the IIEF [24] and the FSFI [33] have been adapted for both men who have sex with men and women who have sex with women, respectively, further studies need to be conducted in order to address some of the questions raised above.

Prevalence of Male Sexual Difficulties

Although prevalence of sexual difficulties has been largely studied among heterosexual men, with empirical data being consistent with premature ejaculation as the most frequent complaint in heterosexual men [38–43], little is known regarding prevalence of sexual difficulties among gay and bisexual men.

Empirical studies addressing prevalence of sexual difficulties in gay and bisexual men are fewer compared to studies conducted worldwide with heterosexual samples. Additionally, instruments for assessing sexual functioning were characterized by a heterosexual bias [28], and several methodological limitations were addressed. Duration criterion varies in a range from experiencing once in lifetime to experiencing during 3 months over the last year. Moreover, studies did not consider associated levels of distress. Despite of the methodological limitations, a few studies have focused on assessing prevalence of sexual problems in gay men community. Findings have suggested rates between 75 and 98% of gay men experiencing at least one sexual problem across lifetime. Lower rates were found for current sexual problems, with ranges between 42.5 and 79% [31, 44–47].

One of the first studies that attempted to assessing the prevalence of gay men' sexual problems found that 97.5% experienced at least one sexual problem across lifetime, and 75% currently had at least one sexual problem [31]. If sexual dysfunctions were considered, frequencies were 92 and 52%, respectively [31]. Regarding lifetime sexual problems, 61% reported receptive painful anal sex, 49% referred lack of sexual desire, 46% experienced difficulties in keeping an erection, 44% had premature ejaculation, 40% experienced difficulties in getting an erection, 39% had orgasmic difficulties, and 14% reported insertive painful anal sex. For current sexual problems, 19% had premature ejaculation, 16% experienced lack of sexual desire, orgasmic difficulties, and receptive painful anal sex, 15% had difficulties in keeping an erection, and 13% in getting an erection, and 3% reported insertive painful anal sex [31].

According to a study conducted in Hong Kong, 49.1% of gay men experienced at least one sexual problem across 3 months in the past year, and 36% felt extremely bothered about that problem [45]. Premature ejaculation was the most frequent sexual problem referred, with a range of 21.8%, followed by lack of sexual desire and absence of sexual pleasure, with a range of 20%, performance anxiety, erectile difficulties, orgasmic difficulties, with ranges of 10.9, 9.4, and 9.1%, respectively, and sexual pain, with a range of 3.6% [45]. On a web-based study conducted by the same authors, with men who have sex with men, findings showed that 42.5% experienced at least one sexual problem over 3 months, in the past year [46]. Findings suggested performance anxiety as the most frequent problem (18.7%), followed by sexual pain and absence of sexual pleasure (13.8%), premature ejaculation (10.8%), lack of sexual desire (8.3%), erectile difficulties (6.3%), and orgasmic difficulties (5.6%). Overall, aging was associated to erectile difficulties and fewer sexual desire problems. Also, men aged 25–34 years reported more frequently sexual pain [46].

In a study conducted in Australia, Mao et al. [48] assessed gay men's sexual problems that occurred at least over a month during the last year. Contrary to what was expected, aging was not associated to any sexual problem, while being HIV-positive was positively associated to sexual problems. Regarding frequency rates, 40.0–59.0% reported lack of sexual desire, 38.5–51.6% experienced erectile difficulties, 41.5–47.0% had performance anxiety, 25.5–31.8% revealed absence of sexual pleasure, 21.8–31.3% had orgasmic difficulties, 16.6–20.7% had premature ejaculation, and 6.5–7.8% experienced sexual pain [48].

Previous findings suggested that current sexual problems were less frequent then lifetime sexual problems. According to a study conducted by Seibel et al. [47], 75% of men who have sex with men attending a workshop about sexual health experienced at least one sexual problem across lifetime, while 65.1% had at least one sexual problem currently. Current sexual problems were defined as being experienced recurrently and persistently over the past year, and being associated to distress and life interference. Results suggested that erectile difficulties were experienced by 38.4% as a current sexual problem, and by 40% as a lifetime sexual problem. For orgasmic difficulties percentages were 32.7 and 43.3, lack of sexual desire was experienced by 26.4 and 34.3%, premature ejaculation occurred in 19.3 and 30.2%, and sexual pain was reported by 2.2 and 5.7% as a current and a lifetime sexual problem, respectively [47].

Recently, Hirshfield et al. [44] conducted a web-based study with men who have sex with men, with 89% identifying themselves as gay men, 10% as bisexuals, and 1% as heterosexuals. Sexual problems were assessed by asking the participants if they experienced a list of symptoms (low sexual desire, erectile difficulties, premature ejaculation, difficulties in reaching orgasm, sexual pain, absence of sexual pleasure, and performance anxiety), at a given time, over the past year. Results indicated that 57% experienced lack of sexual desire, 45% erectile difficulties, 44% performance anxiety, 37% absence of sexual pleasure, 36% orgasmic difficulties, 34% premature ejaculation, and 14% sexual pain. Younger men who have sex with men reported more problems related to sexual desire, premature ejaculation, absence of sexual pleasure and sexual pain [44].

More recently, a study conducted in Portugal indicated anal sex pain was the most frequent sexual difficulty in gay men, followed by lack of sexual desire, retarded and premature ejaculation, and erectile difficulties [49]. When associated levels of distress were considered, anal sex pain remains as the most frequent sexual complaint, followed by lack of sexual desire, retarded ejaculation, erectile difficulties, and premature ejaculation. Moreover, significant differences in prevalence were found when levels of personal distress were considered, with gay men reporting significantly less sexual difficulties when associated distress was assessed [49].

According to a recent study conducted in Croatia, regarding prevalence of sexual difficulties among gay and bisexual men, findings suggested that 60.2% reported at least on sexual difficulty in the previous year, and 52.3% reported at least one sexual dysfunction [50]. The most frequent sexual difficulty was lack of sexual interest, followed by felling anxiety before having sex, erectile difficulties, premature ejaculation, absence of sexual pleasure, and retarded ejaculation. The sexual difficulties with more associated distress were erectile difficulties, performance anxiety and retarded ejaculation [50].

Overall, lifetime sexual problems suggested receptive anal sex pain, lack of sexual desire and erectile difficulties as the most frequent sexual problems [31, 47]. For current sexual problems findings were contradictory, and some studies suggested lack of sexual desire as the most frequent sexual problem [44, 48], while others indicated premature ejaculation [31, 45], erectile difficulties [47], and sexual pain [46] as the most frequent sexual problem.

Concerning sociodemographic predictors of sexual problems in gay men, studies indicated that older gay men reported fewer sexual problems compared to younger men, with exception for erectile difficulties [44, 48, 51]. Contrary to erectile difficulties, highly reported by older gay men, sexual pain was extremely common among younger gay men [46].

Premature ejaculation as a clinical condition refers to latency time about ejaculation after vaginal penetration. Therefore, it is not possible to establish this clinical diagnosis in gay men [52]. Additionally, vaginal intercourse is very common among heterosexual couples, while gay couples reported other sexual behaviors, namely masturbation, oral and anal sex. Therefore, it is important to understand how this difference among sexual behavior affects the ejaculatory function. According to Jern et al. [52], sexual orientation does not seem to have a significant effect on delayed or premature ejaculation. Moreover, a previous study has found no differences between gay men and heterosexuals regarding premature ejaculation [53].

Sexual Difficulties and HIV Status

The treatment for HIV, including antiretroviral therapy may be associated with increased risk of sexual dysfunction in men [54, 55]. Additionally, HIV-positive gay men presenting significantly more complaints related to sexual functioning compared to HIV-negative men [27, 48]. More specifically, HIV-positive gay men reported more complaints about lack of sexual desire and erectile difficulties compared to HIV-negative [55–58]. However, it is not possible to infer whether these difficulties are associated directly to the clinical condition or to other factors, including the use of condoms or regarding the fear of contracting HIV [56]. Furthermore, clinical depression is more common in HIV-positive individuals [55]. Therefore, other psychosocial factors should mediate the relationship between HIV status and sexual problems. HIV-positive gay men state that psychological factors and side effects from HIV treatments can promote sexual problems [55, 57].

Sexual Difficulties and Sex Roles

Gay men who engage in anal sex can adopt three distinctive roles: "top"; "bottom"; or "versatile" [59–62]. Gay men who usually penetrate their partners and engage in penetrative behavior are considered "top," while gay men who frequently are penetrated by their partners and engage in receptive behavior are labeled as "bottom." Finally, gay men who involved in the two previous described behaviors are labeled as "versatile." "Tops" more frequently prefer engage in a sexual relationship where they were dominant and in control, tend to select partners that worship their bodies during sexual intercourse, and partners with a more female body; while "bottoms" prefer a submissive sexual relationship [59]. Also, empirical data suggested that self-sex labels regarding gay men were good predictors of sexual behavior [61]. Consequently, a new complaint associated to painful receptive anal sex, known as *anodyspareunia*, should be considered [29–32].

Rosser et al. [31] studied sexual problems experienced by gay men and found out that about 61% reported painful anal sex. Given this remarkable result, they decided to assess severity and frequency of anal sex pain, and main results suggested that 63% of gay men reported occasional pain, with mild to moderate severity, and 12% experienced persistent pain with extreme severity [32]. The main factors associated to painful anal sex were lubrication, followed by psychological factors such as anxiety, previous stimulation, penis size and confidence level of sexual arousal [32]. Therefore, the authors proposed a new sexual dysfunction-"*anodyspareunia*"—characterized by recurrent or persistent sexual pain felt during receptive anal sex. More recently, Damon and Rosser [29] conducted a study where they studied painful anal sex using a behavioral criterion and a clinical criterion. On one hand, the behavioral criterion was based on frequency and severity of pain. On the other hand, the clinical criterion was based on: (1) if experienced sexual pain very often, (2) if experienced distress and/or interpersonal difficulties due to pain and, finally, (3) if no sexual pain experienced was due to an involuntary spasm of the anus muscle, lack of adequate lubrication, use of drugs/medication, or medical condition. Overall, the results indicated that 14% of the sample met criteria for behavioral painful anal sex and 10% met the clinical criteria. More specifically, 21% of the sample reported that their pain occurred across lifetime, and about 60% considered the pain as problematic. Regarding the distress associated, 25% of the sample reported extreme levels, and 18% experienced extreme interpersonal difficulties. Consequences were avoidance of anal sex for a period of time (82%) and restriction of anal sex as the penetrating partner (49%). Participants attributed the pain to psychological factors, penis size, to specific anus health problems, and no use of drugs.

Prevalence of Female Sexual Difficulties

Across worldwide, new studies emerge concerning female sexual problems, but very little is known regarding lesbian women sexual problems. Specificities regarding lesbian women's sexuality should be addressed, such as sexual behaviors, namely tribadism (genital contact), mutual masturbation, oral sex, or finger–vaginal penetration [63]. Nevertheless, both lesbian women and heterosexuals defined vaginal penetration as sexual intercourse [64]. Research regarding lesbian women's sexuality is mainly focused on frequency of sexual activity, sexual satisfaction, and intimacy [65, 66].

Regardless of lack of empirical data about sexual problems in lesbian women, evidence suggested that, overall, lesbian women reported fewer sexual difficulties when compared to heterosexuals [67–69]. According to a study conducted by

Beaber and Werner [67], lesbian women reported better levels of sexual arousal and orgasmic function [67]. Additionally, a negative association was found for heterosexuals regarding sexual functioning and anxiety levels. No significant association was found for lesbian women, which was explained due to their good communication pattern [67]. Likewise, a previous study also suggested that lesbian women reported fewer difficulties in reaching orgasm, when compared to heterosexuals [68]. Despite of methodological limitations, according to Matthews, Hughes and Tartaro [69], in a study assessing sexual problems with a dichotomy scale "yes or no", sexual dysfunction index was calculated by the presence of two or more sexual difficulties. Findings suggested a lower sexual dysfunction index for lesbian women. More specifically, heterosexuals had more complaints associated to sexual pain, while lesbian women referred more difficulties in reaching orgasm [69]. No significant differences were found for sexual activity frequency [69, 70].

According to Lau, Kim, and Tsui [45], in a study with women who engage in same-sex relationships, over the last year, 75.6% reported at least one sexual problem, and about 45% felt extremely bothered about that sexual difficulty. Lubrication difficulties were the most frequent sexual concern (39.3%), followed by lower sexual desire (30.7%) and absence of sexual pleasure (30.3%), difficulties in reaching orgasm (24.7%), sexual pain (23.6%), and performance anxiety (16.9%). Also, lubrication difficulties increase with aging [45]. Regarding self-reported sexual problems, according to a study conducted by Meana, Rakipi, Weeks, and Lykins [71], 28% of lesbian women reported difficulties in reaching orgasm, 15% experienced arousal difficulties, and 12% referred lack of sexual desire. Findings from a web-based study with women who have sex with women (74.5% were lesbian women and 17.5% self-defined themselves as bisexuals) indicated that 24.8% of the sample scored for high risk for sexual dysfunction [72].

Studies concerning the role of associated levels of distress of sexual problems were also scarce with lesbian women. Nevertheless, associated levels of distress were a crucial variable concerning sexual dysfunctions. According to Burri et al. [66], when distress levels were controlled, 9.9% of non-heterosexual women reported lack of sexual desire, 8.4% experienced difficulties in reaching orgasm, 6.5 and 6.4% referred arousal and lubrication difficulties, respectively, and 5.9% reported sexual pain.

According to a very recent study conducted with lesbian women, in Portugal, lack of sexual desire represents the most frequent sexual complaint, followed by sex pain, difficulties in reaching orgasm, and arousal difficulties. When the same prevalence analysis was conducted with associated distress levels the most frequent sexual difficulty was sex pain, followed by lack of sexual desire and difficulties in reaching orgasm, and sexual arousal difficulties. Consistent with findings among gay men, also with lesbian women sample was found a significant decreasing in prevalence of sexual difficulties when associated distressed levels were considered [73].

As lack of empirical evidence was found for sexual difficulties in lesbian women, also a gap was found regarding the role of age in sexual problems. According to a web-based study conducted with 456 lesbian women with 50 years or more, findings suggested that more than 40% of the sample did not engage in sexual activity over the past year, while 11% referred engage in sexual activity once a week [74]. Lesbian women in steady relationships and with a regular sexual partner reported higher sexual activity frequency. However, in regards to sexual satisfaction, data was heterogeneous. About 17% of the sample referred being very satisfied, 21% reported moderate satisfaction, and 18% was dissatisfied with their sex lives. About 45% of the women considered sexual activity very important under age of 55, while only 22% considered equally important after 55 years. Overall, Averett et al. [74] found that older lesbian women appreciated emotional stability over physical and sexual intimacy.

An interesting phenomenon found on lesbian women literature was the idea that lesbian women report significantly less frequency of sexual activity, when compared to heterosexuals or gay men. According to van Rosmalen-Nooijens, Vergeer and Lagro-Janssen [75], data from a qualitative study suggested that lesbian women reported a decrease of sexual activity frequency as a common phenomenon. An emotional fusion can be conceptualized in lesbian women' relationships [23, 75]. Also, women were socially raised for being sexually passive, which can promote these lower levels of sexual activity [75–79]. Additionally, internalized homonegativity can also contribute for lower levels of sexual interaction [23]. In a patriarchal society, lesbian women had a double discrimination [80].

Lesbian couples appear to be satisfied with their relationships. Similarity between partners in relationship was one of the major issues. More important than individual characteristics, were the characteristics of the relationship, such as closeness [81]. Sexual satisfaction among lesbian couples was half explained by emotional intimacy [82]. Lower sexual desire in lesbian women was not necessarily associated to sexual dissatisfaction. According to Bridges and Horne [83], dissatisfaction to sexual life exists when sexual desire discrepancy is perceived as a problem by one of the couples' element.

"Lesbian Bed Death"

A controversial approach for intimate and sexual relationship among lesbians was discussed in the literature. Described as a "*notorious drop-off in sexual activity about two years into long-term lesbian relationships*" ([77]; p.112), "Lesbian Bed Death" lacks scientific evidence. Even so, empirical data suggest that women had less sexual desire than men, and are more submissive in sexual interactions [75–78, 84, 85].

Despite of the controversy, van Rosmalen-Nooijens et al. [75] interviewed lesbian couples without explaining the phenomenon of "lesbian bed death". The majority of couples described spontaneously a decreased in sexual activity frequency as a common phenomenon in their intimate relationship. According to this qualitative research, lesbian relationships appear to develop to a fusional relationship, where intimacy is the main focus, with sexual contact being secondary for relationship satisfaction. A possible explanation can be the social and cultural pressure women suffer for being sexual submissives and do not engage spontaneously in sexual activity. Other possible explanation is the fact that women reported lower levels of sexual desire compared to men [75–79]. Although little is known about "lesbian bed death," the combination of lower levels of sexual desire in women with the searching for intimacy may help explain the occurrence of decreased levels of sexual activity in lesbian couples.

Psychological Approaches for Sexual Problems in Same-Sex Couples

Regarding psychological variables affecting sexual functioning, both depressed mood and anxiety have been described as associated to a decrease in both male and female sexual functioning (e.g., [86–91]). The prevalence of depressed mood and anxiety states in sexual minority groups is increased, when compared to heterosexual groups (e.g., [92–94]). Therefore, Bancroft et al. [95] explore the relationship between mood (depressive and anxiety states) and sexual functioning in gay men. Findings were consistent with previous results with heterosexual samples. For more than half of the sample, both depressive and anxiety states appear to be associated to a decreased in sexual functioning, while a small percentage reported an increase in their sexual performance when depressed or when feeling anxiety [95].

Cognitive variables have been largely introduced in sex therapy and sex research by D. Barlow [86]. Although most of the studies have been conducted with heterosexual samples, more recently studies with samples of sexual minorities can be found. According to a study conducted by Shires and Miller [22], both heterosexual and gay men reported distress associated to erectile difficulties. Nevertheless, gay men tend to express more feelings of "I'm a sexual failure," while heterosexual men reported higher levels of performance anxiety, when facing erectile difficulties during sexual intercourse. During this failure sexual episodes, heterosexual men reported more frustration, while gay men experienced more inadequacy and fear of being infected with HIV [22].

Non-erotic thoughts constitute a strong resource of cognitive distraction, which impairs sexual functioning and satisfaction, in both men and women [96, 97]. Globally, sexual minorities, such as gay men and lesbian women, reported non-erotic thoughts as heterosexual men and women. However, being afraid of having own sexual orientation revealed constitute an additional source of cognitive distraction during sexual activity for sexual minorities [97]. According to the pioneer study conducted by Lacefield and Negy [97], both gay men and lesbian women reported more non-erotic distractions during sexual intercourse, when compared to heterosexual men and women. Cognitive distractions related to body-image, sexual performance, and IST infections were more frequent in the sexual minority sample.

The Cognitive-Emotional Model for Sexual Dysfunction [98] has been developed for heterosexual men and women sexual dysfunction. According to empirical studies conducted by Nobre and colleagues, individuals with sexual disorders present a personality profile characterized by higher levels of neuroticism and lower levels of extraversion, when compared to sexually health individuals [98–115]. Also, acting as dispositional variables for sexual disorders development, are sexual beliefs about sexual performance, sexual satisfaction and attitudes related to sexual activity [98, 115]. In addition to the dispositional variables, the author also described episode-related variables, elicited by negative sexual events, such as cognitive schemas, automatic thoughts, and emotional responses [98, 116].

Findings with gay men and lesbian women samples have suggested more similarities between heterosexual and gay men, and between heterosexual and lesbian women (e.g., [117, 118]). Moreover, personality profiles of gay men with distressing sexual difficulties are characterized by higher levels of neuroticism [119], which is consistent with previous findings with heterosexual men [114]. Lesbian women with distressing sexual difficulties also shown a personality profile characterized by higher levels of neuroticism and lower levels of extraversion, when compared to sexually healthy lesbian women [119]. These findings are also consistent with data collected for heterosexual women with and without distressing sexual difficulties [119]. Concerning personality traits and sexual problems, sexual orientation differences are mostly inexistent, and health professionals and sex therapists should be aware of neuroticism traits, which are highly and positive correlated to negative affect and negative correlated to positive affect.

Along with personality traits, dysfunctional sexual beliefs also act as dispositional variables for the development and maintenance of sexual problems. Demanding sexual performance and unrealistic expectations are the focus of male dysfunctional sexual beliefs. A recent study conducted with gay and heterosexual men, with and without distressing sexual difficulties, assessed the differences between groups regarding the presence of dysfunctional sexual beliefs. The main findings indicated that gay men with distressing sexual difficulties reported more conservative beliefs about sexuality, and more beliefs related to partner's sexual satisfaction and to sex as an abuse of "top" men's power [117]. According to this study, gay men with distressing sexual difficulties have more conservative attitudes towards sexuality, are more concerned about partner's sexual satisfaction, and have more difficulties in dealing with sex roles during penetrative anal sex. Repressive attitudes for women can be described regarding dysfunctional sexual beliefs, with sexual beliefs being related to aging process, body-image concerns, and sexual performance [120]. Findings from the study conducted by Peixoto and Nobre [117] shown that lesbian women with distressing sexual problems struggle with beliefs about sexual desire and pleasure being considered a sin. This finding is consistent with some previous studies suggesting that lesbian women in committed relationships have less sexual desire and less sexual contact [75–78].

Dysfunctional sexual beliefs, or sexual myths, have been studied over three decades, with the work of Zilbergeld [121] being considered a pioneer study. Based on clinical work with men facing sexual disorders, Zilbergeld [121] illustrated several sexual myths reported by men, mainly related to sexual performance demands and unrealistic expectations about sexual performance and sexual intercourse. Heiman and Lo Piccolo [120] also described sexual beliefs reported by women with sexual difficulties, suggesting that gender roles can also be found in myths related to sexuality. According to the authors, women more frequently are concerned and have dysfunctional attitudes towards sexuality related to being submissive in sexual context and to aging process or to physical appearance [120]. Empirical research about sexual beliefs with gay men or lesbian women is almost inexistent. Hart and Schwartz [122] described possible sexual beliefs reported by gay men with erectile disorder, which have been related to sexual performance demands, to sexual scripts, and to sex roles during penetrative sexual intercourse. Besides beliefs related to sex roles adopted by gay men during penetrative sexual intercourse, dysfunctional sexual beliefs presented by gay and heterosexual men are focused on sexual performance demands and unrealistic expectations. For women, only one empirical study was found, and findings only indicated beliefs related to sexual desire and pleasure as a sin as a common sexual belief for lesbian women with sexual difficulties. No evidence was found for sexual beliefs related to conservative attitudes, and related to aging process or to physical appearance. Some hypothesis could be draw according to these findings. It is possible that lesbian women were not so affected by body-image concerns, such as heterosexual women, for instance.

Other vulnerability factors for the development and maintenance of sexual dysfunction are cognitive schemas activated in sexual context, when individuals face negative sexual episodes [98]. According to the Cognitive-Emotional Model for Sexual Dysfunction [98, 116], incompetence schemas constitute the core schema activated in sexual context when men and women face an unsuccessful sexual episode. In sex research, cognitive schemas may be one of the psychological variables less studied. Only a couple of studies have been found, and data is consistent for heterosexual samples, with incompetence schemas receiving major attention [105, 111, 113, 115]. So far, only one empirical study has been conducted regarding the role of sexual orientation on cognitive schemas activated in sexual context. According to Peixoto & Nobre [118], negative cognitive schemas are activated in sexual context, by gay men and lesbian women, when facing unsuccessful sexual episodes. Moreover, for gay men with distressing sexual difficulties, the cognitive schemas more frequently activated in sexual context, when negative sexual episodes occur are difference/loneliness schemas and undesirability/rejection schemas. Curiously, although incompetence schemas were more frequent in gay men with distressing sexual difficulties, compared to sexually healthy gay men, no significant statistical differences were found [118]. Data from women revealed that lesbian women with distressing sexual difficulties activate more schemas related to incompetence, difference/loneliness, and undesirability/rejection, when compared to sexually healthy lesbian women [118], which is congruent with previous data with heterosexual women [111, 113].

Finally, during sexual activity both automatic thoughts and emotional responses help to maintain sexual difficulties [108–110, 123–126]. Empirical research focusing on non-erotic thoughts and cognitive distraction with gay men and lesbian women has been conducted [97], but assessing frequent negative automatic thoughts during sexual activity reported by heterosexual men and women in samples of gay men and lesbian women is a very recent topic of research. According to a very recent published study about negative automatic thoughts during sexual activity in gay men and lesbian women, the main findings suggested that gay men with distressing sexual difficulties more frequently reported, during sexual intercourse, failure anticipation and erection concern thoughts, as well as lack of erotic thoughts [127]. These results are consistent with data from heterosexual samples ([102, 103, 105, 108, 109]; Nobre and Pinto-Gouveia 2003). For women, data suggested that lesbian women presenting distressing sexual difficulties reported more frequently thoughts related to sexual abuse, to failure and disengagement, to partner's lack of affection, to sexual passivity and control, and less erotic thoughts, when compared to sexually healthy lesbian women [127]. Regarding emotional responses during sexual activity, previously studies suggested that heterosexual men and women with sexual dysfunction reported more negative emotions and less positive emotions [101, 103, 104, 109]. Data from a recent study with gay men and lesbian women partially supported these hypotheses. For lesbian women with distressing sexual difficulties, a similar pattern was found regarding emotional responses during sexual activity, but that pattern was not found for gay men [128]. Altogether, data suggested that during sexual activity, gay men and lesbian women with distressing sexual problems tendentiously reported more negative automatic thoughts, less erotic thoughts, and form women's sample more negative and less positive emotions. For gay men, the thoughts content was mainly related to sexual performance, which is also consistent with more dispositional variables, like dysfunctional sexual beliefs. For lesbian women, the thoughts content was mainly the same as for heterosexual women.

Psychological Interventions for Sexual Problems with Same-Sex Couples

According to empirical research on same-sex couples and sexuality, similarities and differences have been found. Therefore, psychological interventions for sexual problems with same-sex couples should address those specificities. Addressing relationship types (e.g., monogamy; non-monogamy), sexual behaviors (e.g., anal sex in gay couples), internalized homophobia, among other characteristics previously described is a major concern for health professionals working with same-sex couples.

Randomized clinical trials for sexual dysfunction can be found for heterosexual men and women (cf. [129]). Until now, no studies regarding treatment efficacy have been conducted for sexual problems with same-sex couples. Nevertheless, an article with two case-studies addressing cognitive-behavioral intervention for erectile dysfunction in gay men couples has been published recently [122].

Cognitive-behavioral intervention for erectile dysfunction is mainly based on sexual beliefs addressing sexual performance expectancies [121]. According to Hart and Schwartz [122], sexual beliefs related to erectile difficulties in heterosexual men can be found in gay men couples, for instance "*I must always be ready for sex.*" Nevertheless, specific sexual beliefs can be associated to gay men and act as vulnerability factors for developing sexual disorders, such as erectile dysfunction (e.g., "*If I am not ready for anal sex, I am a bad partner*"; [122]). Although no clinical trials assessing the efficacy of psychological interventions for erectile dysfunction in gay men, according to the clinical work conducted by the authors, cognitive-behavioral approaches, focusing on performance anxiety management can produce good outcomes [122].

Empirical data supporting psychological interventions for working clinically with lesbian couples with sexual difficulties is also inexistent. Therefore, paying attention to specificities regarding sexual beliefs, cognitive distraction, types of relationship and sexual behaviors is also a main concern.

Although no (randomized) clinical trials assessing the efficacy of psychological interventions for sexual dysfunctions among same-sex couples can be found, the main findings from recent sex research have shown that cognitive-behavioral approaches may lead to good outcomes (e.g., [122]). Being aware of specificities on sexual behaviors, types of relationships, sex roles, or cognitive distraction will allow health professionals to conduct coherent and consistent interventions with same-sex couples.

References

1. Garnets L, Kimmel D. Lesbian and gay male dimensions in the psychological study of human diversity. In: Garnets L, Kimmel D, editors. Psychological perspectives on lesbian and gay male experiences. New York: Columbia University Press; 1993. p. 1–51.
2. Herek GM, Garnets LD. Sexual orientation and mental health. Annu Rev Clin Psychol. 2007;3:353–75. doi:10.1146/annurev.clinpsy.3.022806.091510.
3. Young RM, Meyer IH. The trouble with "MSM" and "WSW": erasure of the sexual-minority person in public health discourse. Am J Public Health. 2005;95:1144–9. doi:10.2105/AJPH.2004.046714.
4. Bogaert AF. Asexuality: prevalence and associated factors in a national probability sample. J Sex Res. 2004;41:279–87.
5. Van Houdenhove E, Gijs L, T'Soen G, Ezlin P. Asexuality: a multidimensional approach. J Sex Res. 2015;52:669–78. doi:10.1080/00224499.2014.898015.
6. Gressgard R. Asexuality: from pathology to identity and beyond. Psychol Sex. 2013;4:179–92. doi:10.1080/19419899.2013.774166.
7. Prause N, Graham CA. Asexuality: classification and characterization. Arch Sex Behav. 2007;36:341–56. doi:10.1007/s10508-006-9142-3.
8. McCormick NB. Sexual scripts: social and therapeutic implications. Sex Relationsh Ther. 2010;25:96–120. doi:10.1080/14681990903550167.
9. Masters NT, Casey E, Wells EA, Morrison DM. Sexual scripts among young heterosexually active men and women: continuity and change. J Sex Res. 2013;50:409–20. doi:10.1080/00224499.2012.661102.
10. Meyer IH. Minority stress and mental health in gay men. J Health Soc Behav. 1995;36:38–56.
11. Szymanski DM, Chung YB. Internalized homophobia in lesbians. J Lesbian Stud. 2002;7:115–25. doi:10.1300/J155v07n01_08.
12. Williamson IR. Internalized homophobia and health issues affecting lesbians and gay men. Health Educ Res. 2000;15:97–107.
13. American Psychological Association. Avoiding heterosexual bias in language. Committee on Lesbian and Gay Concerns. Am Psychol. 1991;46:973–4.

14. Balsam KF, Beauchaine TP, Rothblum ED, Solomon SE. Three-year follow-up of same-sex couples who had civil unions in Vermont, same-sex couples not in civil unions, and heterosexual married couples. Dev Psychol. 2008;44:102–16. doi:10.1037/0012-1649.44.1.102.
15. Hoff CC, Beougher SC, Chakravarty D, Darbes LA, Neilands TB. Relationship characteristics and motivations behind agreements among gay male couples: differences by agreement type and couples serostatus. AIDS Care. 2010;22:827–35. doi:10.1080/09540120903443384.
16. Moskowitz D, Hart TA. The influence of physical body traits and masculinity on anal sex roles in gay and bisexual men. Arch Sex Behav. 2011;40:835–41. doi:10.1007/s10508-011-9754-0.
17. Carballo-Diéguez A, Dolezal C, Nieves L, Díaz F, Decena C, Balan I. Looking for a tall, dark, macho man … sexual-role behaviour variations in Latino gay and bisexual men. Cult Health Sex. 2004;6:159–71. doi:10.1080/13691050310001619662.
18. Kaplan HS. Disorders of sexual desire. New York: Brunner/Mazel; 1979.
19. Masters WH, Johnson VE. Human sexual response. Boston: Little, Brown; 1966.
20. Mills T, Paul J, Stall R, Pollack L, Canchola J, Chang Y, Moskowitz JT, Catania J. Distress and depression in men who have sex with men: the urban men's health study. Am J Psychiatry. 2004;161:278–85.
21. Sandfort TG, Keizer M. Sexual problems in gay men: an overview of empirical research. Annu Rev Sex Res. 2001;12:93–120.
22. Shires A, Miller D. A preliminary study comparing psychological factors associated with erectile dysfunction in heterosexual and homosexual men. Sex Relationsh Ther. 1998;131:37–49. doi:10.1080/02674659808406542.
23. Spitalnick J, McNair L. Couples therapy with gay and lesbian clients: an analysis of important clinical issues. J Sex Marital Ther. 2005;31:43–56. doi:10.1080/00926230590475260.
24. Rosen R, Riley A, Wagner G, Osterloh I, Kirkpatrick J, Mishra A. The international index of erectile function (IIEF): a multidimensional scale for assessment erectile dysfunction. Urology. 1997;49:822–30.
25. Rosen RC, Cappelleri JC, Gendrano N. The International Index of Erectile Function (IIEF): a state-of-the-science review. Int J Impot Res. 2002;14:226–44. doi:10.1038/sj.ijir.3900857.
26. Coyne K, Mandalia S, McCullough S, Catalan J, Noestlinger C, Colebunders R, Asboe D. The international index of erectile function: development of an adapted tool for use in HIV-positive men who have sex with men. J Sex Med. 2010;7:769–74. doi:10.1111/j.1743-6109.2009.01579.x.
27. Shindel AW, Vittinghoff E, Breyer BN. Erectile dysfunction and premature ejaculation in men who have sex with men. J Sex Med. 2012;9:576–84. doi:10.111/j.1743-6109.2011.02585.x.
28. McDonagh L, Bishop CJ, Brockman M, Morrison TG. A systematic review of sexual dysfunction measures for gay men: how do current measures, measure up? J Homosex. 2014;61:781–816. doi:10.1080/00918369.2014.870452.
29. Damon W, Rosser B. Anodyspareunia in men who have sex with men: prevalence, predictors, consequences and the development of DSM diagnostic criteria. J Sex Marital Ther. 2005;31:129–41. doi:10.1080/00926230590477989.
30. Hollows K. Anodyspareunia: a novel sexual dysfunction? An exploration into anal sexuality. Sex Relationsh Ther. 2007;22:429–42. doi:10.1080/14681990701481409.
31. Rosser B, Metz M, Bockting W, Buroker T. Sexual difficulties, concerns, and satisfaction in homosexual men: an empirical study with implications for HIV prevention. J Sex Marital Ther. 1997;23:61–73. doi:10.1080/00926239708404418.
32. Rosser B, Short B, Thurmes P, Coleman E. Anodyspareunia, the unacknowledged sexual dysfunction: a validation study of painful receptive anal intercourse and its psychosexual concomitants in homosexual men. J Sex Marital Ther. 1998;24:281–92. doi:10.1080/00926239808403963.
33. Rosen RC, Brown C, Heiman J, Leiblum S, Meston C, Shabsig R, et al. The Female Sexual Function Index (FSFI): a multidimensional self-report instrument for the assessment of female sexual function. J Sex Marital Ther. 2000;26:191–208.
34. Wiegel M, Meston C, Rosen R. The female sexual function index (FSFI): cross-validation and development of clinical cutoff scores. J Sex Marital Ther. 2005;31:1–20. doi:10.1080/00926230590475206.
35. Tracy JK, Junginger J. Correlates of lesbian sexual functioning. J Womens Health. 2007;16:499–509. doi:10.1089/jwh.2006.0308.
36. Blumstein P, Schwartz P. American couples: money, work, sex. 1st ed. New York: William Morrow & Company; 1983. ISBN: 0688037720.
37. Loulan J. Lesbian sex. San Francisco: Spinsters Ink; 1984.
38. Buvat J, Glasser D, Neves RC, Duarte FG, Gingell C, Moreira Jr ED. Sexual problems and associated help-seeking behavior patterns: results of a population-based survey in France. Int J Urol. 2009;16:632–8. doi:10.1111/j.1442-2042.2009.02316.x.
39. Laumann EO, Nicolosi A, Glasser DB, Paik A, Gingell C, Moreira E, Wang T. Sexual problems among women and men aged 40–80 y: prevalence and correlates identified in the Global Study of Sexual Attitudes and Behaviors. Int J Impot Res. 2005;17:39–57.
40. Laumann EO, Paik A, Rosen RC. Sexual dysfunction in the United States. JAMA. 1999;281:537–44. doi:10.1001/jama.281.6.537.
41. Mitchell KR, Mercer CH, Ploubidis GB, Jones KG, Datta J, Field N, et al. Sexual function in Britain: findings from the third National Survey of Sexual Attitudes and Lifestyles (Natsal-3). Lancet. 2013;382:1817–29.
42. Quinta-Gomes A, Nobre P. Prevalence of sexual problems in Portugal: pesults of a population-based study using a stratified sample of men aged 18 to 70 years. J Sex Res. 2014;51:13–21. doi:10.1080/00224499.2012.744953.
43. Read S, King M, Watson J. Sexual dysfunction in primary medical care: prevalence, characteristics and detection by the general practitioner. J Public Health Med. 1997;19:387–91.
44. Hirshfield S, Chiasson M, Wagmiller R, Remien R, Humberstone M, Scheinmann R, Grov C. Sexual dysfunction in an internet sample of U.S. men who have sex with men. J Sex Med. 2010;7:3104–14. doi:10.1111/j.1743-6109.2009.01636.x.
45. Lau J, Kim J, Tsui H. Prevalence and factors of sexual problems in Chinese males and females having sex with the same-sex partner in Hong-Kong: a population-based study. Int J Impot Res. 2006;1:130–40. doi:10.1038/sj.ijir.3901368.
46. Lau J, Kim J, Tsui H. Prevalence and sociocultural predictors of sexual dysfunction among Chinese men who have sex with men in Hong Kong. J Sex Med. 2008;5:2766–79. doi:10.1111/j.1743-6109.2008.00892.x.
47. Seibel S, Rosser B, Horvath K, Evans C. Sexual dysfunction, paraphilias and their relationship to childhood abuse in men who have sex with men. Int J Sex Health. 2009;21:79–86. doi:10.1080/19317610902773062.
48. Mao L, Newman C, Ridd M, Saltman D, Rogers G, Kippax S. Self-reported sexual difficulties and their association with depression and other factors among gay men attending high HIV-caseload general practices in Australia. J Sex Med. 2009;6:1378–85. doi:10.1111/j.1743-6109.2008.01160.x.
49. Peixoto MM, Nobre P. Prevalence of sexual problems and associated distress among gay and heterosexual men. Sex Relation Ther. 2015;30:211–25. doi:10.1080/14681994.2014.986084.
50. Ivanković I, Šević S, Štulhofer A. Distressing sexual difficulties in heterosexual and non-heterosexual Croatian men: assessing the role of minority stress. J Sex Res. 2015;52:647–58. doi:10.1080/00224499.2014.909381.

51. Cove J, Boyle M. Gay men's self-defined sexual problems, perceived causes and factors in remission. Sex Relation Ther. 2002;17:137–47. doi:10.1080/14681990220121257.
52. Jern P, Santtila P, Johansson A, Alanko K, Salo B, Sandnabba N. Is there an association between same-sex sexual experience and ejaculatory dysfunction? J Sex Marital Ther. 2010;36:303–12. doi:10.1080/0092623X.2010.488102.
53. Breyer BN, Smith JF, Eisenberg ML, Ando KA, Rowen TS, Shindel AW. The impact of sexual orientation on sexuality and sexual practices in North American medical students. J Sex Med. 2010;7:2391–400. doi:10.1111/j.1743-6109.2010.01794.x.
54. Colson AE, Keller MJ, Sax PE, Pettus PT, Platt R, Choo PW. Male sexual dysfunction associated with antiretroviral therapy. J Acquir Immune Defic Syndr. 2002;30:27–32.
55. Cove J, Petrak J. Factors associated with sexual problems in HIV-positive gay men. Int J STD AIDS. 2004;15:732–6.
56. Bancroft J, Carnes L, Janssen E, Goodrich D, Long JS. Erectile and ejaculatory problems in gay and heterosexual men. Arch Sex Behav. 2005;34:285–97. doi:10.1007/s10508-005-3117-7.
57. Meyer-Bahlburg H, Exner T, Lorenz G, Gruen R, Gorman J, Ehrhardt A. Sexual risk behavior, sexual functioning, and HIV-disease progression in gay men. J Sex Res. 1991;28:3–27.
58. Vansintejan J, Janssen J, Van de Vijver E, Vandevoorde J, Devroey D. The gay men sex studies: prevalence of sexual dysfunctions in Belgian HIV+ gay men. HIV AIDS Res Palliat Care. 2013;5:89–96.
59. Damon W. The relations of power and intimacy motives to genitoerotic role preferences in gay men: a pilot study. Can J Human Sex. 2000;9:15–29.
60. Gil S. A narrative exploration of gay men's sexual practices as a dialectical dialogue. Sex Relationsh Ther. 2007;22:63–75. doi:10.1080/14681990600861057.
61. Hart TA, Wolitski RJ, Purcell DW, Gómez C, Halkitis P, Team SUMS. Sexual behavior among HIV-positive men who have sex with men: what's in a label? J Sex Res. 2003;40:179–88. doi:10.1080/00224490309552179.
62. Moskowitz D, Rieger G, Roloff M. Tops, bottoms and versatiles. Sex Relationsh Ther. 2008;23(3):191–202. doi:10.1080/14681990802027259.
63. Bailey JV, Farquhar C, Owen C, Whittaker D. Sexual behavior of lesbians and bisexual women. Sex Transm Infect. 2003;79:147–50.
64. Horowitz AD, Spicer L. "Having sex" as a graded and hierarchical construct: a comparison of sexual definitions among heterosexual and lesbian emerging adults in the UK. J Sex Res. 2013;50:139–50.
65. Armstrong HL, Reissing ED. Women who have sex with women: a comprehensive review of the literature and conceptual model of sexual function. Sex Relationsh Ther. 2013;28:364–99. doi:10.1080/14681994.2013.807912.
66. Burri A, Rahman Q, Santtila P, Jern P, Spector T, Sandnabba K. The relationship between same-sex experience, sexual distress, and female sexual dysfunction. J Sex Med. 2012;9:198–206. doi:10.1111/j.1743-6109.2011.02538.x.
67. Beaber T, Werner P. The relationship between anxiety and sexual functioning in lesbians and heterosexual women. J Homosex. 2009;56:639–54. doi:10.1080/00918360903005303.
68. Coleman E, Hoon P, Hoon E. Arousability and sexual satisfaction in lesbian and heterosexual women. J Sex Res. 1983;19:58–73.
69. Matthews A, Hughes T, Tartaro J. Sexual behavior and sexual dysfunction in a community sample of lesbian and heterosexual women. In: Omoto A, Kurtzman H, editors. Sexual orientation and mental health: examining identity and development in lesbian, gay, and bisexual people. Washington, DC: American Psychological Association; 2006. p. 185–205.
70. Matthews A, Tartaro J, Hughes T. A comparative study of lesbian and heterosexual women in committed relationships. J Lesbian Stud. 2002;7:101–14. doi:10.1300/J155v07n01_07.
71. Meana M, Rakipi R, Weeks G, Lykins A. Sexual functioning in a non-clinical sample of partnered lesbians. J Couple Relat Ther. 2006;5:1–22. doi:10.1300/J398v05n02_01.
72. Shindel AW, Rowen TS, Lin T-C, Li C-S, Robertson PA, Breyer BN. An internet survey of demographic and health factors associated with risk of sexual dysfunction in women who have sex with women. J Sex Med. 2012;12:1261–71. doi:10.1111/j.1743-6109.2012.02659.x.
73. Peixoto MM, Nobre P. Prevalence of sexual problems and associated distress among lesbian and heterosexual women. J Sex Marital Ther. 2015;41:427–39. doi:10.1080/0092623X.2014.918066.
74. Averett P, Yoon I, Jenkins CL. Older lesbian sexuality: identity, sexual behavior, and the impact of aging. J Sex Res. 2012;49:495–507. doi:10.1080/00224499.2011.582543.
75. van Rosmalen-Nooijens K, Vergeer C, Lagro-Janssen A. Bed death and other lesbian sexual problems unraveled: a qualitative study of the sexual health of lesbian women involved in a relationship. Women Health. 2008;48:339–62. doi:10.1080/03630240802463343.
76. Iasenza S. Lesbian sexuality post-stonewall to post-modernism: putting the "Lesbian Bed Death" concept to bed. J Sex Educ Ther. 2000;25:59–69.
77. Iasenza S. Beyond "Lesbian Bed Death". J Lesbian Stud. 2002;6:111–20. doi:10.1300/J155v06n01_10.
78. Nichols M. Lesbian sexuality/female: rethinking 'lesbian bed death'. Sex Relation Ther. 2004;19:363–71. doi:10.1080/14681990412331298036.
79. Post L, Avery J. Therapeutic approaches to inhibited sexual desire in lesbians. Couns Psychol Q. 1995;8:213–9.
80. Rothblum ED. Lesbians and physical appearance: which model applies? In: Greene B, Herek GM, editors. Lesbian and gay psychology: theory, research, and clinical applications. London: SAGE; 1994. p. 84–97.
81. Peplau LA, Padesky C, Hamilton M. Satisfaction in lesbian relationships. J Homosex. 1982;8:23–35.
82. Eldridge N, Gilbert L. Correlates of relationship satisfaction in lesbian couples. Psychol Women Q. 1990;14:43–62. doi:10.1111/j.1471-6402.1990.tb00004.x.
83. Bridges S, Horne S. Sexual satisfaction and desire discrepancy in same sex women's relationships. J Sex Marital Ther. 2007;33:41–53. doi:10.1080/00926230600998466.
84. Baumeister R, Catanese K, Vohs K. Is there a gender difference in strength of sex drive? Theoretical views, conceptual distinctions, and a review of relevant evidence. Pers Soc Psychol Rev. 2001;5:242–73.
85. Regan PC, Atkins L. Sex differences and similarities in frequency and intensity of sexual desire. SBP J. 2006;34:95–102.
86. Barlow D. Causes of sexual dysfunction: the role of anxiety and cognitive interference. J Consult Clin Psychol. 1986;54:140–8.
87. Beck JG, Barlow DH. The effects of anxiety and attentional focus on sexual responding—I: physiological patterns in erectile dysfunction. Res Ther. 1986;24:9–17.
88. Beck JG, Barlow DH. The effects of anxiety and attentional focus on sexual responding—II: cognitive and affective patterns in erectile dysfunction. Behav Res Ther. 1986;24:19–26.
89. Kennedy S, Dickens S, Eisfeld B, Bagby R. Sexual dysfunction before antidepressant therapy in major depression. J Affect Disord. 1999;56:201–8.
90. Lykins AD, Janssen E, Graham CA. The relationship between negative mood and sexuality in heterosexual college woman and men. J Sex Res. 2006;43:136–43. doi:10.1080/00224490609552308.
91. Mathew R, Weinman M. Sexual dysfunctions in depression. Arch Sex Behav. 1982;11:323–8.

92. Cochran SD, Mays VM, Sullivan JG. Prevalence of mental disorders, psychological distress, and mental health services use among lesbian, gay, and bisexual adults in the United States. J Consult Clin Psychol. 2003;71:53–61.
93. de Graaf R, Sandfort TG, tem Have M. Suicidality and sexual orientation: differences between men and women in a general population-based sample from the Netherlands. Arch Sex Behav. 2006;35:253–62. doi:10.1007/s10508-006-9020-z.
94. Mays VM, Cochran SD. Mental health correlates of perceived discrimination among lesbian, gay, and bisexual adults in the United States. Am J Public Health. 2001;91:1869–76.
95. Bancroft J, Janssen E, Strong D, Carnes L, Vukadinovic Z, Long S. The relation between mood and sexuality in heterosexual men. Arch Sex Behav. 2003;32:217–30.
96. Dove NL, Wiederman MW. Cognitive distraction and women's sexual functioning. J Sex Marital Ther. 2000;26:67–78. doi:10.1080/009262300278650.
97. Lacefield K, Negy C. Non-erotic cognitive distractions during sexual activity in sexual minority and heterosexual young adults. Arch Sex Behav. 2012;41:391–400. doi:10.1007/s10508-011-9792-7.
98. Nobre P. Male sexual dysfunctions. In: Hofmann JG, editor. The Wiley handbook of cognitive behavioral therapy. Part two. Wiley-Blackwell; 2013 New Jersey p. 645–72.
99. Carvalho J, Nobre P. Sexual desire in women: an integrative approach regarding psychological, medical, and relationship dimensions. J Sex Med. 2010;7:1807–15. doi:10.1111/j.1743-6109.2010.01716.x.
100. Carvalho J, Nobre P. Predictors of women's sexual desire: the role of psychopathology, cognitive-emotional determinants, relationship dimensions, and medical factors. J Sex Med. 2010;7:928–37. doi:10.1111/j.1743-6109.2009.01568.x.
101. Carvalho J, Nobre P. Gender issues and sexual desire: the role of emotional and relationship variables. J Sex Med. 2010;7:2469–78. doi:10.1111/j.1743-6109.2009.01689.x.
102. Carvalho J, Nobre P. Biopsychosocial determinants of men's sexual desire: testing an integrative model. J Sex Med. 2011;8:754–63. doi:10.1111/j.1743-6109.2010.02156.x.
103. Carvalho J, Nobre P. Predictors of men's sexual desire: the role of psychological, cognitive-emotional, relational and medical factors. J Sex Res. 2011;48:254–62. doi:10.1080/00224491003605475.
104. Nobre P. Determinants of sexual desire problems in women: testing a cognitive-emotional model. J Sex Marital Ther. 2009;35:360–77. doi:10.1080/00926230903065716.
105. Nobre P. Psychological determinants of erectile dysfunction: testing a cognitive-emotional model. J Sex Med. 2010;7:1429–37. doi:10.1111/j.1743-6109.2009.01656.x.
106. Nobre P, Pinto-Gouveia J. Dysfunctional sexual beliefs as vulnerability factors for sexual dysfunction. J Sex Res. 2006;43(1):68–75.
107. Nobre P, Pinto-Gouveia J. Emotions during sexual activity: differences between sexually functional and dysfunctional men and women. Arch Sex Behav. 2006;35:491–9. doi:10.1007/s10508-006-9047-1.
108. Nobre P, Pinto-Gouveia J. Differences in automatic thoughts presented during sexual activity between sexually functional and dysfunctional men and women. Cognit Ther Res. 2008;32:37–49. doi:10.1007/s10608-007-9165-7.
109. Nobre P, Pinto-Gouveia J. Cognitive and emotional predictors of female sexual dysfunctions: preliminary findings. J Sex Marital Ther. 2008;34:325–42. doi:10.1080/00926230802096358.
110. Nobre P, Pinto-Gouveia J. Cognitions, emotions, and sexual response: analysis of the relationship among automatic thoughts, emotional responses, and sexual arousal. Arch Sex Behav. 2008;37:652–61. doi:10.1007/s10508-007-9258-0.
111. Nobre P, Pinto-Gouveia J. Cognitive schemas associated with negative sexual events: a comparison of men and women with and without sexual dysfunction. Arch Sex Behav. 2009;38:842–51. doi:10.1007/s10508-008-9450-x.
112. Oliveira C, Nobre P. The role of trait-affect, depression, and anxiety in women with sexual dysfunction: a pilot study. J Sex Marital Ther. 2013;39:436–52. doi:10.1080/0092623X.2012.665813.
113. Oliveira C, Nobre P. Cognitive structures in women with sexual dysfunction: the role of early maladaptative schemas. J Sex Med. 2013;10:1755–63. doi:10.1111/j.1743-6109.2012.02737.x.
114. Quinta-Gomes A, Nobre P. Personality traits and psychopathology on male sexual dysfunction: an empirical study. J Sex Med. 2011;8:461–9. doi:10.1111/j.1743-6109.2010.02092.
115. Quinta-Gomes A, Nobre P. Early maladaptive schemas and sexual dysfunction in men. Arch Sex Behav. 2012;41:311–20. doi:10.1007/s10508-011-9853-y.
116. Soares C, Nobre P. Sexual problems, cultural beliefs, and psychosexual therapy in Portugal. In: Hall K, Graham C, editors. The cultural context of sexual pleasure and problems: psychotherapy with diverse clients. New York: Routledge; 2012. p. 278–306.
117. Peixoto MM, Nobre P. Dysfunctional sexual beliefs: a comparative study with heterosexual men and women, gay men, and lesbian women, with and without sexual problems. J Sex Med. 2014;11:2690–700. doi:10.1111/jsm.12666.
118. Peixoto MM, Nobre P. Cognitive schemas activated in sexual context: a comparative study with homosexual and heterosexual men and women, with and without sexual problems. Cognit Ther Res. 2015;39:390–402. doi:10.1007/s10608-014-9661-5.
119. Peixoto MM, Nobre P. Personality traits, sexual problems, and sexual orientation: an empirical study. J Sex Marital Ther. 2016;42:199–213. doi:10.1080/0092623X.2014.985352.
120. Heiman JR, LoPiccolo J. Becoming orgasmic: a sexual and personal growth program for women. Rev. ed. New York: Prentice-Hall; 1988.
121. Zilbergeld B. The new male sexuality. Rev. ed. New York: Batam Books; 1999.
122. Hart TA, Schwartz DR. Cognitive-behavioral erectile dysfunction treatment for gay men. Cogn Behav Pract. 2010;17:66–76.
123. Little CA, Byers ES. Differences between positive and negative sexual cognitions. Can J Hum Sex. 2000;9:167–79.
124. Renaud CA, Byers ES. Exploring the frequency, diversity, and content of university students' positive and negative sexual cognitions. Can J Hum Sex. 1999;8:17–30.
125. Renaud CA, Byers ES. Positive and negative sexual cognitions: subjective experience and relationships to sexual adjustment. J Sex Res. 2001;38:252–62.
126. Rowland DL, Georgoff VL, Burnett AL. Psychoaffective differences between sexually functional and dysfunctional men in response to a sexual experience. J Sex Med. 2011;8:132–9. doi:10.1111/j.1743-6109.2010.01904.x.
127. Peixoto MM, Nobre P. Automatic thoughts during sexual activity, distressing sexual symptoms, and sexual orientation: findings from a web-survey. J Sex Marital Ther. 2016;42:616–34. doi:10.1080/0092623X.2015.1113583.
128. Peixoto MM, Nobre P. Positive and negative affect during sexual activity: differences between sexually dysfunctional and healthy heterosexual and homosexual men and women. J Sex Marital Ther. 2016;42:4–17. doi:10.1080/0092623X.2014.996929.
129. Frühauf S, Gerger H, Munder T, Schmidt H, Barth J. Efficacy of psychological interventions for sexual dysfunctions: a systematic review and meta-analysis. Arch Sex Behav. 2013;42:915–33.

29 Sex and the Heart

Anjali Chandra, Almaz Borjoev, and Ernst R. Schwarz

Introduction

Data extrapolated from various studies have shown that erectile dysfunction is a highly prevalent condition, affecting more than 50% of men over the age of 60. It is estimated that 15–30 million men in the USA report sexual dysfunction [1]. It is further estimated that 10% of men aged 30–39 years have erectile dysfunction with prevalence increasing to over 50% of men aged 70–79 years. Particularly, prevalence of severe erectile dysfunction increases significantly with age, with more than 35% of men over age 70 reporting difficulty in attaining or maintaining erections sufficient for sexual performance [2].

Although multiple epidemiological studies highlight aging as the largest risk factor, erectile dysfunction is a multifactorial problem with vasculogenic, pharmacogenic, neurogenic, hormonal, surgical, medical, and psychogenic factors involved. Recent evidence demonstrates well-established pathophysiologic and epidemiologic links between erectile dysfunction and risk factors for cardiovascular disease [3]. The Massachusetts Male Aging Study identified heart disease, diabetes mellitus, and hypertension as major risk factors for incident erectile dysfunction over 8.8 years of follow-up in men aged 40–69 years [4]. Patients with preexisting cardiovascular disease are at increased risk of experiencing erectile dysfunction. Moreover, research conducted over the past 15 years recognizes erectile dysfunction as a marker of increased cardiovascular risk, notably in younger men. Erectile dysfunction is often an early symptom of systemic vascular disease, which may precipitate cardiac events [5]. Therefore, although erectile dysfunction and cardiovascular disease are different clinical manifestations, the pathophysiology is closely linked.

Vascular Causes of Erectile Dysfunction

The most frequent cause of erectile dysfunction is vasculogenic in nature, involving atherosclerosis and endothelial dysfunction as the underlying mechanism. Normal erectile function is multifactorial, being modulated by neurogenic, hormonal, and psychogenic factors; however, endothelial integrity is an essential factor to the physiology of erections. After the initial release of neurotransmitters, sexual stimulation leads to nitric oxide production and other endothelial factors with subsequent relaxation of arterial smooth muscles supplying erectile tissues, thereby increasing blood flow to the penis. As increased blood flow expands the cavernous sinusoids, simultaneous compression of the venous plexus occurs resulting in occluded venous outflow. As a result, blood is trapped within the corpora cavernosa producing an increase in intracavernous pressure, leading to full and rigid erection.

Erectile dysfunction occurs in the setting of compromised vascular integrity with endothelial dysfunction as the proposed underlying mechanism. Reduced availability of nitric oxide serves as the common pathogenesis of erectile dysfunction and coronary artery disease. Structural vascular abnormalities leading to atherosclerosis and flow-limiting stenosis are a result of impaired endothelial-dependent vasodilation (Figure 29-1).

A commonly proposed mechanism correlating erectile dysfunction and coronary artery disease is the artery-size hypothesis. Common risk factors such as hypertension, diabetes mellitus, obesity and smoking predispose to endothelial dysfunction and flow-limiting stenosis. Atherosclerosis is a generalized process, therefore it is hypothesized that all vascular beds are impacted the same. It is the artery size itself that determines the onset and severity of symptoms. Larger vessels adapt to the same amount of endothelial dysfunction and resulting atherosclerosis better than smaller vessels. Due to the small vessel size of penile arteries (1–2 mm) compared to that of coronary arteries (3–4 mm), atherosclerosis leads to a more significant reduction of blood flow to erectile tissues compared to that seen in coronary arteries. Based on this pathophysiologic mechanism, the penile vascular bed is an indicator of systemic vascular diseases and erectile dysfunction should precede coronary artery disease. In this framework, Montorsi et al. investigated the prevalence

W.W. IsHak (ed.), *The Textbook of Clinical Sexual Medicine*, DOI 10.1007/978-3-319-52539-6_29

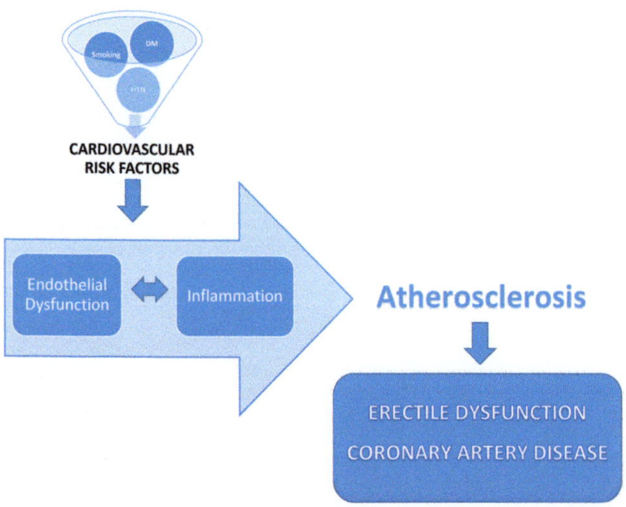

FIGURE 29-1. The relationship of endothelial dysfunction, low-grade chronic inflammation, and atherosclerosis in the pathogenesis of erectile dysfunction and coronary artery diseases.

of erectile dysfunction in patients with coronary artery disease and evaluated the association between the severity of erectile dysfunction and the degree of coronary vessel involvement. One hundred and eighty patients with coronary artery disease confirmed via angiography were divided into three groups: (1) acute coronary syndrome and one-vessel disease, (2) acute coronary syndrome and two- to three-vessel disease, and (3) chronic stable angina. In each group of patients, the extent of erectile dysfunction was determined by the International Index of Erectile Function (IIEF) questionnaire. The key finding of the study demonstrated that erectile dysfunction occurs prior to cardiac symptoms in virtually all patients with chronic coronary syndrome with a time interval of 3 year, whereas patients with acute coronary syndrome have a low prevalence of sexual dysfunction.

Arterial Hypertension and Erectile Dysfunction

Arterial hypertension is a major cardiovascular risk factor that is strongly associated with erectile dysfunction. Erectile dysfunction is frequently encountered in hypertensive men compared to normotensive individuals. The coexistence of arterial hypertension and erectile dysfunction increases with advancing age, the severity and duration of hypertension, and the presence of additional cardiovascular risk factors [6].

Erectile dysfunction is an indicator of asymptomatic coronary artery disease, hence the importance of identifying early symptoms in patients with hypertension. Erectile dysfunction represents a vascular compromise in penile arteries resulting from atheroscelortic lesions. Sexual problems precede cardiovascular symptoms due to the remarkably small diameter of penile arteries in comparison to coronary arteries. Erectile dysfunction is said to appear 3–5 years before the onset of symptomatic coronary artery disease, therefore representing an early diagnostic sign of heart disease. However, despite its clinical significance, erectile dysfunction remains a largely unidentified and undertreated disease entity [7].

Data gathered from multiple studies indicate a positive association between elevated blood pressure and the structural compromise noted in penile arteries. Although arterial hypertension should be treated as a protective measure, reduction in blood pressure attenuates the vascular compromise and thereby worsens erectile function [8]. Many antihypertensive agents further exacerbate erectile dysfunction a drug-specific side effect. The older antihypertensive agents such as thiazide diuretics and beta-adrenergic receptor blockers have the highest incidence of erectile dysfunction [9]. Newer agents such as angiotensin receptor blockers exert neutral effects while agents such as nebivolol provide beneficial effects [10].

Diabetes Mellitus and Erectile Dysfunction

Whether the association of diabetes mellitus with erectile dysfunction is termed vascular-type erectile dysfunction or is summarized as endocrine related remains an academic debate. In any event, diabetes is an established risk factor for sexual dysfunction in men as documented by the Massachusetts Male Aging Study where a threefold increased risk of erectile dysfunction seen in diabetic compared with nondiabetic men [11]. The numerous epidemiological studies do not distinguish between type 1 and type 2 diabetes in being associated with an increased risk of erectile dysfunction [12].

The pathogenesis of erectile dysfunction in diabetes mellitus is multifactorial. Diabetic vasculopathy encompasses macroangiopathy, microangiopathy, and endothelial dysfunction [13]. Macrovascular disease is the result of atherosclerotic damage in the blood vessels, limiting circulation to vascular beds. The endothelial dysfunction caused by the atherosclerotic lesions leads to penile arterial insufficiency, thus the culprit to vascular erectile dysfunction seen in diabetic men.

Similarly, the chronic insult of hyperglycemia on the endothelium results in endothelial dysfunction, linking erectile dysfunction to coronary artery disease. Endothelial dysfunction in diabetes is manifested as the decreased bioavailability of nitric oxide, resulting in insufficient relaxation of the vascular smooth muscle of the corpora cavernosa.

Microvascular disease encompasses ischemic damage in the distal circulation and neuropathic complications. In diabetics, sensory impulses from the penis to the reflexogenic erectile center are impaired, and the reduced or absent parasympathetic activity necessary for relaxation of the smooth muscle of the corpus cavernous contributes to the erectile dysfunction seen in these patients [14].

Due to its multifactorial etiology, the treatment of erectile dysfunction in diabetic men requires a comprehensive approach. For diabetic patients a strong association between glycemic control and the prevalence of erectile dysfunction is well established. Therefore, initial treatment focuses to correct the modifiable risk factors and promote lifestyle changes. Tight glycemic control, achieved by increased physical activity, a Mediterranean diet, and reduced caloric intake, so as to maintain an HbA_{1c} concentration < 7%, is recommended for adults with diabetes to minimize the risk of long-term complications. However, reversal of erectile dysfunction after aggressive treatment of diabetes mellitus has not been compelling. Most likely, treatment must be initiated at a very early stage of the disease process to be effective. Intensified glucose control, along with treatment of associated risk factors, may also prevent sexual dysfunction, even if improvement is not achieved [15].

Heart Failure and Erectile Dysfunction

Heart failure is the leading entity in cardiovascular medicine and the prevalence in the USA is estimated at 5.3 million by the American Heart Association [16].

According to the Massachusetts Male Aging study, in healthy men between the ages of 40 and 70 years, over half reported some degree of erectile dysfunction [4]. Sharing similar risk factors, patients concomitantly present with heart failure and erectile dysfunction. In particular, diabetes mellitus, hypertension, obesity, and smoking are underlying factors in cardiovascular disease and erectile dysfunction. In addition, side effects from drugs such as thiazide diuretics, digoxin, and some beta-adrenergic receptor blockers are reported to induce and worsen erectile dysfunction in men [17]. Moreover, left ventricular dysfunction in advanced stages leads to reduced cardiac capacity, reduced physical functioning, and decreased exercise tolerance secondary to generalized muscle weakness. These combined factors augment the development and worsening of erectile dysfunction in men. Heart failure patients experience symptoms of decreased libido and frequency of sexual intercourse, erectile dysfunction, negative changes in sexual performance, and general dissatisfaction related to their sexual function. The multifactorial causes of sexual dysfunction in heart failure include reduced cardiac capacity, endothelial dysfunction, hormonal imbalances, as well as medication side effects. It is estimated that 60–89% of heart failure patients have some extent of erectile dysfunction [16].

Medications and Erectile Dysfunction

Antihypertensive agents represent one of the most implicated classes of drugs in erectile dysfunction. Older antihypertensive drugs (central-acting, beta-adrenergic receptor blockers, and diuretics) are commonly associated with erectile dysfunction, while the newer agents such as calcium antagonists, angiotensin-converting enzyme (ACE) inhibitors, and angiotensin receptor blockers (ARBs) have demonstrated neutral or possible beneficial effects with regard to sexual function (Table 29-1). Several studies revealed that patients discontinued treatment for hypertension due to erectile dysfunction, albeit real or perceived. Whether the high prevalence of erectile dysfunction seen in hypertensive patients is a result of the disease process, the antihypertensive treatment agents or the combination of both remains to be clarified [26].

Angiotensin Receptor Blockers

As supported by several clinical studies, ARBs have a beneficial effect on sexual function in hypertensive patients. In a cohort of small studies conducted during the past 20 years, patients on ARB therapy showed increased sexual activity and sexual satisfaction. In a study conducted by Llisterri et al., 82 hypertensive patients with erectile dysfunction treated with losartan reported improved sexual satisfaction from an initial 7.3–58.5% ($p = 0.001$). An additional study comparing valsartan with carvedilol on untreated hypertensive patients without erectile dysfunction, demonstrated improved sexual activity with valsartan treatment. During the first month of treatment, sexual activity declined from 8.3 to 6.6 sexual intercourse episodes per month. With ongoing valsartan treatment, sexual activity fully recovered and improved to 10.2 sexual intercourse episodes per month [18].

In a larger study conducted by Della Chiesa et al., hypertensive patients treated with valsartan reported an increase in sexual intercourse per week from 1.0 to 1.6 times during follow-up ($p < 0.0001$). The initial outcomes reporting beneficial effects on erectile function with ARB treatment require further studies to confirm these findings [20].

Angiotensin Converting Enzyme Inhibitors

When compared to ARBs, ACE inhibitors have neutral effects on erectile dysfunction in hypertensive patients. Multiple studies provide data that treatment with ACE

TABLE 29-1. Antihypertensive agents and their effect on erectile function

Antihypertensive drug	Effect on erectile function	Clinical study	Results
Angiotensin receptor blockers			
Losartan	+	Llisterri et al. [18]	Marked increase of self-reported sexual satisfaction; losartan treatment improved sexual satisfaction from an initial 7.3 to 58.5% (chi2; $p = 0.001$)
Valsartan	+	Fogari et al. [19]	Improved sexual activity; 1st month of valsartan treatment, sexual activity declined from 8.3 to 6.6 sexual intercourse episodes (p = NS). With ongoing valsartan treatment, sexual activity fully recovered and improved (10.2 sexual intercourse episodes per month)
		Della Chiesa et al. [20]	Increase in sexual intercourse per week from 1.0 to 1.6 times during follow-up ($p < 0.0001$)
Angiotensin-converting enzyme inhibitors			
Lisinopril	+/–	Fogari et al. [21]	Neutral effects on sexual interest, erectile function, orgasmic ability, and satisfaction. Initial treatment showed significant decline in sexual intercourse episodes per month from 7.1 ± 4.0 to 5.0 ± 2.5, $p < .05$ v placebo. With ongoing lisinopril treatment, sexual activity recovered (7.7 ± 4.0 sexual intercourse episodes per month)
Calcium channel antagonists			
Nifedipine	+/–	Kroner et al. [22]	Neutral effects on sexual function
Beta-adrenergic receptor blockers			
Atenolol	–	Suzuki et al. [23]	Significantly reduced the number of intercourse events per month from 7.8 to 4.2 ($p < 0.01$ compared with pretreatment and placebo)
Carvedilol	–	Kloner et al. [24]	Sexual intercourse episodes per month were reduced from 8.2 to 3.7 ($p < 0.01$ compared with baseline)
x	+	Brixius et al. [25]	Substitution of β adrenergic receptor blockers with nebivolol resulted in significant improvement in erectile function in patients
Thiazide diuretics			
Chlorthalidone	–	Trial of Antihypertensive Interventions and Management (TAIM) trial [27]	Erection-related problems worsened in 28% of men receiving chlorthalidone, compared with 11% of those receiving atenolol and 3% of those receiving placebo ($p < 0.009$)
		Treatment of Mild Hypertension Study (TOMHS)	Participants randomized to chlorthalidone reported a significantly higher incidence of erection problems at 2 years than participants randomized to placebo (17.1% vs. 8.1%; $p = 0.025$). However, the difference between the two groups was not statistically significant at 4 years (chlorthalidone 18.3% and placebo 16.7%)
Aldosterone receptor antagonists	Limited information		
Renin inhibitor	Limited information		
Centrally acting antihypertensives	Limited information		

inhibitors provide no significant impact on sexual interest, erectile function, orgasmic ability, and sexual satisfaction. In examining the quality of life of patients on antihypertensive therapy, Fogari et al. demonstrated the neutral effects seen with ACE inhibitors. Initial treatment with lisinopril showed significant decline in sexual intercourse episodes per month from 7.1 ± 4.0 to 5.0 ± 2.5 ($p < .05$) versus placebo; however, with continued treatment, sexual activity recovered in patients (7.7 ± 4.0 sexual intercourse episodes per month) [21].

Calcium Channel Antagonists

Currently the data regarding the effect of calcium antagonists on erectile function remains inconclusive. The available data, however, establishes a neutral effect. Early studies assessing the effects of nifedipine and diltiazem show no changes in sexual function. Suzuki et al. studied sexual dysfunction induced by antihypertensive agents during a one-year period. Patients self-reported symptoms of reduction in sexual desire, problems in obtaining and maintaining an erection, problems in ejaculation and the number of occasions of sexual intercourse. After initiating daily nifedipine treatment in hypertensive patients, subsequent sexual dysfunction, mainly problems with ejaculation, was reported by patients during the 1-month evaluation. In the long-term follow-up (1-year period), sexual dysfunction resolved and was no longer reported by patients on nifedipine treatment [23].

Beta-Adrenergic Receptor Blockers

Long-standing data has associated beta-adrenergic receptor blocker therapy, primarily older generation beta-blockers, as a major cause of erectile dysfunction. Suzuki et al. demonstrated the negative effect of atenolol on sexual function. Patients reported a reduced number of sexual intercourse events per month from 7.8 to 4.2 ($p < 0.01$ compared with pretreatment and placebo) [23]. Kloner et al. demonstrated similar results obtained with carvedilol therapy; sexual intercourse episodes per month were reduced from 8.2 to 3.7 ($p < 0.01$ compared with baseline) [24].

Conversely, preliminary data from studies conducted on newer beta adrenergic receptor blocker therapies have revealed beneficial effects on erectile function. Brixius et al. found that the substitution of beta-adrenergic receptor blockers with nebivolol resulted in significant improvement in erectile function in hypertensive patients on beta-adrenergic receptor blocker monotherapy [25].

Thiazide Diuretics

When compared to other antihypertensive therapies, thiazide diuretics are commonly thought to disproportionally predispose to erectile dysfunction and sexual dysfunction, as evidenced by two large randomized studies conducted in the USA. In the Trial of Antihypertensive Interventions and Management (TAIM) study, erection-related problems worsened in 28% of men receiving chlorthalidone, compared with 11% of those receiving atenolol and 3% of those receiving placebo ($p < 0.009$). In the Treatment of Mild Hypertension Study (TOMHS), patients randomized to chlorthalidone indicated a significantly higher incidence of erection problems at the 2 year period than patients randomized to placebo (17.1% vs. 8.1%; $p = 0.025$). However, the difference between the two groups was not statistically significant at the 4 year period (chlorthalidone 18.3% and placebo 16.7%). Acebutolol, amlodipine, and enalapril demonstrated effects similar to placebo, while doxazosin exerted positive effects on erectile function (both in patients with and without sexual problems at baseline) [27].

In addition to these larger studies, various studies have been conducted to assess erectile dysfunction, with the majority of available data establishing a negative association between diuretics and erectile function [28].

Although available data on antihypertensive therapy and erectile function demonstrate older generation agents (central-acting, beta-adrenergic receptor blockers, diuretics) negatively affect erectile function, while newer generation agents (calcium antagonists and ACE inhibitors) exert neutral effects, and ARBs exhibit a beneficial effect on erectile function, further, less limiting, studies are warranted to confirm these findings.

Erectile Dysfunction Treatment

Over the years, erectile dysfunction treatment has advanced and continues to be modified with the availability of innovative treatment methods. The treatment comprises of psychosexual therapy, lifestyle modifications, and medical and surgical management. Initially, treatment concentrated on psychotherapeutic approaches alone to treat erectile dysfunction, with limited success. Penile prostheses were subsequently introduced in conjunction with psychotherapy. Later, intracavernosal injections developed as a treatment modality, followed by intraurethral therapy. The introduction of oral phosphodiesterase 5 (PDE5) inhibitors revolutionized the treatment approaches of erectile dysfunction as a nonsurgical approach. Currently, it remains the first-line medical therapy, with three widely available first-generation agents, sildenafil, vardenafil, and tadalafil. Next generation PDE5 inhibitor agents are under development whereas other newer agents, such as avanafil, udenafil, lodenafil, and mirodenafil are not yet approved for use in the USA but have been approved in other countries [29].

Erectile dysfunction remains a challenging entity and improved medications, interventional, and genetic therapies are strongly researched to improve or supplement current treatments. Advancements in medical therapy include guanylate cyclase inhibitors, potassium channel inhibitors, melanocortin system activators, and Rho kinase inhibitors. Surgical approaches include the use of a zotarolimus-eluting stent, benefiting patients with pudendal artery stenosis. Recent studies on gene therapy with the maxi-K potassium channel, given in high doses, showed significant improvement in erectile function. Further research assessing growth factors and cell-based therapies have positive contributions to erectile dysfunction treatments. Likewise, accumulating evidence integrating counseling with new medical and surgical treatments improves efficacy, while simultaneously resulting in patient satisfaction [3]. Figure 29-2 highlights the treatment interventions for erectile dysfunction.

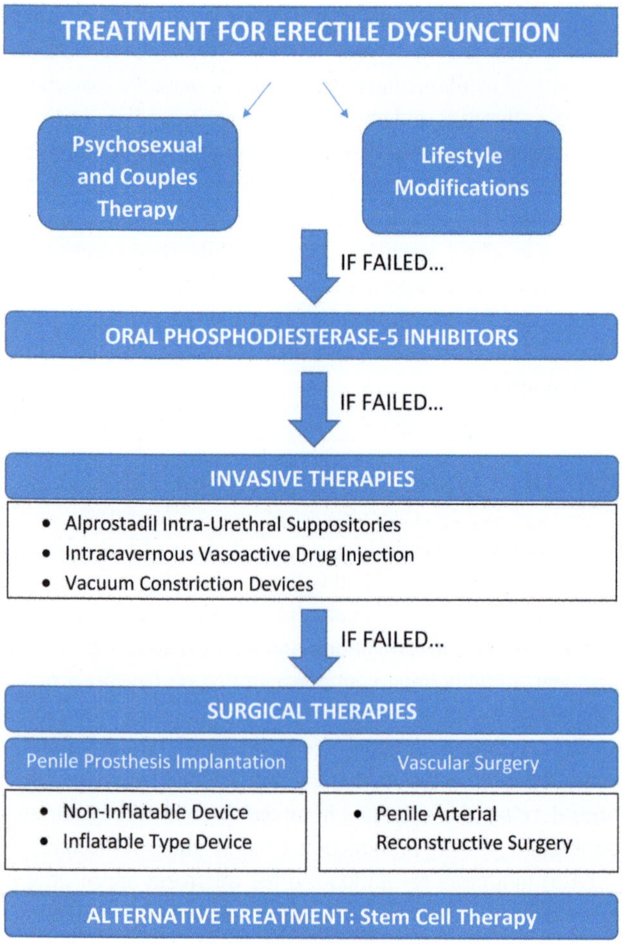

FIGURE 29-2. Treatment for erectile dysfunction.

Stem Cell Therapy for Erectile Dysfunction

Although one of the most widely used options and mainstay treatment for erectile dysfunction, PDE5 inhibitors are limited in their use, namely contraindicated with adjuvant nitrate therapy owing to the synergistic hypotensive effects [30]. PDE5 inhibitors are further limited by the adverse side effect profile, which involve the cardiovascular, digestive, nervous, respiratory, and reproductive systems, rendering them inappropriate for some patients. Moreover, PDE5 inhibitors are limited to and are shown to be partially effective in treating certain types of erectile dysfunction including those associated with diabetes mellitus and nerve injury incurred during surgery, i.e., radical prostatectomy [31]. Consequently, alternative treatment modalities are becoming increasingly appropriate. Recently stem cell therapy has become a focus of experimental and clinical research for the treatment of erectile dysfunction [30].

Numerous studies have explored the ability of stem cells for self-renewal and directed differentiation. Stem cells are understood to differentiate into various cell types including endothelial cells, smooth muscle cells, Schwann cells, and neurons, all key structural and functional components of erectile function [32]. Hence, stem cells represent an emerging therapeutic potential for erectile dysfunction. Several types including bone-marrow mesenchymal stem cells, adipose tissue-derived stem cells, and muscle-derived stem cells, have been investigated for neural, vascular, endothelial, or smooth muscle regeneration in animal models of erectile dysfunction. Limited clinical studies have investigated the potential therapeutic effect of stem cells with differing strategic [30].

A clinical trial of stem cell therapy for erectile dysfunction conducted in Korea included seven type 2 diabetes mellitus (T2DM) men ranging from 57 to 87 years of age, each treated with intracavernous injection of 15 million allogeneic umbilical cord blood stem cells [33]. Three patients reported achieving morning erections within a 1-month period, and six patients within a 3 month period. However, patients were unable to achieve vaginal penetration without sildenafil treatment before sexual intercourse. During an 11-month follow-up, one treated subject reported achieving and maintaining erection adequate for sexual intercourse. Further noted in the study was the ability of stem cell therapy to treat T2DM by reducing blood glucose and glycosylated hemoglobin levels in all patients, with exception to the eldest. This additional finding contributes to the ongoing evidence of the role of stem cell therapy in treating diabetes, as well as systemic therapy achieved by intracavernous injection of stem cells.

Although the current mainstay treatment for erectile dysfunction includes oral PDE5 inhibitors, newer drugs and promising therapeutic approaches in this modern era of medicine are becoming relevant. With the continued clinical challenge of refractory cases of erectile dysfunction, the role of stem cells as a combined therapeutic option in the treatment of erectile dysfunction will gain widespread acceptance as it is the main target for future research endeavors [34].

Female Sexual Dysfunction

Female sexual dysfunction is increasingly attracting more scientific and public interest, and represents a poorly investigated matter. Although sexual dysfunction in females has a higher prevalence compared to males (43% vs. 31%), this phenomenon remains largely under-recognized and rarely investigated by physicians [35]. Female sexual disorders involve multiple aspects including sexual desire, arousal, orgasm, and dyspareunia. The syndromes of clitoral and vaginal vascular insufficiency are directly related to the atherosclerotic process and subsequent decrease genital blood flow of the hypogastric and pudendal arteries. Although female sexual dysfunction has a multifactorial etiology resulting in decreased clitoral engorgement, vascular insufficiency is a main cause [36]. Martins e Silva et al. recently evaluated the incidence of sexual dysfunction in 23 overweight and obese women, using the Female Sexual Function Index (FSFI) [37]. Among the patients with increased risk for sexual dysfunction, all had at least one risk factor for sexual dysfunction, including hypertension, diabetes mellitus, dyslipidemia, cardiovascular disease, and smoking. Dyslipidemia and hypertension showed a higher prevalence, with 61.1% and 33.3%, respectively. Although no clear association can be established between obesity and female sexual dysfunction, it does impact various aspects of sexuality, and the result analysis seen in this investigation demonstrates the need for further research and attention of physicians for patients with female sexual dysfunction.

References

1. Braun M, Wassmer G, Klotz T, Reifenrath B, Mathers M, Engelmann U. Epidemiology of erectile dysfunction: results of the 'Cologne Male Survey'. Int J Impot Res. 2000;12(6):305–11.
2. Lindau ST, Schumm LP, Laumann EO, Levinson W, O'Muircheartaigh CA, Waite LJ. A study of sexuality and health among older adults in the United States. N Engl J Med. 2007;357(8):762–74.
3. Pastuszak AW. Current diagnosis and management of erectile dysfunction. Curr Sex Health Rep. 2014;6(3):164–76. doi:10.1007/s11930-014-0023-9.
4. Feldman HA, Goldstein I, Hatzichristou DG, et al. Impotence and its medical and psychosocial correlates: results of the Massachusetts Male Aging Study. J Urol. 1994;151:54–61.
5. Hackett G, Krychman M, Baldwin D, Bennett N, El-Zawahry A, Graziottin A, Lukasiewicz M, McVary K, Sato Y, Incrocci L. Coronary heart disease, diabetes, and sexuality in men. J Sex Med. 2016;13(6):887–904. doi:10.1016/j.jsxm.2016.01.023.
6. Doumas M, Tsakiris A, Douma S, et al. Factors affecting the increased prevalence of erectile dysfunction in Greek hypertensive compared with normotensive subjects. J Androl. 2006;27:469–77.
7. Sai Ravi Shanker A, Phanikrishna B, Bhaktha Vatsala Reddy C. Association between erectile dysfunction and coronary artery disease and it's severity. Indian Heart J. 2013;65(2):180–6. doi:10.1016/j.ihj.2013.02.013.
8. Doumas M, Viigimaa M, Papademetriou V. Combined antihypertensive therapy and sexual dysfunction: terra incognita. Cardiology. 2013;125(4):232–4.
9. Manolis A, Doumas M. Antihypertensive treatment and sexual dysfunction. Curr Hypertens Rep. 2012;14:285–92.
10. Doumas M, Tsakiris A, Douma S, et al. Beneficial effects of switching from beta-blockers to nebivolol on the erectile function of hypertensive patients. Asian J Androl. 2006;8:177–82.
11. Giugliano F, Maiorino M, Bellastella G, Gicchino M, Giugliano D, Esposito K. Determinants of erectile dysfunction in type 2 diabetes. Int J Impot Res. 2010;22(3):204–9.
12. Maiorino MI, Bellastella G, Esposito K. Diabetes and sexual dysfunction: current perspectives. Diabetes Metab Syndr Obes. 2014;7:95–105. doi:10.2147/DMSO.S36455.
13. Esposito K, Giugliano F, Martedì E, et al. High proportions of erectile dysfunction in men with the metabolic syndrome. Diabetes Care. 2005;28(5):1201–3.
14. Nehra A, Moreland RB. Neurologic erectile dysfunction. Urol Clin North Am. 2001;28(2):289–308.
15. Turek SJ, Hastings SM, Sun JK, King GL, Keenan HA. Sexual dysfunction as a marker of cardiovascular disease in males with 50 or more years of type 1 diabetes. Diabetes Care. 2013;36(10):3222–6.
16. Rosamond W, Flegal K, Furie K, Go A, Greenlund K, Haase N, et al. Heart disease and stroke statistics—2008 update: a report from the American Heart Association Statistics Committee and Stroke Statistics Subcommittee. Circulation. 2008;117:e25–146.
17. Rastogi S, Rodriguez JJ, Kapur V, Schwarz ER. Why do patients with heart failure suffer from erectile dysfunction? A critical review and suggestions on how to approach this problem. Int J Impot Res. 2005;17:S25–36.
18. Llisterri JL, Lozano Vidal JV, Aznar Vicente J, Argaya Roca M, Pol Bravo C, Sanchez Zamorano MA, Ferrario CM. Sexual dysfunction in hypertensive patients treated with losartan. Am J Med Sci. 2001;321(5):336–41.
19. Fogari R, Zoppi A, Poletti L, Marasi G, Mugellini A, Corradi L. Sexual activity in hypertensive men treated with valsartan or carvedilol: a crossover study. Am J Hypertens. 2001;14(1):27–31.
20. Della Chiesa A, Pfiffner D, Meier B, Hess OM. Sexual activity in hypertensive men. J Hum Hypertens. 2003;17(8):515–21.
21. Fogari R, Zoppi A, Corradi L, Mugellini A, Poletti L, Lusardi P. Sexual function in hypertensive males treated with lisinopril or atenolol: a cross-over study. Am J Hypertens. 1998;11(10):1244–7.
22. Kroner BA, Mulligan T, Briggs GC. Effect of frequently prescribed cardiovascular medications on sexual function: a pilot study. Ann Pharmacother. 1993;27(11):1329–32.
23. Suzuki H, Tominaga T, Kumagai H, Saruta T. Effects of first-line antihypertensive agents on sexual function and sex hormones. J Hypertens Suppl. 1988;6(4):S649–51.
24. Kloner RA, Mullin SH, Shook T, Matthews R, Mayeda G, Burstein S, Peled H, Pollick C, Choudhary R, Rosen R, Padma-Nathan H. Erectile dysfunction in the cardiac patient: how common and should we treat? J Urol. 2003;170(2 Pt 2):S46–50 .discussion S50
25. Brixius K, Middeke M, Lichtenthal A, Jahn E, Schwinger RH. Nitric oxide, erectile dysfunction and beta-blocker treatment (MR NOED study): benefit of nebivolol versus metoprolol in hypertensive men. Clin Exp Pharmacol Physiol. 2007;34(4):327–31.
26. Kupelian V, Hall SA, McKinlay JB. Common prescription medication use and erectile dysfunction. Results from the Boston Area Community Health (BACH) Survey. BJU Int. 2013;112(8):1178–87. doi:10.1111/bju.12231.
27. Nicolai MPJ, Liem SS, Both S, et al. A review of the positive and negative effects of cardiovascular drugs on sexual function: a proposed table for use in clinical practice. Neth Heart J. 2014;22(1):11–9. doi:10.1007/s12471-013-0482-z.
28. Javaroni V, Neves MF. Erectile dysfunction and hypertension: impact on cardiovascular risk and treatment. Int J Hyperthermia. 2012;2012:627278. doi:10.1155/2012/627278.
29. Al-Ameri H, Kloner RA. Erectile dysfunction and heart failure: the role of phosphodiesterase type 5 inhibitors. Int J Impot Res. 2009;21(3):149–57. doi:10.1038/ijir.2009.11.
30. Lin C-S, Xin Z-C, Wang Z, et al. Stem cell therapy for erectile dysfunction: a critical review. Stem Cells Dev. 2012;21(3):343–51.
31. Dorsey P, Keel C, Klavens M, Hellstrom WJ. Phosphodiesterase type 5 (PDE5) inhibitors for the treatment of erectile dysfunction. Expert Opin Pharmacother. 2010;11:1109–22.
32. Lin CS, Xin ZC, Deng CH, Ning H, Lin G, Lue TF. Recent advances in andrology-related stem cell research. Asian J Androl. 2008; 10:171–175v.
33. Bahk JY, Jung JH, Han H, Min SK, Lee YS. Treatment of diabetic impotence with umbilical cord blood stem cell intracavernosal transplant. preliminary report of 7 cases. Exp Clin Transplant. 2010;8:150–60.
34. Ismail EA, El-Sakka AI. Innovative trends and perspectives for erectile dysfunction treatment: a systematic review. Arab J Urol. 2016;14(2):84–93. doi:10.1016/j.aju.2016.04.002.

35. Küçükdurmaz F, Efe E, Malkoç Ö, Kolus E, Amasyalı AS, Resim S. Prevalence and correlates of female sexual dysfunction among Turkish pregnant women. Turk J Urol. 2016;42(3):178–83.
36. Pérez-López FR, Chedraui P, Gilbert JJ, Pérez-Roncero G. Cardiovascular risk in menopausal women and prevalent related co-morbid conditions: facing the post-Women's Health Initiative era. Fertil Steril. 2009;92(4):1171–86.
37. Martins e Silva B, Rêgo LM, Galvão MA, Florêncio TM, Cavalcante JC. Incidence of sexual dysfunction in patients with obesity and overweight. Rev Col Bras Cir. 2013;40(3):196–202.

30 Sex and Cancer

Erica Marchand and Andrea Bradford

Introduction

An estimated 14 million new cases of cancer occur each year worldwide, with an estimated 1.7 million new cases annually in the United States alone [1, 2]. Better detection and treatment have improved survival dramatically in recent decades, and currently more than 15 million people in the US are cancer survivors [3]. For many survivors, navigating life after cancer—or with cancer—presents challenges in multiple life domains. Reintegrating sexuality and intimacy is a challenge for many survivors and is the focus of this chapter.

The two most common cancers in the US, breast and prostate cancers, directly affect sexual organs, and many other common cancers have direct or indirect effects on sexuality and sexual function. Treatment providers at all levels of oncology care have a role in assessing and addressing concerns related to sex and intimacy. Given the sensitive nature of the topic, both patients and providers may be hesitant to broach sexuality. Research indicates that patients do want to discuss sexual concerns with providers, but are often embarrassed or unsure whether it is appropriate to bring them up [4, 5]. Patients may rely on providers to ask about sexual concerns [6]. Providers therefore have a crucial role in identifying and treating sexual problems, as patients may only divulge them if asked.

Why Talk About Sex?

In the life and death struggle of cancer treatment and survival, sexual concerns may be an afterthought. However, cancer severely disrupts sexual functioning and satisfaction for many patients [7, 8]. Sexual function and satisfaction are consistently associated with overall quality of life and well-being for adults [9] and are important components of relationship satisfaction for many couples [10, 11]. As cancer survivors recover from illness and rebuild their lives, sexuality is an important area to address.

Recent studies in oncology settings indicate a discrepancy between patients' interest in addressing sexual concerns with their providers, and actually receiving care for such concerns. For example, over 40% of gynecologic and breast cancer survivors surveyed in a large oncology practice reported wanting to discuss sexual health care with their providers, and yet only 7% had done so [4]. Even routine screening for sexual problems is no guarantee of a clinical response. In a recent study of sexual health screening in a long-term breast cancer survivorship clinic, about one in five respondents endorsed one or more sexual problems, but only a minority of these patients had clinical documentation of any further assessment or intervention [12].

Why Don't We Talk About Sex?

What accounts for the difference between patient interest in addressing sexual concerns, and actually discussing them? Reasons patients report for not asking about sexual concerns include embarrassment, fear of offending providers, uncertainty about appropriateness of questions, and uncertainty about which providers to ask questions of. Barriers reported by providers include lack of knowledge, embarrassment, uncertainty of appropriateness of topic, assumption that patient will bring it up, and perceived lack of treatment options [6]. This chapter addresses these barriers and suggests language, resources, and treatment options and referrals that will allow providers to feel more comfortable in discussing sexual topics.

How Does Cancer Affect Sexuality?

Cancer and cancer treatment affect sexuality and sexual function in a multitude of ways, including physical, psychological, emotional, and relationship effects. In the short term, many (but not all) patients undergoing cancer treatment experience a singular focus on understanding and treating the disease that

W.W. IsHak (ed.), *The Textbook of Clinical Sexual Medicine*, DOI 10.1007/978-3-319-52539-6_30

pushes aside many other concerns, including sexual concerns. Patients may experience fatigue, fear, and concern about the outcome of treatment, physical pain, side effects from chemotherapy and radiation, and other experiences that overshadow or diminish sexual concerns or desires [7].

Most of the major categories of primary and adjuvant treatments for cancer have the potential to affect sexuality and sexual function. The effects of these treatments may or may not resolve on their own with time. Surgery, chemotherapy, radiation, and hormone therapy may cause long-term changes in sexual function as follows:

Surgery: Surgical removal of genital or gonadal tissue (e.g., oophorectomy, penectomy, vulvectomy) can have a direct and profound impact on sexual function. However, surgery to other parts of the body can also affect sexual functioning by way of disfigurement, disability, sensory changes, and pain. For example, surgical management of some head and neck cancers may entail some degree of facial disfigurement, resulting in significant body image concerns.

Chemotherapy: Chemotherapy is toxic not only to malignant cells but also to normal cells that grow or divide rapidly (e.g., skin, hair, and bone marrow). Common side effects of chemotherapy include hair loss, mucositis (inflammation of mucosal tissue such as that in the lining of the mouth and vagina), fatigue, neuropathy, and gastrointestinal symptoms. Some specific classes of chemotherapy (e.g., alkylating agents) have especially potent effects on gonadal tissue and can cause short-term or long-term infertility.

Radiation therapy: Ionizing radiation is well known to cause both acute inflammation and long-term scarring of epithelial tissue. Radiation therapy also causes acute and chronic vascular damage, leading to late complications including telangiectasia, atherosclerosis, and tissue ischemia. Radiation exposure to normal tissues adjacent to the tumor site, and to surrounding tissues outside the targeted field ("scatter"), can result in long-term tissue damage. Sexual dysfunction is a common side effect of radiation to the central nervous system, gonads, genitals, and other pelvic organs.

Hormone therapy: Hormonal treatments, common in the treatment of breast and prostate cancers, disrupt the hormonal milieu to discourage growth of hormone-sensitive tumors, often with substantial impact on sexual desire and function.

Sexual Concerns and Intervention Strategies

This section reviews common sexual concerns for men and women surviving cancer. Concerns are organized by gender and discussion of each concern is further divided into risk factors, assessment, and physical/medical and psychosocial intervention strategies. All patients who have been treated for cancer should be screened for sexual concerns at follow-up medical visits.

Cultural Competency

Experiences of sexuality and intimacy are deeply personal for many people, and are influenced by gender, culture, sexual orientation, religion, nationality, family, and other aspects of patients' social context. Assessment and intervention with sexual concerns are ideally grounded in cultural awareness and sensitivity. Cultural norms about sex, sexual behavior, and discussing sexual topics, vary widely among groups and among individuals within groups. Culturally competent practice includes the following considerations [13]:

Self-awareness: What are the provider's own beliefs about sex, its importance, and the appropriateness of discussing it with patients? How do patients' age, gender, ethnicity, sexual orientation, religion, and other characteristics affect provider comfort in broaching sexual topics? It is common to be more comfortable with some aspects of sexuality than others, and more comfortable with some patients than others. Self-awareness about areas of comfort and discomfort can help providers to know when to look out for discomfort getting in the way of effective patient interaction, and when consultation or referral might be appropriate.

Scientific-mindedness: This refers to forming hypotheses about the experience of culturally different patients and gathering more information to support or refute the hypothesis, rather than making assumptions or viewing patients through the lens of the provider's own cultural expectations.

As an example, consider the following case. Peter, a thoughtful, quiet 67-year-old African-American man, retired from a career at the postal service, returns to his urologist's office for a follow-up visit 1 year after radical prostatectomy. He and his wife have had difficulty resuming sexual activity, as Peter has experienced only sporadic erectile function since his surgery and is not sure what to do to address the issue. His urologist's office is some distance from his home in a part of town he does not often drive to. He has found the entire process of prostate cancer stressful, uncomfortable, at times painful, and often embarrassing, and is not particularly looking forward to the visit, though he would like to learn what can be done to improve things sexually. He is not accustomed to sharing so much personal information with anyone, including doctors. When the nurse practitioner, Laura, a friendly, efficient 34-year-old woman who is conducting the patient interview, asks in general terms about his sexual function, he stammers, "Well, it's mostly fine." She notes his answer and indicates "no concerns" in that area of his patient chart. When the urologist, Dr. Smith, a White man in his late

40s, comes into the room to conduct the follow-up examination, he skims the physician assistant's notes and asks, "No sexual concerns?" along with a string of other questions while conducting a physical exam. The patient nervously answers, "Not really;" the doctor congratulates him on healing just fine, and asks him to make a follow-up appointment in 6 months. Peter leaves, relieved it is over but frustrated that he did not ask for the information he wanted.

What happened? Everyone acted with good intentions and asked seemingly appropriate questions. However, Peter was unable to share his concerns, even with a team of competent medical providers. What could the medical office have done differently? They could have been more aware of their hypotheses. When Peter nervously denied sexual problems, the providers may have hypothesized, "He is uncomfortable talking about this and I should not delve further," or "If he had concerns he would bring them up."

These are both valid hypotheses, but could have been tested against the hypothesis, "He is uncomfortable and talking to people both younger and culturally different than him. He might be holding back from embarrassment." To test which hypothesis was true, Laura or Dr. Smith might have said something like, "A lot of people have sexual concerns after prostate cancer and many people find it hard to talk about them. Are there any concerns that you wanted to discuss? This would be an appropriate place to do so." In order to do this, providers have to be aware of their own cultural assumptions (e.g., patients will proactively broach concerns) and be able to take the patient's perspective and create hypotheses about what his or her experience might be.

Acknowledge culture without stereotyping: Another cultural competence skill is to know when is it more helpful to prioritize cultural generalizations (e.g., church and religious faith are important to many Black patients and therefore they may hold conservative beliefs about sex) and when is it more helpful to prioritize individual characteristics (e.g., Peter's reticence about sex has little to do with religion and more to do with discomfort in broaching a personal topic) in understanding patient interactions. Multicultural research [13] has proposed that culturally competent providers engage in a process called *dynamic sizing*—flexibility in deciding when to generalize and when to individualize when conceptualizing patients. In this example, the provider might hold general knowledge as a hypothesis to be tested until further information about the individual patient is available.

Culture-specific knowledge: Cultural groups share history and experiences that shape their beliefs and behavior, and it is often helpful to have some basic knowledge of the experience of cultural groups different than one's own. In this example, Peter is a Black man who grew up in the USA in the 1950s and in his lifetime has had multiple experiences with people in positions of power, including doctors, which have engendered caution in his interactions with them. With this culture-specific knowledge, a provider can make more informed hypotheses—for example, that Peter's reticence may be due to discomfort or fear of being misunderstood rather than the actual absence of concerns.

Cultural awareness, sensitivity, and skill ideally underlie all patient interactions, and are particularly important with personal or culturally influenced domains like sexuality.

Sexual Difficulties in Men with Cancer

Erectile Dysfunction

Risk Factors

Erectile dysfunction (ED) can result from treatment for many cancers, especially when surgery or radiation to the pelvic area damage nerves or tissues related to erectile function. Common cancers with this side effect include prostate, bladder, and colorectal cancers. For some men, treatment of bone marrow or lymphatic cancers can result in genital graft-vs.-host disease with associated scarring, pain, and penile curvature with erections.

Prostate cancer is the most commonly diagnosed cancer among men in the United States [2], Most forms of treatment for prostate cancer—prostatectomy, radiation, and androgen deprivation therapy—carry the risk of ED.

Prostatectomy and other surgeries: Radical prostatectomy (RP), even using nerve-sparing procedures, is associated with at least temporary ED for 30–87% of patients [14]. Estimates range widely due in part to differences in measurement instruments, specified outcomes, and timing of postoperative assessment of erectile function. Prostatectomy leads to ED by damaging the nerves on the surface of the prostate that create erections, and sometimes by damage to penile arteries. In addition to these factors, loss of regular erections causes further deterioration of erectile tissues. Figure 30-1 illustrates multiple contributors to the development of ED after radical prostatectomy.

Many men regain some amount of erectile function within 6–24 months after prostatectomy, with better outcomes observed in men who use some form of "penile rehabilitation"—use of oral phosphodiesterase type-5 inhibitors (PDE-5i) or intracavernosal injections to maintain penile blood flow and/or to assist erectile function during sexual activity [14]. Recovery of erectile function without any pharmacologic intervention 6–12 months after nerve-sparing RP ranges from 4% (recovery of preoperative erectile function) to 29% of men reporting erectile function sufficient for vaginal penetration. With some form of penile rehabilitation, estimates range from 29% to 86% of men reporting erectile function sufficient for vaginal penetration at 6–12 months post-surgery [14]. Unfortunately, little research exists with

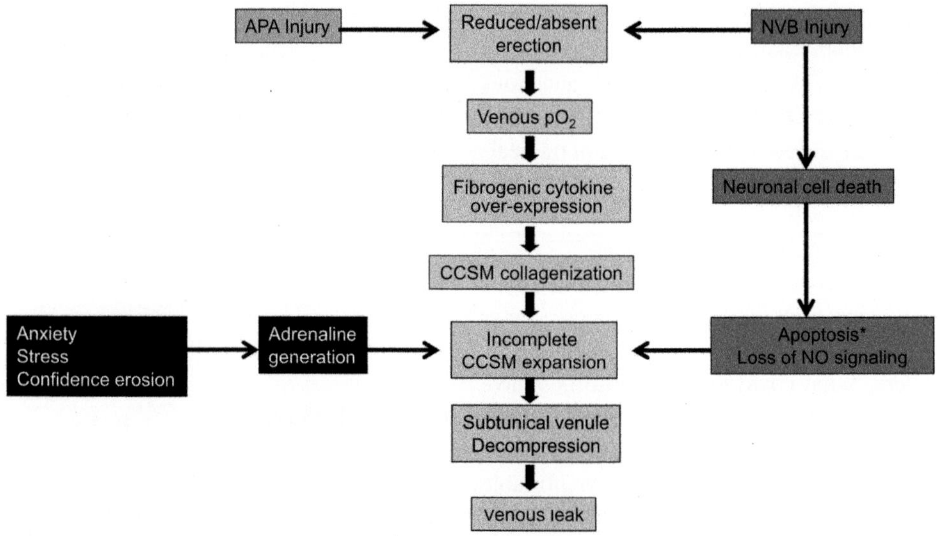

FIGURE 30-1. Schematic representing the pathophysiology of erectile dysfunction after radical prostatectomy. *Apoptosis occurs in nerves, smooth muscle, and endothelium as a result of neural trauma. *APA* accessory pudendal artery, *CCSM* corpora cavernosa smooth muscle, *NVB* neurovascular bundle, pO_2 partial pressure of oxygen. [Reprinted from Mulhall JP, Bivalacqua TJ, Becher EF. Standard operating procedure for the preservation of erectile function outcomes after radical prostatectomy. Journal of Sexual Medicine. 2013;10(1):195–203 with permission from Elsevier].

men for whom penile-vaginal intercourse is not a primary outcome (e.g., men who have sex with men, single men, or men in relationships in which vaginal penetration is not part of sex for some other reason). Variation in reported outcomes is due in part to differing medications, dosages, treatment protocols, and measured outcomes across studies. Table 30-1 summarizes erectile function outcomes from trials of penile rehabilitation after radical prostatectomy. Variability in erectile function post-RP is also influenced by premorbid erectile function, patient age (with younger patients recovering greater function), and surgical variables such as surgeon skill and preservation of nerves [15].

Radical cystectomy for bladder cancer also involves removal of the prostate and seminal vesicles, and has similar risks for erectile function. For some men, treatment of bone marrow or lymphatic cancers with bone marrow transplants can result in genital graft-vs.-host disease with associated scarring, pain, and penile curvature with erections.

Radiation. Both external-beam and seed implant radiation to the prostate are also associated with ED, though onset is later than with prostatectomy [15]. The type of external-beam radiation matters, with more precisely targeted methods such as three-dimensional conformal radiation therapy (3D-CRT) and intensity-modulated radiation therapy (IMRT) causing less damage to erectile function. Similarly, more precise placement of radioactive seeds is associated with fewer sexual side effects [15].

Radiation contributes to ED by damaging the lining of blood vessels in and near the penis, damaging the nerves that create erections, and, in some cases, damaging erectile tissues so that they are unable to hold blood in the penis to maintain erection (a condition called venous leak). Erection problems show up, on average, 1 year after radiation, though the peak negative effects on erections often occur 3–5 years post-treatment. Problems associated with venous leak may occur shortly after radiation. Long-term studies of erectile function post-radiation provide estimates of 37–59% incidence of erectile problems at 3-year follow-up [15].

Assessment

The most common written assessment tool for ED is the International Index of Erectile Function (IIEF) [16]. The brief 5-item version of the scale (IIEF-5 [17]) is a reliable self-report measure of erectile function. One limitation of the IIEF-5 is that it was designed to assess erectile function during penile–vaginal intercourse, and some items may not be applicable to men who have sex with men, or those who are not attempting intercourse. Alternatively, a briefer, validated one-item checklist questionnaire assessing multiple domains of sexual function may be used to screen for sexual problems including ED [18]. For more comprehensive written assessment or for research purposes, the Patient-Reported Outcomes Measurement Information System Sexual Function and Satisfaction measure (PROMIS SexFS) [19] includes items assessing various domains of sexual function and has been validated with individuals with cancer.

Conducting a clinical interview is also an appropriate way to screen for ED, with the advantage of being more personal

Table 30-1. Pharmacological erectile rehabilitation studies

Author	Year	N[a]	Design	Intervention	Outcomes summary
Montorsi	1997	27	Single-center, non-PC, RCT	IC alprostadil vs. no treatment	Natural erection (unassisted) at 6 months 67% ICI vs. 20% non-treatment
Mulhall	2005	132	Single-center, non-R, comparative analysis (rehab vs. no rehab)	Sildenafil nonresponders used ICI	Erectile function recovery at 18 months Natural erection: 52% rehab vs. 19% non-rehab Sildenafil response: 64% rehab vs. 24% non-rehab ICI response: 95% rehab vs. 76% non-rehab
Bannowsky	2008	41	Single center non-R, comparative analysis in patients with preserved nocturnal erections (rehab vs. no rehab)	25 mg sildenafil (s) nightly vs. no treatment (c)	SHIM score: (s) Pre: 20.8 at 12 months: 14.1 (c) Pre: 21.2; at 12 months: 9.3 Erections sufficient for vaginal penetration: 47 (s) vs. 28% (c) without sildenafil on demand 86 (s) vs. 66% (c) with sildenafil on demand
Padma- Nathan	2008	76	Multicenter, DB, PC-RCT	Sildenafil 100 mg vs. sildenafil 50 mg vs. placebo	Return to baseline erectile function at 11 months Sildenafil 27% vs. placebo 4% RigiScan "responders": 100 mg: 33%, 50 mg: 24%, placebo: 5%
Montorsi	2008	423	Multicenter, DB, PC-RCT	Vardenafil 10 mg nightly + placebo for sex (N); Vardenafil 10 or 20 mg for sex + placebo nightly (OD); Placebo for sex and placebo nightly (P)	Proportion EFD ≥ 22 At 9 months: N 32%, OD 48%, P 25% At 11 months: N 24%, OD 29%, P 29% At 13 months: N 53%, OD 54%, P 48% % with "yes" response to SEP 3[b] At 9 months: N 34%, OD 46%, P 25% At 11 months: N 32%, OD 42%, P 34% At 13 months: not reported

NO nitric oxide, *RCT* randomized controlled trial, *Non-R* non-randomized, *PC* placebo-controlled, *DB* double-blind, *ICI* intracavernosal injection, *SHIM* Sexual Health Inventory for Men, *SEP 3* Sexual Encounter Profile (3-item version). [Reprinted from Mulhall JP, Bivalacqua TJ, Becher EF. Standard operating procedure for the preservation of erectile function outcomes after radical prostatectomy. Journal of Sexual Medicine. 2013;10(1):195–203. with permission from Elsevier].

[a]*N*: number of completers.

[b]Data derived from Figures 3 and 4 of REINVENT paper.

and specific to an individual than a written assessment. Verbal screening questions might include whether the patient has any sexual concerns he would like to discuss. Further assessment questions might include whether the patient is sexually active with a partner and partner gender; during the last sexual encounter, whether the patient was able to get some amount of erection, and how much (e.g., percentage of full erection); level of satisfaction with the hardness of erection; whether the erection was sufficient for desired sexual activities; and overall satisfaction with the sexual encounter.

Patients who report ED should also have a thorough physical assessment, including examination of genital appearance and health, test for testosterone levels, and prostate exam (if applicable).

Intervention Strategies

Physical/medical: Men diagnosed with cancers whose treatment may impact sexual function should be counseled about sexual effects *prior* to treatment, and should be advised of alternative treatments, if any, and strategies to minimize sexual side effects or aid sexual recovery. When pelvic surgery is necessary, patients should be counseled to ask—or advised about—whether nerve-sparing procedures are available.

After nerve-sparing radical prostatectomy, regaining erectile function is often improved by a process of penile rehabilitation, which includes daily use of PDE-5 inhibitors (PDE-5i) to increase blood flow and oxygenation to erectile tissues, maintain endothelial health, and prevent collagenation of smooth muscle tissues after prostatectomy [14, 15]. Some experts recommend beginning PDE-5i prior to surgery and then continuing afterward, so patients should be counseled prior to treatment about rehabilitation possibilities in order to make informed decisions [14]. Many trials of penile rehabilitation have shown better recovery of erectile function, better response to on-demand PDE-5i, and better response to intracavernosal injections post-prostatectomy, though one large randomized controlled trial showed benefit of PDE-5i at 9 months post-prostatectomy, but no significant benefit over placebo at 13 months [14].

Vacuum erection devices (VEDs) were often prescribed for the same purpose in the past—to increase blood flow to penile tissues—though PDE-5i are preferred nowadays. While VEDs do draw blood into the penis, this blood is not as oxygen-rich as blood circulated to the penis by PDE-5i, and therefore may not be as beneficial in promoting tissue health and erectile function [15].

Psychosocial: Many men experience embarrassment, shame, frustration, and a sense of not being masculine, manly, or potent with erectile dysfunction [20]. Additionally, while many men regain erectile function after cancer treatment, others do not, depending on type of treatment and individual differences in physiology and recovery. Psychosocial intervention is an integral part of sexual recovery for anyone surviving cancer, but particularly for those for whom full physical recovery is not possible.

Support groups. Support groups for men surviving cancer can provide space for acknowledging feelings of grief and loss with changes in sexual function, normalizing the experience, and providing validation for feelings. Anecdotally, many cancer survivors and their partners report that sexuality is an infrequent topic in support groups, if it comes up at all. Group leaders may be instrumental in broaching the topic or dedicating certain group sessions to discussion of sexuality.

Sex therapy. Sex therapy for ED can help in adjusting to the loss of previous erectile function, identifying and changing unhelpful thoughts and behaviors about sex or sexuality, clarifying goals and desires for sex and intimacy, expanding repertoire of sexual activity with existing sexual function, and identifying conditions under which arousal and erectile function are likely to be best [21]. Research supports the efficacy of sex therapy for ED in improving sexual satisfaction, and recent meta-analyses suggest that a combination of PDE-5i and psychological intervention produces the best outcomes for men with ED, though these studies were not specific to cancer survivors [22, 23].

Individual therapy: Single men with ED as a result of cancer may feel in the minority, as much of the content in this area is directed to couples. Sexual function and self-concept are critical areas to address for men who are dating or looking for a relationship. Individual or group counseling can help to normalize and validate concerns. Information to help navigate dating with ED can be integral to approaching this area. Counseling on interpersonal issues might help with identifying potential dating partners, talking to a dating partner about sex, identifying sexual possibilities within existing sexual function, and coping with risk and rejection [24].

Couples therapy: In addition to individual distress, ED can contribute to distance or conflict in an intimate relationship, or may serve as a barrier to developing intimate relationships with new partners. Couples counseling can help to improve communication about sex and intimacy, decrease shame or embarrassment between partners, and enhance understanding about partners' desires for current sex life. Incorporating relationship-oriented content into existing support groups or workshops may be helpful in settings where formal couples counseling may not be available. Similarly, including partners in follow-up visits can be helpful in addressing partners' questions and concerns, and opening dialogue between partners about ED [25, 26].

Changes in Ejaculation and Orgasm

Here we differentiate between the specific process of ejaculation—the expulsion of semen—and the larger process of orgasm—the collection of physical and mental processes often including pelvic floor muscle contraction, ejaculation, and subjective sense of pleasure and release, that often results from sexual arousal and stimulation. A man can experience orgasm without ejaculation. Further, an erection is not needed to experience orgasm or ejaculation.

Risk Factors

Men who have been treated for many types of pelvic cancers can experience anejaculation (no semen is expelled with orgasm) and changes in the subjective experience of orgasm, with some describing it as less intense, less pleasurable, or just "different." Less commonly, a surgical procedure or medication may cause retrograde ejaculation, in which semen is pushed into the bladder, rather than out through the urethra, at the time of ejaculation. These changes are concerning for many men who are struggling to cope with multiple changes related to the experience of cancer [27, 28].

Anejaculation. Cancer treatment can cause anejaculation in two broad ways (a) through removal or damage to semen-producing structures including the testicles, prostate, and seminal vesicles, or (b) by damage to the nerves that control emission of semen. The seminal vesicles and prostate produce seminal fluid that mixes with sperm cells from the testicles to make semen, and the prostate is involved in the expulsion of semen at the time of ejaculation. Radical prostatectomy (removal of the prostate and seminal vesicles), radical cystectomy (removal of the bladder, prostate, seminal vesicles, and part of the urethra), and radiation therapy to the prostate result in anejaculation or "dry" orgasms, in which men typically have the sensation of orgasm but without release of semen.

Nerve damage from surgery can also affect ejaculation. Nerves from the spinal cord to the pelvis govern emission of semen at the time of orgasm. These nerves are distinct from the nerves that govern erections, and can be damaged during some types of surgery, including retroperitoneal lymphadenectomy in testicular cancer, and abdominoperitoneal resection or sigmoidectomy in colorectal cancer [24].

Retrograde ejaculation. Retrograde ejaculation occurs when the valve that normally closes off the path to the bladder at the time of ejaculation (the internal sphincter) is damaged, and semen shoots back into the bladder rather than being expelled out the end of the urethra with ejaculation. Certain surgical procedures cause retrograde ejaculation, including transurethral resection of the prostate (TURP). This common procedure for an enlarged prostate gland involves hollowing out the core of the prostate via the urethra, and often damages the internal sphincter. Men with retrograde ejaculation experience orgasm, though may report changes in the sensation or intensity of orgasm [15, 24].

Changes in orgasm. Changes in the sensation of orgasm, or ability to reach orgasm, are common with changes in ejaculation. With anejaculation, some men report a difference in the sensation of "fullness" or inevitability preceding orgasm, as semen is not building up to be released. Some men report less intense orgasms as a result. In a recent survey of men's sexual side effects post-prostatectomy, 60% reported decreased orgasm intensity, 57% reported delayed orgasms, 5% reported anorgasmia, and 10% had experienced pain during orgasm [27].

In addition to prostatectomy, hormonal treatment and pelvic radiation can also cause changes in orgasm. Androgen-blocking therapies are associated with delayed orgasm or anorgasmia, as testosterone has a role in orgasmic function. Some men experience sharp pain with orgasm after radiation treatment for prostate cancer, which may be a result of irritation to the urethra or spasms in the pelvic floor muscles [15, 27, 28]. Sometimes the pelvic floor muscles, which contract during ejaculation and orgasm, are damaged during pelvic surgery. This can also create changes in reaching orgasm, or in the feeling or intensity of orgasm. Finally, though not part of cancer treatment per se, many patients going through cancer treatment may be prescribed antidepressant medication. SSRI antidepressants are associated with delayed or absent orgasm, so men complaining of these symptoms should be asked about antidepressant use.

Assessment

For screening purposes, the single-item screener for sexual problems mentioned previously is an appropriate starting point for assessing problems related to ejaculation and orgasm [18]. One of the checklist items relates to problems with orgasm. For more comprehensive assessment or for research purposes, the PROMIS SexFS [19] includes items assessing ejaculation and orgasm and has been validated with patients with cancer. Conducting a clinical interview can also assess concerns about ejaculation and orgasm. Providers may ask patients whether they have experienced any problems with ejaculation and orgasm, the nature of those problems, onset, history and frequency of concerns, and interventions attempted. Physical assessment for concerns related to ejaculation and orgasm may include visual examination of the genitals, tests of penile tactile sensitivity, pelvic floor muscle tone, testosterone level, and prostate examination (if applicable).

Intervention Strategies

Physical/medical: Anejaculation resulting from surgery or radiation is, unfortunately, permanent, as part of the machinery for making or expelling semen has been permanently altered or removed. Though changes to ejaculation may be permanent, changes in orgasm may be amenable to treatment. If pelvic floor muscles have been damaged or weakened by surgery, physical therapy can help to restore proper muscle tone, which can improve orgasmic ability and sensation. For men who experience difficulty reaching orgasm as a result of changes in sensation, muscle tone, or new and unfamiliar physical functioning, increasing penile stimulation may help [24, 28]. This can be achieved by using a vibrator to stimulate the head of the penis, or by exploring different types of manual, oral, or other types of stimulation.

Pharmacologic interventions may help with reaching orgasm. Taking the hormone oxytocin intra-nasally during sexual activity, shortly before desired time of orgasm, helps some men with achieving orgasm [29, 30], though larger randomized controlled trials have not found consistent evidence for efficacy [31]. The drug cabergoline may also help orgasmic function by interfering with the release of prolactin, a hormone that has a role in governing a man's refractory period, or time between orgasms [32, 33]. A recent pilot study [32] of 131 men reported about 66% of those treated with cabergoline for anorgasmia or delayed orgasm experienced subjective improvement in orgasm. Participants included 23 men with prior prostatectomy, and no difference was observed in response to cabergoline between this group and men without prostatectomy. However, cabergoline efficacy appeared to be improved with concomitant testosterone therapy, which is contraindicated for survivors of hormone-sensitive cancers [32].

Psychosocial: Men experiencing changes to ejaculation and orgasm may report a sense of loss of valued aspects of sexual experience, fear or anxiety about partner response to changes, decrease in pleasure from sex, changes in sense of masculinity, low mood, and sexual avoidance [7, 27].

Brief consultation: It may be important for providers to ask specifically about ejaculation and orgasm, as men may not themselves broach the topic even in general discussions of sexual function. Providers can be helpful in normalizing the experience (e.g., many men with this type of treatment report this issue), answering questions, and directing the client to additional resources. Providers can also provide psychoeducation about relationship concerns. Brief consultation may help men to identify concerns they might like to discuss with their partners, and providers can normalize and encourage discussion about these matters. Alternatively, partners can be included in patient visits. This allows providers to provide information and answer questions related to sexual changes.

Men for whom ejaculation or fertility are important parts of sexual activity for having children, or for cultural or religious reasons may have particular difficulty with changes to these functions. Fertility and fertility preservation are discussed in the upcoming section on Infertility. Providers might ask about men's comfort in continuing sexual activity without ejaculation, and with exploring alternative sexual activities. In addition, men from many backgrounds might share the cultural experience of ejaculation symbolizing potency, masculinity, and virility. It may be helpful to acknowledge the meaning and importance of the loss of this function and take care not to minimize its value in attempting to reassure patients; for example, avoiding statements like, "An orgasm is mostly mental anyway," or "your partner probably doesn't mind."

Sex therapy. Sex therapy can address men's concerns about sexual function and partner response, help to process feelings of grief and loss for previous sexual functioning, and help to regain a healthy sexual self-concept and decrease feelings of embarrassment, shame, or inadequacy about changes. Cognitive and behavioral strategies can help to reduce anxiety and cognitive distraction and increase focus on sexual stimulation, which may improve delayed or absent orgasm [34]. Sex therapy can also help to identify strategies for increasing sexual arousal, and for maximizing enjoyment of current sexual function.

Case Study: Karl S. Karl is a 62-year-old White male with a busy professional life and history of good sexual function and high sexual satisfaction, who presented for sex therapy after undergoing radical prostatectomy 2 years prior. He reported having regained good erectile function post-treatment with use of PDE-5i and reported overall positive sexual recovery. Karl had recently begun dating a new female partner and reported distress and anxiety about his anejaculation and "dependence" on PDE-5i for erectile function. He was particularly concerned about his partner's reaction and feared she would perceive him as less masculine or less sexually satisfying than other partners she'd had. Since appropriate medical intervention was already in place, counseling focused on improving communication between Karl and his partner, specifically in talking with her about his concerns and having the opportunity to hear her reaction. In this case, his partner reassured him of her desire and attraction for him, and the lack of importance to her of his PDE-5i use or absence of semen with orgasm. Counseling additionally focused on helping him to prioritize her feedback as evidence for his sexual function being satisfactory to her, and to de-prioritize his own fears. Finally, we discussed cognitive and behavioral methods for stopping his tendency to compare himself to idealized versions of her past sexual partners. Karl's anxiety was reduced and sexual satisfaction in their relationship improved.

Couples therapy: Like ED, changes to ejaculation and orgasm can affect relationships as well as individuals. Couples therapy can help partners openly discuss sexual matters, feelings about loss of ejaculation or changes in orgasm, and their impact on sex in the relationship. For couples who have difficulty or conflict in coping with sexual changes, or additional relationship problems that affect sex and intimacy, couples counseling can be especially helpful.

Low Sexual Desire

Risk Factors

Low desire is an extremely common complaint among both men and women facing cancer [7, 8]. During cancer diagnosis and the active phase of treatment, loss of desire can stem from fear, stress, and anxiety about having cancer, or fatigue, pain, nausea, or illness associated with treatment. Many people in the active phase of treatment focus temporarily on survival, with other concerns, including sex, taking a back seat.

Androgen deprivation therapy. Some cancer treatments have direct effects on sexual desire. For men, androgen deprivation therapy (ADT) has an especially dulling effect on sexual desire. Androgen-blocking drugs and, less commonly, orchiectomy (removal of testicles) are used to reduce testosterone levels in order to prevent certain prostate cancers from growing or spreading. The resulting drop in testosterone results in significant decrease or altogether loss of sexual desire for many men. Other side effects that may not directly impact sex drive, but which may harm body image and sexual self-concept, include hot flashes, decreased energy and motivation, erectile dysfunction, delayed orgasm, weight gain, and breast enlargement [15]. Together, these changes create distress, frustration, relationship difficulties, and an altered sense of masculinity for many men. Men who experience such changes may feel anxious about approaching sexual situations, which can also lead to reduced desire and avoidance of sexual situations. ADT is also associated with depression, which may further diminish sexual desire [35].

Surgery or radiation to the testicles. The testicles produce about 95% of testosterone in men's bodies [15]. In most cases of testicular cancer, only one testicle must be removed, and the other continues to produce enough testosterone to maintain adequate levels. Rarely though, cancer has spread to both testicles, or a remaining testicle does not function properly, and a man's testosterone levels drop after orchiectomy [24]. Radiation can also affect testicular production of testosterone. Pelvic radiation to other organs can scatter to the testicles, temporarily damaging testosterone production. Direct radiation to the testicles is more likely to cause permanent damage.

Endocrine tumors. Pituitary gland tumors can alter hormone levels. For example, some types of pituitary adenoma can cause excess secretion of prolactin, leading to a condition called hyperprolactinemia. Excess prolactin is associated with low sexual desire [36].

Other medications. Narcotic pain medications, anti-nausea drugs, anxiolytics, beta-blockers (for blood pressure reduction), and antidepressants can all decrease libido. While these drugs are not specific to the treatment of cancer, they are often used to treat side effects or concerns that frequently co-occur in cancer patients.

Assessment

For screening purposes, the single-item screener for sexual problems mentioned previously is a good starting point [18]. One of the checklist items relates to problems with sexual desire, or wanting to have sex. For more comprehensive assessment or for research purposes, the PROMIS SexFS [19] includes items assessing sexual interest. A clinical interview can also be used to assess concerns about sexual desire. Providers may ask patients whether they have experienced any changes in sexual desire—including masturbation, sexual initiation or receptivity, sexual fantasies, feelings of sexual drive—along with history and course of the problem, any notable exceptions, current medications, and aspects of the sexual relationship that may be contributing. Patients should also be asked about related aspects of sexual function that may indirectly contribute to low desire, including erectile dysfunction, ejaculatory or orgasm problems, or pain with sex. Physiologic assessment should include tests for testosterone, prolactin, and thyroid function, along with assessment for comorbid sexual problems and psychological concerns [36].

Intervention Strategies

Physical/medical. Medical treatment depends to some extent on the cause of the problem. When anxiety, fatigue, depression, pain, or nausea related to treatment are barriers to sexual desire, treating these conditions with antianxiety, antidepressant, painkiller, or anti-nausea medication may improve sexual interest, though this is a delicate balance as all of these medications may also have the side effect of dulling sexual desire, as discussed previously. In the case of antidepressants, some have better sexual side effect profiles than others. Bupropion has the fewest reported sexual side effects, and for some patients it seems to improve sexual interest and function [15].

Hormonal adjustments can also help. Testosterone therapy, if appropriate for the patient, can improve sexual desire that stems from low testosterone [36]. If androgen deprivation is the culprit, unfortunately this is not an option, but psychosocial intervention can help in reducing the impact of low desire on a patient's sex life. If low desire stems from hyperprolactinemia, high prolactin levels can be treated with bromocriptine or cabergoline [36].

For men who are struggling with changes in sexual function and associated dampening in sexual desire, helping to treat underlying concerns can help. Testosterone therapy and/or PDE-5 inhibitors can improve erectile function for some men, and thereby decrease anxiety about approaching sexual situations. Similarly, treating changes in ejaculation or orgasm that are causing distress can reduce sexual avoidance and improve desire.

Finally, lifestyle behaviors like exercise, adequate sleep, healthy diet, stress reduction, social interaction, fun and pleasure, and smoking cessation are foundational to physical health and therefore to sexual desire.

Psychosocial: Psychosocial intervention can help men to identify existing sexual desire that may not be as intense or frequent as before, find strategies to kindle desire, and improve communication between partners so that lack of desire presents less of a problem.

Behavioral management. Patients can be counseled on ways of managing low sexual desire to ameliorate negative effects on their sex life. One strategy may be for men become more aware of spontaneous desire throughout the day and make a note of when and where it happened, what sparked it, and what was done about it, if anything, in a "desire journal." [28] This can provide clues as to when and under what circumstances desire manifests itself, and identify opportunities to act on desire when appropriate.

Another strategy is for men to "start from neutral" with sexual activity and let desire follow a conscious choice to engage in sexual activity. For many people, desire can follow arousal even if spontaneous desire was not there to begin with [37].

It can also help to identify "turn ons"—situations or activities that assist with becoming aroused from a starting point of feeling neutral. Turn-ons might include using erotic material to become aroused, engaging in longer foreplay with a partner, or increasing variety of sexual activities.

Sex therapy and couples therapy. If behavioral management strategies are insufficient, sex therapy can also help in managing or improving low desire. Particularly if treatment-related low desire is complicated by other factors like difficult past sexual experiences, relationship problems, or other psychological issues like anxiety or depression, sex therapy can provide in-depth and personalized intervention.

Couples therapy can help to improve communication about sexual issues between partners, resolve conflict or misunderstanding, and help partners to work together on creating a plan for improving their sex life. For many heterosexual couples, both partners may be accustomed to their sex life being driven by the man's desire. Absent that, partners may struggle with rebuilding satisfying sexual contact. Partners of men with changes in sexual function are often careful about not pressuring their partners, and not "making them feel bad" by bringing up the topic of sex before they may be ready. Many couples find it helpful to talk about changes in sexual function and discuss fears and desires about their sex life going forward.

Both sex therapy and couples therapy have evidence for effectiveness in treating low sexual desire, and are recommended as components of best-practice treatment for low sexual desire in men [36].

Infertility

Risk Factors

Certain types of radiation, chemotherapy, and surgery can affect fertility. Whole-body radiation (e.g., for leukemia) and external-beam radiation to the abdominal and pelvic areas (e.g., for abdominal tumors, prostate cancer, or testicular cancer) can damage sperm-producing cells in the testicles. Further, some types of radiation to the brain affect the pituitary gland, which sends hormonal signals throughout the body. In some cases, damage to this gland can result in infertility [24, 28].

Some types of chemotherapy drugs also damage sperm-producing cells. These cells are especially vulnerable because they divide rapidly as do cancer cells, and rapidly dividing cells are targets of chemotherapy. Some drugs cause temporary infertility during and after treatment, and some, particularly at high doses, are known to cause permanent infertility [24, 28].

Surgery can lead to infertility by removing semen-producing structures (testicles and prostate), interfering with semen getting to the urethra, or damaging nerves that are necessary for erection or ejaculation. Surgery for testicular cancer often involves removing one or, more rarely, both testicles. Removal of one testicle should still allow for sperm production, as long as the remaining testicle is healthy and not affected by radiation. Radical prostatectomy for prostate cancer removes the prostate and seminal vesicles, which are responsible for making seminal fluid that mixes with the sperm to make semen. Surgery for some types of bladder cancer can involve removal of the bladder as well as the prostate and seminal vesicles. Without the prostate and seminal vesicles, sperm are still produced in the testicles but not able to be expelled [15, 24, 28]. Surgical removal of pelvic lymph nodes—for example, in some cases of testicular or colon cancer—can damage spinal nerves that are involved in ejaculation and orgasm. In these cases, semen may be produced but is unable to be expelled.

Assessment

All men who will receive a type of cancer treatment that is known to affect fertility should be assessed for interest in fathering children and, if interested, counseled about the risks involved and advised of fertility preservation options. It is important not to assume, due to patient age or other characteristics, that a man is not interested in fertility preservation. All patients should be assessed for these concerns. Health care providers can assess concerns about fertility either verbally or, for more extensive assessment or research purposes, a written inventory such as the Reproductive Concerns Scale [38].

Intervention Strategies

Physical/medical: Preventive measures. Men who will receive external-beam radiation to the pelvis may reduce risk of infertility by shielding the testicles from radiation. If infertility is a concern with chemotherapy, oncologists may be able to work with patients to find a chemotherapy regimen that is least likely to be toxic to sperm. With surgical intervention, nerve-sparing procedures, when feasible, provide the best opportunity for continued erectile and ejaculatory functioning and, therefore, fertility.

Sperm banking. Sperm banking may be an option for men undergoing treatment that will impair fertility. Briefly, sperm banking entails collecting semen from a patient prior to treatment and freezing it for later use in egg fertilization. This allows men to father biological children even if cancer treatment damages fertility.

Sperm retrieval. In cases in which sperm are still produced in the testicles but are unable to be expelled, there are surgical procedures for retrieving sperm cells from the testicles. When nerves that control ejaculation have been damaged, sometimes ejaculation can be stimulated by medication (usually ephedrine sulfate) or, more rarely, electrical stimulation. For men with retrograde ejaculation, sometimes sperm can be retrieved from the urine after ejaculation [24].

Psychosocial: Patient counseling. Given the possibility of permanent infertility following some cancer treatments, it is imperative that patients be counseled about risks and fertility preservation options prior to treatment. Unfortunately, some patients undergoing fertility-damaging treatment report that no one discussed fertility risks or preservation with them [39]. Whose job is it to do so? This depends on the medical center and treatment team involved. Anecdotally, some providers have noted that a barrier to discussing fertility with patients is lack of clarity about who is supposed to do so, and during which patient visit it should happen. It is helpful to clarify these details within an oncology department or treatment team so that protocol is clear.

What if fertility preservation is not possible for some reason, or if a patient discovers after treatment that he will be unable to have children? Appropriate empathy from treatment providers is helpful. It can also be helpful to acknowledge regret or anger about the loss of fertility. Support groups and individual or couples counseling can help patients come to terms with the loss of fertility, changes to anticipated life course, and any relationship concerns that arise as a result. If patients are interested, counseling can also help explore options for sperm retrieval, if possible, adoption or other ways of having children in their lives.

Fatigue

Risk Factors

The experience of cancer and treatment is a profoundly fatiguing process for many patients. Fatigue is associated with decreased sexual interest and problems with sexual function [7], and is a common contributor to low sexual desire. Some amount of fatigue is normal with illness and treatment. Chemotherapy creates fatigue for many patients, especially immediately following treatment. Surgery and radiation are also associated with fatigue, as the body directs its resources to healing. Simply having and fighting cancer engages the immune system on an ongoing basis and may result in fatigue. In addition to these factors, the stress of having cancer, fear and uncertainty about the treatment and outcome, and balancing cancer treatment with other life roles can create fatigue for many patients. Fatigue can also be a sign of depression, also common with cancer and its treatment.

Assessment

Clinical interview can be used to inquire about energy level, daytime fatigue, somnolence, ability to perform daily activities, and bother or distress due to low energy or fatigue. For more extensive assessment or research, the PROMIS Cancer Item Bank v. 1.0—Fatigue questionnaire (available from healthmeasures.net) assesses experience of and impairment due to fatigue. Patients complaining of fatigue should also be screened for depression.

Intervention Strategies

Physical/medical: Treatment to reduce correlates of fatigue like pain, nausea, or stress can help to reduce associated fatigue. Patients may consider talking to doctors about adjusting doses of painkillers or anti-nausea drugs if symptoms are inadequately controlled. Stress, anxiety, and worry can be sources of fatigue as well, which may be treated in part with anti-anxiety medication. For depression-related fatigue, antidepressant medication may help. Bupropion has some evidence for ameliorating fatigue as well as treating depression [40]. The stimulants methylphenidate and modafinil have some evidence for efficacy in treating fatigue among cancer patients [41], as does the practice of qi gong [42, 43].

Psychosocial: Psychoeducation. Sometimes the best treatment for fatigue is rest, especially following medical procedures from which the body needs to heal. Extended periods of needing rest can be emotionally challenging, especially for people accustomed to being busy or who derive pleasure, satisfaction, worth, or identity from their work, parenting, or other life roles. Men in particular may struggle with resting or reducing effort, as men are often socialized to work hard, take action, and be instrumental in getting things done for themselves and their families. Brief counseling can help to reassure men that fatigue and needing rest are normal, temporary, and necessary parts of cancer treatment.

Behavioral management. Counseling or brief consultation can also help to identify how to allocate limited energy, how to work around bouts of fatigue related to treatment schedule, and to prioritize valued activities. For fatigue related to stress, anxiety, or depression, counseling can be extremely helpful in identifying underlying causes and coping strategies for managing these feelings.

Counseling can also help to identify strategies for maintaining sexual activity or intimacy, if desired, through treatment-related fatigue. Patients (and their partners, if applicable) might be asked to identify a range of sexual or intimate activities they typically enjoy, and rank them from easiest (requiring least energy) to most demanding (requiring most energy). Men and their partners might then focus on the "easiest" activities in their repertoire while fatigue is present, in order to stay sexually connected during treatment.

Another strategy for coping with fatigue that comes and goes with a treatment schedule is to plan sexual activities for times that a person reliably has more energy. For example, if fatigue tends to occur after chemotherapy treatment but energy is good in the week prior to that, a couple might plan a date with sexual or intimate activity during that time.

Body Image and Sexual Self-Image

Risk Factors

During and after cancer treatment, many men experience their bodies differently than before. Men may have weight loss, hair loss due to chemotherapy, weight gain from hormonal therapy, scars, body parts removed, changes in continence or other bodily functions, ostomies or other medical devices, and changes in body appearance from surgery and radiation. These physical changes can profoundly impact a man's view of himself, his attractiveness and desirability, "normalcy," and sense of masculinity. Changes in body image and associated self-concept can cause a man to withdraw from sexual contact, fearing his partner's reaction to his physical changes or not wanting to be reminded of them himself.

Particularly difficult are changes to sexual organs after treatment. Many men report shortening of penile length, and associated distress, after radical prostatectomy. One study of 126 men found average shortening of 1.3 cm in flaccid penile length, and 2.3 cm in stretched length, at 1 year post-prostatectomy [15]. Men with testicular cancer undergoing orchiectomy often experience distress associated with loss of a testicle. A silicone prosthesis can be implanted at the time of surgery to restore look and feel of the testicles, which may improve body image. The incidence of penile curvature, or Peyronie's disease, is elevated after radical prostatectomy. About 15% of men will experience curvature after this procedure, compared to incidence of 3–9% in the general population [15]. Most men experience at least mild distress related to such changes, and many will experience clinically significant levels of anxiety and/or depression as a result.

Assessment

Clinical interview questions can be used to screen for body image concerns that are interfering with sexual or other activities; e.g., 'are you having any concerns about your body appearance or function that get in the way of intimacy?' The single-item screener by Flynn and colleagues [18] may also be used to indirectly screen for body image concerns. One checklist item inquires about anxiety related to sexual situations.

Intervention Strategies

Physical/medical: Physical management of bodily changes can help with sexual difficulties or embarrassment. For example, a man who experiences incontinence after prostatectomy might use a constriction band during sex to stop leakage during sexual activity or orgasm [15]. Someone with an ostomy following bladder or colon cancer might be instructed on how to empty and cover the ostomy pouch and appliances to make them less intrusive during sex [24]. Penile curvature may be treated with a variety of therapies. While no specific medical intervention exists to address body image concerns, lifestyle factors can help patients feel more positively about their bodies. Healthy diet and regular physical activity are associated with more positive mood and body image. Depression can contribute to negative self-assessment, so treating existing depression may help to address body image concerns as well.

Psychosocial: Individual or group counseling can help men to adjust to body changes and develop healthy self-concept that incorporates new aspects of physical appearance and function. Counseling can help to identify strategies to practice alone or with a partner may help patients to restore feelings of kindness, acceptance, and appreciation toward their bodies. Some strategies for body image improvement may include allowing time to grieve the loss of the pre-cancer body, desensitization to body changes through visual exposure, cultivating positive self-concept, or eliciting and accepting partners' positive feedback.

Pain

Risk Factors

Physical pain can dampen sexual desire and limit physical capacity to engage in sexual activity. Pain may result from cancer itself or from any aspect of cancer treatment, and is often able to be diminished or controlled with medication or other modifications. Pain often subsides with healing. Genital pain in particular may result from certain cancers or their treatments.

For men, the most common type of genital pain is associated with ejaculation and orgasm [24]. Sharp pain in the urethra during ejaculation may result from irritation to the urethra due to use of a catheter or scope during medical procedures or from pelvic radiation, or may result from pelvic floor muscle spasms during orgasm. Surveys estimate that 10–14% of men experience pain with orgasm after radical prostatectomy [15, 27]. This pain is usually not severe, and often temporary. If a man has had pelvic surgery, he may experience pain at the site of surgery as his body heals. Some people form adhesions internally after pelvic surgery or radiation, which can cause pain. Adhesions are thin films of scar tissue that can form between internal organs. With sexual activity or orgasm, these internal adhesions can pull and cause pain [24].

Assessment

Clinical interview (e.g., "do you have any pain with sexual stimulation or activity?") or written questionnaire such as the PROMIS Cancer Item Bank v. 1.1—Pain Interference questionnaire can be used (available from healthmeasures.net).

Intervention Strategies

Physical/medical: For general physical pain associated with cancer or its treatment, most patients will be prescribed painkillers either temporarily or in an ongoing fashion to manage chronic pain. Painkillers can dull sexual interest and response for some people, so patients should be advised of this. Genital pain associated with ejaculation and urethral irritation often resolves on its own as the urethra heals [24, 28].

Psychosocial: Mindfulness strategies can help to manage and reduce pain [44]. Patients might be referred to a mindfulness or meditation class, book, or audio or video recording on mindfulness practice, ideally one that is specifically designed for pain management.

For genital pain in particular, sexual exploration alone or with a partner can help to identify activities and positions that are more comfortable, and those that provoke pain. It can be helpful to make a list of more comfortable activities and rely on those until pain goes away. It is often helpful for men to communicate about pain to their partners, so that partners are aware of what is and is not comfortable, and so they can be allies in creating a pleasurable sexual experience.

Sexual Difficulties in Women with Cancer

Overview

Today, approximately 3.5 million female cancer survivors are living in the United States; this figure is expected to increase by an additional million within 10 years. The most common types of cancer in women are cancers of the breast, uterus, and colon/rectum [3]. The typical treatment regimens for these diseases, and for many other types of cancer, confer significant risk for sexual dysfunction. If left untreated, sexual dysfunction in female cancer survivors tends to have a chronic course.

Effects of Cancer Treatment on Sexual Self-Image

The effects of cancer on women's sexual function do not always map directly onto the conventional response phase-specific classification of sexual dysfunctions. Cancer is often experienced as life altering, regardless of clinical outcome, and may be life limiting as well. Women tend to report higher distress related to cancer than men, and they may find it especially difficult to shift roles when they have been strongly socialized as caregivers.

Appearance and sexual attractiveness have been conceptualized as performative aspects of sexuality in heterosexual women [45]. Not surprisingly, body image disturbance is reliably and independently associated with sexual difficulties in female cancer survivors [46–51]. The literature in this area focuses predominantly on breast cancer survivors, and mainly on the effects of mastectomy versus breast-conserving therapy. Despite some variability among studies, the general consensus is that sexual outcomes are enhanced with preservation of breast tissue, and that breast reconstructive surgery does not reliably attenuate the effects of total mastectomy on body image and sexual function [47, 52–55]. Appearance-related concerns may also result from scarring, disfigurement, hair loss, and changes in hair or skin texture.

Despite the disproportionate focus of the literature on breast surgery, body image is a broad construct that goes beyond appearance alone. Other qualities associated with being "feminine," such as having intact or functional reproductive organs, is also relevant to how many women view their sexual selves [56–58]. In one survey almost half of breast cancer survivors under 50 years endorsed feeling less feminine and/or less sexually attractive [59]. Body image concerns may also pertain to bodily function. For instance, in a recent study of anal cancer survivors gastrointestinal symptom severity was associated with body image disturbance, and in turn with multiple domains of sexual function [46]. Cancer-related infertility is often distressing to survivors of childbearing age and may influence women's sexual self-image both directly and indirectly [39, 60].

Sexual adjustment after cancer is highly variable, even when taking into account the presence or absence of treatment-related risk factors. The concept of a "sexual self schema," a cognitive representation of one's sexuality and sexual attributes [61], offers a way of conceptualizing individual risk and resilience to sexual changes resulting from cancer treatment [62, 63]. For instance, in studies of breast and gynecologic cancer survivors, more negative sexual self schemas (as measured by a validated questionnaire) were found to predict poorer sexual outcomes and more restricted sexual behavior, even after taking into account sexual history and disease-related factors [62, 64]. The sexual self schema thus appears to exert a moderating influence on the effects of treatment on sexual function and behavior. To the extent that one's sexual self schema can be modified, the schema may be a reasonable target of treatment, especially in longitudinal interventions.

In summary, the image a woman has of herself as a sexual person is susceptible to the negative effects of cancer and cancer treatment. Changes in sexual self-image can manifest in nearly all aspects of sexual behavior and sexual function. Whereas the following sections pertain to specific problems common to female cancer survivors, the reader is cautioned to consider the global and pervasive influence of sexual self-image on sexuality.

Low Sexual Desire

A loss of interest in sex is the most common type of sexual problem reported by women with cancer. Low sexual desire is challenging to conceptualize and treat due to the multitude of etiological factors that can be present in any given individual. Complicating matters further, many contributing factors to low sexual desire are not specific to cancer. In fact, studies in some populations have found no differences in rates of low sexual desire between people with and without a history of cancer [65, 66], although several specific risk factors confer vulnerability to long-term changes in sexual desire.

Most studies of sexual desire in female cancer survivors do not distinguish between reduced spontaneous sexual desire, reduced receptivity to sexual stimuli, and aversion to sexual activity. Although sexual aversion disorder was eliminated from the nomenclature for sexual dysfunctions in the most recent version of the *Diagnostic and Statistical Manual of Mental Disorders* [67], from a clinical perspective it remains useful to differentiate reduced or absent interest in sex from fearful or aversive reactions in women with cancer. For instance, in a population of women seen in an oncology sexual health clinic over a period of 2 years, approximately 50% of consultations were related to low or absent interest in sex, whereas 10% of consultations were related to fear or concern about resuming sexual activity after treatment [68].

Risk Factors

Premature menopause. Women and girls with cancer are susceptible to the effects of premature menopause when exposed to treatments that cause damage to the ovaries (e.g., chemotherapy or pelvic radiation), or when oophorectomy is indicated. Both in cancer survivors and in the general population, bilateral salpingo-oophorectomy in premenopausal women ("surgical menopause") is associated with low sexual desire [49, 69, 70]. Similarly, women who experience premature ovarian failure secondary to cancer treatment report lower sexual desire than to survivors who maintain normal ovarian function [69].

Mood disturbance and fatigue. Depressed mood is common along the trajectory of cancer care and may continue after completion of treatment. Mood changes eventually normalize in most long-term cancer survivors [71, 72], but the course of mood disturbance is highly variable. Studies of breast cancer survivors indicate that changes in sexual desire often accompany symptoms of depressed mood and anhedonia [59, 73–75]. Moreover, use of antidepressant medications is associated with sexual difficulties, including low sexual desire, in women with cancer and in the general population. Fatigue is closely related to depressed mood in adult cancer survivors [76] and may have a further influence on sexual desire in women above and beyond the effects of depressed mood [74].

Fear and stigmatization. For a variety of reasons women and/or their partners may choose to avoid or defer sexual activity after cancer treatment. Although sexual inactivity is commonly attributable to factors such as fatigue, low prioritization of sex, or other constraints, sometimes it is linked directly to fear of causing injury, exacerbation of disease, or recurrence. In our experience, women who are afraid of injury or recurrence with sexual activity typically have undergone treatment for a pelvic or abdominal tumor, although concerns about systemic risks may also be present (e.g., post-stem cell transplant).

A fear of pain or of causing harm can manifest in the woman and/or her partner. For example, after pelvic surgery such as hysterectomy or after mastectomy, both women and their partners may express concern about sex interfering with healing or causing further tissue damage. Often, though not always, there is a corresponding knowledge deficit regarding the procedures or the anatomy of the affected organ(s). Further complicating the picture, in couples with limited sexual communication, one partner's fears or concerns may be easily misconstrued as a loss of interest or attraction.

Fear of causing recurrence appears somewhat less common and may be alleviated with reassurance, though these fears may be more challenging to address in survivors of human papillomavirus (HPV)-related cancers. Women with HPV-related cancers often voice concerns about re-infection and transmission of the virus to future sexual partners. Despite the ubiquity of HPV infection, HPV-related cancers remain widely misunderstood and stigmatized. Some women with HPV-related diseases survivors may begin to avoid sexual activity in an attempt to prevent recurrence [62], or simply to avoid unpleasant associations of sexual activity with cancer. Recent work suggests that perceived and women who internalize HPV-related stigmatization are especially vulnerable to anxiety about sexual activity, avoidance of sexual anxiety, and other sexual problems [77, 78].

Assessment

A clinical interview is usually sufficient to characterize changes in sexual desire. Important points to ascertain are changes in spontaneous versus receptive sexual desire, specific disincentives to sexual activity (e.g., embarrassment, pain), changes in relationship adjustment (if applicable), and the presence or absence of key risk factors including changes in mood and body image. If the woman appears to be avoidant of sexual activity, the clinician should inquire about the survivor's awareness of sexual activity restrictions (if any) associated with treatment, and prior counseling from the oncology team once "cleared" for sexual activity. Typically, survivors will have received little such information. A medical history is also important to establish medical comorbidities that increase the risk of low sexual desire, and to evaluate ovarian function when appropriate.

Multidimensional self-report measures of sexual function such as the Female Sexual Function Index [79] and the Sexual Activity Questionnaire [80] have been administered to cancer survivors and include specific items addressing sexual desire. Although most measures of sexual function have not been specifically validated in cancer survivors, an exception is the recently developed PROMIS Sexual Function scales [19, 81]. The Interest in Sexual Activity scale can be used either alone or in conjunction with other sexual function scales in the PROMIS measures. Finally, the Menopausal Sexual Interest Questionnaire [82] is among the few desire-specific scales that have been used in studies of cancer survivors.

Intervention Strategies

Educational and self-management interventions. Education is a cornerstone of most psychosocial and behavioral interventions for sexual difficulties. Sex education both informs and normalizes. Sexually active women with cancer usually appreciate opportunities to learn about sexual anatomy and physiology, common effects of cancer treatments on sexual function, and typical experiences of women who received similar treatments. Education and reassurance are also appropriate first-line interventions in women who demonstrate fear of sexual pain or other fear-related avoidance behavior. Educational interventions can also influence adaptive behavior by providing information about self-management of sexual problems, communication skills, and sexual skills. In a study of women with breast and gynecologic cancer, an Internet-based educational intervention resulted in improvement on the Menopausal Sexual Interest Questionnaire, particularly when accompanied by brief one-one-one counseling [83]. A half-day psychoeducational workshop followed by in-person telephone counseling calls also appeared to enhance sexual desire and other sexual outcomes in a group of women with *BRCA1* or *BRCA2* mutations who had undergone risk-reducing bilateral salpingo-oophorectomy [84].

In general, cancer survivors tend to endorse greater perceptions of stigma and shame when they associate their diagnosis with a voluntary behavior (e.g., smoking, sexual activity). Not surprisingly, women who are aware that HPV is sexually transmitted express endorse more shame and stigma than those who do not. These feelings appear to be magnified when women regard HPV as a less common infection [85]. Thus, clinicians should emphasize the ubiquity of HPV infection, the natural history of HPV infection, and screening and surveillance as effective prevention strategies. This information may enable survivors to reduce their avoidance in the short-term, laying the groundwork to lower shame and stigma over time. Engaging intimate partners, when possible, may enhance the benefits of education.

Sex therapy. Sex therapy interventions for low sexual desire are distinguished from psychoeducational interventions by their depth, scope, degree of personalization to the individual, and emphasis on skill building and feedback. Sex therapy typically includes multiple components including education, communication skills training, sensate focus, and strategies to counter maladaptive thoughts and behaviors related to sexual activity. Recently, mindfulness and acceptance-based techniques have been incorporated into traditional cognitive behavioral sex therapy [86, 87]. Studies of sex therapy interventions in the general population suggest an overall positive, though modest, effect on sexual desire outcomes [88]. Because low sexual desire may be related to non-cancer-specific etiological factors, these interventions may also be appropriate for cancer survivors. Adherence to "homework" and between-session exercises is an important predictor of sex therapy outcome in the general population; our clinical experience suggests this is no different for cancer survivors.

Relatively few published trials have evaluated structured behavioral interventions that specifically target sexual problems in female cancer survivors, although a number of more broadly focused trials (e.g., those focused on general couple/marital adjustment to cancer) include content on sexuality [89, 90]. One trial evaluated outcomes of a three-session group mindfulness-based sex therapy intervention for women with cancers of the uterine corpus or cervix [91, 92]. Compared to the outcomes of a waitlist control condition, participants in the group intervention showed significant improvement on the Female Sexual Function Index, including Desire subscale scores, both immediately post-treatment and 6 months post-treatment [96]. Other recent trials have examined dyadic interventions that include education, sensate focus, and other behavioral exercises, but the available data do not suggest a significant effect on sexual desire [93, 94].

Exposure-based treatment. Although vaginal dilators are usually employed for prevention or treatment of sexual pain in cancer survivors, we have found some success in recommending dilators for the purpose of desensitization prior to resuming penetrative sexual activity in anxious cancer survivors. Imaginal exposure exercises may be of benefit for this purpose. To the best of our knowledge, these interventions have not been tested empirically.

Medical management of low sexual desire. To date, no randomized trials have established the efficacy of hormonal or non-hormonal medication specifically for low sexual desire in women with cancer. The novel central nervous system drug flibanserin, recently approved in the United States for treatment of low sexual desire in premenopausal women, has yet to be tested in a sample of cancer survivors, although to our knowledge there are no contraindications that are specific to cancer survivors.

Estrogen replacement therapy is effective for management of vasomotor symptoms associated with premature menopause but, for reasons not well understood, does not appear to have a significant effect on sexual desire [70, 95]. One possibility is that the loss of ovarian androgens is responsible for low sexual desire, although this hypothesis is undermined by a lack of clear correlation between serum androgen levels and sexual desire after oophorectomy [96, 97]. A more compelling explanation for low sexual desire in the setting of premature menopause, consistent with research evidence, is discomfort due to vulvovaginal symptoms of menopause [49, 98, 99]. These symptoms are not necessarily managed with systemic estrogen replacement therapy alone. However, when adequately treated, management intervention appeared to result in both decreased sexual discomfort and increased sexual desire in a sample of breast cancer survivors [99].

Vaginal Dryness and Dyspareunia

Pain or discomfort during sexual activity is a common complaint in women seeking help for sexual problems after cancer treatment and is typically related to structural changes in the vulvovaginal mucosa. Increasingly, however, the pelvic floor musculature is considered as a primary or secondary source of pain in some cases. Sexual pain has pervasive effects on other aspects of sexual functioning and, for many survivors, results in complete cessation of sexual activity.

Risk Factors

Estrogen deprivation. In premenopausal women, ovarian follicles produce most of the circulating estradiol in the body. In addition to other functions, estradiol regulates the structure and integrity of vulvovaginal tissues. Removal of the ovaries, or ovarian failure due to the effects of chemotherapy or radiation, causes a dramatic reduction in estradiol, resulting in tissue thinning (atrophy), loss of elasticity, architectural changes in the vulva, and changes in pH. The onset of vaginal dryness and dyspareunia may also follow soon after discontinuation of hormone replacement therapy in women who have been recently diagnosed with a hormone-sensitive cancer. The use of aromatase inhibitors, which further lower estradiol levels, accelerates and exacerbates the process of vulvovaginal changes due to menopause (the selective estrogen receptor modulator [SERM] tamoxifen does not appear to have a comparable effect) [100, 101]. In practice, the severity and course of menopausal vulvovaginal atrophy varies, with some women noticing an abrupt and severe change and others noticing a gradual deterioration.

Chemotherapy-related mucositis. Acute mucositis is a frequently overlooked cause of vulvovaginal pain in women who have recently received chemotherapy. Although mucositis will eventually normalize after discontinuation of chemotherapy, it may persist for weeks.

Radiation vaginitis and vaginal stenosis. Patients who receive radiation to the pelvis or vaginal cuff are at especially high risk for sexual complications due to long-term effects of radiation therapy on vulvovaginal tissue. For instance, cervical cancer survivors treated with radiation therapy have significantly poorer long-term sexual outcomes than those treated with radical hysterectomy [102]. In one longitudinal study, only 63% of patients who were sexually active prior to radiation therapy had resumed sexual activity at 12 months post-treatment [103]. In the most severe cases, radiation can lead to partial or total obliteration of the vagina.

Vulvovaginal graft-versus-*host disease.* Women who undergo allogenic stem cell transplant are vulnerable to vulvovaginal manifestations of graft-versus-host disease, which can lead to acute tenderness and eventual vaginal stenosis. In one clinic-based study, a majority of stem cell transplant recipients who were referred to a gynecology clinic for evaluation of dyspareunia were found to have graft-versus-host disease [104].

Vaginal reconstruction. Although a detailed discussion of vaginal reconstructive surgery is beyond the scope of this chapter, clinicians should be aware that women who undergo partial or total vaginal reconstruction in the course of surgical treatment may have pain at or around the tissue flap site. Stenosis of the neovagina is also an occasional outcome.

Pelvic organ scarring and adhesions. Deep dyspareunia may be related to scarring or adhesions after surgery or radiation therapy. For example, women treated with primary chemoradiation for cervical cancer may experience deep dyspareunia due to fibrotic changes in the irradiated uterus or surrounding organs.

Assessment

A physical examination is warranted in cases of new-onset pain or marked increase in pain severity during or after cancer treatment. Typical findings in cancer survivors include thinning of vulvovaginal tissue, loss of color, elasticity, and rugae, and foreshortening and stenosis of the vagina. When possible, palpation of the pelvic floor muscles may reveal hypertonicity or tenderness. Guarding or other pain behaviors are important to note, especially in relation to the degree of observable tissue change. When possible, and with the patient's consent, clinicians should carefully attempt to reproduce the pain during the examination.

Multidisciplinary sexual function instruments such as the Female Sexual Function Index and PROMIS questionnaires contain useful questions about sexual function for clinical assessment and outcome evaluation. Despite the high prevalence of sexual pain in cancer survivors, to our knowledge only the PROMIS Lubrication and Vaginal Discomfort subscales were specifically developed using data from cancer survivors.

Intervention Strategies

Hormone replacement therapy. Local (topical) estrogen therapy in the form of vaginal tablets, rings, or creams is effective for management of dyspareunia due to estrogen deprivation and for prevention of vaginal scarring and stenosis due to radiation therapy exposure. Although systemic absorption of local estrogen therapy is low, there is nevertheless concern about the potential risks of exogenous estrogen in women with a history of estrogen-sensitive tumors (e.g., common in breast, endometrial, and ovarian cancers). No randomized trials have established the safety of local estrogen therapy in these disease populations, although findings from observational studies have been reassuring [105]. Similarly, while a few breast cancer survivors were included in late phase trials for the SERM ospemifene, risks and benefits in this population are unknown, and it is unclear whether ospemifene is less risky than local estrogen in women with a history of estrogen-sensitive disease.

Non-hormonal vaginal moisturizers and lubricants. Non-hormonal topical gels, creams, and suppositories can be considered as first-line management for women with vulvovaginal dryness and atrophy [106]. A few products, including polycarbophil gel [107], hyaluronic acid [108], and olive oil [109] have been evaluated in clinical trials and found to improve symptoms of vaginal dryness and discomfort. Hyaluronic acid has also been found to promote healing after radiation therapy [110]. Although none of these products are superior to topical estrogen, they can provide adequate relief for many women with mild to moderate symptoms who cannot or prefer not to use hormonal treatment. Water- and silicone-based lubricants are used as needed for vaginal penetration, whereas moisturizers must be used on a regular basis (generally, every 2–3 days) to achieve and sustain their benefits. Figure 30-2 presents a general schematic for conservative management of chronic vaginal dryness and atrophy.

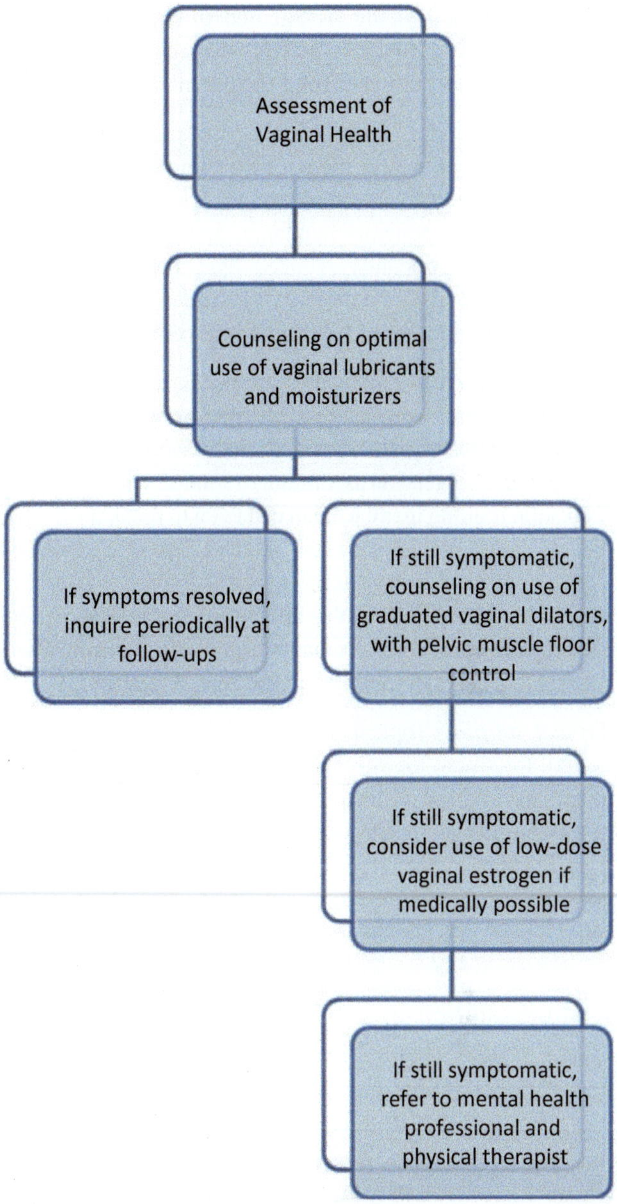

FIGURE 30-2. Treatment algorithm for the oncology team and/or general gynecologist for vaginal health promotion in female cancer survivors. [Reprinted from Carter J, Goldfrank D, Schover LR. Simple Strategies for Vaginal Health Promotion in Cancer Survivors. Journal of Sexual Medicine. 2011; 8(2):549–559 with permission from Elsevier].

Vaginal dilation. Women who receive radiation to the pelvis should be advised to regularly dilate the vagina with the use of a vaginal dilator and/or penile–vaginal intercourse to prevent vaginal stenosis. A vaginal dilator is a rigid or semirigid cylinder that is designed to be inserted and held in the vagina for a brief period of time at regular intervals (3 or more times per week). Although a few studies have demonstrated a preventive effect of regular vaginal dilation on vaginal stenosis [111, 112], the empirical support for this intervention is relatively weak overall [113]. A key challenge in studying the efficacy of vaginal dilators is very poor compliance, although behavioral intervention appears to be somewhat efficacious in improving compliance with dilator use [114]. Clinical experience suggests that vaginal dilation may be highly beneficial in the small percentage of motivated patients who remain compliant over the long term. Dilator use may be also recommended to women with graft-versus-host disease, or to those who are already experiencing moderate to severe vaginal changes due to radiation exposure or menopause. Clinically, dilation is often helpful (though usually not sufficient by itself) in the management of stenosis and severe atrophy. However, to our knowledge there are no randomized trials of vaginal dilation beyond the preventive setting.

Topical anesthetics. Topical lidocaine applied to the vulvar vestibule may be considered for women with dyspareunia due to postmenopausal vulvovaginal atrophy. In an open-label study, 4% aqueous lidocaine, applied shortly before penetration, significantly reduced dyspareunia and sexual distress and enabled the majority of women who were sexually abstinent at baseline to resume intercourse [115].

Pelvic floor exercise. Tension of the pelvic floor muscles is a normal response to repeated provocation of pain that, unfortunately, exacerbates pain. Although many women will experience pelvic floor tension as difficult to control, with pelvic floor relaxation training many women can learn to break the cycle of anxiety, tension, and pain that contributes to dyspareunia. There is no clear consensus on protocols for pelvic floor exercise, although research in this area is emerging [109, 116]. In the case of severe dyspareunia or vaginismus, consultation or referral to a pelvic floor physical therapist is valuable.

Topical steroids. Topical glucocorticoids are a key component of treatment for vulvovaginal graft-versus-host disease. When the disease is localized and diagnosed early, it can often be managed successfully with topical glucocorticoids, topical estrogen, and vaginal dilation [117]. However, severe or widespread manifestations of graft-versus-host disease require systemic management.

Changes in Sensation, Arousal, and Orgasm

Although low sexual desire and dyspareunia are probably the most common presenting complaints in female cancer survivors, and problems with sexual arousal and orgasm often develop secondary to these problems, a notable subset of cancer survivors will present with arousal or orgasm disorders as their primary or only complaint. Typically, survivors report feelings diminished or absent genital sensation, a lack of physiological arousal despite subjective excitement, and/or increased latency to or absence of orgasm. Unfortunately, there is very little literature to guide conceptualization and management of these disorders, as much of the literature is focused on the global sexual dysfunction so often seen in female cancer survivors. Acquired anorgasmia in cancer survivors is less common.

Risk Factors

Menopausal changes in sexual arousal. Hypothetically, decreased vascularization of the vulva and vagina due to menopause would result in reduced genital engorgement secondary to sexual arousal. However, postmenopausal women retain the genital vasocongestive response to sexual stimulation, and this is not clearly distinguishable from responses measured in premenopausal women [118, 119]. Vulvovaginal atrophy appears to be a more important predictor of sexual function, including orgasmic function, than menopausal status per se [120, 121].

Vulvar surgery. The orgasmic response can be surprisingly resilient to many treatments including radical pelvic surgery [102]. However, surgeries that directly affect genital sensory or spongy erectile tissues, such as radical vulvectomy or clitoridectomy, almost invariably result in impaired sexual arousal and orgasm [122].

Chemotherapy. There is a hypothetical risk of damage to genital sensory neurons resulting from neurotoxic chemotherapies, although to date this has been explored little in the clinical literature.

Low sexual excitement. Psychological factors include fatigue, a lack of interest in sex, cognitive distraction due to anxiety or pain, and relationship discord can interfere with arousal and orgasm in women [123].

Non-hormonal medication side effects. Several classes of drugs commonly used by cancer survivors may impair sexual arousal and orgasm. Serotonergic antidepressants are used not only in the treatment of depression, anxiety disorders, and chronic pain but also to manage hot flashes as an alternative to systemic estrogen replacement. It is unclear to what extent the relatively low doses used to treat hot flashes may affect sexual function, however. Other commonly used classes of drugs that may affect sexual function include opioids and anticonvulsants, both used for pain management.

Assessment

For most cancer survivors, low arousal and impaired orgasm occur in the context of other sexual difficulties, other symptoms, and/or the effects of medications. Therefore, a detailed sexual and medical history is necessary to establish risk factors and potential targets of treatment. Beyond this history, clinicians may inquire about changes in the type or intensity of stimulation, especially if treatment has limited the survivor's sexual activities in some way. It is also useful to distinguish between arousal and orgasm problems that occur globally versus in specific situations (especially if there is a different response to partnered sexual activity than masturbation). In general, the dual control model [124, 125] offers a broad but useful perspective in conceptualizing sexual arousal disorders, namely by distinguishing between insufficient excitement/excitability and excessive inhibitory processes.

Intervention Strategies

Behavioral management. Behavioral treatment of arousal and orgasm disorders rests on a careful conceptualization of excitatory and inhibitory processes. Both psychoeducational interventions and cognitive behavioral sex therapy, as described above, may enhance arousal and orgasm in cancer survivors. For some women, increasing the intensity of sexual stimulation (i.e., through direct clitoral stimulation or use of a vibrator) may be an important component of behavioral management. Anxiety management and mindfulness techniques can be used to reduce the effect of cognitive distraction or excessive self-monitoring on sexual response.

Medical. A number of compounds have been evaluated for women who complain of decreased or absent sexual arousal. With few exceptions these are untested in female cancer survivors [126], but results in the general population have been disappointing. For instance, the PDE-5 inhibitors are effective in enhancing genital vasocongestion in women, but this does not appear to enhance their clinical utility in the general population. However, in carefully selected patients with isolated genital-specific arousal complaints, a trial of a PDE-5 inhibitor may be appropriate.

Case Study

Overcoming Pain and Stigma: The Case of Monica

Monica was a 35-year-old woman who had been diagnosed with HPV-related anal cancer about 10 months prior to seeking help for sexual difficulties. Her primary cancer treatment consisted of concurrent chemotherapy and radiation therapy, which resulted in a complete clinical response but at the expense of ongoing fatigue, proctitis, and vulvovaginal dryness and discomfort. Monica was especially bothered by vulvar and perineal burning and itching. She found some relief from increasing the frequency of cleansing her perineal area and using topical creams and ointments, but she remained preoccupied with her symptoms. She reported that intercourse provoked sharp, burning pain despite use of a water-based lubricant, and Monica found it difficult to become aroused and reach orgasm. Gradually, she began to evade her husband's attempts to be physically affectionate, and she began retreating to bed earlier in the evenings due to "exhaustion." After a series of arguments with her husband about her lack of interest in sex, Monica sought help for what she perceived as a hormonal imbalance that caused indifference and aversion to sex.

In most respects, Monica's 6-year marriage was well adjusted. She and her husband, Nicolas, shared a number of values and goals, and they took pleasure in family life and in the care of their 2-year-old son. However, they had long-standing differences in their desire for sex. Throughout their marriage Nicolas typically initiated sex. Whereas in the early years of marriage Monica would accept his advances enthusiastically, she found that her own interest in sex waned over time, especially after the birth of their son. Nevertheless, prior to her cancer diagnosis Monica continued to find sex pleasurable and experienced sexual arousal and orgasm most of the time. Although Monica desired a second child, she understood that her treatment might affect her ability to have another pregnancy. She initiated treatment soon after her diagnosis, and she was not offered fertility preservation.

At the initial consultation with a marital and sex therapist, Monica described a relatively sheltered and conservative moral upbringing in her family of origin. Sexual matters were discussed rarely, and in a mostly negative context. Most of her sexual education came from peers and women's magazines. Monica first engaged in sexual activity during her freshman year of college. She described the experience as exciting and pleasurable, though she admitted to considerable guilt afterward about "giving away her virginity" to a man whom she did not view as a viable long-term partner. Monica revealed a later episode of sexual assault by a dating partner who attempted vaginal intercourse while she was intoxicated. Monica blamed herself for the incident and framed it as a "wake up call" to be more cautious and selective about her partners. Monica appreciated that Nicolas, in contrast to some previous partners, appeared to "cherish" and "honor" her sexuality.

Monica attended the initial consultation alone but brought Nicolas to the next session at the recommendation of the therapist. Nicolas expressed a supportive attitude toward Monica, but admitted to some confusion as to why Monica continued to experience sexual problems nearly a year out from treatment. On providing education to the couple, it became clear that Nicolas did not realize the degree to which Monica experienced pain with intercourse, and Nicolas became upset at the thought of hurting his wife. Monica accepted a referral to a gynecologist who had experience in treating cancer survivors. She was receptive to medical evaluation but had been reluctant to pursue help, believing that little could be done and that she simply needed to "learn to live with it." The therapist offered reassurance to the couple and suggested a temporary prohibition on intercourse while Monica's physical symptoms were being evaluated. Instead, her the therapist suggested that the couple could begin to reconnect with non-sexual, non-coital activity. Monica was cautiously optimistic, and Nicolas was content to take small steps in the service of resuming their sex life.

Monica's gynecologic consultation resulted in three significant outcomes. First, Monica received treatment for her sexual pain with topical estrogen cream that she applied intravaginally and to the perineal area. She also agreed to consult a pelvic floor physical therapist, who recommended an at-home program of exercises to stretch tight perineal tissue and improve her pelvic floor muscle control. Second, Monica learned that the likelihood of a future pregnancy was low as her ovarian function had not returned to normal premenopausal levels and her antral follicle count was low. This came as very disappointing, though not unexpected, news.

Finally, Monica was counseled to continue cervical screening at regular intervals due to her history of HPV-related cancer. Although Monica was aware of her HPV status when she was diagnosed, she had given little thought to the possibility of re-infection up until this point. Monica asked her gynecologist's opinion on using condoms or other methods to prevent re-infection, and remained anxious despite the gynecologist's efforts to reassure her.

Monica and Nicolas continued to attend sex therapy sessions every other week and adhered to sensate focus exercises. Their sexual communication skills improved, and Monica began to feel more comfortable allowing Nicolas to caress and kiss her. In the meantime, she began to notice improvement in her vaginal dryness and discomfort. As they approached the opportunity to have intercourse again, Monica felt hesitant to raise her concerns about HPV infection, having felt dismissed by her gynecologist. Privately, however, her thoughts about having HPV became more frequent and intrusive. She became preoccupied with the question of how she came to contract HPV, despite her understanding of its high prevalence. She began to cast her premarital sexual experiences, previously tinged with guilt but otherwise inconsequential, in a different light as she reflected on the toll of her HPV-related disease. Although she had hoped to look forward to resuming intercourse with Nicolas, her feelings of guilt and shame were stifling.

It was not until Monica and Nicolas did resume intercourse that Monica's HPV-related concerns came to light. Although Monica's pain had improved substantially, she was distracted and tense during intercourse. Nicolas sensed that Monica's distance was more than just nerves, and Monica tearfully admitted to feeling responsible for "devastating" their marriage. Monica and Nicolas shared this revelation in their next sex therapy session. Monica was encouraged to continue therapy focused on modifying her self-punitive and rigid thought patterns. Using a mindfulness and acceptance-based framework, Monica acquired skills for maintaining contact with the present moment, tolerating uncertainty, considering alternatives to her initial thoughts or interpretations of situations, and becoming more aware of her own sources of physical and sexual pleasure. Monica also acquired greater insight into how her early sexual experiences and socialization shaped her somewhat negative perceptions of sexual activity, and this became the impetus for cultivating greater self-compassion. Six months after her first consultation with the sex therapist, Monica reported that she and Nicolas were sexually active, albeit on a less frequent basis than before her cancer diagnosis. Her pain was relatively mild and sometimes minimal. Monica had lingering, but manageable, concerns about HPV re-infection and recurrence, but she perceived a newfound intimacy and openness with Nicolas, and her overall satisfaction with her sexual life was high.

Summary

Cancer and its treatment have significant and broad-ranging effects on sexuality and sexual function. Individuals with cancer and their partners often need help bringing up the topic of sexual difficulty, identifying contributors to sexual concerns, and understanding medical and psychosocial treatment options. Unfortunately, in current practice, assessing and treating cancer patients' and survivors' sexual concerns is the exception rather than the norm. Health care providers at all phases of patient care can help to change this by identifying what can be done to assess and address concerns at each phase of care.

References

1. American Cancer Society. Global cancer facts & figures. 3rd ed. Atlanta: American Cancer Society; 2015. Available at https://www.cancer.org/research/cancer-facts-statistics.html. Accessed on 9 Mar 2017.
2. American Cancer Society. Cancer facts and figures. Atlanta: American Cancer Society; 2016. Available at https://www.cancer.org/research/cancer-facts-statistics.html. Accessed on 9 Mar 2017.
3. American Cancer Society. Cancer treatment and survivorship facts and figures 2016–2017. Atlanta: American Cancer Society; 2016. Available at https://www.cancer.org/research/cancer-facts-statistics.html. Accessed on 9 Mar 2017.
4. Hill EK, Sandbo S, Abramsohn E, Makelarski J, Wroblewski K, Wenrich ER, et al. Assessing gynecologic and breast cancer survivors' sexual health care needs. Cancer. 2011;117:2643–51.
5. Taylor B, Davis S. The extended PLISSIT model for addressing the sexual wellbeing of individuals with an acquired disability or chronic illness. Sex Disabil. 2007;25:135–9.
6. Althof SE, Rosen RC, Perelman MA, Rubio-Aurioles E. Standard operating procedurs for taking a sexual history. J Sex Med. 2013;10:26–35.
7. Bober SL, Varela VS. Sexuality in adult cancer survivors: challenges and intervention. J Clin Oncol. 2012;30(30):3712–9.
8. Sadovsky R, Basson R, Krychman M, Morales AM, Schover L, Wang R, et al. Cancer and sexual problems. J Sex Med. 2010;7:349–73.
9. Rosen RC, Bachmann GA. Sexual well-being, happiness, and satisfaction in women: the case for a new conceptual paradigm. J Sex Marital Ther. 2008;34:291–7.
10. Byers ES. Relationship satisfaction and sexual satisfaction: a longitudinal study of individuals in long-term relationships. J Sex Res. 2005;42(2):113–8.
11. Santtila P, Wager I, Witting K, Harlaar N, Jern P, Johansson A, et al. Discrepancies between sexual desire and sexual activity: gender differences and associations with relationship satisfaction. J Sex Marital Ther. 2007;34(1):31–44.
12. Bradford A, Fellman B, Urbauer D, Bevers T. Effect of routine screening for sexual problems in a breast cancer survivorship clinic. Psychooncology. 2016;25(11):1375–8.
13. Sue S. Cultural competency: from philosophy to research and practice. J Community Psychol. 2006;34:237–45.
14. Mulhall JP, Bivalacqua TJ, Becher EF. Standard operating procedure for the preservation of erectile function outcomes after radical prostatectomy. J Sex Med. 2013;10:195–203.
15. Mulhall JP. Saving your sex life. Bethesda, MD: C-I-Act Publishing; 2010.

16. Rosen RC, Riley A, Wagner G, Osterloh IH, Kirkpatrick J, Mishra A. The international index of erectile function (IIEF): a multidimensional scale for assessment of erectile dysfunction. Urology. 1997;49(6):822–30.
17. Rosen RC, Cappelleri JC, Smith MD, Lipsky L, Pena BM. Development and evaluation of an abridged, 5-item version of the International Index of Erectile Function (IIEF-5) as a diagnostic tool for erectile dysfunction. Int J Impot Res. 1999;11:319–26.
18. Flynn KE, Lindau ST, Lin L, Reese JB, Jeffrey DD, Carter J, et al. Development and validation of a single-item screener for self-reporting sexual problems in U.S. adults. J Gen Intern Med. 2015;30(10):1468–75.
19. Flynn K, Lin L, Cyranowski JM, et al. Development of the NIH PROMIS Sexual Function and Satisfaction measures in patients with cancer. J Sex Med. 2013;10(Suppl. 1):43–52.
20. Bokhour BG, Clark JA, Inui TS, Silliman RA, Talcott JA. Sexuality after treatment for early prostate cancer: exploring the meanings of "erectile dysfunction". J Gen Intern Med. 2001;16:649–55.
21. Zilbergeld B. The new male sexuality. New York: Bantam; 1999.
22. Melnik T, Soares B, Nasello AG. The effectiveness of psychological interventions for the treatment of erectile dysfunction: systematic review and meta-analysis, including comparisons to sildenafil treatment, intracavernosal injection, and vacuum devices. J Sex Med. 2008;5:2562–74.
23. Schmidt HM, Munder T, Gerger H, Fruhauf S, Barth J. Combination of psychological intervention and phosphodiesterase-5 inhibitors for erectile dysfunction: a narrative review and meta-analysis. J Sex Med. 2014;11(6):1376–91.
24. Schover LR. Sexuality and fertility after cancer. New York: Wiley; 1997.
25. Aubin S, Heiman JR, Berger RE, Murallo AV, Yung-Wen L. Comparing sildenafil alone vs. sildenafil plus brief couple sex therapy on erectile dysfunction and couples' sexual and marital quality of life: a pilot study. J Sex Marital Ther. 2009;35:122–43.
26. Manne SL, Kissane DW, Nelson CJ, Mulhall JP, Winkel G, Zaider T. Intimacy-enhancing psychological intervention for men diagnosed with prostate cancer and their partners: a pilot study. J Sex Med. 2011;8(4):1197–209.
27. Frey A, Sonksen J, Jakobsen H, Fode M. Prevalence and predicting factors for commonly neglected sexual side effects to radical prostatectomies: results from a cross-sectional questionnaire-based study. J Sex Med. 2014;11(9):2318–26.
28. American Cancer Society. Sexuality for the man with cancer. American Cancer Society. 2016. http://www.cancer.org/treatment/treatmentsandsideeffects/physicalsideeffects/sexualsideeffectsinmen/sexualityfortheman/index.
29. IsHak WW, Berman DS, Peters A. Male anorgasmia treated with oxytocin. J Sex Med. 2008;5(4):1022–4.
30. MacDonald K, Feifel D. Dramatic improvement in sexual function induced by intranasal oxytocin. J Sex Med. 2012;9(5):1407–10.
31. Abdel-Hamid IA, Elsaied MA, Mostafa T. The drug treatment of delayed ejaculation. Transl Androl Urol. 2016;5:576–91.
32. Hollander AB, Pastuszak AW, Hsieh TC, Johnson WG, Scovell JM, Mai CK, Lipshultz LI. Cabergoline in the treatment of male orgasmic disorder—a retrospective pilot analysis. Sex Med. 2016;4(1):e28–33.
33. Nickel M, Moleda D, Loew T, Rother W, Gil FP. Cabergoline treatment in men with psychogenic erectile dysfunction: a randomized, double-blind, placebo-controlled study. Int J Impot Res. 2007;19(1):104–7.
34. McMahon CG, Jannini E, Waldinger M, Rowland D. Standard operating procedures in the disorders of orgasm and ejaculation. J Sex Med. 2013;10(1):204–29.
35. Walker LM, Robinson JW. Sexual adjustment to androgen deprivation therapy: struggles and strategies. Qual Health Res. 2012; 22(4):452–65.
36. Rubio-Aurioles E, Bivalacqua TJ. Standard operational procedures for low sexual desire in men. J Sex Med. 2013;10(1): 94–107.
37. Basson R. Women's sexual dysfunction: revised and expanded definitions. Can Med Assoc J. 2005;172(10):1327–33.
38. Gorman JR, Su HI, Pierce JP, Roberts SC, Dominick SA, Malcarne VL. A multidimensional scale to measure the reproductive concerns of young adult female cancer survivors. J Cancer Surviv. 2014;8(2):218–28.
39. Canada AL, Schover L. The psychosocial impact of interrupted childbearing in long-term female cancer survivors. Psychooncology. 2012;21(2):134–43.
40. Moss EL, Simpson JS, Pelletier G, Forsyth P. An open-label study of the effects of bupropion SR on fatigue, depression and quality of life of mixed-site cancer patients and their partners. Psychooncology. 2006;15(3):259–67.
41. Spathis A, Dhillan R, Booden D, Forbes K, Vrotsou K, Fife K. Modafinil for the treatment of fatigue in lung cancer: a pilot study. Palliat Med. 2009;23(4):325–31.
42. Campo RA, Agarwal N, LaStayo PC, O'Connor K, Pappas L, Boucher KM, Gardner J, Smith S, Light KC, Kinney AY. Levels of fatigue and distress in senior prostate cancer survivors enrolled in a 12-week randomized controlled trial of Qigong. J Cancer Surviv. 2014;8(1):60–9.
43. Larkey LK, Roe DJ, Weihs KL, Jahnke R, Lopez AM, Rogers CE, Oh B, Guillen-Rodriguez J. Randomized controlled trial of Qigong/Tai Chi easy on cancer-related fatigue in breast cancer survivors. Ann Behav Med. 2015;49(2):165–76.
44. Kabat-Zinn J. Full catastrophe living: using the wisdom of your body and mind to face stress, pain, and illness. New York: Bantam Books.
45. Dove NL, Wiederman MW. Cognitive distraction and women's sexual functioning. J Sex Marital Ther. 2000;26(1):67–78.
46. Benedict C, Philip EJ, Baser RE, Carter J, Schuler TA, Jandorf L, et al. Body image and sexual function in women after treatment for anal and rectal cancer. Psychooncology. 2016;25(3):316–23.
47. Aerts L, Christiaens MR, Enzlin P, Neven P, Amant F. Sexual functioning in women after mastectomy versus breast conserving therapy for early-stage breast cancer: a prospective controlled study. Breast. 2014;23(5):629–36.
48. Burwell SR, Case LD, Kaelin C, Avis NE. Sexual problems in younger women after breast cancer surgery. J Clin Oncol. 2006;24(18):2815–21.
49. Rosenberg SM, Tamimi RM, Gelber S, Ruddy KJ, Bober SL, Kereakoglow S, et al. Treatment-related amenorrhea and sexual functioning in young breast cancer survivors. Cancer. 2014;120(15):2264–71.
50. Rhondali W, Chisholm GB, Daneshmand M, Allo J, Kang D-H, Filbet M, et al. Association between body image dissatisfaction and weight loss among patients with advanced cancer and their caregivers: a preliminary report. J Pain Symptom Manage. 2013;45(6):1039–49.
51. Panjari M, Bell RJ, Davis SR. Sexual function after breast cancer. J Sex Med. 2011;8(1):294–302.
52. Metcalfe KA, Cil TD, Semple JL, Li LDX, Bagher S, Zhong T, et al. Long-term psychosocial functioning in women with bilateral prophylactic mastectomy: does preservation of the nipple-areolar complex make a difference? Ann Surg Oncol. 2015;22(10):3324–30.
53. Rowland JH, Desmond KA, Meyerowitz BE, Belin TR, Wyatt GE, Ganz PA. Role of breast reconstructive surgery in physical and emotional outcomes among breast cancer survivors. J Natl Cancer Inst. 2000;92(17):1422–9.

54. Schover LR, Yetman RJ, Tuason LJ, Meisler E, Esselstyn CB, Hermann RE, et al. Partial mastectomy and breast reconstruction. A comparison of their effects on psychosocial adjustment, body image, and sexuality. Cancer. 1995;75(1):54–64.
55. Avis NE, Crawford S, Manuel J. Psychosocial problems among younger women with breast cancer. Psychooncology. 2004; 13(5):295–308.
56. Juraskova I, Butow P, Robertson R, Sharpe L, McLeod C, Hacker N. Post-treatment sexual adjustment following cervical and endometrial cancer: a qualitative insight. Psychooncology. 2003; 12(3):267–79.
57. Ussher JM, Perz J, Gilbert E. Changes to sexual well-being and intimacy after breast cancer. Cancer Nurs. 2012;35(6):456–65.
58. Bowes H, Jones G, Thompson J, Alazzam M, Wood H, Hinchliff S, et al. Understanding the impact of the treatment pathway upon the health-related quality of life of women with newly diagnosed endometrial cancer—a qualitative study. Eur J Oncol Nurs. 2014;18(2):211–7.
59. Fobair P, Stewart SL, Chang S, D'Onofrio C, Banks PJ, Bloom JR. Body image and sexual problems in young women with breast cancer. Psychooncology. 2006;15(7):579–94.
60. Carter J, Raviv L, Applegarth L, Ford JS, Josephs L, Grill E, et al. A cross-sectional study of the psychosexual impact of cancer-related infertility in women: third-party reproductive assistance. J Cancer Surviv. 2010;4(3):236–46.
61. Andersen BL, Cyranowski JM. Women's sexual self-schema. J Pers Soc Psychol. 1994;67:1079–100.
62. Carpenter KM, Andersen BL, Fowler JM, Maxwell GL. Sexual self schema as a moderator of sexual and psychological outcomes for gynecologic cancer survivors. Arch Sex Behav. 2009;38(5):828–41.
63. Andersen BL, Woods XA, Copeland LJ. Sexual self-schema and sexual morbidity among gynecologic cancer survivors. J Consult Clin Psychol. 1997;65:221–9.
64. Yurek D, Farrar W, Andersen BL. Breast cancer surgery: comparing surgical groups and determining individual differences in postoperative sexuality and body change stress. J Consult Clin Psychol. 2000;68(4):697–709.
65. Marino JL, Saunders CM, Emery LI, Green H, Doherty DA, Hickey M. Nature and severity of menopausal symptoms and their impact on quality of life and sexual function in cancer survivors compared with women without a cancer history. Menopause. 2014;21(3):267–74.
66. Recklitis CJ, Sanchez Varela V, Ng A, Mauch P, Bober S. Sexual functioning in long-term survivors of Hodgkin's lymphoma. Psychooncology. 2010;19(11):1229–33.
67. American Psychiatric Association. Diagnostic and statistical manual of mental disorders. 5th ed. Arlington, VA: American Psychiatric Association; 2013.
68. Bradford A, Nebgen D, Keeler E, Milbourne A. A comprehensive program to meet the sexual health needs of women with cancer. 7th Biennial Cancer Survivorship Research Conference; June, 2014; Atlanta, GA2014.
69. Ford JS, Kawashima T, Whitton J, Leisenring W, Laverdiere C, Stovall M, et al. Psychosexual functioning among adult female survivors of childhood cancer: a report from the childhood cancer survivor study. J Clin Oncol. 2014;32(28):3126–36.
70. Dennerstein L, Koochaki P, Barton I, Graziottin A. Hypoactive sexual desire disorder in menopausal women: a survey of Western European women. J Sex Med. 2006;3(2):212–22.
71. Zhao G, Okoro CA, Li J, White A, Dhingra S, Li C. Current depression among adult cancer survivors: findings from the 2010 Behavioral Risk Factor Surveillance System. Cancer Epidemiol. 2014;38(6):757–64.
72. Krebber AMH, Buffart LM, Kleijn G, Riepma IC, de Bree R, Leemans CR, et al. Prevalence of depression in cancer patients: a meta-analysis of diagnostic interviews and self-report instruments. Psychooncology. 2014;23(2):121–30.
73. Ganz PA, Desmond KA, Belin TR, Meyerowitz BE, Rowland JH. Predictors of sexual health in women after a breast cancer diagnosis. J Clin Oncol. 1999;17(8):2371–80.
74. Webber K, Mok K, Bennett B, Lloyd AR, Friedlander M, Juraskova I, et al. If I am in the mood, I enjoy it: an exploration of cancer-related fatigue and sexual functioning in women with breast cancer. Oncologist. 2011;16(9):1333–44.
75. Milbury K, Badr H. Sexual problems, communication patterns, and depressive symptoms in couples coping with metastatic breast cancer. Psychooncology. 2013;22(4):814–22.
76. Brown LF, Rand KL, Bigatti SM, Stewart JC, Theobald DE, Wu J, et al. Longitudinal relationships between fatigue and depression in cancer patients with depression and/or pain. Health Psychol. 2013;32(12):1199–208.
77. Mortensen GL. Long-term quality of life effects of genital warts—a follow-study. Dan Med Bull. 2010;57(4):A4140.
78. Foster LR, Byers ES. Predictors of the sexual well-being of individuals diagnosed with herpes and human papillomavirus. Arch Sex Behav. 2016;45(2):403–14.
79. Rosen R, Brown C, Heiman J, Leiblum S, Meston C, Shabsigh R, et al. The Female Sexual Function Index (FSFI): a multidimensional self-report instrument for the assessment of female sexual function. J Sex Marital Ther. 2000;26(2):191–208.
80. Thirlaway K, Fallowfield L, Cuzick J. The Sexual Activity Questionnaire: a measure of women's sexual functioning. Qual Life Res. 1996;5(1):81–90.
81. Flynn KE, Reeve BB, Lin L, Cyranowski JM, Bruner DW, Weinfurt KP. Construct validity of the PROMIS (R) sexual function and satisfaction measures in patients with cancer. Health Qual Life Outcomes. 2013;11.
82. Rosen RC, Lobo RA, Block BA, Yang HM, Zipfel LM. Menopausal Sexual Interest Questionnaire (MSIQ): a unidimensional scale for the assessment of sexual interest in postmenopausal women. J Sex Marital Ther. 2004;30(4):235–50.
83. Schover LR, Yuan Y, Fellman BM, Odensky E, Lewis PE, Martinetti P. Efficacy trial of an internet-based intervention for cancer-related female sexual dysfunction. J Natl Compr Canc Netw. 2013;11(11):1389–97.
84. Bober SL, Recklitis CJ, Bakan J, Garber JE, Patenaude AF. Addressing sexual dysfunction after risk-reducing salpingo-oophorectomy: effects of a brief, psychosexual intervention. J Sex Med. 2015;12(1):189–97.
85. Waller J, Marlow LAV, Wardle J. The association between knowledge of HPV and feelings of stigma, shame and anxiety. Sex Transm Infect. 2007;83(2):155–9.
86. Brotto LA, Basson R, Luria M. A mindfulness-based group psychoeducational intervention targeting sexual arousal disorder in women. J Sex Med. 2008;5(7):1646–59.
87. Brotto LA, Basson R. Group mindfulness-based therapy significantly improves sexual desire in women. Behav Res Ther. 2014;57:43–54.
88. Bradford A. Inhibited sexual desire in women. In: Grossman LR, Walfish S, editors. Translating psychological research into practice. New York: Springer; 2013. p. 515–8.
89. Brotto LA, Yule M, Breckon E. Psychological interventions for the sexual sequelae of cancer: a review of the literature. J Cancer Surviv. 2010;4(4):346–60.
90. Candy B, Jones L, Vickerstaff V, Tookman A, King M. Interventions for sexual dysfunction following treatments for cancer in women. Cochrane Database Syst Rev. 2016;2:CD005540.
91. Brotto LA, Erskine Y, Carey M, Ehlen T, Finlayson S, Heywood M, et al. A brief mindfulness-based cognitive behavioral intervention improves sexual functioning versus wait-list control in

women treated for gynecologic cancer. Gynecol Oncol. 2012;125(2):320–5.
92. Brotto LA, Heiman JR, Goff B, Greer B, Lentz GM, Swisher E, et al. A psychoeducational intervention for sexual dysfunction in women with gynecologic cancer. Arch Sex Behav. 2008;37(2):317–29.
93. Scott JL, Halford WK, Ward BG. United we stand? The effects of a couple-coping intervention on adjustment to early stage breast or gynecological cancer. J Consult Clin Psychol. 2004;72(6):1122–35.
94. Kalaitzi C, Papadopoulos VP, Michas K, Vlasis K, Skandalakis P, Filippou D. Combined brief psychosexual intervention after mastectomy: effects on sexuality, body image, and psychological well-being. J Surg Oncol. 2007;96(3):235–40.
95. Madalinska JB, van Beurden M, Bleiker EM, Valdimarsdottir HB, Hollenstein J, Massuger LF, et al. The impact of hormone replacement therapy on menopausal symptoms in younger high-risk women after prophylactic salpingo-oophorectomy. J Clin Oncol. 2006;24(22):3576–82.
96. Everhov ÅH, Flöter Rådestad A, Nyberg T, Smedby KE, Bergmark K, Lindén HA. Serum androgen levels and sexual function before and one year after treatment of uterine cervical cancer: a pilot study. J Sex Med. 2016;13(3):413–24.
97. Aziz A, Brannstrom M, Bergquist C, Silfverstolpe G. Perimenopausal androgen decline after oophorectomy does not influence sexuality or psychological well-being. Fertil Steril. 2005;83(4):1021–8.
98. Schover LR. Premature ovarian failure and its consequences: vasomotor symptoms, sexuality, and fertility. J Clin Oncol. 2008;26(5):753–8.
99. Ganz PA, Greendale GA, Petersen L, Zibecchi L, Kahn B, Belin TR. Managing menopausal symptoms in breast cancer survivors: results of a randomized controlled trial. J Natl Cancer Inst. 2000;92(13):1054–64.
100. Baumgart J, Nilsson K, Evers AS, Kallak TK, Poromaa IS. Sexual dysfunction in women on adjuvant endocrine therapy after breast cancer. Menopause. 2013;20(2):162–8.
101. Schover LR, Baum GP, Fuson LA, Brewster A, Melhem-Bertrandt A. Sexual problems during the first 2 years of adjuvant treatment with aromatase inhibitors. J Sex Med. 2014;11(12):3102–11.
102. Frumovitz M, Sun C, Schover LR, Munsell MF, Jhingran A, Wharton JT, et al. Quality of life and sexual functioning in cervical cancer survivors. J Clin Oncol. 2005;30:7428–36.
103. Jensen PT, Groenvold M, Klee MC, Thranov I, Petersen MA, Machin D. Longitudinal study of sexual function and vaginal changes after radiotherapy for cervical cancer. Int J Radiat Oncol Biol Phys. 2003;56(4):937–49.
104. Chung CP, Sargent RE, Chung NT, Lacey Jr JV, Wakabayashi MT. Graft-versus-host disease-associated vulvovaginal symptoms after bone marrow transplantation. Biol Blood Marrow Transplant. 2016;22(2):378–9.
105. Dew JE, Wren BG, Eden JA. A cohort study of topical vaginal estrogen therapy in women previously treated for breast cancer. Climacteric. 2003;6(1):45–52.
106. Carter J, Goldfrank D, Schover LR. Simple strategies for vaginal health promotion in cancer survivors. J Sex Med. 2011;8(2):549–59.
107. Loprinzi CL, Abu-Ghazaleh S, Sloan JA, van Haelst-Pisani C, Hammer AM, Rowland Jr KM, et al. Phase III randomized double-blind study to evaluate the efficacy of a polycarbophil-based vaginal moisturizer in women with breast cancer. J Clin Oncol. 1997;15(3):969–73.
108. Ekin M, Yasar L, Savan K, Temur M, Uhri M, Gencer I, et al. The comparison of hyaluronic acid vaginal tablets with estradiol vaginal tablets in the treatment of atrophic vaginitis: a randomized controlled trial. Arch Gynecol Obstet. 2011;283(3):539–43.
109. Juraskova I, Jarvis S, Mok K, Peate M, Meiser B, Cheah BC, et al. The acceptability, feasibility, and efficacy (phase I/II study) of the OVERcome (Olive Oil, Vaginal Exercise, and MoisturizeR) intervention to improve dyspareunia and alleviate sexual problems in women with breast cancer. J Sex Med. 2013;10(10):2549–58.
110. Markowska J, Madry R, Markowska A. The effect of hyaluronic acid (Cicatridine) on healing and regeneration of the uterine cervix and vagina and vulvar dystrophy therapy. Eur J Gynaecol Oncol. 2011;32(1):65–8.
111. Decruze SB, Guthrie D, Magnani R. Prevention of vaginal stenosis in patients following vaginal brachytherapy. Clin Oncol. 1999;11(1):46–8.
112. Law E, Kelvin JF, Thom B, Riedel E, Tom A, Carter J, et al. Prospective study of vaginal dilator use adherence and efficacy following radiotherapy. Radiother Oncol. 2015;116(1):149–55.
113. Miles T, Johnson N. Vaginal dilator therapy for women receiving pelvic radiotherapy. Cochrane Database Syst Rev. 2010(9).
114. Jeffries SA, Robinson JW, Craighead PS, Keats MR. An effective group psychoeducational intervention for improving compliance with vaginal dilation: a randomized controlled trial. Int J Radiat Oncol. 2006;65(2):404–11.
115. Goetsch MF, Lim JY, Caughey AB. A practical solution for dyspareunia in breast cancer survivors: a randomized controlled trial. J Clin Oncol. 2015;33(30):3394–400.
116. Mercier J, Morin M, Lemieux MC, Reichetzer B, Khalife S, Dumoulin C. Pelvic floor muscles training to reduce symptoms and signs of vulvovaginal atrophy: a case study. Menopause. 2016;23(7):816–20.
117. Stratton P, Turner ML, Childs R, Barrett J, Bishop M, Wayne AS, et al. Vulvovaginal chronic graft-versus-host disease with allogeneic hematopoietic stem cell transplantation. Obstet Gynecol. 2007;110(5):1041–9.
118. Brotto LA, Gorzalka BB. Genital and subjective sexual arousal in postmenopausal women: influence of laboratory-induced hyperventilation. J Sex Marital Ther. 2002;28(Suppl 1):39–53.
119. van Lunsen RH, Laan E. Genital vascular responsiveness and sexual feelings in midlife women: psychophysiologic, brain, and genital imaging studies. Menopause. 2004;11(6 Pt 2):741–8.
120. Avis NE, Stellato R, Crawford S, Johannes C, Longcope C. Is there an association between menopause status and sexual functioning? Menopause. 2000;7(5):297–309.
121. Levine KB, Williams RE, Hartmann KE. Vulvovaginal atrophy is strongly associated with female sexual dysfunction among sexually active postmenopausal women. Menopause. 2008;15(4 Pt 1):661–6.
122. Aerts L, Enzlin P, Vergote I, Verhaeghe J, Poppe W, Amant F. Sexual, psychological, and relational functioning in women after surgical treatment for vulvar malignancy: a literature review. J Sex Med. 2012;9(2):361–71.
123. Meston CM, Bradford A. Sexual dysfunctions in women. Annu Rev Clin Psychol. 2007;3:233–56.
124. Bancroft J, Graham CA, Janssen E, Sanders SA. The dual control model: current status and future directions. J Sex Res. 2009;46(2/3):121–42.
125. Milhausen RR, Graham CA, Sanders SA, Yarber WL, Maitland SB. Validation of the sexual excitation/sexual inhibition inventory for women and men. Arch Sex Behav. 2010;39(5):1091–104.
126. Greven KM, Case LD, Nycum LR, Zekan PJ, Hurd DD, Balcueva EP, et al. Effect of ArginMax on sexual functioning and quality of life among female cancer survivors: results of the WFU CCOP Research Base Protocol 97106. J Community Support Oncol. 2015;13(3):87–94.

31
Sex and Chronic Physical Illness

Marika Hess, Trisha A. Hicks, and Sigmund Hough

Introduction to Sex and Chronic Physical Illness

Chronic physical illness can have a devastating impact for the individual, family, and significant others. The fact is that illness over time carries an additional burden upon the individual and one's psychosocial world. At times, a person's life desires and expectations are pushed aside. Fortitude and strength are now channeled into finding one's resiliency to endure and carry out day-to-day activities of daily living. A psychophysiological approach to chronic physical illness embraces the understanding that sexuality can be an important part of living. Thus, it is a necessary part of assessment and intervention, and a crucial element for integrated holistic health care to maximize function and quality of living is needed.

The chapter broadens health care's responsibility to address the physical consequences of the health condition and to assess how these physical impairments impact personal attributes (e.g., sense of self-worth, confidence, mood, and self-esteem), relationships and sexual participation. Sexual participation should not just refer to intercourse but rather comprise a more broad definition to include grooming, flirting, engaging with partners, intimacy, mutual permission, and satisfaction. Personal attributes such as resiliency, cognition, coping mechanisms, gender orientation, ethnicity, culture, religion, life-style preference, and psychosocial political-economic environmental factors should be taken into account when assisting the individual achieve one's goals.

Physical Illnesses

Overview of Physical Illness

Health is a state of complete physical, mental, and social well-being and not merely the absence of disease or infirmity. Before we can discuss the impact of medical illness and disease on sexual functioning, it is important to define "disease" as a pathological process, deviation from a biological norm [1]. This definition, however, is very limited without functional or psychosocial context. As clinicians we strive to help bring our patient as close to "health" as possible and need to consider the wide range of consequences a disease might have on an individual and their ability to function in their personal, societal, work, and cultural context. The International Classification of Functioning (ICF) is a useful framework to use when addressing a patient's disease state because it addresses all aspects of functioning and integrates the physical, mental, and social aspects of disease. The main broad components that are considered are body function, activities, and participation. The dynamic interplay between personal, environmental factors and health conditions are critical elements that drive the outcome.

The most benign disease course is a self-limited illness which has a restricted course or can be cured. Other times the illness may present as a single occurrence or result in significant life altering disability (e.g., spinal cord injury or cerebrovascular accident). Chronic illnesses may have a prolonged gradual decline (e.g., dementia), a trajectory with gradual decline, punctuated by episodes of acute deterioration and some recovery (e.g., multiple sclerosis); or a course with steadily progressive trajectory (e.g., amyotrophic lateral sclerosis).

There is generally a positive relationship between informed sexual education, empowerment and sexual activity [2]. Depending on the diagnosis and the trajectory of the illness, the accompanying sexual needs may also change over time. Health care professionals must remain vigilant to assess, monitor, and assist their patients in maintaining sexual health during the entire disease process.

Sexual Difficulties Common to Diagnoses

Over the last century, Americans have experienced dramatic gains in life expectancy. As the diagnosis and management of diseases improve, there is a growing prevalence of chronic

W.W. IsHak (ed.), *The Textbook of Clinical Sexual Medicine*, DOI 10.1007/978-3-319-52539-6_31

diseases. Not only does the illness often result in its own disability, but the treatment of the primary disease often results in secondary health conditions. For example, an individual treated for cancer may develop neuropathy, incontinence, and obesity as a product of the treatment. The resultant multi-morbidity has a cumulative impact on exercise capacity, quality of life, and survival as well as interest in and ability to have and enjoy sexual activity [3].

Chronic illness and its treatments usually have a negative impact on relationships and sexual satisfaction of both patients and partners, either directly as a result of the illness itself or indirectly due to secondary physical, functional, or psychological ramifications. Individuals with chronic illness may develop misconceptions about their ability and the safety of having sex. They may either feel that their illness precludes sexual activity or have experienced sexual "failure" (e.g., erectile dysfunction, anorgasmia) that then reinforces perception of their inability to engage in meaningful sexual activity.

Biopsychosocial Factors

Biological Effects

The effects of chronic illness on sexuality can be classified into biopsychosocial categories [4]. Nonspecific systemic causes limiting sexual activity include reduced cardiovascular and pulmonary reserve, weakness, fatigue, or pain. Anemia and deconditioning are common to chronic illnesses and amplify these problems. Treatments such as surgery, radiation therapy, chemotherapy, and immunotherapy can result in exhaustion, nausea, loss of appetite, and dehydration. When treatment is time limited (e.g., radiation therapy for cancer) these symptoms are expected to improve. However, in many illnesses, the gradual disease progression is associated with increasing symptom burden.

The medical illness and its treatment often directly interfere with the ability to experience arousal and orgasm. Neurological and vascular effects such as neuropathy, accelerated atherosclerosis, and endothelial dysfunction negatively affect ability to appreciate sexual stimulation and stymie the physiological response of arousal. Bladder incontinence due to urinary stress incontinence or detrusor instability can cause shame and embarrassment and interferes with sexual motivation and expression. Similarly, bowel incontinence from neurological or surgical sequelae can have a devastating impact on sexual engagement.

Endocrine abnormalities such as alterations in gonadal hormones result in loss of sexual interest, erectile dysfunction, retrograde and premature ejaculation in men and loss of libido, hot flashes, vaginal tightness or dryness, and anorgasmia in women. Furthermore, medications used to treat the primary and associated conditions may impair sexual function.

Psychological Effects

The expression and practice of sexuality are affected by self-esteem, body image, and interpersonal relationships. Body image can be negatively affected by medical illness and loss or disfigurement of parts of the body. Surgical procedures and medical treatments may result in altered bodily appearance (e.g., scarring, amputation, tracheostomy, mastectomy, ostomy, hair loss). Bodily changes and the loss of a body part, such as a limb, the uterus, ovaries, or genitalia, can have a profound impact on self-esteem, defined as an individual's self-perception of his/her abilities, skills, and overall qualities that guides cognitive processes and behaviors. Individuals with medical illness can experience depression, fatigue, pain, stress, and anxiety which may further contribute to sexual dysfunction. The psychological distress that often accompanies altered body image causes a person to feel devalued and incomplete. This situation can limit patients' or their partners' sexual satisfaction and their motivation to engage in intimacy and sexual activities.

Fear of sexual intercourse is comorbid with decreased desire, satisfaction, and sexual frequency among male and female patients. Patients and their partner may feel apprehensive about engaging in sex fearing that sexual activity may be medically contraindicated or may hurt the partner experiencing the medical illness. In individuals with heart disease, sexual partners may fear that the physical exertion of intercourse could place too great of a strain on the heart and result in sudden death during sex [5].

Chronic medical illness is consistently associated with an increased prevalence of anxiety, depressive symptoms and disorders [6]. Patients with chronic medical illnesses have been found to have two- to threefold higher rates of major depression compared with age- and gender-matched primary care patients. Depression can result from the either direct biologic effects of chronic medical illness (e.g., multiple sclerosis) or be a result of the functional changes and stressors resulting from their medical illness. Not only is depression a common consequence of chronic medical illness, but it is itself a risk factor for the development of chronic illnesses such as diabetes and coronary heart disease and adversely affects the course, complications, and management of chronic medical illness. Risk factors for depression include worsening condition, unrelieved pain, functional impairment, social isolation, and history of mood disorders [7].

Social Effects

Even though views on sexuality vary enormously between different cultures and religions, many societies are uncomfortable with the notion that medically compromised and individuals with disabilities have sexual needs and desires. Pervasive social and cultural norms, standards, and expectations create negative attitudes toward the disabled population and perpetuate a culture of undesirability and inability [8]. Current issues within the sexuality field and the disability movement include the misconceptions about sexual desires and potential expression of sexuality from individuals with disability. Such misconceptions rooted in culture and media, have resulted in the sexual concerns of individuals with disabilities being ignored [9]. Such cultural and societal norms further constrain the initiation and sexual engagement of individuals with complex medial disease and disability.

Education is vital to interrupting the cycle of stigmatization which needs to start with health care providers. However, sexuality is often overlooked by medical personnel who often do not feel comfortable addressing sexual concerns and lack knowledge regarding the impact medical illness has on sexual functioning. Furthermore, many professionals wrongly regard decline of sexual function as an inevitable consequence of ageing and disability.

Medical Conditions

In this section we will review select medical conditions that are common and highly associated with sexual dysfunction, which broadly refers to a disturbance in a person's ability to respond sexually or to experience sexual pleasure during any stage of normal sexual activity resulting in extreme distress and interpersonal strain for a minimum of 6 months. This list is by no means intended to be all inclusive but rather to capture commonly occurring medical illnesses or illnesses that invariably result in sexual dysfunction.

Cerebrovascular Disease

Cerebrovascular diseases are the third leading cause of death and one of the major causes of long-term disability in western countries. Strokes can result in a myriad of physical, autonomic and cognitive impairments that can interfere with sexual satisfaction. Twenty to 75% of patients with stroke suffer some form of sexual dysfunction [10]. The most common sexual problems after stroke are decline in sexual desire and intercourse frequency for both genders, decline in vaginal lubrication and orgasm in females, and decline in erection and ejaculatory function in males.

Post-stroke sexual dysfunction is thought to result from multiple factors, both psychosocial (i.e., depression, anxiety, fear of stroke recurrence, loss of self-esteem, role changes) and/or organic (i.e., stroke lesion, comorbidity, and medications). Additionally, patients who have had a stroke often have comorbidities such as hypertension, diabetes mellitus, atherosclerosis that not only put them at risk for the stroke itself but also cause reduction in blood flow to end organs including genitalia.

Physical limitations were cited by a majority of patients with stroke as having a negative impact on sexual functioning. The extent of sexual dysfunction often parallels the extent of motor disability and the level of independence in activities of daily living can be used as a predictor of sexual activity after stroke [11]. Physical barriers to sexual function after stroke include spasticity, weakness, sensory loss and pain which can restrict mobility, compromise comfort, and interfere with positioning. Flexor spasms can be disruptive and cause pain. Drooling and bladder and bowel incontinence are associated with social stigma and heavily impact social acceptance, and ability to engage intimately with partners. Sensory and perceptual impairments diminish an individual's ability to perceive pleasure with tactile stimulation. Post-stroke fatigue, manifesting as both physical and mental lack of energy, is another common symptom which can impact libido and motivation. Fatigue is likely the culmination of multiple factors, including organic brain lesion, psychosocial stress, altered sleep–wake cycles, and contributions from sedating medications. Nevertheless, nearly half of patients following stroke with no or mild physical disability also experience a decrease in libido, coital frequency, sexual arousal, orgasm, and sexual satisfaction [12].

While most individuals describe decreased sexual activity after a stroke, hypersexuality was reported in 10% of 192 stroke patients in one study [13]. This condition appears to occur in younger individuals and is most commonly associated with temporal lobe lesions but can also occur in subthalamic or bilateral thalamic infarctions [14].

Even though the sidedness of the stroke (right versus left) has not been shown to influence the extent of sexual impairments, it is clear that stroke location determines the physical and cognitive deficits that, in turn, affect sexual functioning. Patients with right sided cerebral strokes are likely to experience hemispatial neglect resulting in an inability to attend to and perceive stimuli from the contralateral side of the body or environment. Neglect can result in an individual's inability to groom and care for one's self as well as extinction of sexual and sensual stimuli emanating from the neglected hemi-body. Left sided lesions located in the middle cerebral artery territory can result in receptive and expressive aphasia which can have detrimental effects on ability to communicate with partners. Loss of effective communication can lead to difficulty with forming and maintaining social and sexual relationships and inability in expressing one's sexual needs and desires.

Persons who had a stroke commonly take medications that have a dampening effect on libido and sexual performance. Many antihypertensive medications, notably beta blockers, calcium channel blockers as well as diuretics reduce libido and result in erectile dysfunction. Antidepressants that are commonly used after stroke for depression and recovery are also associated with sexual side effects.

Even though most strokes do not usually cause significant hormonal changes that influence sexual functioning, aneurysmal subarachnoid hemorrhage is associated with a high risk for hypothalamic–pituitary dysfunction, given the proximity of the pituitary gland to the arterial circle of Willis. The most common neuroendocrine changes resulting from subarachnoid hemorrhage are deficiencies in growth hormone and hypogonadism. Thus, screening of pituitary function is recommended in this patient population.

The prevalence of major depression after stroke is reported to range from 12% to 60% with an estimated pooled frequency of 33% [15, 16]. Post-stroke depression is more commonly associated with left sided lesions and can result in severe apathy and social withdrawal as well as decrease in motor disability and sexual activity.

The effects of stroke on psychological and social functioning may be equally, if not more important in the decline of sexual activity in stroke survivors. Various psychosocial factors such as changes in body image, loss of self-esteem, role changes, and spousal relationships, partner availability, and fear of suffering another stroke may become barriers to healthy sexual functioning [17]. Furthermore patients may lack privacy due to their living arrangements (such as living with a caregiver or residing in a long-term care facility) and encounter negative attitudes towards sexuality.

Chronic Kidney Disease

Sexual dysfunction is highly prevalent in individuals with chronic kidney disease (CKD), especially those receiving dialysis. The etiology of sexual dysfunction in chronic kidney disease is multifactorial: abnormalities in gonadal–pituitary system, autonomic nervous system dysfunction, endothelial dysfunction, anemia and erythropoietin deficiency, secondary hyperparathyroidism, drugs, and psychological problems have been implicated [18]. Sexual dysfunction is inversely associated with glomerular filtration rate [19] and some studies have reported improvements following renal transplantation [20] suggesting that chronic kidney disease may directly contribute to sexual dysfunction.

CKD leads to dysfunction of the hypothalamic–pituitary–gonadal axis in both sexes resulting in loss of the pulsatile release of gonadotropin-releasing hormone (GnRH), low testosterone, and elevated luteinizing hormone (LH) and follicle-stimulating hormone (FSH) levels. CKD is also associated with autonomous production and reduced clearance of prolactin resulting in hyperprolactinemia which reduces gonadal responses to gonadotrophins and has been implicated in impotence, hypogonadism, and reduced desire. The severity of endocrine dysfunction is proportional to the degree of renal impairment and worsens with progression of renal disease. Decreased libido, difficulty with arousal and orgasm, erectile and ejaculatory dysfunction, lack of vaginal lubrication, menstrual irregularities, and amenorrhea are common problems in patients with CKD [21, 22]. Men with CKD experience impaired spermatogenesis, testicular atrophy, hypospermatogenesis, and infertility. Testosterone deficiency occurs in 26–66% of individuals [23]. Approximately 70–80% of men with chronic renal failure endorse ED, due to the effects of renal disease as well as comorbid vascular disease, diabetes, or uremic toxicity to the autonomic nervous system [21].

Women with CKD experience decreased libido and difficulties with arousal and orgasm. Up to 65% of women on hemodialysis report problems with sexual function, and up to 40% no longer engage in sexual intercourse [24]. Reduced ovarian function and hyperprolactinemia result in diminished estrogen production causing pubic hair loss, atrophic vaginitis, dyspareunia, and premature menopause. Menstrual irregularities with anovulation and infertility are common [25].

Treatment includes dialysis, optimization of nutritional intake, discontinuation of offending medications and correcting anemia of chronic renal disease. Vitamin D supplementation helps reduce incidence of secondary hyperparathyroidism, which promotes prolactin production. In some studies, zinc deficiency has been implicated in gonadal failure, and supplementation led to improved libido, sperm counts, and testosterone levels [26].

The administration of recombinant human erythropoietin to raise the hematocrit to 33–36% may enhance physical and sexual function as well as health-related quality of life [27].

There is some evidence that human erythropoietin administration normalizes the pituitary gonadal axis, lowering FSH, LH, and prolactin levels and raising serum testosterone [28].

A trial of hormone replacement therapy can be considered in a patient with CKD and hypogonadism. Unfortunately, testosterone supplementation in uremic men generally fails to restore libido or potency, despite normalized serum testosterone and reduced LH and FSH. Women with low estradiol levels may benefit from estradiol replacement which can be helpful in treating vaginal atrophy and dyspareunia. Women with CKD who suffer from chronic anovulation and lack of progesterone secretion can be treated with progesterone to restore menstrual cycles. Correction of hyperprolactinemia with dopaminergic agonists such as bromocriptine and cabergolide can yield improved sexual function but treatment is often limited by side effects.

Phosphodiesterase inhibitors result in improvements in sexual satisfaction and erectile dysfunction in men with CKD [26]. No single phosphodiesterase inhibitor (PDEi) has been identified as being superior in this population. Sildenafil, the most widely used agent, is mainly metabolized in the liver and excreted in the feces; therefore, its pharmacokinetics do not appear to be affected by mild to moderate renal impairment, but clearance is reduced in patients with creatinine clearance <30 mL/min [29]. Therefore, a lower starting dose is recommended for patients with creatinine clearance <30 mL/min or on hemodialysis. The occurrence of side effects is similar to that in other patients. Hypotension can be severe in a patient on hemodialysis but these effects can be limited by administering PDEi on nondialysis days [30].

Even though renal transplantation is associated with normalization of hormonal and metabolic profiles, its therapeutic effect on libido, erectile function, and sexual satisfaction remains debated [31]. Several studies suggest that rates of erectile dysfunction remain very high even after kidney transplant [32]. Sexual function after renal transplantation may be affected by graft malfunction, duration of dialysis prior to transplant, comorbid conditions, and side effects of immunosuppressive or hypertension therapy. Erectile dysfunction is caused by many other factors and thus, can be highly prevalent in patients with renal insufficiency even after kidney transplantation.

Cardiovascular Disease, Angina, and Myocardial Infarction

Sexual dysfunction is usually thought to be a consequence of cardiovascular disease, though ED and vaginal dryness may actually be presenting signs of heart disease [33]. As the ability to achieve erectile dysfunction is dependent on a robust vascular supply to the genitals, risk factors that compromise genital blood flow are similar to those that cause cardiovascular disease. Consequently, ED occurs commonly in individuals with occult cardiovascular and peripheral vascular disease and the degree of ED appears to correlate with the severity of cardiovascular disease [34–36]. ED and vaginal dryness may be presenting signs of heart disease and may appear 1–3 years before the onset of cardiovascular symptoms. A number of studies have estimated the interval between the onset of ED symptoms and the occurrence of coronary artery disease (CAD) symptoms as 2–3 years and a cardiovascular event as 3–5 years [37–39].

The coexistence and link between ED and CAD should prompt health care providers to inquire about the presence of one if the other has declared itself. Routine assessment of sexual problems should be a component of rehabilitation and management of patients with cardiovascular disease [33].

Patients who have experienced a cardiac event often experience physiological and psychological barriers to sexual activity including general anxiety, and fear of having angina or another myocardial infarction (MI). Fewer than 1% of myocardial infarctions occur during sexual intercourse, and only about 0.6% of sudden cardiac deaths may be related to sexual activity [40]. Even if associated with a very low absolute risk, sexual MI in patients with known cardiac disease [41]. Regular physical activity and cardiovascular risk factor modification might further reduce the risk [42, 43].

Sexual dysfunction after a myocardial infarction is estimated to occur in 50–75% of patients. Both men and women have less sexual activity and less satisfaction with sexual activity after an MI and there appear to be no gender differences in the quantity and quality of sexual activity after MI [44, 45]. Similarly, most patients with heart failure (HF) experience decreased libido, decreased sexual performance and frequency as well as a general dissatisfaction with their sexual function. ED occurs in 69.3% in patients with HF and is exceptionally high in patients with ischemic HF, with a prevalence of 81.1% [46]. A significant relation exists between a patient's sexual function and their New York Heart Association (NYHA) functional class [47]. A patient's exercise tolerance should be evaluated when counseling patients, as the increased exertion associated with sexual activity may increase the risk of another cardiovascular event.

The standard clinical measure of exertion is the metabolic equivalent of oxygen consumption (MET), where 1 MET is equivalent to the resting state. Sexual activity is often equated with an exercise workload of 2–3 METs in the pre-orgasmic stage and 3–4 METs during the orgasmic stage. The metabolic cost of sex in middle-aged married men is no more than 5 METS. If a person with coronary artery disease can achieve an energy expenditure of ≥3–5 METs without demonstrating ischemia during exercise testing, then the risk of an event associated with sexual activity is very low. Patients able to climb two flights of stairs without limiting symptoms and those who can complete stage II of a standard Bruce treadmill test (equivalent to 6–7 METs) are generally free of cardiovascular symptoms during sexual activity. Therefore, exercise testing is often used to assess both exercise tolerance and ability to safely return to sexual activity. The incidence of exertional angina and MI during sexual activities is believed to be reduced by revascularization and optimized medical treatment using aspirin, β-blockers, and lipid-lowering strategies [48–50].

A risk stratification algorithm was developed by the Third Princeton Consensus Panel to evaluate the degree of cardiovascular risk associated with sexual activity for men with varying degrees of cardiovascular disease. The risk stratification is also the basis for treatment recommendations of sexual dysfunction in men and women with known cardiovascular disease. Patients are assigned to three categories based on cardiovascular risk factors and exercise capacity: low, indeterminate (including those requiring further evaluation), and high risk. Those at low risk can resume sexual activity and be treated for sexual dysfunction. Most patients with cardiovascular disease are categorized as low risk and can safely resume sexual activities and receiver phosphodiesterase inhibitors for erectile dysfunction. Patients with uncertain cardiac conditions are at indeterminate risk. It is recommended that these individuals undergo further evaluation and be re-stratified into low or high risk groups before resuming sexual activity. This is often achieved by stress testing, particularly in patients with a sedentary lifestyle. Patients in the high-risk group are deemed to have a potentially significant risk associated with sexual activity, and should undergo cardiac assessment and be appropriately treated before resuming sexual activity and considered for PDE inhibitors. Patients need to be educated about the interaction of phosphodiesterase inhibitors and nitrates.

Epilepsy

Epilepsy is a central nervous system disorder characterized by a predisposition to generate epileptic seizures which is frequently associated with cognitive, psychological, and social consequences. A significant number of individuals have some degree of sexual dysfunction, including problems with libido, arousal, and orgasm [51]. Epileptiform discharges may cause disruption of pathways in the limbic system which plays an essential role in human sexual behavior. Sexual dysfunction can be caused by recurrent seizures as well as neurological, endocrine, psychiatric, and psychosocial factors [52, 53]. The most common sexual dysfunction is hyposexuality, defined as a global reduction in sexual interest, awareness, and activity due to altered neuroendocrine regulation, and effects of antiepileptic medications [54]. Right sided temporal lobe epilepsy has also been associated with other sexual behaviors such as sexual auras, ictal orgasms, and sexual automatisms.

Endocrine abnormalities are more common in people with epilepsy due to hypothalamic dysfunction. Hypogonadotropic hypogonadism is one of the more common endocrine abnormalities described in patients with epilepsy, commonly presenting as sexual dysfunction and lower fertility rates. Seizures of temporal lobe origin are particularly associated with reproductive and endocrine abnormalities as well as sexual dysfunction, with right sided temporal lobe seizures having greater impact than left sided ones. Sexual dysfunction occurs more frequently in persons with temporal lobe epilepsy than other seizure types [55].

Males with epilepsy have been found to have an increased risk of ED of up to 57% compared to 3–9% in the general population [56] and report dissatisfaction with their sexual life [57]. Diminished libido, arousal, and orgasm have also been reported in women with epilepsy. Hirsutism, menstrual cycle irregularities, anovulatory cycles, polycystic ovarian syndrome, and premature menopause are more common than in the general population [58].

Another common complaint in females is decreased sexual interest as well as painful intercourse because of vaginal dryness and vaginismus. In fact, genital blood flow was significantly decreased in women with epilepsy compared with controls during erotic visual stimulation [59].

The contribution of the social and psychological stresses of living with epilepsy may be an important factor in the higher rates of sexual dysfunction. Poor self-esteem, fear of rejection, and fear of having seizures during intercourse may interfere with the development of normal sexual interactions and lead to avoidance of sexual activity. This can make sexual partners feel rejected resulting in relationship problems in existing relationships.

Since antiepileptic agents are known to lower serum testosterone levels and have a significant impact on sexual function, the American Academy of Neurology (AAN) issued a practice parameter advocating single-drug therapy at the lowest possible dose that effectively controls seizures.

Parkinson's Disease

Parkinson's disease (PD) is a neurodegenerative disorder whose cardinal features are tremor, bradykinesia, and rigidity. Pathologically, it is characterized by a loss of nigrostriatal dopaminergic neurons and widespread accumulation of Lewy bodies. The cause of PD is probably multifactorial, with contributions from hereditary predisposition, environmental toxins, and aging. In contrast to Parkinson's disease, Parkinson's Plus syndrome constitutes a group of neurodegenerative disorders that have overlapping clinical symptoms of Parkinson's disease and do not respond to dopamine. The most common Parkinson's plus syndromes are multiple system atrophy (MSA), progressive supranuclear palsy (PSP), cortico-basal ganglionic degeneration (CBGD), and Lewy body dementia.

Parkinson's disease is progressive causing mounting physical disability over time. Most people with PD lose independent function between 3 and 7 years after the onset of symptoms. Motor symptoms include bradykinesia, resting tremor, rigidity and akinesia, impairment of postural reflexes, and loss of fine motor skills. Non-motor symptoms include neuropsychiatric disorders such as anxiety, depression, hallucinations, impaired impulse control, cognitive impairment, and depression as well as autonomic dysfunction, which may present as gastrointestinal, urinary, and sexual disturbances. The combination of motor and non-motor symptoms in PD can result in a host of problems in sexual functioning.

Sexual dysfunction is common in patients with PD and results in depression and disruption in relationships. Males experience decreased libido, erectile dysfunction, premature or no ejaculation, and inability to achieve an orgasm. Erectile dysfunction has been reported in 54–79% of men with PD [60, 61].

Similarly, most women with PD report decreased libido and difficulties reaching orgasm [61]. Women are more likely to report vaginal tightness, loss of lubrication, involuntary urination, anxiety, and inhibition than in matched controls [62].

Loss of normal dopamine levels in the brain may be a primary cause of decreased libido in some persons with PD. Dysfunction of dopamine transmission in the reward circuit in PD is associated with anhedonia, apathy, and dysphoria which results in diminished sexual motivation and difficulty experiencing sexual pleasure and orgasm. PD can result in apathy and lack of sexual drive even in the absence of erectile dysfunction. Profound fatigue, cognitive and psychiatric factors, and hypogonadism have a profoundly negative impact on sexual drive and function. A pilot study reported that nearly 50% of the men with Parkinson's disease studied were testosterone deficient which correlated with apathy [63]. Testosterone deficiency can cause depression, fatigue, decreased libido, and erectile dysfunction which responds to treatment with testosterone replacement therapy [64].

Depression and anxiety are common causes of sexual dysfunction and decreased motivation that can respond to antidepressants and anxiolytics.

Common autonomic manifestations of PD can affect sexual function and sense of self-worth. Sialorrhea is caused by a combination of dysphagia and head posture. It can respond to speech therapy, anticholinergic medications and botulinum toxin injections to the salivary glands. The most common cardiovascular features of PD are hypotension and orthostatic hypotension caused by loss of sympathetic innervation to end-organs. Hypotension and orthostatic hypotension can be associated with fatigue, dizziness, lightheadedness, and generalized weakness which can impact sexual motivation and energy. Sympathomimetic agents such as ephedrine and midodrine increase peripheral vascular resistance and are useful in the treatment of symptomatic hypotension. In PD, degeneration of the substantia nigra, which normally has an inhibitory effect on the micturition reflex [65, 66], leads to hyperreflexia of the detrusor muscle, with involuntary or uninhibited contractions and urinary urgency. Urinary urgency, frequency, and incontinence become more common as the disease progresses.

The treatment of PD can result in improvement in sexual dysfunction. The use of dopaminergic drugs sometimes results in improvement of sexual desire or function [67] and deep brain stimulation of the subthalamic nucleus (STN) has been found to have a small, albeit positive influence on sexual well-being [68]. Compulsive hypersexual behavior with or without mania has been described with the use of dopamine agonists as well as with therapeutic deep brain stimulation [69].

If no medical or psychological reason appears to be causing impotence, medications used for erectile dysfunction can be instituted. Phosphodiesterase inhibitors are effective treatment options for ED in patients with PD. Delayed gastrointestinal motility often seen in PD may result in delayed drug absorption of drugs and patients with MSA, in particular, may be predisposed to symptomatic hypotension as a side effect of this class of medications. Sublingual apomorphine is another therapeutic option for PD patients with ED. The action is through a dopaminergic effect in the hypothalamus and can cause nausea in some patients.

Cerebral Palsy

Cerebral palsy (CP) is the most common cause of physical disability in childhood with a prevalence of 1.5–3.3 per 1000 live births. It is a chronic, non-progressive disorder of movement and posture caused by abnormal brain development or damage to the immature newborn brain. Posture and movement disorders in CP are often accompanied by disturbances in perception, cognition, communication, and behavior, as well as epilepsy.

Cerebral palsy can affect the motor system, resulting in weakness and spasticity. This can result in limb contractures, hip dislocations and scoliosis. Oromotor weakness and incoordination can result in dysarthria, dysphagia, sialorrhea, and aspiration and may necessitate a feeding tube placement. Motor and expressive language impairments can result in significant social and communication difficulties. Behavioral disorders including attention deficit hyperactivity disorder, frustration, aggression, and mood disturbances are more prevalent in children with CP. All of these impairments can have a negative impact on self-perception and self-esteem and interfere with social integration, peer interactions, and formation of romantic and sexual relationships.

The development of secondary sexual characteristics in children with cerebral palsy starts earlier and ends later compared with children in the general population. In girls, menarche occurs an average of 1.3 years later than for the general population [70].

Adolescents and young adults with CP exhibit normal psychosexual development with similar sexual interests as able bodied peers. Despite their interest, they are less likely to attain sexual milestones and attain these milestones at a later age than their peers. At the age of 16–20 years, adolescents with CP are less focused on sexuality and have significantly less sexual experience compared with their age matched peers [71].

Young adults with CP not only have to deal with the difficulties of finding their sexual identity and maturing as sexual and social beings, but they have to overcome the additional hurdle of learning to overcome physical and emotional barriers. It is unclear what effect motor functioning has on the likelihood of forming intimate sexual relationships though ambulatory individuals are more likely to engage in intercourse and are more likely to experience sexual satisfaction than their non-ambulatory counterparts [72, 73].

Children and adolescent with CP have difficulty with achieving social milestones as they mature and transition into adulthood. They have fewer friendships, exhibit fewer social behaviors, and are more isolated and victimized by their peers than classmates without disability [74, 75]. Furthermore, dependence on parents and caregivers can make it difficult for children with cerebral palsy to transition into adulthood and assume the adult roles that are important for building relationships. When engaging in intimate relationships, adults with physical disabilities worry about receiving personal care from potential partners. Their dependence may make them feel different from their peers and more vulnerable to physical, emotional and financial abuse. Psychological adjustment, self-efficacy, and sexual self-esteem are important factors in the development of social and sexual relationships. In fact, high sexual self-esteem can facilitate meeting and engaging with people, flirting and dating, resulting in a higher likelihood of engaging in romantic and sexual relationships.

It is important for family members, care providers, and other contacts to facilitate discussions about sexual questions and interests and provide acceptance of a child's maturing sexual identity.

Spinal Cord Injury

Spinal cord injury (SCI) is a traumatic, life-altering event that is usually associated with loss of motor and sensory function, disruption in autonomic innervation resulting in sexual impairment. The normal sexual response depends on a very intricate interaction between the peripheral somatic and autonomic nervous system, spinal reflexes, and the brain. The location and extent of a spinal cord injury as well as remaining neurological function are major determinants of sexual functioning and can be used to predict sexual responses.

For men, the ability to experience erections is preserved more frequently than the ability to experience ejaculation [76]. A study examining outcomes in 193 men at least 10 years after their spinal cord injury reported that 75% reported achieving an erection, 44% reported being able to achieve ejaculation [77]. There are two areas in the spinal cord that play a central role in controlling sexual function. The sacral cord (S2–4) mediates reflex erections which are erections elicited by penile stimulation. These erections occur reflexively and may or may not be associated with arousal. Genital stimulation triggers reflexogenic erections and the erections last as long as the stimulus is delivered. The erections in spinal cord injured males are usually less rigid and may not allow penetration. Men are generally able to achieve reflex erection if their spinal cord injury spares the sacral spinal cord segments. Largely, injuries higher in the spinal cord predict better likelihood for achieving reflex erections while injuries to the sacral cord segments and the cauda equine impair reflex activity and abolish reflex erection [78].

On the other hand, psychogenic erections are mediated by the brain and depend on cerebral and spinal cord integrity extending to the hypogastric plexus (T10 to L2 spinal cord levels). Lesions above T10 substantially impair the capacity for psychogenic erections. Psychogenic arousal can be predicted by the ability to perceive sensation to pinprick and light touch in the T11–L2 dermatomes.

The majority of men with SCI are unable to ejaculate, with the exception of men with incomplete paraplegia of whom 75% could ejaculate. Despite this, about half of men with SCI are able to experience orgasm. However; the quality of their orgasm may be different [79, 80].

Orgasm is more common among individuals with incomplete injuries (versus complete) and among individuals with upper motor lesions (versus lower motor lesions). The use of oral midodrine to encourage ejaculation may improve likelihood of orgasm but is associated with a significant increase in blood pressure, and can cause autonomic dysreflexia [81].

The location of spinal cord injuries has similar effects on the female sexual responses. The counterpart to an erection in males is vaginal and clitoral vasocongestion and lubrication. Reflexive vaginal lubrication is likely to occur when sacral segments S2–S5 are spared. Women with sacral preservation can utilize manual and vibratory self-stimulation to augment this response.

Women with complete SCIs above T10 are unable to experience psychogenically based genital vasocongestion, even if subjective sexual arousal is present. The ability to recognize light touch and pinprick sensation in the T11–L2 dermatomes predicts a women's ability to experience psychogenically induced genital arousal. Similar to men, women can experience orgasm after spinal cord injury, even if their spinal cord injury is complete (i.e., an injury resulting in a loss of ability to send sensory and motor nerve impulses beyond the level of injury). Approximately one-half of women with spinal cord injury experience orgasm by self-report in the laboratory setting. Women with complete injuries to the S2–S5 spinal segments are less likely to achieve orgasm than women with other levels of spinal cord injury. The latency to orgasm is increased, but the qualitative description of orgasm is indistinguishable from non-injured controls [82].

Audiovisual stimulation leads to similar subjective and autonomic responses found in women without injury, and can be utilized in conjunction with other methods to facilitate arousal.

In both men and women sexual frequency decreases after SCI and sexual expression often changes. Individuals become more open and likely to engage in sexual fantasies. The frequency of hugging, kissing, manual stimulation, and use of oral–genital stimulation is not statistically different than in couples without spinal cord injury. Relationship factors such as partner satisfaction and relationship quality as well as mood and independence appear to be more important predictors of sexual satisfaction than genital functioning in both men and women [83, 84].

Amputation

Individuals who undergo amputations often have diseases that not only result in the amputation itself, but also put them at risk for erectile dysfunction (e.g., diabetes mellitus, vascular disease). Amputations performed for oncological reasons may be associated with decreased libido, and erectile dysfunction due to simultaneous treatment with chemotherapy and/or radiation therapy. Therefore changes in sexual behavior are often difficult to attribute to the amputation alone [85].

The site and level of amputation can result in limitations to physical activities affecting movement, positioning, stability, balance, hand control, and dexterity [86]. Sexual positions may need adaptation to accommodate these changes; after a major limb amputation side lying or bottom position may be preferable. Transfemoral amputees tend to experience a greater decline in sexual function and frequency than transtibial amputees [86, 87].

Ensuing pain is another factor that negatively impacts sexual function after amputation. While nearly all patients experience some degree of phantom limb sensation after an amputation, 55–85% experience phantom limb pain [88]. Amputees who suffered from amputation related pain or discomfort related to their prosthetic device experience more significant sexual dysfunction compared with those who did not have phantom phenomena [87, 89]. Amputation related pain may negatively impact sexual desire and thereby reduce sexual activity.

Other factors that negatively affected sexual functioning include single marital status, older age, and male gender [90].

Apart from these physical factors, psychological consequences of an amputation such as depression, performance anxiety, and an altered body image have been shown to influence sexual adjustment after amputation.

Human Immunodeficiency Virus Infection

The diagnosis of human immunodeficiency virus infection (HIV) is often associated with considerable distress with changes in body image, social stigma, and fear of rejection from friends, family, and society.

In addition, individuals may experience feelings of anxiety or guilt as well as fear of infecting others after HIV diagnosis. Furthermore, the need for adherence to safe sex practices may have an added negative impact on sexual functioning [91]. The use of condoms reduces penile sensitivity and contributes to erectile dysfunction in males [92]. Generally, individuals are more likely to experience sexual dysfunction as disease severity worsens with rates of sexual dysfunction being higher in patients with AIDS than in patients who are HIV infected but do not have AIDS. The most prevalent sexual problems in females are low sexual desire, orgasmic dysfunction, and dyspareunia [93, 94].

Sexual dysfunction in men includes reduced libido, erectile dysfunction (ED), ejaculation disorders, lower orgasmic function, and depressed sexual satisfaction. The likelihood of developing sexual problems is not only increased by the chronic illness but by the comorbidities that are frequently associated with HIV including excessive consumption of alcohol, recreational drug use, and smoking. Metabolic disorders and cardiovascular disease are other risk factors that are more common in HIV infected individuals. Since the prevalence of ED increases with age, its occurrence among HIV-infected persons will likely rise with increasing life expectancy and the increasing prevalence of HIV among those older than 50 years.

Hypothalamic–pituitary function can also be affected resulting in higher rates of hypogonadism in HIV-infected men than in age-matched controls. The premature decline of serum testosterone levels is associated with inappropriately low or normal levels of luteinizing hormone and increased visceral adiposity [95]. The prevalence of hypogonadism has been lowered with the introduction of Highly Active Antiretroviral Therapy (HAART), but it still remains the most common endocrine disorder of HIV-infected men [96]. Estimated rates of hypogonadism in HIV-infected men are as high as 20–25% and 25–62% of HIV-infected men report ED in the post-HAART era [97, 98]. Hypogonadism can be effectively treated with testosterone replacement therapy which not only restores sexual drive and performance, but also enhances PDE-5 inhibitor effectiveness. Testosterone replacement provides multiple benefits beyond improved sexual function, including heightened erythropoiesis, weight gain, and prevention of bone loss, increased energy, and improved mood. However, since most men with ED have normal serum testosterone levels, erectile dysfunction is likely related to other factors.

Other contributing causes for sexual dysfunction in HIV infected individuals are neurological sequalae of the infection and treatment. In many patients with HIV infection or AIDS, sexual desire decreases because of fatigue, generalized wasting, muscle aches, pains, paresthesias, and depression. Body-image concerns also worsen with symptomatic disease. Reports of the prevalence of depression over the course of HIV infection vary widely however; one meta-analysis found that the diagnosis of major depressive disorder is nearly twice as likely in HIV-infected persons as compared to those without HIV [99].

The role of HAART in the pathogenesis of ED is still controversial. Although both protease inhibitors and nonnucleoside reverse transcriptase inhibitors are associated with sexual dysfunction, most studies are retrospective and a direct causal relationship has not been established. HAART treatment is known to contribute to metabolic and hormonal changes as well as alterations in body composition which together might have an adverse effect on erectile function. Specifically, HAART treatment results in lipodystrophy, a syndrome characterized by peripheral fat loss and central fat accumulation which is frequently, but not invariably, associated with alterations of lipid metabolism and derangement of insulin sensitivity and diabetes mellitus. These metabolic changes promote endothelial dysfunction which results in vascular compromise and cause changes in body habitus that can negatively impact self-esteem. Augmented peripheral conversion of androgens to estrogens in lipodystrophic fat tissue is thought to cause elevated estradiol levels in HIV infected men, though its impact on sexual function is not clear. Furthermore, peripheral neuropathy is another complication of both HAART and HIV infection which is associated with both erectile dysfunction and delayed ejaculation.

Current treatment approaches include management of underlying medical and psychological conditions, and testosterone replacement therapy for men with documented hypogonadism. PDE-5 inhibitors are the mainstay of pharmacologic treatment of ED when serum testosterone is normal. When used simultaneously with protease inhibitors which decrease cytochrome P450 efficiency it is important to reduce the dose and increase the interval between PDE-5 inhibitor administrations.

Chronic Respiratory Illness

Chronic respiratory illness or chronic obstructive pulmonary disease (COPD) is a group of illnesses that cause breathing problems, such as emphysema and chronic bronchitis. The overall incidence of ED is 1.88-fold greater in the COPD cohort than in the non-COPD cohort and individuals with more severe disease have higher rates of ED [100].

Individuals with poor COPD control who require more emergency room visits and admissions are more likely to have ED. Sexual dysfunction tends to be worse in individuals with more severe pulmonary function impairments as assessed by pulmonary function tests, blood gases, and exercise tests [101].

Sexual dysfunction and erectile impotence occur in patients with COPD in the absence of other known causes of sexual problems [101]. The mechanism by which COPD results in higher rates of ED is likely multifactorial. Increased arterial stiffness in COPD is related to the severity of airflow obstruction and may be a factor in the excess risk for erectile dysfunction [102]. Hypoxemia itself is likely a cause for ED both by reducing functional capacity as well as its effects on endothelial function. Hypoxia increases sympathetic activation causing vasoconstriction and a significant reduction in nitric oxide synthase activity, the rate-limiting factor for nitric oxide production in the penile corpus cavernosum necessary for erectile function [103]. Tissue hypoxia also contributes to systemic inflammation in COPD which is related to the presence and severity of ED [104]. Long-term treatment with oxygen therapy has been shown to result in modest improvement in arterial pO2, serum testosterone, and erectile function [105].

Dyspnea is prevalent in patients with COPD and the high energy demands of sexual activity can result in increased dyspnea, generalized weakness, and compromised stamina for sexual activity [106]. The fear and anticipation of dyspnea and reduced exercise tolerance may further limit sexual activity [107]. Cough, muscular weakness, and the associated reduction of physical activity are important causes of reduced sexual activity in COPD patients [107]. Fatigue, a perception of mental or physical exhaustion due to exertion, is another frequent and distressing symptom. Furthermore, cardiovascular disease, diabetes mellitus, metabolic syndrome, and hypertension are common conditions coexisting with COPD which are themselves associated with high rates of sexual dysfunction [108].

Individuals with COPD often have progressive weight loss, and loss of lean body mass which has been linked to skeletal muscle dysfunction and debility. Hypogonadism with lower testosterone levels in males with COPD may further exacerbate lean body weight loss and contribute to decreased libido, ED, and reduced ejaculation [109]. Androgen deficiency can also induce depression, anxiety, anger, fatigue, and sleep disorders which negatively impact sexual functioning.

Cancer

With improvements in cancer diagnosis and treatment, life expectancy after cancer is increasing with more cancer survivors living with the effects of cancer.

Sexual dysfunction represents a long-term complication among cancer survivors with a wide range of manifestations and a huge impact on quality of life [110]. Most sexual problems are not caused by the cancer itself, but by toxicities of cancer treatment [111]. Cancer and its treatment result in a host of problems including physical disfigurement, pain, and neurovascular and organ injury which often lead to significant and long-term disruption in sexual function and intimacy, regardless of cancer type [112].

Problems after cancer can be categorized as disorders of sexual response (e.g., arousal, erectile dysfunction, ejaculatory dysfunction, reduced lubrication in females, chronic dyspareunia, orgasmic dysfunction), and disorders of sexual desire and motivation (e.g., hypoactive sexual desire, reduced sexual motivation, body image disturbances, loss of sexual self-esteem) [113].

Pelvic surgeries are among the most common causes of organic sexual dysfunction in men and women. Radical prostatectomies and cystectomies and low anterior or abdominoperineal resections for rectal cancer are associated with considerable rates of erectile dysfunction [114]. If nerve sparing technique is used to perform radical prostatectomies, recovery from erectile dysfunction may occur within the first year following the procedure. External beam radiation therapy induces ED in 30–40% of the patients, between 1 and 2 years of treatment [115]. Even though the reported incidence of erectile dysfunction varies widely, the rate of ED is quite high. Brachytherapy was originally introduced to limit the detrimental effects of external beam radiation therapy on bowel and bladder function and sexual function In contrast to radical prostatectomy, the onset of erectile dysfunction following brachytherapy is gradual and can occur over years with stabilization occurring after approximately 3 years [116, 117].

Penile rehabilitation attempts to address loss of erections by improving oxygen delivery to preserve erectile tissue. Treatment options include PDE inhibitors, intraurethral alprostadil, intracavernosal injections, and vacuum erection devices though no consensus has been reached on an optimal treatment protocol.

Similarly, radical cystectomies, and hysterectomy for cancers of the cervix and endometrium are associated with sexual dysfunction in women. Gynecological surgeries frequently result in vaginal dryness, a shortened and fibrosed vaginal vault and loss of libido. These complications are further aggravated when accompanied by bilateral oophorectomy which causes premature menopause symptoms or treatment with endocrine therapy. Commonly used endocrine therapies that cause estrogen deprivation often have extensive sexual side effects that affect quality of life [118]. The risk of developing more severe sexual problems increases when radiation or chemotherapy is used in addition to surgery. As in men, pelvic radiation therapy contributes to the risk of sexual dysfunction, from a combination of ovarian failure and direct tissue damage to genital areas in the radiation field [119].

Loss of libido is often the result of fatigue and general malaise. In addition, it can be due to "de-prioritization" of sexual activity. Chemotherapy is associated with a loss of desire and decreased frequency of intercourse. Common side effects of chemotherapy such as nausea, vomiting, diarrhea, constipation, mucositis, weight loss or gain, and alopecia can affect self-image. Psychosocial ramifications of the cancer itself and cancer treatments affect mood, self-esteem, sexual drive, and sexual identity posing another layer of challenges [111, 120].

Problems with sexual function, unlike other side effects of cancer therapy, often do not resolve with time [121, 122]. The most common reasons cited for sexual dysfunction in cancer patients have been poorly controlled pain, chronic nausea, anxiety, fatigue, and treatment-related effects such as the cytotoxic effects of certain types of chemotherapy. Chronic opioid use, as an independent factor, can lead to sexual dysfunction, decreased libido, increased fatigue, and generally poor function. Studies have shown that sexual health concerns impose a considerable negative effect on patients' health-related quality of life (HRQoL).

Medications

Brief Summary of Hormones and Neurotransmitters That Play a Role in Sexual Behavior

Libido in both sexes depends on an interplay between hormonal levels, balance of neurotransmitter actions, and social cues. Both men and women depend on the androgen dehydroepiandrosterone (DHEA), a precursor to testosterone and estrogen, for arousal. Decreased libido can be observed with decreased androgen levels (testosterone and DHEA), increased estrogen or an increased estrogen: testosterone ratio.

Dopamine and serotonin are important neurotransmitters that help regulate libido and sexual function. Dopamine is a vital neurotransmitter in the limbic area associated with pleasure and reward and is implicated in heightening sexual motivation. Stimulation of dopaminergic receptors in the hypothalamus is important in obtaining erections. Dopamine in the tuberoinfundibular dopaminergic system of the hypothalamus also has a strong inhibiting influence on hypothalamic prolactin synthesis and secretion. In contrast, serotonin and thyrotrophin releasing hormone increase prolactin release which has an inverse effect on libido, and erectile function. Although the mechanism by which selective serotonin reuptake inhibitors (SSRIs) impair sexual functioning is not fully understood, it is generally agreed that serotonin exerts an inhibitory effect on sexual function, including sexual motivation, orgasm, and ejaculation. In addition, serotonin inhibits nitric oxide production, which has an important role in relaxing the vasculature in erectile tissue.

The autonomic nervous system regulates the peripheral aspects of sexual function with the parasympathetic nervous system causing vasodilation and engorgement of sexual organs while the sympathetic nervous system is active during orgasm. Orgasm and male ejaculation is controlled by the sympathetic autonomic division and utilizes the neurotransmitter acetylcholine. Many antidepressants have some efficacy at cholinergic and alpha1-adrenergic receptors, thereby inhibiting the autonomic nervous system and consequently inhibiting normal sexual function.

Medications that affect libido and sexual functioning mediate their side effects by altering levels of hormones and neurotransmitters in the brain and/or peripheral targets.

Medications

Many antidepressants have been linked to sexual dysfunction. Selective serotonin reuptake inhibitors (SSRIs) and selective norepinephrine reuptake inhibitors (SNRIs) increase serotonin levels and cause sexual dysfunction. Erectile dysfunction and delayed ejaculation or anejaculation are observed in men and reduced sexual desire and difficulty reaching orgasm in women. Monoamine oxidase inhibitors can also depress libido. Tricyclic antidepressants have adverse sexual effects due to their anticholinergic effects and can cause decreased ability to achieve orgasm in both sexes, erectile dysfunction in men and breast enlargement in women.

Fortunately, some antidepressants do not affect libido and sexual function to the same extent as most SSRIs and SNRIs. Medications that promote dopamine activity have a beneficial effect on libido. A much lower incidence of sexual dysfunction is reported for the newer 5-HT2 blockers. These types of antidepressants, which include nefazodone and mirtazapine encourage dopamine activity. Bupropion, unlike the majority of antidepressants, has less serotonergic effects and is a mild dopamine agonist. Therefore, bupropion can actually have a positive influence on sexual desire and can be prescribed to counter the sexual side effects seen with SSRIs and SNRIs.

When starting a patient on an antidepressant, sexual concerns and history should be elicited with goal of choosing an antidepressant that has the best individualized side effect profile. If an individual is on a medication which has sexual side effects, there are several options one can explore short of discontinuing the medication altogether. Since sexual dysfunction associated with serotonergic activity is dose-dependent decreasing the dosage of the antidepressant may improve libido while maintaining adequate treatment of depression. The only evidence about drug holidays comes from a small, open study in which findings suggest that 1- to 2-day holidays from the shorter half-life SSRIs (i.e., sertraline, paroxetine) may be helpful. This effect did not apply to fluoxetine. All antidepressants require adequate trials of at least 6 weeks before a change in dose or medication is considered.

Antipsychotics and lithium also contribute to depressed libido and sexual function, with a reported prevalence of 45–80% in males and 30–80% in females [123]. Antipsychotics have multiple mechanisms by which they disrupt sexual functioning: their anti-dopaminergic effects can cause hyperprolactinemia resulting in galactorrhea, erection disorders, and reduced libido. Most antipsychotics block noradrenergic receptors, which can cause erectile and ejaculatory problems and decreased lubrication in women [124]. Finally, they have generalized sedating properties which reduce energy and sexual motivation. First-generation classical antipsychotics are associated with a very high incidence of sexual dysfunction [125].

Olanzapine, paliperidone, risperidone, and ziprasidone are atypical antipsychotics that increase prolactin to a much lesser extent than typical antipsychotics. Atypical antipsychotics such as aripiprazole, clozapine, and quetiapine do not elevate prolactin levels and therefore have a more benign side effect profile in regards to libido and sexual function [126].

Anticonvulsants have been associated with sexual dysfunction due to increased prolactin levels and reduced sex hormones. In particular, enzyme-inducing antiepileptic drugs (AEDs) such as phenobarbital, phenytoin, and carbamazepine influence the metabolism of sex hormones and their binding. This results in abnormalities in sex hormone profiles (increased sex hormone-binding globulin, low estradiol, low testosterone, low dehydroepiandrosterone), resulting in sexual dysfunction. Newer antiepileptic agents that are not enzyme inducing such as oxcarbazepine, levetiracetam, and lamotrigene appear to have a better side effect profile [127, 128].

The use of long-term opioid therapy has been associated with androgen deficiency referred to as opioid associated androgen deficiency which persists even after cessation of treatment and can last months to years. Opioid associated androgen deficiency is thought to result from the inhibitory action of morphine on hypothalamic gonadotropin-releasing hormone secretion. The syndrome is characterized by the presence of inappropriately low levels of gonadotropins (follicle stimulating hormone and luteinizing hormone) leading to inadequate production of sex hormones, particularly testosterone. Symptoms include reduced libido, erectile dysfunction, fatigue, hot flashes, and depression [129]. There should be a high index of suspicion for the development of opioid associated androgen deficiency when treatment duration is longer than a few weeks [130]. Doses exceeding approximately 100 mg of oral morphine equivalents daily may be more likely to cause androgen deficiency than lower opioid doses [131].

Antihypertensive drugs represent one of the most implicated classes of drugs in causing sexual dysfunction. Even though antihypertensive agents are used in patients who likely have coexisting small vessel disease that would affect erectile ability, the observation that sexual problems occur more frequently in patients receiving antihypertensive medication than in those with untreated hypertension underscores the separate effect antihypertensive medications have on erectile potential [132]. Diuretics, methyldopa, clonidine, and β blockers (especially nonselective ones), are well known to cause sexual problems or exacerbate existing problems. One of the proposed mechanisms by which β-blockers may cause sexual dysfunction is inhibition of the sympathetic nervous system, which is involved during sexual arousal and in the regulation of luteinizing hormone and testosterone secretion [133]. Of the beta blockers on the market, metoprolol and especially nebivolol appear to have a very low risk of sexual side effects compared with other agents in its class.

Spironolactone, a diuretic commonly used in congestive heart failure also has a detrimental side effect profile causing gynecomastia, impotence, and decreased libido [134]. Spironolactone is structurally similar to sex hormones and acts as an androgen receptor blocker which results in these side effects.

Thiazide diuretics are associated with an exceptional high risk for erectile dysfunction, likely due to their link to vascular and metabolic abnormalities, including endothelial dysfunction, insulin resistance, and diabetes mellitus. Thiazide diuretics including hydrochlorothiazide and chlorthalidone cause decreased libido, erectile dysfunction, and anejaculation with an incidence that varies from 3% to 32%, and may be associated with decreased vaginal lubrication [135]. Loop diuretics might have a more favorable side effect on sexual functioning than thiazides [136].

On the other hand, calcium channel blockers, alpha-blockers, ACE inhibitors and angiotensin II receptor antagonists (ARBs) generally have relatively neutral effects on erectile function in hypertensive patients [137, 138].

Statins and lipid-lowering medications also appear to improve erectile function in patients who have no cardiovascular risks other than erectile dysfunction. It is thought that statins may provide sexual benefit due to antioxidant effects. However, in patients with cardiovascular risk factors such as smoking or diabetes, erectile dysfunction was more likely to occur after statin initiation [138].

Physiology of Sexuality

Sexual function is a very intricate process that relies on a complex network of peripheral and central pathways involving the autonomic and somatic nerves and the integration of spinal and supraspinal sites in the central nervous system with the hypothalamic and limbic regions. Sexual functions are governed centrally by the anteromedial and medial-tuberal zones of the hypothalamus which receive input from cortical and subcortical structures concerned with emotion and memory. Although they remain poorly understood, these nuclei act as integrative centers for sexual responses and are also thought to be involved in more complex aspects of sexuality, such as sexual preference and gender identity.

Spinal reflexes are regulated by highly integrated somatic and autonomic pathways in the spinal cord and brain. Normally, spinal cord reflexes mediating genital arousal are under tonic inhibition by higher brain centers. When there is an interruption between the brain and the sacral spinal cord, such as exists in spinal cord injuries or multiple sclerosis affecting the spinal cord, there is release of this tonic inhibition, resulting in heightened spinal reflexes. This can be harnessed to enhance sexual experience.

Reflexogenic excitement refers to genital vasocongestion resulting in penile and clitoral erection in response to direct genital stimulation (e.g., tactile, oral, vibratory). The afferent, sensory component of the reflex enters the spinal cord through the pudendal nerve where it activate parasympathetic efferent fibers which then leave the spinal cord in the cauda equine forming the pelvic nerves.

Sensation

The genitals receive a rich supply of sensory nerve endings that mediate vasocongestion and erotic sensation. The density of sensory nerve endings is highest in the penis in males and clitoris in females though there is considerable variation in their distribution between individuals. Sensory nerve cells reside in the second and third sacral segments and their axons form the pudendal nerve. The pudendal nerve contains the primary afferent sensory and motor pathways to the genitals and the cavernous nerve contains the primary parasympathetic contribution.

Following sexual stimulation, neurogenic and endothelial release of nitric oxide (NO) plays an important role in relaxation of the clitoral and cavernosal arteriolar smooth muscles resulting in engorgement of the genitalia. This results in enhanced genital sensitivity and genital lubrication. Neurological injury along the entire neuraxis can result in decreased genital and body sensation. When sensation is impaired, pleasurable sensation derived from stimulation of erotic body part is either partially or completely disrupted. All senses should be harnessed to achieve a heightened sexual state including smell, vision, taste, and touch. Music, lighting, and sexual props may contribute to a heightened romantic mood. Sensory input can be further augmented by using masturbation, mirrors, vibrators, dildos, and penile sheaths. Partners can enjoy sexually erotic images and movies together and explore each other's body parts for sensual and sexually heightened sensations. Sensate areas that have preserved sensation such as the nipples, neck, or inner thighs may be perceived as erogenous. Patients and their partners should be encouraged to explore their bodies and utilize their environment to achieve sexual fulfillment.

Movement/Mobility

Physical deficits such as hemiparesis, hemiplegia, paraplegia, tetraplegia, or monoplegia as well as spasticity may limit body positioning and movement. Activities such as undressing, positioning, cuddling, embracing, stroking, stimulating, and engaging in intercourse can be cumbersome, difficult and require assistance. This can put significant emotional strain on the individual as well as their partner. Care attendants can be recruited to help with self-care tasks, transfers, and positioning.

Range of motion can improve flexibility and be incorporated into foreplay. Often, spasticity can be managed with spasticity medication with and without injections of neurotoxins, such as botulinum toxin into affected muscles. Most spasmolytics, with the exception of dantrolene, cause sedation and may interfere with motivation and arousal. Illnesses that result in upper motor neuron injury can cause hip flexion and adduction spasticity which interferes with positioning necessary for intercourse. This can often be treated satisfactorily with neurolysis to the obturator nerve or upper lumbar rami supplying the iliopsoas muscles. Nerve blocks can result in improved hip joint movement, pain control, spasticity, and hygiene.

Props and positioning devices can assist with positioning for people with functional limitations. Wedges, pillows, and cushions can be purchased through internet retailers or at sexuality shops. Pillows behind the lower back and knees can reduce lower back pain, decrease spasms, and improve access to the genital area. Thigh slings support the thighs in an elevated and abducted position facilitating genital access. Sexual pleasure should be explored on surfaces other than the bed including wheelchairs or shower chairs. Some couples find that a stream of water can enhance their sexual pleasure when performing sexual acts in the shower. When hand function is compromised and weakened, occupational therapists can be involved to design alternate methods of holding enhancement devices. For example, Velcro closures can be applied to gadgets to improve grasp ability and devices can be attached to the mouth and tongue if extremities are too weak.

Even when the sequelae of medical illness make intercourse impossible, individuals and their partners should be encouraged to explore other ways of providing each other with sexual satisfaction such as reciprocal masturbation, oral sex, and non-genital touching [139]. Communication between sexual partners should be promoted to help partners discover what is sexually pleasurable. Sexual adjustment after injury is closely and positively correlated to frequency of intercourse, and willingness to experiment with alternative sexual expressions [84].

Fatigue

Fatigue is one of the most common reported causes for loss of sexual desire and needs to be addressed in the rehabilitation of persons with medical illness [140]. Timing sexual activities during periods of the day when fatigue is at its lowest can minimize its detrimental effects. Most people feel more energetic in the morning, the beginning of the week and on quiet, less stress-filled days. Sufficient amount of sleep promotes libido and genital arousal in healthy women and likely has a similar effect in persons with disabilities [141]. Strengthening and endurance training as part of the overall rehabilitation program can help improve physical function and endurance during sexual relations. Energy conservation techniques, such as taking naps, using ambulation aids, and getting assistance for activities of daily living can preserve energy for sexual activities. Couples should be encouraged to experiment with various positions that may be less fatiguing. For example, an individual might find assuming the bottom or side to side position less strenuous. A conditioning program should address mental and physical stress reduction, as well as energy conservation during sexual activities.

Pain

Pain management is very important in chronic illness and should focus on identifying the source of pain to better target analgesic interventions. Pain may be chronic or just related to sexual activities. Chronic pain may be nociceptive or neuropathic and the description of pain usually indicates the etiology and helps with the treatment choices. Nociceptive pain is related to direct tissue injury with resultant stimulation of pain fibers and can further be subdivided into somatic pain involving skin, soft tissue, muscle, and bone and visceral pain which stems from autonomic transmission of pain stimuli from the organs. In neuropathic pain, signals are generated as a result of changes in the nervous system that sustain pain signals even after the inciting injury resolves. It is frequently observed in conditions affecting the nervous system such as multiple sclerosis or strokes.

The initial treatment of neuropathic pain involves either antidepressants (e.g., tricyclic antidepressants or serotonin noradrenaline reuptake inhibitors) or antiepileptic medications (e.g., gabapentin and pregabalin). A meta-analysis of pharmacotherapy for neuropathic pain in adults provided strong recommendations for the use of gabapentin, pregabalin, duloxetine, and venlafaxine as well as tricyclic antidepressants [142].

The pharmacologic approach to nociceptive pain primarily involves nonnarcotic and, if severe, opioid analgesics. Acetaminophen and nonsteroidal anti-inflammatory drugs are first line agents that have been shown to be more effective than placebo and can be useful for arthritis and low back pain. These agents, however, are associated with risks, particularly in older patients, pregnant patients, and patients with certain comorbidities such as cardiovascular, renal, gastrointestinal, and liver disease. While the use of opioids to manage cancer pain is well accepted, the role of opioids in chronic non-cancer pain is controversial because of concerns about efficacy, safety, and the possibility of addiction or abuse. Opioid therapy should be reserved for those who have chronic intractable pain which is inadequately managed with other methods. Opioids should not be considered first line agents in managing chronic pain. When opioids are used, they should be combined with nonpharmacologic therapy and nonopioid pharmacologic therapy for maximal effect.

Behavioral and psychological interventions such as relaxation and guided imagery, biofeedback, and cognitive behavioral therapy address psychosocial contributors to pain and can help modify cognitive processing of pain [143]. Stretching and strengthening exercises, ergonomics, and posture training can improve physical function and improve physiological and psychological adaptation to chronic pain [144, 145].

Physical treatments utilizing heat, ice, and electroanalgesia modify pain signal processing and improve pain perception. Some patients have good results in pain and sense of well-being with non-allopathic pain strategies including acupuncture, yoga, and massage therapy.

If sexual activity causes pain, individuals may benefit from the use of an analgesic, including nonsteroidal anti-inflammatory medications, acetaminophen, or opioids approximately 30 min before sexual activity.

Pain caused by dyspareunia can be controlled with topical analgesic creams, including lidocaine jelly or ointment, as well as amitriptyline and baclofen creams that can be applied to the genitals prior to sexual intercourse to relieve discomfort. Many creams cause a burning sensation and anesthetic creams have a numbing effect that can reduce genital sensation and interfere with achieving pleasure. Dyspareunia due to vaginal atrophy, usually presenting in postmenopausal women occurs as a result of declining estrogen levels and can be managed with estrogen preparations [146]. Ospemifene, a novel selective estrogen receptor modulator that was approved by the Food and Drug Administration in 2013 for postmenopausal dyspareunia is an oral alternative that is taken once daily [147].

Neurogenic Bowel and Bladder

Diseases involving the entire nervous system can result in bowel and bladder dysfunction. Bowel and bladder control depends on the intricate and coordinated interplay between the peripheral nerves, spinal cord, brainstem, and cerebral cortex.

Neurogenic bowel refers to loss of sensory and/or motor control of the bowels that results in incontinence and constipation. Depending on the location of the pathology individuals present with decreased bowel sensation, slowed bowel transit time, and constipation, with reduced or absent voluntary control of defecation. Similarly, neurogenic bladder refers to bladder dysfunction due to a neurological process resulting in difficulty controlling urination and incontinence.

Bowel Management

Most of the literature on managing neurogenic bowel stems from the spinal cord injured population. A bowel program refers to a method of evacuating bowels on a predictable schedule in order to minimize fecal incontinence and should be customized to an individual's preference and neurological impairment. Stool softeners, laxatives, and fluid intake should be adjusted to maintain optimal stool consistency and foods that cause flatulence or adversely affect stool bulk should be avoided. In the presence of neurological disorders where sacral reflexes are preserved, defecation can be triggered with manual stimulation or suppository insertion. Individuals who have lost their rectal tone and reflexes are best managed with digital evacuation. Digital evacuation has been shown to reduce the duration of a bowel program and the frequency of fecal incontinence in the spinal cord injury population [148–150].

The increased pressure in the abdominal compartment caused by voluntary and involuntary muscle contractions in the later stage of arousal [151] can trigger a bowel movement. A rise in oxytocin levels which occurs during arousal and orgasm [152–154] is another cause for fecal incontinence as oxytocin is known to stimulate colonic activity [155]. The bowel program should be tailored to avoid incontinence and is often performed before sexual activity.

Bladder Management

The importance of timed hygiene prior to sexual intimacy to avoid accidents should be emphasized. Many individuals will empty their bladder right before sexual activity and decrease fluid intake several hours prior to intimacy. Diuretics and caffeinated beverages should be avoided.

If a person has an indwelling catheter the catheter can either be removed for intercourse or taped to the side. Generally men are more likely than women to maintain continence when the catheter is removed because of a longer urethra. A bladder relaxant can be trialed before sexual activity if bladder leakage occurs despite timed emptying. As bladder retention may precipitate autonomic dysreflexia in spinal cord injured individuals, the bladder should not be left undrained for a long period of time. If the catheter is left in place, it can be run along the penis and covered by a condom catheter, but it should be anchored down in a slack position to allow for penile engorgement. Care should be taken to ensure adequate urinary drainage to prevent urinary retention.

Autonomic Dysreflexia

Autonomic dysreflexia (AD) is an abnormal and uncontrolled sympathetic reflexive response to noxious or other strong stimuli below the level of a spinal cord injury [156]. While it is usually seen in individuals who have an injury at or above the sixth thoracic spinal level, it has been reported in individuals with lesions lower in the spinal cord. Autonomic dysreflexia is considered a medical emergency because it regularly results in severe blood pressure elevations that can be life threatening [157]. Systolic and diastolic blood pressures as high as 300 mmHg have been reported [158].

The most common trigger is bladder distention or irritation; however, erection, ejaculation and sexual stimulation are well recognized precipitants. The experience of sexual climax itself is associated with enhanced sympathetic activity resulting in elevated blood pressures. This sympathetic surge modulated poorly in individuals with higher spinal cord lesions resulting in AD during sexual climax in these individuals. In fact, orgasmic experience in men with SCI may be, in part, a result of the sympathetic outpouring inherent to autonomic dysreflexia [159]. Usually the rise in blood pressure occurs during the stimulus exposure, but ensuing blood pressure variability may persist for hours and, sometimes days and weeks [160]. Rarely, protracted, persistent, and debilitating autonomic dysreflexia associated with sexual activity has been described. As the subjective symptoms of autonomic dysreflexia during sexual activity poorly correlate with objective blood pressure measurements, blood pressure needs to be checked during any symptoms in a susceptible individual [160].

As outlined in the Guidelines of the Consortium for Spinal Cord Medicine [161], initial management with nonpharmacological measures including assuming an upright position, removal of constrictive clothing, and causes for bowel and bladder irritation should be investigated. If these measures fail, pharmacological agents such as nifedipine, nitrates, and captopril should be given with close monitoring of blood pressure [162].

When sexual activity is thought to precipitate autonomic dysreflexia, aborting sexual stimulation should result in its resolutions within minutes in the vast majority of cases. However, Elliott et al. have documented three cases of "malignant autonomic dysreflexia" referring to protracted progressively worsening AD following ejaculation [159].

Treatment of Erectile Dysfunction

Conservative Management

Individuals with erectile dysfunction should be counseled on the association between cardiovascular risk factors such as obesity, smoking, hyperlipidemia, and erectile dysfunction. Modifiable risk factors for ED include smoking, lack of physical activity, obesity, metabolic syndrome, and excessive alcohol consumption. The importance of lifestyle changes need to be discussed with individuals suffering from ED [163]. Obesity and smoking both double the risk of ED [164, 165] and modest weight reduction combined with regular exercise improved erectile function in obese males [166]. There is some evidence that lipid-lowering drugs themselves have beneficial effects on erectile function [167]. The presence of contributing conditions such as hyperlipidemia, diabetes mellitus, hyperthyroidism and hypothyroidism, uremia, hypertension, and alcohol and drug use needs to be evaluated.

Hormone Replacement

Individuals with certain neurological conditions (including epilepsy, multiple sclerosis, spinal cord injury), obesity, hypertension, hyperlipidemia, osteoporosis, AIDS wasting syndrome, and COPD appear to have a higher incidence of testosterone deficiency than the general population [168–171]. Furthermore, iatrogenic hypogonadism is observed in men following testicular surgery for cancer, and individuals treated with radiation, chemotherapy with anti-mitotic drugs and opioids [172]. Checking testosterone levels should be included in standard screening for erectile dysfunction. Luteinizing hormone and follicle stimulating hormone levels can be used to differentiate primary from secondary hypogonadism. As there is individual variation in testosterone secretion and levels at which symptoms appear, a low testosterone measurement should be reconfirmed prior to therapeutic intervention [173]. Testosterone replacement may improve libido, sexual function, and other health outcomes such as lean body mass, bone health, well-being, mood, energy, and quality of life [172].

Testosterone therapy is contraindicated in patients with prostate or breast cancer and should be used cautiously in patients with benign prostatic hypertrophy, sleep apnea, peripheral edema, congestive heart failure, polycythemia, and hepatic disease.

Vacuum Erection Devices

Vacuum Erection Devices (VED) offer a noninvasive, safe means to achieve an erection in individuals with erectile dysfunction regardless of the underlying cause. Penile engorgement is achieved by placing the penis in a cylinder while negative pressure is introduced via a vacuum pump that draws arteriolar blood into the corpora cavernosa resulting in penile engorgement and tumescence. Tumescence is maintained by placing a constriction band at the base of the penis preventing venous outflow. The ring, which acts like a tourniquet, should not be left on longer than 30 min to avoid ischemia. VEDs with a battery powered pump can be beneficial in individuals with impaired hand dexterity. Side effects include penile hematoma and pain and individuals with significant sensory loss are at risk for ischemic gangrene. Drawbacks are a long time to onset (approximately 30 min) and lack of spontaneity.

Vacuum erection devices are contraindicated in individuals who have sickle cell anemia and blood dyscrasias and should be used with caution in individuals who take anticoagulants. VEDs have a high effectiveness in up to 90% in individuals with spinal cord injury [174]. The combination of a VED with intracavernosal or intraurethral alprostadil is associated with a higher efficacy rate than use of the VED alone. VEDs in general have great success in the neurogenic population. Limitations that may affect use are limited manual dexterity, lack of spontancity, obesity, and anticoagulant use.

Intracavernosal Injection

Intracavernosal injection therapy should be used cautiously by patients at risk for priapism, including patients with sickle cell disease, leukemia, or multiple myeloma and patients who may develop bleeding complications secondary to injections, such as individuals with thrombocytopenia or those taking anticoagulants.

Alprostadil

Alprostadil, also known as prostaglandin E1, is the only FDA approved penile injection therapy approved for erectile dysfunction. It is available commercially as EDEX, or Caverject. Intracavernosal alprostadil is preferred over its intraurethral formulation because of greater effectiveness.

Alprostadil stimulates adenyl cyclase, resulting in increased production of cyclic adenosine monophosphate (cAMP), causing smooth muscle relaxation of the arterial blood vessels and sinusoidal tissues in the corpora. This results in enhanced blood flow. Unlike many other agents on the market, alprostadil does not require nitric oxide as a substrate, making it a lucrative agent in patients with erectile dysfunction due to diseases that are associated with an impaired nitric oxide pathway (e.g., diabetes mellitus, post-radical prostatectomy). The usual dose of intracavernosal alprostadil is 10–20 μg, with a maximum recommended dose of 60 μg. The effect is seen within 5–10 min of injection and the response and duration of action are dose dependent.

The most common adverse event is penile pain, which is usually self-limited. Despite a high initial response rate of more than 70% [175]. 20–50% of patients discontinue therapy. Common reasons for discontinuation include lack of effectiveness, inconvenience, dissatisfaction with the method, and cost [176].

Papaverine

Papaverine is a nonspecific PDE inhibitor resulting in corporal smooth muscle relaxation that is not FDA approved for erectile dysfunction. Papaverine has a reported efficacy of 54% with a faster onset of action and more side effects than alprostadil [173]. It is more effective in men with psychogenic and neurogenic erectile dysfunction than in men whose ED is due to vascular causes [177].

Due to its high side effect profile including priapism, corporal fibrosis, hypotension, and hepatotoxicity and long half-life it is not used as a single agent for erectile dysfunction. Rather, it is administered in lower doses in combination with phentolamine and/or alprostadil. A variety of formulas have been used, but no combination has been proven superior.

Phentolamine

Phentolamine is a competitive nonselective α-adrenergic blocking agent resulting in smooth muscle dilation causing vasodilation. Hypotension is the most common adverse. Other reported side effects are nasal congestion (10%), headache (3%), dizziness (3%), and tachycardia (3%) [178]. Like papaverine, phentolamine is not administered as a single agent due to its hypotensive effects but is administered in combination with other vasoactive agents such as papaverine and/or alprostadil.

Vasoactive Intestinal Peptide

Vasoactive intestinal peptide (VIP) is a neurotransmitter that is found in the male genital tract and may act together with nitric oxide to evoke erections [179, 180]. VIP has a stimulatory effect on adenylyl cyclase leading to an increase in cAMP, causing an increase in arterial blood flow, decrease in venous outflow, and sinusoidal relaxation [181]. In healthy men VIP induces tumescence but not erection [182]. Due to its role in mediating erectile congestion it is a natural target for the treatment of ED.

Although VIP is not FDA approved in the USA, a combination of vasoactive intestinal polypeptide and phentolamine mesylate is available in the United Kingdom and Europe for the management of ED and has been shown to have similar success to other intracavernosal therapies on the market with few untoward effects [174, 183].

Combination Therapy

Phentolamine, papaverine, PGE1, and VIP are the vasoactive agents most commonly used in combination therapy to treat ED and are not FDA approved for their use in erectile dysfunction. Multiple combinations of intracavernosal therapy exist and none is superior. Theoretically, combination formulations are safer and are associated with fewer serious adverse effects than high doses of any single agent.

The combination of VIP with phentolamine, only available in European markets, has been shown to result in erections suitable for intercourse in 84% of respondents with maintenance of good response over a 6–12-month period [184, 185].

The combination therapies most commonly used in the USA are the bimixture (a combination of phentolamine and papaverine) and trimixture (a combination of papaverine, phentolamine, and PGE1). In addition, a quadmixture of phentolamine, papaverine, prostaglandin E1, and atropine has also been tried.

Most practitioners start with prostaglandin E1 (Caverject or Edex) and switch to combination therapy when patients experience significant penile pain, a lack of efficacy, or high cost. No differences in rigidity, pain and self-satisfaction were demonstrated between trimix and prostaglandin E1 injections, though trimix does cause longer erections and is associated with a higher incidence of priapism than PgE1 [186].

Transurethral Therapy

Intraurethral alprostadil is a synthetic form of prostaglandin E1 that stimulates adenyl cyclase, resulting in increased production of cAMP, causing smooth muscle relaxation of the arterial blood vessels and sinusoidal tissues in the corpora. Alprostadil may be delivered in the form of a urethral pellet (in addition to intracavernosal delivery) and is the only agent administered via this route that is approved by the FDA for ED. In two large clinical trials intraurethral alprostadil was effective in 43% of men with erectile dysfunction from various organic causes [187, 188].

The major disadvantages are penile pain (32%) and urethral pain or burning (12%), a low response rate, and inconsistent efficacy. The initial dose of intraurethral alprostadil is 125 μg, and onset of action is seen within 5–10 min, with a duration of 30–60 min. The first dose should be administered by a health care provider because of the potential complications of urethral bleeding, vasovagal reflex, hypotension, syncope, and priapism. Patients who have unsatisfactory results from intraurethral suppositories can use it in combination with an adjustable penile constriction band, but adverse effects may increase.

PDE Inhibitors

Due to their effectiveness, convenient dosing, oral availability, and benign side effect profile phosphodiesterase inhibitors (PDEi) are considered first-line therapy for erectile dysfunction [189]. Normally penile erection occurs through the release of nitric oxide (NO), which causes dilation of the blood vessels of the corpus cavernosum via an accumulation of cyclic guanosine monophosphate (cGMP). The vasodilatory effect of cGMP can be enhanced when its breakdown by PDE is inhibited and thereby the vasodilatory effect of NO is enhanced. There are many types of PDEi, with type 5 being most prevalent in penile tissue. Phosphodiesterase inhibitors reversibly inhibit penile-PDE-5, thereby increasing nitric oxide availability in the penis, allowing maintenance of an erection with sexual stimulation. All commercially available phosphodiesterase inhibitors are considered to be equally effective but some patients may respond to one PDE inhibitor better than others [190]. The overall efficacy rate of these drugs is approximately 60–70% [190] but is considerably lower in certain patient populations, in which ED is caused by neurological damage, radical prostatectomy, diabetes, or severe vascular disease [191]. The choice of a PDE inhibitor depends on effectiveness, safety, cost, insurance coverage, frequency of intercourse, and personal experience [192].

There are four FDA-approved PDE inhibitors in the USA: avanafil (Stendra®), sildenafil (Viagra®), tadalafil (Cialis®), and vardenafil (Levitra®). Each medication varies slightly in its dosing, onset, and duration. Sildenafil and vardenafil have similar onsets and duration of action, and both demonstrate a decreased efficacy with the intake of high-fat foods. Avanafil, sildenafil, and vardenafil are taken "on demand" at least 30 min before sexual activity. Tadalafil has a longer half-life, which allows for both daily and "on demand" dosing. Daily dosing can increase spontaneity but also increase duration of side effects. All currently available PDE inhibitors are effective and safe [191].

Adverse effects are usually dose related and due to vasodilation or inhibition of other PDE enzymes. The most common adverse effects reported in patients taking PDE inhibitors are headache (10–30%), rhinitis (1–11%), flushing (10–20%), dyspepsia (3–16%), myalgia and back pain (0–10%), and dizziness (up to 5%) [190]. All PDE inhibitors weakly inhibit PDE6 located in retinal rod and cone photoreceptors resulting in mild and transient visual manifestations. The most common symptoms are a blue tinge to vision, increased light sensitivity, and reversible problems with color discrimination. Even though the use of phosphodiesterase type 5 inhibitors has been associated with nonarteritic anterior ischemic optic neuropathy (NAION), an acute optic neuropathy with sudden vision loss, their role in the development of NAION remains unknown. Up to 6% of patients report muscle and back pain with tadalafil, the exact cause of which is unknown [193, 194]. Vardenafil should be avoided in patients with preexisting QT prolongation and in those taking class I antiarrhythmic drugs, which can cause QT prolongation.

Co-administration of alpha-blockers and PDE inhibitors may result in orthostatic hypotension. Therefore, patients should be stable on α-blocker therapy before the combination therapy is initiated, and the initial dose of PDE-inhibitors should be the lowest possible.

PDE inhibitors should be initiated at the lowest possible dose in patients already stable on alpha-blockers. Uroselective alpha-blockers such as tamsulosin and alfuzosin are preferred in patients with benign prostatic to reduce the risk of significant hypotension.

The usage of PDE inhibitors with nitrates is absolutely contraindicated due to potential of fatal hypotension-related cardiac or cerebrovascular injury. Although a safe time interval between the use of nitrates and PDE inhibitors has not been determined, a suggested time interval is 24 h for sildenafil [195] and 48 h for tadalafil [196].

Lower doses of PDE inhibitors are recommended for the elderly and those with renal and hepatic impairment. PDE5 levels may be reduced in patients taking cytochrome P450 enzyme inducers, such as phenytoin, rifampin, phenobarbital, and carbamazepine, requiring an increase in dose to achieve efficacy.

Penile Implant Surgery

Penile implants are usually recommended when other treatments have not resulted in satisfactory results. Implants allow individuals to achieve an on-demand erection but have no effect on ability to achieve ejaculation or orgasm. There are two broad categories of penile implants: the semirigid rods and the inflatable devices. Semirigid rods are paired, solid cylinders that are implanted into the corpora cavernosa that can be adjusted into position for sexual activity. Their advantages are low mechanical failure rate, ease of operation requiring minimal manual dexterity, and relative inexpensiveness. However, their drawback is that the penis is maintained in an erect state which can be difficult to conceal. On the other hand, inflatable devices are hollow cylinders which are also implanted into the corpora cavernosa and are connected to a reservoir that is implanted into the scrotum.

Inflatable implants are further subdivided according to the design of the prosthesis: a two-piece inflatable prosthesis consists of two cylinders attached to a scrotal pump, while a three-piece inflatable prosthesis consists of two cylinders attached to a scrotal pump and a separate reservoir. In the resting state the penis is flaccid; however, the cylinders can be inflated to produce penile rigidity when an erection is desired by releasing a valve mechanism in the pump that transfers saline solution from the reservoir into the cylinders.

Complications of penile implants are infections and device malfunctions, but also include device erosions, reservoir herniation, penile deformity, and cylinder migration.

The incidence of infection is reported to be approximately 4% for first time implants and 10% for revision implants [197]. Five-year mechanical failure rates range from 0% to 9% [198].

Penile implants are very effective treatment options for patients with refractory erectile dysfunction and are associated with high patient satisfaction. Satisfaction appears to be higher for inflatable penile prostheses than malleable penile prostheses [199].

Women

Topical Creams

Topical analgesic creams, including lidocaine jelly or ointment, as well as amitriptyline, and baclofen cream can be applied to the genitals prior to sexual intercourse and relieve the discomfort of dyspareunia. Depending on hand dexterity, creams can be applied by the individual or their partner. Many creams can cause a burning sensation and anesthetic creams have a numbing effect on both the individual and their partner and interfere with achieving genital pleasure.

A 2006 Cochrane review of 19 trials involving more than 4000 women found that estrogen preparations were associated with a statistically significant reduction in dyspareunia caused by vaginal atrophy compared with placebo [200]. The US Food and Drug Administration has approved local hormone therapy for use in moderate to severe vulvovaginal atrophy and dyspareunia. Current practice recommendations from professional organizations advise that individuals be treated with the lowest effective dose of estrogen for the shortest amount of time to achieve satisfactory results [200]. Ospemifene, a novel selective estrogen receptor modulator that increases vaginal epithelial cells can be used as an alternative to vaginal estrogen.

Vaginal lubricants provides external lubrication to minimize discomfort during sexual activity. These lubricants can be applied to the labia, clitoris, penis, or object intended for insertion in order to facilitate intromission. Water-based gels that lack perfumes, coloring, spermicides, or flavors are preferable to minimize irritation of delicate genital tissues. Petroleum, skin lotions, and other oil-based lubricants may raise the risk of yeast infection; petroleum products can also cause damage to latex condoms.

Flibanserin, sold under the trade name Addyi, is a medication approved for the treatment of premenopausal women with hypoactive sexual desire disorder (HSDD). HSDD refers to a woman's chronic lack of interest in sex with absence of sexual fantasies or desire for sexual activity resulting in personal distress or relationship problems.

Phosphoidiesterase Inhibitors

Based on their ability to enhance genital blood flow phosphodiesterase inhibitors have been studied in women with sexual dysfunction. Since sexual dysfunction is such a broad term encompassing many etiologies leading to sexual dissatisfaction, this entity is more difficult to study in women who do not experience genital erection like their male counterparts. Based on conflicting results and small, suboptimal designed studies, the impact of phosphodiesterase inhibitors on female sexual function remains inconclusive, but they appear to enhance blood flow and sexual arousal [201].

Sexuality in Rehabilitation Health Care

Interdisciplinary Team

Following a new medical diagnosis, many individuals will spend several weeks in a rehabilitation setting. These include: inpatient acute rehabilitation hospitals, sub-acute rehabilitation hospitals, skilled in-home care, and outpatient therapy. The initial diagnosis or injury period is often followed by a short stay in an acute rehabilitation hospital setting. There are various individuals involved in a person's care while in acute rehabilitation: case manager, chaplain, nurse, occupational therapist, physical therapist, physician, psychologist, recreation therapist, rehabilitation counselor, social worker, speech and language pathologist, vocational/educational specialist. In some settings, either on staff or as a consultant, a sex therapist may also be available to address sexuality concerns.

The physician often leads the team in directing the individual's care plan and treatment while in rehabilitation. Most physicians that work in acute rehabilitation hospitals specialize in physical medicine and rehabilitation. There may be other specialists or generalists that also follow patients while in acute rehabilitation. The role of the physician is to initiate conversations regarding sexuality, provide medical information related to sexuality (e.g., orthopedic clearances for sexual activity), and discuss the role of medications in relation to sexuality. Regarding sexuality, physicians often discuss sexual function, reproduction, and medications. Some individuals may be hesitant to discuss sexuality with their physician. All members of the interdisciplinary team can introduce sexuality and give permission for the individual to discuss any thoughts or concerns with the appropriate person.

The psychologist, social worker, and rehabilitation counselor focus on providing social and emotional interventions with the patient and their partner or family. These sessions are often done in private, with the psychologist, social worker, and rehabilitation counselor completing a biopsychosocial assessment, which may include taking a sexual history and developing a treatment plan. Common issues discussed include: adjustment to disability, coping, relationship changes, role changes, body image, self-esteem, pain and stress management, and sexuality education.

Physical and occupational therapists provide hands-on therapy related to mobility and function in daily life. For many individuals with physical disabilities, sexuality can be greatly impacted due to functional changes in mobility. Therapy sessions may address secondary impacts on sexuality due to a disability, such as bladder incontinence. Nurses are also important in providing specific and overarching educational information and normalizing questions and concerns. Physical and occupational therapy can address common areas impacted by a disability such as: mobility, sensation, bowel and bladder management, and pain. Both therapies utilize education and physical "practice" to maximize function and assist patients in regaining as much independence as possible.

There are several recommendations for all rehabilitation team members to consider when discussing sexuality with patients and their partners [202–204]. It is recommended that health care professionals maintain an open dialogue with patients, including a nonjudgmental attitude that maintains privacy and confidentiality. Asking open-ended questions and tailoring the discussion to the patient's interests can help to elicit more information. Assess each individual's readiness to discuss and learn about sexuality and provide information several times through both formal and informal mediums. Encourage individuals to actively seek out information about sexual issues and to explore the various ways sexuality may present in their lives.

Addressing Sexuality

Soon after a new diagnosis, patients and families will have many questions. Some may be about sexuality but many are related to the individuals' new diagnosis and prognosis. Many providers find it helpful to utilize a treatment framework when addressing sexuality to improve consistency across patient diagnoses and demographics. At the minimum, sexuality should be part of a discussion and basic education should be provided.

Professionals may choose to utilize a treatment framework, such as the EX-PLISSIT model. The Ex-PLISSIT model expands upon the original PLISSIT model proposed by Jack Annon [204]. The PLISSIT acronym follows four different stages for discussing sexuality and sexual health.

"EX-P" stands for explicit permission-giving, which involves directly asking about sexuality and allowing patients the opportunity to discuss any concerns they may have. Additionally, it is understood that each and every interaction involves giving permission. "LI" stands for limited information, which may include education on how sexuality may be impacted by a diagnosis, dispelling myths and misinformation, and giving limited information about sexuality. "SS" stands for specific suggestions, recommendations that can focus on the individual patient, their diagnosis, and specific concerns they may have. "IT" stands for intensive therapy, which is often recommended for individuals who have concerns that cannot be addressed adequately by the health care professional based on experience, training, or time restraints.

Using the Ex-PLISSIT model, education may be provided at various stages following a diagnosis. Sexuality education can be both formal and informal. Information should be provided through several mediums: verbal, written, and visual. Many individuals will receive their initial education while they are in an acute or sub-acute rehabilitation setting, followed by ongoing education through home care or outpatient therapy. Timing is also important in delivering sexuality education. Some individuals may not be comfortable discussing sexuality initially, or may not have questions until they have been home for a few months and have been sexually active, either with themselves or another person or persons.

While in inpatient rehabilitation, many health care professionals offer formal education groups. These groups should be run by a trained health care professional who is comfortable and knowledgeable in discussing sexuality. This can be supplemented with written material or individual discussions with staff members. Individual and couples counseling should also be offered. Research shows that educational content provided by health care professionals varies and can be inconsistent in its delivery [205]. There is no standardized assessment and intervention tool used consistently in rehabilitation settings. Individual health care professionals follow models that align with their conceptions of sexuality and their role in the patient's care. Physicians may prioritize different areas than a psychologist or social worker. However, there are common components that should be included in addressing sexuality for each patient. Three possible models are outlined below; although slightly different, there are large overlaps in content between all three models.

Bancroft's Model [206] focuses on three main areas: direct physical effects, psychological effects, and the effects of treatment on sexuality. Direct physical effects includes any changes specific to the genitals or other sexual responses and other nonspecific effects such as pain, fatigue, or changes in desire. Psychological effects include changes on the individual, the relationship, and concerns about how sexual activity will impact the condition/diagnosis.

Another model focuses on primary, secondary, and tertiary effects of a disability. Primary effects include neurological changes that directly affect sexual feelings or sexual responses. Examples include altered or impaired genital sensation, decreased vaginal lubrication, and decreased intensity of orgasm. Secondary effects address physical changes that indirectly affect sexual feelings and sexual responses. Examples of secondary effects include fatigue, spasticity, decreased coordination, and bowel and bladder dysfunction.

Tertiary effects include the psychological, social, emotional, and cultural aspects that impact sexuality and may include changes in body image and self-esteem, concerns about sexual performance, and feelings of dependency.

A third model, adapted from Stevenson and Elliot [207] proposes four areas for assessment, education, and intervention. Direct effects address the motor, sensory, and autonomic pathways affected by a disability that alter sexual response. Indirect effects include changes due to a disability where the changes may impact sexuality. For example, fatigue, pain or bowel and bladder incontinence. Iatrogenic effects address factors related to treatments, such as medication side effects or surgical side effects. Contextual influences include the effects of a disability on an individual and their relationships, and one's roles and responsibilities within the family.

There are many areas of sexuality to be addressed for individuals with disabilities. The interdisciplinary nature of rehabilitation allows multiple health care providers to address sexuality based on their knowledge, training, and expertise. To improve consistency, formalized groups or protocol for disseminating education can be developed. Education should be age-appropriate; an individual's age of initial injury should also be considered [205]. The use of explicit materials as education should be used after an individual's readiness has been evaluated. For individuals under 18 years of age, parental consent may be required based on individual state laws.

Relational Changes

A new disability can be life-altering. Many individuals may spend weeks, even months, beginning to adjust to their disability. For those individuals in relationships, their partner is also experiencing changes. Couples often face new challenges to their relationship and life at home following a life-altering disability. For many, disabilities do not exist in a silo. Individuals and couples have a history prior to hospitalization that will impact their recovery and response to a new disability. Tensions in a relationship can be exacerbated by a disability.

Disabilities also vary in their presentation. An individual with a spinal cord injury may have a difficult adjustment initially and then be medically and functionally stable for several years. For someone with multiple sclerosis, their functional level may improve and then worsen with flare-ups. As changes occur, whether due to fluctuating medical issues or aging, clear communication is necessary between partners and can improve relationship quality.

Many couples report feeling nervous before their first sexual encounter after a life impacting injury/medical condition. For couples who were together prior to hospitalization, there is a previously established sexual relationship. Often, this sexual relationship becomes the baseline to which individuals and couples will compare any future sexual interactions. Health care professionals can help to teach individuals that although sexual activity may look and feel different, it can still be pleasurable for both parties involved. Couples will often have several concerns about what their first sexual encounter will be like. They may have questions about whether their partner still finds them desirable or if they will be able to satisfy their partner. Some express concerns about becoming a parent or becoming pregnant. Many newly disabled individuals are unsure of how their body will work; some may expect it to be the exact same as prior to their disability. Many individuals also express concern about hurting their partner physically during sex. Given medical clearance, most individuals are able to resume sexual activity. Open communication about positioning and pain may help to ease a partner's concerns. Exploring sexual activity with a partner following a disability is often a process of trial and error; certain positions may work better than others, pain may be less early in the morning, or muscle spasms may be less frequent in certain positions.

Knowledge of available sexual assistive devices can help couples to enhance their bedroom routine. If an individual is unable to maintain an erection, a strap-on device may be an appropriate alternative. For individuals with impaired bed mobility, positioning wedges can help provide options for a variety of positions. Altered sensation may respond well to a vibrator. There are resource manuals written for consumers that offer quick breakdowns of available products, including purchasing information, cleaning recommendations, and cost [208].

It can be helpful to discuss the concepts of pleasure with individuals and their partners. Education should include information on the sexual response cycle, including a differentiation between sexual response and sexual pleasure, orgasm and ejaculation, and orgasm and lubrication. Often, pleasure is not discussed based on assumptions that people with disabilities are child-like and asexual or not physically capable of experiencing pleasure [209]. It may also stem from beliefs that sex should be for the purpose of procreation, not pleasure [210].

Many individuals are "goal-oriented" and focused on orgasm as the ultimate goal to any sexual encounter. Pleasure can be derived from a number of other intimate activities including kissing, cuddling, manual stimulation, mutual masturbation, oral sex, anal play, and exploration with sex toys. It is recommended to assess a couple's prior sexual history and history as a couple, including use of and interest in sex toys. For example, some couples may benefit from sensate focus exercises if they experience changes in sensation due to a disability or are having a difficult time reconnecting emotionally and physically with their partner.

Communication

With any new changes, communication is key to sustaining a healthy dialogue between partners. After a disability, much has changed in an individual's life: physical functioning, loss of independence, financial instability, and increased stress. For individuals with tetraplegia, communication becomes essential—asking a nurse for a sip of water or asking a partner to adjust your pillow. Some individuals will also use augmentative and alternative communication devices to make their needs, wishes, and desires known.

There are four basic steps to communicating successfully, as outlined by Hernandez [211]. The first is to know what you want to communicate. For newly diagnosed individuals, self-exploration can help an individual to relearn their body to help communicate physical and emotional changes to their partner. Knowing what to communicate is based in self-awareness. The second step is figuring how to communicate the message. This can include verbal and nonverbal communication. Encourage couples to think about how they best communicate and when they feel the most comfortable and confident. The third step is communication. The final step involves listening and being open and receptive to your partner's response.

Health care professionals can assist patients and their partners by encouraging communication and providing alternative ways of communication. For patients with altered sensation or pain, a sensation map can be a helpful tool to visualize altered sensation and open dialogue around pleasurable activities.

Partner as Caregiver

Secondary to functional deficits, many individuals will require assistance to complete some activities of daily living (e.g., toileting, bathing, dressing). Many people do not have the financial means or insurance coverage to hire an aide or nurse to assist them at home. For these people, their partner often becomes their primary caregiver. Caregiver duties may include assistance with getting dressed and undressed, help toileting, completing wound care, and help bathing. For example, patients with spinal cord injuries complete daily bowel routines, which often includes several medications, possibly an enema or suppository, and digital stimulation.

For patients who are unable to reach or turn, they will need someone to help them with an enema, suppository, or digital stimulation every day. This can make intimacy harder to maintain as the roles blur between partner and caregiver. It is recommended that for couples where one partner is a caregiver, that they outline possible times of day for caregiving and for intimacy. It can be challenging to switch back and forth from being a care-giver to being a partner. For individuals with spinal cord injury, some choose to complete their bowel routines in the morning and be intimate in the evenings with their partner. This allows several hours to pass between role duties.

For individuals with newly acquired disabilities, the transition from independence to some level of dependence can be challenging. Many patients report decreased self-esteem. Societal views prominently display individuals with disabilities in a child-like manner or needing pity. Often, these views can be internalized, making it difficult for individuals with disabilities to still see themselves as sexy and desirable. Patient's partners may also struggle vacillating between taking care of an individual and being intimate or sexually active with the same person a few hours later.

Adjustment to Disability

Acquiring a disability is life-changing. Many individuals struggle with a loss of independence. Independence often is not the only loss that people grieve after a disability. People may lose sensation, movement, the ability to communicate, jobs/careers, financial stability, financial savings, relationships, and the privilege of being able-bodied. It is normal for individuals to take weeks, even months, grieving the losses they have experienced. Many will also experience depression. Some individuals may voice regret, guilt, anger with their situation.

For newly "disabled individuals," the positive development of identity as a person with a disability correlates with empowerment [211]. Gill [212] proposed a model that outline four types of integration that influence disability identity development: integration into society, integration into the disability community, internally integrating similarities and differences with others, and integrating how one feels with how one presents oneself. Internally integrating similarities and differences with others focuses on how individuals are able to recognize and accept their disability as being part of themselves.

An individual's beliefs and values will impact their adjustment following a disability, both in general and in relation to sexuality. People have beliefs and values about sexuality before they become disabled. For example, some individuals report that sexual activity was a large part of their lives. They spent several hours a day masturbating and enjoyed having sex with a partner multiple times a day. For others, sex and sexuality does not cross their minds until someone else initiates the conversation. An individual's beliefs about sexuality prior to an injury may impact their response to sexuality following their disability.

Based on common societal beliefs, many individuals view people with disabilities as asexual. Asexual can have several meanings based around absence of sexual behavior, absence of sexual attraction, or asexual self-identification [213]. For most of history, individuals with disabilities have been affected by the damaging myth that they are asexual [214]. Many have fought to be seen as sexual beings, capable of having sexual desires and needs. This also marginalizes and invalidates those who identify as being asexual. Most important is to recognize that individuals with disabilities may have sexual desires, attractions, and needs or they may not and both are healthy and normal.

In adjusting to a new disability, many individuals face physical and functional changes. Some may lose or gain weight, use a wheelchair, wear a prosthetic device, or have a colostomy. This can negatively impact one's body image and self-esteem. While some individuals may adjust to their new body fairly quickly, others may take longer. Encourage them to discuss their concerns with someone they feel comfortable with, whether that be a health care professional or close friend or family member. While in the hospital, individuals often do not continue their same grooming routine at home. If wearing makeup or shaving helped the individual to feel better about themselves prior to their disability, it may help after as well. Remember, it can take time for individuals to feel comfortable asking for help.

Raising Children

Becoming a parent can be a rewarding and challenging experience for any individual. For individuals with disabilities, there are additional layers and societal views that impact parenting with a disability. Common concerns of couples include: fertility, genetic testing, childbirth, active involvement in parenting, adjustment of children to a person with disability [215].

Many individuals struggle with concerns about reproduction and whether they will be able to safely have healthy children. The ability to procreate may be impacted by a disability but as technology advances, many times reproduction is possible. Many couples may have to seek specialized services in a fertility clinic or with a urologist or obstetrician who is familiar with their disability.

Societal views on parenting for individuals with disabilities has a storied past. At times in the recent past, individuals with intellectual and physical disabilities were involuntarily sterilized. There is a bias about the appropriateness of individuals with disabilities becoming parents. This bias has led to legal discrimination where parents who use wheelchairs were denied custody of their children. Several states have child welfare laws that state that a parent with a disability is grounds for removing the child from the home and terminating parental rights [216].

Being a parent can be an active job. Individuals with physical limitations may face some common challenges, despite the type of disability they have. Effects of one's own disability, such as pain, limited strength, and fatigue can make the physical aspects of parenting a unique demand that requires some creative problem solving. Disciplining children can be a challenge for individuals with physical and communication barriers.

Social issues can also prove to be arduous. Individuals with disabilities may not have transportation and may rely on paratransit services, which will often not allow children on. Other people may need someone to drive them or be able to drive but may have difficulties with car seats. Additionally, many families where one parent is disabled are often on a fixed income. This can make it difficult to afford certain products and technologies designed to make parenting more accessible. Without these products and technologies, individuals are required to hire additional help, rely on other family members more, or increase risk of stress or personal injury [217].

Conclusion

Tragedy, obstacles, and unplanned events can bring people together to face life challenges. Health care continues to experience the opportunity to do as much as we can to help and improve. Much has been and continues to be accomplished in the area of sexuality, which shows promise for the needed efforts that lie ahead.

References

1. Boyd KM. Disease, illness, sickness, health, healing and wholeness: exploring some elusive concepts. J Med Humanit. 2000;26(1):9–17.
2. Hess MJ, Hough S. Impact of spinal cord injury on sexuality: broad based clinical practice intervention and practical application. J Spinal Cord Med. 2012;35(4):211–8.
3. Appa AA, et al. The impact of multimorbidity on sexual function in middle-aged and older women: beyond the single disease perspective. J Sex Med. 2014;11(11):2744–55.
4. McInnes RA. chronic illness and sexuality. Med J Aust. 2003;179(5):263–6.
5. Kazemi-Saleh D, Pishgou B, Assari S, Tavallaii SA. Fear of sexual intercourse in patients with coronary artery disease: a pilot study of associated morbidity. J Sex Med. 2007;4(6):1619–25.
6. Wells K, Golding JM, Burnam MA. Psychiatric disorder in a sample of the general population with and without chronic medical conditions. Am J Psychiatry. 1988;145:976–81.
7. Clarke D, Currie KC. Depression, anxiety and their relationship with chronic diseases: a review of the epidemiology, risk and treatment evidence. Med J Aust. 2009;190(7):54–60.
8. Milligan MS, Neufeldt AH. The myth of asexuality: a survey of social and empirical evidence. Sex Disabil. 2001;19(2):91–109.
9. Fiduccia BW. Current issues in sexuality and the disability movement. Sex Disabil. 2000;18(3):167–74.
10. Jong-Ho P, Ovbiagele B, Feng W. Stroke and sexual dysfunction—a narrative review. J Neurol Sci. 2015;350(1–2):7–13.
11. Rosenbaum T, Vadas D, Kalichman L. Sexual function in post-stroke patients: considerations for rehabilitation. J Sex Med. 2014;11(1):15–21. doi:10.1111/jsm.12343.
12. Cheung RTF. Sexual functioning in Chinese stroke patients with mild or no disability. Cerebrovasc Dis. 2002;14:122–8.
13. Korpelainen JT, Nieminen P, Myllyla VV. Sexual functioning among stroke patients and their spouses. Stroke. 1999;30:715–9.
14. Monga TN, Monga M, Raina MS, Hardjasudarma M. Hypersexuality in stroke. Arch Phys Med Rehabil. 1986;67:415–7.
15. Paolucci S. Epideniology and treatment of post-stroke depression. Neuropsychiatr Dis Treat. 2008;4:145–54.
16. Hackett ML. Frequency of depression of observational studies after stroke: a systematic review. Stroke. 2005;36:1330–40.
17. Stein J, Hillinger M, Clancy C, Bishop L. Sexuality after stroke: patient counseling preference. Disabil Rehabil. 2013;35(21):1842–7.
18. Suzuki E, et al. Chronic kidney disease and erectile dysfunction. World J Nephrol. 2014;3(4):220–9.
19. Bellinghieri G, Santoro D, Mallamace A, Savica V. Sexual dysfunction in chronic renal failure. J Nephrol. 2008;21:s113–7.
20. Mehrsai A, et al. Improvement of erectile dysfunction after kidney transplantation: the role of the associated factors. Urol J. 2006;3(4):240–4.
21. Finkelstein SH, Finkelstein FO. Evaluation of sexual dysfunction in dialysis patients. In: Nissenson AR, Fine RN, editors. Dialysis therapy. 3rd ed. Philadelphia, PA: Hanley and Belfus; 2002. p. 368–73.
22. Manish R, Ramachandran R. Sexual and gonadal dysfunction in chronic kidney disease: pathophysiology. Indian J Endocrinol Metab. 2012;16(2):214–9.
23. Iglesias P, Carrero JJ, Díez JJ. Gonadal dysfunction in men with chronic kidney disease: clinical features, prognostic implications and therapeutic options. J Nephrol. 2012;25(1):31–42.
24. Milde FK. Sexuality and fertility concerns of dialysis patients. ANNA J. 1996;23:307–31.
25. Weisinger JR, Bellorin-Font E. Outcomes associated with hypogonadism in women with chronic kidney disease. Adv Chronic Kidney Dis. 2004;11:361–70.
26. Vecchio M. Treatment options for sexual dysfunction in patients with chronic kidney disease: a systematic review of randomized controlled trials. Clin J Am Soc Nephrol. 2010;5(6):985–95.
27. Delano BG. Improvements in quality of life following treatment with r-HuEPO in anemic hemodialysis patients. Am J Kidney Dis. 1989;14(2 Suppl 1):14.
28. Anantharaman P, Schmidt RJ. Sexual function in chronic kidney disease. Adv Chronic Kidney Dis. 2007;14(2):119–25.
29. Grossman EB, et al. The pharmacokinetics and hemodynamics of sildenafil citrate in male hemodialysis patients. Kidney Int. 2004;66:367–3.
30. Mohamed EA, MacDowall P, Coward RA. Timing of sildenafil therapy in dialysis patients-lessons following an episode of hypotension. Nephrol Dial Transplant. 2000;15(6):926.
31. Pourmand G. Does renal transplantation improve erectile dysfunction in hemodialysed patients? What is the role of associated factors? Transplant Proc. 2007;39:1029–32.
32. Antonucci M, et al. Male sexual dysfunction in patients with chronic end-stage renal insufficiency and in renal transplant recipients. Arch Ital Urol Androl. 2016;87(4):299–305.
33. Steinke E. Sexual counselling for individuals with cardiovascular disease and their partners. Eur Heart J. 2013;34(41):3217–35.

34. Chiurlia E, et al. Subclinical coronary artery atherosclerosis in patients with erectile dysfunction. J Am Coll Cardiol. 2005;46:1503–6.
35. Billups KL, et al. Relation of C-reactive protein and other cardiovascular risk factors to penile vascular disease in men with erectile dysfunction. Int J Impot Res. 2003;15:231–6.
36. Roumeguere T, et al. Erectile dysfunction is associated with a high prevalence of hyperlipidemia and coronary heart disease risk. Eur Urol. 2003;44:355–9.
37. Montorsi P, et al. Association between erectile dysfunction and coronary artery disease. Role of coronary clinical presentation and extent of coronary vessels involvement: the COBRA trial. Eur Heart J. 2006;27:2632–9.
38. Baumhakel M, et al. Erectile dysfunction correlates with left ventricular function and precedes cardiovascular events in cardiovascular high-risk patients. Int J Clin Pract. 2007;61:361–6.
39. Hodges LD, et al. The temporal relationship between erectile dysfunction and cardiovascular disease. Int J Clin Pract. 2007;61:2019–25.
40. Muller JE, et al. Triggering myocardial infarction by sexual activity: low absolute risk and prevention by regular physical exertion. JAMA. 1996;275:1405–9.
41. DeBusk R, et al. Management of sexual dysfunction in patients with cardiovascular disease: recommendations of the Princeton consensus panel. Am J Cardiol. 2000;86:175–81.
42. Stein RA, et al. The effect of exercise training on heart rate during coitus in the post myocardial infarction patient. Circulation. 1977;55:738–40.
43. DeBusk R, et al. Sexual activity triggering myocardial infarction. One less thing to worry about. JAMA. 1996;275(18):1447–8.
44. Bloch A, et al. Sexual problems after myocardial infarction. Am Heart J. 1975;90:536–7.
45. Drory Y, et al. Comparison of sexual activity of women and men after a first acute myocardial infarction. Am J Cardiol. 2000;85:1283–7.
46. Apostolo A, et al. Erectile dysfunction in heart failure: correlation with severity, exercise performance, comorbidities, and heart failure treatment. J Sex Med. 2009;6:2795–805.
47. Jaarsna T, et al. Sexual function in patients with advanced heart failure. Heart Lung. 1996;25(4):262–70.
48. Jackson G, et al. Sexual dysfunction and cardiovascular disease: a transatlantic consensus. Int J Clin Pract. 2000;54(8):483.
49. Ueno M. The so-called coital death. Nippon Univ. J Med. 1965;7:235–42.
50. Jackson G, et al. Stable angina: drugs, angioplasty or surgery? Eur Heart J. 1997;18:B2–B10.
51. Harden CL. Sexuality in men and women with epilepsy. CNS Spectr. 2006;11(Suppl 89):13–8.
52. Lambert MV. Seizures, hormones and sexuality. Seizure. 2001;10:319–40.
53. Duncan S, et al. Erectile function, sexual desire and psychological well-being in men with epilepsy. Epilepsy Behav. 2009;15(3):351–7.
54. Toone BK. Sexual disorders in epilepsy. In: Pedley TA, Meldrum BS, editors. Recent advances in epilepsy. 3 Edinburgh: Churchill Livingstone; 1986. p. 233–59.
55. Kolarsky A. Male sexual deviation: association with early temporal lobe damage. Arch Gen Psychiatry. 1967;17:735–43.
56. Smaldone M, et al. Epilepsy and erectile dysfunction: a review. Seizure. 2004;13:453–9.
57. Braun M, Wassmer G, Klotz T, Reifenrath B, Mathers M, Engelmann U. Epidemiology of erectile dysfunction: results of the 'Cologne Male Survey'. Int J Impot Res. 2000;12(6):305–11.
58. Morell MJ. Self-reported sexual function and sexual arousal in women with epilepsy. In: Harden CL (ed) Seizure frequency is associated with age at menopause in women with epilepsy. Neurology. 2003;61(4):451.
59. Morrell MJ, Sperling MR, Stecker M, Dichter MA. Sexual dysfunction in partial epilepsy: a deficit in physiologic sexual arousal. Neurology. 1994;44:243–7.
60. Singer C, et al. Sexual function in patients with Parkinson's disease. J Neurol Neurosurg Psychiatry. 1991;54:942.
61. Bronner G. Sexual dysfunction in Parkinson's disease. J Sex Marital Ther. 2004;30(2):95–105.
62. Welsh M. Sexuality in women with Parkinson's disease. Mov Disord. 1997;12(6):923–7.
63. Ready RE. Testosterone deficiency and apathy in Parkinson's disease: a pilot study. J Neurol Neurosurg Psychiatry. 2004;75(9):1323–6.
64. Okun MS, et al. Testosterone therapy in men with Parkinson DISEASE. JAMA Neurol. 2006;63(5):729–35.
65. Lewin RJ, et al. Extrapyramidal inhibition of the urinary bladder. Brain Res. 1967;4:301–7.
66. Yoshimura N, et al. Dopaminergic mechanisms underlying bladder hyperactivity in rats with a unilateral 6-hydroxydopamine (6-OHDA) lesion of the nigrostriatal pathway. Br J Pharmacol. 2003;139:1425–32.
67. Bronner G. Management of sexual dysfunction in Parkinson's disease. Ther Adv Neurol Disord. 2011;4(6):375–83.
68. Castelli L, et al. Sexual well being in parkinsonian patients after deep brain stimulation of the subthalamic nucleus. Neurol Neurosurg Psychiatry. 2004;75(9):1260–4.
69. Romito LM, et al. Transient mania with hypersexuality after surgery for high frequency stimulation of the subthalamic nucleus in Parkinson's disease. Mov Disord. 2002;17(6):1371–4.
70. Worley G. Secondary sexual characteristics in children with cerebral palsy and moderate to severe motor impairment: a cross-sectional survey. Pediatrics. 2002;110:897–902.
71. Wiegerink DJHG, et al. Personal and environmental factors contributing to participation in romantic relationships and sexual activity of young adults with cerebral palsy. Disabil Rehabil. 2012;34(17):1481–7.
72. Wiegerink DJHG, et al. Development of romantic relationships and sexual activity in young adults with Cerebral Palsy: a longitudinal study. Arch Phys Med Rehabil. 2010;91(9):1423–8.
73. Cho SR, et al. Characteristics of psychosexual functioning in adults with cerebral palsy. Clin Rehabil. 2004;18(4):423–9.
74. Wadsworth J, et al. The social needs of adolescents with cerebral palsy. Dev Med Child Neurol. 1993;35(11):1019–22.
75. Wiegerink DJ, et al. Social and sexual relationships of adolescents and young adults with cerebral palsy: a review. Clin Rehabil. 2006;20(12):1023–31.
76. Courtois FJ, et al. Sexual function in spinal cord injury men. I. Assessing sexual capability. Paraplegia. 1993;31(12):771–84.
77. Biering-Sorenson I, et al. Sexual function in a traumatic sci population 10–45 years after injury. J Rehabil Med. 2012;44(11):926–31.
78. Courtois FJ, et al. Post-traumatic erectile potential of spinal cord injured men: how physiologic recordings supplement subjective reports. Arch Phys Med Rehabil. 1999;80:1268.
79. Phelps G, et al. Sexual experience and plasma testosterone levels in male veterans after spinal cord injury. Arch Phys Med Rehabil. 1983;64(2):47–52.
80. Dahlberg A, et al. Sexual activity and satisfaction in men with traumatic spinal cord lesion. Rehabil Med. 2007;39(2):152–5.
81. Courtois FJ, et al. Blood pressure changes during sexual stimulation, ejaculation and midodrine treatment in men with spinal cord injury. BJU Int. 2008;101(3):331–7.
82. Sipski ML, et al. Sexual arousal and orgasm in women: effects of spinal cord injury. Ann Neurol. 2001;49(1):35–44.

83. Kreuter M, et al. Sexual adjustment and quality of relationship in spinal paraplegia: a controlled study. Arch Phys Med Rehabil. 1996;77(6):541–8.
84. Siosteen A, et al. Sexual ability, activity, attitudes and satisfaction as part of adjustment in spinal cord-injured subjects. Paraplegia. 1990;28(5):285–9.
85. Manucharian SR. Changes in sexual functioning in persons with limb amputation. J Prosthet Orthot. 2013;25:177–83.
86. Kegel B, et al. Functional capabilities of lower extremity amputees. Arch Phys Med Rehabil. 1978;59:109–20.
87. Reinstein L, et al. Sexual adjustment after lower extremity amputation. Arch Phys Med Rehabil. 1978;59(11):501–4.
88. Flor H, et al. Phantom limb pain: a case of maladaptive CNS plasticity? Nat Rev Neurosci. 2006;7(11):873–81.
89. Williamson GM, Walters AS. Perceived impact of limb amputation on sexual activity: a study of adult amputees. J Sex Res. 1996;33(3):249–56.
90. Geertzen JH, et al. Sexuality and amputation: a systematic literature review. Disabil Rehabil. 2009;31(7):522–7.
91. Newshan B, et al. Sexual functioning in ambulatory men with HIV/AIDS. Int J STD AIDS. 1998;9(11):672–6.
92. Graham CA, et al. Erection loss in association with condom use among young men attending a public STI clinic: potential correlates and implications for risk behaviour. Sex Health. 2006;3:255–60.
93. Hijazi L, et al. Medical management of sexual difficulties in HIV-positive individuals. Int J STD AIDS. 2002;13(9):587–92.
94. Luzi K, et al. Body image is a major determinant of sexual dysfunction in stable HIV-infected women. Antivir Ther. 2009;14:85–92.
95. Rochira V, et al. Premature decline of serum total testosterone in HIV-infected men in the HAART-Era. PLoS One. 2011;6(12):e28512.
96. Cum NF, et al. A review of hypogonadism and erectile dysfunction among HIV-infected men during the pre- and post-HAART eras: diagnosis, pathogenesis, and management. AIDS Patient Care STDS. 2005;19(10):655–71.
97. Lamba H, et al. Antiretroviral therapy is associated with sexual dysfunction and with increased serum oestradiol levels in men. Int J STD AIDS. 2004;15:234–7.
98. Lallemand F, et al. Sexual dysfunction in 156 ambulatory HIV-infected men receiving highly active antiretroviral therapy combinations with and without protease inhibitors. J Acquir Immune Defic Syndr. 2002;30:187–90.
99. Ciesla JA, et al. Meta-analysis of the relationship between HIV infection and risk for depressive disorders. Am J Psychiatry. 2001;158:725–30.
100. Shen T-C, et al. The risk of erectile dysfunction in chronic obstructive pulmonary disease: a population-based cohort study in Taiwan. Medicine. 2015;94(14):e448.
101. Fletcher EC, et al. Sexual dysfunction and erectile impotence in chronic obstructive pulmonary disease. Chest. 1982;81(4):413–21.
102. Sabit R, et al. Arterial stiffness and osteoporosis in chronic obstructive pulmonary disease. Am J Respir Crit Care Med. 2007;175:1259–65.
103. Verratti V, et al. The role of hypoxia in erectile dysfunction mechanisms. Int J Impot Res. 2007;19:496–500.
104. Vlachopoulos C, et al. Inflammation, metabolic syndrome, erectile dysfunction and coronary artery disease: common links. Eur Urol. 2007;52:1590–600.
105. Ulf A, et al. Reversal of sexual impotence in male patients with chronic obstructive pulmonary disease and hypoxemia with long term oxygen therapy. J Steroid Biochem Mol Biol. 1993;46(6):79.
106. Vincent EE, et al. Review article: addressing the sexual health of patients with COPD: the needs of the patient and implications for health care professionals. Chron Respir Dis. 2007;4(2):111–5.
107. Schönhofer B, et al. Sexuality in patients with restricted breathing. Med Klin. 2002;97:344–9.
108. Fabbri LM, et al. Complex chronic comorbidities of COPD. Eur Respir J. 2008;31:204–12.
109. Laghi F, et al. Hypogonadism in men with chronic obstructive pulmonary disease: prevalence and quality of life. Am J Respir Crit Care Med. 2005;171(7):728–33.
110. Goldfarb J, et al. Sexual and reproductive health in cancer survivors. Semin Oncol. 2013;40(6):726–44.
111. Sadovsky R, et al. Cancer and sexual problems. J Sex Med. 2010;7:349–73.
112. McKee AL, et al. Sexuality rehabilitation. Cancer. 2001;92:1008–12.
113. Basson R, et al. Sexual sequelae of general medical disorders. Lancet. 2007;369:409–24.
114. Gacci M, et al. Quality of life and sexual health in the aging of PCa survivors. Int J Endocrinol. 2014;2014:470592.
115. Pinkawa M, et al. Erectile dysfunction after external beam radiotherapy for prostate cancer. Eur Urol. 2009;55(1):227–34.
116. Akbal C, et al. Erectile dysfunction following radiotherapy and brachytherapy for prostate cancer: pathophysiology, prevention and treatment. Int Urol Nephrol. 2008;40(2):355–63.
117. Merrick GS, et al. Management of sexual dysfunction after prostate brachytherapy. Oncology (Williston Park). 2003;17(1):52–62. discussion 62, 67–70, 73.
118. Goldfarb S. Endocrine therapy and its effect on sexual function. Am Soc Clin Oncol Educ Book. 2015;2015:575–81.
119. Lind H. Late symptoms in long-term gynaecological cancer survivors after radiation therapy: a population-based cohort study. Br J Cancer. 2011;104:737–45.
120. Bober SL, Varela VS. Sexuality in adult cancer survivors: challenges and intervention. J Clin Oncol. 2012;30:3712–9.
121. Taylor KL, et al. Long-term disease-specific functioning among prostate cancer survivors and noncancer controls in the prostate, lung, colorectal, and ovarian cancer screening trial. J Clin Oncol. 2012;30(22):2768–75.
122. Bakewell RT, et al. Sexual dysfunction related to the treatment of young women with breast cancer. Clin J Oncol Nurs. 2005;9:697–702.
123. Yeon WP, et al. Antipsychotic-induced sexual dysfunction and its management. World J Mens Health. 2012;30(3):153–9.
124. Knegtering H, et al. What are the effects of antipsychotics on sexual dysfunctions and endocrine functioning? Psychoneuroendocrinology. 2003;28(Suppl 2):109–23.
125. Montejo AL, et al. Frequency of sexual dysfunction in patients with a psychotic disorder receiving antipsychotics. J Sex Med. 2010;7(10):3404–13.
126. Geriatric Lexi-Drugs Online. Atypical antipsychotics. http://online.lexi.com/crlsql/servlet/crlonline. Accessed on 28 August 2008.
127. Gil-Nagel A, et al. Effect of lamotrigine on sexual function with epilepsy. Seizure. 2006;15(3):142 9.
128. Yang Y, et al. Sexual dysfunction related to antiepileptic drugs in patients with epilepsy. Expert Opin Drug Saf. 2016;15(1):31–42.
129. Smith HS, et al. Opioid-induced androgen deficiency (OPIAD). Pain Physician. 2012;15:ES145–56.
130. Elliott JA, et al. The endocrine effects of long-term oral opioid therapy: a case report and review of the literature. J Opioid Manag. 2011;7:145–54.
131. Colamenco C, Coren JS. Opioid-induced endocrinopathy. J Am Osteopath Assoc. 2009;109:20–5.
132. Ferrario CM, et al. Sexual dysfunction in patients with hypertension: implication for therapy. J Clin Hypertens. 2002;4(6):424–32.
133. Barksdale JD, et al. Review. The impact of first-line antihypertensive drugs on erectile dysfunction. Pharmacotherapy. 1999;19(5):573–81.

134. Bansal S, et al. Sexual dysfunction in hypertensive men. A critical review of the literature. Hypertension. 1988;12:1–10.
135. Duncan L, et al. Review. Sexual function in women. Do antihypertensive drugs have an impact? Drug Saf. 1993;8(3):225–3.
136. Carvajal A, et al. ACE inhibitors and impotence: a case series from Spanish drug monitoring system. Drug Saf. 1995;13:130–1.
137. Neaton JD, et al. Treatment of mild hypertension study. Final results. Treatment of Mild Hypertension Study Research Group. JAMA. 1993;270(6):713–24.
138. Nicolai A. Review of the positive and negative effects of cardiovascular drugs on sexual function: a proposed table for use in clinical practice. Neth Heart J. 2014;22:11–9.
139. Rowen TS. Sexual health care for people with physical disabilities. J Sex Med. 2015;12(3):584–9.
140. Holloway V, et al. Sex drive and sexual desire. Curr Opin Psychiatry. 2015;28(6):424–9.
141. Kalmbach DA, et al. The impact of sleep on female sexual response and behavior: a pilot study. J Sex Med. 2015;12(5):1221–32.
142. Finnerup NB, et al. Pharmacotherapy for neuropathic pain in adults: as systematic review and meta-analysis. Lancet Neurol. 2015;2:162–73.
143. Williams AC, et al. Psychological therapies for the management of chronic pain (excluding headache) in adults. Cochrane Database Syst Rev. 2012;(11):CD007407.
144. Koele R, et al. Multidisciplinary rehabilitation for chronic widespread musculoskeletal pain: results from daily practice. Musculoskeletal Care. 2014;12:210–20.
145. Ambose K, et al. Physical exercise as non-pharmacological treatment of chronic pain: why and when. Best Pract Res Clin Rheumatol. 2015;29(1):120–30.
146. Suckling J, et al. Local estrogen for vaginal atrophy in postmenopausal women. Cochrane Database Syst Rev. 2006;(4):CD001500.
147. Portman DJ, et al. Ospemifene, a novel selective estrogen receptor modulator for treating dyspareunia associated with postmenopausal vulvar and vaginal atrophy. Menopause. 2013;20(6):623–30.
148. Solomons J, et al. Digital removal of faeces in the bowel management of patients with spinal cord injury: a review. Br J Neurosci Nurs. 2013;9:216–22.
149. Haas U, et al. Bowel management in patients with spinal cord injury—a multicentre study of the German speaking society of paraplegia (DMGP). Spinal Cord. 2005;43(12):724–30.
150. Reynolds MR, et al. Sexual intercourse and cerebral aneurysmal rupture: potential mechanisms and precipitants. J Neurosurg. 2011;114:969–77.
151. Masters WH, et al. Human sexual response. Boston, MA: Little, Brown and Co.; 1996. p. 273–93.
152. Ohlsson B, et al. Oxytocin stimulates colonic motor activity in healthy women. Neurogastroenterol Motil. 2004;16:33–40.
153. Moreno J, et al. Improved quality of life and sexuality with continent urinary diversion in quadriplegic women with umbilical stoma. Arch Phys Med Rehabil. 1995;76(8):758–62.
154. Khan Z, et al. Urinary incontinence during orgasm. Urology. 1988;31(3):279–82.
155. Karlsson AK, et al. Review autonomic dysreflexia. Spinal Cord. 1999;37(6):383–91.
156. Wan D, et al. Life-threatening outcomes associated with autonomic dysreflexia: a clinical review. J Spinal Cord Med. 2014;37(1):2–10.
157. Mathias CJ, et al. Autonomic disturbances in spinal cord lesions Autonomic failure, a textbook of clinical disorders of the autonomic nervous system. New York, NY: Oxford Medical Publications; 2002. p. 839–81.
158. Courteous F, et al. Perceived physiological and orgasmic sensation at ejaculation in spinal cord injured men. J Sex Med. 2008;5(10):2419–30.
159. Elliott S, et al. Malignant autonomic dysreflexia in spinal cord injured men. Spinal Cord. 2006;44:386–92.
160. Krassioukov A, et al. A systematic review of the management of autonomic dysreflexia following spinal cord injury. Arch Phys Med Rehabil. 2009;90(4):682–95.
161. Consortium for Spinal Cord Medicine. Sexuality and reproductive health in adults with spinal cord injury: a clinical practice guideline for health-care providers. Palo Alto, CA: Paralyzed Veterans of America; 2012.
162. Maiorino M, et al. Lifestyle modifications and erectile dysfunction: what can be expected? Asian J Androl. 2015;17(1):5–10.
163. Bacon CG, et al. Sexual function in men older than 50 years of age: results from the health professionals follow up study. Ann Intern Med. 2003;139(3):161–8.
164. Johannses CB, et al. Incidence of erectile dysfunction in men 40 to 69 years old: longitudinal results from the Massachusetts male aging study. J Urol. 2000;163(2):460–3.
165. Esposito K, et al. Effect of lifestyle changes on ED in obese men: a randomized controlled trial. JAMA. 2004;291(24):2978–84.
166. Cai X, et al. The role of statins in erectile dysfunction: a systematic review and meta-analysis. Asian J Androl. 2014;16(3):461–6.
167. Alsemari A, et al. Hypogonadism and neurological diseases. Neurol Sci. 2013;34(5):629–38.
168. Safarinejad MR. Evaluation of endocrine profile, hypothalamic-pituitary-testis axis and semen quality in multiple sclerosis. J Neuroendocrinol. 2008;20(12):1368–75.
169. Durga A, et al. Prevalence of testosterone deficiency after SCI. PM R. 2011;3(10):929–32.
170. Mulligan T, et al. Prevalence of hypogonadism in males aged at least 45 years: the HIM study. Int J Clin Pract. 2006;60:762–9.
171. Kalyani RR, et al. Male hypogonadism in systemic disease. Endocrinol Metab Clin North Am. 2007;36(2):333–48.
172. Dandona P, et al. A practical guide to male hypogonadism in the primary care setting. Int J Clin Pract. 2010;64(6):68.
173. Lue TF, et al. Erectile dysfunction. N Engl J Med. 2000;342:1802–13.
174. Porst H. The rationale for prostaglandin E1 in erectile failure: a survey of worldwide experience. J Urol. 1996;155(3):802–15.
175. Tsai YS, et al. Safety and efficacy of alprostadil sterile powder in diabetic patients with erectile dysfunction. Eur Urol. 2000;38(2):177–83.
176. Chen JK, et al. Comparison of effects following the intracorporeal injection of papaverine and prostaglandin E1. Br J Urol. 1992;69:404–7.
177. Goldstein I. Oral phentolamine: an alpha-1, alpha-2 adrenergic antagonist for the treatment of erectile dysfunction. Int J Impot Res. 2000;12(S1):S75–80.
178. Willis E, et al. Vasoactive intestinal polypeptide (VIP) as a possible neurotransmitter involved in penile erection. Acta Physiol Scand. 1981;113(4):545–7.
179. Willis EA, et al. Vasoactive intestinal polypeptide (VIP) as a putative neurotransmitter in penile erection. Life Sci. 1983;33:383–91.
180. Juenemann KP, et al. The role of vasoactive intestinal polypeptide as a neurotransmitter in canine penile erection: a combined in vivo and immunohistochemical study. J Urol. 1987;138(4):871–7.
181. Wagner G, et al. Intracavernosal injection of vasoactive intestinal polypeptide (VIP) does not induce erection in man per se. World J Urol. 1987;5:171–2.
182. Dinsmore WW, et al. Vasoactive intestinal polypeptide/phentolamine for intracavernosal injection in erectile dysfunction. BJU Int. 2008;102(8):933–7.
183. Dinsmore WW. Treating men with predominantly nonpsychogenic erectile dysfunction with intracavernosal vasoactive intestinal polypeptide and phentolamine mesylate in a novel auto-injector system: a multicentre double-blind placebo-controlled study. BJU Int. 1999;83(3):274–9.

184. Sandhu DA, et al. A double blind, placebo controlled study of intracavernosal vasoactive intestinal polypeptide and phenotolamine mesylate in a novel auto-injector for the treatment of non-psychogenic erectile dysfunction. Int J Impot Res. 1999;11(2):91–7.
185. Seyam R, et al. A prospective randomized study to optimize the dosage of trimix ingredients and compare its efficacy and safety with prostaglandin E1. Int J Impot Res. 2005;17(4): 346–53.
186. Padma-Nathan H, et al. Treatment of men with erectile dysfunction with transurethral alprostadil. N Engl J Med. 1997;336:1–7.
187. Williams G, et al. Efficacy and safety of transurethral alprostadil therapy in men with erectile dysfunction. Br J Urol. 1998;81:889–94.
188. Hatzimouratidis K, et al. Guidelines on male sexual dysfunction: erectile dysfunction and premature ejaculation. Eur Urol. 2010;57(5):804–14.
189. Montague DK, et al. Chapter 1: The management of erectile dysfunction: an AUA update. J Urol. 2005;174:230–9.
190. Hatzimouratidis K, et al. A comparative review of the options for treatment of erectile dysfunction: which treatment for which patient? Drugs. 2005;65:1621–50.
191. Mirone V, et al. Tadalafil and vardenafil vs sildenafil: a review of patient-preference studies. BJU Int. 2009;103(9):1212–7.
192. Corona G, et al. Phosphodiesterase type 5 (PDE5) inhibitors in erectile dysfunction: the proper drug for the proper patient. J Sex Med. 2011;8(12):3418–32.
193. Pomeranz HD. The relationship between phosphodiesterase-5 inhibitors and nonarteritic anterior ischemic optic neuropathy. J Neuroophthalmol. 2016;36(2):193–6.
194. Hellstrom WG, et al. Tadalafil has no detrimental effect on human spermatogenesis or reproductive hormones. J Urol. 2003;170:887–91.
195. Cheitlin MD, et al. Use of sildenafil (Viagra) in patients with cardiovascular disease. Technol Pract Execut Comm Circ. 1999;99:168.
196. Kloner RA, et al. Cardiovascular effects of tadalafil. Am J Cardiol. 2003;92(9A):37M–46M.
197. Henry GD, et al. Penile prosthesis cultures during revision surgery: a multicenter study. J Urol. 2004;172:153–6.
198. Hellstrom WJ, et al. Implants, mechanical devices, and vascular surgery for erectile dysfunction. J Sex Med. 2010;7:501.
199. Bozkurt IH, et al. Does the etiology affect the outcome and satisfaction rates of penile prosthesis implantation surgery? Kaohsiung J Med Sci. 2014;30(11):570–3.
200. Kingsberg SA, et al. Treating dyspareunia caused by vaginal atrophy: a review of treatment options using vaginal estrogen therapy. Int J Women Health. 2009;1:105–11.
201. Gao L, et al. Systematic review and meta-analysis of phosphodiesterase type 5 inhibitors for the treatment of female sexual dysfunction. Int J Gynaecol Obstet. 2016;133(2):139–45.
202. Dasgupta R, et al. Efficacy of sildenafil in the treatment of female sexual dysfunction due to multiple sclerosis. J Urol. 2004;171(3):1189–93.
203. Alexander MS, et al. Sildenafil in women with sexual arousal disorder following spinal cord injury. Spinal Cord. 2011;49:273–9.
204. Taylor B, et al. Using the extended PLISSIT model to address sexual healthcare needs. Nurs Stand. 2006;21(11):35–40.
205. Tepper MS. Providing comprehensive sexual health care in spinal cord injury rehabilitation: implementation and evaluation of a new curriculum for health care professionals. Sex Disabil. 1997;15:131–65.
206. Bancroft J. Human sexuality and its problems. 2nd ed. New York, NY: Churchill Livingstone; 1989. p. 745.
207. Stevenson R, et al. Sexuality and medical illness in principles and practice of sex therapy. 4th ed. New York, NY: Editor Sandra Leiblum Guilford Press; 2007. p. 313–49.
208. MacHattie E, et al. Pleasure ABLE: sexual device manual for persons with disabilities. Disabilities health research network; 2009.
209. Tepper MS. Sexuality and disability: the missing discourse of pleasure. Sex Disabil. 2000;18(4):283–90.
210. Kaufman M, et al. The ultimate guide to sex and disability: for all of us who live with disabilities, chronic pain, and illness. San Francisco, CA: Cleis Press Inc.; 2007.
211. Hernandez B. A voice in the chorus: perspectives of young men of color on their disabilities, identities, and peer mentors. Disabil Soc. 2005;20(2):117–33.
212. Gill C. Four types of integrations in disability identity development. J Voc Rehabil. 1997;9:39–46.
213. Houdenhove EV, et al. Asexuality: few facts, many questions. J Sex Marital Ther. 2014;40(3):175–92.
214. Kim E. Asexuality in disability narratives. Sexualities. 2011;14(4):479–93.
215. Ducharme SH, et al. Sexuality after spinal cord injury. Baltimore, MD: Paul H. Brookes Publishing Company Inc.; 1997.
216. United Spinal Association. The effects of spinal cord injury on parenting. Life in Action Magazine; 2013.
217. Through the Looking Glass. Babycare assistive technology for parents with physical disabilities: relational, systems, and cultural perspectives. AFTA Newsl. 1997;1997:20–6.

32 Sex and Chronic Psychiatric Illness

Anna Klimowicz, Adriana Janicic, and Waguih William IsHak

Introduction

It is estimated that one in five adults in the USA—43.6 million people—experiences mental illness in a given year, and approximately one in 25 experiences a serious mental illness that significantly impairs major life activities [1]. Most psychiatric disorders are associated with markedly lower quality of life (QOL) [2–5], including global deficits in social and interpersonal functioning. Impairments in sexuality, with its complex interplay of biopsychosocial factors, are more prevalent in the psychiatric population [6] and seem to be the most severely affected QOL domain [7]. Despite this, clinicians often fail to attend to sexual problems in psychiatric patients [8], while patients themselves feel too embarrassed to initiate conversations or share concerns about sexual dysfunctions [6].

The relationship between chronic mental illness and sexual dysfunction is bidirectional and multifactorial (Figure 32-1)—sexual impairments can both cause or exacerbate and result from mental illness, with biological, psychological, and sociocultural influences as underlying and modulating influences. From a biological perspective, several neurotransmitters such as dopamine, norepinephrine, and serotonin, are implicated in both sexual functioning and the pathophysiology and pharmacological treatment of the major psychiatric disorders [9]. For example, dopamine is involved in such sexual behavior as arousal, erection, and orgasm, and is also a common psychopharmacological target [9]. Antipsychotic medications antagonize dopaminergic systems, and are known to suppress sexual functioning, while other medications, such as L-dopa used in the treatment of Parkinson's disease, can have the opposite effect. The influence of psychiatric medications on sexual functioning is a major factor in treatment compliance and calls for clinician necessity to discuss sexual problems with psychiatric patients. For an in-depth discussion, please refer to the chapter "Evaluation and Treatment of Substance/Medication-Induced Sexual Dysfunction."

Psychosocial and interpersonal dimensions play an important role in sexual functioning in both the psychiatric and the general populations. However, people with mental disorders face exceptional challenges in the social domain due to sexual isolation resulting from stigma [10]. Experiences of being stereotyped, discriminated against and excluded can lead to internalized stigma [11] which may reduce self-esteem and provide further obstacles in forming intimate relationships. Additionally, some evidence suggests that social stigma leads to risky sexual behaviors, due to interference with the ability to negotiate safe sex behaviors [12]. In spite of social and interpersonal barriers, people with mental illness do desire intimate relationships and view sexually and emotionally intimate relationships as a key facilitator and indicator of recovery [13]. Interpersonal domain is a significant factor in both mental illness and sexual dysfunction, and is an important component of therapeutic framework for treatment of either condition.

This chapter provides an overview of sexual functioning in people with major chronic psychiatric illness. It discusses psychopathology as related to sexual dysfunction, gender differences, and clinical considerations. Sections follow the DSM-V [14] order: Neurodevelopmental Disorders, Schizophrenia Spectrum and Other Psychotic Disorders, Bipolar and Related Disorders, Depressive Disorders, Anxiety Disorders, Obsessive-Compulsive and Related Disorders, Trauma- and Stressor-Related Disorders, Dissociative Disorders, Somatic Symptom and Related Disorders, Feeding and Eating Disorders, Substance-Related and Addictive Disorders, Neurocognitive Disorders, and Personality Disorders.

Neurodevelopmental Disorders

Neurodevelopmental disorders comprise a heterogeneous group of conditions producing personal, social, or occupational deficits due to a disruption in the normal course of human development.

W.W. IsHak (ed.), *The Textbook of Clinical Sexual Medicine*, DOI 10.1007/978-3-319-52539-6_32

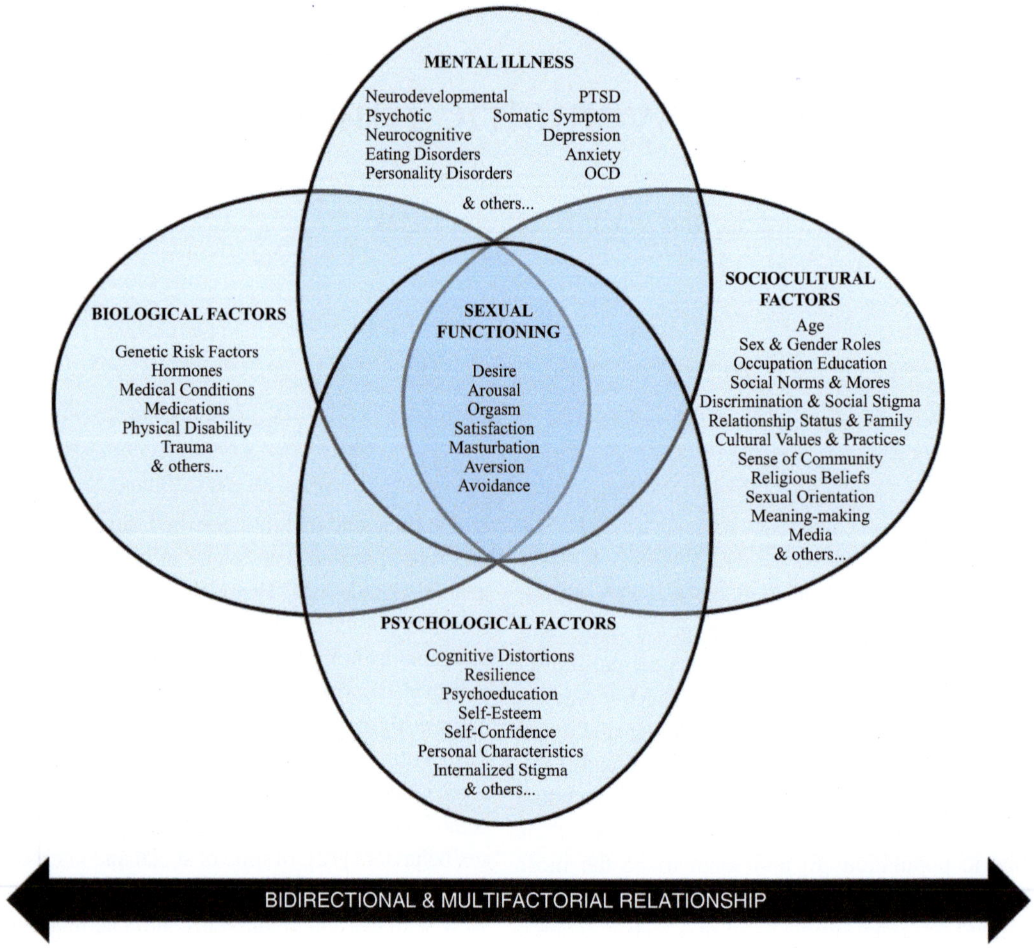

FIGURE 32-1. The relationship between mental illness and sexual functioning is bidirectional and multifactorial [Courtesy of Anna Klimowicz, Adriana Janicic, and Waguih William IsHak].

Intellectual Disability

Intellectual disability (ID) is characterized by mild to severe impairments in general cognitive abilities and adaptive functioning, leading to a decrease in the capacity for personal independence [14]. Due to reliance on others for care and daily functioning, many life domains of people with IDs have historically been restricted, including the right to sexuality and parenting [15]. Despite advances in human rights for individuals with IDs, academic research focuses mostly on sexual abuse, sexual perpetration, and societal attitudes towards sexual activity in individuals with ID, giving much less attention to positive experiences of sexuality.

People with intellectual disabilities are more likely than their peers to be victims of sexual abuse [16], with the rate being significantly higher for women, who also tend to have more negative feelings about the abuse [17]. Murphy and O'Callaghan [18] point to the delicate balance between empowering individuals with IDs to express their sexual rights and protecting them from unwanted sexual contact, as adults with IDs had difficulty distinguishing between consensual and abusive sexual relationships. However, this capacity significantly increased with sexual education and higher IQ [18].

Notably, there is insufficient sexual and intimacy education and training for individuals with IDs and their parents/caregivers, respectively. Only about half of adolescents with disabilities ever talked about sex with their parents [19]. Staff carers, despite holding generally positive attitudes, could benefit from more targeted training on how to support sexuality in persons with ID [20, 21].

Qualitative research has provided a window into the subjective sexual experiences of people with IDs, indicating that the majority of women with IDs could not conceptualize themselves as sexual beings, had negative attitudes about sex, believed others did not permit them to engage in sex [22], and remained abstinent due to fears based on misconceptions about sex [23]. Additionally, young people with IDs of both genders face stigma related to their ID, which can overshadow their developing sexual identity [24, 25].

Despite many barriers to a sexual well-being, persons with IDs do desire intimate relationships and consider them important [26]. The increasing social awareness of sexual needs in this population and the accompanying emergence of sexual educational programs are promising for lowering sexual abuse rates and increasing sexual well-being among persons with IDs.

Autism Spectrum Disorder

Autism spectrum disorder (ASD) is a complex condition, presenting as social interaction deficits in multiple domains as well as a restrictive, repetitive behavioral pattern [14]. The number of children diagnosed with the disorder is rising, with a 2016 report citing 23.6 boys and 5.3 girls per 1000 children aged 8 years meeting the diagnostic criteria [27]. Recent years have seen substantial attention given to autism both by academia and the general public; however, many aspects of pathophysiology and psychology of autism remain poorly understood. Studies on the well-being of autistic individuals show generally lowered quality of life [28, 29]. However, investigation of sexual functioning specifically is limited by small sample sizes, focuses on high functioning samples only, and groups lower functioning autistic individuals with other intellectually disabled populations. For these and other reasons, many reports on sexual satisfaction and sexual behaviors show contradictory conclusions.

Persons with ASD are shown to generally desire romantic relationships and sexual experiences [30–32], but may face difficulty engaging in romance and sexual activities due to deficits in social communication [33, 34]. Lower sexual satisfaction tends to be correlated with autistic symptom severity [35, 36]. Additionally, higher satisfaction with romantic relationship was shown among individuals whose partners were also diagnosed with ASD [30].

There are significant gender differences in sexual functioning of autistic men and women. Higher prevalence of ASD in males, as well as relatively strong social skills "masking" ASD diagnosis in females, leads to an underrepresentation of autistic girls and women in research. In Byers et al. [35] study of 68 women and 61 men with ASD, women reported significantly higher sexual anxiety, more frequent sexual problems, and lower sexual arousability. In a different study, Byers [37] found that autistic men reported better solitary sexual well-being, more sexual thoughts and desires, despite having lower sexual knowledge. Although most research points to normative sexual behaviors in individuals with ASD, some report increased presence of paraphilias [32, 38] and sensory fascination with a sexual connotation [31].

Attention-Deficit/Hyperactivity Disorder (ADHD)

Attention-deficit/hyperactivity disorder (ADHD) is characterized by a persistent pattern of attention deficits and/or hyperactivity-impulsivity that causes impairments in functioning or development [14]. It is a neurodevelopmental disorder with childhood onset that persists into adulthood, with a prevalence of 2.5% in adults and 5% in children [14].

Symptoms related to hyperactivity and excitability have brought about investigations into the link between ADHD and increased sexual impulsivity. Both male and female adolescents typically report having more romantic partners in comparison with their peers [39, 40], with Rokeach et al. citing double the number of lifetime sexual partners. Individuals with ADHD are more likely to engage in risky sexual activities [41] and are being treated for STDs more often [42]. They also report having earlier dating experiences [43], more partner pregnancies [40] and become parents earlier than the general population [42]. However, high prevalence of comorbidities such as addiction and conduct disorders pose several methodological limitations, as risky sexual behaviors may be attributable to comorbid conduct disorder, substance or alcohol use [44], rather than ADHD.

Although some studies report good overall quality of romantic relationships in adolescents with ADHD [39], others report higher incidence of verbal aggression and violence towards partners [45] and lower relationship quality, possibly mediated by hostile relationship conflicts [46]. Adults with ADHD symptomatology may also experience more fear of intimacy, despite lack of sexual anxiety [47].

Other Neurodevelopmental Disorders

Neurodevelopmental disorders also include communication disorders, specific learning disorder, as well as motor disorders. Research on sexual functioning in individuals with Communication Disorders is severely lacking. Learning disorders are often included in studies sampling populations with intellectual disabilities and share some of the same limitations as research on IDs, such as inclusion of participants with vastly different symptomatology. Inappropriate sexual behaviors, exhibitionism, and copropraxia are common symptoms of Tourette's syndrome [48, 49]. However, research on pharmacological treatment is based mostly on case studies [50, 51] and there is a lack of investigation into psychotherapy and psychological factors involved in sexual symptoms of this disorder.

Schizophrenia Spectrum and Other Psychotic Disorders

Schizophrenia spectrum and other psychotic disorders are characterized by delusions, hallucinations, disorganized thinking, abnormalities in motor behavior, as well as negative symptoms such as diminished emotional expression and anhedonia [14]. The lifetime prevalence of schizophrenia is estimated to be 0.3–0.7% [14]. Individuals suffering from this spectrum of disorders are known to have a significantly impaired quality of life [52–55] and are likely to suffer from internalized stigma [56, 57]. Sexual functioning impairments can be found in both females and males with schizophrenia or schizoaffective disorder [58] and are believed to be more prevalent than in patients treated for other mental disorders [59], with between 45% and 95% of patients reporting sexual impairments [58, 60, 61]. Problems with sexuality are significant factors lowering the quality of life in this population [61, 62]. Sexual dysfunction in men is most typically reported as lower libido, erectile dysfunction, premature ejaculation, and lesser intensity of orgasms [63], while research on women often uses more vague categories [64] such as lesser enjoyment of sex and organism dysfunctions [63, 65].

Sexual dysfunction in patients with schizophrenia is a complex phenomenon, with multiple factors contributing to its etiology: the pathophysiology of schizophrenia itself, socioeconomic impact of the disease, and side effects of treatment [59]. The impact of antipsychotic medications and adjunct pharmacological treatments is covered in Chapter X, "Evaluation and Treatment of Substance/Medication-Induced Sexual Dysfunction" and is arguably the most studied topic on sexuality in schizophrenic patients, which can be partly attributable to the fact that medication-induced sexual dysfunctions lead to poor treatment compliance [65, 66]. However, treatment-naïve patients also report decreased satisfaction with their sexuality [67]. Aizenberg et al. [68] found decreased desire and increased masturbatory activity in both treated and untreated schizophrenic patients; however, the untreated group also reported reduction in the frequency of sexual thoughts. It has thus been suggested that the pathophysiology of schizophrenia is involved in sexual dysfunction, possibly due to lower estrogen levels in females [69, 70] and testosterone in males [71, 72].

Overall reduction in quality of life, institutionalization, stigma, and other social repercussions of the disease negatively contribute to schizophrenic patients' ability to form and sustain fulfilled romantic and sexual relationships [73–75]. Despite the evident negative effects of sexual dysfunctions, psychiatrists routinely underestimate the prevalence of sexual problems such as loss of libido or impotence in this population [60, 73]. In-depth interviews with schizophrenic patients reveal that they often feel overlooked by psychiatric services as sexual beings [74]. Avoidance of the topic by healthcare provides not only fails to address an important aspect of well-being but it may also lead to inadequate reproductive health care and poor treatment compliance. Discussion of sexuality should be included whenever assessing a patient with psychotic disorders.

Bipolar and Related Disorders

Bipolar and related disorders are characterized by manic or hypomanic states with a history of major depressive disorder, although depression is no longer a necessary diagnostic criterion for Bipolar I in the DSM-V [14]. Mania includes symptoms such as elevated and expansive mood, grandiosity, increased energy, and risky behaviors for at least 1 week. Mood fluctuations, cognitive impairments, and interpersonal difficulties accompanying this disorder lead to a markedly lower quality of life [2].

A number of studies have shown that, compared to both the general and psychiatric populations, bipolar males and females have sex with more partners [76–79], are less likely to use condoms [76–78], have more STIs [80, 81], and are more likely to engage in sex with people of unknown HIV status [82, 83]. Women with bipolar disorder are more likely to have adverse reproductive outcomes such as unplanned pregnancies and abortions [81], with rates increased especially for bipolar adolescents [84]. Special consideration should be given to women in postpartum period due to increased risk of manic or depressive episodes [85–87] and a higher likelihood of symptom relapse [88].

Bipolar disorder is associated not only with risky sexual behaviors but also with an elevated sexuality in general, commonly referred to as "hypersexuality." Akiskal et al. [79] studied over 1000 patients with Bipolar II disorder and found that they reported increased frequency of various sexual behaviors, including intramarital and extramarital sex, visiting prostitutes, and masturbation. Although the authors suggest that any patient with depression exhibiting such heightened sexuality should be evaluated for bipolarity, they propose that those sexual symptoms may not necessarily be pathological but rather a result of evolutionary advantage. It seems that hypomanic patients themselves, while recognizing the risks and consequences of hypersexuality, might not deem treatment necessary [78]. Additionally, a recent review of literature on hypersexuality, couples relationship and bipolar disorder reveals that bipolar patients are more similar to control group rather than other psychiatric patients when it comes to establishing and maintaining romantic relationships [77].

Other studies point to the positive correlation between sensation seeking, low effortful self-control and hypersexuality [89]. Diagnostic problems may arise especially in adolescents and children with hypersexuality, due to overlaps with ADHD and difficulty in identifying grandiose or pathologically elevated mood in such young population [90, 91]. Although there is no consensus on whether hypersexuality is pathological [92], some psychodynamic issues such as seeking validation through sexual attention may be present in adolescents and successfully addressed through cognitive behavioral therapy [93].

Depressive Disorders

Depressive disorders are characterized by the presence of sad, empty, or irritable mood, and somatic and cognitive changes that impede functioning [14]. They include Disruptive Mood Dysregulation Disorder, Major Depressive Disorder, Persistent Depressive Disorder, and Premenstrual Dysphoric Disorder, which all differ in duration, timing, or presumed etiology [14]. No evidence of sexual dysfunction within Premenstrual Dysphoric Disorder was documented, perhaps due to the nascence of this disorder in the nomenclature. The majority of available literature on sexual functioning clusters together the depressive disorders or only focuses on Major Depressive Disorder (MDD) [14].

Major Depressive Disorder

The cardinal features of MDD include depressed, low mood and/or anhedonia (decreased pleasure in activities previously enjoyed), causing significant distress and impair functioning [14]. MDD is one of the most common psychiatric disorders, with a 7% 12-month prevalence rate in the USA [14], with the highest rates of sexual dysfunction among other common mental disorders [94].

The DSM-5 states that for some individuals the diminished interest or pleasure in activities may be experienced as a loss of sexual interest or desire [14]. Therefore, sexual dysfunction is built into the criteria of MDD and significant impairment in marital adjustment and sexual functioning frequently accompany the negative symptoms of this diagnosis [95, 96]. MDD is associated with loss of libido for both men and women [96], which may be among the most distressing symptoms of depression and contributed to deteriorated quality of life [97]. Besides lower sexual drive, MDD is also correlated with decreased interest in sexually explicit material, and reduced sexual fantasizing for males and females alike [96, 97]. Masturbation rates among depressed individuals have received inconsistent findings, with some studies showing reductions and others purporting increases in solitary sexual experiences [96]. Ramrahka et al. [98] established that diagnosis of depressive disorders among young people predicted risky sexual intercourse, contraction of sexually transmitted infections, and first sexual intercourse prior to age 16. Laurent and Simons [96] maintain that the relationship between depression and sexual functioning is complex, with sexual and depressive symptoms often co-occurring.

Sexual arousal concerns are also common in men with depression, with erectile dysfunction and nocturnal penile tumescence being the most frequently reported and studied [96]. Less research is available on female sexual arousal and depression; still, more sexual arousal issues and vaginal dryness is noted for depressed versus non-depressed females [99], and compared to women without any history of MDD [100]. Increased rates of sexual pain or intercourse difficulty (functional dyspareunia) and inhibited orgasm (anorgasmia) in women, and premature as well as delayed ejaculation in men have been linked to emotional problems and depression [96]. While sexual satisfaction among depressed individuals has insufficient research, it is lower for depressed individuals than controls [96]. Laumann et al. [101] found that sexual well-being was substantially lower in depressed women than depressed men, paralleling the gender discrepancy in prevalence of depression. Overall, Laurent and Simons [96] contend that sexual dysfunction should be considered as part of internalizing disorders, which include depression and anxiety, due to the degree of interconnectedness between their symptoms and impact on one another.

Some medications used to treat depression, particularly selective serotonin reuptake inhibitors (SSRIs), have common adverse effects on sexual functioning, which are poorly tolerated and may exacerbate existing sexual dysfunction caused by depression [9, 102]. Please refer to the chapter on *Evaluation and Treatment of Substance/Medication-Induced Sexual Dysfunction* for a thorough discussion of these effects. Hence, sexual functioning needs to be assessed prior to the commencement of medication in order to fully understand the impact of both depressive disorders and medications on sexual functioning.

Anxiety Disorders

Anxiety disorders are characterized by persistent and excessive fear or anxiety in anticipation of a future threat. They include separation anxiety disorder, selective mutism, specific phobia, social anxiety disorder, panic disorder, agoraphobia, generalized anxiety disorder (GAD), as well as anxiety due to substance or medical condition. Although anxiety disorders are not uncommon—lifetime morbidity of GAD is 9.0% [14]—their effect on sexual functioning has been researched by a very small number of studies.

Due to activation of the sympathetic nervous system during anxious states, researchers have wondered whether anxiety may increase sexual arousal. Some experimental studies on women demonstrated that the state of anxiety does in fact increase genital arousal, however, it does not affect subjective perception of sexual arousal [103, 104]. In fact, women with anxiety disorders report worse sexual functioning than healthy controls, despite no change in desire, lubrication, and pain [105, 106]. Sexual inhibition, mostly caused by concern over sexual performance, is markedly higher in women with anxiety disorders [105], with over 60% of women with panic disorder reporting sexual avoidance [107]. Similarly, men with anxiety disorders are more likely than controls to experience performance anxiety related to sex [108].

Among different anxiety disorders, panic disorder seems to be associated with exceptionally high number of comorbid sexual disorders for both men and women [109–111]. Social phobia is also related to such impairments as lower arousal, lower sexual enjoyment, or orgasmic dysfunctions, with women reporting more severe impairments than men [112]. Additionally, men with social phobia are more likely to pay for sex, whereas women report fewer sexual partners than healthy controls [112]. Premature ejaculation (PE) and erectile dysfunction are often present in men with anxiety disorders [108, 113], in particular with social phobia. It is suggested that adrenergic hyperactivity that is common to both PE and social phobia might be responsible for the high comorbidity [114].

Anxiety disorders may be risk factors for lower sexual functioning in men and women and it is recommended that patients with anxiety should be asked about their sexual lives. Likewise, sexual impairments might be caused by sexual performance anxiety, which may be a symptom of an underlying anxiety disorder that patients should be screened for.

Obsessive-Compulsive and Related Disorders

Obsessive-compulsive and related disorders comprise a range of conditions that frequently overlap associated with developmentally inappropriate and excessive preoccupations and rituals, including obsessive-compulsive disorder (OCD), body dysmorphic disorder (BDD), hoarding disorder, trichotillomania, and excoriation [14]. Research examining the relationship between both trichotillomania and excoriation, and sexual functioning was severely lacking and require further research.

Obsessive-Compulsive Disorder

Obsessive-compulsive disorder (OCD) is characterized by the presence of persistent, distressing, and time-consuming intrusive thoughts, urges, or images (obsessions) and/or repetitive unrealistically related or excessive behaviors or mental acts that individuals feel impelled to perform (compulsions) in response to their obsessions or rigid rules to impart temporary relief [14]. Sexual dysfunction in OCD is a complex phenomenon that cannot be simply explained by the impact of the disorder itself, or the pharmacological treatment of it [115]. Despite methodological limitations of poor generalizability [116, 117], the available literature converges on the presence of high rates of sexual dysfunction among both men and women with OCD, with 54–73% reporting sexual dissatisfaction and sexual avoidance [115]. Individuals with OCD's capacity for intimacy is impeded by their excessive need for control, need to control their thoughts, high disgust sensitivity, and concealing of obsessional beliefs due to shame or fears of increased probability of occurrence with disclosure [118], resulting in increased interpersonal impairment and distress [115]. Further, cognitive biases and inflexible rules present in OCD are implicated in reduced sexual satisfaction and functioning [115].

In exploring the role of disgust in sex, de Jong and colleagues [119] discuss that the mouth and vagina, while playing a central role in sexual activity, also display the highest disgust sensitivity. This, paired with the high correlation between bodily secretions and disgust may perpetuate contamination fears, chronic sexual disgust, and avoidance of sexual behavior [119]. Intuitively, individuals with OCD and sexual dysfunction experience significantly more distress than those without sexual concerns [117]. Sexual dysfunction occurs in 39% of females with OCD, including sexual disgust, lack of sexual desire, reduced sexual arousal, anorgasmia, and increased avoidance of sexual intercourse [107, 117]. Further, sexual infrequency was observed among 57.1% of men and 63.6% of women with OCD [107].

Sexual obsessions are under-reported, frequently misdiagnosed, and often involve the thought-action fusion cognitive bias, leading to increased distress [120, 121]. Common OCD clinical features of contamination fears and sexual taboo obsessions are related to impaired sexual performance and satisfaction [122]. A subset of sexual obsessions, sexual orientation preoccupation, is often easily misperceived as sexual identity confusion, resulting in inappropriate treatment planning [115].

Additionally, there is some clinical overlap between OCD features and compulsive-impulsive sexual behavior [115]. Inconsistencies over the association between OCD and paraphilias exist in the literature; yet, sexual obsessions within OCD tend to be ego-dystonic, unpleasurable, and unbearable, as differentiated from the ego-syntonic, exciting thoughts observed in paraphilic and compulsive sexual behaviors [115]. Further, when thoughts are perceived as unacceptable and unwanted (e.g., non-consensual, aggressive, or incestuous), as often noted by individuals with OCD, sexual activity tends to be avoided [115]. However, the research also cautions that relying on the distressing versus non-distressing differential alone leaves much room for misdiagnosis, potential exacerbation of symptoms [123], and iatrogenic treatment [124].

With the presence of additional psychiatric diagnoses, such as depression, the phenomenology of sexual dysfunction in OCD becomes more complex and multidirectional [117].

Body Dysmorphic Disorder

Body dysmorphic disorder (BDD) involves distressing preoccupation with one or more perceived or slight defect or flaw in physical appearance, and engaging in repetitive behaviors or mental acts in response to appearance concerns [14]. BDD also includes muscle dysmorphia, which is defined by the belief that one's body build is too small or not muscular enough [14].

The emphasis on physical appearance dissatisfaction has received more attention than the diagnosis of BDD with regard to sexual functioning research. Overall self-image and body image are significant predictors of sexual activity, including orgasm, initiating sex, comfort undressing in front of partners, having sex with the lights on, trying new sexual behaviors, and pleasing their partners sexually [125]. Yet positive body esteem and self-perceived sexual attractiveness are not consistently correlated with sexual satisfaction for women across the literature [125–127]. Pujols et al. [126] suggest that distress and cognitive distractions over appearance and body image predict sexual satisfaction, even after accounting for sexual dysfunction. Women who experienced cognitive distractions during sexual activity report proportionately lower sexual esteem and sexual satisfaction, less consistent orgasms, and higher incidence of faking orgasm [128]. More recent research adds that cognitions, evaluations, and self-consciousness also interfere with sexual avoidance and risky sexual behavior among females [129].

Due to the high frequency of individuals with BDD pursuing various cosmetic procedures to improve their body esteem [126, 130, 131], the literature on BDD and cosmetic procedures offers possible avenues for further empirical investigation. A descriptive study by Veale et al. [132] indicates that the women presenting for labiaplasty endorsed reduced sexual satisfaction, interference with quality of life, greater avoidance of sexual intimacy and intercourse, as well as greater probability of BDD diagnosis related to their body image, compared to controls. Moreover, sexual dysfunction was identified as one of the motivators for seeking genital modification procedures [132]. In another small-sampled psychosexual outcome study following labiaplasty, Veale et al. [133] also report that of the nine women that met criteria for BDD pre-operation, eight showed full remission of BDD and enhanced sexual satisfaction at three months, with 26% reporting minor side effects. More research with larger studies is required to determine actual connections between sexual functioning and genital dissatisfaction.

Penile dysmorphic disorder (PDD) has been used to distinguish men who have BDD with predominant preoccupations about their penis size [134]. Veale and colleagues [134] reveal that men with BDD were more likely to experience erectile dysfunction, orgasmic dysfunction, and reduced sexual intercourse satisfaction, compared to controls and men with small penis anxiety; however, all three groups maintained their sexual desire/libido. Additionally, BDD has been closely linked to EDs due to the presence of similar clinical variables including body image disturbance [135, 136].

Trauma- and Stressor-Related Disorders

Trauma- and stressor-related disorders encompasses a range of disorders that enlist exposure to a traumatic or stressful event as a core feature, including reactive attachment disorder, disinhibited social engagement disorder, posttraumatic stress disorder, acute stress disorder, adjustment disorders [14].

Posttraumatic Stress Disorder

Posttraumatic stress disorder (PTSD) is characterized by direct exposure to a traumatic or stressful event to self or close other, recurrent and distressing intrusive symptoms, persistent avoidance of triggers associated to traumatic event, negative alterations in cognitions and mood, hyperarousal, and reactivity associated to traumatic event [14].

Significantly poorer sexual functioning was found across all domains (desire, arousal, orgasm, activity, and satisfaction) for patients with treated and untreated PTSD, in comparison to controls without PTSD [137]. Indeed, Yehuda and colleagues [138] propose that post-traumatic sexual dysfunction is possibly mediated by PTSD-related biological, cognitive, and affective processes. Letourneau et al. [139] assert that PTSD serves as a moderator for the development of sexual dysfunction for both sexually and non-sexually traumatized women.

The sexual functioning of individuals with histories of sexual trauma has received relatively greater empirical attention, compared to other types of trauma or abuse [140]. Noll and colleagues [141] studied the impact of childhood sexual trauma (CSA) on sexuality, finding that history of CSA was correlated with anxiety, sexual aversion, sexual ambivalence, and dissociation. The authors [141] also imply that sexual abuse by biological father may be related to higher sexual aversion and ambivalence. Shaaf and McCanne [142] note that women who experienced not only sexual but also physical abuse in childhood faced the greatest risk for sexual victimization in adulthood, which then exposed them to increased risk of developing PTSD. In addition, CSA increases risk of being sexually exploited [143] and PTSD-related symptoms can both precede and accompany sexual exploitation [144]. Sexually exploited populations also are at greater risk for sexually transmitted diseases and HIV/AIDS, posing a grave public health concern [145, 146]. The impact of sexual exploitation on sexual dysfunction may include hypersexuality, preoccupation with sex, younger age at initial intercourse, teen pregnancies, anorgasmia, vaginal pain, as well as other emotional vulnerabilities pertinent to sexual functioning [143, 147].

While the connection between PTSD and intimate relationship problems for combat veterans is well documented in the literature [148] the exploration of sexual functioning of this population has received less attention. Combat veterans with PTSD experience higher rates of sexual dysfunction compared to veterans without PTSD, and demonstrate impaired overall sexual satisfaction, orgasmic function, intercourse satisfaction, and erectile dysfunction or vaginal pain [149–151]. Greenberg [149] suggests that PTSD symptoms co-occur with intimacy and sexual dysfunction, such as impotency and/or hypersexuality. Joannides [152] further emphasizes that due to the powerful physical sensations and emotional vulnerability of sex, PTSD symptoms (i.e., flashbacks) can be triggered for veterans and hence, impair sexual relationships. The author [152] specifically highlights the combat imagery and language in sexual activity, paralleling explosion with the sensation of orgasm and the sounds made amid sexual pleasure and release that could sound like cries of pain. Also, the fluctuation between sexual urgency and sexual disinterest often experienced by combat veterans may be confusing for their spouses, leading their spouses to avoid intimate interactions and complicating sexual relationships further [149]. Additionally, extramarital affairs are reportedly high among combat veterans with PTSD due to potential sexual acting out, experience of sexual activities as mundane compared to the intensity of combat, discomfort sharing sexual fantasies or desires with spouses, or the spouses' inability to sustain their sexual intensity [149].

From a neurobiological stance, sexual dysfunction among veterans with PTSD was not resultant from an organic disorder, and has been associated with plasma DHEA and cortisol, urinary catecholamines, and glucocorticoid sensitivity, even after accounting for concurrent depressive symptoms [153]. Additionally, PTSD predicted higher levels of dihydrotestosterone, which is connected to sexual dysfunction [153].

Dissociative Disorders

Dissociative disorders are characterized by global impairments in integrating consciousness, memory, identity, emotion, body representation, and behavior [14] and comprise of dissociative identity disorder (DID), depersonalization/derealization disorder, and dissociative amnesia as the major disorders in this group. The etiology of these disorders is closely linked to trauma, especially severe neglect or CSA [14, 154, 155] with over 70% of patients reporting physical or sexual abuse [156, 157]. However, sexual trauma as a cause of pathological dissociation remains controversial [158, 159].

In a 2004 review, Piper and Merskey [160] found no consistent evidence that DID results from childhood trauma. A recent study by Vissia et al. [154] tested the Trauma Model, supporting trauma as etiology of DID, vs. Fantasy Model, which posits that DID can be simulated and is mediated by high susceptibility and fantasy proneness. They found that patients with genuine DID were no more fantasy prone or susceptible than healthy controls or patients with selected other psychiatric diagnoses [154]. Additionally, it seems that childhood sexual trauma is linked to dissociative symptoms without the mediation of depression, anxiety, or mood swings [161]. Recognizing sexual trauma as a strong predictor of dissociative disorders warrants screening patients with dissociative symptoms for sexual abuse.

Female adolescents with dissociative disorders and history of sexual abuse are at a higher risk of self-injurious behavior [162]. Women who experience intimate partner violence are more likely to experience dissociative symptoms that may interfere with their ability to protect themselves from STIs/HIV [163]. It has been noted that patients with DID might themselves become perpetrators of intimate partner violence, as dissociation might allow them to distance themselves from the victim [164], however, there is not enough evidence to establish a definite link.

Despite sexual trauma being established as one of the causes of dissociative disorders, very little is known about sexual functioning and well-being of patients with this diagnosis. In a study on women with and without a history of CSA, no measure of dissociation was significantly associated with sexual response [165]. Additionally, for women in both groups, more derealization was related to higher sexual arousal [165]. It is suggested that some level of dissociation during sex might be a common, rather than pathological, experience [166].

Somatic Symptom and Related Disorders

Somatic symptom and related disorders is a new category of disorders in the DSM-5 and include somatic symptom disorder, illness anxiety disorder, and factitious disorder, among others. These disorders are characterized by the prominence of somatic symptoms associated with significant distress and impairment [14]. The DSM-5 emphasizes that affective, cognitive, and behavioral presentation of somatic symptoms are at the core of these disorders, rather than the lack of medical explanation for them [14]. Prevalence in the general adult population is 5–7% [14] and these patients typically present in primary care or other non-psychiatric medical settings.

Sexual functioning in patients with somatic symptoms disorders has been studied primarily with regards to chronic pelvic pain in women and erectile dysfunction in men. Psychogenic pelvic pain can be a sign of feeling trapped in marriage, job, or other interpersonal aspects of life [167]. Although there is no definitive evidence establishing sexual trauma as etiology of pelvic somatization [168, 169], there is a strong positive correlation between history of sexual abuse and somatic symptoms [170–172]. History of non-sexual violence is less strongly but still significantly related to somatization [173]. Women with pelvic venous congestion, which is not associated with pain, are also more likely to have experienced CSA, thus suggesting that pain alone is not responsible for somatization in these patients [174]. Although there is little research on somatic disorders and sexual functioning in women, sexual abuse as a moderating factor can predict lower sexual satisfaction [175–177]. Given that women with somatic pelvic symptoms often feel stigmatized and stereotyped by doctors and are worried that their condition is perceived an excuse to avoid intercourse [178], sensitivity in clinical interview is required.

A recent large scale study investigating biochemical, clinical, and psychological parameters of sexual functioning, found that somatization was the most important factor determining or worsening male sexual dysfunction [179]. Another study looking into erectile dysfunction in men with different psychiatric disorders such as depression, anxiety, and OCD, reported that patients with somatization symptoms showed the worst erectile dysfunctions [179]. The extant literature thus supports somatization as a significant factor affecting sexuality in both men and women.

Feeding and Eating Disorders

Feeding and eating disorders (FEDs) entail a range of eating-related behavioral disturbances causing significant impairment to physical health and/or psychological functioning [14]. These include pica, rumination disorder, avoidant/restrictive food intake disorder (ARFID), anorexia nervosa (AN), bulimia nervosa (BN), binge-eating disorder (BED), other specified feeding or eating disorder, and unspecified feeding or eating disorder [14].

The prevailing literature tends to address the sexual functioning of AN, BN, and BED collectively under eating disorders (EDs). As frequently observed in the overarching EDs literature, the examination of sexuality in EDs presents a female sampling bias [180], potentially perpetuating unsubstantiated stereotypical views of EDs and contributing to the underestimation of male vulnerability to EDs [181]. Indeed, Kelly et al. [182] demonstrate that contrary to other eating disorders, BED occurs at similar rates among men (8%) and women (10%) prevalence in community samples.

EDs are commonly accompanied by sexual dysfunction [183, 184]. Castellini and colleagues [183] found four pervasive themes at the cross section of EDs pathology and sexuality: puberty, CSA, sexual orientation, and sexual dysfunction. A significant relationship between body dissatisfaction and severity of sexual dysfunction has been established [185–187], with reduced female sexual functioning associated with greater body shape concerns across AN, BN, and BED [185, 187].

Further, specific EDs psychopathology (preoccupation with with body shape and weight) may serve as maintaining factors of sexual dysfunction in EDs [183]. Consequent to the impact of EDs, women frequently face numerous obstetric/gynecologic complications, including infertility, unplanned pregnancies, poor perinatal nutrition, negative attitudes towards pregnancies, increased risk of abortions and miscarriages, postpartum depression and anxiety, and sexual dysfunctions [183, 188].

Anorexia Nervosa

Anorexia nervosa (AN) is defined by three fundamental features: persistent energy intake restriction resulting in significantly low body weight relative to age, sex, developmental trajectory, and physical health; intense fear of gaining weight or becoming fat, or persistent behavior that interferes with weight gain; and a disturbance in self-perceived weight, shape, or pursuit of thinness [14]. Further, AN tends to have a long-lasting, chronic course, significant functional impairments, and high suicidality and mortality rates [14]. The subtypes differentiate between predominantly restricting or binge/purging type at current diagnostic evaluation, as the individual may migrate across subtypes or diagnoses over time [14, 189]. Although amenorrhea is no longer a defining diagnostic criterion of AN due to its exclusion of males, prepubertal and postmenopausal females, as well as females taking hormonal contraceptives, it may ensue as a physiological sequela of AN in some individuals [190].

The relationship between severity of low weight and sexual dysfunction is unclear, but worsened sexual dysfunction is evidenced among individuals with AN compared to healthy controls [186, 187, 191]. As a result of hypogonadism and emaciation [192] individuals with AN experience decreased sexual interest; once weight is restored, libido tends to increase [193]. Low libido, commonly observed in AN, is linked to both low concentrations of circulating sex hormones and psychological factors, such as body dissatisfaction and depleted self-esteem [183]. Zemishlany and Weizman [9] highlight that patients with AN suffer from low sexual interest, inhibited sexual behavior, sexual disgust, and intimacy fears. The authors [9] observe a pattern of normal or advanced sexual development in adolescence prior to the manifestation of AN, and a significant decline in sexual interest and need for intimacy during AN. Non acceptance of their sexuality, low sexual desire, sexual aversion, and anorgasmia likely continue post AN recovery [9]. Moreover, sexual dysfunction may ensue due to the physiological effects of starvation seen in AN and/or development of depressive symptoms [191] and fertility problems [183].

A few studies demonstrate AN subtype differences in sexuality, with decreased sexual drive [187, 194] and limited sexual fantasy [192] among restricting anorectics compared to purging anorectics. Also, purging anorectics have higher rates of multiple sexual partners than restricting subtype anorectics [187]. Further, Castellini et al. [187] suggest that varying levels of sexual dysfunction correspond with pathological eating behavior, as restricting anorectics report lower arousal, lubrication, orgasm, satisfaction, and more pain, compared to purging type AN and BN.

Bulimia Nervosa

The essential features of bulimia nervosa (BN) include recurrent episodes of uncontrollable binge eating and repeated inappropriate compensatory behaviors to prevent weight gain (purging), accompanied by self-evaluation that is disproportionately driven by body shape and weight [14]. Notably, a subset of individuals with BN continue to engage in binge eating, but discontinue purging behaviors—resulting in a change in diagnosis to BED or other category [14, 182].

Sexual dysfunction in BN is correlated with impulsive behaviors, including excessive drinking, sexual disinhibition, bullying, truancy, and binge/purge practices [183]. Indeed, individuals with EDs who have low self-control and emotional dysregulation reported increased impulsive and chaotic sexual functioning [194]. Similarly to results for binge/purging subtype anorectics, individuals with BN also had higher rates of multiple sexual partners compared to restricting anorectics [187]. Further, individuals with BN display increased risk for induced abortion compared to controls [183]. Gonidakis and colleagues [191] indicate that sexual functioning in BN is associated with level of depression.

Binge Eating Disorder

The novel inclusion of binge eating disorder (BED) in DSM-5 allows for the diagnosis of recurrent episodes of uncontrollable binge eating, causing marked distress, without engagement in any repeated inappropriate compensatory behavior [14, 182]. Individuals with BED commonly experience social role adjustment issues, reduced health-related quality of life, increased healthcare utilization, and poor life satisfaction, along with higher morbidity and mortality compared to BMI-matched controls [14].

Provided that BED is a relatively new diagnosis, the research on BED is often grouped with findings on obesity, with expectations of similar sexual functioning impairments [183, 185]. Individuals with BED are at elevated risk for weight gain and developing obesity, which has been demonstrated to have multiple effects on sexual functioning [195]. The role of weight or perception of body shape and size may be critical in sexual functioning for individuals with BED, as BMI modification has been hypothesized to affect sexual dysfunction within individuals with BED [183]. In the same vein, research shows that post-bariatric surgery weight loss was associated with significantly improved hormonal profiles and sexual functioning in both males [196] and females [197]. Notably, diagnosis of BED is correlated with higher risk of miscarriage [183].

Substance-Related and Addictive Disorders

The substance-related disorders are characterized by excessive use of drugs that enhance the brain reward system, for example, alcohol, caffeine, cannabis, hallucinogens, or opioids [14]. Additionally, gambling disorder shares similar behavioral patterns and underlying mechanism, and is included in this disorder category.

The relationship between substance abuse and sexual functioning appears to be bidirectional—sexual dysfunctions may arise as a consequence of substance dependence and may also be the reason for substance use [198, 199]. Despite having different physiological effects, many addictive substances such as alcohol [200], ecstasy [201], amphetamines [202], or nicotine [203] seem to increase subjective sexual arousal. However, long term use and development of substance dependence disorder leads to lower sexual functioning [203]. Domains of sexual functioning that are most commonly affected through substance addiction are erectile dysfunction, orgasm impairments, and painful sex, while desire seems less commonly implicated [204]. Patients with dependent on opioids [205, 206] nicotine [203], amphetamines [202], cocaine [207], and alcohol [207, 208] have a higher prevalence of sexual dysfunctions. Importantly, it has been shown that sexual dysfunctions in men may be present even after a year of abstinence from the addictive substance [209].

Substance abuse is positively correlated with risky sexual behaviors. People with alcohol dependence are less likely to delay intercourse in order to find a condom [210], thus increasing risk of contracting STIs and HIV. Ecstasy users are also more likely to have unprotected sex with multiple partners [211, 212]. Cocaine [213, 214] and amphetamine [215] abuse is likewise related to higher risk of HIV and other STD infections.

There is limited research on sexual functioning and pathological gambling. However, given evidence of overall lower quality of life in this population [216], patients should be assessed for sexual dysfunctions and inquired about sexual risky behaviors.

Neurocognitive Disorders

The neurocognitive disorders (NCDs) comprise a large group of disorders characterized primarily by mild to major cognitive deficits. They are often of known etiology, such as NCD with Lewy bodies, frontotemporal NCD, NCD due to Alzheimer's disease or NCD due to Parkinson's disease.

Sexual dysfunctions such as decreased libido, erectile dysfunction, difficulty reaching orgasm, and sexual dissatisfaction are common among people with dementias [217, 218]. Despite their marginalization as sexual beings, these patients do maintain intimate relationships [219], with about 70% of Alzheimer's disease patients initiating intimate activities such as kissing, hugging or intercourse [220]. It is noted, however, that sexuality that does not include intercourse is often preferred [219, 220] and sexual satisfaction in married couples affected by the disease is significantly lower [221]. Patients with frontotemporal dementia may exhibit more prominent hyposexual symptoms in comparison to those with Alzheimer's disease or semantic dementia [222]. The pathophysiological causes of sexual dysfunctions are multifactorial; pain, sensory loss, motor impairments, autonomic dysfunctions, and cognitive deficits themselves are cited as contributing factors [217].

Hypersexuality alone or with inappropriate sexual behavior (ISB) is estimated to be present in 2.9–8% of patients living at home and in 3.8–7% of patients in institutions [223]. Such behaviors are generally considered a result of global disinhibition rather than a separate neuropsychiatric symptom [224]. Damage to the frontal and temporal lobes, as well as the medial striatum of the basal ganglia, are commonly involved is producing hypersexuality or ISB, as seen in Alzheimer's disease, frontotemporal dementia, and Huntington disease [219, 225]. Symptoms of both hypo- and hyper-sexuality are documented in patients with Parkinson's disease [226, 227]. Hypersexuality and ISB have been mostly reported through case studies and there is no consensus on successful clinical management, although a variety of pharmacological and non-pharmacological treatments may help in symptom reduction [228].

Personality Disorders

Personality disorders (PDs) are characterized by a pattern of enduring, inflexible, and pervasive inner experience and behavior that is culturally incongruent and stable over time, with an onset in adolescence or early adulthood, that result in distress and impairment [14]. These patterns are grouped into clusters based on descriptive similarities. Cluster A PDs refer to paranoid, schizoid, and schizotypal PDs; individuals with these disorders usually appear odd or eccentric [14]. Cluster B PDs include antisocial, borderline, histrionic, and narcissistic PDs, who often present as dramatic, emotional, or erratic [14]. Cluster C PDs are comprised of avoidant, dependent, and obsessive-compulsive PDs; individuals with these disorders often appearing anxious or fearful [14]. In spite of the pervasive impact of PDs on interpersonal impairment, very little research addresses the influence on sexual functioning, much less so on male sexuality or cultural diversity.

Cluster A: Social avoidance and isolation in Schizoid and Schizotypal Personality Disorders is common, leading to limited interpersonal relationships and lack of sexual experience [229].

Cluster B: Women with histrionic personality disorder have decreased sexual assertiveness, sexual drive, and self-esteem, as well as increased sexual preoccupation, sexual boredom, negative response to sexual cues, and orgasmic dysfunction, yet report higher sexual esteem [230]. They also report more marital dissatisfaction and extramarital affairs compared to their partners [230]. Narcissistic personality disorder is associated with exhibitionism and voyeurism [231] unrestricted sexual attitudes and behavior and hence, low relationship commitment [232]. Individuals with antisocial personality disorder (ASPD) tend to be irresponsible and exploitative in their sexual relationships, lacking remorse and distress due to the ego-syntonic nature of the pathology [14] ASPD in both men and women is also linked to CSA, physical trauma, and crime-related trauma [233–235] as well as with high instances of risky sexual behavior, contraction of sexual diseases [98] and sex offending [234, 236, 237]. The lack of empathy and exploitative nature that accompanies ASPD may overlap with some sadistic sexual behavior and paraphilic disorders [236, 238].

The majority of the extant literature focuses on borderline personality disorder (BPD), characterized by intense abandonment fears and unstable interpersonal relationships [14]. Patients with BPD have significantly more sexual relationship difficulties than other PDs patients (61% versus 19%) [239], attesting to the important role of interpersonal problems in this population [9, 240, 241]. Patients with BPD indicate that consenting sex as well as avoiding sex can trigger BPD symptoms, such as dissociation, suicidality, and self-harm, which dissipate markedly over time [239].

Notably, childhood abuse and neglect are significant predictors of BPD [240]. Zanarini et al. [239] suggest that patients with BPD with histories of CSA and rape in adulthood show greater patterns of sexual dysfunction, and predisposition to sexual avoidance due to fears of triggering BPD symptoms, being re-traumatized, or both. Furthermore, Mangassarian et al. [241] maintain that women with BPD are at elevated risk for engaging in sexually impulsive high-risk behaviors, exposing them to HIV/AIDS and other chronic medical conditions [242]. Women with BPD are hypothesized to engage in sexual impulsivity as maladaptive attempts to cope with chronic feelings of emptiness and fears of abandonment (BPD symptoms) [241]. Additionally, individuals with BPD report higher instances of being coerced into sexual encounters, rape, as well as younger age at sexual exposure [242]. In exploring the sexuality of women with BPD, Hurlbert et al. [243] found significantly higher sexual assertiveness, sexual esteem, and increased positive response to sexual cues. However, women with BPD also display significantly higher sexual preoccupation, sexual depression, and sexual dissatisfaction [244]. In this way, sexuality within individuals with BPD can be conceptualized as oscillating between impulsivity and victimization [242].

Cluster C: The development of avoidant personality disorder is also related to CSA, leading to intimacy avoidance, and ensuing interpersonal problems [244]. Moreover, individuals with dependent personality disorder tend to have greater emotional and/or economic dependency that lead to disruptive interactions with others, increased risk of male and female-perpetrated intimate partner violence and difficulty leaving victimizing relationships [245], causing detrimental consequences for the individual, close others, and greater society [246]. Additionally, Cain and colleagues [247] indicate that individuals with obsessive-compulsive personality disorder (OCPD) report lower empathic perspective taking, high interpersonal distress, sensitivity to interpersonally warm behavior by others, and controlling and hostile interpersonal patterns, compared to healthy controls.

Conclusion

Sexual functioning is an important quality of life factor that is often compromised in individuals living with chronic psychiatric illness. Given the biopsychosocial nature of both sexuality and mental disorders, these two domains are closely correlated with each other and are often influenced by one's sociodemographic, cultural, familial, and uniquely psychological characteristics. Global assessment of a patient's functioning in multiple life domains is thus recommended for providing better reproductive, psychiatric, and psychological care (Figure 32-2). Overall, the implications for integrating sexual health into both medical and mental health care practices are supported by the findings of the extant literature.

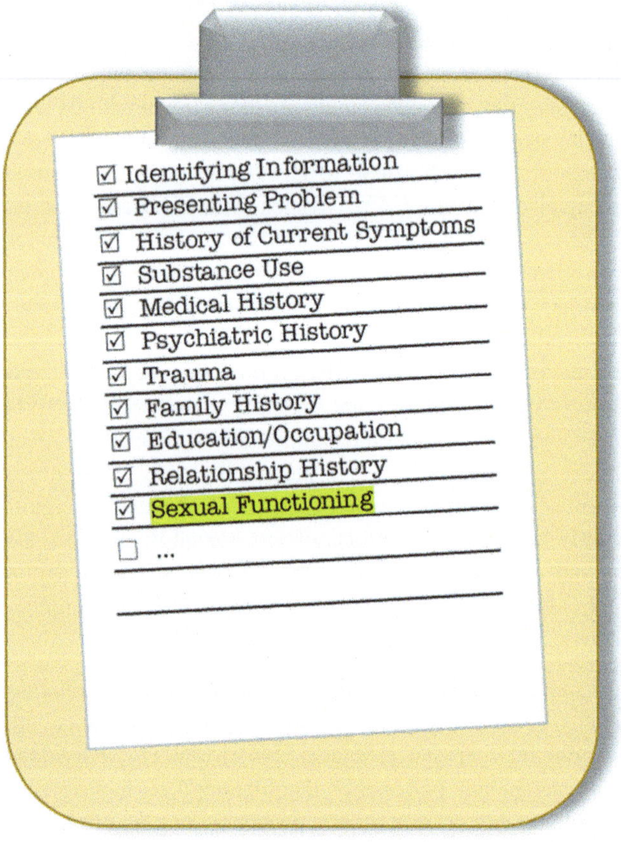

FIGURE 32-2. Sexual functioning should be an integral component of a comprehensive psychological and medical assessment [Courtesy of Anna Klimowicz, Adriana Janicic, and Waguih William IsHak].

It should be noted that the research represented in this chapter reflects the available literature on sexual functioning and psychiatric disorders, which was not found to be diverse in terms of age, sex, or ethnicity and did not account for variations in cultural beliefs, practices, or healing surrounding sexuality. Additionally, psychiatric and medical comorbidities may further complicate real life clinical practice and cause exacerbation of sexual symptoms. Direct inquiry into the patient's sexual well-being is always recommended for patients presenting with any psychiatric symptoms and vice versa.

References

1. Hedden SL (Ed). Behavioral health trends in the United States: results from the 2014. Natl Surv Drug Use Health. 2015;15:4927.
2. IsHak WW, Greenberg JM, Balayan K, Kapitanski N, Jeffrey J, Fathy H, Fakhry H, Rapaport MH. Quality of life: the ultimate outcome measure of interventions in major depressive disorder. Harv Rev Psychiatry. 2011;19(5):229–39.
3. IsHak WW, Brown K, Aye SS, Kahloon M, Mobaraki S, Hanna R. Health-related quality of life in bipolar disorder. Bipolar Disord. 2012;14(1):6–18.
4. Davidoff J, Christensen S, Khalili DN, Nguyen J, IsHak WW. Quality of life in panic disorder: looking beyond symptom remission. Qual Life Res. 2012;21(6):945–59.
5. Macy AS, Theo JN, Kaufmann SC, Ghazzaoui RB, Pawlowski PA, Fakhry HI, Cassmassi BJ, IsHak WW. Quality of life in obsessive compulsive disorder. CNS Spectr. 2013;18(01):21–33.
6. Laumann EO, Paik A, Rosen RC. Sexual dysfunction in the United States: prevalence and predictors. JAMA. 1999;281(6):537–44.
7. Östman M. Low satisfaction with sex life among people with severe mental illness living in a community. Psychiatry Res. 2014;216(3):340–5.
8. Nnaji RN, Friedman T. Sexual dysfunction and schizophrenia: psychiatrists' attitudes and training needs. Psychiatrist. 2008;32(6):208–10.
9. Zemishlany Z, Weizman A. The impact of mental illness on sexual dysfunction. Sex Dysfunct. 2008;29:89–106.
10. Wright ER, Wright DE, Perry BL, Foote-Ardah CE. Stigma and the sexual isolation of people with serious mental illness. Soc Probl. 2007;54(1):78–98.
11. Link BG, Struening EL, Neese-Todd S, Asmussen S, Phelan JC. Stigma as a barrier to recovery: the consequences of stigma for the self-esteem of people with mental illnesses. Psychiatr Serv. 2001;52(12):1621–6.
12. Wainberg ML, González MA, McKinnon K, Elkington KS, Pinto D, Mann CG, Mattos PE. Targeted ethnography as a critical step to inform cultural adaptations of HIV prevention interventions for adults with severe mental illness. Soc Sci Med. 2007;65(2):296–308.
13. Boucher ME, Groleau D, Whitley R. Recovery and severe mental illness: the role of romantic relationships, intimacy, and sexuality. Psychiatr Rehabil J. 2016;39(2):180.
14. American Psychiatric Association. DSM 5; 2013.
15. McCabe MP, Schreck A. Before sex education: an evaluation of the sexual knowledge, experience, feelings and needs of people with mild intellectual disabilities. Aust N Zeal J Dev Disabil. 1992;18(2):75–82.
16. Reiter S, Bryen DN, Shachar I. Adolescents with intellectual disabilities as victims of abuse. J Intellect Disabil. 2007;11(4):371–87.

17. McCarthy M, Thompson D. A prevalence study of sexual abuse of adults with intellectual disabilities referred for sex education. J Appl Res Intellect Disabil. 1997;10(2):105–24.
18. Murphy GH, O'Callaghan AL. Capacity of adults with intellectual disabilities to consent to sexual relationships. Psychol Med. 2004;34(07):1347–57.
19. Isler A, Tas F, Beytut D, Conk Z. Sexuality in adolescents with intellectual disabilities. Sex Disabil. 2009;27(1):27–34.
20. Rushbrooke E, Murray CD, Townsend S. What difficulties are experienced by caregivers in relation to the sexuality of people with intellectual disabilities? A qualitative meta-synthesis. Res Dev Disabil. 2014;35(4):871–86.
21. Meaney-Tavares R, Gavidia-Payne S. Staff characteristics and attitudes towards the sexuality of people with intellectual disability. J Intellect Dev Disabil. 2012;37(3):269–73.
22. Fitzgerald C, Withers P. 'I don't know what a proper woman means': what women with intellectual disabilities think about sex, sexuality and themselves. Br J Learn Disabil. 2013;41(1):5–12.
23. Bernert DJ, Ogletree RJ. Women with intellectual disabilities talk about their perceptions of sex. J Intellect Disabil Res. 2013;57(3):240–9.
24. Burns J. Gender identity and women with learning difficulties: the third sex. Clin Psychol Forum. 2000;137:137–9.
25. Wilkinson VJ, Theodore K, Raczka R. 'As normal as possible': sexual identity development in people with intellectual disabilities transitioning to adulthood. Sex Disabil. 2015;33(1):93–105.
26. Rushbrooke E, Murray C, Townsend S. The experiences of intimate relationships by people with intellectual disabilities: a qualitative study. J Appl Res Intellect Disabil. 2014;27(6):531–41.
27. Christensen DL. Prevalence and characteristics of autism spectrum disorder among children aged 8 years—autism and developmental disabilities monitoring network, 11 sites, United States, 2012. MMWR Surveill Summ. 2016;65.
28. Kamio Y, Inada N, Koyama T. A nationwide survey on quality of life and associated factors of adults with high-functioning autism spectrum disorders. Autism. 2013;17(1):15–26.
29. de Vries M, Geurts H. Influence of autism traits and executive functioning on quality of life in children with an autism spectrum disorder. J Autism Dev Disord. 2015;45(9):2734–43.
30. Strunz S, Schermuck C, Ballerstein S, Ahlers CJ, Dziobek I, Roepke S. Romantic relationships and relationship satisfaction among adults with asperger syndrome and high-functioning autism. J Clin Psychol. 2016. doi:10.1002/jclp.22319.
31. Hellemans H, Colson K, Verbraeken C, Vermeiren R, Deboutte D. Sexual behavior in high-functioning male adolescents and young adults with autism spectrum disorder. J Autism Dev Disord. 2007;37(2):260–9.
32. Fernandes LC, Gillberg CI, Cederlund M, Hagberg B, Gillberg C, Billstedt E. Aspects of sexuality in adolescents and adults diagnosed with autism spectrum disorders in childhood. J Autism Dev Disord. 2016;46(9):3155–65.
33. Howlin P, Mawhood L, Rutter M. Autism and developmental receptive language disorder—a follow-up comparison in early adult life. II: social, behavioural, and psychiatric outcomes. J Child Psychol Psychiatry. 2000;41(05):561–78.
34. Mehzabin P, Stokes MA. Self-assessed sexuality in young adults with high-functioning autism. Res Autism Spectr Disord. 2011;5(1):614–21.
35. Byers ES, Nichols S, Voyer SD. Challenging stereotypes: sexual functioning of single adults with high functioning autism spectrum disorder. J Autism Dev Disord. 2013;43(11):2617–27.
36. Byers ES, Nichols S. Sexual satisfaction of high-functioning adults with autism spectrum disorder. Sex Disabil. 2014;32(3):365–82.
37. Byers ES, Nichols S, Voyer SD, Reilly G. Sexual well-being of a community sample of high-functioning adults on the autism spectrum who have been in a romantic relationship. Autism. 2013;17(4):418–33.
38. Hellemans H, Roeyers H, Leplae W, Dewaele T, Deboutte D. Sexual behavior in male adolescents and young adults with autism spectrum disorder and borderline/mild mental retardation. Sex Disabil. 2010;28(2):93–104.
39. Rokeach A, Wiener J. The romantic relationships of adolescents with ADHD. J Atten Disord. 2014;pii:1087054714538660.
40. Flory K, Molina BS, Pelham Jr WE, Gnagy E, Smith B. Childhood ADHD predicts risky sexual behavior in young adulthood. J Clin Child Adolesc Psychol. 2006;35(4):571–7.
41. Brown LK, Hadley W, Stewart A, Lescano C, Whiteley L, Donenberg G, DiClemente R. Psychiatric disorders and sexual risk among adolescents in mental health treatment. J Consult Clin Psychol. 2010;78(4):590.
42. Barkley RA, Fischer M, Smallish L, Fletcher K. Young adult outcome of hyperactive children: adaptive functioning in major life activities. J Am Acad Child Adolesc Psychiatry. 2006;45(2): 192–202.
43. Canu WH, Carlson GL. Differences in heterosocial behavior and outcomes of ADHD-symptomatic subtypes in a college sample. J Atten Disord. 2003;6(3):123–33.
44. Sarver DE, McCart MR, Sheidow AJ, Letourneau EJ. ADHD and risky sexual behavior in adolescents: conduct problems and substance use as mediators of risk. J Child Psychol Psychiatry. 2014;55(12):1345–53.
45. Wymbs BT, Molina B, Pelham W, Cheong J, Gnagy E, Belendiuk K, Walther C, Babinski D, Waschbusch D. Risk of intimate partner violence among young adult males with childhood ADHD. J Atten Disord. 2011;1087054710389987.
46. Bruner MR, Kuryluk AD, Whitton SW. Attention-deficit/hyperactivity disorder symptom levels and romantic relationship quality in college students. J Am Coll Health. 2015;63(2):98–108.
47. Marsh LE, Norvilitis JM, Ingersoll TS, Li B. ADHD symptomatology, fear of intimacy, and sexual anxiety and behavior among college students in China and the United States. J Atten Disord. 2012;pii:1087054712453483.
48. Cavanna AE, Servo S, Monaco F, Robertson MM. The behavioral spectrum of Gilles de la Tourette syndrome. J Neuropsychiatry Clin Neurosci. 2009;21(1):13–23.
49. Robertson MM. Tourette syndrome, associated conditions and the complexities of treatment. Brain. 2000;123(3):425–62.
50. Sandyk R. Naltrexone suppresses abnormal sexual behavior in Tourette's syndrome. Int J Neurosci. 1988;43(1-2):107–10.
51. McDougle CJ, Southwick SM, Rohrbaugh RM. Tourette's disorder and associated complex behaviors: a case report. Yale J Biol Med. 1990;63(3):209.
52. Eack SM, Newhill CE. Psychiatric symptoms and quality of life in schizophrenia: a meta-analysis. Schizophr Bull. 2007;33(5): 1225–37.
53. Maat A, Fett AK, Derks E. Group Investigators. Social cognition and quality of life in schizophrenia. Schizophr Res. 2012; 137(1):212–8.
54. Karow A, Bullinger M, Lambert M. Quality of life as an outcome and a mediator of other outcomes in patients with Schizophrenia. In: Awad A, Voruganti G, Lakshmi NP, editors. Beyond assessment of quality of life in Schizophrenia. New York, NY: Springer; 2016. p. 123–44.
55. Bobes J, Garcia-Portilla MP, Bascaran MT, Saiz PA, Bousono M. Quality of life in schizophrenic patients. Dialogues Clin Neurosci. 2007;9(2):215.
56. Park SG, Bennett ME, Couture SM, Blanchard JJ. Internalized stigma in schizophrenia: relations with dysfunctional attitudes, symptoms, and quality of life. Psychiatry Res. 2013;205(1):43–7.
57. Temilola MJ, Adegoke AO, Olaolu AT, Adegboyega O, Olaide AK. Self-stigma, quality of life and schizophrenia: an outpatient

clinic survey in Nigeria. Int J Soc Psychiatry. 2013; 0020764013491738.
58. Fan X, Henderson DC, Chiang E, Briggs LB, Freudenreich O, Evins AE, Cather C, Goff DC. Sexual functioning, psychopathology and quality of life in patients with schizophrenia. Schizophr Res. 2007;94(1):119–27.
59. Baggaley M. Sexual dysfunction in schizophrenia: focus on recent evidence. Hum Psychopharmacol Clin Exp. 2008;23(3):201–9.
60. Dossenbach M, Hodge A, Anders M, Molnár B, Peciukaitiene D, Krupka-Matuszczyk I, Tatu M, Bondar V, Pecenak J, Gorjanc T, McBride M. Prevalence of sexual dysfunction in patients with schizophrenia: international variation and underestimation. Int J Neuropsychopharmacol. 2005;8(2):195–201.
61. Olfson M, Uttaro T, Carson WH, Tafesse E. Male sexual dysfunction and quality of life in schizophrenia. J Clin Psychiatry. 2005;66(3):331–8.
62. Stephens DM. Sexual behavior and quality of life in persons with schizophrenia in an outpatient population (Doctoral dissertation, Fielding Graduate University).
63. Macdonald S, Halliday J, MacEwan T, Sharkey V, Farrington S, Wall S, McCreadie RG. Nithsdale schizophrenia surveys 24: sexual dysfunction. Br J Psychiatry. 2003;182(1):50–6.
64. Kelly DL, Conley RR. Sexuality and schizophrenia: a review. Schizophr Bull. 2004;30(4):767–79.
65. Malik P, Kemmler G, Hummer M, Riecher-Roessler A, Kahn RS, Fleischhacker WW, EUFEST Study Group. Sexual dysfunction in first-episode schizophrenia patients: results from European First Episode Schizophrenia Trial. J Clin Psychopharmacol. 2011;31(3):274–80.
66. La Torre A, Conca A, Duffy D, Giupponi G, Pompili M, Grözinger M. Sexual dysfunction related to psychotropic drugs: a critical review part II: antipsychotics. Pharmacopsychiatry. 2013;46(06): 201–8.
67. Chiesa A, Leucci V, Serretti A, De Ronchi D. Antipsychotics and sexual dysfunction: epidemiology, mechanisms and management. Clin Neuropsychol. 2013;10(1):31–6.
68. Aizenberg D, Zemishlany Z, Dorfman-Etrog P, Weizman A. Sexual dysfunction in male schizophrenic patients. J Clin Psychiatry. 1995;56(4):137–41.
69. Huber TJ, Rollnik J, Wilhelms J, Von Zur MA, Emrich HM, Schneider U. Estradiol levels in psychotic disorders. Psychoneuroendocrinology. 2001;26(1):27–35.
70. Huber TJ, Borsutzky M, Schneider U, Emrich HM. Psychotic disorders and gonadal function: evidence supporting the oestrogen hypothesis. Acta Psychiatr Scand. 2004;109(4):269–74.
71. Ozcan DD, Banoglu R. Gonadal hormones in schizophrenia and mood disorders. Eur Arch Psychiatry Clin Neurosci. 2003;253(4):193–6.
72. Huber TJ, Tettenborn C, Leifke E, Emrich HM. Sex hormones in psychotic men. Psychoneuroendocrinology. 2005;30(1):111–4.
73. de Boer MK, Castelein S, Wiersma D, Schoevers RA, Knegtering H. The facts about sexual (dys) function in schizophrenia: an overview of clinically relevant findings. Schizophr Bull. 2015;41(3):674–86.
74. Östman M, Björkman AC. Schizophrenia and relationships: the effect of mental illness on sexuality. Clin Schizophr Relat Psychoses. 2013;7(1):20–4.
75. Redmond C, Larkin M, Harrop C. The personal meaning of romantic relationships for young people with psychosis. Clin Child Psychol Psychiatry. 2010;15(2):151–70.
76. Downey J, Friedman RC, Haase E, Goldenberg D, Bell R, Edsall S. Comparison of sexual experience and behavior between bipolar outpatients and outpatients without mood disorders. Psychiatry J. 2016;2016.
77. Kopeykina I, Kim HJ, Khatun T, Boland J, Haeri S, Cohen LJ, Galynker II. Hypersexuality and couple relationships in bipolar disorder: a review. J Affect Disord. 2016;195:1–4.
78. Fletcher K, Parker G, Paterson A, Synnott H. High-risk behaviour in hypomanic states. J Affect Disord. 2013;150(1):50–6.
79. Akiskal HS. Searching for behavioral indicators of bipolar II in patients presenting with major depressive episodes: the "red sign," the "rule of three" and other biographic signs of temperamental extravagance, activation and hypomania. J Affect Disord. 2005;84(2):279–90.
80. Hariri AG, Karadag F, Gokalp P, Essizoglu A. Risky sexual behavior among patients in Turkey with bipolar disorder, schizophrenia, and heroin addiction. J Sex Med. 2011;8(8):2284–91.
81. Marengo E, Martino DJ, Igoa A, Fassi G, Scápola M, Baamonde MU, Strejilevich SA. Sexual risk behaviors among women with bipolar disorder. Psychiatry Res. 2015;230(3):835–8.
82. Coverdale JH, Turbott SH. Risk behaviors for sexually transmitted infections among men with mental disorders. Psychiatr Serv. 2000;51(2):234–8.
83. Carey MP, Carey KB, Maisto SA, Schroder KE, Vanable PA, Gordon CM. HIV risk behavior among psychiatric outpatients: association with psychiatric disorder, substance use disorder, and gender. J Nerv Ment Dis. 2004;192(4):289.
84. Heffner JL, DelBello MP, Fleck DE, Adler CM, Strakowski SM. Unplanned pregnancies in adolescents with bipolar disorder. Am J Psychiatry. 2012;169(12):1319.
85. Freeman MP, Gelenberg AJ. Bipolar disorder in women: reproductive events and treatment considerations. Acta Psychiatr Scand. 2005;112(2):88–96.
86. Battle CL, Weinstock LM, Howard M. Clinical correlates of perinatal bipolar disorder in an interdisciplinary obstetrical hospital setting. J Affect Disord. 2014;158:97–100.
87. Khan SJ, Fersh ME, Ernst C, Klipstein K, Albertini ES, Lusskin SI. Bipolar disorder in pregnancy and postpartum: principles of management. Curr Psychiatry Rep. 2016;18(2):1–1.
88. Doyle K, Heron J, Berrisford G, Whitmore J, Jones L, Wainscott G, Oyebode F. The management of bipolar disorder in the perinatal period and risk factors for postpartum relapse. Eur Psychiatry. 2012;27(8):563–9.
89. Dvorak RD, Wray TB, Kuvaas NJ, Kilwein TM. Mania and sexual risk: associations with behavioral self-regulation. J Affect Disord. 2013;150(3):1076–81.
90. Craney JL, Geller B. A prepubertal and early adolescent bipolar disorder-I phenotype: review of phenomenology and longitudinal course. Bipolar Disord. 2003;5(4):243–56.
91. Geller B, Zimerman B, Williams M, DelBello MP, Frazier J, Beringer L. Phenomenology of prepubertal and early adolescent bipolar disorder: examples of elated mood, grandiose behaviors, decreased need for sleep, racing thoughts and hypersexuality. J Child Adolesc Psychopharmacol. 2002;12(1):3–9.
92. Adelson S. Psychodynamics of hypersexuality in children and adolescents with bipolar disorder. Psychodyn Psychiatry. 2010;38(1):27.
93. Basco MR, Celis-de Hoyos CE. Biopsychosocial model of hypersexuality in adolescent girls with bipolar disorder: strategies for intervention. J Child Adolesc Psychiatr Nurs. 2012;25(1):42–50.
94. Kendurkar A, Kaur B. Major depressive disorder, obsessive-compulsive disorder, and generalized anxiety disorder: do the sexual dysfunctions differ. Prim Care Companion J Clin Psychiatry. 2008;10(4):299–305.
95. Munir A, Muhsin H. Difference between anxiety and depression with respect to marital adjustment and sexual functioning. World Appl Sci J. 2013;28(12):2147–51.
96. Laurent SM, Simons AD. Sexual dysfunction in depression and anxiety: conceptualizing sexual dysfunction as part of an internalizing dimension. Clin Psychol Rev. 2009;29(7):573–85.
97. Thakurta RG, Singh OP, Bhattacharya A, Mallick AK, Ray P, Sen S, Das R. Nature of sexual dysfunctions in major depressive disorder and its impact on quality of life. Indian J Psychol Med. 2012;34(4):365.

98. Ramrakha S, Caspi A, Dickson N, Moffitt TE, Paul C. Psychiatric disorders and risky sexual behaviour in young adulthood: cross sectional study in birth cohort. BMJ. 2000;321(7256):263–6.
99. Dunn KM, Croft PR, Hackett GI. Association of sexual problems with social, psychological, and physical problems in men and women: a cross sectional population survey. J Epidemiol Community Health. 1999;53(3):144–8.
100. Cyranowski JM, Bromberger J, Youk A, Matthews K, Kravitz HM, Powell LH. Lifetime depression history and sexual function in women at midlife. Arch Sex Behav. 2004;33(6):539–48.
101. Laumann EO, Paik A, Glasser DB, Kang JH, Wang T, Levinson B, Moreira Jr ED, Nicolosi A, Gingell C. A cross-national study of subjective sexual well-being among older women and men: findings from the Global Study of Sexual Attitudes and Behaviors. Arch Sex Behav. 2006;35(2):143–59.
102. Kennedy SH, Dickens SE, Eisfeld BS, Bagby RM. Sexual dysfunction before antidepressant therapy in major depression. J Affect Disord. 1999;56(2):201–8.
103. Palace EM, Gorzalka BB. The enhancing effects of anxiety on arousal in sexually dysfunctional and functional women. J Abnorm Psychol. 1990;99(4):403.
104. Bradford A, Meston CM. The impact of anxiety on sexual arousal in women. Behav Res Ther. 2006;44(8):1067–77.
105. Dèttore D, Pucciarelli M, Santarnecchi E. Anxiety and female sexual functioning: an empirical study. J Sex Marital Ther. 2013;39(3):216–40.
106. Van Minnen A, Kampman M. The interaction between anxiety and sexual functioning: a controlled study of sexual functioning in women with anxiety disorders. Sex Relation Ther. 2000;15(1):47–57.
107. Aksoy UM, Aksoy ŞG, Maner F, Gokalp P, Yanik M. Sexual dysfunction in obsessive compulsive disorder and panic disorder. Psychiatr Danub. 2012;24(4):381–5.
108. Rajkumar RP, Kumaran AK. Depression and anxiety in men with sexual dysfunction: a retrospective study. Compr Psychiatry. 2015;60:114–8.
109. Figueira I, Possidente E, Marques C, Hayes K. Sexual dysfunction: a neglected complication of panic disorder and social phobia. Arch Sex Behav. 2001;30(4):369–77.
110. Mercan S, Karamustafalioglu O, Ayaydin EB, Akpinar A, Goksan B, Gonenli S, Guven T. Sexual dysfunction in female patients with panic disorder alone or with accompanying depression. Int J Psychiatry Clin Pract. 2006;10(4):235–40.
111. Sbrocco T, Weisberg RB, Barlow DH, Carter MM. The conceptual relationship between panic disorder and male erectile dysfunction. J Sex Marital Ther. 1997;23(3):212–20.
112. Bodinger L, Hermesh H, Aizenberg D, Valevski A, Marom S, Shiloh R, Gothelf D, Weizman A. Sexual function and behavior in social phobia. J Clin Psychiatry. 2002;63(10):874–9.
113. Mourikis I, Antoniou M, Matsouka E, Vousoura E, Tzavara C, Ekizoglou C, Papadimitriou GN, Vaidakis N, Zervas IM. Anxiety and depression among Greek men with primary erectile dysfunction and premature ejaculation. Ann Gen Psychiatry. 2015;14(1):1.
114. Corretti G, Pierucci S, De Scisciolo M, Nisita C. Comorbidity between social phobia and premature ejaculation: study on 242 males affected by sexual disorders. J Sex Marital Ther. 2006;32(2):183–7.
115. Real E, Montejo Á, Alonso P, Manuel MJ. Sexuality and obsessive-compulsive disorder: the hidden affair. Neuropsychiatry. 2013;3(1):23–31.
116. Vulink NC, Denys D, Bus L, Westenberg HG. Sexual pleasure in women with obsessive–compulsive disorder? J Affect Disord. 2006;91(1):19–25.
117. Thakurta RG, Dhar OP, Sarkar S, Ray P, Mallick AK. Prevalence and nature of sexual dysfunctions in OCD in a tertiary medical college. East J Psychiatry. 2016;17(2):20–30.
118. Newth S, Rachman S. The concealment of obsessions. Behav Res Ther. 2001;39(4):457–64.
119. de Jong PJ, van Overveld M, Borg C. Giving in to arousal or staying stuck in disgust? Disgust-based mechanisms in sex and sexual dysfunction. J Sex Res. 2013;50(3-4):247–62.
120. Rachman S. Obsessions, responsibility and guilt. *Behav Res Ther.* 1993;31(2):149–54.
121. Wetterneck CT, Smith AH, Burgess AJ, et al. Distress from sexual thoughts; do religiosity, emotions, and thought appraisal matter? J Cogn Psychother. 2011;25(3):189–202.
122. Aksaray G, Yelken B, Kaptanoglu C, et al. Sexuality in women with obsessive compulsive disorder. J Sex Marital Ther. 2001;27(3):273–7.
123. Vella-Zarb RA, Cohen JN, McCabe RE, Rowa K. Differentiating sexual thoughts in obsessive-compulsive disorder from paraphilias and nonparaphilic sexual disorders. Cogn Behav Pract 2016. http://www.sciencedirect.com/science/article/pii/S1077722916300578. Accessed 23 Nov 2016.
124. Gordon WM. Sexual obsessions and OCD. Sex Relation Ther. 2002;17(4):343–54.
125. Ackard DM, Kearney-Cooke A, Peterson CB. Effect of body image and self-image on women's sexual behaviors. Int J Eat Disord. 2000;28(4):422–9.
126. Pujols Y, Meston CM, Seal BN. The association between sexual satisfaction and body image in women. J Sex Med. 2010;7(2pt2):905–16.
127. Koch PB, Mansfield PK, Thurau D, Carey M. "Feeling frumpy": the relationships between body image and sexual response changes in midlife women. J Sex Res. 2005;42(3):215–23.
128. L. Dove, Michael W. Wiederman N. Cognitive distraction and women's sexual functioning. J Sex Marital Ther 2000;26(1): 67-78.
129. Woertman L, van den Brink F. Body image and female sexual functioning and behavior: a review. J Sex Res. 2012;49(2-3): 184–211.
130. Crerand CE, Franklin ME, Sarwer DB. Body dysmorphic disorder and cosmetic surgery. Plast Reconstr Surg. 2006;118(7):167–80.
131. Gladfelter J, Murphy D. Breast augmentation motivations and satisfaction: a prospective study of more than 3,000 silicone implantations. Plast Surg Nurs. 2008;28(4):170–4.
132. Veale D, Eshkevari E, Ellison N, Costa A, Robinson D, Kavouni A, Cardozo L. Psychological characteristics and motivation of women seeking labiaplasty. Psychol Med. 2014;44(03):555–66.
133. Veale D, Naismith I, Eshkevari E, Ellison N, Costa A, Robinson D, Abeywickrama L, Kavouni A, Cardozo L. Psychosexual outcome after labiaplasty: a prospective case-comparison study. Int Urogynecol J. 2014;25(6):831–9.
134. Veale D, Miles S, Read J, Troglia A, Wylie K, Muir G. Sexual functioning and behavior of men with body dysmorphic disorder concerning penis size compared with men anxious about penis size and with controls: a cohort study. Sex Med. 2015;3(3):147–55.
135. Hartmann AS, Greenberg JL, Wilhelm S. The relationship between anorexia nervosa and body dysmorphic disorder. Clin Psychol Rev. 2013;33(5):675–85.
136. Higgins MK, Choukas-Bradley S, Crowder EE, Bardone-Cone AM. Examining moderators of the relation between body consciousness during sexual activity and disordered eating. Adv Eat Disord. 2016;4(1):31–46.
137. Kotler M, Cohen H, Aizenberg D, Matar M, Loewenthal U, Kaplan Z, Miodownik H, Zemishlany Z. Sexual dysfunction in male posttraumatic stress disorder patients. Psychother Psychosom. 2000;69(6):309–15.
138. Yehuda R, Lehrner A, Rosenbaum TY. PTSD and sexual dysfunction in men and women. J Sex Med. 2015;12(5):1107–19.
139. Letourneau EJ, Resnick HS, Kilpatrick DG, Saunders BE, Best CL. Comorbidity of sexual problems and posttraumatic stress disorder in female crime victims. Behav Ther. 1996; 27(3):321–36.

140. Seehuus M, Clifton J, Rellini AH. The role of family environment and multiple forms of childhood abuse in the shaping of sexual function and satisfaction in women. Arch Sex Behav. 2015;44(6):1595–608.
141. Noll JG, Trickett PK, Putnam FW. A prospective investigation of the impact of childhood sexual abuse on the development of sexuality. J Consult Clin Psychol. 2003;71(3):575.
142. Schaaf KK, McCanne TR. Relationship of childhood sexual, physical, and combined sexual and physical abuse to adult victimization and posttraumatic stress disorder. Child Abuse Negl. 1998;22(11):1119–33.
143. Lalor K, McElvaney R. Child sexual abuse, links to later sexual exploitation/high-risk sexual behavior, and prevention/treatment programs. Trauma Violence Abuse. 2010;11(4):159–77.
144. Gerassi L. From exploitation to industry: definitions, risks, and consequences of domestic sexual exploitation and sex work among women and girls. J Hum Behav Soc Environ. 2015;25(6):591–605.
145. Zimmerman C, Hossain M, Watts C. Human trafficking and health: a conceptual model to inform policy, intervention and research. Soc Sci Med. 2011;73(2):327–35.
146. Willis BM, Levy BS. Child prostitution: global health burden, research needs, and interventions. Lancet. 2002;359(9315):1417–22.
147. Muftić LR, Finn MA. Health outcomes among women trafficked for sex in the United States: a closer look. J Interpers Violence. 2013;0886260512469102.
148. Monson CM, Taft CT, Fredman SJ. Military-related PTSD and intimate relationships: from description to theory-driven research and intervention development. Clin Psychol Rev. 2009;29(8):707–14.
149. Greenberg JH. Post-traumatic stress disorder and sexual intimacy. In: Ritchie EC, editor. Intimacy post-injury: combat trauma and sexual health. Oxford: Oxford University Press; 2016. p. 73.
150. Tran JK, Dunckel G, Teng EJ. Sexual dysfunction in veterans with post-traumatic stress disorder. J Sex Med. 2015;12(4):847–55.
151. Cosgrove DJ, Gordon Z, Bernie JE, Hami S, Montoya D, Stein MB, Monga M. Sexual dysfunction in combat veterans with post-traumatic stress disorder. Urology. 2002;60(5):881–4.
152. Joannides P. Guide to getting it on. Walport, OR: Goofy Foot Press; 2014.
153. Lehrner A, Flory JD, Bierer LM, Makotkine I, Marmar CR, Yehuda R. Sexual dysfunction and neuroendocrine correlates of posttraumatic stress disorder in combat veterans: preliminary findings. Psychoneuroendocrinology. 2016;63:271–5.
154. Vissia EM, Giesen ME, Chalavi S, Nijenhuis ER, Draijer N, Brand BL, Reinders AA. Is it trauma- or fantasy-based? Comparing dissociative identity disorder, post-traumatic stress disorder, simulators, and controls. Acta Psychiatr Scand. 2016;134(2):111–28.
155. Bozkurt H, Duzman Mutluer T, Kose C, Zoroglu S. High psychiatric comorbidity in adolescents with dissociative disorders. Psychiatry Clin Neurosci. 2015;69(6):369–74.
156. Sar V, Yargic LI, Tutkun H. Structured interview data on 35 cases of dissociative identity disorder in Turkey. Am J Psychiatry. 1996;153(10):1329.
157. Foote B, Smolin Y, Kaplan M, Legatt ME, Lipschitz D. Prevalence of dissociative disorders in psychiatric outpatients. Am J Psychiatry. 2006;163(4):623–9.
158. Mulder RT, Beautrais AL, Joyce PR, Fergusson DM. Relationship between dissociation, childhood sexual abuse, childhood physical abuse, and mental illness in a general population sample. Am J Psychiatry. 1998;155(6):806–11.
159. Wolf MR, Nochajski TH. Child sexual abuse survivors with dissociative amnesia: what's the difference? J Child Sex Abus. 2013;22(4):462–80.
160. Piper A, Merskey H. The persistence of folly: a critical examination of dissociative identity disorder. Part I. The excesses of an improbable concept. Can J Psychiatry. 2004;49(9):592–600.
161. Thompson A, Marwaha S, Nelson B, Wood SJ, McGorry PD, Yung AR, Lin A. Do affective or dissociative symptoms mediate the association between childhood sexual trauma and transition to psychosis in an ultra-high risk cohort? Psychiatry Res. 2016;236:182–5.
162. Lev-Wiesel R, Zohar G. The role of dissociation in self-injurious behavior among female adolescents who were sexually abused. J Child Sex Abus. 2014;23(7):824–39.
163. Sutherland MA, Fantasia HC, Adkison L. Sexual health and dissociative experiences among abused women. Issues Ment Health Nurs. 2014;35(1):41–9.
164. Webermann AR, Brand BL, Chasson GS. Childhood maltreatment and intimate partner violence in dissociative disorder patients. Eur J Psychotraumatol. 2014;5:10.3402/ejpt.v5.24568.
165. Bird ER, Seehuus M, Clifton J, Rellini AH. Dissociation during sex and sexual arousal in women with and without a history of childhood sexual abuse. Arch Sex Behav. 2014;43(5):953–64.
166. Hall JM. Dissociative experiences of women child abuse survivors a selective constructivist review. Trauma Violence Abuse. 2003;4(4):283–308.
167. Wood DP, Wiesner MG, Reiter RC. Psychogenic chronic pelvic pain: diagnosis and management. Clin Obstet Gynecol. 1990;33(1):179–95.
168. Fry RP, Crisp AH, Beard RW. Sociopsychological factors in chronic pelvic pain: a review. J Psychosom Res. 1997;42(1):1–5.
169. Fry RP, Crisp AH, Beard RW, McGuigan S. Psychosocial aspects of chronic pelvic pain, with special reference to sexual abuse. A study of 164 women. Postgrad Med J. 1993;69(813):566–74.
170. Nijenhuis ER, Van Dyck R, Ter Kuile MM, Mourits MJ, Spinhoven P, Van der Hart O. Evidence for associations among somatoform dissociation, psychological dissociation and reported trauma in patients with chronic pelvic pain. J Psychosom Obstet Gynecol. 2003;24(2):87–98.
171. Hahn L. Chronic pelvic pain in women. A condition difficult to diagnose--more than 70 different diagnoses can be considered. Lakartidningen. 2001;98(15):1780–5.
172. Bonvanie IJ, van Gils A, Janssens KA, Rosmalen JG. Sexual abuse predicts functional somatic symptoms: an adolescent population study. Child Abuse Negl. 2015;46:1–7.
173. Halpern CT, Tucker CM, Bengtson A, Kupper LL, McLean SA, Martin SL. Somatic symptoms among US adolescent females: associations with sexual and physical violence exposure. Matern Child Health J. 2013;17(10):1951–60.
174. Fry RP, Beard RW, Crisp AH, McGuigan S. Sociopsychological factors in women with chronic pelvic pain with and without pelvic venous congestion. J Psychosom Res. 1997;42(1):71–85.
175. Dunlop BW, Hill E, Johnson BN, Klein DN, Gelenberg AJ, Rothbaum BO, Thase ME, Kocsis JH. Mediators of sexual functioning and marital quality in chronically depressed adults with and without a history of childhood sexual abuse. J Sex Med. 2015;12(3):813–23.
176. Leclerc B, Bergeron S, Binik YM, Khalifé S. History of sexual and physical abuse in women with dyspareunia: association with pain, psychosocial adjustment, and sexual functioning. J Sex Med. 2010;7(2pt2):971–80.
177. Staples J, Rellini AH, Roberts SP. Avoiding experiences: sexual dysfunction in women with a history of sexual abuse in childhood and adolescence. Arch Sex Behav. 2012;41(2):341–50.
178. Nguyen RH, Turner RM, Rydell SA, MacLehose RF, Harlow BL. Perceived stereotyping and seeking care for chronic vulvar pain. Pain Med. 2013;14(10):1461–7.
179. Fanni E, Castellini G, Corona G, Boddi V, Ricca V, Rastrelli G, Fisher AD, Cipriani S, Maggi M. The role of somatic symptoms in

sexual medicine: somatization as important contextual factor in male sexual dysfunction. J Sex Med. 2016;13(9):1395–407.

180. Striegel-Moore RH, Rosselli F, Perrin N, DeBar L, Wilson GT, May A, Kraemer HC. Gender difference in the prevalence of eating disorder symptoms. Int J Eat Disord. 2009;42(5):471–4.
181. Sweeting H, Walker L, MacLean A, Patterson C, Räisänen U, Hunt K. Prevalence of eating disorders in males: a review of rates reported in academic research and UK mass media. Int J Men Health. 2015;14(2):10.3149/jmh.1402.86.
182. Kelly NR, Cotter EW, Tanofsky-Kraff M, Mazzeo SE. Racial variations in binge eating, body image concerns, and compulsive exercise among men. Psychol Men Mascul. 2015;16(3):326.
183. Castellini G, Lelli L, Ricca V, Maggi M. Sexuality in eating disorders patients: etiological factors, sexual dysfunction and identity issues. A systematic review. Horm Mol Biol Clin Investig. 2016;25(2):71–90.
184. Kang Y, Zheng L, Zheng Y. Sex and eating: relationships based on wanting and liking. Front Psychol. 2016;6:2044. doi:10.3389/fpsyg.2015.02044.
185. Castellini G, Mannucci E, Mazzei C, Lo Sauro C, Faravelli C, Rotella CM, Maggi M, Ricca V. Sexual function in obese women with and without binge eating disorder. J Sex Med. 2010;7(12):3969–78.
186. Pinheiro AP, Raney TJ, Thornton LM, Fichter MM, Berrettini WH, Goldman D, Halmi KA, Kaplan AS, Strober M, Treasure J, Woodside DB. Sexual functioning in women with eating disorders. Int J Eat Disord. 2010;43(2):123–9.
187. Castellini G, Lelli L, Lo Sauro C, Fioravanti G, Vignozzi L, Maggi M, Faravelli C, Ricca V. Anorectic and bulimic patients suffer from relevant sexual dysfunctions. J Sex Med. 2012;9(10):2590–9.
188. Kimmel MC, Ferguson EH, Zerwas S, Bulik CM, Meltzer-Brody S. Obstetric and gynecologic problems associated with eating disorders. Int J Eat Disord. 2016;49(3):260–75.
189. Fairburn CG, Bohn K. Eating disorder NOS (EDNOS): an example of the troublesome "not otherwise specified"(NOS) category in DSM-IV. Behav Res Ther. 2005;43(6):691–701.
190. Kenny MC, Ward-Lichterman M, Abdelmonem MH. The expansion and clarification of feeding and eating disorders in the DSM-5. Prof Counsel. 2014;4:246–56.
191. Gonidakis F, Kravvariti V, Varsou E. Sexual function of women suffering from anorexia nervosa and bulimia nervosa. J Sex Marital Ther. 2015;41(4):368–78.
192. Rothschild BS, Fagan PJ, Woodall C, Andersen AE. Sexual functioning of female eating-disordered patients. Int J Eat Disord. 1991;10(4):389–94.
193. Meguerditchian C, Samuelian-Massat C, Valéro R, Begu-Le Corroller A, Fromont I, Mancini J, Sparrow JD, Poinso F, Vialettes B. The impact of weight normalization on quality of recovery in anorexia nervosa. J Am Coll Nutr. 2009;28(4):397–404.
194. Westen D, Harnden-Fischer J. Personality profiles in eating disorders: rethinking the distinction between axis I and axis II. Am J Psychiatry. 2001;158(4):547–62.
195. Kolotkin RL, Zunker C, Østbye T. Sexual functioning and obesity: a review. Obesity. 2012;20(12):2325–33.
196. Sarwer DB, Spitzer JC, Wadden TA, Rosen RC, Mitchell JE, Lancaster K, Courcoulas A, Gourash W, Christian NJ. Sexual functioning and sex hormones in men who underwent bariatric surgery. Surg Obes Relat Dis. 2015;11(3):643–51.
197. Sarwer DB, Spitzer JC, Wadden TA, Mitchell JE, Lancaster K, Courcoulas A, Gourash W, Rosen RC, Christian NJ. Changes in sexual functioning and sex hormone levels in women following bariatric surgery. JAMA Surg. 2014;149(1):26–33.
198. Palha A, Esteves M. Drugs of abuse and sexual functioning. Adv Psychosom Med. 2008;29:131–49.
199. La Pera GI, Franco Giannotti CE, Taggi F, Macchia T. Prevalence of sexual disorders in those young males who later become drug abusers. J Sex Marital Ther. 2003;29(2):149–56.
200. Beckman LJ, Ackerman KT. Women, alcohol, and sexuality. In: Marc G, editor. Recent developments in alcoholism. New York, NY: Springer; 2002. p. 267–85.
201. Theall KP, Elifson KW, Sterk CE. Sex, touch, and HIV risk among ecstasy users. AIDS Behav. 2006;10(2):169–78.
202. Chou NH, Huang YJ, Jiann BP. The impact of illicit use of amphetamine on male sexual functions. J Sex Med. 2015;12(8):1694–702.
203. Costa RM, Peres L. Smoking is unrelated to female sexual function. Subst Use Misuse. 2015;50(2):189–94.
204. Johnson SD, Phelps DL, Cottler LB. The association of sexual dysfunction and substance use among a community epidemiological sample. Arch Sex Behav. 2004;33(1):55–63.
205. Ramdurg S, Ambekar A, Lal R. Sexual dysfunction among male patients receiving buprenorphine and naltrexone maintenance therapy for opioid dependence. J Sex Med. 2012;9(12):3198–204.
206. Venkatesh K, Mattoo SK, Grover S. Sexual dysfunction in men seeking treatment for opioid dependence: a study from India. J Sex Med. 2014;11(8):2055–64.
207. Cocores JA, Miller NS, Pottash AC, Gold MS. Sexual dysfunction in abusers of cocaine and alcohol. Am J Drug Alcohol Abuse. 1988;14(2):169–73.
208. Zaazaa A, Bella AJ, Shamloul R. Drug addiction and sexual dysfunction. Endocrinol Metab Clin North Am. 2013;42(3):585–92.
209. Vallejo-Medina P, Sierra JC. Effect of drug use and influence of abstinence on sexual functioning in a Spanish male drug-dependent sample: a multisite study. J Sex Med. 2013;10(2):333–41.
210. Johnson PS, Sweeney MM, Herrmann ES, Johnson MW. Alcohol increases delay and probability discounting of condom-protected sex: a novel vector for alcohol-related HIV transmission. Alcohol Clin Exp Res. 2016;40(6):1339–50.
211. Dunn M, Day C, Bruno R, Degenhardt L, Campbell G. Sexual and injecting risk behaviours among regular ecstasy users. Addict Behav. 2010;35(2):157–60.
212. Sterk CE, Klein H, Elifson KW. Young adult ecstasy users and multiple sexual partners: understanding the factors underlying this HIV risk practice. J Psychoactive Drugs. 2008;40(3):237–44.
213. DeHovitz JA, Kelly P, Feldman J, Sierra MF, Clarke L, Bromberg J, Wan JY, Vermund SH, Landesman S. Sexually transmitted diseases, sexual behavior, and cocaine use in inner-city women. Am J Epidemiol. 1994;140(12):1125–34.
214. Wilson TE, Minkoff H, DeHovitz JA, Feldman J, Landesman S. The relationship of cocaine use and human immunodeficiency virus serostatus to incident sexually transmitted diseases among women. Sex Transm Dis. 1998;25(2):70–5.
215. Buchacz K, McFarland W, Kellogg TA, Loeb L, Holmberg SD, Dilley J, Klausner JD. Amphetamine use is associated with increased HIV incidence among men who have sex with men in San Francisco. AIDS. 2005;19(13):1423–4.
216. Grant JE, Kim SW. Quality of life in kleptomania and pathological gambling. Compr Psychiatry. 2005;46(1):34–7.
217. Bronner GI, Aharon-Peretz JU, Hassin-Baer SH. Sexuality in patients with Parkinson's disease, Alzheimer's disease, and other dementias. Handb Clin Neurol. 2015;130:297–323.
218. Momtaz YA, Hamid TA, Ibrahim R. The impact of mild cognitive impairment on sexual activity. Am J Alzheimers Dis Other Demen. 2013;28(8):759–62.
219. Abdo CH. Sexuality and couple intimacy in dementia. Curr Opin Psychiatry. 2013;26(6):593–8.
220. Davies HD, Sridhar SB, Newkirk LA, Beaudreau SA, O'Hara R. Gender differences in sexual behaviors of AD patients and their relationship to spousal caregiver well-being. Aging Ment Health. 2012;16(1):89–101.
221. Simonelli C, Tripodi F, Rossi R, Fabrizi A, Lembo D, Cosmi V, Pierleoni L. The influence of caregiver burden on sexual intimacy

and marital satisfaction in couples with an Alzheimer spouse. Int J Clin Pract. 2008;62(1):47–52.
222. Ahmed RM, Kaizik C, Irish M, Mioshi E, Dermody N, Kiernan MC, Piguet O, Hodges JR. Characterizing sexual behavior in frontotemporal dementia. J Alzheimers Dis. 2015;46(3):677–86.
223. Ibrahim C, Reynaert C. Hypersexuality in neurocognitive disorders in elderly people-a comprehensive review of the literature and case study. Psychiatr Danub. 2014;26(Suppl 1):36–40.
224. Bartelet M, Waterink W, van Hooren S. Extreme sexual behavior in dementia as a specific manifestation of disinhibition. J Alzheimers Dis. 2014;42(s3):S119–24.
225. Cipriani G, Ulivi M, Danti S, Lucetti C, Nuti A. Sexual disinhibition and dementia. Psychogeriatrics. 2016;16(2):145–53.
226. Bronner G, Royter V, Korczyn AD, Giladi N. Sexual dysfunction in Parkinson's disease. J Sex Marital Ther. 2004;30(2):95–105.
227. Bronner G, Hassin-Baer S. Exploring hypersexual behavior in men with Parkinson's disease: is it compulsive sexual behavior? J Parkinson Dis. 2012;2(3):225–34.
228. Tucker I. Management of inappropriate sexual behaviors in dementia: a literature review. Int Psychogeriatr. 2010;22(05):683–92.
229. Widiger TA. Personality disorders. In: Barone DF, editor. Advanced personality. New York, NY: Springer; 1998. p. 335–52.
230. Apt C, Hurlbert DF. The sexual attitudes, behavior, and relationships of women with histrionic personality disorder. J Sex Marital Ther. 1994;20(2):125–34.
231. Lodi-Smith J, Shepard K, Wagner S. Personality and sexually deviant behavior. Personal Individ Differ. 2014;70:39–44.
232. Foster JD, Shrira I, Campbell WK. Theoretical models of narcissism, sexuality, and relationship commitment. J Soc Pers Relation. 2006;23(3):367–86.
233. Luntz BK, Widom CS. Antisocial personality disorder in abused and neglected children grown up. Am J Psychiatry. 1994;151(5):670–4.
234. Strickland SM. Female sex offenders: exploring issues of personality, trauma, and cognitive distortions. J Interpers Violence. 2008;23(4):474–89.
235. Gobin RL, Reddy MK, Zlotnick C, Johnson JE. Lifetime trauma victimization and PTSD in relation to psychopathy and antisocial personality disorder in a sample of incarcerated women and men. Int J Prison Health. 2015;11(2):64–74.
236. Berger P, Berner W, Bolterauer J, Gutierrez K, Berger K. Sadistic personality disorder in sex offenders: relationship to antisocial personality disorder and sexual sadism. J Pers Disord. 1999;13(2):175.
237. Schroeder M, Iffland JS, Hill A, Berner W, Briken P. Personality disorders in men with sexual and violent criminal offense histories. J Pers Disord. 2013;27(4):519.
238. Turco RN, Geberth VJ. Antisocial personality disorder, sexual sadism, malignant narcissism, and serial murder. J Forensic Sci. 1997;42(1):49–60.
239. Zanarini MC, Parachini EA, Frankenburg FR, Holman JB, Hennen J, Bradford Reich D, Silk KR. Sexual relationship difficulties among borderline patients and axis II comparison subjects. J Nerv Ment Dis. 2003;191:479–82.
240. Bierer LM, Yehuda R, Schmeidler J, Mitropoulou V, New AS, Silverman JM, Siever LJ. Abuse and neglect in childhood: relationship to personality disorder diagnoses. CNS Spectr. 2003;8(10):737–54.
241. Mangassarian S, Sumner L, O'Callaghan E. Sexual impulsivity in women diagnosed with borderline personality disorder: a review of the literature. Sex Addict Compuls. 2015;22(3):195–206.
242. Sansone RA, Sansone LA, Wiederman M. The prevalence of trauma and its relationship to borderline personality symptoms and self-destructive behaviors in a primary care setting. Arch Fam Med. 1995;4(5):439–42.
243. Hurlbert DF, Apt C, White LC. An empirical examination into the sexuality of women with borderline personality disorder. J Sex Marital Ther. 1992;18(3):231–42.
244. Alden LE, Capreol MJ. Avoidant personality disorder: interpersonal problems as predictors of treatment response. Behav Ther. 1993;24(3):357–76.
245. Goldenson J, Geffner R, Foster SL, Clipson CR. Female domestic violence offenders: their attachment security, trauma symptoms, and personality organization. Violence Vict. 2007;22(5):532–45.
246. Bornstein RF. Illuminating a neglected clinical issue: societal costs of interpersonal dependency and dependent personality disorder. J Clin Psychol. 2012;68(7):766–81.
247. Cain NM, Ansell EB, Simpson HB, Pinto A. Interpersonal functioning in obsessive–compulsive personality disorder. J Pers Assess. 2015;97(1):90–9.

33 Sexual Emergencies

Asbasia A. Mikhail

Introduction

It is believed that of the 2.3 million injuries filed in the last 6 years, less than 0.5% were due to sex injuries. However, it is also believed that most sex injuries go unreported [1]. This may be due to a number of reasons, shame and degree of seriousness to name a few. Some of the more common and less serious injuries that patients sustain during sex are muscle strains, bites/scratches, rug burns, and broken or sprained bones due to accidentally falling (especially on a slippery floor) or bumping into furniture. While these are all legitimate emergencies, these injuries are not specific to intercourse and are usually widely treated without much difficulty [2]. Subsequently, this chapter focuses on the injuries that are more specific to sex and are more emergent requiring more specific and complex care. It is important to emphasize that this chapter does not discuss non-consensual intercourse/sexual behaviors, but these cases need to be dealt with and reported appropriately. While some may argue (even patients themselves) over what is the most emergent sexual complication, sexual emergencies in this chapter are listed in the following order: 1) sexual emergencies pertaining to men only, specifically priapism and penile fractures, 2) those pertaining to women only, namely hemorrhage due to vaginal tears, foreign body entrapment in the vagina, and hemoperitoneum usually due to ruptured ovarian cysts, and 3) those applicable to both men and women such as anorectal perforation, foreign body entrapment in the rectum, postcoital headaches, and complications of sexual enhancing medication. There is also a brief discussion on a few very rare sexual emergencies that were found to be of interest.

Sexual Emergencies in Men

Priapism

Epidemiology

Although this is a rare condition overall, it is estimated that there are over 10,000 visits/year to all EDs for priapism (but not necessarily due to a sexual complication). Priapism is defined as a sustained erection that lasts for over an hour and is beyond sexual stimulation.

Clinical Presentation

There are essentially two types of priapism. There is *ischemic* VS *non-ischemic* priapism.

Ischemic Priapism

The penis is very PAINFUL and RIGID. In this form, there is almost little to no blood flow to the corpora cavernosa (see Figure 33-1) also known as a veno-occlusive disorder. It has also been referred to as a "compartment syndrome." Blood gas of cavernous blood during priapism usually reveals acidosis. There is also a condition known as stuttering priapism, which is a form of ischemic priapism. It occurs when patients experience recurrent and unwanted painful erections. It does eventually resolve spontaneously, but because it does recur, it can have a negative impact on quality of life [3].

Non-ischemic Priapism

Usually not painful and the penis is not as rigid. It is often a result of trauma or nonsexual causes. It is also known as a high flow disorder in which there is increased arterial blood flow. This type of priapism does **not** require emergent treatment [3].

W.W. IsHak (ed.), *The Textbook of Clinical Sexual Medicine*, DOI 10.1007/978-3-319-52539-6_33

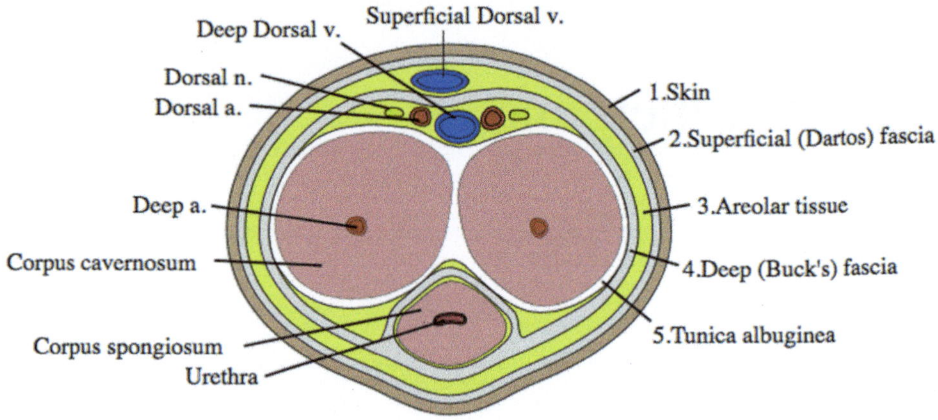

FIGURE 33-1. Penis: cross section [Reprinted from https://commons.wikimedia.org/wiki/File:Penis_cross_section.svg#. With permission from Creative Commons].

Diagnosis

In order to treat ischemic priapism, a clinician must first determine what type of priapism they are dealing with. In order to differentiate which type of priapism you are dealing with, there are a few requirements that need to be met. If the patient's penis is very painful and rigid, and its cavernous blood gas is acidotic, hypercarbic, and hypoxic, then it is clearly the ischemic form. A cavernous blood gas is obtained by needle aspiration of blood from the corpus cavernosa.

It is important to note that there are other causes of ischemic priapism, like sickle cell disease, leukemia, and platelet abnormalities that must also be ruled out during the workup. One must also determine if certain drugs may have been the culprit (e.g. sexual enhancers, psychoactive drugs, and illicit drugs).

The imaging of choice used to confirm ischemic priapism is color duplex ultrasonography in which no blood flow will be seen in the corpora cavernosa [3].

Treatment

Given that *ischemic* priapism is a true emergency and that it is a complication of sexual activity as well as sexual drug enhancers, we will primarily focus on the treatment of this form of priapism. Because this is a rare condition, guidelines on how to treat this complication is based largely on multiple case reports and review of all previous literature.

The goal of treatment is to preserve erectile dysfunction. The initial treatment modality of choice for ischemic priapism (no matter what the etiology) is therapeutic aspiration with or without irrigation in conjunction with injection of a sympathomimetic into the corpora cavernosa (see Figure 33-2). Sympathomimetic injections may be repeated if initial results are not optimal. The most recommended sympathomimetic is phenylephrine due to its minimal cardiovascular risk. Once treated with sympathomimetic injection, the patient must be monitored appropriately for any adverse effects like hypertension, headache, bradycardia, and tachycardia vs. arrhythmias [3].

If patient's priapism has been present for about 48 h or more, studies have shown that phenylephrine is far less effective primarily because smooth muscle relaxation in the corpora cavernosa is impaired by ischemia and acidosis.

Most importantly, the clinician must also treat any underlying systemic disease that may be contributing to patient's priapism (acute sickle cell crisis, leukemia, etc.). By performing the above three treatment modalities, the majority of patients (~80%) will not sustain any erectile dysfunction. If after the above methods have been successfully executed and there is still no resolution of symptoms, then surgical treatment should be instituted [3, 4].

Surgical treatment should be the **last resort**. Surgical treatment entails a shunting procedure. The American Urology Association (AUA) recommends the cavernoglanular shunt as the first shunting procedure of choice (see Figure 33-3). However, a more difficult shunt procedure known as the "Al-Gorab" procedure (also known as the T-shunt, which is the third method seen in Figure 33-3) is very effective and can be performed even if the first two shunt procedures have failed [5–8].

Prognosis

There are many factors that affect overall prognosis. These are: (1) time to treatment, (2) preexisting comorbidities such as sickle cell and leukemia, (3) type of treatment chosen to relieve ischemic priapism, and (4) location of surgical shunting (proximal vs. distal). However, about 70–80% of patients who receive appropriate therapy will regain full sexual function [3, 4, 9].

Prevention

Alpha adrenergic agonists like Etilefrine injected intra-cavernously has been shown to prevent recurrence about 70% of the time [3].

Penile Fracture

Epidemiology/Etiology

Penile fractures are the result of an unnatural bend of the erect penis, which then results in an abrupt tear of the tunica albuginea. There may also be an associated rupture of the corpus

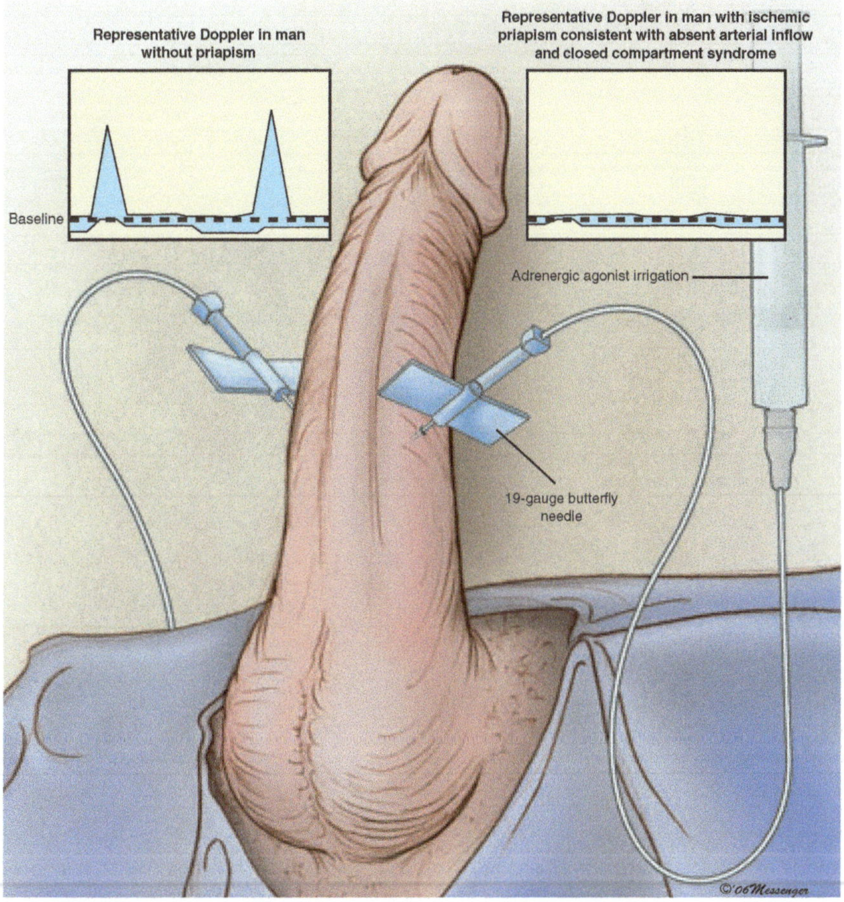

FIGURE 33-2. Aspiration + adrenergic agonist combination after a reasonable dosage and duration (e.g., 20 mg of diluted phenylephrine over 1 h) [Reprinted from Lue TF, Pescatori ES. Distal cavernosum-glans shunts for ischemic priapism. J Sex Med. 2006;3(4), 749–52. With permission from Elsevier].

spongiosum and/or the urethra. While it is considered to be a rare occurrence, experts believe that it happens far more than it is actually reported due to the shame associated with this injury. Studies have shown that about half of all penile fractures (of those reported) occur during enthusiastic intercourse. During intercourse, the male misses entering the vagina and accidentally hits the hard region of the perineum or pubic symphysis. Circumstances leading to such an event could be due to stressful sex (like in an extramarital affair) or due to awkward positions/locations as couples experiment sexually. Other etiologies include the act of aggressive masturbation and a direct blow or bend to the penis to eradicate an undesired erection [10].

Some men are more predisposed to penile fractures than others. For instance, a man who is overly excited and using excessive force is more at risk. Also, men who have a history of fibrosclerosis of the tunica albuginea, or a history of chronic urethritis are also at higher risk for penile fractures [10].

Clinical Presentation

Patients with a penile fracture will usually present with an edematous, painful, and bruised penis that is often bent or deformed (see Figure 33-4). About half of the time, patients will come in stating that their injury occurred after intercourse while the other half of the time the etiology is not clear, but usually they were either aggressively masturbating or fighting off an undesired erection (although patients may deny the latter two reasons). They will generally state that they heard a loud pop at the time of injury with loss of erection soon after the popping sound is heard [11].

Diagnostic Testing

Diagnosis is made primarily by history and visual inspection of the penis. However, a color-Doppler ultrasound may be a very efficient and a noninvasive test to assist in diagnosing a penile fracture. However, once the diagnosis is made, further investigation is needed to determine the extent of the injury. The surgeon may opt to do an MRI or an urethrography or cavernosography prior to surgical repair to determine the exact site of the tear as well as the extent of the tear. For both urethrography and cavernosography, a radiographic study performed with contrast media is used to evaluate the urethra and the corpus cavernosum [12, 13].

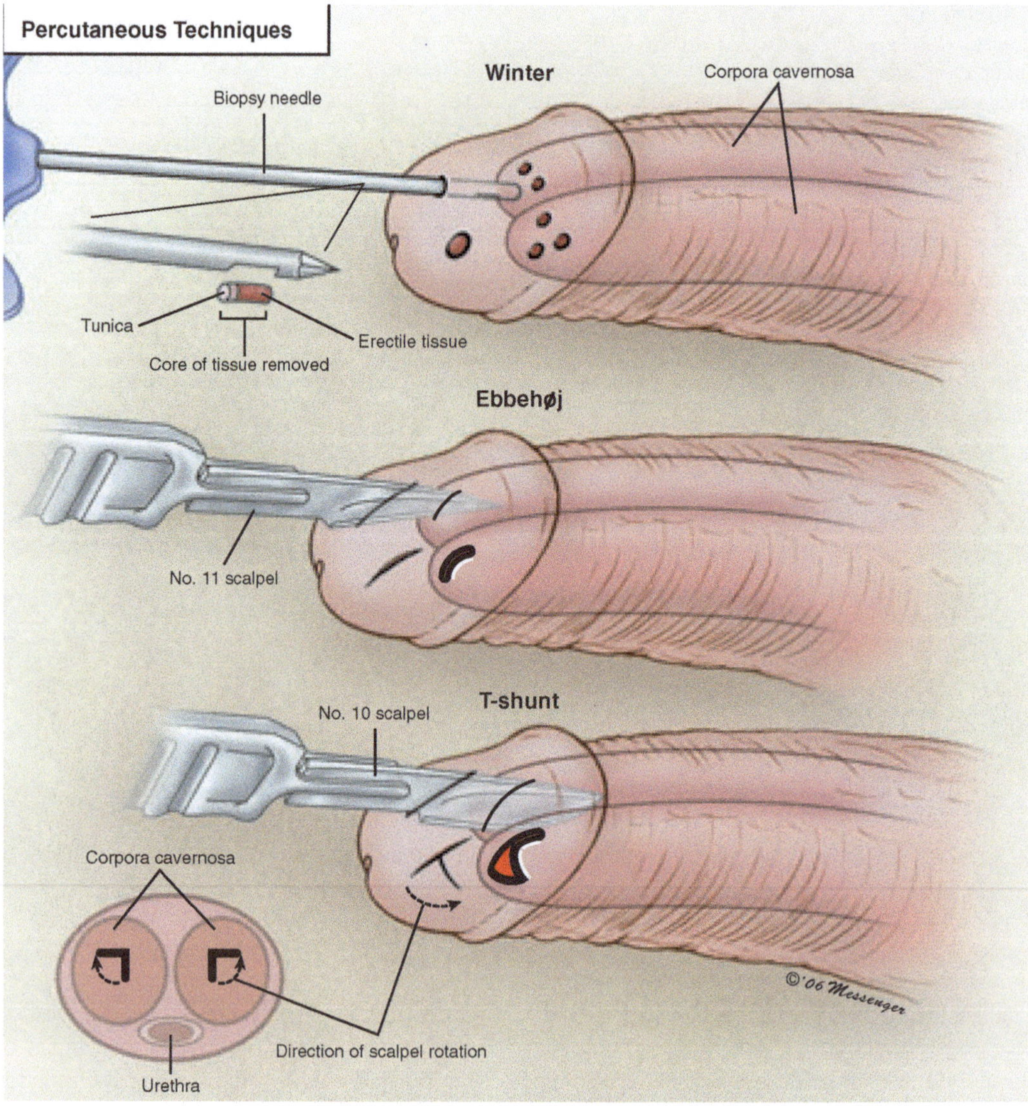

FIGURE 33-3. Visual description of each form of caverno-glanular shunting, also referred to as distal shunts [Reprinted from Lue TF, Pescatori ES. Distal cavernosum-glans shunts for ischemic priapism. J Sex Med. 2006;3(4), 749–52. With permission from Elsevier].

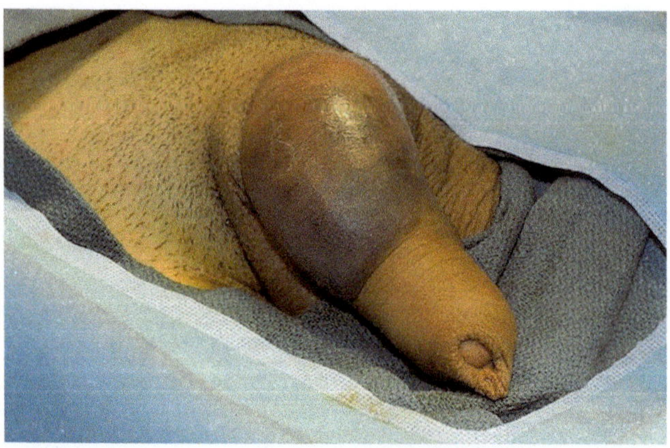

FIGURE 33-4. Penile fracture [Courtesy of Dr. Joel Gelman, Center for Reconstructive Urology, used with permission].

Treatment

In the past, it was acceptable to resort to conservative treatment, which entailed cold compresses, pressure dressings, oral anti-inflammatory drugs, and in some instances, fibrinolytics and anti-androgens. Complications include erectile dysfunction, penile curvature, painful erections, missed urethral injuries, and penile nodules and fistulas. Subsequently, surgical correction has become the standard of care. In fact, research studies have shown that surgical treatment significantly reduced the incidence of erectile dysfunction and painful erections [11, 14].

Prognosis

Prognosis is overall good if the patient with penile fracture seeks medical attention soon and if their fracture is treated surgically. However, even if a patient has a delayed presentation, erectile dysfunction is still improved with surgical treatment [15, 16].

Sexual Emergencies in Women

Trauma to Female Genitalia

Epidemiology

Most injuries to the vagina are caused by forceful blunt trauma either by the penis, fingers/hands, or foreign bodies. However, these injuries are more common in women who do not have adequate lubrication of their vagina before intercourse. Inadequate lubrication can be the result of menopause, lack of sufficient foreplay, and previous history of sexual abuse. Experts have also hypothesized that certain positions during intercourse make a woman more vulnerable for genital trauma, primarily when their male counterpart is on top. The same can be postulated about those females who are having sexual toys being forcefully inserted into their vaginas since certain positions can also make them more vulnerable for injury [17].

Clinical Presentation

The typical presentation of a woman with a vaginal tear is that of a burning and painful sensation in their vagina. There is usually minimal bleeding. If the vaginal laceration is more complex, the patient will most likely complain of more pain and more bleeding. There have even been a few case reports of women who have bled to the point of shock because of deep vaginal tears, but these presentations are rare. Subsequently, a deeper laceration of the vagina could mean that the vagina has been perforated. There have also been reports of vaginal–rectal fistulas that have occurred as a result of forceful sex. Vaginal tears have also been the result of oral sex as the piercings on their partner's tongue/lips may lacerate the external genitalia. If a patient presents with the above presentation, the clinician must use their clinical judgment and investigate/report the case if warranted [18].

Diagnostic Testing

In addition to obtaining a proper history, the primary manner in diagnosing a vaginal tear is by careful examination of the external (labia majora and minora) and the internal genitalia (the vaginal vault). Most importantly, the extent and depth of the injury should be determined so as not to miss a vaginal perforation and/or simultaneous rectal perforation [19, 20].

Treatment

Treatment usually consists of repairing and suturing the laceration. Care must be taken in suturing more complex lacerations, as each layer that is breached must be sutured separately. In the case of a rectovaginal tear, three different layers must be repaired; the vaginal mucosa, the rectovaginal septum and the rectal mucosa. Some tears involving the rectum can be so severe that they have to be repaired in the operating room for primary repair of the tear and diverting colostomy. It is also prudent to send the patient home with oral antibiotics for prophylaxis [19, 20].

Prognosis

Prognosis is improved with early treatment. The longer one waits, the more susceptible they are to complications, i.e., delayed healing/closure, infections, and in some cases, death.

Prevention

The most logical way to approach prevention is by reviewing the cause for such tears. Naturally, the better the lubrication, the less risk there is of sustaining such tears. There are numerous synthetic lubricants available for women in menopause to use just before sex. There are also different types of hormonal therapy that can be used but these become more risky for older women. As for younger women, they may want to have their partners engage in longer foreplay to achieve appropriate lubrication. Experts have also recommended that a women may consider changing her positioning. For instance, by putting herself on top of her partner, she, in theory, is in more control in regards to the force of intercourse.

Most importantly, two consenting adults engaging in any kind of sexual activity should communicate with each other and be able to express freely what gives them pleasure and vice versa [17].

Vaginal Foreign Body Entrapment

Epidemiology

The two most common locations for Foreign Body (FB) entrapment to occur are the vagina and the rectum (foreign bodies in the rectum are discussed later in the chapter).

The most common retained vaginal foreign body after intercourse is a condom. However, there have been case reports of objects such as sex toys and other plastic objects (used to enhance sexual pleasure) that have been retained [21].

Clinical Presentation

For women presenting with a retained vaginal FB, their usual complaints are persistent malodorous vaginal discharge, vaginal spotting, and vaginal irritation/itching. It is also not uncommon for women to complain of dysuria and a genital rash. Many times, the patient will not suspect the possibility of having a retained vaginal FB [21].

Diagnostic Testing

Diagnosis of retained foreign bodies is primarily made by history and physical. Visual inspection via pelvic speculum exam will usually be sufficient for the clinician to locate the foreign body. Ultrasound of the pelvis has also been shown to be useful in locating a vaginal foreign body. In the case of a foreign body that has perforated the vaginal vault, a plain film of the torso may be obtained to look for free air, but an abdominal/pelvic CT may reveal a more definitive diagnosis [21].

For those patients for whom radiation is a concern, an MRI has also been used as a diagnostic tool but an MRI is absolutely contraindicated if the FB entrapped is known to have metal properties [22].

Treatment

Once the clinician has located the foreign body, forceps may be used to pull the foreign body out. There are those rare instances in which a vaginal foreign body may be too large or it may have even perforated into the peritoneal cavity. In those cases, a gynecologist must be consulted immediately as these injuries require immediate surgery. There have also been case reports of foreign bodies leading to vesico-vaginal fistulas (communication between the bladder and the vagina) and to colo-uterine fistulas (communication between the colon and the uterus). These injuries are rare and may have occurred at the time of penetration into the vaginal vault or as a result of a foreign body left in the vaginal vault for an extended period of time. Such complications ultimately require surgical repair [23, 24].

Prognosis

These patients will do well if they are treated appropriately. However, for those women who present much later, they may sustain long-term complications [25].

Ruptured Ovarian Cysts and Hemoperitoneum

Epidemiology

While ruptured ovarian cysts are relatively common among women, it is unclear exactly what percent of these ruptured cysts are due to intercourse. None the less, intercourse has been known to be a cause of ruptured ovarian cysts. Very rarely, these ruptured cysts lead to a hemoperitoneum, which can lead to hemorrhagic shock. The data is scant on the rate at which these ruptured ovarian cysts occur as a result of sexual intercourse and there are only a handful of case reports describing patients who suffered hemorrhagic shock as a result of hemoperitoneum caused by a ruptured ovarian cyst after sexual intercourse [26].

Clinical Presentation

Women presenting with ruptured ovarian cysts will usually complain of sudden onset of severe lower abdominal pain localized to one side. This acute onset of pain may be associated with nausea, vomiting, and diaphoresis. The pain is usually the worst in the first hours after the cyst ruptures, but gradually, the pain lessons but is still felt with movement and ambulation. Patients with hemoperitoneum, however, will have persistent severe pain and they may even be hypotensive on arrival [27, 28].

Diagnosis

A good history from the patient is often helpful, but diagnosis is usually made by visualization of free fluid in the pelvis via ultrasonography. A pelvic ultrasound yields the best results if performed trans-vaginally. After a cyst has ruptured, the ultrasound (US) technician may or may not see an ovarian cyst, but seeing some free fluid in the pelvis may indicate that a cyst has ruptured. The technician is usually able to tell if the free fluid is consistent with blood or not. If a pelvic US is inconclusive or if a patient is found to have a hemoperitoneum, then a CT scan of the abdomen and pelvis with IV contrast should be considered to rule out other emergent causes of free fluid and hemoperitoneum in the pelvis. The contrast will allow visualization of extravasation and source of bleeding. For instance, a case was reported of a hemoperitoneum being found in a female after sexual activity which happened to be a result of a laceration of their round ligament rather than a ruptured ovarian cyst [29]. If the patient's pain is in the right lower quadrant of the abdomen, there is always concern that the cause of pain could be due to appendicitis. Therefore, in some cases, a CT is necessary to differentiate whether or not a patient's pain is due to appendicitis especially since management is completely different for both. Keep in mind that a CT scan of the abdomen does expose a patient to a considerable amount of radiation and this should always be taken into account when ordering a CT scan, especially since ruptured ovarian cysts can be a recurrent problem and may put a patient at risk for having more CT scans (i.e., more radiation exposure) in the future [27, 28].

A urine pregnancy test should always be performed because if positive, an ectopic pregnancy must be ruled out. Blood work may be diagnostic in the sense that an elevated white blood cell count (WBC) with a left shift may suggest something other than a ruptured cyst. However, it is not uncommon to see an elevated WBC with a simple ruptured ovarian cyst. A low hemoglobin (HgB) may suggest that a patient has had significant amount of blood loss indicating that a patient may require a blood transfusion and emergent surgical intervention [27, 28].

Treatment

Treatment of a ruptured ovarian cyst where there is minimal free fluid in the pelvis requires usually only pain control. Ketorolac (Toradol) 30 mg IVP or 60 mg IM (intramuscular) is usually very effective for pain control. Oral Ibuprofen (Motrin) 600 mg per oral (PO) is also helpful but must be taken with food. Many times these patients come in nauseated and have to be given antiemetics first. Some common antiemetics include Zofran (odansetron) 4 mg PO or IVP, Metoclopramide (Reglan) 5–10 mg PO, IVP, or IM, and Promethazine (Phenergan) 12.5–25 mg IM or IVP. Note that romethazine has a tendency to cause sedation and sometimes may affect respiratory drive (especially in older patients and children). If Toradol is not enough to control the pain, then IV or IM opiates should be considered. If a patient has vomited several times, then a liter of IVFs (normal saline) may be administered [28].

Treatment of a ruptured ovarian cyst resulting in a large hemoperitoneum and shock is a true emergency and a gynecologist on duty should be called emergently. The patient should be hemodynamically stabilized with IVFs (usually normal saline), but type and cross-matched blood may need to be administered if patient's low blood pressure is not responding to IVFs or if the patient's HgB is less than 7 (or less than 8 and patient is symptomatic). If a hemoperitoneum due to a ruptured cyst is diagnosed, then a gynecologist is needed emergently to take the patient to the Operating Room (OR) to perform an emergent laparotomy [29].

Prevention

It is very difficult to predict who will develop ovarian cysts. However, a patient who has a history of a known ovarian cyst is at higher risk of having recurring cysts and subsequently a higher likelihood of suffering from a recurring ruptured ovarian cyst. Very often, females who develop recurrent cysts are started on birth control pills in order to prevent the formation of ovarian cysts and ultimately, the complications of having these ovarian cysts (e.g. chronic pain and ruptured ovarian cysts) [27].

Prognosis

Most of these patients do well especially if it was a simple ovarian cyst that ruptured. However, Patients who develop a hemoperitoneum are at risk for exsanguinating and dying. For this reason, if diagnosis is made in a timely manner and source of bleeding is detected and stopped, then the patient will also recover without any negative sequelae.

Sexual Emergencies Pertaining to Men and Women

Anal Tears and Perforation

Epidemiology

While anal injuries are rare, they do occur more frequently than one might think. Injuries of the anus and rectum can range from a small tear also know as a fistula to a complete perforation. Anal and rectal injuries are caused by forceful anal intercourse, anal foreign bodies, and handballing (also known as fisting in which primarily gay men place their fists into their partners' anus) [30–32].

Clinical Presentation

Clinical presentation of a patient with an anal injury will vary based on the complexity of the injury. For instance, a patient who sustains an anal fistula will more likely present with pain in the rectum, anal bleeding, and pain upon sitting/defacating. The patient may also have mild lower abdominal pain. A patient with an anal perforation, however, will present with severe abdominal pain, or with rectal bleeding and pain being secondary [33].

Diagnostic Testing

A good history from the patient can usually be sufficient to hone in on the diagnosis. However, patients who have engaged in anal intercourse or other forms of anal eroticism may not be so forth coming with how they sustained their injuries. Even worse is that patients may hold off on seeking treatment due to their being embarrassed of having engaged in such activities. Unfortunately, the longer these patients wait before seeking treatment, the higher the risk that they are likely to suffer severe morbidity and even mortality.

Once the patient presents to the ED, visual inspection, and even anal endoscopy may be needed to diagnose an anal tear/fistula. However, if anal perforation is suspected, then abdominal and chest X-rays may be obtained to look for free air in the peritoneum (see Figure 33-5). Some tears and lacerations are difficult to locate, but studies have shown that the use of certain dyes like toluidine blue can be helpful. Toluidine blue binds to cells in the deeper layers of tissue and therefore any region that retains the dye is usually consistent with a tear [34].

Treatment

A surgeon, primarily a colorectal surgeon, should be consulted emergently. Patient should be started on appropriate antibiotics. If perforation has occurred, then a laparotomy is usually mandatory. Decision not to do a laparotomy is specifically up to the surgeon.

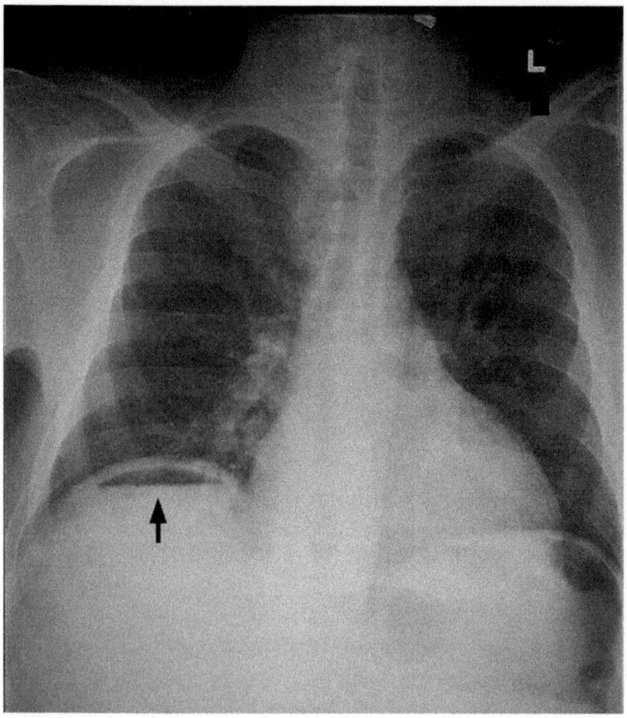

FIGURE 33-5. Pneumoperitoneum seen as lucency between the diaphragm and the liver as pointed out by the *arrow*. [Reprinted from https://commons.wikimedia.org/wiki/File:Pneumoperitoneum_modification.jpg. With permission from Creative Commons].

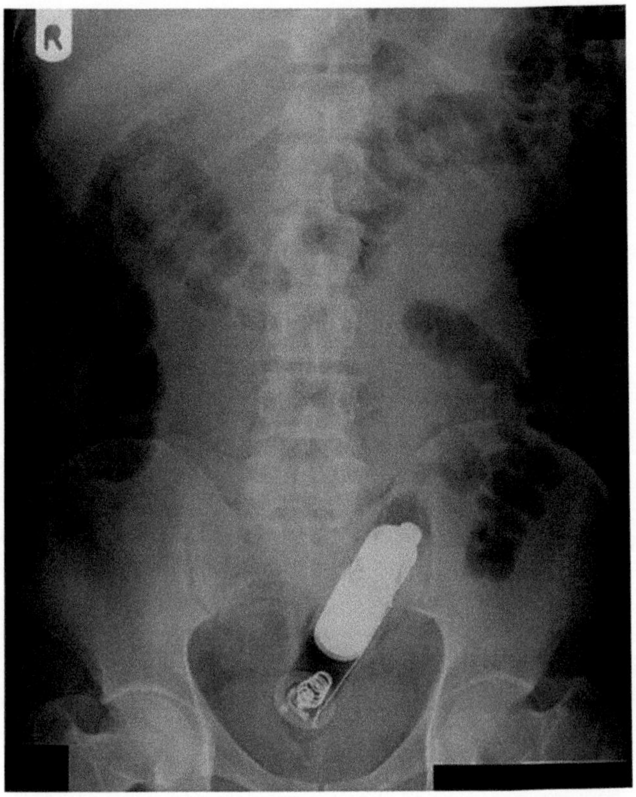

FIGURE 33-6. X-ray of an abdomen, which reveals a foreign body (sex toy) in the rectum [Reprinted from https://commons.wikimedia.org/wiki/File:CAVibrator.jpg. With permission from Creative Commons].

Prognosis

In the past, these injuries were usually associated with a poor recovery rate. However, with the advent of new treatment approaches discovered from experience with patients sustaining similar injuries in recent wars, prognosis has significantly improved. Additionally, the sooner the patient seeks treatment, the better the prognosis. However, death from anal perforation is still a realistic possibility.

Prevention

As with most sexual complications, abstinence is the most surefire way to avoid such complications. However, if patients insist on engaging in anal eroticism, then one must know that they are putting themselves at risk for the above complications.

Rectal Foreign Body Entrapment Rectal Foreign Body Entrapment

Epidemiology

Retained foreign bodies in the rectum can range from sex toys to an array of household products (bottles, toothbrushes, utensils, etc.).

While retained vaginal foreign bodies are only pertinent to females, retained rectal foreign bodies can be a problem for both men and women. However, they are far more common of a problem for male patients [35–37].

Clinical Presentation

In regards to patients presenting with a retained rectal FB, these patients almost always know they have got a retained FB in the rectum. They will usually complain of rectal pain and fullness. Additionally, if perforation has occurred, then patient will also present with severe abdominal pain [35–37].

Diagnostic Testing

Diagnosis of retained foreign bodies is primarily made by history and physical. Visual inspection and rectal examination via anal endoscopy will usually be sufficient for the clinician to locate the foreign body. Plain films of the abdomen are not only helpful in determining the presence of a rectal foreign body, but they are also very useful for assessing for rectal perforation (see Figure 33-6). However, a CT scan of the abdomen and pelvis will provide a definitive diagnosis of perforation as well as location of the foreign body [35–37].

Treatment

Once the clinician has located the foreign body, forceps may be used to pull the foreign body out. Anal blocks and sedation may ease the removal of rectal foreign bodies. However, certain rectal foreign bodies must be removed surgically, especially if perforation or impaction has occurred. Once the foreign body has been removed, the rectum must be inspected carefully for any tears or perforation. This can be done endoscopically. However, there are small tears that could be missed. One study revealed that Toluidine blue has been useful in locating small tears. Once the tear has been repaired, antibiotics (targeting intestinal flora) are administered to those with any evidence of external infection or peritonitis [34–37].

Prognosis

Like the other emergencies already mentioned, the sooner the foreign body is retrieved, the better the prognosis [38].

Postcoital Headaches

Epidemiology

Headaches associated with sexual activity account for about 3% of all headaches reported. These types of headaches are known as exertional headaches and occur either during sexual activity/climax or immediately after. Surprisingly, researchers have found that they are more common in males [39].

Clinical Presentation

These headaches (HA's) are described as general and throbbing (even pulsating) usually coming on acutely. They are categorized as primary or secondary. They are distinguished by several qualities. Primary headaches usually do not last for more than 48 h and they are usually gradual and throbbing. Typically, there are no associated neurologic deficits and can be both unilateral or at times, bilateral. On the other hand, coital headaches have been known to be secondary and triggered by another underlying comorbidity (i.e., migraine HA's, malignancy, intracerebral space-occupying lesions, and vascular abnormalities). These headaches have a sudden onset and are usually bilateral. Although both categories entail nausea, vomiting is primarily associated with secondary headaches and they are very severe in nature.

Researchers have described three types of headaches associated with sexual activity:

Type 1: Pressure-like Headache (HA) that involves the occipital region bilaterally and it usually comes on gradually and increases as sexual excitement is heightened.

Type 2: This is more of a sudden type of HA that feels explosive in nature and occurs just before or during orgasm. This is not to be confused with the acute thunderclap HA of a ruptured cerebral aneurysm (subarachnoid hemorrhage). This is the most common of all and unfortunately is the most concerning. Subsequently, other secondary underlying conditions need to be considered. Most of these were already mentioned above, but they include: subarachnoid hemorrhage (SAH), hemorrhagic stroke, certain drugs (contraceptives/illicit drugs/cardiac meds/ephedrine-containing meds), and a rare tumor known as pheochromocytoma.

Type 3: Headaches of this type are general and involve the entire head. They are worsened by certain positions. They are very similar to post-spinal headaches where CSF pressure is considered to be low [39].

Diagnosis

Patients who present with coital/postcoital HAs should be ruled out for other causes like those already mentioned. Neuro-imaging like a CT scan of the head should be performed. If however, patient's headache persists despite negative head CT and appropriate treatment, a lumbar puncture should be performed to rule out microscopic bleeding that may have occurred, but may no longer be visible on the head CT scan due to the change in blood properties over time [39].

Patients that present weeks later with symptoms after their last sexual encounter may need to have a more elaborate workup performed which may include an MRI with or without contrast, and a lumbar puncture if warranted [39].

Treatment

Usually treated with Ibuprofen (Indomethacin is the drug of choice) once intracerebral hemorrhage is ruled out. Initially, intravenous ibuprofen (Toradol) or opiates (Morphine) may be used for immediate relief. Patients may also be advised to pretreat each sexual encounter with propranolol (40–200 mg/day) or indomethacin (25–225 mg/day) [40, 41].

Prognosis and Prevention

The occurrence of one postcoital headache does not necessarily guarantee the same one will occur with every sexual encounter. Most of these headaches resolve. A patient could be advised to engage in less strenuous sexual activity. They may also be advised to pretreat with certain medications as mentioned above if they have recurrent symptoms. Those who have underlying disease processes must seek treatment for their underlying condition [40, 41].

Complications of Sexually Enhancing Medications

Introduction

While there is a separate chapter addressing sexual enhancers, we focus in this chapter on the possible emergencies that can arise from using certain sexual enhancers. Most of the discussion around emergencies due to sexual enhancers will occur regarding male sexual enhancers given how numerous they are in comparison to female sexual enhancers. There are a few female sexual enhancers available, but the FDA, has only approved one in particular. Subsequently, because of the relative newness of these medications, there is not a significant amount of scientific data to refer to. However, here is what we know so far. There are four types of sexual enhancers [42]. They are:

1. Prescription Medications

   There are three prescription drugs in particular that are used most frequently as male sexual enhancers. They are: Viagra, Cialis, and Levitra. These medications work by increasing blood flow to the penis.

   (a) Sildenafil (Viagra) was initially used to treat pulmonary hypertension. Serendipitously, it was found that male patients who used sildenafil also sustained an unintentional erection. Ultimately studies revealed that it did, indeed, substantially improve erectile dysfunction. Sildenafil is a vasodilator and it can lead to severe hypotension especially if taken with certain cardiac medications like nitroglycerine or other alpha antagonists. It is usually taken just prior to sexual activity [43, 44].
   (b) Tadalafil (Cialis) works like Viagra, but lasts longer and may be taken daily without regard to sexual activity since it lasts for about 24 h (higher doses will last longer for up to 72 h) [45].
   (c) Vardenafil (Levitra) works similarly to Viagra. The main difference is that it could be taken with alcohol and food [46].
   (d) There are also a couple of other sexual enhancers sold in the Black Market known as Spontane-ES and Stamina-RX, however, side effects and bad outcomes due to these meds may even be worse because they are said to contain even higher doses of the actual active ingredients found in the prescription medications [47, 48].
   (e) As for women, the FDA recently approved a drug called flibanserin (Addyi) for low Libido in women (also known as hypoactive sexual desire disorder) [49]. Flibanserin is a serotonin 1A receptor agonist and a serotonin 2A receptor antagonist. However, it is unclear by which mechanism this medication actually improves sexual function. Unlike sexually enhancing meds for men, flibanserin has to be taken daily and not only when improved sexual enhancement is desired. Additionally, a patient is not allowed to consume alcohol while taking this medication as it will potentiate the effects of flibanserin and ultimately lead to serious complications like severe hypotension or sedation [50, 51].

2. Herbal Supplements
   (a) Maca root is a starchy Andean root that is said to increase libido by increasing male testosterone. It also happens to be a nutritional staple of the Peruvian diet. However, there are no significant studies that prove that it does increase libido [52].
   (b) Tongkat Ali is an herb found in Malaysia, which is known to increase male testosterone levels. Unlike the Maca root, there have been a few studies out of Malaysia revealing that Tongkat Ali does indeed increase testosterone and erectile function, leading to enhanced libido [53].
   (c) Horny Goat Weed (Epimedium) is an herb originating in China and has been used for erectile dysfunction. Experts have suggested that it may even work better than prescription drugs and have fewer side effects. Its chemical property and its mechanism of action are very similar to the already existing prescriptions medications that currently exist for erectile dysfunction [54].
   (d) Muira Puama (also known as Potency Wood) is extracted from the bark and root of a plant found in South America. It is known as an aphrodisiac. Its GABA inhibitory properties are what were deemed to be the reason for sexual arousal [55].
3. Essential oils

   There are two oils in particular that are known to enhance sexual activity. These oils are known as Ylang Ylang and Jasmine. Either one is rubbed all over the body and are said to excite the body leading to enhanced sexual activity. There have not been any serious side effects from using such oils. These oils can be used on either men or women [56].
4. Natural enhancers

   Natural enhancers include stress reduction, regular exercise, a healthy diet, a secure sexual relationship, and use of erotic materials such as clothing, videos, and toys [42].

Epidemiology

Since the advent of male prescription sexual enhancers a little over a decade ago, far more men have found relief for their erectile dysfunction. There are, however, serious side effects that can occur as a result of their use.

The most common significant medical emergencies arising from sexual enhancers are severe hypotension, which can lead to syncope and stroke, priapism, and anaphylactic allergic reactions.

Clinical Presentation

There are three significant side effects that clinicians should be aware of:

(a) Syncope and Stroke: Patients may present to the Emergency department after having had a syncopal episode and their blood pressure will usually be low. Some patients whose blood pressure has dropped may complain of dizziness and near syncope. In some cases, a patient's blood pressure may have gotten so low that their cerebral blood pressure drops significantly, thereby leading to an ischemic stroke [57, 58]. A patient presenting with an ischemic stroke may have altered mental status, partial paralysis, or an expressive aphasia. If a stroke is suspected, emergent evaluation and treatment is essential.

(b) Priapism: Patients may come in complaining of prolonged and painful erection. Please refer to section on priapism above.

(c) Anaphylactic Reaction: Patients may come in complaining of a fullness in the throat and feeling like they cannot breathe and they may even have stridor on exam. Their blood pressure may be very low and they may present with a generalized erythematous rash, scattered hives, or both.

Diagnosis

Diagnosis of serious side effects is usually made by careful history and methodical review of a patient's entire medication list as certain side effects are worsened by the concurrent use of certain medications. There are currently no methods to detect oral sexual enhancing medications in the blood. Once the etiology of patient's symptoms is determined, the patient's treatment is targeted appropriately.

If a patient is suspected of having suffered a stroke, then a CT of the Head or even an MRI of the brain will be needed to make the diagnosis and rule out other causes for altered mental status/paralysis. More importantly, the patient's stroke may actually be due to a thromboembolic occlusion of the cerebral arteries which may necessitate the need for treatment with a thrombolytic like tissue plasminogen activator (TPA) [59].

Treatment

For low blood pressure and syncope, the treatment is to increase blood pressure mainly with intravenous fluids (IVFs). However, because some of these patients may also have comorbidities like heart disease, administration of IVFs should be done judiciously. The treating clinician should administer about 500 cc of fluid at a time and reassess each time for any fluid overload. If patient has not responded to a total of 2 L of IVF, then starting a continuous intravenous drip of a pressor like norepinephrine should be considered. Similar treatment would also apply to a patient presenting with an ischemic stroke due to a severe drop in blood pressure [59]. For treatment of priapism, please refer to the above section on priapism. For a patient presenting with an anaphylactic reaction, the treatment consists of Epinephrine 0.3 mg subcutaneously or intravenous (IV) push, Diphenhydramine (Benadryl) 50 mg IV push, Methylprednisolone (Solu-Medrol) 125 mg IV push, and Famotidine (Pepcid) 20 mg IV push. Patients usually show improvement within minutes of starting this treatment regimen. There are those rare occasions, however, where a repeat dose of epinephrine may need to be administered if the patient fails to respond to the first dose.

Prognosis

Most of these patients will do well with appropriate treatment, but it is difficult to predict outcome for those who have sustained an ischemic stroke as their prognosis may vary.

Prevention

There are a number of things that could be done in order to avoid any of the above complications. The most important form of prevention is to avoid the concomitant use of any medications that cause vasodilation, primarily nitroglycerine/alpha agonists. Patients should also stay well hydrated and it is prudent for patients to stand up gradually when getting up out of a bed or chair.

Researchers have also found that older patients appear to be at higher risk for these more serious complications. Clinicians are encouraged to take extra caution when prescribing these medications to older patients

Other Rare Sexual Complications

Air Embolism

While this is an extremely rare sexual complication, clinicians should be aware of an air embolism that results from cunnilingus (oral sex performed on a women). Somehow, air enters the circulation and ultimately leads to an air embolism. There have only been a little over a dozen cases reported and all of these women were pregnant and never made it to the hospital alive. There was one woman, however, that was not pregnant, who developed an air embolism after having air blown into her vagina. Interestlingly, this women did have an IUD in place, and it was thought that the IUD seemed to aid in the formation of the air embolism [60, 61].

If a patient happens to make it to the hospital, the treatment is to place the patient in Trendelenburg position or in left lateral decubitus position and administer high flow oxygen to the patient. Most of these patients, however, do not ever make it to a hospital in time as they die within minutes if the air embolism is large enough. Their prognosis is obviously very poor [60, 61].

Oculolinctus

There is a peculiar sexual fetish that seems to have become popular in Japan known as oculolinctus (also known as eye-ball licking). While it may seem harmless, the act can be associated with eye infections. When treating such infections, a clinician must also have to take into account pathogens that are usually associated with sexually transmitted diseases (e.g. Chlamydia) [62].

.

Conclusion

This chapter covers most of the more serious sexual emergencies that we are bound to see in the Emergency Department. However, it is very difficult to get an accurate count of how many sexual emergencies that do actually occur. Most patients have some level of shame associated with sexual injuries. Depending on the intensity of their shame will also depend on which patients will be forthcoming with the truth. As an emergency medicine physician, we hear a plethora of stories daily, some of them true, and others embellished, and others are not true at all. I once had a patient tell me that the rectal laceration he/she sustained was the result of his/her falling and landing on a knife that had been propped up in the door of his/her open dishwasher only to find out later that this was not the case at all.

Many times, the key to helping out patients whose presentations match those mentioned above is to obtain a very good history. It is advantageous to try to develop an immediate rapport with the patient. In some cases, this may be a very difficult task. However, in doing so, a clinician allows for the patient to trust their doctor and ultimately give them an honest story. By obtaining a precise history, it allows for a patient to receive appropriate and timely care. Subsequently, the patient's overall prognosis is improved.

References

1. Sydney L. 2016 Gross anatomy: you can't put that in there-nearly 450 sex injuries found in federal database. MedPage Today. http://www.medpagetoday.com/Blogs/GrossAnatomy/56174. Accessed 21 Oct 2016
2. Pfortmueller CA, Koetter JN, Zimmermann H, Exadaktylos AK. Sexual activity-related emergency department admissions: eleven years of experience at a Swiss university hospital. Emerg Med J. 2013;30(10):846–50. doi:10.1136/emermed-2012-201845.
3. Montague DK, Jarow J, Broderick GA, Dmochowski RR, Heaton JP, Lue TF, Nehra A, Sharlip ID, Members of the Erectile Dysfunction Guideline Update Panel; American Urological Association. American urological association guideline on the management of priapism. J Urol. 2003;170(4 Pt 1):1318–24.
4. Melman A, Serels S. Priapism. Int J Impot Res. 2000;12(Suppl 4):S133–9.
5. Ebbehoj J. A new operation for priapism. Scand J Plast Reconstr Surg. 1974;8(3):241–2.
6. Ercole CJ, Pontes JE, Pierce Jr JM. Changing surgical concepts in the treatment of priapism. J Urol. 1981;125(2):210–1.
7. Winter CC. Cure of idiopathic priapism: new procedure for creating fistula between glans penis and corpora cavernosa. Urology. 1976;8(4):389–91.
8. Lue TF, Pescatori ES. Distal cavernosum-glans shunts for ischemic priapism. J Sex Med. 2006;3(4):749–52.
9. Okpala I, Westerdale N, Jegede T, Cheung B. Etilefrine for the prevention of priapism in adult sickle cell disease. Br J Haematol. 2002;118(3):918–21.
10. Amer T, Wilson R, Chlosta P, AlBuheissi S, Qazi H, Fraser M, Aboumarzouk OM. Penile fracture: a meta-analysis. Urol Int. 2016;96(3):315–29.
11. Özorak A, Hoşcan MB, Oksay T, Güzel A, Koşar A. Management and outcomes of penile fracture: 10 years' experience from a tertiary care center. Int Urol Nephrol. 2014;46(3):519–22.
12. Buyukkaya R, Buyukkaya A, Ozturk B, Kayıkçı A, Yazgan Ö. Role of ultrasonography with color-Doppler in the emergency diagnosis of acute penile fracture: a case report. Med Ultrason. 2014;16(1):67–9.
13. Agarwal MM, Singh SK, Sharma DK, Ranjan P, Kumar S, Chandramohan V, Gupta N, Acharya NC, Bhalla V, Mavuduru R, Mandal AK. Fracture of the penis: a radiological or clinical diagnosis? A case series and literature review. Can J Urol. 2009; 16(2):4568–75.
14. Morey AF, Brandes S, Dugi III DD, Armstrong JH, Breyer BN, Broghammer JA, Erickson BA, Holzbeierlein J, Hudak SJ, Pruitt JH, Reston JT, Santucci RA, Smith III TG, Wessells H, American Urological Assocation. Urotrauma: AUA guideline. J Urol. 2014;192(2):327–35.
15. Pavan N, Tezzot G, Liguori G, Napoli R, Umari P, Rizzo M, Chiriacò G, Chiapparrone G, Vedovo F, Bertolotto M, Trombetta C. Penile fracture: retrospective analysis of our case history with long-term assessment of the erectile and sexological outcome. Arch Ital Urol Androl. 2014;86(4):359–70.
16. Gamal WM, Osman MM, Hammady A, Aldahshoury MZ, Hussein MM, Saleem M. Penile fracture: long-term results of surgical and conservative management. J Trauma. 2011;71(2):491–3.
17. EverydayHealth.com. How to Avoid Vaginal Cuts http://www.everydayhealth.com/sexual-health/avoiding-vaginal-cuts.aspx. Accessed 21 Oct 2016.
18. Jeng CJ, Wang LR. Vaginal laceration and hemorrhagic shock during consensual sexual intercourse. J Sex Marital Ther. 2007;33(3):249–53.
19. Symeonidis N, Ballas K, Micha A, Psarras K, Pavlidis T. Consensual intercourse resulting in an extensive rectovaginal tear: an extremely rare occurrence. J Sex Med. 2015;12(2):572–5.
20. Ugurel V, Özer DP, Varol F. A rare case of rectovaginal fistula following consensual vaginal intercourse. J Sex Med. 2014;11(5):1345–8.
21. Webmd.com. Vaginal foreign bodies. http://www.webmd.com/women/guide/foreign-body-vagina#1. Accessed 21 Oct 2016.
22. Kihara M, Sato N, Kimura H, Kamiyama M, Sekiya S, Takano H. Magnetic resonance imaging in the evaluation of vaginal foreign bodies in a young girl. Arch Gynecol Obstet. 2001;265(4):221–2.
23. Islam A, Arif S. Colouterine fistula with a foreign body. J Ayub Med Coll Abbottabad. 2010;22(2):205–7.
24. Bansal A, Kumar M, Goel S, Aeron R. Vesicovaginal fistula following insertion of a foreign body in the vagina for sexual gratification: could it be catastrophic pii: bcr2016214705? BMJ Case Rep. 2016;2016:9.
25. Miklos M, Moore M. Vesicovaginal fistula. http://www.miklosandmoore.com/vesicovaginal-fistula-atlanta/?gclid=CKro89zm388CFUONfgodBZEDeQ. Accessed 21 Oct 2016.
26. Mohamed M, Al-Ramahi G, McCann M. Postcoital hemoperitoneum caused by ruptured corpus luteal cyst: a hidden etiology pii rjv. J Surg Case Rep. 2015;2015(10):120.
27. Mayo Clinic Staff. Ovarian cysts. www.Mayoclinic.org. Accessed 21 Oct 2016.

28. Sharp H, Levine D, Falk S. FACOG evaluation and management of ruptured ovarian cyst. http://www.uptodate.com/contents/evaluation-and-management-of-ruptured-ovarian-cyst. Accessed 21 Oct 2016.
29. McColgin SW, Williams LM, Sorrells TL, Morrison JC. Hemoperitoneum as a result of coital injury without associated vaginal injury. Am J Obstet Gynecol. 1990;163(5 Pt 1):1503–5.
30. Reiner SC. Colorectal laceration after manual-anal intercourse. Ann Emerg Med. 1984;13(2):130–2.
31. Waraich NG, Hudson JS, Iftikhar SY. Vibrator-induced fatal rectal perforation. N Z Med J. 2007;120(1260):U2685.
32. Cohen C, Giles A, Nelson M. Sexual behavior, sexual trauma associated with fisting and recreational drugs. Sex Transm Infect. 2004;80:469–70.
33. Lohsiriwat V. Anorectal emergencies. World J Gastroenterol. 2016;22(26):5867–78.
34. Zink T, Fargo JD, Baker RB, Buschur C, Fisher BS, Sommers MS. Comparison of methods for identifying ano-genital injury after consensual intercourse. J Emerg Med. 2010;39(1):113–8.
35. Givel JC, Mortensen NJ, Roche B. Anorectal and colonic diseases: a practical guide to their management. 3rd ed. Berlin: Springer Verlag; 2010.
36. Cologne KG, Ault GT. Rectal foreign bodies: what is the current standard? Clin Colon Rectal Surg. 2012;25(4):214–8.
37. Coskun A, Erkan N, Yakan S, Yıldirim M, Cengiz F. Management of rectal foreign bodies. World J Emerg Surg 2013;8(1):11.
38. Al-Qurayshi ZH, Hauch AT, Slakey DP, Kandil E. Retained foreign bodies: risk and outcomes at the national level. J Am Coll Surg. 2015;220(4):749–59.
39. Cutrer MF. Headaches associated with exertion and sexual activity. Mayo Clinic. https://americanheadachesociety.org/wp-content/uploads/2016/07/F._Michael_Cutrer_-_Headaches_Associated_with_Exertion_and_Sexual_Activity.pdf. Accessed 21 Oct 2016.
40. Frese A, Rahmann A, Gregor N, Biehl K, Husstedt I-W, Evers S. Headache associated with sexual activity: prognosis and treatment options. Cephalalgia. 2007;27:1265–70.
41. Pascual J, Inglesias F, Oterino MD, Vazquez-Barquero MD, Bericano J. Cough, exertional, and sexual headaches: an analysis of 72 benign and symptomatic cases. Neurology. 1996;46:1520–4.
42. Len B. Male sexual enhancers—4 types of sexual enhancers for men. http://www.sooperarticles.com/health-fitness-articles/sexual-health-articles/male-sexual-enhancers-4-types-sexual-enhancers-men-4514.html. Accessed 21 Oct 2016.
43. Loran OB, Ströberg P, Lee SW, Park NC, Kim SW, Tseng LJ, Collins S, Stecher VJ. Sildenafil citrate 100 mg starting dose in men with erectile dysfunction in an international, double-blind, placebo-controlled study: effect on the sexual experience and reducing feelings of anxiety about the next intercourse attempt. J Sex Med. 2009;6(10):2826–35.
44. Sabourin G. Potentially deadly: warning about Revatio (sildenafil) taken with nitroglycerine. Perspect Infirm. 2010;7(5):42.
45. Eardley I, Cartledge J. Tadalafil (Cialis) for men with erectile dysfunction. Int J Clin Pract. 2002;56(4):300–4.
46. Porst H, Rosen R, Padma-Nathan H, Goldstein I, Giuliano F, Ulbrich E, Bandel T. The efficacy and tolerability of vardenafil, a new, oral, selective phosphodiesterase type 5 inhibitor, in patients with erectile dysfunction: the first at-home clinical trial. Int J Impot Res. 2001;13(4):192–9.
47. WebMD. Stamina-Rx supplements recalled-FDA finds products contain an unapproved drug that may pose health risks. http://www.webmd.com/erectile-dysfunction/news/20090617/stamina-rx-supplements-recalled. Accessed 21 Oct 2016.
48. AssociatedPress. Popping herbal sex pills linked to increased risk of stroke, headaches, vision problems. Published 13 Nov 2007. http://www.foxnews.com/story/2007/11/13/report-popping-herbal-sex-pills-linked-to-increased-risk-stroke-headaches.html. Accessed 21 Oct 2016.
49. Puppo G, Puppo V. U.S. Food and Drug Administration approval of Addyi (Flibanserin) for treatment of hypoactive sexual desire disorder. Eur Urol. 2016;69(2):379–80.
50. Terrier C, Terrier JE. Efficacy and safety of flibanserin "new female Viagra(®)"? Literature review. Prog Urol. 2016;pii:S1166–7087(16)30415–8.
51. Fantasia HC. Nurs Womens Health. Flibanserin Female Sex Desire 2016;20(3):309–314.
52. Shin BC, Lee MS, Yang EJ, Lim HS, Ernst E. Maca (*L. meyenii*) for improving sexual function: a systematic review. BMC Complement Altern Med. 2010;10:44.
53. Kotirum S, Ismail SB, Chaiyakunapruk N. Efficacy of Tongkat Ali (Eurycoma longifolia) on erectile function improvement: systematic review and meta-analysis of randomized controlled trials. Complement Ther Med. 2015;23(5):693–8.
54. Corazza O, Martinotti G, Santacroce R, Chillemi E, Di Giannantonio M, Schifano F, Cellek S. Sexual enhancement products for sale online: raising awareness of the psychoactive effects of yohimbine, maca, horny goat weed, and *Ginkgo biloba*. Biomed Res Int. 2014;2014:841798.
55. Adimoelja A. Phytochemicals and the breakthrough of traditional herbs in the management of sexual dysfunctions. Int J Androl. 2000;23(Suppl 2):82–4.
56. Tan LT, Lee LH, Yin WF, Chan CK, Abdul Kadir H, Chan KG, Goh BH. Traditional uses, phytochemistry, and bioactivities of *Cananga odorata* (Ylang-Ylang). Evid Based Complement Alternat Med. 2015;2015:896314.
57. Strandgaard S, Olesen J, Skinhoj E, Lassen NA. Autoregulation of brain circulation in severe arterial hypertension. Br Med J. 1973;1(5852):507–10.
58. Hoshide S, Eguchi K, Ishikawa J, Murata M, Katsuki T, Mitsuhashi T, Shimada K, Kario K. Can ischemic stroke be caused by acute reduction of blood pressure in the acute phase of cardiovascular disease? J Clin Hypertens (Greenwich). 2008;10(3):195–200.
59. Powers WJ, Derdeyn CP, Biller J, Coffey CS, Hoh BL, Jauch EC, Johnston KC, Johnston SC, Khalessi AA, Kidwell CS, Meschia JF, Ovbiagele B, Yavagal DR, American Heart Association Stroke Council. 2015 American Heart Association/American Stroke Association focused update of the 2013 guidelines for the early management of patients with acute ischemic stroke regarding endovascular treatment: a guideline for healthcare professionals from the American Heart Association/American Stroke Association. Stroke. 2015;46(10):3020–35.
60. Marc B, Chadly A, Durigon M. Fatal air embolism during female autoerotic practice. Int J Leg Med. 1990;104(1):59–61.
61. Aronson ME, Nelson PK. Fatal air embolism in pregnancy resulting from an unusual sexual act. Obstet Gynecol. 1967;30(1):127–30.
62. Herbenick D. Semen in the eye: is it dangerous? What should i do if i get sperm in my eye? My sex professor, April 15, 2009. http://mysexprofessor.com/how-to-have-sex/semen-in-the-eye-is-it-dangerous-what-should-i-do/. Accessed 21 Oct 2016

34 Sex and Quality of Life

Jared Matt Greenberg, Kyle P. Smith, Tae Y. Kim, Lancer Naghdechi, and Waguih William IsHak

Defining Quality of Life and Measuring Sexual Quality of Life

The World Health Organization (WHO) defined "Quality of life" (QoL) as the "individuals' perception of their position in life in the context of the culture and value systems in which they live and in relation to their goals, expectations, standards and concerns," which is further broken down into three elements: (1) subjective evaluation, (2) cultural, social, and environmental context, and (3) assessment of specific life domains such as health, work, family, and social relations, and leisure activities [1] (Figure 34-1). QoL is often used in a generic fashion in reference to general health and well-being, and is frequently used in literature interchangeably with terms like functioning, functional impairment, or psychosocial functioning [2]. It is important to this discussion to define terminology and to be as explicit as possible. Functioning is defined as one's *performance* in activities such as work, love, and play as rated by self or observers, whereas QoL refers to one's *satisfaction* and *perception* with the aforementioned by self-report [2].

Lastly, the WHO defines sexual health as "a state of physical, emotional, mental and social well-being in relation to sexuality; [...] not merely the absence of disease, dysfunction or infirmity. Sexual health requires a positive and respectful approach to sexuality and sexual relationships, as well as the possibility of having pleasurable and safe sexual experiences, free of coercion, discrimination and violence. For sexual health to be attained and maintained, the sexual rights of all persons must be respected, protected and fulfilled" [3].

Sex is a key function of human beings. Its physical, emotional, psychological, and social aspects permeate into many parts of our lives. Thus it is not difficult to see how sexual health and functioning plays a crucial role in one's QoL, nor is it surprising to learn that QoL worsens in the presence of sexual dysfunction as has been shown by numerous studies on various disorders and dysfunctions [4].

We begin our discussion on sexual QoL with measurements of sexual function and QoL and how the two are interrelated. In a nationally representative sample consisting of 3515 sexually active US adults, 62.2% of men and 42.8% of women considered sexual health as "highly important" to QoL [5]. There are many direct and indirect methods of assessing sexual function in females and males using questionnaires, devices, and/or lab values. In men, erectile functioning can be directly measured using Nocturnal Penile Tumescence devices, intracavernosal injections with prostaglandin E1, penile brachial pressure indices, Doppler studies, and sacral evoked potentials. In women, genital blood peak systolic velocity, vaginal pH, intravaginal compliance, and genital vibratory perception thresholds can assess sexual function directly. Useful lab values indirectly assessing sexual function can include testosterone, luteinizing hormone (LH), estrogen, and/or prolactin levels. Given the various methods of assessing sexual function, it should be noted that there is no "best" measurement since many are not well researched and almost none are used in clinical practice [6].

In addition to these measurements, self-reports can be used to assess the psycho-physiological aspects of sex looking at desire or satisfaction, as described by Kaplan and Levine, respectively [7]. Arrington et al. performed a literature review looking at 62 questionnaires measuring sexual function to determine the domains most commonly assessed and to examine evidence for their usefulness in different populations. Their results showed six commonly represented domains: interest and desire, satisfaction/quality of experience, excitement/arousal, performance, attitude/behavior (attitudes or behaviors of the respondent and his or her partner such as feelings of avoidance, embarrassment, and change in frequency of sexual intercourse), and impact of sexual functioning on relationship. Of note, their results also showed that only nine of the questionnaires had evidence for both adequate reliability and validity and that no single questionnaire was universally useful for researchers or clinicians to measure sexual function [6].

W.W. IsHak (ed.), *The Textbook of Clinical Sexual Medicine*, DOI 10.1007/978-3-319-52539-6_34

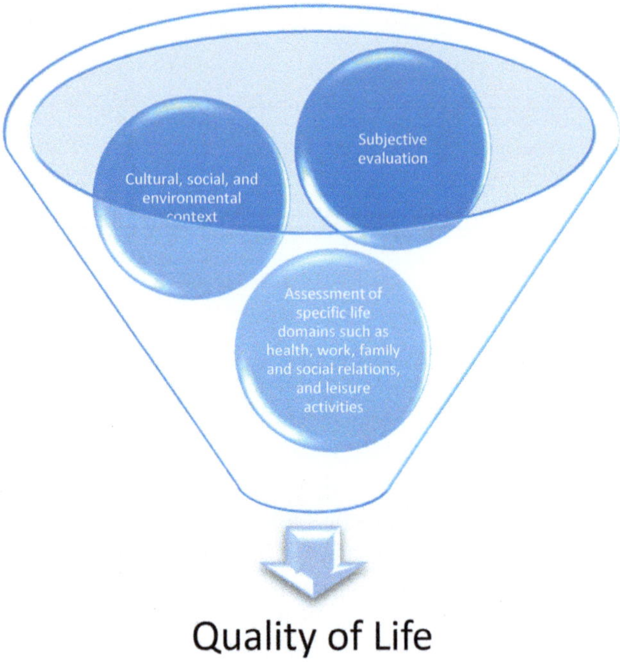

FIGURE 34-1. Quality of life elements.

Several studies have demonstrated the effects of sexual dysfunction on QoL. For example, Helgason et al. developed a questionnaire they called "Radiumhemmets Scale of Sexual Functioning" which measures sexual desire, erectile capacity, orgasm, and to what extent a decrease in any of these aspects of sexual functioning affects QoL. Of the 53 men treated with radiation therapy for localized prostate cancer who were sent this questionnaire, 48 men answered the question regarding the extent to which decreased function affected QoL. Fifty percent of those men stated that decreased erectile capacity affected their QoL "much" or "very much." Decreased orgasm function was reported to reduce QoL as much in 46% of cases and decreased sexual wishes in 33% [8].

In a Brazilian study of 56 women undergoing hemodialysis for end stage renal disease, 46 women with sexual dysfunction had worse QoL (especially physical aspects of QoL) when compared to women without sexual dysfunction. Sexual function was measured using the 19-item validated Female Sexual Function Index (FSFI) and QoL was measured using the Brazilian version of the Medical Outcomes Study 36-Item Short Form Health Questionnaire (SF-36), a well-validated 36-item questionnaire covering eight dimensions of QoL: physical functioning, role-physical, bodily pain, general health, vitality, social functioning, role-emotional, and mental health [9].

Similarly, a Korean study including 137 women who had been treated with surgery or radiotherapy for cervical cancer showed that sexual function (measured using FSFI) had a negative relationship with depression while having a positive relationship with QoL, as measured by Functional Assessment of Cancer Therapy-General Version 4. This scale is composed of a total of 26 items with four subcategories, with a five-point Likert scale ranging from 0 (*never*) to 4 points (*always*) for each item: physical well-being, social well-being, emotional well-being, and functional well-being. Results showed that physical well-being, social well-being, and functional well-being, but not psychological well-being were positively correlated to sexual dysfunction [10].

A Turkish study assessing sexual function and QoL (using the FSFI and the SF-36, respectively) of 67 women with dyspareunia that were matched to 87 sexually healthy women showed that in the dyspareunia group, not only was sexual dysfunction more prevalent and severe than expected, but QoL was lower, specifically with regard to the domains of physical role, social function, bodily pain, and vitality.

In a 2010 study, 33 men and nine women who had undergone heart transplantation were evaluated for QoL (using the Quality of Life Enjoyment and Satisfaction Questionnaire—Short Form and the Short Form 12 Health Survey Questionnaire) and sexual dysfunction (using the International Index of Erectile Dysfunction and the Female Sexual Function Index). The authors reported that the overall prevalence of sexual dysfunction among participants was 61%, with 78% of men and 50% of women being affected, and no significant difference in measures between genders. Heart transplant recipients with sexual dysfunction reported significantly worse QoL on measures of physical health when compared to those without sexual dysfunctions. [11]

It should be noted that by using sexual function to predict QoL, one could fail to recognize the psychological aspects of patients' subjective experiences. This is evident in erectile dysfunction as it can be a physiological and/or psychological condition.

Several questionnaires exist having to do with sexual function and QoL, some broad (having to do with general health and well-being) such as WHO's Health Related QoL, and some disease specific. When evaluating the sexual aspect of QoL, though, it is important to have a tool that is more sensitive to change (as opposed to general QoL questionnaires) that can be used to compare different populations and disease processes [12].

This was the goal when Symonds et al. created the SQOL-F, a questionnaire that specifically assesses the relationship between female sexual dysfunction and QoL. The SQOL-F is based on Spitzer's Quality of Life model involving physical, emotional, psychological, and social components. Interviews with 82 women ages 19–65 from the UK, USA, Australia, France, Denmark, Holland, and Italy were used to generate the items in the questionnaire. The questionnaire consists of 18 items rated on a six-point scale, ranging from "completely agree" to "completely disagree" which can be scored 1–6 or 0–5, generating scores of 18–108 or 0–90, respectively, with higher scores indicating better sexual QoL in females. The SQOL-F defines sexual life as "both the physical sexual activities and the emotional sexual relationship that the individual has with their partner" and sexual activity as "any activity which may result in sexual stimulation or sexual pleasure, e.g. intercourse, caressing, foreplay, masturbation (i.e. self-masturbation or partner masturbation) and oral sex" [13].

Validity of the SQOL-F was first shown in the UK and USA where internal consistency was 0.95 and intraclass correlation coefficient was reported to be 0.85 [14]. More recently, an Iranian version of the SQOL-F showed that the questionnaire is a valid and reliable instrument for evaluation of female sexual QoL [14]. In addition, the SQOL-F showed good convergent validity with the 28 item Sexual Functioning Questionnaire (SFQ28) [15].

Following in the footsteps of the SQOL-F came the Sexual Quality of Life-Male (SQOL-M) questionnaire, containing 11 items (seven less than the SQOL-F), each with a six-point Likert-like response scale ranging from "completely agree" to "completely disagree." To allow easy comparisons with other measures, raw scores were transformed into a standardized scale of 0–100. The SQOL-M has seven fewer items than the SQOL-F: two on relationship, one related to emotional well-being, three related to frequency and avoidance of sexual activity, and one on overall enjoyment [12].

The importance of obtaining a subjective measure such as QoL in patients with sexual dysfunctions, as opposed to solely one of sexual function, lies in the fact that many, if not all, sexual dysfunctions are composed of both a physiologic (functional) aspect and a psychological aspect. Satisfaction with one's sexual life may not be related to their physiologic functioning as can be seen with psychogenic erectile dysfunction, or any other psychogenic sexual dysfunction.

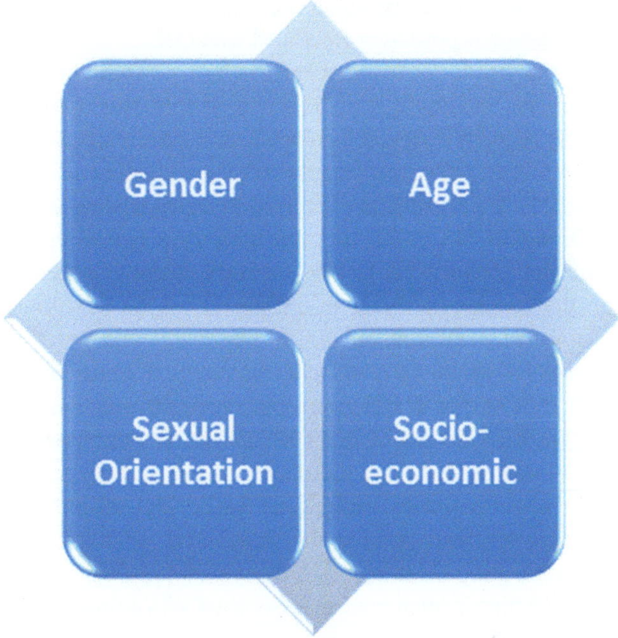

FIGURE 34-2. Nonclinical demographic groups.

Sex and Quality of Life in Nonclinical Populations

Introduction

Analysis of literature on sexual health and QoL confirms what people implicitly understand—that having good sexual health or sexual quality of life (SQoL) is integral to having a high QoL [16]. According to Hawkes (1996), our society's heavy biomedical emphasis on sexuality indicates that we consider healthy sexuality to be synonymous with good health [17]. Since good health is the single most important factor in determining QoL across all age groups [18–20], there is a significant correlation between good sexual health and QoL [21].

The vast majority of studies on sex and QoL have been done on clinical populations with specific pathological conditions in order to understand how those specific conditions affect the patients' sexual health. Studies on sex and QoL on nonclinical populations (Figure 34-2), or rather on a broader concept of sex and QoL, are sparse in comparison and can often seem outdated, perhaps due to the dynamic nature of the subject itself.

Sexual health is multifactorial. It cannot be measured purely objectively or purely physically, but instead, subjective interpretations of one's sexual health play an important role in how we understand the quality of one's sexual health [20, 22, 23]. Given that subjective idealization of sex is heavily influenced by one's cultural upbringing, cultural context becomes another important factor in our understanding of sex and QoL [24]. For example, the sexual revolution of the 1960s was initiated by the changing economical and geopolitical realm of the preceding decades [25]. Also, the practice and interpretation of sex and QoL in the Medieval period was dictated by the dominant religious culture [26]. Cultures are ever-changing and so are the values of sexual normality associated within a specific culture. It seems prudent to point out that different individuals experience different aspects of the dominant culture, which may distinctively impact each individual's sexual health and QoL. Therefore, different groups of people vary widely in their interpretation and understanding of good sexual health. Because of this variation caused by the subjectivity of SQoL, it is important to examine how good sexual health differs among people and what the characteristic features of those differences are. Regardless of the differences, the literature draws a common conclusion, which is that good sexual health is positively correlated with QoL.

Sexual health is often perceived as just the ability to have intercourse, but multiple studies point out that it also depends heavily on body image, sexual behavior, reproductive health, different forms of sexual expression [27], and even education level [21]. Such variability involved in understanding sexual health points to the idea that the interplay between physiologic and psychosocial factors is a key element in determining the context in which sexual health can be monitored, determined, measured, or studied. Especially when examining sexual health in a nonclinical population where the decline of sexual health is not pathologically induced, the psychosocial aspects of one's sexual health must take the central role in furthering our understanding of the relationship between sexual health and QoL. The relationship between sex and QoL among nonclinical populations is harder to grasp than in clinical populations. Their sexual health decline is often gradual, associated with aging [21, 24, 28–31], and in some cases is hidden due to subclinical depression. Furthermore, the lack of a clinical diagnosis makes it harder for these individuals to evaluate their sexual health and thus correlate it to their general QoL.

In most of the studies on sexual health and QoL reviewed in this section, data was collected using validated questionnaires for measuring QoL, such as those created by the World Health Organization (WHO) or variations developed for use in specific populations. Other questionnaires used include the Comprehensive Quality of Life Scale (COMQOL), the Sexual Knowledge, Experience, and Needs Scale [20], and the Sexual Quality of Life–Female (SQOL-F) questionnaire [13]. In these cases, study participants are asked to use a scale to rate satisfaction with various aspects of their life including sexuality. The WHO questionnaires cover six domains of life including social relationships, psychology, and physical domains [32]. It is within these three domains that sexual health plays a particularly important role and demonstrates a positive correlation with QoL [18]. In Daker-White and Donovan's studies on heterosexual relationships and QoL, due to the variety of circumstances that effect the testing subjects' sex and QoL, detailed responses regarding their sexual life, rather than a scale, were recorded and analyzed to reach a conclusion [28]. According to WHO, having standardized questionnaires that can measure QoL is important for helping to determine treatment decisions, fund allocation and policy research, and gain an anthropological understanding of various cultures [32].

Gender Differences

To fully understand the relationship between sexual health and QoL among nonclinical populations, first considering clinical populations and their pathological sexual dysfunction can give insights into the nature of normal sexual health. Normal sexual health is dependent on a complex interplay between the physical and psychosocial facets of an individual, while sexual dysfunction is contingent upon a person's previous sexual experiences before they started noticing problems. The American Psychiatric Association places an emphasis on requiring "clinically significant distress" to define sexual dysfunction [33], meaning it relies on a subjective interpretation. In addition, WHO categorizes sexual health in the social domain rather than in the physical domain [28, 32], meaning it is subjected to environmental influences. Hence, we must be aware of the different psychosocial reasons that cause distress and be cautious about how we use the term sexual dysfunction [34].

In studies conducted by Daker-White and Donovan [28] on heterosexual British hospital patients experiencing the sexual dysfunction due to physical causes, distinct differences between males and females emerged in terms of what constitutes as having "normal" sexual health. In general, the interviewees' descriptions of what distressed them most about their sexual health showed that for women normal sexual health means having the ability to fulfill expected sexual work as someone who is supposed to receive sexual satisfaction, and abnormal sexual health occurs when they have issues related to fulfilling that work. Their inability to fulfill expectations was usually caused by two issues. One was a concern about their physical appearances not being able to stimulate their partners. This indicates the presence of issues related to the quality of the relationship with their sexual partners or their confidence level, which is influenced by societal norms and psychological conflicts. The second cause was physical pain during intercourse. In contrast, for men, sexual dysfunction was distressing mainly due to their inability to perform the expected work of sex. The "work" was to perform and accomplish sexual intercourse, and their physical limitations prevented them from satisfying their urges and accomplishing sexual intimacy. In summary, this study points to the notion that female sexual health is more contingent on external influences.

There have been many other studies that examined physical sexual health in male populations. Erectile dysfunction (ED), premature ejaculation (PE), and hypogonadism have all been associated with poor QoL in both mental and physical domains [35–37]. Other studies that focused exclusively on females showed that sexual health satisfaction was based on a combination of sexual function, psychological well-being, and strength of their relationship with their partner [38, 39]. Hawton et al. found that among middle aged women with partners, the quality of their marriage had the highest correlation to the frequency of intercourse, orgasm, and sexual satisfaction, while all other factors such as age, gynecological, and psychiatric symptoms made little difference [40]. More reviews of studies on gender differences are discussed within the context of demographic differences.

Age Differences

Young Populations

A large number of studies have been conducted to assess sexual health and QoL in different age groups. Most of the studies were focused on either middle aged (40–60 years old) or elderly populations (>60 years old), with very few studies on the young adult and adolescent populations. The reason for this might be the relatively recent development of effective treatment for male sexual dysfunction that may come with aging which, given increasing longevity, makes addressing sex and QoL in older adults an ever more important topic.

The few studies on young adult populations further support our understanding that sex and QoL are deeply affected by psychosocial influences. In comparison to the data that was collected in the 1960s and 1970s, more young adults in the 1980s and 1990s linked sex with love and relationships [41]. A study conducted on Australian university students revealed that sex was understood as a natural part of a developing relationship and that relationships were considered to be a very important part of maintaining high subjective QoL [20]. Sex-related issues that had a negative association with QoL were anxieties caused by peer pressure and unrealistic expectations related to sex among the sexually inexperienced [42]. Anything that detracted from school, friends, and dating, such as pregnancy, also negatively impacted QoL. Overall, studies revealed that sex in the context of love and relationships was associated with both a higher objective and subjective assessment of QoL. Although the studies on young adults and adolescents seem to focus on sexual behavior and how sex and QoL change over time due to cultural influences, there does not seem to be an equal amount of research interest in sex and QoL when there is physical sexual dysfunction. Most likely it is due to the fact that sexual dysfunction is more associated with aging, but such a study would help us understand how sex and QoL in young adult and adolescent populations suffering from sexual dysfunction differ in the way they are influenced by cultural norms on sex.

Middle-Aged and Older Adults

When reviewing studies regarding sex and QoL in middle-aged populations, we find that physical dysfunction starts to play a bigger role in determining SQoL than in younger populations. But the studies also show that subjective assessment of SQoL is intertwined with not only physical but also psychosocial influences. In a study that was conducted on middle-aged male and female populations in Korea [21], body image, depression, education level, SQoL, and stress levels were all strong predictors influencing QoL. A study done exclusively on midlife females showed that depression and negative body image were considered the strongest negative influences on QoL, replicating the Korean study and at the same time differentiating what is most crucial in QoL between the genders [43]. In another study conducted in a middle-aged female population, healthy relationships with sexual partners were considered the strongest positive influence on sexual satisfaction, while feelings about body or attractiveness had no effect [39]. Other studies in female populations also shared similar findings: self-reported physical sexual dysfunction did not always coincide with low SQoL [39, 44]. This meant that when evaluating SQoL, other sexual health concerns such as emotional satisfaction and self-esteem achieved through sexual intercourse, emotional and physical well-being, and healthy relationships with partners should all be addressed instead of focusing solely on sexual satisfaction through physical contact.

Increasing life expectancy has directed much focus on examining QoL in elderly populations [45–47]. One study indicates that sexual desire and activity are widespread among middle-aged and elderly populations [22], and many older men and women are physically capable of enjoying orgasm and sexual excitement well into their 70s and beyond [29, 31]. Yet, the prevalence of sexual dysfunction is high among this population [22], contributing to poorer QoL. Many studies also show that as in the middle-aged populations, psychosocial factors of sexual health are a crucial part of SQoL in the elderly. It is generally agreed that sexual activity and the frequency of it are associated with psychological and physical health, and positively correlate with satisfaction in life and marriage [48], and also with QoL [47]. This makes sexual activity and its link to QoL an especially important factor to consider for the older population [31, 49]. Older adults are more likely to suffer from sexual dysfunction that is physical in nature [50] and so it makes sense to conclude that in these populations, particularly in men, the most important predictor of sexual activity is physical health. Interestingly though, for the older female population, the most important predictor of frequency of sex was still the quality of the relationship [31]. Overall, sexual activity in older populations was related to their previous level of sexual activity, sexual interest between the partners, and physical health [51]. It is easy to understand how deficiency in any of these factors can lead to poor sexual health and QoL.

The physical and psychosocial aspects of sexual health and QoL were also emphasized in a study conducted on a rural older Indonesian population [24]. This study highlights the importance of culture and age in association with sex and QoL. Akin to other studies, infrequency of sexual activity and sexual dysfunction were associated with poor QoL in both men and women. Among this population, the main reason couples did not engage in sexual activity was due to lack of a partner's interest, which could either be due to physical or psychosocial reasons, but the study did not clarify the cause of the disinterest. Physical limitation was a main reason for the sexual dysfunction and thus caused a negative impact on QoL, but the study also showed that married men with sexual dysfunction had a significantly higher subjective assessment of QoL than unmarried men. The author theorized that this difference was probably due to the heightened social and emotional support that comes with marriage in this specific culture, indicating that different cultural norms surrounding marriage affects sex and QoL differently.

Sexual Orientation Differences

The impact of psychosocial factors on SQoL is especially pronounced when reviewing sex and QoL studies done in LGBT populations. Sexuality is often described as having three dimensions: sexual attraction, sexual behavior, and sexual identification [52–54]. Sexual attraction and behavior are mostly physically dictated, but sexual identification is largely influenced by the culture and how people define their physical attraction in their own psychosocial context. Sexual identification can become problematic to psychological and general health, SQoL and overall QoL when it is not in agreement with one's sexual behavior or attraction.

A study that was conducted in the Netherlands with LGBT populations found that homosexual men, but not homosexual women, had lower QoL in various domains of QoL assessments than their heterosexual counterparts [55]. The authors conclude that the differences in QoL between homosexual men and women validate the theory that there are other factors influencing QoL than purely sexual attraction or behavior. A similar finding that sexual behavior alone is not directly linked to QoL was also noted in a study conducted by Horowitz, Weis, and Laflin [56]. In the Netherlands study, homosexual men had less-positive evaluations of their general health, mental health, and emotional health, and they were also assessed to have more comorbid psychiatric conditions than their heterosexual counterparts. It is generally well accepted that such a finding is due to the stigma and discrimination felt by LGBT populations, which creates psychological distresses [57–59] and the eventual demise of general QoL. It is important to point out that low QoL was associated with riskier sexual behavior such as unprotected anal sex [60, 61]. Traeen et al. compared QoL of LGBT college age populations across different countries and showed that in cultures that had a more accepting attitude towards homosexuality, LGBT individuals had better QoL [23]. The article points out that for women living in a culture where homosexuality is more accepted, having sex with another woman can be interpreted as an "expression of self-realization and social competence." This, as well as the fact that women tend to be better at forming a community for social support [52], may explain the reason why in the Netherlands study, homosexual women did not suffer lower QoL than their heterosexual counterparts. Data from a Norwegian university age population showed that homosexual and bisexual women actually scored higher on the personal growth scale than heterosexual women [23].

So far the concept of how sexual identification relates to QoL has been discussed. But just as straight women were found to have specific physical concerns associated with their SQoL that were different from men, there are physical sexual concerns for homosexual men and women that are different from their straight counterparts. For both gay men and women, the heterosexual assumption of their sexual orientation by the larger society becomes problematic, especially as they seek health care. They can fear rejection of their sexual orientation or have their particular gender orientation–related sexual needs ignored by their caretakers. A study by Rose, Ussher, and Perz on gay and bisexual men with prostate cancer investigates this particular issue. They point out that in current medical practice, support for sexual rehabilitation after prostate cancer surgery focuses solely on restoring men's erectile function just enough to achieve vaginal intercourse, all while ignoring the alternative anal intercourse practiced by gay and bisexual men where a stiffer erection is often required [62]. One important aspect of anal intercourse and pleasure is also addressed in this study. The notion among many homosexual men that the prostate is "the male G-spot" is completely ignored during prostate cancer treatment, so that this important pleasure center is disregarded as significant to the well-being of the patient following treatment [63].

Waite conducted a study of lesbian women which found that double discrimination due to both female gender and sexual orientation, also referred to as lesbophobia, was found to have a negative impact on QoL. Lesbians are frequently subjected to microaggression by the dominant culture, where comments about them not having children or not having a man, messages that invalidate their lived experiences and identity, position them as inferior or inadequate [64, 65]. It is also clinically relevant to note that more than half of older lesbians are found to have the highest number of risk factors for breast cancer due to their age, in some cases having never had children, and possibly having never breast-fed [66], a pathophysiological perspective often overlooked by healthcare professionals.

Socioeconomic Differences

Data on socioeconomic factors (SEF) related to sex and QoL are limited, but a few studies provide insight into how they can affect sexual health and QoL. In a study conducted by Aytaç et al. [67] in a male popuation in Massachussetts, it was found that men with blue-collar occupations had a much higher likelihood of developing ED. The author did not investigate if ED had a direct negative effect on their QoL, but as shown in previous studies of sex and QoL in men, having any kind of demise in sexual function can adversely affect SQoL and overall QoL. Although the explanation for this correlation between blue-collar occupations and ED is unclear, the data seems to decline in overal general health as a possible cause. People with low socioeconomic status (SES), specifically those having income lower than $40,000 per year, were twice as likely to experience depression, and populations with low education were more likely to suffer from diabetes and hypertension. It is a well-accepted medical concept that depression, hypertension, and diabetes contribute to sexual dysfunction in men [28, 43, 68]. The Massachusetts study concluded that besides age, occupation had the highest association with ED of any SEF, accounting for 47% of the variance in ED risk. The author interestingly theorized that perhaps the demise of general health and sexual dysfunction in populations with lower SES could be due to the numerous social inequalities—and related levels of stress—they encounter that cannot directly be measured [67].

Similar findings with regard to sexual dysfunction were also noted in studies conducted on other highly stressed populations. Medical residents and students spend long hours working and studying in highly stressed environments with overwhelming responsibilities and lack of free time. It was found that these stressors have a negative effect on sexual function in female populations but not in male populations, and on sexual dissatisfaction in both male and female populations [69]. Such an observation again supports the notion that, first, negative psychosocial factors lower SQoL, and second, that perhaps for women, sexual function and health is more dependent on psychosocial influences than for their male counterparts.

Among women, it is important to note that although relationship status was the most important factor in sexual satisfaction, SES also had a positive influence on the frequency of sex and satisfaction [40]. As suggested by Aytaç et al., low SES is a source of stress, which affects psychosocial function, and this in turn affects SQoL to varying degrees [67].

Conclusion

The interface between sexuality and QoL is an evolving field of study. Our understanding and practice of sex are contexual in that they change with the passage of time and shifting cultural influences such as the economy, belief systems, and science. Griffin's sociological study [70] on the rapid rise of illegitimacy revealed that the industrial revolution has brought a new sense of sexual freedom that did not exist in the preindustrial era. Currently, as we go through the internet revolution, we are already seeing signs of change in how we define and address sexual health. Searching through a list of peer reviewed articles found using the keywords *internet* and *sex*, there are numerous studies on pathologic internet behavior of sex seeking and viewing of pornography [71–74]. The studies mostly examine risks associated with such behaviors and try to determine the extent of the negative effects internet usage can have on general well-being. As internet usage evolves further, it will be important to study the potential the internet has to help individuals improve their sexual health and QoL. By doing quick "how to" searches on various forums related to sex, there are already signs of some positive impacts of the internet on SQoL. Just as the industrial revolution brought us economic freedom which allowed people to enjoy and practice sex the way they wanted to, the internet revolution is in the process of giving us the informational freedom [75] to be able to identify sexual problems, find out about available remedies, and seek help.

Sex and Quality of Life in Medical and Surgical Disorders and Their Treatments

Introduction

A wide variety of medical conditions, and physical health in general, can impact sexual function to varying degrees, and this in turn can affect sex-related QoL as well as overall QoL (Figure 34-3). Furthermore, this is an area that is often overlooked by clinicians relative to other symptomatic and functional consequences of disease.

It is important to recognize that the impact of medical illness on sexuality and related QoL is multidimensional. For example, Tierney describes multiple etiologies for sexual dysfunction among cancer survivors: (1) direct effects of illness; (2) psychological distress due to illness; (3) treatment for illness; (4) side effects of treatment for illness; (5) psychological distress after treatment; (6) changes in relationships due to illness [76].

These sources of sexual dysfunction can be applied to any medical condition, not just cancer. Notably, they affect QoL at all stages of illness, from onset, to diagnosis, to chronic management, remission, or cure. Furthermore, these sources of sexual dysfunction include psychological and social factors in addition to physical health, demonstrating that patients are best served by clinicians who address not just progression of illness, but associated QoL challenges, those related to sexuality in particular. To that end, this section reviews what is known about relationships between certain categories of medical and surgical illness, sexual function, and QoL.

Circulatory

A review of the literature suggests that sexual dysfunction is more prevalent among people who have hypertension than in controls, with such sexual dysfunction contributing to impaired QoL [77]. Some antihypertensive drugs, including beta-

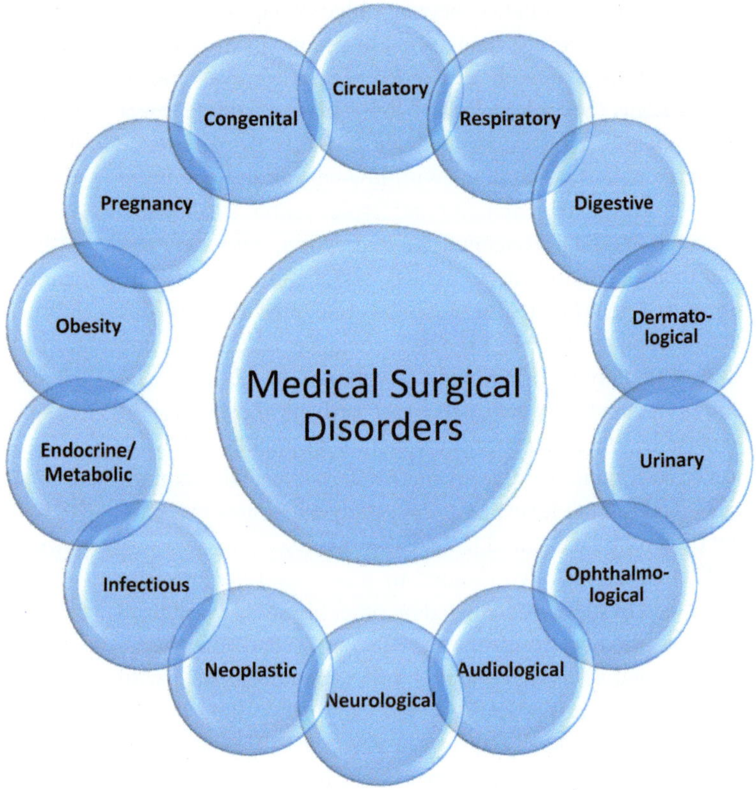

FIGURE 34-3. Medical and surgical disorders.

blockers and diuretics, contribute to sexual dysfunction, impairing QoL and leading to treatment non-adherence [77].

For patients undergoing coronary artery bypass grafting (CABG), the data shows impaired sexuality despite improvements in QoL overall, with one study showing up to 71% of patients reporting no improvement in sexual function post-surgery [78]. Other studies demonstrate increased erectile dysfunction (ED), decreased sexual frequency, and decreased sexual satisfaction overall post-CABG [78]. A study of 66 patients after CABG found that fear of resuming sexual activity was associated with decreased sexual interest and frequency, but there was no association between fear and sexual satisfaction [78].

A study of sexuality and QoL in 39 heart transplant recipients found sexual dysfunction in 61% of participants [11]. The patients with impaired sexual function also reported worse QoL than those without sexual dysfunction in physical domains including general health, physical health, physical functioning, and physical role limitation. Of note, this was despite a lack of any significant differences in mental health or depression in patients with and without sexual dysfunction. Research on left ventricular assist devices has given contradictory results regarding their impact on sexuality and QoL, with fear of damaging the unit during sexual activity emerging as one concern [79].

Respiratory

Sexual dysfunction is common in chronic obstructive pulmonary disease COPD. One study of 90 men with moderate-to-severe COPD found that 74% had at least one problem, most commonly ED (72%) [80]. Still, a lower proportion of men with COPD than in the community said that their QoL was impaired by ED (76% vs. 90%) or loss of libido (58% vs. 65%), which the authors hypothesize may be due to reduced expectations for sexual functioning in the COPD group. At the same time, the groups reported that anorgasmia impaired their QoL at similar rates (77% vs. 73%). ED was independently associated with depressive symptoms and low testosterone in the study, but not with dyspnea or all-cause mortality.

Women with asthma have greater impairments in sexuality and QoL than controls, according to a study of 31 women with asthma aged 18–45 [81]. The women with asthma had impairments in arousal, lubrication, orgasm, sexual satisfaction, and pain compared to controls, although causality remains unclear. Sexual dysfunction was associated with duration of illness in the study, but not with treatment or severity of symptoms. There was also no association between sexuality and severity of symptoms in a study of 55 men and women with asthma and COPD, with the authors suggesting that psychosocial factors such as coping mechanisms and social supports play a role in preserving sexual function [82].

Men with COPD had more sexual dysfunction and more dissatisfaction with sexual activity than women with COPD in the study. Women with asthma had more sexual dysfunction and more dissatisfaction with sexual activity than men with asthma in the study.

Digestive

The impact of sexuality on QoL in inflammatory bowel disease (IBD) remains understudied, despite a review demonstrating that patients find it a primary concern [83]. The review cites four studies analyzing sexuality and QoL in patients with IBD post-surgery, with results supporting an association between the two variables; it also examines three studies analyzing body image and QoL in patients with IBD post-surgery, with results also suggesting an association. Still, the review found that the most important predictor of QoL in IBD was actually disease severity, while the most important risk factor for sexual dysfunction was not any disease-specific concern, but instead depression, which is common in IBD.

Dermatological

In vitiligo, a condition that is primarily cosmetic, a study of 50 women showed an association between impaired sexuality and QoL, including impairments in genital self-image, in addition to impaired desire, arousal, lubrication, and overall satisfaction [84]. Research on psoriasis also shows that the psychosocial impact, including perception of stigmatization, causes impairments in sexuality and QoL [85]. A study of 354 patients with psoriasis found genital involvement in a majority, which corresponded to even greater impairments in sexuality and QoL than for those without genital involvement; symptoms such as itch, pain, stinging, and dyspareunia contributed [85]. Women with lichen sclerosus were also shown to have impairments in QoL associated with sexual dysfunction, especially dyspareunia due to psychological, anatomical, and dermatological changes caused by the condition [86]. A study of 300 patients with hidradenitis suppurativa found that women suffered worse sexual dysfunction than men, and that sexual dysfunction was associated with impaired QoL in women only [87].

Urinary

A comparison of subtypes of urinary incontinence in 111 women found that, among them, stress incontinence most impairs sexual function, but that urge incontinence and mixed incontinence cause greater impairments in QoL [88]. A study of 66 couples in which the female partner had stress incontinence showed greater impairments than in controls for both sexual function and QoL (the latter was measured only in the women), including decreases in sexual frequency and satisfaction for both women and men, more avoidance of sex in women, and more ED in men [89]. Still, the study found no association between the impairments in sexual function and QoL. In men, an enlarged prostate can cause lower urinary tract symptoms that impair sexuality and QoL [90]. Numerous options exist for pharmacotherapy and surgical treatment of enlarged prostate, each with different benefits and risks for urinary symptoms, sexuality, and the QoL associated with both domains [90].

Ophthalmological

A review of the literature shows that age-related vision loss has wide prevalence and significantly impairs QoL, irrespective of the cause of vision loss [91]. However, the degree to which impaired sexuality due to age-related vision loss impairs QoL represents a gap in the literature.

Audiological

A study of adult onset bilateral sensorineural hearing loss in 76 young and middle-aged men found impaired erectile function, intercourse satisfaction, and overall satisfaction compared to controls, with impaired QoL in the domains of social functioning and physical role difficulty, but not physical functioning, bodily pain, general health perception, vitality, emotional role difficulty, or mental health [92]. The impairments on sexuality were independent of degree of hearing loss, although the study excluded people who had severe hearing loss.

Musculoskeletal

A systematic review of research on hip replacement found an overall improvement in sexual QoL in both functional and psychosocial domains post-surgery, although it did not examine its relation to general QoL [93]. A study of 1082 people with chronic musculoskeletal pain reported impaired sexuality and QoL compared to controls, although people with chronic pain actually reported better satisfaction with partner relationships than controls and their level of pain was not found to be associated with their sexual satisfaction [94]. Sexuality is not routinely part of questionnaires that assess QoL in rheumatic diseases, even though these conditions are widely known to cause sexual dysfunction [95].

Neurological

A study of 120 people with spinal cord injuries found no association between sexual satisfaction and QoL, though there was an association between relationship satisfaction and QoL [96]. Although less than half of the patients in the study were satisfied with their sex lives, more than three-quarters were satisfied with their overall QoL, which the authors theorize may be due to resignation or shift in priorities after injury. In multiple sclerosis, a study of 6,183 people found that sexual dysfunction significantly impaired mental aspects of health-related QoL and in fact the impairment was much greater than that attributable to disability level, age, gender, or employment status [97]. A study of 70 survivors of stroke showed an association between impairments in libido and QoL, but found that impaired libido was associated with depression, which is common after stroke, rather than functional disability [98]. Another study examining 121 survivors of stroke found an association between impairments in sexuality and health-related QoL, but found that the impaired QoL was a consequence of functional disability [99].

Neoplastic

A study of 100 patients who took chemotherapy found that loss of sexual interest was ranked sixth among factors that negatively impact QoL. Subgroup analysis showed that young people ranked it second among factors negatively impacting QoL, that women ranked it higher than men, and that partnered patients ranked it higher than single ones [100]. A different group of 752 cancer survivors also ranked sexual dysfunction sixth among factors that negatively affect their QoL, with over 40% of those surveyed calling it an issue for them [101]. The study found that sexual dysfunction was the only factor negatively affecting QoL that was reported more often among men than women and partnered people over single ones. Additionally, sexual dysfunction was the number one factor negatively affecting QoL noted by survivors of prostate cancer in the sample. Prior research found that, among different types of cancer, sexual problems were most prevalent in survivors of breast, testicular, and prostate cancer [101].

Infectious

Studies on genital herpes shows that difficulty with sexual relationships and related psychological sequelae (isolation, anxiety, fear of rejection) cause significant negative impact on QoL, but that antiviral therapy has significant beneficial effect on QoL for those with frequent outbreaks [102]. A study of 895 people who had genital warts showed that decreases in QoL were most often due to anxiety and depression (37%), followed by pain and discomfort (26%) [103]. A study of 112 men with chronic hepatitis C infection showed impaired QoL compared to controls. Among men with hepatitis C, QoL was significantly lower for those who had sexual dysfunction compared to those who did not [104]. The study also specifically found that the sexual dysfunction was independent of depression. In a focus group on tuberculosis and QoL, a majority of the six male patients remarked that fatigue from the illness and its treatment resulted in loss of libido or ED, with normal function returning only sometime after completion of treatment [105].

In one study of 237 people living with HIV, psychosocial factors, including satisfaction with sex life, had more impact on health-related QoL than clinical measures [106]. Another study of 1194 people living with HIV found that less sexual activity in middle-aged to older people (ages 50–81) compared to younger ones was the main factor accounting for lower scores in the social domain of QoL for the older group [107]. A review focusing on QoL and antiretroviral therapy in HIV found that some patients attributed sexual dysfunction to their medication, with the QoL impairment contributing to treatment non-adherence [108].

Endocrine/Metabolic

In people with type 1 diabetes, sexual dissatisfaction was shown to be associated with impairments in mental aspects of QoL, while sexual dysfunction and metabolic parameters were not. Of note, sexual dysfunction in women with diabetes has been more strongly associated with anxiety and depression than with diabetes itself [109]. A study of 126 men with type 2 diabetes showed an association between impaired QoL and both low testosterone and ED that was independent of age, body mass index, and hemoglobin A1c, with worse erectile function associated with worse QoL [110]. A study using testosterone in 92 men with type 2 diabetes found improvements in QoL and in all tested domains of sexual function compared to men taking placebo, with greatest benefits in less obese men and men over 60, and reduced benefit in men who also had depression [111].

In people with growth hormone deficiency, arousal and subjective view of body shape were found to be impaired during the transition phase compared to controls, but there was no corresponding impairment in QoL. The impairments in arousal and body shape improved with growth hormone treatment [112]. A review of QoL in adrenal insufficiency was inconclusive as to whether dehydroepiandrosterone sulfate (DHEA-S) replacement therapy in women positively affects sexuality and QoL [113]. In a study of 59 patients with either Graves' disease or toxic nodular goiter, both groups showed significant improvements in QoL after thyroidectomy. Only the Graves' disease group had impaired sexuality prior to surgery, which improved after the procedure [114]. Likewise, a study of 143 patients divided into those with Hashimoto's thyroiditis and those with other benign goiters found significant improvements in QoL for both groups after thyroidectomy. In this case, only the Hashimoto's thyroiditis patients had impaired sexuality prior to surgery, which improved after the procedure [115].

Obesity

A study of 95 adults with obesity showed an association between impaired sexuality and QoL, with further associations between sexual dysfunction and body mass index (BMI), waist circumference, psychological distress, obesity-related disability, and female gender [116]. In contrast, another study showed that among 334 obese adults, impaired QoL caused by obesity-related sexual dysfunction had limited importance to men and non-African American women [117].

Pregnancy

Impaired sexuality during pregnancy is associated with reduced QoL, with depression as the best predictor of sexual dysfunction, according to a study of 150 pregnant women [118]. Safarinejad et al. found that delivery of the first child by planned caesarean section resulted in greater frequency of intercourse, sexual satisfaction, and QoL in women than other methods (spontaneous vaginal delivery, vaginal delivery with episiotomy, operative vaginal delivery, and emergency caesarean section) at both three and 12 months post-delivery, as well as lower frequency of ED in men over the same period [119].

Congenital

A study of 144 adults with disorders of sex development (46,XX and 46,XY; both social genders) showed comparable QoL between the chromosomal genders, which in turn were comparable to the general population [120]. The study showed that higher age at initiation of treatment was associated with impaired QoL as an adult, and there was a significant mean difference in QoL between patients with adequate and inadequate sexual performance. Still, sexual performance explained only 4% of variability in QoL; influencing QoL far more were general health (18%), positive feelings (18%), and spirituality, religion, and personal beliefs (18%). Women with Turner's syndrome have impaired sexual arousal compared to controls and impaired QoL in domains of physical functioning and role physical functioning, according to one small study. However, sexually active and non–sexually active women in the study had comparable levels of QoL [121]. The same study examined 21 women with other congenital hypogonadisms and found impairments in desire, lubrication, orgasm, and pain compared to controls, and impaired QoL in domains of physical functioning and bodily pain. Finally, a study of 32 men with congenital adrenal hyperplasia showed that they were less sexually active than controls, but had similar sexual satisfaction and QoL [122].

Conclusion

The studies reviewed here illustrate the many associations between physical health, sexual health, and a healthy QoL. At the same time, this review shows that effects on QoL differ across conditions and cannot simply be assumed to fit an expected pattern, as evidenced by certain conditions or subpopulations in which sexual function had little or no impact on QoL. Such instances may in some cases represent pockets of resilience that warrant further study. In any event, this serves to underscore the importance of clinical inquiry about a patient's well-being to guide treatment of medical conditions which affect sexual health, and of further research into this complex three-way relationship so as to inform intervention design and implementation.

Sex and Quality of Life in Psychiatric and Substance Use Disorders

Introduction

As with many other types of illness, people living with a wide variety of psychiatric and substance use disorders experience sexual dysfunctions at a higher rate than the general population. In fact, nearly all psychiatric conditions have been associated with some degree of sexual dysfunction [123] (Figure 34-4). Reasons for this are complex and include physiological, psychological, social, and even demographic factors [123]. This impairment in sexual health contributes to additional illness burden in terms of impact on QoL, which for many people with psychiatric conditions is already substantial [2, 124]. Compounding this is the widespread under appreciation of, inattention to, and discomfort with this problem on the part of clinicians [125], creating a missed opportunity to intervene on a treatable problem and therefore improve patients' overall QoL irrespective of improvement in other aspects of an illness. No less significant in this equation is the well-recognized fact that psychiatric medications can themselves be a cause of sexual dysfunction [123, 125, 126]. This requires astute and nuanced assessments by providers in order to tease out causes and enact appropriate remedies. This section reviews what is known about the relationship between sexual dysfunction and QoL in a number of prevalent psychiatric and substance use disorders and their treatments.

Depression

There is evidence for a bidirectional relationship between sexual dysfunction and depression. That is to say, a depressed state can entail or result in sexual impairments and, conversely,

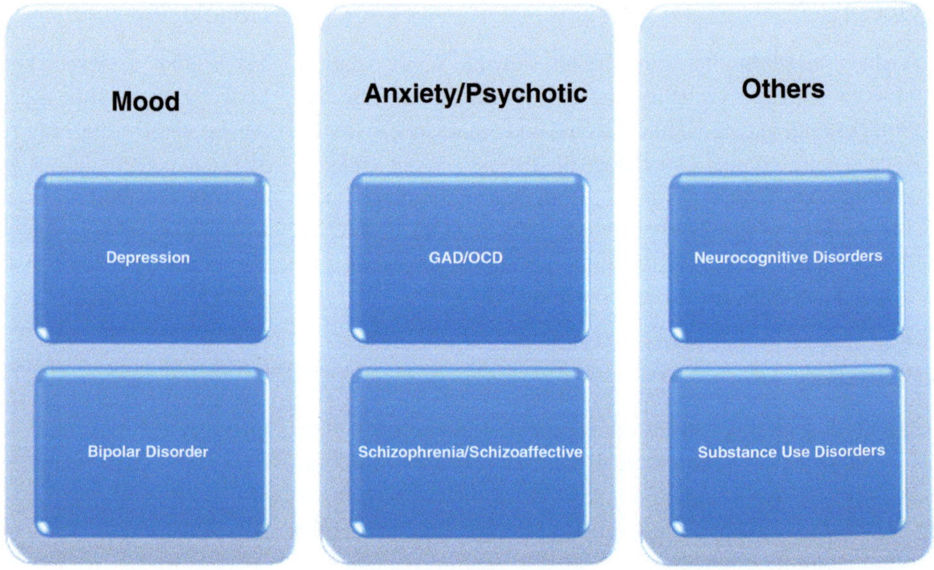

FIGURE 34-4. Psychiatric disorders.

impaired sexual functioning can contribute to depression, which could conceivably result in a mutually reinforcing cycle. While causality in this relationship is a matter of some debate, the association itself is well established in both men [127, 128] and women [129]. In a cross-sectional sample of 600 men across four countries, Nicolosi et al. showed that depressive symptoms were more prevalent among men with erectile dysfunction (ED), and that participants with moderate or complete erectile dysfunction were 2.3 times more likely to have a history of diagnosed depression than those without ED. Additionally, frequency of intercourse was associated with degree of satisfaction with sexual life in all age groups; men with ED had a reduced coital frequency; and depressive symptoms were correlated with sexual satisfaction in a linear (or "dose-dependent") fashion. This led the authors to infer that the link between ED and depression is mediated by reduced sexual activity and dissatisfaction with one's sexual life, suggesting a causal association [130]. At least two clinical trials have demonstrated that depressive symptom burden was reduced following successful treatment of ED [131, 132]. One such trial included a measure of ED-specific QoL, Erectile Dysfunction Effect on Quality of Life (ED-EQoL), and found that it also improved with treatment [131]. In the reverse direction, depression has been proposed as one among many potential factors leading to the development of sexual dysfunction [133–135], with one explanation positing depression, anxiety, and other stress reactions as "cognitive interferences" that distract attention from erotic stimuli, inhibiting arousal [135]. Shindel et al. found an association between sexual dysfunction and depression in a cross-sectional sample of 1241 North American female medical students. Specifically, those below a cutoff value on the Female Sexual Function Index (FSFI) designated as having "high risk of female sexual dysfunction" were 2.25 more likely to report depressive symptoms, with the most strongly associated sexual function domains being orgasmic impairments, interference in sex life from stress or lack of a partner, and lower overall life satisfaction (one aspect of QoL). [129]

As in the case of depression and sexual dysfunction, IsHak et al. have pointed out that depressive symptoms and QoL are bidirectionally related: depression can lead to QoL impairment (but is not merely synonymous with it) and vice versa [2]. This makes for an especially complex three-way relationship between depression, sexual functioning and satisfaction, and overall QoL. Adding to this complexity is the fact that serotonergic medications, the most common treatments for depression, frequently and infamously cause sexual side effects [136–140]. Such antidepressant medications include monoamine oxidase inhibitors (MAOIs, e.g., amitriptyline, desipramine), serotonin-selective reuptake inhibitors (SSRIs, e.g., fluoxetine, paroxetine, citalopram), and serotonin-norepinephrine reuptake inhibitors (SNRIs, e.g., duloxetine, venlafaxine) [136, 137, 139], and have been implicated in reduced libido, impaired arousal (vaginal lubrication or penile erection), and orgasmic dysfunctions (delay in or inability to achieve climax) [138, 140]. Sexual side effects are a common cause of nonadherence to antidepressant treatment [137, 139]. Depressed patients therefore often find themselves in the "double bind" of experiencing sexual problems due to their depression, antidepressant medications, or both. The result is that individuals living with depressive disorders often contend with sexual problems, which reduce their QoL, whether or not their depression is "successfully" treated.

Thakura et al. sought to characterize the nature of sexual dysfunctions in Major Depressive Disorder (MDD) and their impact on QoL, specifically enrolling only patients not on antidepressants so as to examine impacts of the disorder itself. There was no comparison group in the study. A majority rural sample of 60 patients with MDD in India completed the Hamilton Rating Scale for Depression (HAM-D), Arizona Sexual Experience Scale (ASEX) assessing sexual interest and function, and the Quality of Life Enjoyment and Satisfaction Questionnaire–Short Form (QLES-Q-SF). Two-thirds of the men and three fourths of the women reported sexual dysfunction. Problems frequently reported by men were low desire (33%) and erectile dysfunction (29%), whereas problems with orgasm and orgasmic satisfaction were about half as common. Female subjects similarly reported low desire (42%) followed by excitement (22%) and vaginal lubrication (19%) problems, and lastly problems with orgasm and orgasmic satisfaction (11% each). HAM-D (depression) scores correlated positively with total ASEX (sexual dysfunction) scores as well as all individual ASEX items except arousal. Meanwhile, subjects with sexual dysfunction (defined categorically based on ASEX scores) reported substantially lower QoL on average than those without sexual dysfunction, with means of 31% and 65% of maximum possible QLES-Q-SF score, respectively. Notably, the mean differences between groups were significant for all QLES-Q-SF items, not only total score, indicating widespread impact of sexual dysfunction on multiple domains of QoL: social, physical, mental, occupational, daily functioning, leisure, financial, overall satisfaction, and overall well-being domains in addition to sexual QoL. In a further analysis, both total HAM-D scores and total ASEX scores correlated negatively with all QoL domains as well as QLES-Q-SF total score. In light of these correlations, and despite the design limitations precluding definitive causal conclusions, the authors proposed the likelihood that "depressive symptoms and sexual problems are linked in a cyclic fashion with one contributing to the other." On this basis they urged early recognition of sexual dysfunctions in order to guide choice of antidepressant medication and treatment plan, and to prevent progression in illness severity [141]. Returning to the notion that QoL impairment can lead to or prolong depression, it becomes all the more important to address sexual dysfunctions lest they lead to a lower QoL and, in turn, worsening depression.

IsHak et al. analyzed sexual satisfaction and QoL data in patients with MDD before and after treatment with a common SSRI, citalopram. The study examined data from 2280 patients diagnosed with MDD who participated in the Sequenced Treatment Alternatives to Relieve Depression (STAR*D) trial, the largest-ever clinical trial of treatments for MDD. Measures of interest were the Quick Inventory of Depressive Symptomatology–Self Report (QIDS-SR); Quality of Life Enjoyment and Satisfaction Questionnaire (Q-LES-Q), a self-reported measure of QoL; and a single item from the Q-LES-Q which queries satisfaction with "sexual drive, interest, and/or performance." Impaired sexual satisfaction (ISS, based on a score threshold on the sexual satisfaction item) was highly prevalent in this sample before treatment—64% overall—and occurred more frequent in women, whose rate was 67% compared to 59% for men. After 12 weeks of treatment with citalopram, this rate fell to 47% overall, 47% among women, and 48% among men. This paralleled a reduction in depressive symptom scores following treatment, with depression severity increasing the odds of ISS by 13% at pretreatment and 19% at post-treatment. Furthermore, ISS was significantly more prevalent in those who did not achieve remission following treatment than in remitted patients (61% vs. 21%). These findings led to the conclusion that depressive symptoms "outweigh" the sexual side effects associated with citalopram in terms of contribution to ISS, and that this may be related to an increase in libido, boosting the case for SSRI treatment. These finding were consistent with other studies that have shown that sexual dysfunction seemed to be more closely related to depression than side effects of SSRIs or SNRIs [142–145] (although, of note, in one smaller study of 25 subjects taking sertraline or paroxetine, this held true for women but not for men [145]). On the other hand, the same study by IsHak et al. found that among patients whose symptoms remained moderate to severe following treatment, citalopram demonstrated a direct and negative effect on sexual satisfaction. Gelenberg et al. reached the same conclusion in a study of venlafaxine and fluoxetine [143]. In other words, for patients who did not get better from taking the antidepressant, it appears the side effect burden compounded the ISS they were already experiencing due to their depression [146].

In terms of impact on QoL, the IsHak et al. study found that Q-LES-Q scores (excluding the sexual satisfaction item) were lower in those with ISS than in those without, both before and after treatment. As with mood symptoms and sexual satisfaction, QoL improved following treatment in the overall sample as well as in the subset of subjects both with and without ISS. A multivariate regression analysis showed a substantial effect of ISS on overall QoL, with regression coefficients of –5.0 pretreatment and –8.1 post-treatment, after adjusting for age, gender, ethnicity, marital status, and depression severity; similar results were found using continuous score on the sexual satisfaction item rather than categorically defined ISS. Patients with poor symptomatic response to citalopram had lower QoL than would be expected from depression severity alone, suggesting the role of ISS in further QoL reduction. This was not true of those with a favorable treatment response. The principal recommendations made by the authors were that clinicians treat depression thoroughly until remission and recognize the importance of sexual satisfaction for QoL, and that investigators conduct randomized controlled trials in this area [146].

Bipolar Disorder

Research on sexual health in individuals living with bipolar disorders has been relatively scant, with much of the literature focusing on the contribution of childhood sexual abuse (and other types of abuse) to the development and course of bipolar disorders [147–154]. In that regard, a 2013 systematic review concluded that prevalence of sexual abuse was higher in persons with bipolar disorder than among healthy individuals, but not higher than people with other forms of psychiatric illness [151]. A separate systematic review by the same author found that a history of sexual abuse was weakly associated with a number of signs of illness severity—suicide attempts, substance use disorders, psychotic symptoms, and early age of illness onset—though the author raised the possibility that these were indirect effects [152].

Much of the remaining literature on sexuality in bipolar disorder has focused on sexual risk behaviors, which can occur during manic and hypomanic phases of the condition [155–158] or even in euthymic states between mood episodes [159]. These behaviors can include more frequent casual or non-monogamous sexual activity [159, 160], having sex with partners whose HIV status is unknown [159], and having sex without using a condom [160] (though one study found this was no more common in women with bipolar disorder than controls [159]). As McCandless and Sladen have pointed out, such behaviors have the potential to create painful consequences that range from strained or severed relationships when sexual indiscretion is involved, to contraction of sexually transmitted infections, increased risk of sexual exploitation (especially among women), and unplanned pregnancy [157], all of which have been associated with reduced QoL, either directly [161–163] or indirectly (e.g., via increased risk of depression in the case of unplanned pregnancies [164]). In a particularly striking finding, Dell'Osso et al. found that bipolar participants, as compared to unipolar depressed participants and healthy controls, were more sexually active and promiscuous, and that among the bipolar group a history of periods in which sexual partners changed frequently was linked to increased thoughts of death. The same study found that impairments in all phases of the sexual response cycle had a higher lifetime prevalence among people with bipolar disorder (as well as unipolar depression) than those without [165]. McCandless and Sladen have argued for sexual health promotion measures in this population while decrying a death of evidence to guide such efforts [157].

An interesting study by Lam et al. assessed the marital and sexual satisfaction of 37 heterosexual spouses of people living with bipolar disorder using semi-structured interviews and standardized instruments. On average, partners' sexual satisfaction and marital satisfaction suffered when patients were either manic or depressed relative to when they were well, and this was true for both men and women. Not surprisingly, marital dissatisfaction was associated with sexual dissatisfaction. The difference in partners' sexual satisfaction levels when patients were manic vs. depressed was not statistically significant, but overall marital satisfaction was lower when patients were manic rather than depressed. A number of specific problems were reported to be more frequent when patients were experiencing a mood episode. For male partners these included avoidance of sexual contact, dissatisfaction with the sexual side of their relationships, and difficulty communicating sexual needs. For female partners, vaginismus was more prevalent when patients were either manic or depressed, and sexual dissatisfaction was also greater during their partners' episodes. Female partners complained of sexual infrequency during patients' depressed phases more so than during their manic phases. The authors discussed possible mechanisms for the reductions in sexual satisfaction among partners, such as difficulty adjusting to a patient's changes in sexual interest, responsiveness, sensitivity, or affection. They concluded by recommending interventions involving education, problem-solving strategies, and sex therapy to help to reduce marital dissatisfaction [166].

There is limited data regarding the effects of treatments for bipolar disorder on sexual functioning. Lithium has long been a mainstay of treatment of bipolar disorder, although this has changed in recent years with the rise in use of certain anticonvulsant mood stabilizers and, increasingly, atypical (also known as second-generation) antipsychotics [167, 168]. A 2014 study by Grover et al. found that among 100 clinically stable patients receiving lithium for at least 2 years, one third reported sexual dysfunction as measured by ASEX, including problems with desire, sexual drive, arousal, and erectile dysfunction/vaginal lubrication. In most cases, more than one domain was affected. Prevalence of sexual dysfunction did not differ by gender, nor was it affected by sociodemographic variables, clinical variables including residual mood symptoms, or lithium dose. Those who experienced sexual dysfunction as a group had a greater number of additional side effects of lithium, lower Global Assessment of Functioning (GAF) scores, and worse medication adherence [169]. Ghadirian et al. studied sexual functioning in a sample of 104 outpatients with bipolar disorder taking lithium alone or in combination with other medications. Nearly half (49%) of patients taking a combination of lithium and benzodiazepines reported deficits in sexual functioning, as compared to 14% of those taking lithium alone and 17% of those taking lithium in combination with other drugs. In contrast to Grover et al., this led the authors to attribute problems with sexual function to concomitant use of benzodiazepines rather than lithium, which they concluded had no "major effect" on sexual function [170]. Lastly, a study of antipsychotic treatment in 108 men with remitted bipolar I disorder found that 66% of participants reported dysfunction in either sexual desire, arousal, attainment of orgasm, or a combination thereof. ED was the most commonly reported type of dysfunction with a rate of 42%, and was more prevalent in users of typical (first-generation) than atypical (second-generation) antipsychotics [171]. Although none of the above studies of bipolar treatments included an unmedicated control group so as to compare prevalence rates, it is clear based on absolute rates alone that clinicians should be attentive to medication-induced sexual dysfunction in this population, given important ramifications for illness management, adherence, and QoL.

Anxiety and Obsessive Compulsive Disorder

Sexual functioning in anxiety disorders is understudied and to date has not included explicit assessment of QoL. Kendurkar and Kaur administered the ASEX to groups of men and women with MDD, Generalized Anxiety Disorder (GAD), and Obsessive-Compulsive Disorder (OCD) as well as healthy individuals, in order to compare rates of sexual dysfunction. Study participants had not taken psychiatric medications during at least the preceding month. Sexual dysfunction was more prevalent in participants with GAD (64%) and OCD (50%) than in healthy participants, but less than in those with MDD (76%). Whereas participants with MDD were nearly three times as likely to have sexual dysfunction as controls, the odds ratios for GAD and OCD were 2.0 and 1.5, respectively, and were similar among women and men. The most frequent complaints among men with GAD were low desire (31%) and ED (28%), and among women with GAD were orgasmic dysfunction (44%) followed by poor orgasmic satisfaction and low desire (both 39%). The most common sexual complaint among both male and female participants with OCD was orgasmic dysfunction (46% and 45%, respectively). In men, participants with OCD had the highest rates of orgasmic dysfunction among the four groups, whereas in women rates were similar among the three clinical groups. All three diagnostic groups reported similar mean levels of severity (as opposed to prevalence) for penile erection/vaginal lubrication, orgasmic function, and orgasmic satisfaction, and mean scores on all ASEX items were similar between GAD and OCD [172]. The study results were generally consistent with the few other published studies on this topic [173–177]. Of note, severity of sexual dysfunction in this study did not depend on psychiatric symptom burden as measured by standard scales for depression, anxiety, and OCD [172]. This speaks to the importance of gauging domains beyond psychiatric symptoms in considering the overall impact of illness on a person's life, with sexual functioning being one important dimension.

Medication treatments for GAD and other forms of anxiety as well as OCD overlap greatly with those for depression, namely the use of serotonergic medications described previously. Therefore, the same sexual side effect considerations discussed in the Depression section above apply in those cases. At least two studies have focused on sexual issues related to medications for GAD not previously mentioned in the context of depression. Notwithstanding potential conflicts of interest disclosed by the authors, Clayton et al. found that GAD patients prescribed vilazodone, a newer SSRI, had a similar sexual functioning profile to those receiving placebo [178]. Othmer and Othmer found that sexual function normalized over a four-week period in a small sample of GAD patients receiving buspirone who reported sexual dysfunction prior to treatment [176]. Effects of treatment on QoL were not explicitly assessed.

Schizophrenia and Schizoaffective Disorder

Individuals with schizophrenia and schizoaffective disorder suffer disproportionately from a range of sexual problems relative to the general population. At the same time, contrary to common perceptions, studies have found that a large proportion of people with schizophrenia and schizoaffective disorder are sexually active, supporting the importance of determining the impact of sexual dysfunction on QoL in individuals with these disorders. While there are some conflicting findings, the preponderance of evidence supports an association between sexual dysfunction and reduced QoL in this population.

It is first important to recognize that people living with schizophrenia and schizoaffective disorder as a group are interested in sex and to a great extent are sexually active. In a small study of 23 chronically institutionalized women with schizophrenia, 18 of 23 responded that they would like to have an active sex life, 16 indicated they would not hesitate to have sex with a man they found attractive, and 15 reported having had intercourse within the preceding 3 months despite being hospitalized [179]. Aizenberg et al. found that among 122 men with schizophrenia, the majority reported being sexually active despite a high frequency of sexual dysfunction [180]. Additionally, in a study by Lyketsos et al. comparing 113 individuals with schizophrenia to 104 healthy controls, the groups did not differ in the proportion of participants with sexual dreams and fantasies, and those with the diagnosis reported having intercourse more than once per week [181].

Numerous studies have shown that sexual dysfunction is extremely prevalent in both treated and untreated individuals with psychotic disorders. Although a detailed discussion of mechanisms is beyond the scope of this chapter, it is generally agreed that both the illness itself and side effects of antipsychotic medications used to control psychotic symptoms are responsible for these problems, albeit possibly with differential effects [180, 182–188]. Unsurprisingly, medications that tend to increase prolactin levels, in particular, have been implicated in sexual dysfunction in men, whereas prolactin-sparing medications have been shown to cause fewer such problems [189].

Macdonald et al. compared responses to self-reported gender-specific surveys regarding sexual dysfunction from 135 persons with schizophrenia and 114 controls. One or more types of sexual dysfunction were reported by 82% of men and 96% of women in the schizophrenia group. Specifically, men with the diagnosis had reduced sexual desire, increased ED and PE, and less satisfaction with orgasm intensity. Relative to controls, female patients reported reduced sexual enjoyment [187]. Other studies have found very high rates of sexual dysfunction in this population, ranging from 50–88% in men and 30–94% in women depending on the study, according to literature review conducted by Bushong et al. [190].

Aizenberg et al. [180] compared 51 patients on long-acting injectable antipsychotics, 20 nonmedicated patients, and 51 healthy controls with regard to sexual dysfunction using a detailed structured interview. Sexual dysfunction was highly prevalent in both treated and untreated patients, with levels of sexual desire being reduced in both groups. However, problems with arousal (erection) and orgasm during sex were reported mainly by the medicated group, as was overall dissatisfaction with sexual functioning, while reduction in the frequency of sexual thoughts was found only in those not receiving medication. Subjects with schizophrenia were more involved in masturbatory activity than control subjects, consistent with at least one other study which found that the primary sexual activity of persons with schizophrenia is auto-erotic in nature [188].

Given the importance of sexuality to people living with schizophrenia, the very high prevalence of sexual problems in this population begs an understanding of how such problems impact patients' QoL. However, as several authors have pointed out, the subject of sexuality is often neglected by clinicians treating individuals with psychosis. This may have many causes: clinicians failing to realize that many people with schizophrenia are sexually active [191]; clinicians underestimating the prevalence of sexual problems in this population [189]; discomfort among both providers and patients around the topic of sexuality [182, 186]; a belief that discussion of sexual matters will trigger or worsen symptoms [192]; or simply an assumption that myriad other concerns (such as amelioration of psychotic symptoms) take precedence. In reality, in one telling example, Finn et al. found that patients rated impotence as more bothersome than any positive psychotic symptom [193]. It is not surprising, then, that sexual side effects of antipsychotic medications are one important (and underappreciated) cause of nonadherence to treatment [194, 195].

Irrespective of degree of attention from clinicians, a number of investigators have posed the question of whether sexual dysfunction is associated with reduced QoL in people living with psychotic disorders, and the weight of evidence supports such an association. Olfson and colleagues examined cross-sectional associations between sexual dysfunction, psychiatric symptoms, global function, and QoL among 139 male outpatients meeting criteria for schizophrenia or schizoaffective disorder. The authors were especially interested in the effect of sexual dysfunction on the ability to form and sustain intimate relationships in this population. Sexual function was assessed using the Changes in Sexual Functioning Questionnaire (CSFQ), which covers sexual desire/frequency, desire/interest, pleasure, arousal, and orgasm. Items from the Quality of Life Interview were used to assess QoL. Nearly half (45.3%) of the subjects exceeded the CSFQ threshold indicating sexual dysfunction. Of note, while neither symptom burden, global functioning, nor proportion with substance use disorders differed significantly between those with and without sexual dysfunction, the groups did separate with respect to QoL. After controlling for age and race/ethnicity, those with current sexual dysfunction reported lower general QoL as well as less satisfaction with the amount of enjoyment in their lives. Furthermore, subjects with sexual dysfunction were only about one-third as likely to have a romantic partner. Those who did have partners reported lower satisfaction with the quality of those relationships, by an average of slightly more than one full point on a seven-point scale. Relationship satisfaction suffered, relative to those without sexual dysfunction, not only in terms of sexual satisfaction but extending to include a reduced likelihood of talking to their partners about their illness, sharing personal thoughts, being praised by their partners, and being reminded by their partners to take medications (with this last finding approaching but not reaching significance). The authors concluded that sexual dysfunction is an important contributor to reduced QoL in this population, and one that merits improved recognition and attention as well as further research. While acknowledging that relatively little is currently known about how to ameliorate sexual dysfunction in this population, they recommend that clinicians have open discussions about sexuality with patients, provide sex education and rehabilitative interventions to build intimacy skills where appropriate, and consider pharmacologic approaches (dose reduction, medication switching, or specific drug therapies) when antipsychotics are implicated in the dysfunction [196].

In contrast to the preceding study conducted in men, a study by Fan and colleagues of men and women with schizophrenia and schizoaffective disorder did not find a significant association between any subscale measures of the CSFQ (see preceding paragraph) and two instruments intended to measure QoL, Heinrichs's Quality of Life Scale (QLS) and the Behavior and Symptom Identification Scale (BASIS) [186]. It should be noted, however, that Heinrichs's QLS, an observer-rated instrument developed by Heinrich et al. in 1984, was designed to measure "deficit symptoms" (i.e., negative symptoms) of schizophrenia, and therefore includes such items as social initiative, withdrawal, role function items, motivation, anhedonia, and emotional interaction. For this reason, despite its name this scale likely does not adequately assess QoL as now commonly defined and as conceived in this chapter (at the very least, an observer-rated scale cannot measure a participant's subjective QoL). Similarly, the BASIS, a self-report scale, asks respondents to rate "how much difficulty [they] have been having" in a variety of functional (e.g., work, school, social, household, leisure) and symptomatic (e.g., depression, anxiety, suicidality, concentration/memory) domains and therefore serves more properly as a measure of global functioning rather than QoL per se. Even so, the association between sexual desire/frequency dysfunction and higher BASIS score (indicating greater global functioning deficit) approached significance. With these clarifications in mind and despite the authors' interpretations, the above findings are in fact consistent with, rather than contradictory to, the Olfson et al. study in that both studies showed that neither symptoms (negative symptoms in the case of the present study) nor global functioning were significantly associated with sexual dysfunction; conclusions about QoL arguably cannot be drawn from the Fan study in the absence of a suitable measure of QoL [197].

A more recent study conducted in China also failed to find a significant association between sexual dysfunction (as measured by the ASEX) and QoL (as measured by the SF-12) among 607 primary care patients with schizophrenia, a finding the authors considered surprising. The authors conjectured that the brevity and generality of the SF-12, as opposed to a measure which includes items specific to QoL related to sexual function, makes it probable that the instrument was not sufficiently sensitive to detect QoL changes [198].

Another relatively large study by Bushong et al. [190] surveyed 238 adult outpatients who met criteria for either schizophrenia or schizoaffective disorder and were being treated with risperidone, quetiapine, or olanzapine. Among the measures collected were the ASEX for sexual dysfunction and a single item querying general life satisfaction from the Quality of Life Interview developed by Lehman et al. The authors found a negative relationship between ASEX total score and general life satisfaction for the overall sample, after adjusting for potential covariates. (There was no significant association, however, when running the analysis for men and women as separate groups.) As noted by the authors, while a small effect size was observed, the correlation was of comparable strength to that between subjective QoL and both positive ($r = -0.15$) and negative ($r = -0.12$) symptoms of psychosis reported in a 2007 meta-analysis by Eack and Newhill [199]. Additionally, associations were seen between general life satisfaction and each of the five items of the ASEX individually. The strongest among these was with the "physical arousal" item querying vaginal lubrication or penile erection. Among several limitations mentioned by the authors, the lack of a non-medicated or pretreatment group precluded the ability to determine whether the sexual dysfunction and related QoL deficit were characteristic of the illness itself, medication side effects, or both. Regardless, the authors recommended that clinicians screen their patients on antipsychotic medications for sexual side effects and, if present, considering switching medications. Underscoring this recommendation is the finding by Adrianzen et al. that sexual dysfunction was the treatment-emergent adverse event most strongly associated with reduced health-related QoL for patients on neuroleptics, stronger than both extrapyramidal symptoms and tardive dyskinesia, two conditions which clinicians screen for regularly [200].

In summary, evidence suggests that people living with schizophrenia and schizoaffective disorders are interested in sex and are sexually active but suffer from a very high burden of sexual dysfunction, owing both to the disorders themselves and to medications used to treat them, and this is associated with reduced overall QoL as well as reduced treatment adherence. There is little if any evidence basis, however, for recommending interventions that specifically improve sexuality-related QoL in this population. Nonetheless, expert opinion has centered on the following recommendations: (1) Increased awareness among clinicians about sexual problems in this population [182, 186, 188, 189, 196]; (2) Provision of sex education whenever possible, including the incorporation of sex education into rehabilitative programs [182, 196]; (3) Inquiry and open discussions with patients about sexual matters with the aim of tailoring treatment accordingly [182, 186, 196]; (4) Consideration of dose reduction or change in medications where applicable, particularly to an agent not associated with significant prolactin elevation [189, 196]; (5) Use of other pharmacologic approaches (e.g., PDE-5 inhibitors for erectile dysfunction) [187, 196]; (6) Further research into sexual dysfunction and QoL in this population [196].

Neurocognitive Disorders

Dementia (the term used in DSM-IV and earlier editions, and therefore in most existing studies), also known as Major Neurocognitive Disorder (the DSM-5 term) is, generally speaking, a disorder of old age, with a prevalence of about 14% of people in the United States over the age of 71 [201]. As such those living with this condition are subject to some misconceptions regarding old age in general, namely that sexuality is reserved for the young [202]. In fact, sexuality is a part of human nature throughout the life cycle [203]. Furthermore, although sexual frequency often decreases with advancing age [202], older people remain sexually active, at a rate of 50–80% of adults over the age of 60 [204]. Similarly, despite common assumptions to the contrary, couples affected by dementia continue to be interested in sex and maintain physical intimacy in their relationships [203]. In a study of male nursing home residents with dementia, intimacy was strongly associated with life satisfaction and contributed to QoL [205]. However, the cognitive, physical, and environmental impairments experienced by people with dementia can interfere with the ability to express and experience sexuality [206]. In some individuals living with dementia, sex may represent a form of compensation for the cognitive and functional losses, which erode self-esteem. Those living in nursing facilities may experience an increased psychological need for intimacy due to the lack of physical closeness in those environments [207], which for a variety of reasons including privacy and staff attitudes are usually not conducive to sexual expression [208, 209]. This in turn can contribute to the well-known hypersexual or sexually inappropriate behaviors of some patients with dementia which, although rare, can impact the QoL of everyone involved [207], and have been the focus of a great deal of research [207, 210–214]. Benbow and Beeston presented a model, modified from an earlier version by Roach [215], of "proactive protection" in managing difficult sexual behaviors of nursing home residents, characterized by supporting and educating staff while showing regard for residents' needs, dignity, and autonomy. Notably, improved QoL for residents serves as a central hub in the model, with a number of the other components flowing into it (e.g., positive resident–staff interactions) or out from it (e.g., greater job satisfaction for staff) [202].

Mild Neurocognitive Disorder is a DSM-5 diagnosis that is similar to Major Neurocognitive Disorder but is less severe and is not associated with inability to carry out activities of daily living. Although not included as a diagnosis in DSM-IV, this was referred to in the pre-DSM-5 literature as mild cognitive impairment (MCI) or, when memory is primarily affected, mild memory impairment (MMI). A very important consideration surrounding both Major and Mild Neurocognitive Disorders is their impact on caregivers and their QoL. Davies et al. conducted a comparative study of spousal caregivers of individuals with MMI and dementia. Focus group discussions of sexuality and intimacy revealed the themes of communication, marital cohesion, expression of affection, caregiver burden, and ambiguity concerning the future of the relationship. Dementia caregivers described more problems with communication, cohesion, and caregiver burden than MMI caregivers. Both groups reported reduced sexual activity due to physical limitations. In this regard, "substitute" activities such as hand-holding, massaging, and hugging were mentioned. Difficulty anticipating the future of the relationship was an issue for both groups, but while dementia caregivers were able to consider sexual relationships with others in the future, MMI caregivers mainly considered future relationships for companionship and emotional intimacy only. The authors hoped that this work would inform interventions to modify couples' activities, behaviors, and expectations with the aim of improving relationship satisfaction and QoL [216], a worthy goal in this vulnerable population whose general QoL is both significantly compromised and often undervalued [217].

Substance Use Disorders

The intersection of substance use and sexuality produces a variety of considerations, some of which seem to diverge. On the one hand, alcohol and several illicit drugs can cause impairment in sexual function, while on the other, they are sometimes used in order to enhance sexual desire, performance, or pleasure [218, 219]. Drug and alcohol use can greatly increase the likelihood of risky sexual behavior and vulnerability to sexual coercion or assault [220], the latter of which is associated with severe negative effects on mental health [221], QoL [221], and such domains as self-esteem, relationships, social life, work life, perceived reputation, and sexual health [222]. Even when not directly contributing to sexual dysfunction, substance use disorders can lead to physical health problems which in turn cause impaired sexual health [223]. Lastly, given the strong associations between mental health problem and drug abuse [224–226], when sexual dysfunctions lead to a deteriorating mood and impaired QoL, the risk of substance use disorders in affected individuals increases. Sexual dysfunction and substance use disorders therefore represent another case with the potential for a mutually reinforcing cyclic relationship, much to the detriment of the individual, thereby warranting particular clinical attention (Figure 34-5).

Alcohol

Alcohol use disorder is among the most common mental disorders worldwide [227]. In the immediate timeframe, alcohol consumption suppresses the physiological sexual response while at the same time disinhibiting psychological

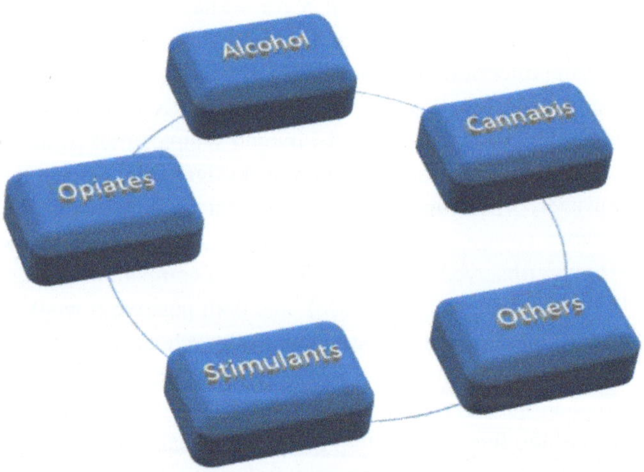

FIGURE 34-5. Substance use disorders.

arousal. Crowe and George conducted a review of this topic and concluded that the psychological disinhibition effect is strong at lower alcohol doses while the physiological suppression is stronger at higher doses. Furthermore, the disinhibition effect appears to have both a pharmacological dimension, via interference with cognition, and a psychological dimension related to learned expectancies. These two dimensions can operate together or separately [228]. Whatever the etiology, Mandell and Miller found that during heavy drinking, 59% of men interviewed experienced ED, 48% had problems ejaculating, and 84% reported at least one type of sexual dysfunction [229].

In the long term, chronic heavy alcohol use has a well-documented negative impact on sexual functioning. In severe cases, sequelae of alcoholic liver disease and chronic alcohol overuse itself can include infertility, sterility, gonadal atrophy, hypoandrogenization, and feminization. These changes have been attributed to a number of physiological mechanisms entailing the hypothalamic–pituitary axis, specifically hyperprolactenemia-increased estrogen-stimulated neurophysin levels, suppressed secretion of plasma gonadotropins, and loss of gonadotropin reserve [223]. However, several studies have shown that sexual dysfunction is prevalent in this population even in the absence of such changes. In one study, Fahrner found that a full three-quarters of men with alcohol addictions had ED, loss of libido, and premature or delayed ejaculation; this was unchanged after 9 months of inpatient treatment for alcohol addiction. Testosterone levels of all participants were normal at both time points [230]. Another study by the same author found that a behavioral treatment for addicts with sexual dysfunction resulted in significantly less sexual dysfunction compared to untreated controls, suggesting that the dysfunctions were not purely physiologically determined [230]. Gluud et al. surveyed 221 men with alcoholic liver cirrhosis participating in a clinical trial of oral testosterone for liver disease. At study entry, two-thirds reported sexual dysfunction. Unlike in the Fahrner study above, Gluud et al. found that dysfunction was significantly associated with lower levels of testosterone, including protein-bound and unbound forms, but some of these associations were eliminated upon adjusting for age, alcohol consumption, and severity of liver disease. Although sexual dysfunction improved significantly at 6-, 12-, and 24-month time points as participants reduced their alcohol consumption, testosterone treatment was not observed to play a role in these improvements [231].

While the preceding studies did not include comparison groups, Jensen et al. used matched groups to compare men with alcohol use disorders with and without overt liver disease, insulin-dependent diabetic men, and men without chronic disease. Roughly consistent with Gluud et al.'s finding above, 61% of men with alcoholic cirrhosis reported sexual dysfunction, a rate similar to the 56% of both non-cirrhotic alcoholic men and insulin-dependent diabetic men, and substantially greater than the 11% of healthy controls. Types of sexual dysfunction were similar across the three clinical samples (and in fact any differences were statistically nonsignificant), with ED being the most common (50% of cirrhotic participants), followed by reduced desire and PE. Notably, a number of physical parameters including testicular atrophy, testosterone, gynecomastia, and liver function did not different significantly between those with and without sexual dysfunction in the overall sample, while prevalence of psychological problems necessitating treatment was four times higher in those reporting sexual dysfunction [232]. It should also be noted that alcohol might amplify other risks of sexual dysfunction in some populations; for example, one study found that alcohol use increases the risk of sexual dysfunction five-fold in men with physical disabilities [233]. While the impact of alcohol-related male sexual dysfunction on QoL have not been explicitly studied as of the date of publication, one can infer a deleterious effect based on what is known about male sexual dysfunction and QoL in general and in other contexts. Thankfully, evidence suggests that with attainment of sobriety, male sexual function can rebound [234]. Further, there is evidence that treatments aimed at sexual dysfunction can help in this population [219].

Alcohol use disorders also have well-established negative effects on sexual health in women, and this is associated with poor QoL. Although consumption of alcohol increases subjective sexual desire, arousal, and pleasure for many women [235], it has been associated with reductions in genital blood flow and arousal, vaginal lubrication, sexual sensation, orgasmic function, and sexual satisfaction [236–239]. Psychosocially, alcohol use is correlated with earlier age of sexual activity, unplanned adolescent pregnancy, marital problems, and increase in sexual victimization [235, 236]. Dissiz et al. conducted a study of 71 women with alcohol dependence as well as 183 healthy women in Turkey. They measured QoL using the World Health Organization Quality of Life Scale–Brief Form (WHOQOL-BREF), sexual function using the Female Sexual Function Index (FSFI), and depressive symptoms using the Beck Depression Inventory (BDI). Compared to healthy controls, alcohol-dependent women had lower scores on all QoL subdomains (physical, psychological, social, environmental, and national), higher prevalence of sexual dysfunction (83% exceeded cutoff score on FSFI, vs. 44% of controls), and higher prevalence of depression (70% exceed cutoff score on BDI, vs. 10% of controls). Furthermore, all subdomain scores of WHOQOL-BREF except national subdomain were positively correlated with FSFI, albeit weakly so, and this was true for both alcohol-dependent and healthy women; that is, as sexual function improved, so did QoL. In a multivariate analysis, psychological and social subdomains of WHOQOL-BREF accounted for 27% of variance in sexual functioning as measured by FSFI. Given the cross-sectional nature of the study, causal direction cannot be determined; after all, it is not unreasonable to posit that better QoL could contribute to better sexual functioning, although the converse is more intuitive. Also uncertain given the study design is the role of depression as a possible mediator: BDI scores were also correlated with WHOQOL-BREF subdomains, and depression has known relationships with QoL and sexual dysfunctions (as described above) as well as addiction [240]. Nonetheless, in light of the implications for QoL revealed by their study, the authors recommended monitoring QoL, sexual function, and depression in alcohol-dependent women using understandable measurement tools, responding to any changes, and providing education and guidance regarding available treatments and services [241].

Opioids

Opioid use disorders have been associated with elevated rates of sexual dysfunction in men and women. A review conducted by Grover et al. found rates of sexual dysfunction ranging from 34 to 85% among people living with heroin addiction, 14–81% among individuals on methadone maintenance, 36–83% for those on buprenorphine maintenance, and 90% for those on naltrexone maintenance, depending on the study [242]. Venkatesh et al. found that among a sample of 100 men seeking treatment for opioid dependence, all phases of the sexual response cycle as well as overall sexual satisfaction were impaired relative to healthy controls, with a remarkable 92% of opioid-dependent men reporting dysfunction in at least one domain on the International Index of Erectile Function (IIEF), compared to 16% of controls [243]. Women who chronically abuse heroin may experience reduced sexual desire and performance, irregular menstrual cycles, and, less commonly, amenorrhea, owing to the suppression of pituitary hormones by the drug. Some women may misinterpret such changes and conclude that they have been rendered sterile. Interestingly, while sexual dysfunction in people with substance use disorders can lead to poor treatment adherence and relapse [242], it has also been reported as a motivating factor for attaining sobriety [244].

The few existing studies of sex-related QoL in this population have focused primarily on treatments for opioid addiction. For example, a recent study from China found that sexual dysfunction complicated the course of methadone maintenance treatment. Patients perceived methadone to cause greater sexual dysfunction than heroin, particularly in terms of reduced desire and pleasure. This led to a reduction in QoL and damage to intimate relationships, thereby negatively impacting the stability of the treatment. Moreover, patients with sexual dysfunction did not receive professional assistance for this problem and lacked pertinent coping skills. The study results highlight the need for awareness among clinicians and attention to this important problem in order to enhance treatment success and improve QoL [245]. Byrne et al. evaluated the impact of sexuality on self-rated unmet need and QoL in 190 people on methadone treatment, using WHOQOL-BREF to measure QoL. Compared to men, women in the study had a greater number of unmet needs and lower QoL in the domains of physical health, environmental well-being, social relationships, and, especially, psychological well-being [246].

Yee et al. compared a group receiving methadone to another receiving buprenorphine with respect to sexual functioning and QoL measured, again, with WHOQOL-BREF. The methadone group had lower sexual desire, orgasmic function, and overall sexual satisfaction than the buprenorphine group, and this paralleled lower QoL in all four WHOQOL-BREF domains (physical health, psychological health, social relationships, and environment). In the buprenorphine group, intercourse function and erectile function were significantly correlated with all QoL domains, and sexual desire with the psychological and social relationships domains. In the methadone group, overall satisfaction was strongly correlated with both the psychological and social relationships QoL domains. It is worthwhile to highlight the degree of impact of sexual dysfunction on social relationships. In the combined sample, sexual dysfunction accounted for 21% of the variance in the social relationships QoL domain, as compared to 16% in physical health, 11% in psychological health, and 8% in the environmental domain. These results underscore the importance of considering sexual dysfunction and QoL when making treatment decisions in this population, and provide evidence supporting the use of buprenorphine, particularly when sexual dysfunction is a concern [247]. Finally, the Sexual Concerns and Substance Abuse Project reported on by Smith et al. recommends screening for sexual dysfunction when patients enter treatment for opiate use disorders, followed by additional evaluation, education, and referral to a sex therapist where indicated, with the aim of reducing the rate of relapse and improving QoL [248].

Cannabis

The relationship between cannabis use and sexual health has been called paradoxical [249]. Many people report enhancement of both sexual performance and satisfaction from cannabis use [249–252]. Proposed mechanisms have included slowing of time perception allowing prolonged enjoyment [253], disinhibition and relaxation [254], and facilitation of sensate focus [255]. These observations have even led to calls for further research into the therapeutic use of cannabis for individuals with sexual dysfunctions [251]. At the same time, there is some inconsistent evidence that cannabis use can negatively affect sexual functioning. Among men, daily users were found to have higher rates of inability to reach orgasm, delayed orgasm, or premature orgasm, although the same study found no associations with sexual problems in women [256]. Evidence for ED in cannabis users is mixed: according to a 2011 review by Shamloul et al., different studies have shown that cannabis either enhances erectile function [252], inhibits it [249] (via effects on endothelial function [257], receptors in the hypothalamus [258], or both), or has no appreciable effect [256, 259]. A possible explanation for this discrepancy may be the finding that small amounts of cannabis can enhance sexual activity, while larger amounts may interfere with sexual motivation [250]. Shamloul et al. noted a dearth of high-quality evidence, including lack of use of validated measures of sexual dysfunction in this population, and encouraged a renewal of research in this important area given the high rates of cannabis use [250]. Additionally, studies of sex-related QoL in cannabis users have yet to be undertaken and are therefore warranted.

Psychostimulants

Psychostimulants such as cocaine and methamphetamine, both of which entail increased activity of the neurotransmitter dopamine in reward centers of the brain, represent perhaps the quintessential example of a drug often used to enhance the sexual experience. Acute cocaine use can induce a hypersexual state which is sometimes but not always accompanied by increased sexual performance [260]. However, chronic cocaine abuse can cause depletion of dopamine with or without hyperprolactinemia (due to dopamine's inhibition of prolactin). This, in addition to other mechanisms, can result in sexual dysfunction [261] including decreased libido and performance, reduced sperm count in men, and infertility [260]. Henderson et al. interviewed 100 female users of crack cocaine with regard to their sexual feelings and functioning. Interestingly, the data did not support the common perception that crack cocaine is an aphrodisiac for women and causes women to want sex. Additionally, sexual dysfunction in this sample was found to be higher than that of women who used alcohol [262].

A number of studies have focused on high-risk sexual behaviors among cocaine and methamphetamine users [263–266]. One such study by Edelman et al. in female users of crack cocaine and opioids found that two-thirds of sexually active participants reported having had sex that could lead to pregnancy during the preceding month. More than half had been forced to have sex against their will at some point in their lives. These women also had high rates of sexually transmitted infections, pregnancy terminations, miscarriages, and abnormal (i.e., precancerous) cervical cells [266]. The potential negative effects of such consequences and experiences on well-being seem obvious, but QoL as related to sexuality in psychostimulant users has not been formally studied, representing yet another gap in the literature on QoL.

Quality of Life in Sexual Dysfunctions

Introduction

Irrespective of etiology and comorbidity, the sexual disorders covered in Part II of this book can affect the overall QoL of those who experience them as well as their sexual partners. This section discusses what is known about the relationship between QoL and several forms of sexual dysfunction (Figures 34-6 and 34-7), as well as how their treatment affects QoL in cases where that question has been studied.

Erectile Disorder or Dysfunction

Erectile dysfuction (ED), also known as erectile disorder, is one of the most common sexual problems in men [267] and is associated with QoL impairment. Abolfotough and al-Helali found that two-thirds of a sample of 388 patients with ED reported poor QoL. Notably, among a number of variables including age, exercise, substance use, smoking, and cardiovascular disease, severe ED was the only significant predictor of QoL, and was not an indicator for comorbidities [267]. National Health and Social Life Survey data show that

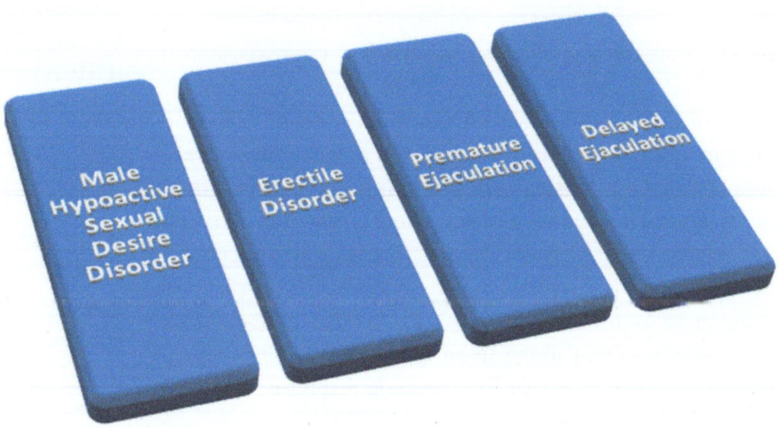

FIGURE 34-6. Male sexual dysfunctions.

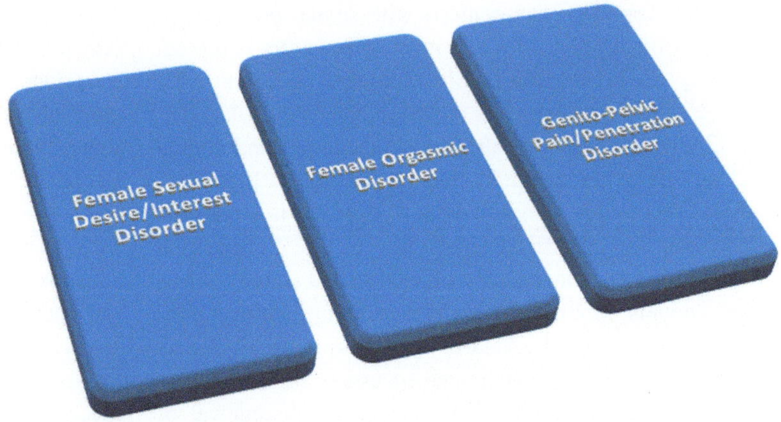
Female Sexual Desire/Interest Disorder
Female Orgasmic Disorder
Genito-Pelvic Pain/Penetration Disorder

FIGURE 34-7. Female sexual dysfunctions.

ED is associated with declining QoL and has strong associations with low physical satisfaction, low emotional satisfaction, and low general happiness domains [268]. Treatment of ED has the potential to improve QoL. In particular, a number of PDE-5 inhibitors have been shown to improve both ED symptoms and QoL. Treatment with sildenafil was found to result in an increase in all subscales of the SF-36, with physical functioning, general health, and role–emotional functioning subscales being statistically significant. Additionally, those who reported erectile outcomes as "excellent" had the biggest increases in three SF-36 subscales, demonstrating an association between degree of clinical improvement and QoL [269]. Other studies have found that sildenafil treatment was associated with improved emotional well-being [270] and quality of relationship [271].

To study the effects of treatment on QoL in men with ED and their female partners, Rubio-Aurioles and colleagues compared ED patients treated with tadalafil for 12 weeks to a placebo group. The treated group showed significant improvement with regard to erectile function as compared to the placebo group. Patients and their partners completed the Sexual Quality of Life (SQOL) domain of the Sexual Life Quality Questionnaire (SLQQ) before and after treatment. Treatment with tadalafil improved sexual QoL for patients as well as their partners to a greater extent than placebo. Of note, the size of this post-treatment difference was even greater for female partners than for the patients themselves. Furthermore, the superiority of sexual QoL improvements in the treated group held for every SQOL item—frequency of sex, duration of sex, ease of insertion, ease of achieving orgasm, ease of initiating sex, pleasure of anticipation, carefree feelings during sex, pleasure of orgasm, pleasure overall, and partner's overall pleasure—and this was true for both patients and their partners. Lastly, following treatment with tadalafil but not placebo, SQOL scores were on par with those prior to the onset of ED [272]. Another PDE-5 inhibitor, vardenafil, was found in an industry sponsored trial to improve quality of sexual life based on response to an item on the Fugl-Meyer QoL questionnaire [273].

Male Hypoactive Sexual Desire Disorder

Male hypoactive sexual desire disorder (Male HSDD) is defined in DSM-5 by having at least 6 months of a "persistently or recurrently deficient (or absent) sexual/erotic thoughts or fantasies and desire for sexual activity" causing "clinically significant distress in the individual" [33]. Meuleman and van Lankveld have argued that, in part due to stereotypes surrounding male sexuality, male HSDD is grossly under-recognized and often misinterpreted as ED, but in fact is more prevalent in men than women [274]. Along with the many other proposed causes and contributors including low testosterone and high prolactin levels [274], poor or fair health and emotional problems or stress—two salient aspects of QoL—both increase the probability of having low sexual desire more than threefold. Daily drinkers of alcohol and men who have had any history of same-sex activity also have greater risk of low desire compared to the general population, by more than a twofold difference in both cases [268]. At the same time, as with ED, low sexual desire in men is associated with reduction in the QoL dimensions of physical satisfaction, emotional satisfaction, and general happiness. QoL impairment for men with low desire is less than that for men with ED in the domains of physical satisfaction and emotional satisfaction, but slightly greater than in ED in the domain of general happiness [268]. QoL has rarely been taken into consideration in treatment studies for Male HSDD, but one study of dehydroepiandrosterone (DHEA) treatment in men and women found that, for men only, well-being as measured by the Mental Health Inventory improved with treatment, as did several clinical variables including sexual drive [275]. A study of testosterone and letrozole (an aromatase inhibitor) for low desire caused by highly active antiretroviral therapy (HAART) among HIV-positive men measured mood, anxiety, and stress using the Depression Anxiety Stress Scale-21 (DASS-21). Both substances increased levels of desire, but there were no corresponding changes in mood, anxiety, or stress scores across the sample [276].

Female Sexual Interest/Arousal Disorder

Female Sexual Interest/Arousal Disorder (FSIAD) entails reduced or absent sexual interest, thoughts, fantasies, activity, arousal, pleasure, or sensation, with at least three features required for diagnosis. The disorder was introduced in DSM-5 [33], published in 2013, and there has been scant research on this newly defined condition to date. However, the diagnosis subsumes within it criteria for two DSM-IV-TR disorders, hypoactive sexual desire disorder (HSDD), in which sexual fantasies and desire are reduced or absent, causing marked distress or interpersonal difficulty, and female sexual arousal disorder (FSAD), in which there is an inadequate lubrication-swelling response of sexual excitement [277]. The psychological toll of female HSDD has been widely reported, including the finding that women meeting DSM-IV-TR criteria for HSDD are more likely than women with normal desire to agree with statements expressing such negative emotional states as frustration, hopelessness, anger, loss of femininity, and low self-esteem [278]. Affected women experience reduced QoL, as do their partners [279]. A 2009 study by Biddle et al. examined health-related QoL (HRQoL) and overall health burden in 1189 postmenopausal women with HSDD, using SF-12 to measure QoL and EuroQol (EQ-5D) to measure general health status. Women with HSDD had significantly lower HRQoL and poorer health status than women without the condition. The SF-12 domains for which this effect was greatest were mental health, vitality, social function, and bodily pain. HRQoL in the HSDD group was similar to that of adults with other chronic conditions including diabetes and back pain, and rates of physical impairment and general health were comparable to individuals with depression [280].

As detailed in the chapter on treatment of FSIAD, treatment options for low sexual desire in women include lifestyle changes, treatment of comorbid medical or psychiatric conditions, switching or discontinuing offending medications, hormone therapies, non-hormonal medications (including flibanserin, an FDA-approved treatment with mixed results in terms of efficacy [281–283]), and marital therapy [284]. Most of these treatments have yet to be studied in terms of direct effects on QoL, with a few exceptions. Among the many studies of hormone (e.g., testosterone) treatments showing positive clinical effects, one study found that daily application of intravaginal DHEA resulted in an increase in Menopause Specific Quality of Life (MENQoL) Sexual Desire score and a decrease in avoidance of intimacy [285]. In contrast, another study of DHEA supplementation in perimenopausal women found that DHEA did not have a significant effect on libido, mood, or well being [286]. Shifren showed that treatment with transdermal testosterone resulted in positive changes relative to placebo on the Psychological General Well-Being Index total score and subscales of vitality, positive well-being, depressed mood, and anxiety [287]. Yet another study found that treatment with a testosterone patch, in addition to symptomatic improvement, caused reduction in personal distress [288]. Finally, in a Taiwanese study of tibolone (a synthetic steroid with hormonal activity) compared to standard hormone replacement therapy (HRT) in postmenopausal women, tibolone was found to be superior in treating problems with desire/interest, arousal, orgasm, and satisfaction, and was at least as effective as HRT in improving QoL measured by the Greene Climacteric Scale.

Female Orgasmic Disorder

After low sexual desire, orgasmic dysfunction is the second most common sexual problem in women [289], affecting between 11 and 41% of women worldwide [290]. DSM-5 defines female orgasmic disorder (FOD) as at least 6 months of "marked delay in, marked infrequency of, or absence of orgasm" or "markedly reduced intensity of orgasmic sensations" during most or all occasions of sexual activity, causing significant impairment or distress [33]. Given that one definition of orgasm includes the induction of a state of well-being and contentment [291], it stands to reason that a lack of orgasmic adequacy would entail reduction in well-being, and indeed the disorder is known to negatively impact QoL [290]. One study found rates of distress from orgasmic difficulties to be around 5% of the general female population, and interestingly this rate was found to be similar for all age groups even though rates of the dysfunction were seen to increase dramatically with age [292]. As with other sexual disorders, there is a strong relational component to FOD. Communication within couples seems to be impaired when a female partner has FOD [293], with greater use of blame language found in one study [294]. It is no wonder, then, that relationship distress—an important correlate of QoL—has been associated with female orgasmic dysfunction (although directionality has not been established), while positive orgasmic functioning has been correlated with marital satisfaction, happiness, and stability [295]. It stands to reason, then, that restoration of the ability to achieve high-quality orgasms in women with FOD would be accompanied by a better QoL. Despite this, clinical trials of the myriad pharmacologic and non-pharmacologic treatments for FOD that have been studied (see Chap. 15) have yet to include assessments of QoL.

Premature Ejaculation

In men, premature ejaculation (PE) has been associated with poor QoL as well as such negative psychological effects as anxiety, depression, and distress in affected men as well as their female partners [296]. Despite the long-accepted view that PE is less distressing to men than are other sexual dysfunctions, particularly ED, Rowland and colleagues found that distress levels related to PE were on par with those due to ED [297]. Seven studies reviewed by Rosen and Althof showed high levels of personal distress in men with PE compared to those without, and three studies found that this was also true for female partners [296]. Two studies have found moderate correlations between the distress levels of both partners in a couple [298, 299]. It has been suggested that female partners of men with PE are as affected as patients, if not more so [296].

In terms of validated QoL measures, McCabe found that compared to men without the dysfunction, men living with PE reported lower levels of satisfaction in all areas of life assessed by the Comprehensive Quality of Life Scale (ComQol): material well-being, health, productivity, intimacy, safety, place in the community, and emotional well-being. By comparison, men with ED had lower levels of satisfaction in the above areas except productivity, and men lacking sexual desire had lower levels in intimacy and safety domains only. Similarly, Rowland et al. found that men with PE scored significantly lower on overall health-related QoL than men without PE. This included all mental component domains of the SF-36 as well as physical role functioning. They also scored lower on the Self Esteem and Relationship (SEAR) scale [297]. Indeed, at least eight studies have found that PE is associated with interpersonal difficulties between affected men and their partners [296]. Compounding these problems is the infrequency with which men with PE seek treatment. In addition to embarrassment and perception that no effective treatment is available, there is evidence that partner influence plays a major role in treatment-seeking behavior in this population [296].

Numerous treatments, both pharmacologic and nonpharmacologic, have demonstrated efficacy in PE. However, among 103 clinical trials reviewed by Cooper et al. in 2005, only a small few assessed effects of treatment on QoL issues beyond sexual satisfaction [300]. Behavioral therapy was found to increase sexual self-confidence compared to a wait-list control, despite a lack of clinical efficacy in one trial [301]. A few treatments such as tramadol [302], lidocaine-prilocaine (also called EMLA) cream [303], and lidocaine-prilocaine spray [300, 303] were found to reduce distress, though one study found no difference in sexual QoL with lidocaine-prilocaine spray at 4 weeks [304]. Another trial suggested that self-confidence and depression were improved with both acupuncture and paroxetine relative to placebo [305]. Clearly, more research is needed into the effects of treatment on QoL in men with PE.

Delayed Ejaculation

Delayed ejaculation (DE) as defined in DSM-5 is characterized by at least 6 months of "marked delay in ejaculation" or "marked infrequency or absence of ejaculation" on most or all occasions, causing significant distress [33]. According to Althof, it is the least common, least understood, and least studied of the male sexual dysfunctions [306]. Among the many hormonal, neurological, psychological, and relational factors thought to contribute to development of DE, some factors related to life quality, such as stress at work and psychiatric distress, have been shown to increase the risk for the condition [307]. In turn, having DE is associated with significant reductions in HRQoL, self-esteem, and sexual satisfaction, and increases in anxiety, depression, and relationship dissatisfaction and discord [308]. In terms of impact on partners of affected men, while in some cases they may enjoy the extended coital duration, they will often engage in self-blame such as feeling they are not attractive enough, experience a sense of rejection, or in some cases experience physical pain due to the longer duration of intercourse [306]. Despite a long list of compounds under investigation, the quest for effective drug treatments for DE is considered to be in its infancy [308]. Likewise, psychological interventions, which stem from diverse theoretical underpinnings and diverge into a variety of approaches with insufficient conclusive evidence, are in great need of further research [306]. Therefore it is not surprising that effects of treatments for DE on QoL have yet to be determined.

Genito-Pelvic Pain/Penetration Disorder

According to DSM-5, genito-pelvic pain/penetration disorder (GPPPD) in women entails distressing difficulties with vaginal penetration during intercourse, vulvovaginal or pelvic pain during intercourse or penetration attempts (i.e., dyspareunia), fear or anxiety about such pain, or marked tensing of the pelvic floor muscles with attempted penetration (i.e., vaginismus) [33]. The prevalence of dyspareunia, one facet of the disorder, has been estimated to be between 8 and 40% depending on the study, and the condition is known to impose a significant burden on women's health, relationships, and QoL [309]. A Turkish study of the relationship between dyspareunia, other female sexual dysfunctions, and QoL found that other sexual dysfunctions were much more common in dyspareunic women (87%) than controls (37%). Specifically, dyspareunic women had relative impairments in sexual desire, arousal, lubrication, orgasm, and satisfaction. Where QoL is concerned, the group with dyspareunia had lower scores in physical role function, social function, bodily pain, and vitality domains of the SF-36 [310]. In a study of women with endometriosis, chronic pelvic pain and depression were the only two among nine putative factors found to be independent risk factors for poor QoL measured by the SF-12 [311]. As for effect of the condition on partners, it is has been shown that sexual functioning is unaffected in male partners of women with dyspareunia [311]. On the other hand, partners' attitudes and responses toward dyspareunia can influence the affected women's experience of the condition, with less catastrophic partner responses being associated with decreased pain [312]. Research into the effects of treatment on QoL in this disorder is generally lacking. However, a study of prasterone treatment for sexual dysfunctions in postmenopausal women showed that having dyspareunia did not affect the treatment-emergent improvements in desire, avoidance of intimacy, vaginal dryness, and SQoL measured by the Menopause Specific Quality of Life (MENQoL) questionnaire [313].

Vaginismus—the spastic contraction of vaginal muscles with contact—constitutes another facet of genito-pelvic pain/penetration disorder. Among treatments tested for vaginismus, botulinum toxin has been shown to improve QoL as well as such outcomes as the ability to have intercourse and scores on the Female Sexual Function Index (FSFI) in otherwise refractory patients [314]. Another recent treatment development pertinent to genito-pelvic pain/penetration disorder is the adjunctive use of transcutaneous electrical nerve stimulation (TENS) for refractory cases of provoked vestibulodynia, which is pain in the entrance of the vagina when touched. One study found that use of TENS resulted in reduced vulvar pain, improved sexual functioning measured by the FSFI, and reduced levels of sexually related personal distress, an analog of SQoL [315].

Conclusion

The preceding review of sexual disorders and their relationship to QoL is notable for the consistency of findings that, wherever examined, sexual health and QoL go hand-in-hand. The design of most studies does not allow us to make causal statements, but one can nonetheless conceive of ways in which QoL factors might influence the development of sexual disorders, in contrast to those ways in which sexual dysfunction might impinge on QoL. Equally apparent is the relative lack of research into the effects of treatments for sexual disorders on QoL, even as evidence builds for the clinical efficacy of many treatments. It is hoped that as new treatments emerge and existing ones undergo further study, measures of QoL will be routinely included in outcomes research. In this way we can assure that our interventions are aimed at important goals beyond symptomatic relief, namely the well-being and overall life satisfaction of our patients.

Enhancing Quality of Life: Interventions to Improve Quality of Life in General and in Sex in Particular

Introduction

As previously discussed, it has been shown that sexual function and QoL are interrelated. That is, when sexual function is sub-par, so too is QoL. Naturally, the next step would be to determine if treating the disorder and restoring sexual function results in an improved QoL. It was this issue that led researchers to create instruments such as the sexual life quality questionnaire (SLQQ), a questionnaire that takes into account sexual QoL and satisfaction with treatments associated with erectile dysfunction (ED) for patients and their partners [316]. In this section we discuss various interventions that have shown to increase sexual and overall QoL in patients with sexual dysfunctions.

Enhancing Sexual QoL in Men

We begin our discussion with interventions aimed at treating ED including phosphodiesterase-5 (PDE-5) inhibitors, injections, implants, and vacuum devices. PDE-5 inhibitors such as sildenafil, tadalafil, and vardenafil have revolutionized the treatment of ED. They work by increasing blood flow to the penis via decreased breakdown of C-GMP by PDE-5, leading to vasodilation. Numerous studies including different populations of men with ED being treated with sildenafil have all clearly demonstrated an increase in QoL measures [317]. Vardenafil was shown to improve QoL in a Phase III, multicenter, randomized, double-blind, placebo-controlled, parallel-group study conducted at 54 centers in the USA and Canada involving 805 men with ED using the Fugl-Meyer QoL questionnaire. Results showed that improvement in sexual life indicated statistically significant superiority for all doses of vardenafil vs. placebo treatment [273]. A study by Rubio-Aurioles et al. using the SLQQ to measure QoL in 342 patients taking tadalafil and their female partners showed that 5 mg tadalafil once daily not only significantly improved QoL in patients, but also in their partners [272].

Intracavernosal injections exist for the treatment of ED in addition to the well-known PDE-5 inhibitors. Prostaglandin E1 (PGE1) is the standard treatment when treatment with PDE-5 inhibitors fails. PGE1's mechanism of action is to potentiate C-AMP, which ultimately leads to a decrease in intracellular calcium levels and therefore causes vasodilation. Research involving 596 questionnaires sent to patients with ED taking PGE1 intracavernosal injections for at least three months showed that 70.1% of patients noted improvements in their sex life, 50% noted improvements in their relationship with their partner, 44.8% noticed improved QoL, and 80.3% noticed improved confidence in attempting sexual intercourse [318]. Previous studies showed that prostaglandin injections also improved mental health, social health, and self-esteem [317]. In addition to intracavernosal injections, PGE1 can also be self-administered as a transurethral pellet. A multicenter European study of 249 men with ED using transurethral PGE1 (the Medicated Urethral System for Erection [MUSE] study) showed that 34% of patients showed improvement in the "relationship with partner" domain, a 70% improvement in the "quality of erection" domain, and statistically significant improvements in personal wellness, contentment, and self-esteem were also noted. Other vasoactive forms of intracavernosal injections besides PGE1 include phentolamine (alpha-adrenergic blocker), papaverine (smooth muscle relaxant), and combined formulations according to a treatment algorithm [319]. In a study of 20 post-radical prostatectomy men with ED being treated with intracavernosal therapy, results showed that in addition to improvements to erectile function, patients exhibited improved scores in sexual self-esteem, confidence in the sexual relationship, and satisfaction with treatment, but there was no significant increase in general health perceptions and overall QoL. The author notes however that results should be interpreted with caution given the small sample size, as scores indicated that patients were experiencing a high QoL and remained stable, with the exception of the psychological/spiritual domain which increased (though not statistically significantly) [320]. Two other studies involving intracavernosal therapy showed that 80% of men satisfied with intracavernosal treatment indicated that it had improved their life, in response to the question "Has treatment improved your QoL?" [319]. Other therapies for treating ED include penile prosthesis implants and vacuum devices. A study involved 69 patients that received a three-component hydraulic prosthesis and were given the QoL and Sexuality with Penile Prosthesis (QoLSPP) questionnaire which the authors developed to examine general and sexual QoL in four domains: functional, personal, relational, and social. Results showed high satisfaction levels in all QoL domains [321]. Penile prosthesis is offered to those who have contraindications to other forms of treatment. Two studies, one of 94 patients that received the Dura II malleable penile prosthesis implant and the other of 80 patients that received the AMS 700CX inflatable penile implant both showed excellent results in terms of functional outcome and increased QoL [322, 323].

Interventions for treating premature ejaculation (PE) include SSRIs, TCA, topical anesthetic agents, PDE-5 inhibitors, and behavioral therapies. Topical local anesthetics such as lidocaine-prilocaine cream and aerosolized forms have been used to treat PE. Although these treatments have been shown to be effective, they have not been widely used due factors such as onset time and the need for condoms [324]. A randomized double-blind, placebo-controlled study of 54 patients with PE and their partners treated with a metered-dose aerosol spray containing a eutectic mixture of lidocaine and prilocaine showed improvements in SQOL-M and SQOL-F scores (of patients and their partners, respectively). Although the improvements in sexual QoL were not significant, the authors note that the treatment was only administered four times and that longer duration studies are warranted as the results look promising [324]. Unfortunately, because there are few randomized, double-blind, placebo-controlled studies on treatment options for PE, little is known about the effect of PE treatment on measures of QoL [325]. Interestingly though, a recently published prospective, multicenter, phase I–II study involving 91 patients with lifelong PE given oral tablets of a phytotherapeutic combination of Rhodiola rosea, folic acid, biotin, and zinc (EndEP®) showed significantly improved ejaculatory control and quality of sexual life (using the SF-36) [326].

Enhancing Sexual QoL in Women

Moving onto therapies for female sexual dysfunctions, we again encounter a paucity of research looking specifically at measures of QoL, and thus only those treatments with research containing QoL outcomes are discussed. According to the DSM-5, female sexual dysfunctions include female sexual interest/arousal disorder (FSIAD), female orgasmic disorder (FOD), and genito-pelvic pain/penetration disorder (GPPPD). Hormonal therapy is the primary therapy for FSIAD, and can be used in the other dysfunctions as well. In a randomized double blind study by Blumel et al. aiming to evaluate changes in QoL and sexual function via questionnaires (Female Sexual Function Index [FSFI] and the menopause-specific quality of life questionnaire [MENQOL]) in 47 healthy postmenopausal women receiving hormonal replacement therapy, they found that of the 40 diagnosed with sexual dysfunction, the group taking 0.625 mg conjugated estrogens plus 1.25 mg of methyl-testosterone and 100 mg of micronized progesterone daily showed significantly improved QoL scores of vasomotor, psychological, physical and sexual symptoms compared with no change in the placebo group. Interestingly, 68.7% of subjects did not meet criteria for sexual dysfunction per the FSFI by the end of the study [327]. Although used off label, PDE-5 inhibitors can be used in female arousal disorders as it has the same mechanism of increased blood flow in women as it does in men. A study of 5 mg daily tadalafil on 32 premenopausal women affected by sexual genital arousal disorder showed improvements in the physical role, bodily pain, emotional role, mental health, and general health categories of the SF-36 questionnaire used to investigate QoL. The categories for physical function, vitality, and social function improved as well, though not statistically significantly [328]. With regard to GPPPD, several antinociceptive therapies have shown promise in terms of QoL improvement. Danielsson et al. conducted a prospective randomized study where 46 women with vulvar vestibulitis were randomized to receive either electromyographic biofeedback or topical lidocaine treatment for four months. QoL was measured using the SF-36 and showed similar statistically significant improvements in all outcome measures [329]. Pelletier et al. evaluated QoL and sexual function (Dermatology Life Quality Index and sexual function by the Female Sexual Function

Index) in 20 patients with provoked vestibulodynia receiving 50 U of botulinum toxin. Results showed that the efficacy of the treatment on pain was associated with a significant beneficial effect on sexual function and QoL [330].

Chapter Conclusion

Sexual QoL is a vital component of an individual's overall QoL. As we can see, there is a need to include measures of QoL and sexual QoL in future research regarding the treatments of medical, surgical, psychiatric, and sexual disorders. More importantly, clinicians should be aware of important disease process and iatrogenic factors that could impair QoL and sexual QoL. Clinicians should work diligently to develop personalized plans to improve sexual QoL and overall QoL.

References

1. The WHOQOL Group. The World Health Organization Quality of Life assessment (WHOQOL): position paper from the World Health Organization. Soc Sci Med. 1995;41(10):1403–9.
2. IsHak WW, et al. Quality of life: the ultimate outcome measure of interventions in major depressive disorder. Harv Rev Psychiatry. 2011;19(5):229–39.
3. World Health Organization. Defining sexual health, report of a technical consultation on sexual health 28–31 January 2002. http://www.who.int/reproductive-health/gender/sexual_health.html#3. Accessed October 3, 2016.
4. Fugl-Meyer AR, et al. On life satisfaction in male erectile dysfunction. Int J Impot Res. 1997;9(3):141–8.
5. Flynn KE, et al. Sexual satisfaction and the importance of sexual health to quality of life throughout the life course of U.S. adults. J Sex Med. 2016;13(11):1642–50.
6. Arrington R, Cofrancesco J, Wu AW. Questionnaires to measure sexual quality of life. Qual Life Res. 2004;13(10):1643–58.
7. Conte HR. Development and use of self-report techniques for assessing sexual functioning: a review and critique. Arch Sex Behav. 1983;12(6):555–76.
8. Helgason AR, et al. Decreased sexual capacity after external radiation therapy for prostate cancer impairs quality of life. Int J Radiat Oncol Biol Phys. 1995;32(1):33–9.
9. Santos PR, et al. Quality of life among women with sexual dysfunction undergoing hemodialysis: a cross-sectional observational study. Health Qual Life Outcomes. 2012;10:103.
10. Bae H, Park H. Sexual function, depression, and quality of life in patients with cervical cancer. Support Care Cancer. 2016;24(3):1277–83.
11. Phan A, et al. Persistent sexual dysfunction impairs quality of life after cardiac transplantation. J Sex Med. 2010;7(8):2765–73.
12. Abraham L, Symonds T, Morris MF. Psychometric validation of a sexual quality of life questionnaire for use in men with premature ejaculation or erectile dysfunction. J Sex Med. 2008;5(3):595–601.
13. Symonds T, Boolell M, Quirk F. Development of a questionnaire on sexual quality of life in women. J Sex Marital Ther. 2005;31(5):385–97.
14. Maasoumi R, et al. The sexual quality of life-female (SQOL-F) questionnaire: translation and psychometric properties of the Iranian version. Reprod Health. 2013;10:25.
15. Symonds T, et al. Sexual function questionnaire: further refinement and validation. J Sex Med. 2012;9(10):2609–16.
16. Fallowfield L. The quality of life: the missing measurement in health care. London: Souvenir; 1993.
17. Hawkes G. Sociology of sex and sexuality. London: McGraw-Hill Education; 1996.
18. Flynn TJ, Gow AJ. Examining associations between sexual behaviours and quality of life in older adults. Age Ageing. 2015;44(5):823–8.
19. Bean EJ, Mazur T, Robinson AD. Mayer-Rokitansky-Kuster-Hauser syndrome: sexuality, psychological effects, and quality of life. J Pediatr Adolesc Gynecol. 2009;22(6):339–46.
20. McCabe MP, Cummins RA. Sexuality and quality of life among young people. Adolescence. 1998;33(132):761–73.
21. Clayton AH, Kim DH. Hypoactive sexual desire disorder: separating fact from fiction. CNS Spectr. 2016;21(1):9–11.
22. Nicolosi A, et al. Sexual behavior and sexual dysfunctions after age 40: the global study of sexual attitudes and behaviors. Urology. 2004;64(5):991–7.
23. Traeen B, et al. Sexual orientation and quality of life among university students from Cuba, Norway, India, and South Africa. J Homosex. 2009;56(5):655–69.
24. Santosa A, et al. Cross-sectional survey of sexual dysfunction and quality of life among older people in Indonesia. J Sex Med. 2011;8(6):1594–602.
25. Sprague C. Sexual revolution and counter revolution. Pasadena, CA: Salem Press; 2015.
26. Bullough VL, Brundage JA. Handbook of medieval sexuality. New York, NY: Garland; 1996.
27. Yuen Loke AJ. Editorial: sexual health: an integral part of our health and quality of life. J Clin Nurs. 2013;22(23–24):3239.
28. Daker-White G, Donovan J. Sexual satisfaction, quality of life and the transaction of intimacy in hospital patients' accounts of their (hetero)sexual relationships. Sociol Health Illn. 2002;24(1):89.
29. Masters WH, Johnson VE. The sexual response cycle of the human female. III. The clitoris: anatomic and clinical consideration. West J Surg Obstetr Gynecol. 1962;70:248–57.
30. Rüütel K, et al. Factors influencing quality of life of people living with HIV in Estonia: a cross-sectional survey. J Int AIDS Soc. 2009;12(1):1.
31. Dominguez L, Barbagallo M. Ageing and sexuality. Eur Geriatr Med. 2016;7(6):512–8.
32. The WHOQOL Group. The World Health Organization quality of life assessment (WHOQOL): development and general psychometric properties. Soc Sci Med. 1998;46(12):1569–85.
33. American Psychiatric Association. Diagnostic and statistical manual of mental disorders. 5th ed. Arlington, VA: American Psychiatric Publishing; 2013.
34. Potts S, Bhugra D. Classification of sexual disorders. Int Rev Psychiatry. 1995;7(2):166.
35. Schulman CC, et al. Testosterone deficiency: a common, unrecognised syndrome? Eur Urol Suppl. 2009;8:772–7.
36. Khera M, Lipshultz LI. The role of testosterone replacement therapy following radical prostatectomy. Urol Clin North Am. 2007;34:549–53.
37. Moncada I. Testosterone and men's quality of life. Aging Male. 2006;9(4):189–93.
38. Hucker A, McCabe MP. An online, mindfulness-based, cognitive-behavioral therapy for female sexual difficulties: impact on relationship functioning. J Sex Marital Ther. 2014;40(6):561–76.
39. Dundon CM, Rellini AH. More than sexual function: predictors of sexual satisfaction in a sample of women age 40–70. J Sex Med. 2010;7(2pt2):896–904.
40. Hawton K, Gath D, Day A. Sexual function in a community sample of middle-aged women with partners: effects of age, marital,

socioeconomic, psychiatric, gynecological, and menopausal factors. Arch Sex Behav. 1994;23(4):375–95.
41. Schmidt G, et al. Changes in adolescents' sexuality between 1970 and 1990 in West-Germany. Arch Sex Behav. 1994;23(5):489–513.
42. Ellis A. Commentary on the status of sex research. J Psychol Hum Sex. 1990;3(1):5–18.
43. Gavin AR, Simon GE, Ludman EJ. The association between obesity, depression, and educational attainment in women: the mediating role of body image dissatisfaction. J Psychosom Res. 2010;69(6):573–81.
44. Hayes RD, Dennerstein L, Bennett CM, Sidat M, Gurrin LC, Fairley CK. Risk factors for female sexual dysfunction in the general population: exploring factors associated with low sexual function and sexual distress. J Sex Med. 2008;5(7):1681–93.
45. Rowe JW, Kahn RL. Successful aging. Gerontologist. 1997;37(4):433–40.
46. Baltes PB, Baltes MM. Successful aging: perspectives from the behavioral sciences. Cambridge: Cambridge University Press; 1993.
47. Trudel G, Turgeon L, Piché L. Marital and sexual aspects of old age. Sexual and Relationship Therapy. 2000;15(4):381–406.
48. Galinsky AM, Waite LJ. Sexual activity and psychological health as mediators of the relationship between physical health and marital quality. J Gerontol B Psychol Sci Soc Sci. 2014;69(3):482–92.
49. Ni Lochlainn M, Kenny RA. Sexual activity and aging. J Am Med Dir Assoc. 2013;14(8):565–72.
50. Maserejian NN, et al. Sexual arousal and lubrication problems in women with clinically diagnosed hypoactive sexual desire disorder: preliminary findings from the hypoactive sexual desire disorder registry for women. J Sex Marital Ther. 2012;38(1):41–62.
51. Comfort A, Dial LK. Sexuality and aging. An overview. Clin Geriatr Med. 1991;7(1):1–7.
52. Boladale M, et al. Sexual orientation and quality of life among students of Obafemi Awolowo University (OAU). Nigeria Afr Health Sci. 2015;15(4):1065–73.
53. Even L, et al. Long-term outcomes after hypospadias surgery: sexual reported outcomes and quality of life in adulthood. Prog Urol. 2015;25(11):655–64.
54. Saewyc EM, et al. Original article: measuring sexual orientation in adolescent health surveys: evaluation of eight school-based surveys. J Adolesc Health. 2004;35:345e-1–15.
55. Sandfort TG, de Graaf R, Bijl RV. Same-sex sexuality and quality of life: findings from the Netherlands Mental Health Survey and Incidence Study. Arch Sex Behav. 2003;32(1):15–22.
56. Horowitz SM, Weis DL, Laflin MT. Differences between sexual orientation behavior groups and social background, quality of life, and health behaviors. J Sex Res. 2001;38(3):205–18.
57. van Heeringen C, Vincke J. Suicidal acts and ideation in homosexual and bisexual young people: a study of prevalence and risk factors. Soc Psychiatry Psychiatr Epidemiol. 2000;35(11):494–9.
58. Walls EN, Freedenthal S, Wisneski H. Suicidal ideation and attempts among sexual minority youths receiving social services. Soc Work. 2008;53(1):21–9.
59. Hatzenbuehler ML. How does sexual minority stigma "get under the skin"? A psychological mediation framework. Psychol Bull. 2009;135(5):707.
60. Chen JP, et al. HIV-related behaviors, social support and health-related quality of life among men who have sex with men and women (MSMW): a cross-sectional study in Chongqing, China. PLoS One. 2015;10(2):e0118651.
61. Xiao M, et al. Quality of life and sexuality in disease-free survivors of cervical cancer after radical hysterectomy alone: a comparison between total laparoscopy and laparotomy. Medicine (Baltimore). 2016;95(36):e4787.
62. Rose D, Ussher JM, Perz J. Let's talk about gay sex: gay and bisexual men's sexual communication with healthcare professionals after prostate cancer. Eur J Cancer Care (Engl). 2016 ;26(1):e12469. doi:10.1111/ecc.12469.
63. Asencio M, et al. The prospect of prostate cancer: a challenge for gay men's sexualities as they age. Sex Res Soc Policy J NSRC. 2009;6(4):38–51.
64. Waite H. Old lesbians: Gendered histories and persistent challenges. Australas J Ageing. 2015;34(Suppl 2):8–13.
65. Araujo AA, et al. Changes the sexual quality of life of the obeses submitted Fobi-Capella gastroplasty surgery. Rev Col Bras Cir. 2009;36(1):42–8.
66. Brandenburg DL, et al. Breast cancer risk and screening: a comparison of lesbian and heterosexual women. Women Health. 2007;45(4):109–30.
67. Aytaç IA, et al. Socioeconomic factors and incidence of erectile dysfunction: findings of the longitudinal Massachussetts Male Aging Study. Soc Sci Med. 2000;51(5):771–8.
68. Kim JS, Kang S. A study on body image, sexual quality of life, depression, and quality of life in middle-aged adults. Asian Nurs Res (Korean Soc Nurs Sci). 2015;9(2):96–103.
69. Sangi-Haghpeykar H, Ambani DS, Carson SA. Stress, workload, sexual well-being and quality of life among physician residents in training. Int J Clin Pract. 2009;63(3):462–7.
70. Griffin E. Sex, illegitimacy and social change in industrializing Britain. Social History. 2013;38(2):139–61.
71. Melendez-Torres G, Nye E, Bonell C. Internet sex-seeking is inconsistently linked with sexual risk in men who have sex with men: systematic review of within-subjects comparisons. Sex Health. 2015;12(3):183–7.
72. Abdo CH, et al. Hypoactive sexual desire disorder in a population-based study of Brazilian women: associated factors classified according to their importance. Menopause. 2010;17(6):1114–21.
73. Brand M, et al. Watching pornographic pictures on the Internet: role of sexual arousal ratings and psychological–psychiatric symptoms for using Internet sex sites excessively. Cyberpsychol Behav Soc Netw. 2011;14(6):371–7.
74. Bolding G, Davis M, Hart G, Sherr L, Elford J. Gay men who look for sex on the Internet: is there more HIV/STI risk with online partners? AIDS. 2005;19(9):961–8.
75. McMullan M. Patients using the Internet to obtain health information: how this affects the patient–health professional relationship. Patient Educ Couns. 2006;63(1):24–8.
76. Tierney DK. Sexuality: a quality-of-life issue for cancer survivors. Semin Oncol Nurs. 2008;24(2):71–9.
77. Manolis A, Doumas M. Sexual dysfunction: the 'prima ballerina' of hypertension-related quality-of-life complications. J Hypertens. 2008;26(11):2074–84.
78. Reese JB, Shelby RA, Taylor KL. Sexual quality of life in patients undergoing coronary artery bypass graft surgery. Psychol Health. 2012;27(6):721–36.
79. Alonso W, et al. Response to letter to the editor: time to integrate sexual function in the health-related quality of life of patients with left ventricular assist devices. Heart Lung. 2016;45(3):294.
80. Collins EG, et al. Sexual dysfunction in men with COPD: impact on quality of life and survival. Lung. 2012;190(5):545–56.
81. Skrzypulec V, Drosdzol A, Nowosielski K. The influence of bronchial asthma on the quality of life and sexual functioning of women. J Physiol Pharmacol. 2007;58(Supl Pt 2):647–55.
82. Kaptein AA, et al. Sexuality in patients with asthma and COPD. Respir Med. 2008;102(2):198–204.
83. Jedel S, Hood MM, Keshavarzian A. Getting personal: a review of sexual functioning, body image, and their impact on quality of life in patients with inflammatory bowel disease. Inflamm Bowel Dis. 2015;21(4):923–38.

84. Sarhan D, et al. Female genital dialogues: female genital self-image, sexual dysfunction, and quality of life in patients with vitiligo with and without genital affection. J Sex Marital Ther. 2016;42(3):267–76.
85. Ryan C, et al. Genital psoriasis is associated with significant impairment in quality of life and sexual functioning. J Am Acad Dermatol. 2015;72(6):978–83.
86. Van de Nieuwenhof HP, et al. The effect of vulvar lichen sclerosus on quality of life and sexual functioning. J Psychosom Obstet Gynaecol. 2010;31(4):279–84.
87. Janse IC, Deckers IE, van der Maten AD, Evers AW, Boer J, van der Zee HH, Prens EP, Horváth B. Sexual health and quality of life are impaired in hidradenitis suppurativa: a multicenter cross-sectional study. Br J Dermatol. 2016. doi:10.1111/bjd.14975.
88. Asoglu MR, et al. Effects of urinary incontinence subtypes on women's quality of life (including sexual life) and psychosocial state. Eur J Obstet Gynecol Reprod Biol. 2014;176:187–90.
89. Lim R, et al. Effect of stress urinary incontinence on the sexual function of couples and the quality of life of patients. J Urol. 2016;196(1):153–8.
90. Martin DJ, Mulhall JP. Enlarging the scope of managing benign prostatic hyperplasia: addressing sexual function and quality of life. Int J Clin Pract. 2005;59(5):579–90.
91. Wang C-W, Chan CL, Chi I. Overview of quality of life research in older people with visual impairment. Adv Aging Res. 2014;2014.
92. Bakır S, et al. Relationship between hearing loss and sexual dysfunction. J Laryngol Otol. 2012;127(2):142–7.
93. Harmsen RT, et al. Does total hip replacement affect sexual quality of life? BMC Musculoskelet Disord. 2016;17:198.
94. Boonstra AM, et al. Life satisfaction in patients with chronic musculoskeletal pain and its predictors. Qual Life Res. 2013;22(1):93–101.
95. Tristano AG. The impact of rheumatic diseases on sexual function. Rheumatol Int. 2009;29(8):853–60.
96. Reitz A, et al. Impact of spinal cord injury on sexual health and quality of life. Int J Impot Res. 2004;16(2):167–74.
97. Schairer LC, et al. The impact of sexual dysfunction on health-related quality of life in people with multiple sclerosis. Mult Scler. 2014;20(5):610–6.
98. Carod J, et al. Poststroke sexual dysfunction and quality of life. Stroke. 1999;30(10):2238–9.
99. Oyewole OO, et al. Prevalence and impact of disability and sexual dysfunction on health-related quality of life of Nigerian stroke survivors. Disabil Rehabil. 2016;1-6.
100. Carelle N, et al. Changing patient perceptions of the side effects of cancer chemotherapy. Cancer. 2002;95(1):155–63.
101. Baker F, et al. Adult cancer survivors: how are they faring? Cancer. 2005;104(S11):2565–76.
102. Brentjens MH, et al. Recurrent genital herpes treatments and their impact on quality of life. Pharmacoeconomics. 2003;21(12):853–63.
103. Woodhall SC, et al. The impact of genital warts: loss of quality of life and cost of treatment in eight sexual health clinics in the UK. Sex Transm Infect. 2011;87(6):458–63.
104. Danoff A, et al. Sexual dysfunction is highly prevalent among men with chronic hepatitis C virus infection and negatively impacts health-related quality of life. Am J Gastroenterol. 2006;101(6):1235–43.
105. Hansel NN, et al. Quality of life in tuberculosis: patient and provider perspectives. Qual Life Res. 2004;13(3):639–52.
106. Degroote S, et al. Socio-economic, behavioural, (neuro)psychological and clinical determinants of HRQoL in people living with HIV in Belgium: a pilot study. J Int AIDS Soc. 2013;16(1):18643.
107. Monteiro F, Canavarro MC, Pereira M. Factors associated with quality of life in middle-aged and older patients living with HIV. AIDS Care. 2016;28(Suppl 1):92–8.
108. Gakhar H, Kamali A, Holodniy M. Health-related quality of life assessment after antiretroviral therapy: a review of the literature. Drugs. 2013;73(7):651–72.
109. Mellerio H, et al. Long-term impact of childhood-onset type 1 diabetes on social life, quality of life and sexuality. Diabetes Metab. 2015;41(6):489–97.
110. Brooke JC, et al. Testosterone deficiency and severity of erectile dysfunction are independently associated with reduced quality of life in men with type 2 diabetes. Andrology. 2014;2(2):205–11.
111. Hackett G, et al. Testosterone replacement therapy with long-acting testosterone undecanoate improves sexual function and quality-of-life parameters vs. placebo in a population of men with type 2 diabetes. J Sex Med. 2013;10(6):1612–27.
112. Attanasio AF, et al. Quality of life in childhood onset growth hormone-deficient patients in the transition phase from childhood to adulthood. J Clin Endocrinol Metab. 2005;90(8):4525–9.
113. Aulinas A, Webb SM. Health-related quality of life in primary and secondary adrenal insufficiency. Expert Rev Pharmacoecon Outcomes Res. 2014;14(6):873–88.
114. Bukvic B, et al. Improved quality of life in hyperthyroidism patients after surgery. J Surg Res. 2015;193(2):724–30.
115. Zivaljevic VR, et al. Quality of life improvement in patients with Hashimoto thyroiditis and other goiters after surgery: a prospective cohort study. Int J Surg. 2015;21:150–5.
116. Poggiogalle E, et al. Health-related quality of life and quality of sexual life in obese subjects. Int J Endocrinol. 2014;2014:847871.
117. Wee CC, et al. Sex, race, and the adverse effects of social stigma vs. other quality of life factors among primary care patients with moderate to severe obesity. J Gen Intern Med. 2015;30(2):229–35.
118. Nik-Azin A, et al. Evaluation of sexual function, quality of life, and mental and physical health in pregnant women. J Family Reprod Health. 2013;7(4):171–6.
119. Safarinejad MR, Kolahi AA, Hosseini L. The effect of the mode of delivery on the quality of life, sexual function, and sexual satisfaction in primiparous women and their husbands. J Sex Med. 2009;6(6):1645–67.
120. Amaral RC, et al. Quality of life of patients with 46,XX and 46,XY disorders of sex development. Clin Endocrinol (Oxf). 2015;82(2):159–64.
121. Ros C, et al. Turner's syndrome and other forms of congenital hypogonadism impair quality of life and sexual function. Am J Obstet Gynecol. 2013;208(6):4841–6.
122. Falhammar H, Nystrom HF, Thoren M. Quality of life, social situation, and sexual satisfaction, in adult males with congenital adrenal hyperplasia. Endocrine. 2014;47(1):299–307.
123. Perlman CM, et al. Prevalence and predictors of sexual dysfunction in psychiatric inpatients. Psychosomatics. 2007;48(4):309–18.
124. Lam JA, Rosenheck RA. Correlates of improvement in quality of life among homeless persons with serious mental illness. Psychiatr Serv. 2000;51(1):116–8.
125. McClure L. Where is the sex in mental health practice? A discussion of sexuality care needs of mental health clients. J Ethics Mental Health. 2012;7:1–6.
126. Waldinger MD. Psychiatric disorders and sexual dysfunction. Handb Clin Neurol. 2015;130:469–89.
127. Araujo AB, et al. The relationship between depressive symptoms and male erectile dysfunction: cross-sectional results from the Massachusetts Male Aging Study. Psychosom Med. 1998;60(4):458–65.
128. Mak R, et al. Prevalence and correlates of erectile dysfunction in a population-based study in Belgium. Eur Urol. 2002;41(2):132–8.
129. Shindel AW, et al. Sexual function and depressive symptoms among female North American medical students. J Sex Med. 2011;8(2):391–9.

130. Nicolosi A, et al. A population study of the association between sexual function, sexual satisfaction and depressive symptoms in men. J Affect Disord. 2004;82(2):235–43.
131. MacDonagh R, Ewings P, Porter T. The effect of erectile dysfunction on quality of life: psychometric testing of a new quality of life measure for patients with erectile dysfunction. J Urol. 2002;167(1):212–7.
132. Muller MJ, Benkert O. Lower self-reported depression in patients with erectile dysfunction after treatment with sildenafil. J Affect Disord. 2001;66(2–3):255–61.
133. Barlow DH. Causes of sexual dysfunction: the role of anxiety and cognitive interference. J Consult Clin Psychol. 1986;54(2):140–8.
134. Jacobs JA, et al. A multidisciplinary approach to the evaluation and management of male sexual dysfunction. J Urol. 1983;129(1):35–8.
135. Smith AD. Psychologic factors in the multidisciplinary evaluation and treatment of erectile dysfunction. Urol Clin North Am. 1988;15(1):41–51.
136. Bet PM, et al. Side effects of antidepressants during long-term use in a naturalistic setting. Eur Neuropsychopharmacol. 2013; 23(11):1443–51.
137. Carvalho AF, et al. The safety, tolerability and risks associated with the use of newer generation antidepressant drugs: a critical review of the literature. Psychother Psychosom. 2016;85(5): 270–88.
138. Clayton AH, Croft HA, Handiwala L. Antidepressants and sexual dysfunction: mechanisms and clinical implications. Postgrad Med. 2014;126(2):91–9.
139. Keks NA, Hope J, Culhane C. Management of antidepressant-induced sexual dysfunction. Australas Psychiatry. 2014;22(6): 525–8.
140. Serretti A, Chiesa A. Treatment-emergent sexual dysfunction related to antidepressants: a meta-analysis. J Clin Psychopharmacol. 2009;29(3):259–66.
141. Thakurta RG, et al. Nature of sexual dysfunctions in major depressive disorder and its impact on quality of life. Indian J Psychol Med. 2012;34(4):365–70.
142. Baldwin D, Bridgman K, Buis C. Resolution of sexual dysfunction during double-blind treatment of major depression with reboxetine or paroxetine. J Psychopharmacol. 2006;20(1):91–6.
143. Gelenberg AJ, et al. Sexual functioning in patients with recurrent major depressive disorder enrolled in the PREVENT study. J Nerv Ment Dis. 2013;201(4):266–73.
144. Montejo AL, et al. Sexual function during long-term duloxetine treatment in patients with recurrent major depressive disorder. J Sex Med. 2011;8(3):773–82.
145. Piazza LA, et al. Sexual functioning in chronically depressed patients treated with SSRI antidepressants: a pilot study. Am J Psychiatry. 1997;154(12):1757–9.
146. Ishak WW, et al. Sexual satisfaction and quality of life in major depressive disorder before and after treatment with citalopram in the STAR*D study. J Clin Psychiatry. 2013;74(3):256–61.
147. Du Rocher Schudlich T, et al. Physical and sexual abuse and early-onset bipolar disorder in youths receiving outpatient services: frequent, but not specific. J Abnorm Child Psychol. 2015;43(3):453–63.
148. Duarte DG, et al. Sexual abuse and suicide attempt in bipolar type I patients. Rev Bras Psiquiatr. 2015;37(2):180–2.
149. Hyun M, Friedman SD, Dunner DL. Relationship of childhood physical and sexual abuse to adult bipolar disorder. Bipolar Disord. 2000;2(2):131–5.
150. Leverich GS, et al. Early physical and sexual abuse associated with an adverse course of bipolar illness. Biol Psychiatry. 2002;51(4):288–97.
151. Maniglio R. Prevalence of child sexual abuse among adults and youths with bipolar disorder: a systematic review. Clin Psychol Rev. 2013;33(4):561–73.
152. Maniglio R. The impact of child sexual abuse on the course of bipolar disorder: a systematic review. Bipolar Disord. 2013;15(4):341–58.
153. Post RM, et al. Verbal abuse, like physical and sexual abuse, in childhood is associated with an earlier onset and more difficult course of bipolar disorder. Bipolar Disord. 2015;17(3):323–30.
154. Romero S, et al. Prevalence and correlates of physical and sexual abuse in children and adolescents with bipolar disorder. J Affect Disord. 2009;112(1–3):144–50.
155. Downey JI. Driven sexual behavior in bipolar spectrum patients: psychodynamic issues. J Am Acad Psychoanal Dyn Psychiatry. 2011;39(1):77–92.
156. Mazza M, et al. Sexual behavior in women with bipolar disorder. J Affect Disord. 2011;131(1-3):364–7.
157. McCandless F, Sladen C. Sexual health and women with bipolar disorder. J Adv Nurs. 2003;44(1):42–8.
158. Meade CS, et al. The relationship of manic episodes and drug abuse to sexual risk behavior in patients with co-occurring bipolar and substance use disorders: a 15-month prospective analysis. AIDS Behav. 2011;15(8):1829–33.
159. Marengo E, et al. Sexual risk behaviors among women with bipolar disorder. Psychiatry Res. 2015;230(3):835–8.
160. Downey J, et al. Comparison of sexual experience and behavior between bipolar outpatients and outpatients without mood disorders. Psychiatry J. 2016;2016:5839181.
161. Han KT, et al. Is marital status associated with quality of life? Health Qual Life Outcomes. 2014;12:109.
162. Krakow B, et al. Sleep-disordered breathing, psychiatric distress, and quality of life impairment in sexual assault survivors. J Nerv Ment Dis. 2002;190(7):442–52.
163. Valsangkar S, et al. Impairment of quality of life in symptomatic reproductive tract infection and sexually transmitted infection. J Reprod Infertil. 2014;15(2):87–93.
164. Faisal-Cury A, et al. Unplanned pregnancy and risk of maternal depression: secondary data analysis from a prospective pregnancy cohort. Psychol Health Med. 2016;1-10.
165. Dell'Osso L, et al. Sexual dysfunctions and suicidality in patients with bipolar disorder and unipolar depression. J Sex Med. 2009;6(11):3063–70.
166. Lam D, et al. Burden and marital and sexual satisfaction in the partners of bipolar patients. Bipolar Disord. 2005;7(5):431–40.
167. Miller CJ, et al. The ascendancy of second-generation antipsychotics as frontline antimanic agents. J Clin Psychopharmacol. 2015;35(6):645–53.
168. Mitchell PB, Malhi GS. The expanding pharmacopoeia for bipolar disorder. Annu Rev Med. 2002;53:173–88.
169. Grover S, et al. Sexual dysfunction in clinically stable patients with bipolar disorder receiving lithium. J Clin Psychopharmacol. 2014;34(4):475–82.
170. Ghadirian AM, Annable L, Belanger MC. Lithium, benzodiazepines, and sexual function in bipolar patients. Am J Psychiatry. 1992;149(6):801–5.
171. Nagaraj AK, et al. A comparative study of sexual dysfunction due to typical and atypical antipsychotics in remitted bipolar-I disorder. Indian J Psychiatry. 2004;46(3):261–6.
172. Kendurkar A, Kaur B. Major depressive disorder, obsessive-compulsive disorder, and generalized anxiety disorder: do the sexual dysfunctions differ? Prim Care Companion J Clin Psychiatry. 2008;10(4):299–305.
173. Aksaray G, et al. Sexuality in women with obsessive compulsive disorder. J Sex Marital Ther. 2001;27(3):273–7.
174. Freund B, Steketee G. Sexual history, attitudes and functioning of obsessive-compulsive patients. J Sex Marital Ther. 1989; 15(1):31–41.
175. Lustman PJ, Clouse RE. Relationship of psychiatric illness to impotence in men with diabetes. Diabetes Care. 1990;13(8): 893–5.

176. Othmer E, Othmer SC. Effect of buspirone on sexual dysfunction in patients with generalized anxiety disorder. J Clin Psychiatry. 1987;48(5):201–3.
177. Vulink NC, et al. Sexual pleasure in women with obsessive-compulsive disorder? J Affect Disord. 2006;91(1):19–25.
178. Clayton AH, et al. Characterizing sexual function in patients with generalized anxiety disorder: a pooled analysis of three vilazodone studies. Neuropsychiatr Dis Treat. 2016;12:1467–76.
179. McEvoy JP, et al. Chronic schizophrenic women's attitudes toward sex, pregnancy, birth control, and childrearing. Hosp Community Psychiatry. 1983;34(6):536–9.
180. Aizenberg D, et al. Sexual dysfunction in male schizophrenic patients. J Clin Psychiatry. 1995;56(4):137–41.
181. Lyketsos GC, Sakka P, Mailis A. The sexual adjustment of chronic schizophrenics: a preliminary study. Br J Psychiatry. 1983;143:376–82.
182. Assalian P, Fraser R, Tempier R, Cohen D. Sexuality and quality of life of patients with schizophrenia. Int J Psychiatry Clin Pract. 2000;4(1):29–33.
183. Byerly MJ, et al. Sexual dysfunction associated with second-generation antipsychotics in outpatients with schizophrenia or schizoaffective disorder: an empirical evaluation of olanzapine, risperidone, and quetiapine. Schizophr Res. 2006;86(1–3):244–50.
184. Byerly MJ, Nakonezny PA, Rush AJ. Sexual functioning associated with quetiapine switch vs. risperidone continuation in outpatients with schizophrenia or schizoaffective disorder: a randomized double-blind pilot trial. Psychiatry Res. 2008;159(1–2):115–20.
185. Dossenbach M, et al. Effects of atypical and typical antipsychotic treatments on sexual function in patients with schizophrenia: 12-month results from the Intercontinental Schizophrenia Outpatient Health Outcomes (IC-SOHO) study. Eur Psychiatry. 2006;21(4):251–8.
186. Fan X, et al. Sexual functioning, psychopathology and quality of life in patients with schizophrenia. Schizophr Res. 2007;94(1-3): 119–27.
187. Macdonald S, et al. Nithsdale Schizophrenia Surveys 24: sexual dysfunction. Case-control study. Br J Psychiatry. 2003;182:50–6.
188. Nestoros JN, Lehmann HE, Ban TA. Sexual behavior of the male schizophrenic: the impact of illness and medications. Arch Sex Behav. 1981;10(5):421–42.
189. Dossenbach M, et al. Prevalence of sexual dysfunction in patients with schizophrenia: international variation and underestimation. Int J Neuropsychopharmacol. 2005;8(2):195–201.
190. Bushong ME, Nakonezny PA, Byerly MJ. Subjective quality of life and sexual dysfunction in outpatients with schizophrenia or schizoaffective disorder. J Sex Marital Ther. 2013;39(4):336–46.
191. Abernethy V, et al. Family planning during psychiatric hospitalization. Am J Orthopsychiatry. 1976;46(1):154–62.
192. Pinderhughes CA, Grace EB, Reyna LJ. Psychiatric disorders and sexual functioning. Am J Psychiatry. 1972;128(10):1276–83.
193. Finn SE, et al. Subjective utility ratings of neuroleptics in treating schizophrenia. Psychol Med. 1990;20(4):843–8.
194. Compton MT, Miller AH. Sexual side effects associated with conventional and atypical antipsychotics. Psychopharmacol Bull. 2001;35(3):89–108.
195. Cutler AJ. Sexual dysfunction and antipsychotic treatment. Psychoneuroendocrinology. 2003;28(Suppl 1):69–82.
196. Olfson M, et al. Male sexual dysfunction and quality of life in schizophrenia. J Clin Psychiatry. 2005;66(3):331–8.
197. Heinrichs DW, Hanlon TE, Carpenter Jr WT. The quality of life scale: an instrument for rating the schizophrenic deficit syndrome. Schizophr Bull. 1984;10(3):388–98.
198. Hou CL, et al. Sexual dysfunction and its impact on quality of life in Chinese patients with schizophrenia treated in primary care. Compr Psychiatry. 2016;65:116–21.
199. Eack SM, Newhill CE. Psychiatric symptoms and quality of life in schizophrenia: a meta-analysis. Schizophr Bull. 2007;33(5): 1225–37.
200. Adrianzen C, et al. Relative association of treatment-emergent adverse events with quality of life of patients with schizophrenia: post hoc analysis from a 3-year observational study. Hum Psychopharmacol. 2010;25(6):439–47.
201. Plassman BL, et al. Prevalence of dementia in the United States: the aging, demographics, and memory study. Neuroepidemiology. 2007;29(1–2):125–32.
202. Benbow SM, Beeston D. Sexuality, aging, and dementia. Int Psychogeriatr. 2012;24(7):1026–33.
203. Abdo CH. Sexuality and couple intimacy in dementia. Curr Opin Psychiatry. 2013;26(6):593–8.
204. Marsiglio W, Donnelly D. Sexual relations in later life: a national study of married persons. J Gerontol. 1991;46(6):S338–44.
205. Bullard-Poe L, Powell C, Mulligan T. The importance of intimacy to men living in a nursing home. Arch Sex Behav. 1994;23(2):231–6.
206. Roelofs TS, Luijkx KG, Embregts PJ. Intimacy and sexuality of nursing home residents with dementia: a systematic review. Int Psychogeriatr. 2015;27(3):367–84.
207. Higgins A, Barker P, Begley CM. Hypersexuality and dementia: dealing with inappropriate sexual expression. Br J Nurs. 2004;13(22):1330–4.
208. Ehrenfeld M, et al. Sexuality among institutionalized elderly patients with dementia. Nurs Ethics. 1999;6(2):144–9.
209. Elias J, Ryan A. A review and commentary on the factors that influence expressions of sexuality by older people in care homes. J Clin Nurs. 2011;20(11–12):1668–76.
210. Bartelet M, Waterink W, van Hooren S. Extreme sexual behavior in dementia as a specific manifestation of disinhibition. J Alzheimers Dis. 2014;42(Suppl 3):S119–24.
211. Black B, Muralee S, Tampi RR. Inappropriate sexual behaviors in dementia. J Geriatr Psychiatry Neurol. 2005;18(3):155–62.
212. Cipriani G, et al. Sexual disinhibition and dementia. Psychogeriatrics. 2016;16(2):145–53.
213. De Giorgi R, Series H. Treatment of inappropriate sexual behavior in dementia. Curr Treat Options Neurol. 2016;18(9):41.
214. Murphy K. What to do about sexually inappropriate behavior in patients with dementia. Nursing. 2015;45(9):53–6.
215. Roach SM. Sexual behaviour of nursing home residents: staff perceptions and responses. J Adv Nurs. 2004;48(4):371–9.
216. Davies HD, et al. The impact of dementia and mild memory impairment (MMI) on intimacy and sexuality in spousal relationships. Int Psychogeriatr. 2010;22(4):618–28.
217. Martin-Garcia S, et al. Comorbidity, health status, and quality of life in institutionalized older people with and without dementia. Int Psychogeriatr. 2013;25(7):1077–84.
218. Kumsar NA, Kumsar Ş, Dilbaz N. Sexual dysfunction in men diagnosed as substance use disorder. Andrologia. 2016. doi:10.1111/and.12566.
219. Roehrich L, Kinder BN. Alcohol expectancies and male sexuality: review and implications for sex therapy. J Sex Marital Ther. 1991;17(1):45–54.
220. Messman-Moore TL, et al. Sexuality, substance use, and susceptibility to victimization: risk for rape and sexual coercion in a prospective study of college women. J Interpers Violence. 2008; 23(12):1730–46.
221. Suris A, et al. Mental health, quality of life, and health functioning in women veterans: differential outcomes associated with military and civilian sexual assault. J Interpers Violence. 2007;22(2):179–97.
222. Perilloux C, Duntley JD, Buss DM. The costs of rape. Arch Sex Behav. 2012;41(5):1099–106.
223. Van Thiel DH, Lester R. Alcoholism: its effect on hypothalamic pituitary gonadal function. Gastroenterology. 1976;71(2):318–27.

224. Arias F, et al. Bipolar disorder and substance use disorders. Madrid study on the prevalence of dual disorders/pathology. Adicciones. 2016;782.
225. Mason MJ, et al. Psychiatric comorbidity and complications. Child Adolesc Psychiatr Clin N Am. 2016;25(3):521–32.
226. Searby A, Maude P, McGrath I. Prevalence of co-occurring alcohol and other drug use in an Australian older adult mental health service. Int J Ment Health Nurs. 2016;25(2):151–8.
227. Grant BF, et al. The 12-month prevalence and trends in DSM-IV alcohol abuse and dependence: United States, 1991–1992 and 2001–2002. Drug Alcohol Depend. 2004;74(3):223–34.
228. Crowe LC, George WH. Alcohol and human sexuality: review and integration. Psychol Bull. 1989;105(3):374–86.
229. Mandell W, Miller CM. Male sexual dysfunction as related to alcohol consumption: a pilot study. Alcohol Clin Exp Res. 1983;7(1):65–9.
230. Fahrner EM. Sexual dysfunction in male alcohol addicts: prevalence and treatment. Arch Sex Behav. 1987;16(3):247–57.
231. Gluud C, Wantzin P, Eriksen J. No effect of oral testosterone treatment on sexual dysfunction in alcoholic cirrhotic men. Gastroenterology. 1988;95(6):1582–7.
232. Jensen SB, Gluud C. Sexual dysfunction in men with alcoholic liver cirrhosis. A comparative study. Liver. 1985;5(2):94–100.
233. Owiredu WK, et al. Sexual dysfunction and sexual quality of life among the physically challenged in the Kumasi metropolis. Ghana Health Qual Life Outcomes. 2015;13:3.
234. Schiavi RC, et al. Chronic alcoholism and male sexual function. Am J Psychiatry. 1995;152(7):1045–51.
235. Beckman LJ, Ackerman KT. Women, alcohol, and sexuality. Recent Dev Alcohol. 1995;12:267–85.
236. Bozkurt A. Alcohol and sexuality. J Med Sci. 2005;47:52–5.
237. Farkas GM, Rosen RC. Effect of alcohol on elicited male sexual response. J Stud Alcohol. 1976;37(3):265–72.
238. Flaherty, J.A., K. Kim, and S. Adams 2003. The cause of alcoholism in men and women, In: The principle and practice of addiction in psychiatry, N.S. Miller, W.B. Sounders: Philadelphia, PA.
239. Malatesta VJ, et al. Acute alcohol intoxication and female orgasmic response. J Sex Res. 1982;18(1):1–16.
240. Golding JM, et al. Risk factors for secondary depression among Mexican Americans and non-Hispanic whites. Alcohol use, alcohol dependence, and reasons for drinking. J Nerv Ment Dis. 1993;181(3):166–75.
241. Dissiz M, Beji N, Oskay U. The effects of alcohol dependence on the quality of life and sex life of women. Subst Use Misuse. 2015;50(11):1373–82.
242. Grover S, et al. Sexual dysfunction in patients with alcohol and opioid dependence. Indian J Psychol Med. 2014;36(4):355–65.
243. Venkatesh K, Mattoo SK, Grover S. Sexual dysfunction in men seeking treatment for opioid dependence: a study from India. J Sex Med. 2014;11(8):2055–64.
244. Palha AP, Esteves M. A study of the sexuality of opiate addicts. J Sex Marital Ther. 2002;28(5):427–37.
245. Xia Y, et al. Sexual dysfunction during methadone maintenance treatment and its influence on patient's life and treatment: a qualitative study in South China. Psychol Health Med. 2013;18(3):321–9.
246. Byrne P, Ducray K, Smyth BP. The impact of sex upon needs and quality of life within a population on methadone treatment. J Addict Med. 2016;10(1):60–7.
247. Yee A, et al. Sexual dysfunction in heroin dependents: a comparison between methadone and buprenorphine maintenance treatment. PLoS One. 2016;11(1):e0147852.
248. Smith DE, et al. A clinical guide to the diagnosis and treatment of heroin-related sexual dysfunction. J Psychoactive Drugs. 1982; 14(1–2):91–9.
249. Cohen S. Cannabis and sex: multifaceted paradoxes. J Psychoactive Drugs. 1982;14(1–2):55–8.
250. Shamloul R, Bella AJ. Impact of cannabis use on male sexual health. J Sex Med. 2011;8(4):971–5.
251. Dawley Jr HH, et al. An attitude survey of the effects of marijuana on sexual enjoyment. J Clin Psychol. 1979;35(1):212–7.
252. Halikas J, Weller R, Morse C. Effects of regular marijuana use on sexual performance. J Psychoactive Drugs. 1982;14(1–2): 59–70.
253. Melges FT, et al. Marihuana and the temporal span of awareness. Arch Gen Psychiatry. 1971;24(6):564–7.
254. McKay A. Sexuality and substance use: the impact of tobacco, alcohol, and selected recreational drugs on sexual function. Can J Hum Sex. 2005;14(1–2):47–56.
255. Gawin FH. Pharmacologic enhancement of the erotic: Implications of an expanded definition of aphrodisiacs. J Sex Res. 1978; 14(2):107–17.
256. Smith AM, et al. Cannabis use and sexual health. J Sex Med. 2010;7(2 Pt 1):787–93.
257. Aversa A, et al. Early endothelial dysfunction as a marker of vasculogenic erectile dysfunction in young habitual cannabis users. Int J Impot Res. 2008;20(6):566–73.
258. Argiolas A, Melis MR. Central control of penile erection: role of the paraventricular nucleus of the hypothalamus. Prog Neurobiol. 2005;76(1):1–21.
259. Johnson SD, Phelps DL, Cottler LB. The association of sexual dysfunction and substance use among a community epidemiological sample. Arch Sex Behav. 2004;33(1):55–63.
260. Cocores JA, et al. Sexual dysfunction in abusers of cocaine and alcohol. Am J Drug Alcohol Abuse. 1988;14(2):169–73.
261. Cocores JA, Dackis CA, Gold MS. Sexual dysfunction secondary to cocaine abuse in two patients. J Clin Psychiatry. 1986; 47(7):384–5.
262. Henderson DJ, Boyd CJ, Whitmarsh J. Women and illicit drugs: sexuality and crack cocaine. Health Care Women Int. 1995; 16(2):113–24.
263. Bolin BL, et al. Buspirone reduces sexual risk-taking intent but not cocaine self-administration. Exp Clin Psychopharmacol. 2016;24(3):162–73.
264. Borders TF, et al. Risky sex in rural America: longitudinal changes in a community-based cohort of methamphetamine and cocaine users. Am J Addict. 2013;22(6):535–42.
265. Duff P, et al. Sex-for-crack exchanges: associations with risky sexual and drug use niches in an urban Canadian city. Harm Reduct J. 2013;10:29.
266. Edelman NL, et al. Sexual health risks and health-seeking behaviours among substance-misusing women. J Adv Nurs. 2014;70(12):2861–70.
267. Abolfotouh MA, Al-Helali NS. Effect of erectile dysfunction on quality of life. East Mediterr Health J. 2001;7(3):510–8.
268. Laumann EO, Paik A, Rosen RC. Sexual dysfunction in the United States: prevalence and predictors. JAMA. 1999;281(6):537–44.
269. Fujisawa M, et al. Evaluation of health-related quality of life in patients treated for erectile dysfunction with viagra (sildenafil citrate) using SF-36 score. Arch Androl. 2002;48(1):15–21.
270. Paige NM, et al. Improvement in emotional well-being and relationships of users of sildenafil. J Urol. 2001;166:1774–8.
271. Muller MJ, et al. Quality of partnership in patients with erectile dysfunction after sildenafil treatment. Pharmacopsychiatry. 2001;34:91–5.
272. Rubio-Aurioles E, et al. Impact on erectile function and sexual quality of life of couples: a double-blind, randomized, placebo-controlled trial of tadalafil taken once daily. J Sex Med. 2009;6(5):1314–23.
273. Donatucci C, et al. Vardenafil improves patient satisfaction with erection hardness, orgasmic function, and overall sexual experience, while improving quality of life in men with erectile dysfunction. J Sex Med. 2004;1(2):185–92.

274. Meuleman EJ, van Lankveld JJ. Hypoactive sexual desire disorder: an underestimated condition in men. BJU Int. 2005;95(3):291–6.
275. Bloch M, et al. The use of dehydroepiandrosterone in the treatment of hypoactive sexual desire disorder: a report of gender differences. Eur Neuropsychopharmacol. 2013;23(8):910–8.
276. Richardson D, et al. Letrozole versus testosterone. a single-center pilot study of HIV-infected men who have sex with men on highly active anti-retroviral therapy (HAART) with hypoactive sexual desire disorder and raised estradiol levels. J Sex Med. 2007;4(2):502–8.
277. American Psychiatric Association. Diagnostic and statistical manual of mental disorders: DSM-IV-TR. 4th ed. Washington, DC: American Psychiatric Association; 2000.
278. Leiblum SR, et al. Hypoactive sexual desire disorder in postmenopausal women: US results from the Women's International Study of Health and Sexuality (WISHeS). Menopause. 2006;13(1):46–56.
279. Palacios S, Graziottin A. Patient scenario: a 53-year-old woman with hypoactive sexual desire disorder. Maturitas. 2009;63(2):164–8.
280. Biddle AK, et al. Hypoactive sexual desire disorder in postmenopausal women: quality of life and health burden. Value Health. 2009;12(5):763–72.
281. Jaspers L, et al. Efficacy and safety of flibanserin for the treatment of hypoactive sexual desire disorder in women: a systematic review and meta-analysis. JAMA Intern Med. 2016;176(4):453–62.
282. Joffe HV, et al. FDA approval of flibanserin—treating hypoactive sexual desire disorder. N Engl J Med. 2016;374(2):101–4.
283. Shaughnessy AF. Flibanserin ineffective for hypoactive sexual desire disorder in women. Am Fam Physician. 2016;94(5):384–6.
284. Warnock JJ. Female hypoactive sexual desire disorder: epidemiology, diagnosis and treatment. CNS Drugs. 2002;16(11):745–53.
285. Labrie F, et al. Effect of intravaginal dehydroepiandrosterone (Prasterone) on libido and sexual dysfunction in postmenopausal women. Menopause. 2009;16(5):923–31.
286. Barnhart KT, et al. The effect of dehydroepiandrosterone supplementation to symptomatic perimenopausal women on serum endocrine profiles, lipid parameters, and health-related quality of life. J Clin Endocrinol Metab. 1999;84(11):3896–902.
287. Shifren JL, et al. Transdermal testosterone treatment in women with impaired sexual function after oophorectomy. N Engl J Med. 2000;343(10):682–8.
288. Shifren JL, et al. Testosterone patch for the treatment of hypoactive sexual desire disorder in naturally menopausal women: results from the INTIMATE NM1 Study. Menopause. 2006;13(5):770–9.
289. Catalan J, Hawton K, Day A. Couples referred to a sexual dysfunction clinic. Psychological and physical morbidity. Br J Psychiatry. 1990;156:61–7.
290. Rellini AH, Clifton J. Female orgasmic disorder. Adv Psychosom Med. 2011;31:35–56.
291. Meston CM, et al. Disorders of orgasm in women. J Sex Med. 2004;1(1):66–8.
292. Shifren JL, et al. Sexual problems and distress in United States women: prevalence and correlates. Obstet Gynecol. 2008;112(5): 970–8.
293. Kelly MP, Strassberg DS, Turner CM. Communication and associated relationship issues in female anorgasmia. J Sex Marital Ther. 2004;30(4):263–76.
294. Kelly MP, Strassberg DS, Turner CM. Behavioral assessment of couples' communication in female orgasmic disorder. J Sex Marital Ther. 2006;32(2):81–95.
295. Mah K, Binik YM. The nature of human orgasm: a critical review of major trends. Clin Psychol Rev. 2001;21(6):823–56.
296. Rosen RC, Althof S. Impact of premature ejaculation: the psychological, quality of life, and sexual relationship consequences. J Sex Med. 2008;5(6):1296–307.
297. Rowland DL, et al. The psychological burden of premature ejaculation. J Urol. 2007;177(3):1065–70.
298. Giuliano F, et al. Premature ejaculation: results from a five-country European observational study. Eur Urol. 2008;53(5):1048–57.
299. Patrick DL, et al. Premature ejaculation: an observational study of men and their partners. J Sex Med. 2005;2(3):358–67.
300. Cooper K, et al. Interventions to treat premature ejaculation: a systematic review short report. Health Technol Assess. 2015;19(21): 1–180, v-vi.
301. van Lankveld JJ, et al. Internet-based brief sex therapy for heterosexual men with sexual dysfunctions: a randomized controlled pilot trial. J Sex Med. 2009;6(8):2224–36.
302. Bar-Or D, et al. A randomized double-blind, placebo-controlled multicenter study to evaluate the efficacy and safety of two doses of the tramadol orally disintegrating tablet for the treatment of premature ejaculation within less than 2 minutes. Eur Urol. 2012;61(4):736–43.
303. Carson C, Wyllie M. Improved ejaculatory latency, control and sexual satisfaction when PSD502 is applied topically in men with premature ejaculation: results of a phase III, double-blind, placebo-controlled study. J Sex Med. 2010;7(9):3179–89.
304. Dinsmore W, Wyllie M. Results of a phase III, randomized, placebo-controlled study show that PSD502 improves ejaculatory latency and patient reported outcomes, with benefit maintained over 3 months. J Sex Med. 2009;6:418–9.
305. Sunay D, et al. Acupuncture versus paroxetine for the treatment of premature ejaculation: a randomized, placebo-controlled clinical trial. Eur Urol. 2011;59(5):765–71.
306. Althof SE. Psychological interventions for delayed ejaculation/orgasm. Int J Impot Res. 2012;24(4):131–6.
307. Corona G, et al. Psychobiological correlates of delayed ejaculation in male patients with sexual dysfunctions. J Androl. 2006;27(3):453–8.
308. Abdel-Hamid IA, Elsaied MA, Mostafa T. The drug treatment of delayed ejaculation. Transl Androl Urol. 2016;5(4):576–91.
309. Sung SC, Jeng CJ, Lin YC. Sexual health care for women with dyspareunia. Taiwan J Obstet Gynecol. 2011;50(3):268–74.
310. Artune-Ulkumen B, et al. Sexual dysfunction in Turkish women with dyspareunia and its impact on the quality of life. Clin Exp Obstet Gynecol. 2014;41(5):567–71.
311. De Graaff AA, et al. Dyspareunia and depressive symptoms are associated with impaired sexual functioning in women with endometriosis, whereas sexual functioning in their male partners is not affected. Hum Reprod. 2016;31(11):2577–86.
312. Lemieux AJ, et al. Do romantic partners' responses to entry dyspareunia affect women's experience of pain? The roles of catastrophizing and self-efficacy. J Sex Med. 2013;10(9):2274–84.
313. Labrie F, et al. Lack of influence of dyspareunia on the beneficial effect of intravaginal prasterone (dehydroepiandrosterone, DHEA) on sexual dysfunction in postmenopausal women. J Sex Med. 2014;11(7):1766–85.
314. Bertolasi L, et al. Botulinum neurotoxin type A injections for vaginismus secondary to vulvar vestibulitis syndrome. Obstet Gynecol. 2009;114(5):1008–16.
315. Vallinga MS, et al. Transcutaneous electrical nerve stimulation as an additional treatment for women suffering from therapy-resistant provoked vestibulodynia: a feasibility study. J Sex Med. 2015;12(1):228–37.
316. Woodward JM, Hass SL, Woodward PJ. Reliability and validity of the sexual life quality questionnaire (SLQQ). Qual Life Res. 2002;11(4):365–77.
317. Althof SE. Quality of life and erectile dysfunction. Urology. 2002;59(6):803–10.
318. Alexandre B, et al. Intracavernous injections of prostaglandin E1 for erectile dysfunction: patient satisfaction and quality of sex life on long-term treatment. J Sex Med. 2007;4(2):426–31.
319. Albaugh JA. Intracavernosal injection algorithm. Urol Nurs. 2006;26(6):449–53.

320. Albaugh JA, Ferrans CE. Impact of penile injections on men with erectile dysfunction after prostatectomy. Urol Nurs. 2010;30(1):64–77.
321. Caraceni E, Utizi L. A questionnaire for the evaluation of quality of life after penile prosthesis implant: quality of life and sexuality with penile prosthesis (QoLSPP): to what extent does the implant affect the patient's life? J Sex Med. 2014;11(4):1005–12.
322. Ferguson KH, Cespedes RD. Prospective long-term results and quality-of-life assessment after Dura-II penile prosthesis placement. Urology. 2003;61(2):437–41.
323. Vitarelli A, et al. Long term patient satisfaction and quality of life with AMS700CX inflatable penile prosthesis. Arch Ital Urol Androl. 2013;85(3):133–7.
324. Dinsmore WW, et al. Topical eutectic mixture for premature ejaculation (TEMPE): a novel aerosol-delivery form of lidocaine-prilocaine for treating premature ejaculation. BJU Int. 2007;99(2):369–75.
325. McMahon CG, et al. Efficacy of sildenafil citrate (Viagra) in men with premature ejaculation. J Sex Med. 2005;2(3):368–75.
326. Cai T, et al. Rhodiola rosea, folic acid, zinc and biotin (EndEP(R)) is able to improve ejaculatory control in patients affected by lifelong premature ejaculation: results from a phase I–II study. Exp Ther Med. 2016;12(4):2083–7.
327. Blumel JE, et al. Effect of androgens combined with hormone therapy on quality of life in post-menopausal women with sexual dysfunction. Gynecol Endocrinol. 2008;24(12):691–5.
328. Caruso S, et al. Tadalafil 5 mg daily treatment for type 1 diabetic premenopausal women affected by sexual genital arousal disorder. J Sex Med. 2012;9(8):2057–65.
329. Danielsson I, et al. EMG biofeedback versus topical lidocaine gel: a randomized study for the treatment of women with vulvar vestibulitis. Acta Obstet Gynecol Scand. 2006;85(11):1360–7.
330. Pelletier F, et al. Efficacy of high doses of botulinum toxin A for treating provoked vestibulodynia. Br J Dermatol. 2011;164(3):617–22.

35 Alternative Medicine Approaches in Sexual Medicine

Lucy Postolov

Alternative Medicine in Sexual Performance Enhancement

Cultures around the world have been practicing what Western medicine calls alternative for over 5000 years (Figure 35-1). Traditional oriental medicine, homeopathy, Ayurvedic medicine, aromatherapy and meditation, massages, etc. have long been practiced in China, India, and the European continent. These treatments and techniques have been the mainstay of health in these cultures. Although these traditional medical beliefs differ in language, philosophy, and metaphors, they base their faith on the principle that health is a state of balance or wholeness regulated by a universal life force. This life force is constant with cultures throughout the world. It is called "Qi" in China, "ki" in Japan, "prana" in India, and the ancient Greeks would know it as "pneuma." Medical cultures outside of Western medicine believe any illness results within the body from unbalances that block the aforementioned life force from flowing freely.

The patient interest in alternative medicines in the 1990s grew at a remarkable rate and continues to gain wider interest and recognition. A report from the National Ambulatory Medical Care Survey conducted in 1990 and 1996 released these remarkable numbers [1]. In 1997, visits to all primary care practitioners were 385 million, almost two million less than comparable visits in 1990. Conversely, visits to practitioners of alternative therapies rose dramatically from 427 million in 1990 to 628 million in 1997. It would benefit Western medical practitioners greatly to familiarize themselves with the different modalities available to patients and to be well versed in the underlying principles of those medicines.

The patient who has an interest in some of the techniques mentioned in this chapter, such as acupuncture, homeopathy, Ayurveda, and herbal medicine, must seek a licensed[1] or certified practitioner of these arts. Although considered natural healing remedies, they are not to be practiced by the patient on their own.

Western medical science focuses on human sexuality in terms of anatomy, physiology, and psychology. In Eastern cultures, sex is regarded as an art, science, and a path to a spiritual development. It is a path toward greater intimacy not only with the partner but also with the divine self.

Those who understand the nature of sex will nurture their vigor and prolong their life. Those who treat its principle with contempt will injure their spirit and shorten their life. Tung Hsuan Tzu

The most extensive approaches to sex are those of China (Taoism), India (yoga), and Tibet (tantra) which have drawn upon unique ancient classical texts on sexual practices. These texts include Kama Sutra-Vatsyayana (400 A.D.), Ananga Ranga, Perfumed Garden (fifteenth century), Tao Te Ching-Lao Tzu (fifth century B.C.), The Yellow Emperor Classics-Huang Ti (2697–2598 B.C.), The Secret Art of Bedchamber (590–618 A.D.), and Pillow Book and the Tantric Buddhism (eight century). In the Han dynasty, there were over 165 books on sexual techniques and 8 different schools on the subject.

Eastern metaphysical traditions make use of the mystery of sexuality as a means to the transcendental experience of unity. The feeling of oneness, achieved during or following the sexual act, is the most universally accessible mystical experience. Nik Douglas and Penny Slinger/ Sexual Secrets [2]

[1] In the United States, acupuncture is a licensed practice in most states. Homeopathy, Ayurveda, and aromatherapy are not licensed but are certified by credible schools throughout the country.

W.W. IsHak (ed.), *The Textbook of Clinical Sexual Medicine*, DOI 10.1007/978-3-319-52539-6_35

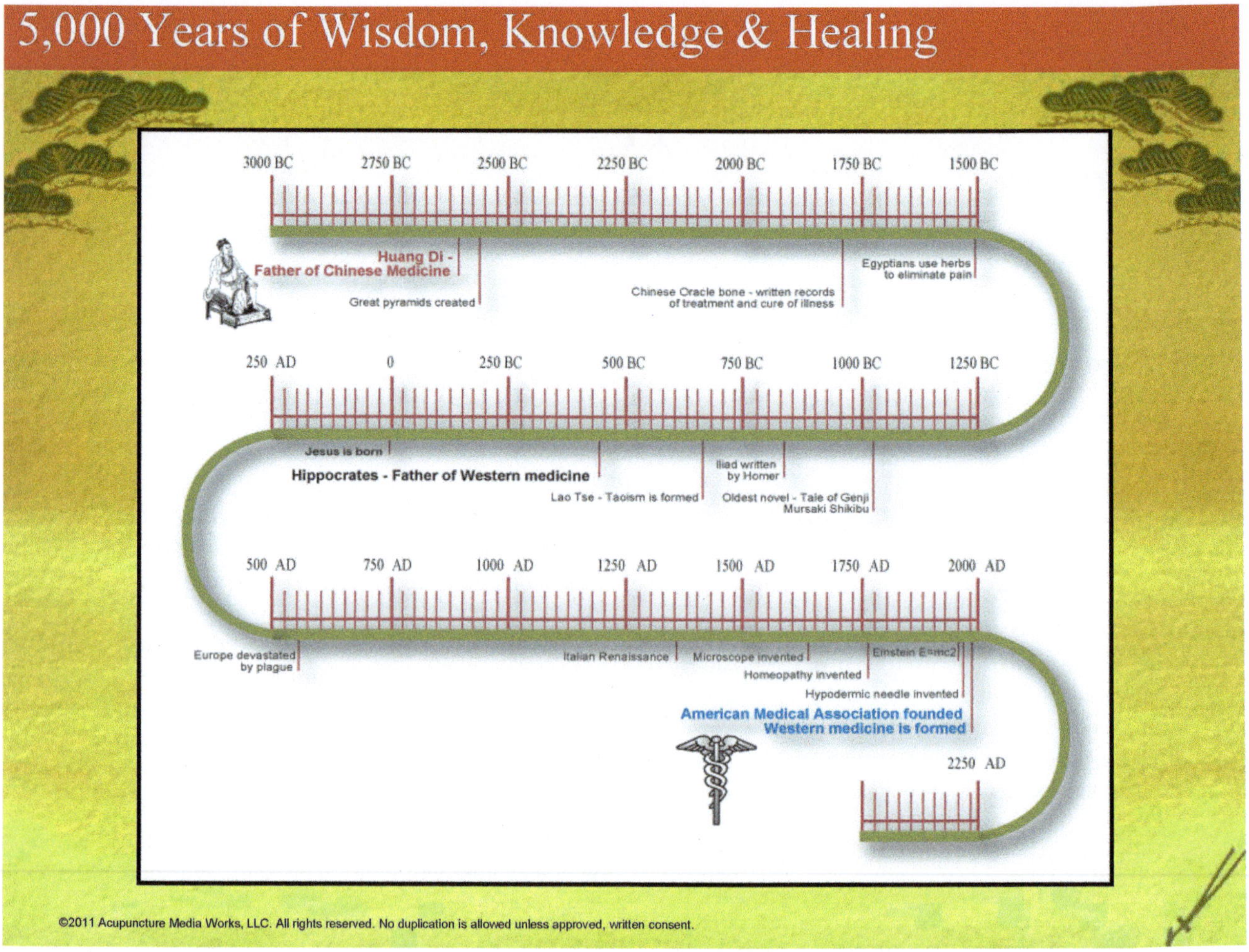

FIGURE 35-1. Five-thousand year timeline slide [Courtesy of Acupuncture Media Works, LLC ©2011].

Traditional Oriental Medicine

A Comprehensive System of Modalities That Includes Herbal Medicine, Acupuncture, Massage, Meditation, and Exercise

Chinese philosophers and healers have studied and practiced human sexuality to enhance relationships and vitality and restore health of the body, mind, and spirit. It is very important to note that this philosophy confirms not only an anatomical or physiological difference between man and woman but also an energetic one.

The feminine energy or "yin" is always receiving or "being and opening" the energy of the spirit. The male energy, or "yang," is the proactive of the two and is giving and doing. With this responsibility, the man is required to perfect his power of retention. The sexual energy of man is like a fire: quick to get hot, quick to boil, and ultimately to explode. The female sexual energy, like water, heats up and boils slowly but staying warm longer.

The Chinese texts "Classics of the Plain Girl" and "Counsels of a Simple Girl" are conversations between the legendary Yellow Emperor and his female advisor, Su Nu. She shares with the Emperor the secret methods of lovemaking called the "Sex Recipes of the Plain Girl" and therapeutic lovemaking, called the "Discourse of the Plain Girl." In these books, the Plain Girl declares, "Woman is superior to man in the way that water is superior to fire [Common translation from The Yellow Emperor's Classic of Medicine/Neijing Suwen written approx. 221 BCE]. People who are experts in the art of love are like excellent cooks who know how to blend the different flavors with a tasty meal. Those who know the art of Yin and Yang can blend the pleasures of the senses, but those who do not know it will have an unexpected death, without ever having enjoyed the art of lovemaking."

The human body has the innate ability to heal itself. It is just a matter of triggering the right mechanisms. Specific points of the body, different breathing techniques, and unique postures channel energy to create balance. Therapeutic lovemaking allows energy to flow freely within the body. Using specific positions in lovemaking helps the energy to be concentrated in specific organs, and at orgasm, the energy is released in this healing way. By using these unique positions, sexual performance will be enhanced and more satisfying to both partners. Sexual problems as well as other health-related issues can also be resolved.

Sexual Positions: Therapeutic Lovemaking

When referring to the ancient texts, you will find many sexual positions named after animals. Taoist masters believed that by imitating the movements of the animals, humans would be more in tune with nature and bring balance to heaven and earth. Here are just a few of the many positions as described in classical texts [3].

Mandarin Duck

This position is beneficial for man who has problems sustaining erection and has difficulties with sexual performance. This also improves the concentration of the man's semen. For the woman this position benefits her sexual organs, uterus and ovaries. The position can relieve the symptoms of premenstrual syndrome. From the Chinese medicine point of view, it benefits the yin of the woman and strengthens the jing (essence) of the man (Figure 35-2).

Pawing Horse

A position that is especially beneficial to the woman who has emotional blockage, mood swings, and inability to reach orgasm. The stretch in the pelvic area allows the release of liver energy at the time of orgasm. Her hand is in the "mudra" position, known to be beneficial in the release of negative emotions. From the Chinese medicine point of view, this position is of benefit for liver Qi stagnation (Figure 35-3).

Overlapping Fish Scale

This position is beneficial to the woman with premenstrual syndrome and fibroid tumors and helps regulate menstruation. For the man it can prevent premature ejaculation and low-back pain. The Chinese medical benefits tonify blood in liver channel for woman and for man tonify kidney yin deficiency (Figure 35-4).

Tiger Attacks

This improves the immune system and bone marrow production and also helps pain in the spine for woman. A position that is beneficial for harmonizing life force (Qi) and balances all five elements (Figure 35-5).

Crane with Two Necks

A position that creates and sustains a harmonious sexual relationship. The couple is seated in close union and learns to give as well as receive sexual energy. From the Chinese medicine point of view, benefits "Three Treasures" being Shen "spirit," Qi "energy," and jing "essence" (Figure 35-6).

Flattering Phoenix

This position is tranquilizing the life force. Helps the woman with PMS and fibroids and harmonizes the joints of the man. From the Chinese medicine point of view beneficial for woman with blood Qi stagnation and man with kidney deficiency (Figure 35-7).

Acupuncture

A treatment that involves puncturing the skin with hair-thin needles inserted into underlying tissue. The word acupuncture originated from the Latin "acus" (needle) and "puncture" (puncture) and originated in China some 5000 years ago. A typical treatment consists of needles inserted at specific

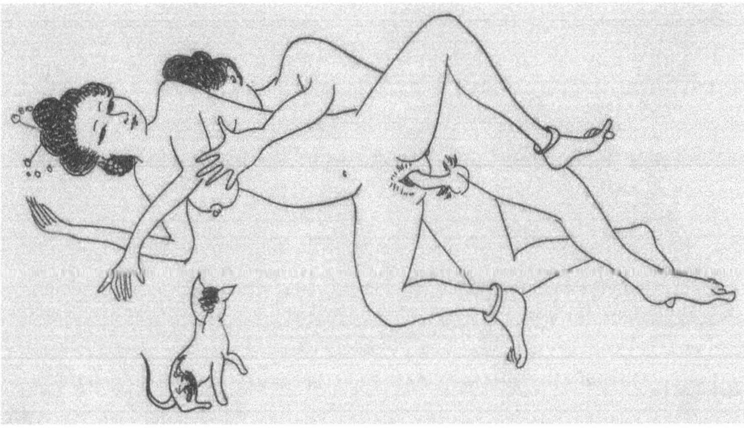

FIGURE 35-2. Mandarin duck [Courtesy of Lucy Postolov, L.Ac].

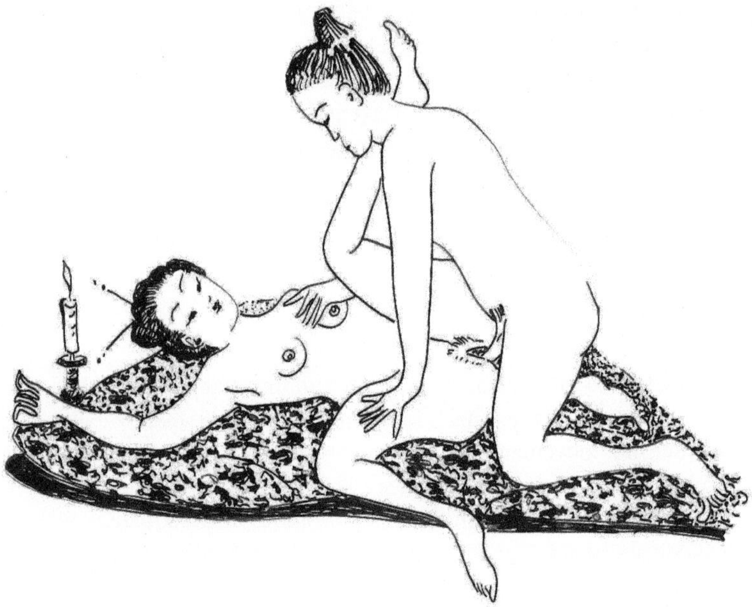

FIGURE 35-3. Pawing horse [Courtesy of Lucy Postolov, L. Ac.].

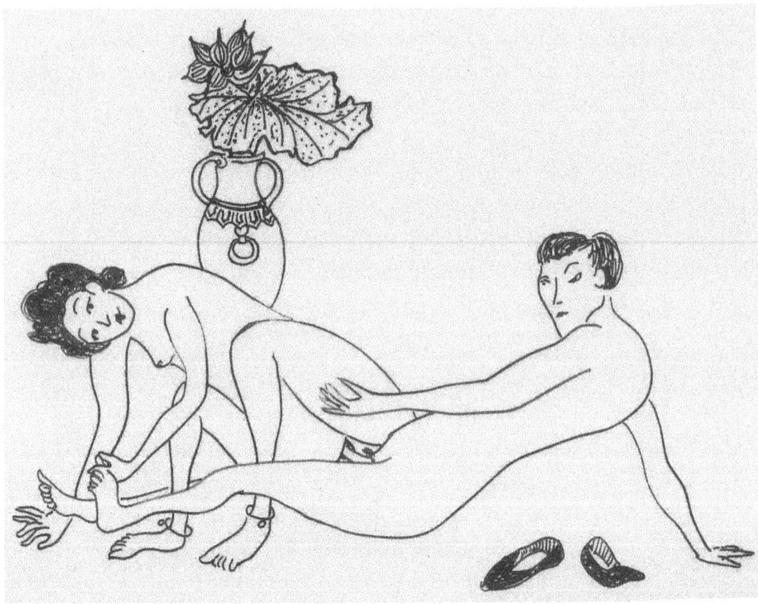

FIGURE 35-4. Overlapping fish scale [Courtesy of Lucy Postolov, L.Ac.].

points in the body, extremities, face, and ears along lines called meridians and channels. These meridians and channels are vessels for the life force or "Qi" to flow freely. Through diagnosis unique to the Chinese medicine practitioner, which is observation of the tongue, palpation of the abdomen and meridians, and traditional pulse palpation, it is determined where blockages, stagnations, or deficiency of energy occurs.

Traditional Chinese Herbal Medicine

One of the most ancient forms of healthcare began with *Shennong Ben Cao Jing* (pharmacopeia of the heavenly husbandman) in the second century B.C.

Chinese herbs are effective when prescribed according with traditional Chinese diagnosis. They work the same way as do conventional pharmaceutical drugs via their chemical reactions.

The Use of Acupuncture and Herbal Medicine to Enhance Sexual Performance

Differentiation and Treatment

1. Lack of sexual desire
2. Sexual anhedonia
3. Impotence

FIGURE 35-5. Tiger attacks [Courtesy of Lucy Postolov, L.Ac.].

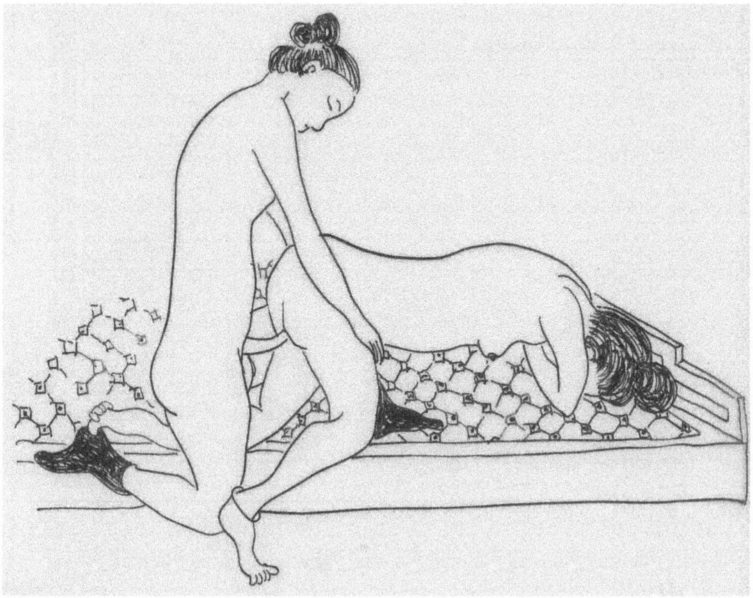

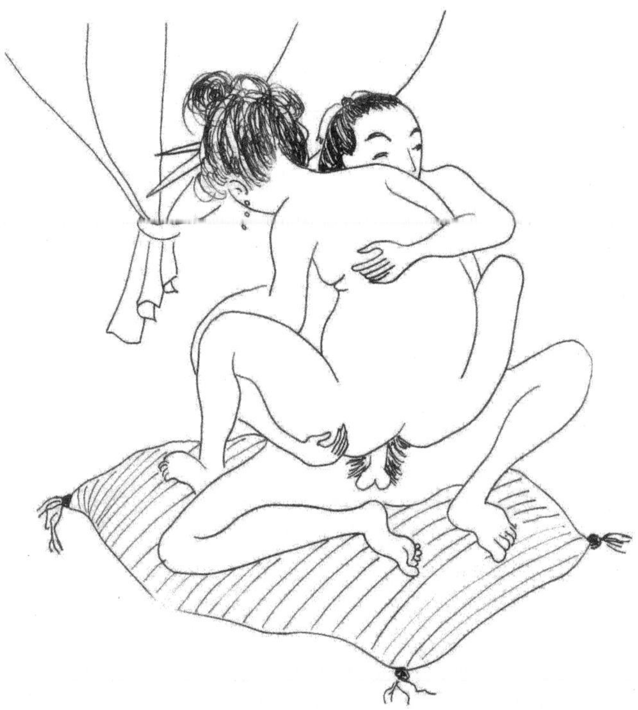

FIGURE 35-6. Crane with two necks [Courtesy of Lucy Postolov, L.Ac.].

Lack of Sexual Desire

From the Chinese point of view, lack of desire could be due to three reasons.

Heart Qi deficiency

Treatment principle:

In the case of heart Qi deficiency, which in some instances is accompanied by spleen Qi deficiency (overcritical of partner or over watchful of themselves), points to use are Bl15, H9, Sp1, and P6. The use of moxa or silver pellets at home on Sp1 is also recommended.

Kidney yin deficiency

Acupuncture treatment:

Points to use: K3,6,10, and BL25

Kidney yang deficiency

Acupuncture treatment:

K2, K7, BL23, and BL52

Sexual Anhedonia

Treatment principle

Patients who can perform but do not enjoy sex. Chinese diagnosis is liver Qi stagnation.

Acupuncture treatment:

Bl22 and Liv 2, 3, 5, 8, 9

Chinese herbal formula:

"xiao yao san"

Impotence

Treatment principle:

Could be due to kidney yin deficiency, kidney yang deficiency, and liver Qi stagnation

Acupuncture points:

Kidney yin deficiency: K3, K6, and K10

Chinese herb:

Shou Di Huang (*Rehmannia glutinosa*, Rx) single herb

Gui Zhi Jia Long Gu Mu Li Tang (cinnamon twig and oyster shell) (formula)

Gui Zhi (Ramulus Cinnamomi)

Bai Shao (Radix Paeoniae Alba)

Long Gu (Os Draconis)

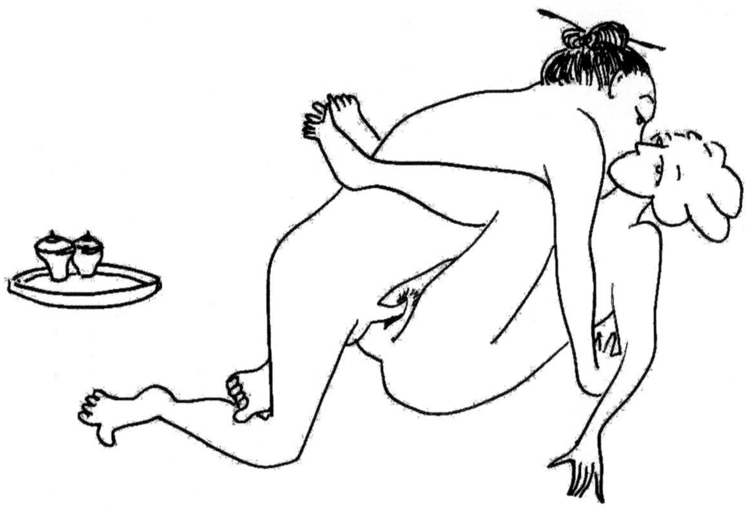

FIGURE 35-7. Flattering PHOENIX [Courtesy of Lucy Postolov, L.Ac.].

Mu Li (Concha Ostreae)
Sheng Jiang (Rm. Zingiberis)
Da Zao (Fructus Zizyphi Jujubae)
Gan Cao (Rx. Glycyrrhiza)
Kidney yang deficiency:
Acupuncture points: K2, 7, and Bl23 Combination of deficiencies: K3, 7, and UB52
Herbal formula:
Rou Cong Rong (Cistances, Hb)
Wu Wei Zhi (Schisandrae, Fr)
Tu Si Zi (Cuscutae, Sm)
Yuan Zhi (Polygalae, Rx)
She Chuang Zi (Cnidii, Sm)
Liver Qi stagnation
Acupuncture points:
Liv 2,3,5,8, and 9
Herbal formula:
Xiao Yao San
Additional herbal formulas and single herbs:
Weak erection/penis strengthening topical application:
Sichuan (Zanthoxyli Fr.)
Wu Wei Zhi (Schisandrae Fr.)
Xi Xin (Asari Hb)
Haizao (Sargassi Hb)
These preceding herbs should be ground, mixed with li dan dao, and applied topically on the penis.
Chinese herbs known to increase testosterone level and sexual drive
yang deficiency:
Yin Yang Huo (Epimedii, Hb)
Ba Gi Tian (Morindae Officinalis, Rx)
Rou Cong Rong (Cistances, Hb)
Qi deficiency:
Huang Qi (Astragalus)
Ren Shen (Ginseng)
Yohimbine, Muira Puama, Damiana

Ear acupuncture points:
Shen Men, Sympathetic, Internal Secretion, Brain, Genital, Kidney, Liver, Heart, Lumbar, Sexual Desire point
Abdominal points to increase sexual performance:
Abdominal Zigong (3 cun lateral to Ren 3), for woman both sides and for men right side only.
ST 30 (needle oblique toward genitals)
Ren 4 (needle downward plus moxa)

Exercises and Techniques to Enhance Sexual Performance

Microcosmic Orbits[2]

With the male's genitals being external and the females internal, the union of the two provides an opportunity for the yin and the yang to mesh and achieve a perfect exchange of energy. Emotionally, the woman is yang energy; it is easier for her to express herself. Physically the woman is yin, while the male is physically yang and emotionally yin. During the act of intercourse, the male, with his external sexual yang energy, is the giver to the female's internal sexual yin energy. Emotionally, vice versa, the female gives through her heart and the male receives. Together, they complement and balance each other's energy, sexually and emotionally [4].

Kegel exercise and its variation from Taoist practice for both men and women [5]:

1. Rapid contraction and release of the pelvic area for 1–2 min
2. Slow contraction and release of the pelvic area for 1–2 min

[2]From the book, *Sexual Reflexology* by Mantak Chia, Destiny Books, 2003.

A woman can improve her sexual experience by strengthening the muscles in the vaginal wall by inserting two fingers in her vagina during these contractions. Also effective would be the Jade Egg, a more traditional device.

Massage the Ears

With the ears each having over 150 acupuncture points, they are an excellent source for stimulation of sexual energy. In Chinese medicine, the ear is an extension of the kidney energy, which is responsible for sexuality. A couple instinctively massages, kisses, and nibbles each other's ears during lovemaking. When the ear is massaged, it stimulates the entire body [6].

Taoist Retention of the Semen Exercise

The Taoist man uses his mind to control his breath, his breath to control his blood, and his blood to control the semen. By mastering breathing techniques and utilizing them during lovemaking, the male can control his heartbeat, which speeds up prior to ejaculation. Using deep, rhythmic abdominal breathing, he is able to control his heartbeat and thus "quiet" the rush of blood to the penis, suppressing the ejaculation [7].

> Of all the things that make mankind prosper, none can be compared to sexual intercourse. It is modeled after Heaven and takes its form by Earth; it regulates Yin and rules Yang…Thus the four seasons succeed each other; man thrusts, woman receives; above there is action; below, receptivity. Taoist Master

Food as Aphrodisiacs

The legend and reality of the existence of aphrodisiacs have been questioned through time. The truth of the matter is that *indeed* there are foods which are rich in minerals, vitamins, and essential fatty acids that in both short and long term can enhance the sexual libido [8].

Foods: Oysters, shrimp, mustard, garlic, leeks, avocado, nuts, seeds, kelp, yogurt, eggs, and beans

Minerals: Iodine, magnesium, manganese, zinc, chromium, and calcium

Essential Fatty Acids: L-Arginine, phenylalanine and tyrosine, and phenylethylamine

Vitamins: Vitamin E, B1, B2, B3, B6, B12, folic acid, and vitamin C

All foods, vitamins, and minerals should be taken in moderation and not exceed the daily dietary requirements.

Aromatherapy

A sense that is frequently overlooked, smell plays an important role in our lives. One of the most primal senses, its power, has only recently begun to be explored. The sense of smell is unique in that it evades the cerebral cortex. Smell receptors in the nose are directly connected to the limbic center, which controls emotions, moods, memories, and sex drive. It is therefore very common to get a whiff of a familiar scent and be nostalgic of a person, place, and time in one's life without the control of our conscious mind.

Aromatherapy uses the power of plant chemicals as well as other smells to arouse the body, elevate emotions and mood, and create a desired ambiance. Specific smells are often used to increase sex drive and sexual arousal, often unconsciously. Aromas are usually contained in essential oils and can be used as inhalants or mixed with base oils and used as massage oil, either way serving as an erotic stimulant.

A number of smells are responsible for triggering sexual memories and excitement and are attainable at most health stores. For example, *ambergris*, a mild, sweet, earthy-smelling aroma continues to be used in Asia as an aphrodisiac. Often coffee would be laced with ambergris to exhibit its aphrodisiac quality when taken orally. In the novel Moby-Dick, *ambergris* was the highly prized, sweet-smelling product of a sperm whale; in reality, it is the vomit of a sperm whale caused by digestive irritation. Although the thought of whale vomit may not seem romantic, the smell is very pleasant. Once their rare power were discovered, not only was it distributed as oil, but perfume manufactures began to incorporate ambergris in fine fragrances, especially those with floral hints.

Both *jasmine* and *rose* have intoxicating smells capable of exciting either sex. Fragrances containing jasmine are very expensive because oil extraction is very laborious as well as tedious. Jasmine has the power to strengthen male sex organs, low libido, as well as treat impotence and prostate problems. It has also been used an antidepressant. The precious fragrance of rose is also esteemed and was once used by kings. If jasmine is the king, rose is its queen. Rose has been the choice in various ceremonies and love potions. It is said that when Cleopatra met Anthony, she layered her floor an inch deep with rose petals an action typical in Rome where rose petals were scattered at weddings as well as bridal beds. Rose oil is also hard to extract and is an expensive oil, however, highly sought after for several reasons. The smell is very sensual and seemingly popular therefore arousing erotic memories. It is also a mood elevator and may contain phenyl ethanol, which has narcotic properties. The sweet smell of rose, like ylang-ylang, is calming and pacifies anxiety and stress.

Perhaps the most provocative fragrance, musk, has been referred to as the "universal" aphrodisiac. Derived from the Sanskrit word for testicle, it is a scent produced my males in nature. Nonetheless, this general term for the erosion of male hormones is rousing for both sexes. Musk oil was the preferred fragrance of Josephine Bonaparte, Napoleon's wife, and when he decided to leave her, she poured the oil all over the bedroom so he would never forget her. Musk has an unmistaken and obstinate smell. Originally acquired from the abdominal gland from the male musk deer, today it is synthesized as galaxolide and Exaltolide. Unlike the other smells discussed, musk provokes the VNO, a special organ identifying pheromones, because it produces alpha-androstenol. For this reason musk is not only erotic through smell but also a hormone-related substance.

Smells from nature have been used to arouse for centuries, but for a long time, natural smell was overlooked. It is evident that animals are sexually stimulated by smells (dogs in heat) and even recognize territories. Can humans have a similar attraction through smells? The VNO (vomeronasal organ) found in the nostrils detects pheromones and chemical messengers similar to hormones, among humans. Dr. David Berliner was researching an unrelated topic and was scraping skin cells from used casts of skiers. He made extracts from the cells in vials. Whenever Berliner left the vials open, the atmosphere of the lab was much friendlier. When they were closed, the labs chaos resumed. Hearing about the discovery of the VNO, Berliner teamed up with Dr. Luis Monti-Bloch to test the human VNO. After puffing pure air, scented air, Berliner's two compounds, air without hormones or pheromones, and fragrant compound, the two men found that the VNO only reacted to Berliner's extracts. In addition, male subjects reacted to female extract and vice versa. When the men tested the olfactory nerves, the subject only responded to the fragrant smell. This evidence gave rise to more questions and initiated the discovery of pheromones as aphrodisiacs.

Pheromones are produced in sweat glands and appear where hair is highly concentrated. Bacteria are trapped in, and as they decompose, pheromones are released. The aroma from pheromones is often called a person's smell and is as individual as fingerprints. Males secrete a musky odor, which is paired with the odor-producing skin bacteria. The female pheromones result from estrogen and progesterone, which control the odor men release and fluctuate during the monthly cycle. While pheromones do not stimulate sexual activity, they arouse an erotic mood. Using synthetic hormones has been reported to make people feel more attractive and romantic. They also explain certain degrees of sexual attraction; when a person cannot understand what they see in someone, it may simply be compatible pheromones. Tight clothes restrict the release of pheromones that are natural sex enhancers. The smell of sweat on a lover's body after a workout is very arousing because that same smell is secreted during lovemaking. Couples sleeping on foreign sides of the bed are the VNO recognizing the pheromones that are still lingering, providing comfort.

Different smells will appeal to different people even though the ingredients are exactly the same. The chemistry of the smell with the individual will vary. The power of smell plays a major role in lovemaking and can enhance the arousal and pleasure.

Ayurvedic Medicine

The origins of Ayurveda can be found in India over 5000 years ago. Ayurvedic (meaning "science of life") medicine places its emphasis on the state of the individual body, mind, and spirit, in equal proportions. As with many alternative approaches to medicine and health, the prominence of prevention is the approach to a patient's health as opposed to curing a disease.

Upon the patient's initial visit to the Ayurvedic practitioner, the individual constitution is determined by determining the metabolic body type or *doshas*. The practitioner will base the diagnosis on physical observation, personal and family history, palpation, and listening to the heart, lungs, and intestines. Particular consideration will be paid to the pulse, tongue, eyes. and nails. In Ayurveda medicine, the concept of metabolic types is categorized in three distinctive doshas. These doshas are known as *vata*, *pitta*, and *kapha*. The characteristics of these doshas include a number of different factors unique to the individual. Some contributing (but not limited to) features are build, hair, skin, temper, appetite, sleeping habits, energy level, personality, and sexual desire.

Most individuals will have predominance in one of the dosha body types, but all three will be present. Equally, the three doshas are located in specific areas of the body. The individual is at most favorable health when all doshas are in balance.

Sexual Balance

Each dosha has characteristics and responsibilities unique to the development of sexuality. Sexual realization is attained when the correct equilibrium is reached among the doshas.

The dosha *vata* is responsible for the movement of the body. If depleted, there will be an adverse reaction in the actual act of sex and retention of the sexual energy.

Pitta is the impetus for sexual drive. When there is an imbalance in the pitta dosha, you will find a lack of initiative in sexual activity. Accompanying this state will be physical manifestations (rashes, herpes outbreaks, acne, odors, etc.) that would make this person less desirable for sexual interest.

Finally, *kapha* takes on the responsibility of sexual potency. An imbalance here will directly affect the fertility and effectiveness of the sexual excretions. Finding exhaustion in the kapha will directly affect the ability to procreate.

Treatment Plan

After diagnosis of the disease or the imbalance of the individual, the practitioner has four methods of management available to obtain the desired results: cleansing and detoxification (*shodan*), palliation (*shaman*), rejuvenation (*rasayana*), and mental hygiene (*satvajaya*).

Improving Sexual Performance with Ayurvedic Medicine

The Ayurvedic practitioner will address the individual's sexual concerns after a systematic management plan is in place to balance the doshas. After the patient has been cleansed and detoxed, the practitioner will look to rejuvenate and enhance the body's ability to function. Herbs are commonly used to address sexual problems and to enhance the sexual abilities of the individual. Here are two recipes (all recipes from *Ayurveda for Life* by Dr. Vinod Verma, Samuel Weiser Inc., 1997) that may be used for specific sexual purpose:

Premature ejaculation: Put a pinch of camphor in 1/8 cup (25 ml) rose essence and mix well. Apply this on the penis in a very small quantity by putting two to three drops of it on your fingers and then smearing it on penis about an hour before intercourse.

Increase desire: This is a very simple preparation with readily available ingredients. You need powdered licorice, ghee, honey, and milk. For one dose, mix 1 tablespoon each: powdered licorice, honey, and ghee. Whip well. You should obtain a kind of paste which should be eaten with some hot milk. It is excellent to increase the sexual urge.

Ayurveda medicine, as many of the "alternative" medicines, has been practiced and utilized by patients around the world for thousands of years. Its popularity and success rate in India and Europe cannot be ignored. As the demand for this technique in the Western countries continues to rise, more clinical research will be conducted and given credence.

Homeopathy

Homeopathy is a form of holistic medicine based on Hippocrates *Law of Similars* (like cures like) with the premise that "through the like, disease is produced, and through the application of the like, it is cured." In order for a homeopathic treatment to cure a disease, it must produce similar symptoms of the disease in a healthy person. This of course is a principle that is the theoretical basis for the vaccines of Edward Jenner, Jonas Salk, and Louis Pasteur. A practice founded in the late eighteenth century by German physician, Samuel Hahnemann, the word homeopathy is derived from the Greek word "homois" meaning similar and "pathos" meaning disease. Hahnemann was translating medical text when he learned about *cinchona*, a Peruvian bark that was used in the treatment of malaria. Hahnemann experimented with the substance and ingested it twice daily. Upon taking his own mixture with Peruvian bark, he began to develop symptoms similar to malaria. The same substance, when taken in a smaller, regulated dose, would stimulate the body to fight the disease. Hahnemann went on to test hundreds of plants, minerals, and animals to discover that many of these produced symptoms similar to the disease that they cured. It is here that Hahnemann formulated the principles of homeopathy.

In addition to the *Law of Similars*, homeopathy is also based on the *Law of the Infinitesimal Dose*. The more a remedy is diluted, the more potent its strength in fighting the disease. Typically, a single dose of a homeopathic substance would be ten drops placed below a "clean" tongue. More is not better, and when an additional dose is taken, it will interfere with the action of the first dose and harm the balance being created. One dose on the other hand will catalyze the body to make a change. Unlike Western medicine, where a higher dosage means increased strength, homeopathy requires the lowest possible dose to stimulate the body's own healing powers. With the effect being similar to an enzyme or a hormone, a small amount results in a large change. In addition, Hahnemann was concerned by the side effects of frequently used medications and found that medications that were diluted reduced side effects and maintained effectiveness. Striking and shaking the homeopathic solution increased the substance's medicinal properties, conveying that diluted and whisked treatments had stronger medicinal effects [9].

The practice of homeopathy works with an individual's self-healing powers. An alternative form of medicine, homeopathy focuses on energy or "chi" and seeing how an individual's body works as a whole. Hahnemann explained that treatments create a stronger force that overpowers the illness and produces a cure. Homeopathy also uses water's power as a solvent to carry information about its solute and become more potent with repeated usage and addition of solute.

The FDA (Food and Drug Administration) recognizes homeopathic remedies as official drugs and regulates the manufacture, labeling, and dispensing. The remedies have their own official compendium, the *Homeopathic Pharmacopoeia of the United States* that was first published in 1897.

There are specific substances, plant, mineral, and animal, which have a history of being effective with sexual enhancement and certain dysfunctions. With the proper guidance of a homeopath, remedies can be both safe and effective.

The following are some homeopathic remedies for various sexual concerns [9]:

Coitus troubles:

Aversion to coitus—*Arnica*, graphites, *lyco*
Suppressed desire—*Conium*
Frequent emissions before erection is complete—*sulfur*
Early ejaculation due to weakness—*titanium*
Erections absent partially/completely—*Conium*
Erections absent entirely and sexual drive lost, involuntarily emissions during stool/urine—*Nuphar*
Absence of enjoyment—*berb V, caust, sepia*

Impotence:

Impotence in old age, partial erection—*lyco IM*
Impotence, absence of desire—*damiana*
Impotence—*berb V, calc C, Conium, graphites, Sabal, calad, lyco IM, staph, phos, selen, acid phos, lecithin*
Sexual weakness due to early emissions—*titanium*
Impotence due to masturbation, and violent sexual desire, erection when half asleep in the morning and ceasing when waking up—*calad*
Impotence due to diabetes—*mosch, cupr met*
Impotence due to neurasthenia—*Yohimbinum*
When due to injury—*Hypericum, Arnica*

Sexual impulse defect in females:

Aversion or reduced desire—*agnus C, aAmm C, berb V, caust, ferr mur, graph, Ign, nat murr, onosm, plb. seb*
Aversion in anemic women plus dry mouth, dry vagina, and painful coitus—*nat murr, ferr mur, arg nit, kreos*
Aversion due to absence of enjoyment during coitus—*brom, caust*
Absence of usual thrill during orgasm—*osmium*
Painful coitus—*apis, bell, Thuja*

Desires for coitus or sexual impulse:

Desire for coitus increased in females—nymphomania—*ambra, asteria, Hyos, Bufo, dulc, kali phos, kali brom, mosch, murex, Origanum, picr-ac, phos-ac, plat, stram, strych, ver V, zinc*
Desire insatiable—craving not satisfied even after coitus—*asterias R*

Conclusion

Homeopathy is a low-cost, safe system of medicine that should be explored further. Millions of people around the world are already using homeopathic remedies effectively and in a self-care environment.

References

1. Ernst E. The desktop guide to complimentary and alternative medicine. London: Harcourt Publishers Limited; 2001.
2. Douglas N, Slinger P. Sexual secrets. Rochester, VT: Destiny Books; 1979.
3. Douglas N, Slinger P. The erotic sentiment in the paintings of China & Japan. Rochester, VT: Park Street Press; 1990.
4. Chia M. Taoist secrets of love. Santa Fe, NM: Aurora Press; 1984.
5. Chia M, et al. The multi-orgasmic couple. San Francisco, CA: Harper Collins; 2009a.
6. Oleson T. Auriculotherapy manual. 4th ed. London: Churchill Livingstone; 1996.
7. Chia M, et al. The multi-orgasmic man. New York, NY: Harper Collins; 2009b.
8. Nickell NL. Nature's aphrodisiacs. Berkeley, CA: Crossing Press, Inc.; 1999.
9. Merani VH. The practitioner's hand book of homoeopathy. New Delhi: B. Jain Publishers Pvt. Ltd.; 1994.

Suggested Reading

American Institute of Homeopathy (Committee of Pharmacopeia). Homeopathic pharmacopoeia of the United States. Boston, MA: O. Clapp; 1897.
Beurdeley M, et al. Chinese erotic art. North Clarendon, VT: Charles E. Tuttle Company Inc.; 1969.
The Burton Goldberg Group. Alternative medicine. Puyallup, WA: Future Medicine Publishing; 1994.
Chia M, Wei WU. Sexual reflexology. Rochester, VT: Destiny Books; 2003.
Dunas F, Goldberg P. Passion play. Riverhead: New York, NY; 1997.
Hahnemann S, Boericke W. Organon of medicine, new translated ed. New Delhi: B. Jain Publishers Pvt. Ltd.; 2002.
Hooper A. Kamasutra. New York, NY: Dorling Kindersley Publishing, Inc.; 1994.
Maciocia G. Obstetrics & gynecology in Chinese medicine. New York, NY: Churchill Livingstone; 1998.
Novey DW. Complementary & alternative medicine. St. Louis, MO: Mosby Inc.; 2000.
Stux G, Pomeranz B. Acupuncture: textbook and atlas. Springer: Berlin; 1987.
Verma V. Ayurveda for life: nutrition, sexual energy & healing. York, ME: Samuel Weiser, Inc.; 1997.

36 Future Directions in Sexual Medicine

Albert Aboseif and Waguih William IsHak

Introduction

Leading up to the twenty-first century, the field of sexual medicine made tremendous strides in the advancement of biological treatments for sexual dysfunction, yet several new challenges still persist. Primarily, the field continues to remain challenged by the limitations of sexual complaint self-report. In the absence of truly objective measures of sexual dysfunction, diagnostic criteria has become more of a subjective guideline for physicians, resulting in a wide variety of response measures, as well as issues with historian reliability. Despite significant efforts spent on revising and refining diagnostic criteria, such as the merging of desire and arousal in women and of dyspareunia and vaginismus in the DSM-5, clinicians and scholars continue to struggle adopting the established criteria in both clinical and research settings. Other clinical categories such as hypersexual behavior [1] and postcoital dysphoria [2] remain without specific diagnostic criteria despite their epidemiological and phenomenological evidence. Furthermore, the field continues to struggle with defining anatomical and physiological genital areas linked to sexual function and dysfunction such as the G-spot, the quantifying of vaginal lubrication as an indicator of arousal [3], as well as the role of "chemosexual communication" through pheromones [4].

Another major challenge is the ongoing conflict between biological and psychosocial practice. Whereas some clinicians rely solely on the "quick fix" pharmacological route to solve the immediate performance problem, other practitioners continue to emphasize the importance in understanding the deep-seated psychosocial issues that may be preventing an increased quality of relationships and an improved physical intimacy [5]. Moreover, there is an increasing expectation and reliance on fast-acting and effective biological interventions with a low side effect profile. This became especially true after the introduction of sildenafil for the treatment of erectile dysfunction (ED), one of the most common sexual dysfunctions in men [6]. An important sequel to this breakthrough pharmaceutical would have been a similar biological intervention for women. However, this did not turn out to be as simple. Flibanserin was approved nearly 20 years later for women, but the skepticism about its potency and clinical efficacy relative to sildenafil continues to be a major point of contention among clinicians and researchers. Nonetheless, the "medicalization of sexuality" [7] and the eventual replacement of psychosocial interventions by pharmacological interventions are becoming the norm. This is especially true in light of a lack of psychosocial advances and an increase in pharmaceutical resources for drug development, testing, and marketing. Nevertheless, there are exciting new directions in the assessment and treatment of specific sexual dysfunctions.

Future Directions in the Assessment of Sexual Dysfunctions

Standardization of Assessment Methods

The International Consultation on Sexual Medicine recently proposed a specific algorithm for the evaluation of sexual dysfunctions in men and women, with clear evidenced-based recommendations for sexual history taking and the use of validated scales and questionnaires [8]. This algorithm is founded on three basic principles that allow for proper evaluation and treatment of sexual dysfunction [8]. The three basic principles include a patient-centered framework that fosters cultural understanding, the application of evidence-based principles in patient care, and a parallel framework between men and women [8]. The committee places a strong emphasis on an integrative biopsychosocial approach to patient care, underscoring the conviction that sexual dysfunction is a multifactorial process rather than a simplistic and generalizable one [8].

W.W. IsHak (ed.), *The Textbook of Clinical Sexual Medicine*, DOI 10.1007/978-3-319-52539-6_36

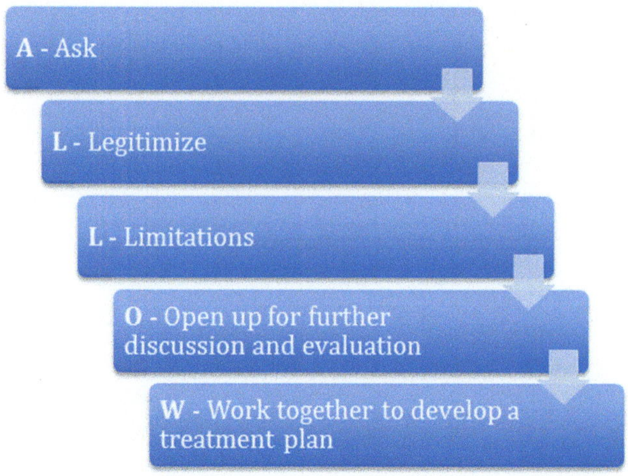

FIGURE 36-1. The five-step "allow" algorithm for managing sexual dysfunction.

The committee recommends a five-step approach for handling sexual dysfunction in patients, beginning with an essential basic evaluation that emphasizes a sexual, medical, and psychosocial patient history [8] as seen in Figure 36-1.

This first step is crucial as it highlights the multifactorial nature of sexual dysfunction and provides the physician with the required information to make an informed decision about the next step in patient management. Once the provider has determined that further investigation is required, the committee recommends that the patient be educated properly on their diagnosis, with a focus on partnering with the patient to share in the decision-making process regarding the treatment. In the recommendation for therapeutic intervention, lifestyle modification is the first category emphasized, followed by psychological intervention, medical treatment, and surgery if appropriate. Finally, step five encourages the physician to continue to follow up with the patient to monitor progress in both symptom relief as well as overall sexual well-being [8]. The five-step approach reflects a trend toward a more holistic view of sexual dysfunction, encouraging the physician to create a more individualized treatment plan for their patient.

Screening checklists and questionnaires have also become a major component in sexual dysfunction diagnostics, and there are both pros and cons to this development. Screening checklists allow for an efficient and simple way to identify potential sexual dysfunction in a patient population. This is especially important as many patients may not come in with a sexual problem as their primary complaint and because patients often may not be completely honest about their problem [8]. Furthermore, screening checklists can be easily integrated into patient check-in and help prime physicians on where the dysfunction may lie. Similar to screening checklists, questionnaires are currently the primary format in which sexual dysfunction is evaluated. While similarly convenient, questionnaires are innately limited due to their brevity and generality and thus should not be used as a substitute for a detailed sexual history performed by the physician. Furthermore, due to their general nature, they may not address specific situational concerns encountered by the patient. This becomes especially true in the context of nonheterosexual patient population, as most questionnaires have been developed to address primarily heterosexual problems. It also presents issues when administering questionnaires in the context of a multicultural patient population, where cultural and linguistic barriers may interfere with proper comprehension and completion of the questionnaire [8]. Thus the future of sexual dysfunction assessment must work toward increased inclusivity as well as a continued integration between screening tools and physician-administered sexual histories.

Technological Advances

Imaging (Local and Brain)

Growing efforts are made using MRI and fMRI [9] both to assess genital internal and external anatomical structures and function with exciting new directions into brain imaging using fMRI and diffusion tensor imaging [10].

Biomarkers

An association between biomarkers such as endothelial nitric oxide synthase (eNOS) polymorphisms and increased risk of erectile dysfunction has been established [11]. More research needs to be performed in correlating biomarker to drug response, as well as discovering new ones for other sexual dysfunctions.

Physiological Studies

EEG has provided emerging evidence in the study of human sexual response and understanding dysfunction [12]. More studies need to be performed to provide evidence for specific links between identifiable patterns and specific sexual dysfunctions. Quantitative sensory testing (QST) is a neurophysiological assessment method for small and large nerve fiber function. Its application to assess genital sensation could add valuable objective information about the assessment of sexual dysfunction in men [13] and women [14]. The roles of plethysmography and thermography in the assessment of sexual dysfunction in both women and men cannot be understated.

Future Directions in Sexual Dysfunction Treatments

Regenerative Medicine and Stem Cells

The goal of stem cell therapy is to regenerate damaged or dysfunctional penile tissue in order to restore functionality [15, 16]. Several forms of stem cell therapy exist, derived

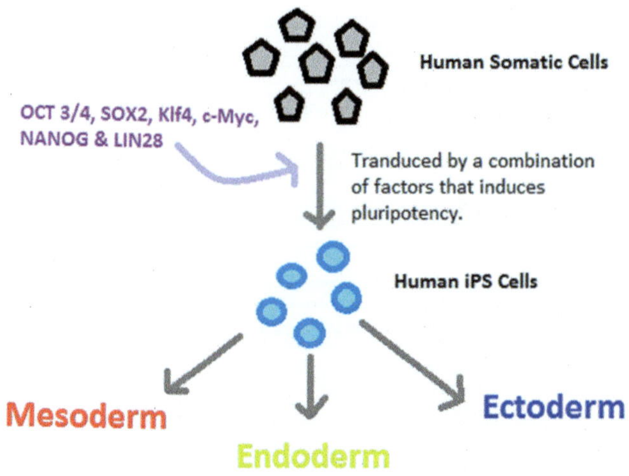

FIGURE 36-2. Somatic cells induction to pluripotent cells then to mesoderm, endoderm, or ectoderm [Reprinted from https://commons.wikimedia.org/wiki/File:Overview_of_iPS_cells.png. With permission from the Creative Commons].

from different forms of progenitor cells including adipose, muscle, and bone marrow tissue-derived stem cells [17].

Stem cell therapy is starting to show beneficial effects in the treatment of erectile dysfunction, especially in the context of diabetes, aging, and hyperlipidemia [18]. More clinical trials are now actively enrolling patients. Growth factor therapy and gene therapy are also acquiring more research presence.

Somatic cells could be induced to pluripotent cells then to mesoderm, endoderm, or ectoderm (Figure 36-2). Adipose tissue-derived stem cells (ADSCs) have been investigated for their potential ability to repair damaged nerve tissue, specifically cavernosal nerve injury-related ED. Chen et al. found that the use of ADSCs was able to repair both the nerve and the penile fibrosis, restoring erectile function in rats [19]. Liu et al. went one step further by modifying ADSCs with hepatocyte growth factor, finding an enhanced curative effect on erectile function in diabetic rats [20].

Additionally exciting is the potential of ADSCs to repair structural abnormalities, such as those found in Peyronie's disease. Gokce et al. experimented with local injections of ADSC into damaged tissue and found attenuation of structural changes associated with Peyronie's disease, resulting in enhanced erectile function in rats [21].

Human umbilical cord blood stem cells (HUCB-MSCs) have also been studied for their therapeutic efficacy. In one of the first human studies exploring the efficacy of stem cell treatment of ED, two patients that were completely unresponsive to oral therapy were able to successfully sustain an erection independently, with a third patient achieving the same results after 3 months [22]. Bone marrow-derived stem cells have also been used, primarily in patients with post-radical prostatectomy ED, with very promising results and minimal side effects [23].

Pharmacological Interventions

The future pharmacological interventions and future uses are summarized in Figure 36-3 and detailed in the following sections.

Male Pharmacological Targets

Future pharmacological interventions for men are highlighted in Figure 36-4.

D4 agonists are currently being looked at as one of the most potent centrally acting treatments for erectile dysfunction [24]. While similar in function to apomorphine, these specific receptor agonists lack the emetic properties that made apomorphine so problematic [25]. However, currently D4 agonists require intravenous administration, which may lessen their favorability. Dopamine agonists may also play an important role in the treatment of hypoactive sexual desire disorder (HSDD), as pathways in the brain related to arousal are affected by dopamine [24].

PT-141 is an alpha-MSH analogue that can function to stimulate MC receptors and increase penile erection in men [26]. MC3 and MC4 receptors have become important targets in pharmaceutical research regarding the treatment of erectile dysfunction and will be an important aspect of future treatment [24].

The stimulation of 5-HT2 serotonin receptors has the ability to delay ejaculation [24]. Thus, SSRIs are currently being studied for their possible therapeutic effect on premature ejaculation). However, due to the fact that prolonged use of SSRIs can reduce sexual activity and lead to HSDD, prophylactic treatment with short half-life SSRIs before intercourse are now being suggested. Clinical trials for this pharmacological treatment are currently underway, but with mixed results [27, 28]. One approach to treatment of PE is a daily administration of an SSRI, with paroxetine showing the strongest ejaculation delay [29]. Adverse effects of this treatment may include mild nausea, fatigue, loose stools or perspiration, and symptoms usually disappear within 2–3 weeks of treatment onset [29]. A second approach to treatment is on-demand use of SSRIs which seems to be well tolerated by slightly less efficacious than daily administration [29].

Dapoxetine, an ejaculo-selective serotonin transport inhibitor, is the first pharmaceutical specifically developed for PE treatment [29]. A potent SSRI, dapoxetine, works by binding and inhibiting 5-HT, dopamine, and norepinephrine reuptake transporters [30]. It has been investigated as a strong candidate for an on-demand treatment of PE based on its pharmacokinetic profile [29]. Thus far, dapoxetine has

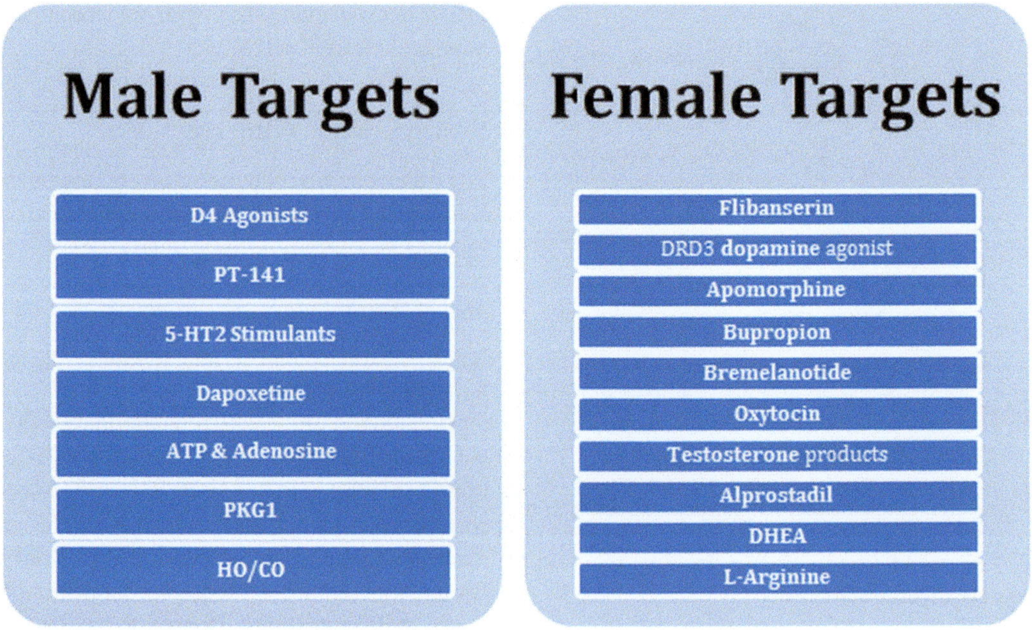

FIGURE 36-3. Future pharmacological interventions and future uses.

FIGURE 36-4. Male pharmacological targets.

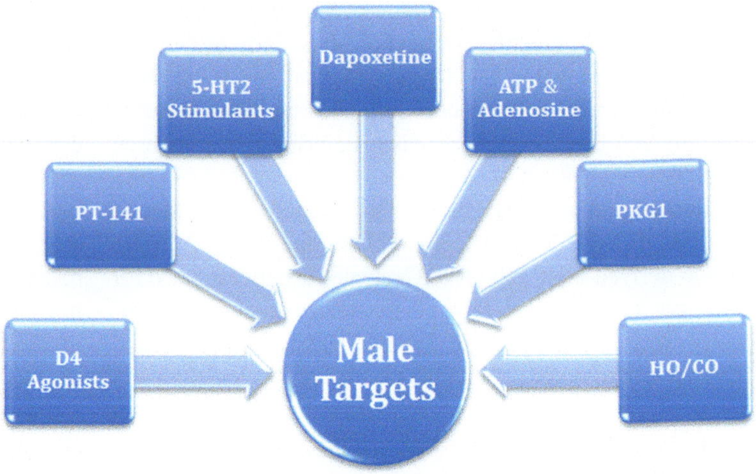

successfully undergone two phase II trials and two phase III trials. Double-blind, placebo-controlled phase III multicenter trials were conducted to assess the efficacy of an on-demand use of dapoxetine, 1–3 h prior to sexual intercourse [29]. Results showed significant increases in intravaginal ejaculatory latency time (IELT) with dapoxetine compared with placebo in both phase III trials [29]. IELT increased from 0.91 min at baseline to 2.78 and 3.32 min for 30 and 60 mg dapoxetine, respectively [29]. Side effects of this treatment included headache, nausea, dizziness, and diarrhea [29].

Both ATP and adenosine are being explored for their potential positive effects on penile erection. ATP has been found to both initiate and maintain penile erections, modulating erectile function rather than acting as a direct neurotransmitter [31, 32]. It has also been found to relax the smooth muscle of the corpus callosum independently of nitric oxide [33]. Adenosine, which is a metabolic product of ATP breakdown, has the ability to act as an effective vasodilator with a very short half-life [34]. Several animal and human studies have revealed the increased penile tumescence with the administration of intracavernous adenosine injections [35, 36]. However, not all forms of erectile dysfunction are due to a problem with adenosine function, and thus treatment efficacy is limited [37].

The role of nitric oxide in vasodilation of smooth muscle of the corpus callosum has been well established. It has been recently discovered that NO stimulation and the corresponding increase in cGMP activate two separate protein kinases within the cell: PKG1a and PKG1b [38]. Diminished functionality of these two kinases has been found in erectile tissue of diabetic rats [38]. However, gene transfer of PKG1a into these diabetic rats resulted in restored erectile function [38]. Researchers are now targeting PKG1a gene transfer as a future treatment for diabetic patients with ED resistant to oral pharmacotherapy [24].

Heme oxygenase/carbon monoxide (HO/CO) is another pro-erectile gas currently being investigated, working similarly to NO in its ability to relax penile smooth muscle via cGMP pathways [24]. While studies thus far have not yet been tried on aging animals, preliminary findings suggest increased male sexual function including erectile function [39]. Further studies are needed to deduce the exact role that HO/CO plays in ED pathophysiology [24].

Female Pharmacological Targets

Due to the difficulty in clearly defining female sexual dysfunction (FSD) as well as objectively measuring sexual dysfunction in the laboratory, pharmacological treatment for females has been more difficult. There is an interplay of several various factors that contribute to FSD, thus selecting one specific target is often insufficient. It has also been suggested that the pathologic process of FSD follows a more circular model rather than a linear one, complicating matters further [40]. In terms of standard laboratory measures of sexual dysfunction, there seems to be a crucial dissociation between physiological measurements of sexual functionality and a woman's subjective experience and satisfaction [41]. Finally, due to the fact that placebo has been determined as most effective treatment of FSD creates difficulty in truly understanding the efficacy of pharmacologic treatment [42, 43]. Nevertheless, there are several pharmacological targets currently being studied for their possible therapeutic effect on FSD as depicted in Figure 36-5.

Flibanserin is a 5-HT 1A agonist, 2A antagonist, initially created as an antidepressant that failed to prove general effectiveness during stage 2 trials. However, researchers found a trend in which almost all of their subjects were free of symptoms of sexual dysfunction [44]. Testing began on flibanserin for its possible efficacy in treating HSDD in females, yet its overall efficacy has proven tenuous. Initial phase III trials using e-Diary to measure daily sexual desire did not show significance over placebo [44]. However, flibanserin did show increases in satisfying sexual events (SSE) as well as an increase in Female Sexual Function Index (FSFI) and a decrease in Female Sexual Distress Scale (FSDS-R) [44]. Yet, despite these positive results, the FDA refused approval of flibanserin in 2009 due to its inability to show statistical significance regarding e-Diary scores as well as its side effect profile [44]. Side effects of flibanserin were found to include vomiting, drowsiness, and vertigo, which were dose dependent [44]. Furthermore, drug-drug interactions with fluconazole as well as its ability to suppress CYP3A4 lead to symptoms of hypotension and syncope [44]. These effects were further increased by an interaction with ethanol [44].

Due its high side effect profile, FDA rejected flibanserin's NDA resubmission in 2013. Another notable concern presented by the FDA regarding flibanserin lies in the diagnostic

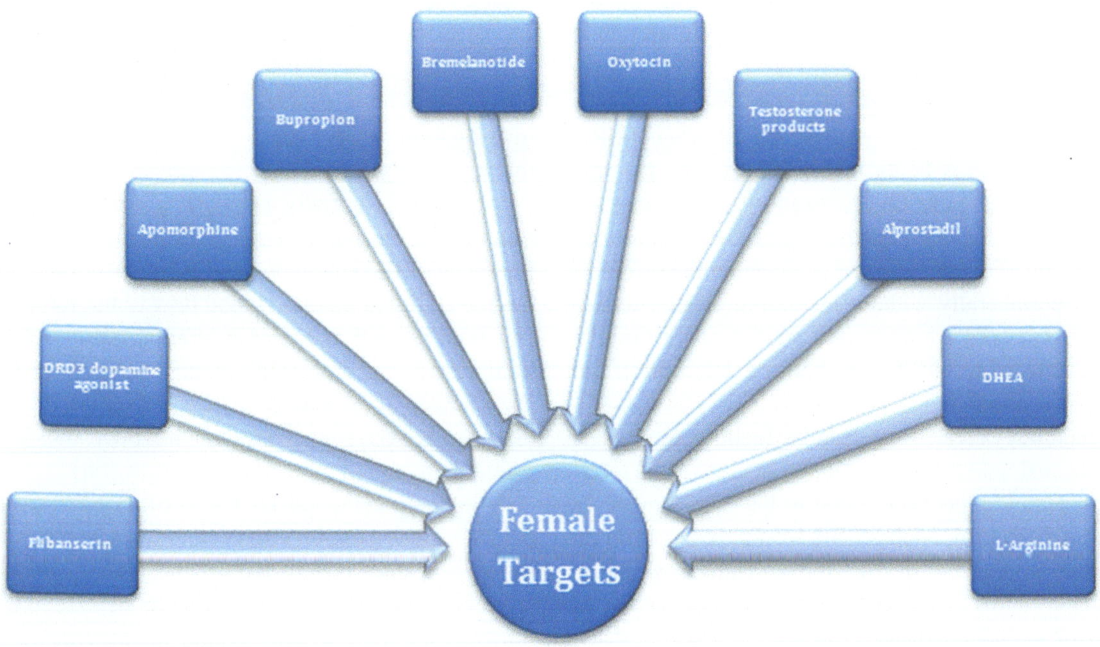

FIGURE 36-5. Female pharmacological targets.

criteria of HSDD and the drug's potential off-label use. Due to the generalized and often subjective criteria for diagnosing HSDD, it is likely that flibanserin might be prescribed to patients who do not necessarily fit the HSDD label [44]. This may lead to a safety hazard, due to Flibanserin's high side effect profile. However, it is important to note that several groups have come out in support of flibanserin, most notably even the score, which argued that disapproval of the drug by the FDA was a matter of gender inequality [44]. Despite these concerns, in 2015, the FDA finally approved flibanserin, under the condition that risk management tools would be enforced [44].

A selective dopamine (DRD3) agonist is currently under investigation by Pfizer for the treatment of FSD [45]. Dopamine agonists work by stimulating dopamine receptors in several dopaminergic pathways in the brain. The stimulation of these receptors can enhance approach behavior, possibly leading to pro-sexual behavior [46–48]. In humans, pro-sexual behavior due to dopamine agonists was first witnessed in patients with Parkinson's disease who showed "hypersexual behavior" in response to treatment with pramipexole, a DA agonist [49, 50].

Apomorphine (APO) is also being studied as a primer for increased sexual function in women. Apomorphine was found to increase subjective arousal, self-reported lubrication, and peak clitoral blood flow velocity in premenopausal women with anorgasmia during vibratory stimulation [51]. APO was administered 40 min prior to vibrational stimulation, thus acting as a primer for sexual function [51]. A second study with APO revealed increased sexual enjoyment as well as an improved orgasm in female participants, without an increase in frequency of sexual encounters [52]. While therapeutic efficacy of APO looks to be promising, there is concern due to reported incidence of nausea, vomiting, and diarrhea, possibly limiting its effectiveness [52].

Bupropion is an atypical antidepressant given to individuals looking to avoid the negative sexual side effects of SSRIs. Currently, bupropion is being investigated for its potential benefit in nondepressed females with anorgasmia and sexual arousal disorder [53, 54]. Furthermore, PDE-5 inhibitors could act as an adjuvant treatment, enhancing the effects of buproprion peripherally without increasing central activity [55]. Currently, there are no human studies confirming the synergistic effect of PDE-5 inhibitors on buproprion, but animal work is promising.

Bremelanotide, created by Palatin Technologies, is an alpha-MSH analogue that preferentially binds to MC4 receptors. Bremelanotide has been found to have efficacy in the treatment of FSD [56]. Alpha-MSH works by targeting the paraventricular nucleus of the hypothalamus, which is thought to play a role in sexual desire [57]. An increase in the frequency of sexual satisfaction, arousal, and sexual desire has been reported in healthy premenopausal women undergoing phase II trials of bremelanotide [58–60]. However, increased blood pressure has been reported as a side effect of drug therapy [61]. Phase III trials will be complete in 2016, and an improved drug with less blood pressure effects will also be created [61].

The hormone oxytocin, released by the posterior pituitary gland, is also being explored as a treatment for FSD. Due to its ability to increase pair bonding as well as to decrease anxiety, it may work to alleviate psychological barrier inhibiting proper sexual function [62]. Several animal studies have been conducted on oxytocin, with findings revealing positive psychosocial effects, specifically female mate approach behavior [63]. Currently, two pharmaceutical compounds are being investigated—an OT receptor agonist and an enzyme inhibitor that slows down OT degradation [64]. However, the unpredictability of OT absorption through the blood-brain barrier limits its efficacy [64]. Future investigation of OT compounds will focus on its ability to reverse vaginal atrophy in female patients with genitopelvic pain [65].

With regard to sex steroid hormone therapy, efficacy has been quite mixed. Androsorb, a testosterone cream created by Novavax, has shown increased libido in postmenopausal women and is currently in early clinical trials [66]. Tefina, is an intranasal testosterone gel which is currently being tested for its efficacy on females with orgasmic disorder [67]. Research subjects have reported feelings of intense arousal, with increased genital response relative to placebo [67]. LibiGel is transdermal testosterone gel specifically aimed at treating HSDD. It is currently being developed by BioSante Pharmaceuticals and has undergone two phase III trials known as BLOOM. However, phase III trials revealed that LibiGel was no more effective than placebo in increasing sexual desire. Currently, BioSante is conducting a phase III trial investigating LibiGel's long-term safety. While testosterone supplementation for FSD looks to be promising, more investigation is necessary before a product is brought to market.

Alprostadil, initially established for male erectile dysfunction, is currently being investigated for its efficacious treatment of FSD. As a prostaglandin vasodilator, alprostadil has the ability to increase blood flow to the female reproductive tract as well as increase afferent nerve sensation [68]. Femprox is an alprostadil cream developed by Apricus Biosciences developed primarily for female sexual arousal disorder (FSAD) [68]. Thus far, it has been shown to increase primary arousal in nine clinical studies [68].

While supplemental DHEA is often used by postmenopausal women, findings indicate that systemic DHEA does not significantly benefit women with FSD. However, there have been positive results with the use of prasterone, an intravaginal DHEA, with reports of increased sexual function and sexual desire [69, 70].

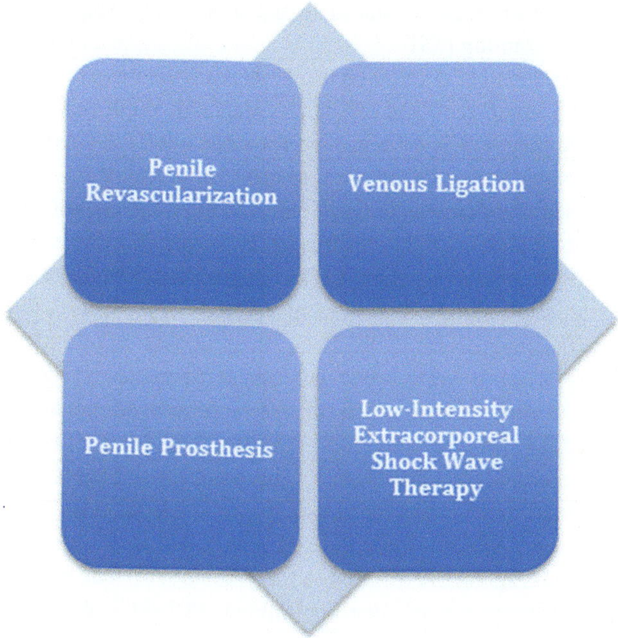

Figure 36-6. Surgical interventions.

Supplemental L-arginine has also been a topic of discussion regarding OTC therapy for FSD, as it has shown promise in its treatment of mild-moderate FSD [71]. Female subjects responded positively to treatment with L-arginine, showing increased sexual satisfaction, clitoral sensitivity, and frequency of intercourse compared with control subjects, in a 4-week placebo-controlled study [72]. Future positive results with L-arginine may result in a wide variety of OTC supplements.

Surgical Interventions

Surgical interventions (Figure 36-6), especially minimally invasive procedures, are gaining more traction for both men and women.

Penile revascularization is a type of surgery performed on the penile arteries in patients with erectile dysfunction. Typically these surgeries are performed on younger patients who have undergone major pelvic trauma, often resulting in a blockage of the internal pudendal arteries [73]. However, this type of surgery is not performed often, due to a high rate of long-term revascularization failure caused by slow runoff into the corpora when the penis is flaccid [74].

Venous ligation is another form of surgical treatment for erectile dysfunction. It has been well established that penile veins play an important role in maintaining erections [75]. These veins maintain erection by providing veno-occlusion, preventing blood from leaving the penis. If this mechanism fails, erectile dysfunction may result [76]. Venous ligation is a method of surgery that aims to reinstate the veno-occlusive mechanism, to prevent venous leakage associated with erectile dysfunction [76]. However, while these surgeries were often performed in the past, they have fallen out of popularity due to their lack of long-term efficacy [75].

Penile prosthetic surgery has been around since the 1970s but has undergone several iterations throughout the years. These surgeries continue to be the mainstay of surgical treatment for erectile dysfunction. Among all therapeutic treatments for ED, penile prosthesis have shown the highest satisfaction rates [77]. However, this treatment is reserved for use after other treatment modalities, such as medication, have failed [77].

Currently, there are two major types of penile prosthesis. The first is the inflatable prosthesis, which features two inflatable cylinders, one in each corporal body, as well as a pump and a fluid-filled reservoir. Fluid is pumped from the reservoir and into the inflatable cylinders when erection is warranted [78]. The inflatable prosthesis tends to be the more popular of the two. The second type of prosthesis is termed semirigid. These devices remain firm in the penis but are often very pliable [78]. Both types of prosthesis come in different lengths and girths, and proper sizing based on corporal body size is very important for patient functionality and satisfaction [78].

It is important to note that because of the invasiveness associated with penis prosthesis, oftentimes surgery will result in the development of scar tissue around the prosthesis [3]. Thus, an important consideration for penile prosthesis is that after surgery, pharmacological therapies will no longer be effective, due to the irreversible damage to the erectile bodies [3]. Furthermore, the patient should be informed that surgery often might result in a shortened penis length [79].

Low-intensity extracorporeal shock wave therapy (Li-ESWT) is a new, minimally invasive, experimental ED treatment. Li-ESWT works to improve ED with vasculogenic origin, often seen in diabetic patients [80]. While the exact mechanism of action is not yet known, Li-ESWT acts on the NO/cGMP signaling pathways to increase erectile function [80]. Lei et al. [80] showed that in a rat model with streptozotocin-induced diabetes, Li-ESWT worked to improve erectile function as well as reduce the diabetes-induced pathologic changes occurring in penile tissue. Li-ESWT promoted eNOS phosphorylation and regenerated nNOS-positive nerves, endothelium, and smooth muscle [80]. Since these early reports, several clinical trials have presented encouraging results. Many of these studies showed that Li-ESWT significantly improved the IIEF and EHS, the main questionnaires used to assess the quality of erectile function in ED patients [81]. A recent study showed the ability of Li-ESWT to shift 50 % of PDE5 inhibitor nonresponders into responders, suggesting a possible benefit even in patients with severe nonresponsive ED [82]. Despite encouraging early reports of this minimally invasive therapy, longer follow-up is needed to establish the place of Li-ESWT in patients with ED [82].

Psychosocial Interventions

As stated earlier, there is currently a heavy emphasis within the field of sexual medicine in treating dysfunction using fast-acting pharmaceuticals. However, pharmaceuticals alone may not be adequate to fully treat patients. Not only can the pharmacological route lead to several negative side effects, oftentimes the sexual dysfunction is complex and intricately related to patient's psychosocial well-being [83]. Sexual dysfunction is often not solely based on biological factors alone, and it is difficult to separate the psychosocial influence on a patient's sexual dysfunction. Thus, it would be prudent to take a more balanced approach to treatment, utilizing both medication and psychotherapy.

While pharmaceuticals have proven their efficacy in treating sexual dysfunction, it has been found that without a reinforcing form of therapy, rates of premature pharmaceutical discontinuation are much higher in patients [83]. Althof suggests an integrative treatment utilizing both medication and therapy in order to help patients increase the success of their sexual functioning [83]. Furthermore, there are several psychosocial benefits associated with psychotherapy that may be integral to returning sexual functionality. Some of these benefits to the patient include empowerment to create change, increased understanding of the nature of the dysfunction, and the creation of realistic expectations [83].

Mindfulness-based cognitive therapy is being studied further for its efficacy in treating sexual dysfunction. Female sexual desire/arousal disorder (SIAD) is one of the most common sexual dysfunctions in women and one in which pharmaceutical treatment has shown inconsistent efficacy [84]. It has been suggested that an increase in cognitive distraction during sex may be a main contributing factor to SIAD in women [85]. Furthermore, other studies have shown a relation between SIAD and an increased predisposition for anxiety, as well as increased judgmental intrusions [86]. These associated psychosocial symptoms related to SIAD make this dysfunction a particularly good candidate for mindfulness-based sex therapy. This specific type of therapy helps the patient to focus attention on the present moment, cultivating an open, nonjudgmental, accepting awareness [87].

In a recent study conducted by Brotto et al., researchers measured the efficacy of mindfulness-based therapy in the treatment of SIAD by measuring concordance between genital sexual arousal and subjective self-reported sexual arousal. Researchers found an increased concordance between genital arousal and subjective arousal, suggesting that mindfulness-based therapy may result in increased integration between physical and mental sexual responses to erotic stimuli in women [84]. It has also been suggested that mindfulness-based therapy may increase sensitivity to sexual stimuli due to its focus on breathing and thought patterns. This finding was demonstrated in a study that found a decrease in reaction time to sexual stimuli following mindfulness training [88].

Sex therapy is another form of psychotherapy that has shown some treatment efficacy in the field. While sex therapy in general has been around for some time, the approach to treatment has changed quite a bit. Initially, sex therapy focused on what was initially believed to be the goal of sexual intercourse—the orgasm [89]. However, in more recent years, the focus has changed, as practitioners have begun to direct treatment goals toward an increase in pleasure, satisfaction, and desire [90]. Thus, practitioners have moved away from a bottom-line biological response and have instead emphasized much of the psychosocial nature of sexuality.

Recently, there has been a movement toward modifying sex therapy in order to make it more efficient, so as to improve symptoms more quickly with less therapy sessions, thus making it more affordable for patients [90]. One method that incorporates this line of thinking, PLISSIT created by Jack Annon, is often used for both men and women being treated for sexual dysfunction [90]. This treatment aims at quick individualized interventions for treating several sexual dysfunctions. The therapist works to give the patient "permission" for the patient's sexual activities, fully educating the patient on their "limited" information about sexual functioning and recommending "specific suggestions" to increase functionality [90]. Only when these three modalities fail to improve outcomes is "intensive therapy" initiated to address more underlying causes of dysfunction [90].

There has also been an emphasis on internet-delivered cognitive behavioral therapy (ICBT) that allows patients to perform several self-help treatment exercises from the comfort of their own home [91]. Again, this form of therapy offers a more cost-effective therapeutic treatment for patients in a space that allows them to be comfortable, honest, and fully expressive [92]. A recent study testing the efficacy of ICBT showed significant improvements in erectile function relative to control [91]. ICBT has also been shown to be effective for treating female sexual dysfunction, often incorporating exercises such as sensate focus and communication skills. In one study measuring these effects, 44 % of women are no longer classified as has having sexual dysfunction after completing the ICBT program [93].

Future Direction of Lifestyle Treatments and Complementary Medicine

While general medical practice has long relied heavily on pharmacological methods of treatment, there is an increasing focus on lifestyle modifications in order to arrest or even reverse a wide variety of disease. It is widely accepted that nutritional balance and physical activity can both prevent as well as treat several noncommunicable lifestyle morbidities such as diabetes, heart disease, and hypertension. A combination of nutritional balance and adequate physical activity may play a significant role in the treatment of sexual dysfunction. Special attention has been given to plant-based diets, which continue to prove their efficacy throughout the literature. Currently, researchers in the field of sexual medicine are exploring the possible link between diseases of lifestyle and their relationship to sexual dysfunction. There seems to be strong evidence that adopting healthier lifestyle choices may not only lead to better cardiovascular health but to increased sexual function as well.

One of the most common sexual dysfunctions affecting men globally is erectile dysfunction. In America, over 18 million men are affected [94]. It has long been known that erectile dysfunction is closely related to several lifestyle diseases such as cardiovascular disease and type II diabetes. This is due to the fact that penile erection is highly dependent on the blood flow to the penis. Thus, risk factors such as a high resting heart rate, decreased blood vessel elasticity, and atherosclerosis, can all contribute to the restriction of proper penile perfusion [94].

Diabetic males are at an increasingly high risk for developing erectile dysfunction [95]. Current estimates suggest that by 2025, the prevalence of ED is expected to double [95]. Much of the increased prevalence in ED may parallel a simultaneous spike in type II diabetes. Conducting a study on the comorbidities in men with ED, Kalter-Lebovici et al. found that the longer a patient lived with diabetes, both prevalence and severity of erectile dysfunction increased [95]. Furthermore, a correlation was found between higher A1C values and the severity of ED. The less controlled the patient's diabetes, the more severe the dysfunction, leading researchers to believe that increased microvascular injury secondary to hyperglycemia may be contributing to decreased perfusion and thus increased severity of dysfunction [95].

For diabetic patients with comorbidity of erectile dysfunction, nutritional intervention may prove to be a powerful treatment choice for both diseases. The latest nutritional research has established that the whole food plant-based diet may be one of the most efficacious lifestyle modifications in the prevention and treatment of diabetes [96]. The development of type II diabetes is thought to be due to increased accumulation of adipose tissue in the body leading to a blockage of insulin receptors and thus increased insulin insensitivity [96]. Thus, individuals with a higher intake of fats will develop increased intramyocellular lipids within their muscle cells, leading to free radical damage of insulin receptors causing insulin resistance [96]. The Adventist Health Study-2, conducted by Fraser et al., assessed BMI as well as the prevalence of diabetes across several different diets. During the study, Fraser assessed nonvegetarians, pesco-vegetarians, lacto-ovo-vegetarians, and vegans. Results found a correlation between diet and BMI, with individuals eating a vegan diet having the lowest average BMI at 23.13.

Furthermore, researchers discovered that while semi-vegetarians, individuals who only eat meat a few days of the week, were able to reduce their risk of developing diabetes by 28 %, vegans were able to reduce their risk of diabetes by 78 % [97]. Researchers postulated that a low BMI coupled with a diet low in animal protein and high in vegetables, fruits, and nuts may result in a significantly decreased risk of diabetes [97]. In another study assessing the specific relationship between animal protein intake and type II diabetes, Evans et al. found that individuals that consumed a higher intake of red meat were at a much higher risk of developing type II diabetes. Furthermore, the effects of red meat on diabetes occurred even in individuals who initially consumed a very low amount, suggesting that the effects of red meat on diabetic pathology develop quickly. These results held true even after researchers adjusted for differences in weight [98]. Thus, one of the initial interventions for treating erectile dysfunction secondary to type II diabetes may be a reduction in weekly animal protein intake.

A high intake of saturated fats has also been linked to the development of type II diabetes. Goff et al. analyzed the relationship between storage of lipids in muscle cells and insulin sensitivity. Since vegans were found to have a much lower intake of saturated fatty acids, they were compared to a sample of omnivores. Vegans were found to have a lower total cholesterol level, lower fasting serum glucose, and improved pancreatic beta cell function compared with omnivores [99]. Results showed that a diet high in unsaturated fats, with a lower intake of saturated fats, might decrease the accumulation of intramyocellular lipids, reducing the risk of insulin resistance ([99, 100]).

Having diabetes also puts patients at a high risk for developing small vessel disease such as atherosclerosis. Furthermore, hyperlipidemia and a diet high in cholesterol are also major contributors to CAD. Kalter-Leibovici found a correlation between hyperlipidemia and erectile dysfunction, noting that the severity of the erectile dysfunction was strongly related to the patient's concentration of plasma triglycerides [95]. Spessoto et al. compared hypertensive patients and normotensive patients, both with CAD. Findings showed that generally, hypertension worsens CAD and thus indirectly decreases erectile function. Over time, hypertension was found to worsen erectile dysfunction, leading to an increase in arteriosclerosis and thus a decrease in blood flow to the penis, along with increasing the risk of several other health problems. [94]. Overall there was a 75 % risk for peripheral artery disease in patients who already had erectile dysfunction [94]. Due to this strong correlation between coronary artery blood flow and erectile function, physicians can now predict the results of a cardiac stress test with 80 %

accuracy based on penile blood flow alone [101]. Since many physicians have come to view erectile dysfunction as an early warning sign for cardiovascular disease, it seems logical that dietary changes that work to increase vascular flow may also increase erectile function.

Atherosclerotic arteries may be affecting female sexual function as well. Esposito et al. studied the effects of hyperlipidemia on the sexual function of females who did not show symptoms of cardiovascular disease. Compared with the control group, women with hyperlipidemia had significantly lower scores on their Female Sexual Function Index (FSFI) [107]. The hyperlipidemia group reported lower lubrication, lower arousal and orgasm, as well as decreased sexual satisfaction relative to control [107]. Researchers hypothesized that increased atherosclerosis of the pelvic arteries were responsible for decreased vaginal engorgement and decreased arousal [107].

Many researchers have found that nutrition may be one of the most effective medicines against arterial damage. Three of the main contributors to high-serum cholesterol are trans fat, saturated fat, and dietary cholesterol [126]. Intake of these metabolic precursors is largely derived from consumption of animal products including meat, dairy, and eggs [126]. A whole food plant-based diet can help to slow down the rate of atherosclerosis and may potentially even reverse the damage that's already been done [96]. One study measuring the effects of a plant-based diet on cholesterol levels found that compared with patients on a statin medication, a plant-based diet alone was able to lower cholesterol to the same degree, without any of the pharmacological side effects that often prevent compliance [110]. Thus the effect that a plant-based diet may have on reversing atherosclerosis may translate to increased penile perfusion and reversal of erectile dysfunction. However, at this time more research must be conducted in order to fully confirm causation.

While hypertension itself has not been directly linked to erectile dysfunction, many antihypertensive drugs have. Specifically, diuretics, prescribed for hypertension are significantly correlated with erectile dysfunction [95]. Seventy-eight million people in the USA alone are currently diagnosed with hypertension, about one in three adults [109]. Furthermore, it has long been established that blood pressure tends to rise with age, paralleling the trend in erectile dysfunction onset. Yet, this trend in increasing the prevalence of hypertension with age does not seem to hold true in more rural populations globally, suggesting that perhaps the onset of hypertension has less to do with age than initially believed. One early study comparing the incidence of hypertension in the US population compared to that of the native Kenyan population found that rates tended to remain equal until about age 60, at which point incidence in the USA began to far surpass that of Kenya [106].

In fact, when researchers looked at the medical records of the 1800 rural Kenyans admitted to the hospital, not a single individual was diagnosed with hypertension [106]. Researchers predicted that these changes were most likely due to the differences in diet between the two populations, as rural Kenyans on average ate a whole plant food diet with much lower sodium intake [129]. While it is now a common knowledge that high sodium intake is one of the major contributors to high blood pressure, a large majority of the population fails to realize that most of their sodium intake is derived from packaged and processed foods, rather than in the salt they themselves add [96]. This has led to an average American sodium consumption of 3500 mg daily, twice the daily amount recommended by the American Heart Association [130]. This massive intake of salt is not only contributing to a hypertension epidemic across the country; it is also altering taste buds, causing healthier foods to taste bland and unappetizing [96].

Several nutritional options have been found to lower blood pressure. Specifically, whole grains may be as effective as antihypertensive medication in combating high blood pressure, without the negative side effects [125]. Three portions of whole grains per day, including oats, whole wheat, and brown rice, were able to lower the risk of both stroke and MI, two risk factors caused by hypertension [111]. In a study mentioned earlier comparing the effects of diet on several health measurements, individuals on a vegan diet had the greatest reduction in the risk for hypertension at 75 % [97]. Flaxseed has also recently been found to have a significant effect on blood pressure. In a double-blind placebo-controlled, randomized trial, hypertensive individuals who consumed flaxseed for a 6-month period were found to lower their diastolic blood pressure by seven points, resulting in 29 % less heart disease and 46 % less stroke [121]. In comparison, calcium channel blockers on average lower diastolic blood pressure by three points, while ACE inhibitors on average lower diastolic blood pressure by two points [119]. Hibiscus tea, with the highest antioxidant content of any tea, has also demonstrated significant antihypertensive effects in prehypertensive patients compared with a placebo beverage [115]. Implementing lifestyle modification in order to reduce blood pressure may allow patients to lower the dosage of their antihypertensive medication and thus mitigate the negative effects on their sexual functioning.

Nitric oxide availability is crucial for proper genital blood flow, and its absence tends to correlate with both cardiovascular disease as well as erectile dysfunction [118]. Both nutrition and lifestyle have been identified as direct contributors to NO production and thus are directly linked to proper erectile functioning [96]. Specifically, inflammation is strongly associated with endothelial dysfunction, leading to low nitric oxide availability. One way to reduce inflammation and thus increase nitric oxide is through exercise.

Physical activity works to increase endothelial-derived NO, as well as decrease oxidative stress, causing a decrease in endothelial dysfunction [96]. In the only meta-analysis yet conducted on the relationship between physical activity and sexual function, results showed that moderate to high physical activity levels correlated with a lower risk of erectile dysfunction [104].

Several nutritional choices can also boost nitric oxide levels. An increased inflammatory state in the body coupled with a high level of free radicals, reduces NO availability and prevents proper cardiovascular function [96]. Thus, a diet high in antioxidant content can lead to an increase in nitric oxide by removing free radicals from the body [96]. Plant foods contain on average, 64 times the antioxidant level that animal foods contain [96]. Foods with the highest antioxidant concentrations include berries, dark chocolate, pomegranate, cinnamon, and several other spices and herbs [96]. Another nutritional method of increasing nitric oxide levels in the body is by consuming foods containing nitrates, which can be converted into NO within the body [96]. Leafy greens such as arugula, cilantro, basil, and chard, as well as beets, were found to have the highest nitrate content of all foods [96]. Increased intake of nitrate-containing foods has been found to have highly beneficial effects on cardiovascular health as well as erectile functioning [103, 128].

A direct relationship has also been found between improved erectile function and the consumption of pistachio nuts. One study found improved erectile function in men who consumed 3–4 handfuls a day of pistachios for 3 weeks [102]. Randomized placebo-controlled studies are needed to explore the specific impact on sexual functioning. Continued research is needed in the field of sexual medicine to further elucidate the relationship between lifestyle changes and improving sexual function and dysfunction. However, the future treatment of sexual dysfunction through lifestyle modification looks to be highly promising.

Future of Sexual Health Education

The education of students on sexual health and dysfunction, especially in undergraduate medical education, has often been sparse and inconsistent. As discussed throughout this chapter, sexual dysfunction is multifactorial and highly associated with all aspects of patient health. Thus, it is important for all physicians and the majority of health professionals to be knowledgeable about a wide variety of topics relating to sexual health and dysfunction. There are several reasons for implementing a standard medical education in sexual health, stemming from the fact that medical school classes are often varied, with a wide range of political, religious, and social attitudes toward human sexuality [116]. For example, studies have shown that individuals with more conservative religious and political convictions tend to report negative attitudes coupled with less knowledge regarding sexuality [116]. Furthermore, introversion and social anxiety among some students may cause them to feel uncomfortable broaching this topic with patients [117]. It is important for all medical students to gain the proper knowledge on sexual health and become aware of their biases toward sexuality, in order to provide appropriate treatment to their patients [123]. Students with the least comfort toward discussing topics of sexuality will often be less likely to supplement their medical education with knowledge on sexual health mandated by the curriculum [112, 113]. Thus, in order to produce a majority of physicians with adequate proficiency in handling problems of sexuality, a medical education in sexual health must become mandatory [105, 124].

The history of sexual health education in medical schools has fluctuated greatly since its initial inclusion into the general curricula [123]. Only after the inception of contraceptives, coupled with a more liberal view on sexuality, did medical schools begin considering implementing sexual health education into the curriculum [131]. While this focus on the importance of sexual health education peaked in the 1970s, it has since seen a modest decline [123]. As of 2008, of the 92 medical schools surveyed in the USA, only 55 % reported having a formal curriculum in sexual health [114]. A global survey found that about 30 % of international medical schools featured no curriculum in sexual health [127]. The vast majority of studies in this field have concluded that no universal standard exists for sexuality education and that medical school graduates are not prepared for future practice relating to sexual health and dysfunction [108].

Several recommendations have been made for the future implementation of a standardized sexual health curriculum. It is important that contributions to this curriculum are representative of several different medical specialties with a variety of viewpoints [123]. Three foundational areas should be emphasized within the sexual health curriculum to allow sufficient understanding of the topic: attitudes, knowledge, and skill [120]. By initially addressing student attitude toward sexuality, students can be made aware of their personal biases which may interfere with proper future care of patients [112, 122]. Knowledge refers to a proper scientific understanding of the anatomy and physiology of sexual function, as well as the variety of sexual experiences that a patient may relay to the physician [123]. Finally, skill refers to psychomotor application of both knowledge and attitude in the clinical setting [123]. It is important to stress that a sufficient medical education in sexual health must also include management options for different sexual dysfunction as well as proper understanding of contributing risk factors

[123]. As discussed earlier, lifestyle factors play a crucial role in sexual function; thus, medical students must familiarize themselves with the effect of diet and exercise on sexual wellness [132].

Conclusion

Sexual dysfunction is a global issue that spans several cultures and economic classes. However, while the disorders are shared, the social causes may differ between regions. The primary social issue leading to sexual dysfunction worldwide seems to be marital/relational issues. Thus, an exclusively biological approach to treatment of sexual dysfunction would not suffice to address the problem experienced. The healthcare professional must work toward understanding the patient's social situation as it relates to biological functioning. Sexual dysfunction disorders represent a crossroad between several aspects of human health and requires a comprehensive treatment of the whole individual. In order to treat sexual dysfunction, the healthcare professional must study the individual's psychological, biological, and social state of being, realizing that all three aspects of the individual are intimately related. Thus, the successful treatment of sexual dysfunction seems to represent a paradigm for the current progress of general medicine toward an integrative whole body personalized treatment of the individual and the couple.

References

1. Kafka MP. Hypersexual disorder: a proposed diagnosis for DSM-V. Arch Sex Behav. 2010;39(2):377–400.
2. Schweitzer RD, O'Brien J, Burri A. Postcoital dysphoria: prevalence and psychological correlates. Sex Med. 2015;3(4):235–43.
3. Levin RJ, Both S, Georgiadis J, Kukkonen T, Park K, Yang CC. The physiology of female sexual function and the pathophysiology of female sexual dysfunction (committee 13A). J Sex Med. 2016;13(5):733–59.
4. Mazzatenta A, De Luca C, Di Tano A, Cacchio M, Di Giulio C, Pokorski M. Swelling of erectile nasal tissue induced by human sexual pheromone. Adv Exp Med Biol. 2016;885:25–30.
5. IsHak W. The Guidebook of Sexual Medicine. Beverly Hills, CA: A & W Publishing; 2008.
6. Guirguis WR. Oral treatment of erectile dysfunction: from herbal remedies to designer drugs. J Sex Marital Ther. 1998;24(2):69–73.
7. Tiefer L. The medicalization of sexuality: conceptual, normative, and professional issues. Annu Rev Sex Res. 1996;7:252–82.
8. Hatzichristou D, Kirana PS, Banner L, Althof SE, Lonnee-Hoffmann RA, Dennerstein L, Rosen RC. Diagnosing sexual dysfunction in men and women: sexual history taking and the role of symptom scales and questionnaires. J Sex Med. 2016;13(8):1166–82.
9. Vaccaro CM. The use of magnetic resonance imaging for studying female sexual function: a review. Clin Anat. 2015;28(3):324–30.
10. Miner MH, Raymond N, Mueller BA, Lloyd M, Lim KO. Preliminary investigation of the impulsive and neuroanatomical characteristics of compulsive sexual behavior. Psychiatry Res. 2009;174(2):146–51.
11. Liu T, Peng Y, Jia C, Fang X, Li J, Zhong W. Hepatocyte growth factor-modified adipose tissue-derived stem cells improve erectile function in streptozotocin-induced diabetic rats. Growth Factors. 2015a;33:282–9.
12. Ortigue S, Patel N, Bianchi-Demicheli F. New electroencephalogram (EEG) neuroimaging methods of analyzing brain activity applicable to the study of human sexual response. J Sex Med. 2009;6(7):1830–45.
13. Salonia A, Saccà A, Briganti A, Del Carro U, Dehò F, Zanni G, Rocchini L, Raber M, Guazzoni G, Rigatti P, Montorsi F. Quantitative sensory testing of peripheral thresholds in patients with lifelong premature ejaculation: a case-controlled study. J Sex Med. 2009;6(6):1755–62.
14. Burke YZ, Lowenstein L. Value of quantitative sensory testing in the evaluation of genital sensation: its application to female sexual dysfunction. Sex Med Rev. 2016;4(2):121–5.
15. Lin CS, Xin ZC, Deng CH, Ning H, Lin G, Lue TF. Recent advances in andrology-related stem cell research. Asian J Androl. 2008;10:171–5.
16. Morrison SJ, Shah NM, Anderson DJ. Regulatory mechanisms in stem cell biology. Cell. 1997;88:287–98.
17. Ismail EA, El-Sakka A. Innovative trends and perspectives for erectile dysfunction treatment: a systematic review. Arab J Urol. 2016;14(2):84–93.
18. Albersen M, Weyne E, Bivalacqua TJ. Stem cell therapy for erectile dysfunction: Progress and future directions. Sex Med Rev. 2013;1:50–64.
19. Chen X, Yang Q, Zheng T, Bian J, Sun X, Shi Y, et al. Neurotrophic effect of adipose tissue-derived stem cells on erectile function recovery by pigment epithelium-derived factor secretion in a rat model of cavernous nerve injury. Stem Cells Int. 2016;2016:5161248.
20. Liu C, Lu K, Tao T, Zhang L, Zhang X, Jiang L, Huang Y, Guan H, Chen M, Xu B. Endothelial nitric oxide synthase polymorphisms and erectile dysfunction: a meta-analysis. J Sex Med. 2015b;12(6):1319–28.
21. Gokce A, Abd Elmageed ZY, Lasker GF, Bouljihad M, Braun H, Kim H, et al. Intratunical injection of genetically modified adipose tissue-derived stem cells with human interferon a 2b for treatment of erectile dysfunction in a rat model of tunica albugineal fibrosis. J Sex Med. 2015;12:1533–44.
22. Levy JA, Marchand M, Iorio L, Cassini W, Zahalsky MP. Determining the feasibility of managing erectile dysfunction in humans with placental-derived stem cells. J Am Osteopath Assoc. 2016;116:e1–5.
23. Yiou R, Hamidou L, Birebent B, Bitari D, Lecorvoisier P, Contremoulins I, et al. Safety of intracavernous bone marrow mononuclear cells for postradical prostatectomy erectile dysfunction: an open dose-escalation pilot study. Eur Urol. 2016;69(6):988–91.
24. Burnett AL, Goldstein I, Andersson KE, Argiolas A, Christ G, Park K, Xin ZC. Future sexual medicine physiological treatment targets. J Sex Med. 2010;7(10):3269–304.
25. Proctor JD, Chremos AN, Evans EF, Wasserman AJ. Apomorphine-induced vomiting model for antiemetic studies in man. J Clin Pharmacol. 1978;18:95–9.
26. Rosen RC, Diamond LE, Earle DC, Shadiack AM, Molinoff PB. Evaluation of the safety, pharmacokinetics, and pharmacodynamic effects of subcutaneously administered PT-141, a melanocortin receptor agonist, in healthy male subjects and in patients with an inadequate response to Viagra. Int J Impot Res. 2004;16:135–42.
27. Hellstrom WJ. Emerging treatments for premature ejaculation: focus on dapoxetine. Neuropsychiatr Dis Treat. 2009;5:37–46.

28. Kendirci M, Salem E, Hellstrom WJ. Dapoxetine, a novel selective serotonin transport inhibitor for the treatment of premature ejaculation. Ther Clin Risk Manag. 2007;3:277–89.
29. Mcmahon CG, Mcmahon CN, Leow LJ. New agents in the treatment of premature ejaculation. Neuropsychiatr Dis Treat. 2006; 2(4):489–503.
30. Gengo RJ, Giuliano F, McKenna KE, et al. Monoaminergic transporter binding and inhibition profile of dapoxetine, a medication for the treatment of premature ejaculation. J Urol. 2005;173(4):230 .abstract 878
31. Tong YC, Broderick G, Hypolite J, Levin RM. Correlations of purinergic, cholinergic and adrenergic functions in rabbit corporal cavernosal tissue. Pharmacology. 1992;45:241–9.
32. Wu HY, Broderick GA, Suh JK, Hypolite JA, Levin RM. Effects of purines on rabbit corpus cavernosum contractile activity. Int J Impot Res. 1993;5:161–7.
33. Filippi S, Amerini S, Maggi M, Natali A, Ledda F. Studies on the mechanisms involved in the ATP-induced relaxation in human and rabbit corpus cavernosum. J Urol. 1999;161:326–31.
34. Dai Y, Zhang Y, Phatarpekar P, Mi T, Zhang H, Blackburn MR, Xia Y. Adenosine signaling, priapism and novel therapies. J Sex Med. 2009;6(3 suppl):292–301.
35. Chiang PH, Wu SN, Tsai EM, Wu CC, Shen MR, Huang CH, Chiang CP. Adenosine modulation of neurotransmission in penile erection. Br J Clin Pharmacol. 1994;38:357–62.
36. Noto T, Inoue H, Mochida H, Kikkawa K. Role of adenosine and P2 receptors in the penile tumescence in anesthetized dogs. Eur J Pharmacol. 2001;425:51–5.
37. Carneiro FS, Giachini FR, Lima VV, Carneiro ZN, Leite R, Inscho EW, Tostes RC, Webb RC. Adenosine actions are preserved in corpus cavernosum from obese and type II diabetic db/db mouse. J Sex Med. 2008;5:1156–66.
38. Bivalacqua TJ, Kendirci M, Champion HC, Hellstrom WJ, Andersson KE, Hedlund P. Dysregulation of cGMP-dependent protein kinase 1 (PKG-1) impairs erectile function in diabetic rats: Influence of in vivo gene therapy of PKG1 alpha. BJU Int. 2007;99:1488–94.
39. Shamloul R. The potential role of the heme oxygenase/carbon monoxide system in male sexual dysfunctions. J Sex Med. 2009; 6:324–33.
40. Basson R. The female sexual response: a different model. J Sex Marital Ther. 2000;26:51–65.
41. van Anders SM, Brotto L, Farrell J, et al. Associations among physiological and subjective sexual response, sexual desire, and salivary steroid hormones in healthy premenopausal women. J Sex Med. 2009;6:739–51.
42. Bradford A. Listening to placebo in clinical trials for female sexual dysfunction. J Sex Med. 2013;10:451–9.
43. Bradford A, Meston CM. Placebo response in the treatment of women's sexual dysfunctions: a review and commentary. J Sex Marital Ther. 2009;35:164–81.
44. Sang JH, Kim TH, Kim SA. Flibanserin for treating hypoactive sexual desire disorder. J Menopausal Med. 2016;22(1):9.
45. Blagg J, Allerton CM, Batchelor DV, et al. Design and synthesis of a functionally selective D3 agonist and its in vivo delivery via the intranasal route. Bioorg Med Chem Lett. 2007;17:6691–6.
46. Da Cunha C, Gomez AA, Blaha CD. The role of the basal ganglia in motivated behavior. Rev Neurosci. 2012;23:747–67.
47. Keeler JF, Pretsell DO, Robbins TW. Functional implications of dopamine D1 vs. D2 receptors: a 'prepare and select' model of the striatal direct vs. indirect pathways. Neuroscience. 2014;282C: 156–75.
48. Sano H, Chiken S, Hikida T, et al. Signals through the striatopallidal indirect pathway stop movements by phasic excitation in the substantia nigra. J Neurosci. 2013;33:7583–94.
49. Moore TJ, Glenmullen J, Mattison DR. Reports of pathological gambling, hypersexuality, and compulsive shopping associated with dopamine receptor agonist drugs. JAMA Intern Med. 2014;174:1930–3.
50. Weintraub D, Koester J, Potenza MN, et al. Impulse control disorders in Parkinson disease: a cross-sectional study of 3090 patients. Arch Neurol. 2010;67:589–95.
51. Bechara A, Bertolino MV, Casabe A, et al. A double-blind randomized placebo control study comparing the objective and subjective changes in female sexual response using sublingual apomorphine. J Sex Med. 2004;1:209–14.
52. Caruso S, Agnello C, Intelisano G, et al. Placebo-controlled study on efficacy and safety of daily apomorphine SL intake in premenopausal women affected by hypoactive sexual desire disorder and sexual arousal disorder. Urology. 2004;63:955–9.
53. Hartmann UH, Ruffer-Hesse C, Kruger TH, et al. Individual and dyadic barriers to a pharmacotherapeutic treatment of hypoactive sexual desire disorders: results and implications from a small-scale study with bupropion. J Sex Marital Ther. 2012;38:325–48.
54. Modell JG, May RS, Katholi CR. Effect of bupropion-SR on orgasmic dysfunction in nondepressed subjects: a pilot study. J Sex Marital Ther. 2000;26:231–40.
55. Socala K, Nieoczym D, Wyska E, et al. Influence of sildenafil on the antidepressant activity of bupropion and venlafaxine in the forced swim test in mice. Pharmacol Biochem Behav. 2012;103:273–8.
56. Pfaus J, Giuliano F, Gelez H. Bremelanotide: an overview of preclinical CNS effects on female sexual function. J Sex Med. 2007;4(Suppl. 4):269–79.
57. Lippert RN, Ellacott KL, Cone RD. Gender-specific roles for the melanocortin-3 receptor in the regulation of the mesolimbic dopamine system in mice. Endocrinology. 2014;155:1718–27.
58. Belkin ZR, Krapf JM, Goldstein AT. Drugs in early clinical development for the treatment of female sexual dysfunction. Expert Opin Investig Drugs. 2015;24:159–67.
59. Portman DJ, Edelson J, Jordan R, Clayton A, Krychman ML. Bremelanotide for hypoactive sexual desire disorder: analyses from a phase 2B dose-ranging study. Obstet Gynecol. 2014; 123:26S.
60. Safarinejad MR. Evaluation of the safety and efficacy of bremelanotide, a melanocortin receptor agonist, in female subjects with arousal disorder: a double-blind placebo-controlled, fixed dose, randomized study. J Sex Med. 2008;5:887–97.
61. Palatin Technologies. PL-6983 for female sexual dysfunction [Internet]. Palatin Technologies: Cranbury, NJ; 2016.
62. Nyuyki KD, Waldherr M, Baeuml S, et al. Yes, I am ready now: differential effects of paced versus unpaced mating on anxiety and central oxytocin release in female rats. PLoS One. 2011;6:e23599.
63. Preckel K, Scheele D, Kendrick KM, et al. Oxytocin facilitates social approach behavior in women. Front Behav Neurosci. 2014;8:191.
64. Macdonald K, Feifel D. Helping oxytocin deliver: considerations in the development of oxytocin-based therapeutics for brain disorders. Front Neurosci. 2013;7:35.
65. Al-Saqi SH, Uvnas-Moberg K, Jonasson AF. Intravaginally applied oxytocin improves post-menopausal vaginal atrophy. Post Reprod Health. 2015;21:88–97.
66. Allahdadi KJ, Tostes RC, Webb RC. Female sexual dysfunction: therapeutic options and experimental challenges. Cardiovasc Hematol Agents Med Chem. 2009;7:260–9.
67. Kingsberg SA, Woodard T. Female sexual dysfunction: focus on low desire. Obstet Gynecol. 2015;125:477–86.
68. Kielbasa LA, Daniel KL. Topical alprostadil treatment of female sexual arousal disorder. Ann Pharmacother. 2006;40:1369–76.
69. Labrie F, Archer D, Bouchard C, et al. Effect of intravaginal dehydroepiandrosterone (Prasterone) on libido and sexual dysfunction in postmenopausal women. Menopause. 2009a;16:923–31.

70. Labrie F, Archer D, Bouchard C, et al. Intravaginal dehydroepiandrosterone (Prasterone), a physiological and highly efficient treatment of vaginal atrophy. Menopause. 2009b;16:907–22.
71. Farmer M, Yoon H, Goldstein I. Future targets for female sexual dysfunction. J Sex Med. 2016;13(8):1147–65. doi:10.1016/j.jsxm.2016.05.016.
72. Ito TY, Trant AS, Polan ML. A double-blind placebo-controlled study of ArginMax, a nutritional supplement for enhancement of female sexual function. J Sex Marital Ther. 2001;27:541–9.
73. Zuckerman JM, McCammon KA, Tisdale BE, Colen L, Uroskie T, McAdams P, et al. outcome of penile revascularization for arteriogenic erectile dysfunction after pelvic fracture urethral injuries. Urology. 2012;80(6):1369–74. doi:10.1016/j.urology.2012.07.059.
74. Molodysky E, et al. Penile vascular surgery for treating erectile dysfunction: current role and future direction. Arab J Urol. 2013;11(3):254–66. doi:10.1016/j.aju.2013.05.001.
75. Hsu G-L, et al. The venous drainage of the corpora cavernosa in the human penis. Arab J Urol. 2013;11(4):384–91. doi:10.1016/j.aju.2013.04.002.
76. Wespes E, Schulman CC. Venous leakage: surgical treatment of a curable cause of impotence. J Urol. 1985;133:796–8.
77. Kucuk EV, et al. Erectile dysfunction patients are more satisfied with penile prosthesis implantation compared with tadalafil and intracavernosal injection treatments. Andrology. 2016;4(5):952–6. doi:10.1111/andr.12237.
78. Henry GD, Laborde E. A review of surgical techniques for impending distal erosion and intraoperative penile implant complications: part 2 of a three-part review series on penile prosthetic surgery. J Sex Med. 2012;9(3):927–36. doi:10.1111/j.1743-6109.2011.02606.x.
79. Levine, LA et al. Penile prosthesis surgery: current recommendations from the international consultation on sexual medicine. J Sex Med 2016;13(4):489–518. doi:10.1016/j.jsxm.2016.01.017.
80. Lei H, et al. Low-intensity pulsed ultrasound improves erectile function in streptozotocin-induced type I diabetic rats. Urology. 2015;86(6):1241. doi:10.1016/j.urology.2015.07.026.
81. Assaly-Kaddoum R, et al. Low intensity extracorporeal shock wave therapy improves erectile function in a model of type II diabetes independently of NO/CGMP pathway. J Urol. 2016;196(3):950–6. doi:10.1016/j.juro.2016.03.147.
82. Kitrey ND, et al. Penile low intensity shock wave treatment is able to shift PDE5i nonresponders to responders: a double-blind, sham controlled study. J Urol. 2016;195(5):1550–5. doi:10.1016/j.juro.2015.12.049.
83. Althof SE, Wieder M. Psychotherapy for erectile dysfunction: now more relevant than ever. Endocrine. 2004;23(2–3):131–4. doi:10.1385/endo:23:2-3:131.
84. Brotto, LA et al. "Mindfulness-based sex therapy improves genital-subjective arousal concordance in women with sexual desire/arousal difficulties." Arch Sex Behav 2015;45(8):1907–1921. doi:10.1007/s10508-015-0689-8.
85. Nobre P, Pinto-Gouveia J. Emotions during sexual activity: differences between sexually functional and dysfunctional men and women. Arch Sex Behav. 2006;35:491–9. doi:10.1007/s10508-006-9047-1.
86. Meston CM. The effects of state and trait self-focused attention on sexual arousal in sexually functional and dysfunctional women. Behav Res Ther. 2006;44:515–32.
87. Bishop SR, Lau M, Shapiro S, Carlson L, Anderson ND, Carmody J. Mindfulness: a proposed operational definition. Clin Psychol Sci Pract. 2004;11:230–41. doi:10.1093/clipsy/bph077.
88. Silverstein RG, Brown AH, Roth HD, Britton WB. Effects of mindfulness training on body awareness to sexual stimuli: implications for female sexual dysfunction. Psychosom Med. 2011;73:817–25. doi:10.1097/PSY.0b013e318234e628.
89. McCarthy B. McCarthy E. Discovering your couple's sexual style. New York: Routledge; 2009.
90. Assalian P. Psychological and interpersonal dimensions of sexual function and dysfunction. Arab J Urol. 2013;11(3):217–21.
91. Anderson G. Using the Internet to provide cognitive behaviour therapy. Behav Res Ther. 2009;47:175–80.
92. Van Lankueld JJ. Self-help therapies for sexual dysfunction. J Sex Res. 2009;46:143–55.
93. Jones L, McCabe M. The effectiveness of an Internet-based psychological treatment for female sexual dysfunction. J Sex Med. 2011;8:2781–92.
94. Spessoto LC, et al. Association of hypertension with erectile function in chronic peripheral arterial insufficiency patients. J Clin Med Res. 2016;8(8):582–4.
95. Kalter-Leibovici O, et al. Clinical, socioeconomic, and lifestyle parameters associated with erectile dysfunction among diabetic men. Diabetes Care. 2005;28(7):1739–44. doi:10.2337/diacare.28.7.1739.
96. Greger M, Stone G. How not to die: discover the foods scientifically proven to prevent and reverse disease. New York, NY: Flatiron Books; 2015.
97. Fraser GE. Vegetarian diets: what do we know of their effects on common chronic diseases? Am J Clin Nutr. 2009;89(5):1607S–12S. doi:10.3945/ajcn.2009.26736k.
98. Evans WJ. Oxygen-carrying proteins in meat and risk of diabetes mellitus. JAMA Intern Med. 2013;173(14):1335–6. doi:10.1001/jamainternmed.2013.7399.
99. Goff LM, et al. Veganism and its relationship with insulin resistance and intramyocellular lipid. Eur J Clin Nutr. 2004;59(2):291–8. doi:10.1038/sj.ejcn.1602076.
100. Wang, Lu et al. "Plasma fatty acid composition and incidence of diabetes in middle-aged adults: the atherosclerosis risk in communities (ARIC) study." Am J Clin Nutr 2003;78:91–98.
101. Corona G, Fagioli G, Mannucci E, et al. Penile Doppler ultrasound in patients with erectile dysfunction (ED): role of peak systolic velocity measured in the flaccid state in predicting arteriogenic ED and silent coronary artery disease. J Sex Med. 2008;5(11):2623–34.
102. Aldemir M, Okulu E, Neşelioğlu S, Erel O, Kayıgil O. Pistachio diet improves erectile function parameters and serum lipid profiles in patients with erectile dysfunction. Int J Impot Res. 2011; 23(1):32–8.
103. Bhupathiraju SN, Wedick NM, Pan A, Manson JE, Rexrode KM, Willett WC, Rimm EB, Hu FB. Quantity and variety in fruit and vegetable intake and risk of coronary heart disease. Am J Clin Nutr. 2013;98(6):1514–23.
104. Cheng JY, Ng EM, Ko JS, Chen RY. Physical activity and erectile dysfunction: meta-analysis of population-based studies. Int J Impot Res. 2007;19:245–52.
105. Coleman E, Elders J, Satcher D, et al. Summit on medical school education in sexual health: Report of an expert consultation. J Sex Med. 2013;10:924–38.
106. Donnison C. Blood pressure in the african native. Lancet. 1929; 213(5497):6–7.
107. Esposito K, Ciotola M, Maiorino MI. Hyperlipidemia and sexual function in premenopausal women. J Sex Med. 2009;6(6): 1696–703.
108. Galletly C, Lechuga J, Layde JB, et al. Sexual health curricula in U.S. medical schools: current educational objectives. Acad Psychiatry. 2010;34:333–8.
109. Go AS, Bauman MA, Coleman-King SM, Fonarow GC, Lawrence W, Williams KA, et al. An effective approach to high blood pressure control. J Am Coll Cardiol. 2014;63(12):1230–8.
110. Jenkins DJ, Kendall CW, Marchie A, Jenkins AL, Connelly PW, Jones PJ, et al. The garden of Eden—plant based diets, the genetic drive to conserve cholesterol and its implications for heart disease in the 21st century. Comp Biochem Physiol A Mol Integr Physiol. 2003;136(1):141–51.

111. Law, M. R., Morris JK., and Wald NJ. Use of blood pressure lowering drugs in the prevention of cardiovascular disease: meta-analysis of 147 randomised trials in the context of expectations from prospective epidemiological studies. BMJ 2009;338:1665.
112. Lief HI. Preparing the physician to become a sex counselor and educator. Pediatr Clin North Am. 1969;16:447–58.
113. Lief HI. Sexual knowledge, attitudes, and behavior of medical students: Implications for medical practice. In: Abse DW, Nash EM, Louden LMR, editors. Marital and sexual counseling in medical practice. New York: Harper & Row; 1974. p. 474–94.
114. Malhotra S, Khurshid A, Hendricks KA, et al. Medical school sexual health curriculum and training in the United States. J Natl Med Assoc. 2008;100:1097–106.
115. Mckay DL, Chen C-Y, Saltzman E, Blumberg JB. *Hibiscus sabdariffa* L. Tea (Tisane) lowers blood pressure in prehypertensive and mildly hypertensive adults. J Nutr. 2010;140(2):298–303.
116. McKelvey RS, Webb JA, Baldassar LV, et al. Sex knowledge and sexual attitudes among medical and nursing students. Aust N Z J Psychiatry. 1999;33:260–6.
117. Merrill JM, Laux LF, Thornby JI. Why doctors have difficulty with sex histories. South Med J. 1990;83:613–7.
118. Meldrum DR, Gambone JC, Morris MA, Meldrum DA, Esposito K, et al. The link between erectile and cardiovascular health: the canary in the coal mine. Am J Cardiol. 2011;108:599–606.
119. Ninomiya T, Perkovic V, Turnbull F. Blood pressure lowering and major cardiovascular events in people with and without chronic kidney disease: meta-analysis of randomised controlled trials. BMJ. 2013;347:5680.
120. Parish SJ, Clayton AH. Sexual medicine education: review and commentary. J Sex Med. 2007;4:259–68.
121. Rodriguez-Leyva D, Weighell W, Edel AL, Lavallee R, Dibrov E, Pinneker R, et al. Potent antihypertensive action of dietary flaxseed in hypertensive patients. Hypertension. 2013;62(6):1081–9.
122. Sandler B. The student and sex education. Lancet. 1957;273:832–3.
123. Shindel AW, Baazeem A, Eardley I, Coleman E. Sexual health in undergraduate medical education: existing and future needs and platforms. J Sex Med. 2016;13(7):1013–26.
124. Shindel AW, Ando KA, Nelson CJ, et al. Medical student sexuality: how sexual experience and sexuality training impact U.S. and Canadian medical students' comfort in dealing with patients' sexuality in clinical practice. Acad Med. 2010;85:1321–30.
125. Tighe P, Duthie G, Vaughan N, Brittenden J, Simpson WG, Duthie S, et al. Effect of increased consumption of whole-grain foods on blood pressure and other cardiovascular risk markers in healthy middle-aged persons: a randomized controlled trial. Am J Clin Nutr. 2010;92(4):733–40.
126. Trumbo PR, Shimakawa T. Tolerable upper intake levels for trans fat, saturated fat, and cholesterol. Nutr Rev. 2011;69(5):270–8.
127. Wagner G. Sexual medicine in the medical curriculum. Int J Androl. 2005;28:7–8.
128. Wang F, Dai S, Wang M, Morrison H. Erectile dysfunction and fruit/vegetable consumption among diabetic canadian men. Urology. 2013;82(6):1330–5.
129. Walker, A. R., and B. Walker F. High high-density-lipoprotein cholesterol in African children and adults in a population free of coronary heart disease. BMJ 1978;2(6148):1336–1337.
130. Whelton PK, Appel LJ, Sacco RL, CAM A, Antman EM, Campbell N, et al. Sodium, blood pressure, and cardiovascular disease: further evidence supporting the American Heart Association Sodium Reduction Recommendations. Circulation. 2012;126(24):2880–9.
131. Wiggers TT, Grover PL, Labrum AH. Some new methods for the evaluation of medical school sex education curricula. Med Educ. 1977;11:385–9.
132. Wittenberg A, Gerber J. Recommendations for improving sexual health curricula in medical schools: results from a two-arm study collecting data from patients and medical students. J Sex Med. 2009;6:362–8.

Appendix A: Rating scales

Compiled by Waguih William IsHak, MD, FAPA

W.W. IsHak (ed.), *The Textbook of Clinical Sexual Medicine*, DOI 10.1007/978-3-319-52539-6

Summary table of selected scales and questionnaires

Questionnaire	Target population	Items	Domains	Published cutoff scores	Level of evidence
Selected sexual functioning scales and questionnaires					
Female Sexual Function Index (FSFI) [1]	Women—heterosexual and homosexual	19 and 6	Sexual function, including desire, arousal, lubrication, orgasm, satisfaction, and pain	Available for pre- and postmenopausal women and women with medical and sexual disorders	A-1
Sexual Functioning Questionnaire (SFQ) [2, 3]	Women—heterosexual and sexually active during past 4 weeks	28	Desire, arousal, orgasm, pain, enjoyment, and partner relationship	Available	B-3
Female Sexual Distress Scale–Revised (FSDS-R) [4]	Women—pre- and postmenopausal dissatisfied with their sexual function	13 and 1	Distress about sexual life	Available	A-1
Sexual Interest and Desire Inventory (SIDI) [5–7]	Women—premenopausal with low desire	15	Hypoactive sexual desire disorder	Available on women with no sexual desire disorder	B-2
International Index of Erectile Function (IIEF) [8–10]	Men from community and medical populations	10 and 5	Erectile function, orgasmic function, sexual desire, intercourse satisfaction, and overall satisfaction	Available	A-1
Male Sexual Health Questionnaire (MSHQ) [11]	Men—middle age or aging with urogenital symptoms of LUTS and sexual dysfunction	25 and 4	Ejaculation, erection, and sexual satisfaction	Available	B-2
Premature Ejaculation Profile (PEP) [12]	Men	4	Satisfaction with sexual intercourse, control over ejaculation, ejaculation-related distress, and interpersonal difficulty	Not available	B-2
Index of Premature Ejaculation (IPE) [13]	Men		Control, sexual satisfaction, and distress	Available	B-2
Sexual function questionnaires for specific patient populations					
PROMIS Sexual Function and Satisfaction (SexFS) [14, 15]	Patients with cancer	79	Interest in sexual activity, lubrication, vaginal discomfort, erectile function, global satisfaction with sex life, orgasm, anal discomfort, therapeutic aids, sexual activities, interfering factors, and screener questions	Available	A-1
European Organization for Research and Treatment of Cancer (EORTC) QLQ-C30 [16]; also disease-specific modules such as prostate cancer [17]	Patients with cancer	30	Quality of life and sexual function	Available	A-2
Multiple Sclerosis Intimacy and Sexuality Questionnaire (MSISQ-19) [18]	Patients with MS	19 and 15	Primary, secondary, and tertiary sexual dysfunction	Not available	B-1

(continued)

(continued)

Questionnaire	Target population	Items	Domains	Published cutoff scores	Level of evidence
Peyronie's disease [19–21]	Men—Peyronie's disease	15	Psychological and physical symptoms, Peyronie's symptom bother, and penile pain	Not available	A-1
Pelvic Organ Prolapse/ Urinary Incontinence Sexual Questionnaire (PISQ) [22]	Women—pelvic organ prolapse, urinary incontinence, fecal incontinence	31 and 12	Behavioral and emotive, physical, and partner related	Not available	B-2
Spinal Cord Injury Secondary Conditions Scale (SCI-SCS) [23]	Patients with spinal cord injury	16	Secondary conditions and dissatisfaction with sexual function	Not available	C-3
Antipsychotics and Sexual Functioning Questionnaire (ASFQ) [24, 25]	Patients under antipsychotic medication	11 + 3 for men and 5 for women, semistructured interview	Sexual functioning	Not available	C-1
Female Genital Self-Image Scale (FGSIS) and Male Genital Self-Image Scale (MGSIS) [26, 27]	Female or male genital self-image on sexual function and behavior	4 women, 5 male	Feelings and beliefs about own genitals	Not available	A-1
Penile Dysmorphic Disorder Scale [28]	Men	9	Penile dysmorphic disorder	Available	B-2
Treatment outcome and sexual quality-of-life scales					
Erectile Dysfunction Inventory for Treatment and Satisfaction (EDITS) [29–31]	Men with ED and their partners	29	Treatment satisfaction (men) and partner satisfaction (women)	Not available	A-1
Treatment Satisfaction Scale [32]	Men with ED and their partner	40 (all modules together)	Satisfaction with medication, ease with erection, satisfaction with erectile function, pleasure from sexual activity, satisfaction with orgasm, and either sexual confidence (for patients) or confidence in completion (for partners)	Not available	A-2
Self-Esteem and Relationship Scale (SEAR) [33]	Men with ED	14	Self-esteem, confidence, and relationships	Not available	A-1
Psychological and Interpersonal Relationship Scale (PAIRS) [34]	Men >65 year old	23	Sexual confidence, spontaneity, time concerns, relative to treatment	Not available	B-1
Sexual Quality of Life for men (SQOL-M) and women (SQOL-F) [35]	Men with ED or PE and women with HSDD or FSAD	11 and 18	Sexual confidence, emotional well-being, and relationship issues	Not available	C-2

ED erectile dysfunction, *FSAD* female sexual arousal disorder, *HSDD* hypoactive sexual desire disorder, *LUTS* lower urinary tract symptoms, *MS* multiple sclerosis, *PE* premature ejaculation. [Reprinted from Hatzichristou D, Kirana PS, Banner L, Althof SE, Lonnee-Hoffmann RA, Dennerstein L, Rosen RC. Diagnosing Sexual Dysfunction in Men and Women: Sexual History Taking and the Role of Symptom Scales and Questionnaires. J Sex Med. 2016;13(8): 1166–82 with permission from Elsevier]

NIH PROMIS Measures

PROMIS Sexual Function Profile v1.0 – Female

Please respond to each question or statement by marking one box per row.

	Interest in Sexual Activity **In the past 30 days...**		**Not at all**	**A little bit**	**Somewhat**	**Quite a bit**	**Very**
SFINT101	How interested have you been in sexual activity?...		☐ 1	☐ 2	☐ 3	☐ 4	☐ 5
			Never	**Rarely**	**Sometimes**	**Often**	**Always**
SFINT102	How often have you felt like you wanted to have sex?..........		☐ 1	☐ 2	☐ 3	☐ 4	☐ 5
	Lubrication **Over the past 4 weeks...**	**No sexual activity**	**Almost always or always**	**Most times (more than half the time)**	**Sometimes (about half the time)**	**A few times (less than half the time)**	**Almost never or ever**
SFLUB001	How *often* did you become lubricated ("wet") during sexual activity or intercourse?	☐ 0	☐ 5	☐ 4	☐ 3	☐ 2	☐ 1
	In the past 30 days...	**Have not tried to get lubricated in the past 30 days**	**Not at all**	**A little bit**	**Somewhat**	**Quite a bit**	**Very**
SFLUB101	How difficult has it been for your vagina to get lubricated ("wet") when you wanted it to?..........	☐ 0	☐ 5	☐ 4	☐ 3	☐ 2	☐ 1
	Vaginal Discomfort **In the past 30 days...**		**Have not had any sexual activity in the past 30 days**	**Very comfortable**	**Comfortable**	**Uncomfortable**	**Very Uncomfortable**
SFVAG101	How would you describe the comfort of your vagina during sexual activity?		☐ 0	☐ 1	☐ 2	☐ 3	☐ 4
		Have not had any sexual activity in the past 30 days	**Never**	**Rarely**	**Sometimes**	**Often**	**Always**
SFVAG102	How often have you had difficulty with sexual activity because of discomfort or pain in your vagina?...	☐ 0	☐ 1	☐ 2	☐ 3	☐ 4	☐ 5
SFVAG103	How often have you stopped sexual activity because of discomfort or pain in your vagina?	☐ 0	☐ 1	☐ 2	☐ 3	☐ 4	☐ 5
	Orgasm **In the past 30 days...**	**Have not tried to have an orgasm/ climax in the past 30 days**	**Excellent**	**Very good**	**Good**	**Fair**	**Poor**
SFORG101	How would you rate your ability to have a satisfying orgasm/climax?.....	☐ 0	☐ 5	☐ 4	☐ 3	☐ 2	☐ 1
	Satisfaction **In the past 30 days...**	**Have not had sexual activity in the past 30 days**	**Not at all**	**A little bit**	**Somewhat**	**Quite a bit**	**Very much**
SFSAT105	When you have had sexual activity, how much have you enjoyed it?	☐ 0	☐ 1	☐ 2	☐ 3	☐ 4	☐ 5
		Have not had sexual activity in the past 30 days	**Not at all**	**A little bit**	**Somewhat**	**Quite a bit**	**Very**
SFSAT106	When you have had sexual activity, how satisfying has it been?..........	☐ 0	☐ 1	☐ 2	☐ 3	☐ 4	☐ 5

PROMIS Sexual Function Profile v1.0 – Male

Please respond to each question or statement by marking one box per row.

	Interest in Sexual Activity **In the past 30 days…**		**Not at all**	**A little bit**	**Somewhat**	**Quite a bit**	**Very**
SFINT101	How interested have you been in sexual activity?...		☐ 1	☐ 2	☐ 3	☐ 4	☐ 5
			Never	**Rarely**	**Sometimes**	**Often**	**Always**
SFINT102	How often have you felt like you wanted to have sex?		☐ 1	☐ 2	☐ 3	☐ 4	☐ 5
	Erectile Function **In the past 30 days…**	**Have not tried to get an erection in the past 30 days**	**Not at all**	**A little bit**	**Somewhat**	**Quite a bit**	**Very**
SFEFN102	How difficult has it been for you to get an erection when you wanted to? (If you use pills, injections, or a penis pump to help you get an erection, please answer this question thinking about the times that you used these aids.)	☐ 0	☐ 5	☐ 4	☐ 3	☐ 2	☐ 1
		Have not had an erection in the past 30 days	**Not at all**	**A little bit**	**Somewhat**	**Quite a bit**	**Very**
SFEFN103	How difficult has it been to keep an erection (stay hard) when you wanted to? (If you use pills, injections, or a penis pump to help you get an erection, please answer this question thinking about the times that you used these aids.).........	☐ 0	☐ 5	☐ 4	☐ 3	☐ 2	☐ 1
	How would you rate the following during the LAST 4 WEEKS…		**Very poor**	**Poor**	**Fair**	**Good**	**Very Good**
SFEFN002	Your ability to have an erection		☐ 1	☐ 2	☐ 3	☐ 4	☐ 5
	Orgasm **In the past 30 days…**	**Have not tried to have an orgasm/ climax in the past 30 days**	**Excellent**	**Very good**	**Good**	**Fair**	**Poor**
SFORG101	How would you rate your ability to have a satisfying orgasm/climax? .	☐ 0	☐ 5	☐ 4	☐ 3	☐ 2	☐ 1
	Satisfaction **In the past 30 days…**	**Have not had sexual activity in the past 30 days**	**Not at all**	**A little bit**	**Somewhat**	**Quite a bit**	**Very much**
SFSAT105	When you have had sexual activity, how much have you enjoyed it?....	☐ 0	☐ 1	☐ 2	☐ 3	☐ 4	☐ 5
		Have not had sexual activity in the past 30 days	**Not at all**	**A little bit**	**Somewhat**	**Quite a bit**	**Very**
SFSAT106	When you have had sexual activity, how satisfying has it been?	☐ 0	☐ 1	☐ 2	☐ 3	☐ 4	☐ 5

PROMIS Sexual Function Profile v1.0 – Male & Female

Please respond to each question or statement by marking one box per row.

	Interest in Sexual Activity **In the past 30 days…**		**Not at all**	**A little bit**	**Somewhat**	**Quite a bit**	**Very**
SFINT101	How interested have you been in sexual activity?...		☐ 1	☐ 2	☐ 3	☐ 4	☐ 5
			Never	**Rarely**	**Sometimes**	**Often**	**Always**
SFINT102	How often have you felt like you wanted to have sex?........		☐ 1	☐ 2	☐ 3	☐ 4	☐ 5
	Orgasm **In the past 30 days…**	**Have not tried to have an orgasm/ climax in the past 30 days**	**Excellent**	**Very good**	**Good**	**Fair**	**Poor**
SFORG101	How would you rate your ability to have a satisfying orgasm/climax?......	☐ 0	☐ 5	☐ 4	☐ 3	☐ 2	☐ 1
	Satisfaction **In the past 30 days…**	**Have not had sexual activity in the past 30 days**	**Not at all**	**A little bit**	**Somewhat**	**Quite a bit**	**Very much**
SFSAT105	When you have had sexual activity, how much have you enjoyed it?	☐ 0	☐ 1	☐ 2	☐ 3	☐ 4	☐ 5
		Have not had sexual activity in the past 30 days	**Not at all**	**A little bit**	**Somewhat**	**Quite a bit**	**Very**
SFSAT106	When you have had sexual activity, how satisfying has it been?...............	☐ 0	☐ 1	☐ 2	☐ 3	☐ 4	☐ 5
			Male	**Female**			
SFSCR103r	Are you...		☐	☐			
			Male→ Go to question SFEN102. Female→ Skip to SFLUB0001.				
	Erectile Function **In the past 30 days…**	**Have not tried to get an erection in the past 30 days**	**Not at all**	**A little bit**	**Somewhat**	**Quite a bit**	**Very**
SFEFN102	How difficult has it been for you to get an erection when you wanted to? (If you use pills, injections, or a penis pump to help you get an erection, please answer this question thinking about the times that you used these aids.)..................	☐ 0	☐ 5	☐ 4	☐ 3	☐ 2	☐ 1

PROMIS Sexual Function Profile v1.0 – Male & Female

	Erectile Function **In the past 30 days…**	**Have not had an erection in the past 30 days**	**Not at all**	**A little bit**	**Somewhat**	**Quite a bit**	**Very**
SFEFN103	How difficult has it been to keep an erection (stay hard) when you wanted to? (If you use pills, injections, or a penis pump to help you get an erection, please answer this question thinking about the times that you used these aids.)	☐ 0	☐ 5	☐ 4	☐ 3	☐ 2	☐ 1
	How would you rate the following during the LAST 4 WEEKS…		**Very Poor**	**Poor**	**Fair**	**Good**	**Very Good**
SFEFN002	Your ability to have an erection..............................		☐ 1	☐ 2	☐ 3	☐ 4	☐ 5
	MALE STOP HERE						
	Lubrication **Over the past 4 weeks…**	**No sexual activity**	**Almost always or always**	**Most times (more than half the time)**	**Sometimes (about half the time)**	**A few times (less than half the time)**	**Almost never or never**
SFLUB001	How *often* did you become lubricated ("wet") during sexual activity or intercourse?	☐ 0	☐ 5	☐ 4	☐ 3	☐ 2	☐ 1
	In the past 30 days…	**Have not tried to get lubricated in the past 30 days**	**Not at all**	**A little bit**	**Somewhat**	**Quite a bit**	**Very**
SFLUB101	How difficult has it been for your vagina to get lubricated ("wet") when you wanted it to?....................	☐ 0	☐ 5	☐ 4	☐ 3	☐ 2	☐ 1
	Vaginal Discomfort **In the past 30 days…**		**Have not had any sexual activity in the past 30 days**	**Very comfortable**	**Comfortable**	**Uncomfortable**	**Very Uncomfortable**
SFVAG101	How would you describe the comfort of your vagina during sexual activity?		☐ 0	☐ 1	☐ 2	☐ 3	☐ 4
		Have not had any sexual activity in the past 30 days	**Never**	**Rarely**	**Sometimes**	**Often**	**Always**
SFVAG102	How often have you had difficulty with sexual activity because of discomfort or pain in your vagina?...	☐ 0	☐ 1	☐ 2	☐ 3	☐ 4	☐ 5
SFVAG103	How often have you stopped sexual activity because of discomfort or pain in your vagina?	☐ 0	☐ 1	☐ 2	☐ 3	☐ 4	☐ 5

References

1. Rosen R, Brown C, Heiman J, et al. The Female Sexual Function Index (FSFI): a multidimensional self-report instrument for the assessment of female sexual function. J Sex Marital Ther. 2000;26:191–208.
2. Quirk FH, Heiman JR, Rosen RC, et al. Development of a sexual function questionnaire for clinical trials of female sexual dysfunction. J Womens Health Gend Based Med. 2002;11:277–89.
3. Quirk F, Haughie S, Symonds T. The use of the sexual function questionnaire as a screening tool for women with sexual dysfunction. J Sex Med. 2005;2:469–77.
4. Derogatis LR, Rosen R, Leiblum S, et al. The Female Sexual Distress Scale (FSDS): initial validation of a standardized scale for assessment of sexually related personal distress in women. J Sex Marital Ther. 2002;28:317–30.
5. Sills T, Wunderlich G, Pyke R, et al. The Sexual Interest and Desire Inventory-Female (SIDI-F): item response analyses of data from women diagnosed with hypoactive sexual desire disorder. J Sex Med. 2005;2:801–18.
6. Clayton AH, Segraves RT, Leiblum S, et al. Reliability and validity of the Sexual Interest and Desire Inventory-Female (SIDI-F), a scale designed to measure severity of female hypoactive sexual desire disorder. J Sex Marital Ther. 2006;32:115–35.
7. Clayton AH, Goldmeier D, Nappi RE, et al. Validation of the sexual interest and desire inventory-female in hypoactive sexual desire disorder. J Sex Med. 2010;7:3918–28.
8. Rosen RC, Riley A, Wagner G, et al. The International Index of Erectile Function (IIEF): a multidimensional scale for assessment of erectile dysfunction. Urology. 1997;49:822–30.
9. Rosen RC, Cappelleri JC, Gendrano III N. The International Index of Erectile Function (IIEF): a state-of-the-science review. Int J Impot Res. 2002;14:226–44.
10. Rosen RC, Cappelleri JC, Smith MD, et al. Development and evaluation of an abridged, 5-item version of the International Index of Erectile Function (IIEF-5) as a diagnostic tool for erectile dysfunction. Int J Impot Res. 1999;11:319–26.
11. Rosen RC, Catania J, Pollack L, et al. Male Sexual Health Questionnaire (MSHQ): scale development and psychometric validation. Urology. 2004;64:777–82.
12. Patrick D, Giuliano F, Ho K, et al. The Premature Ejaculation Profile: validation of self-reported outcome measures for research and practice. BJU Int. 2009;103:358–64.
13. Althof S, Rosen R, Symonds T, et al. Development and validation of a new questionnaire to assess sexual satisfaction, control, and distress associated with premature ejaculation. J Sex Med. 2006;3:465–75.
14. Flynn KE, Lin L, Cyranowski JM, et al. Development of the NIH PROMIS (R) Sexual Function and Satisfaction measures in patients with cancer. J Sex Med. 2013;10(Suppl. 1):43–52.
15. Flynn KE, Reeve BB, Lin L, et al. Construct validity of the PROMIS(R) sexual function and satisfaction measures in patients with cancer. Health Qual Life Outcomes. 2013;11:40.
16. Jeffery DD, Barbera L, Andersen BL, et al. Self-reported sexual function measures administered to female cancer patients: a systematic review, 2008e2014. J Psychosoc Oncol. 2015;33:433–66.
17. O'Leary E, Drummond FJ, Gavin A, et al. Psychometric evaluation of the EORTC QLQ-PR25 questionnaire in assessing health-related quality of life in prostate cancer survivors: a curate's egg. Qual Life Res. 2015;24:2219–30.
18. Sanders A, Foley F, Larocca N, et al. The Multiple Sclerosis Intimacy and Sexuality Questionnaire-19 (MSISQ-19). Sex Disabil. 2000;18:3–26.
19. Hellstrom WJ, Feldman R, Rosen RC, et al. Bother and distress associated with Peyronie's disease: validation of the Peyronie's disease questionnaire. J Urol. 2013;190:627–34.
20. Coyne KS, Currie BM, Thompson CL, et al. Responsiveness of the Peyronie's Disease Questionnaire (PDQ). J Sex Med. 2015;12:1072–9.
21. Coyne KS, Currie BM, Thompson CL, et al. The test-retest reliability of the Peyronie's Disease Questionnaire. J Sex Med. 2015;12:543–8.
22. Rogers RG, Kammerer-Doak D, Villarreal A, et al. A new instrument to measure sexual function in women with urinary incontinence or pelvic organ prolapse. Am J Obstet Gynecol. 2001;184:552–8.
23. Kalpakjian CZ, Scelza WM, Forchheimer MB, et al. Preliminary reliability and validity of a Spinal Cord Injury Secondary Conditions Scale. J Spinal Cord Med. 2007;30:131–9.
24. De Boer MK, Castelein S, Bous J, et al. The Antipsychotics and Sexual Functioning Questionnaire (ASFQ): preliminary evidence for reliability and validity. Schizophr Res. 2013;150:410–5.
25. De Boer MK, Castelein S, Wiersma D, et al. A systematic review of instruments to measure sexual functioning in patients using antipsychotics. J Sex Res. 2014;51:383–9.
26. Herbenick D, Reece M. Development and validation of the female genital self-image scale. J Sex Med. 2010;7:1822–30.
27. Herbenick D, Schick V, Reece M, et al. The Female Genital Self-Image Scale (FGSIS): results from a nationally representative probability sample of women in the United States. J Sex Med. 2011;8:158–66.
28. Veale D, Miles S, Read J, et al. Penile dysmorphic disorder: development of a screening scale. Arch Sex Behav. 2015;44:2311–21.
29. Lewis R, Bennett CJ, Borkon WD, et al. Patient and partner satisfaction with Viagra (sildenafil citrate) treatment as determined by the Erectile Dysfunction Inventory of Treatment Satisfaction Questionnaire. Urology. 2001;57:960–5.

W.W. IsHak (ed.), *The Textbook of Clinical Sexual Medicine*, DOI 10.1007/978-3-319-52539-6

30. Cappelleri JC, Althof SE, Siegel RL, et al. Association between the Erectile Dysfunction Inventory of Treatment Satisfaction and the Self-Esteem and Relationship Questionnaire following treatment with sildenafil citrate for men with erectile dysfunction. Value Health. 2005;8(Suppl. 1):S54–60.
31. Fugl-Meyer A, Althof S, Buvat J, et al. Aspects of sexual satisfaction in men with erectile dysfunction: a factor analytic and logistic regression approach. J Sex Med. 2009;6:232–42.
32. Rosen R, Goldstein I, Huang XY, et al. The Treatment Satisfaction Scale (TSS) is a sensitive measure of treatment effectiveness for both patients and partners: results of a randomized controlled trial with vardenafil. J Sex Med. 2007;4:1009–21.
33. Cappelleri JC, Althof SE, Siegel RL, et al. Development and validation of the Self-Esteem And Relationship (SEAR) questionnaire in erectile dysfunction. Int J Impot Res. 2004;16:30–8.
34. Sharlip ID, Shumaker BP, Hakim LS, et al. Tadalafil is efficacious and well tolerated in the treatment of erectile dysfunction (ED) in men over 65 years of age: results from Multiple Observations in Men with ED in National Tadalafil Study in the United States. J Sex Med. 2008;5:716–25.
35. Symonds T, Boolell M, Quirk F. Development of a questionnaire on sexual quality of life in women. J Sex Marital Ther. 2005;31:385–97.

Appendix B: Evaluation and Treatment Algorithms

W.W. IsHak (ed.), *The Textbook of Clinical Sexual Medicine*, DOI 10.1007/978-3-319-52539-6

Diagnostic and Treatment Algorithm for Sexual Dysfunction in Men and Women

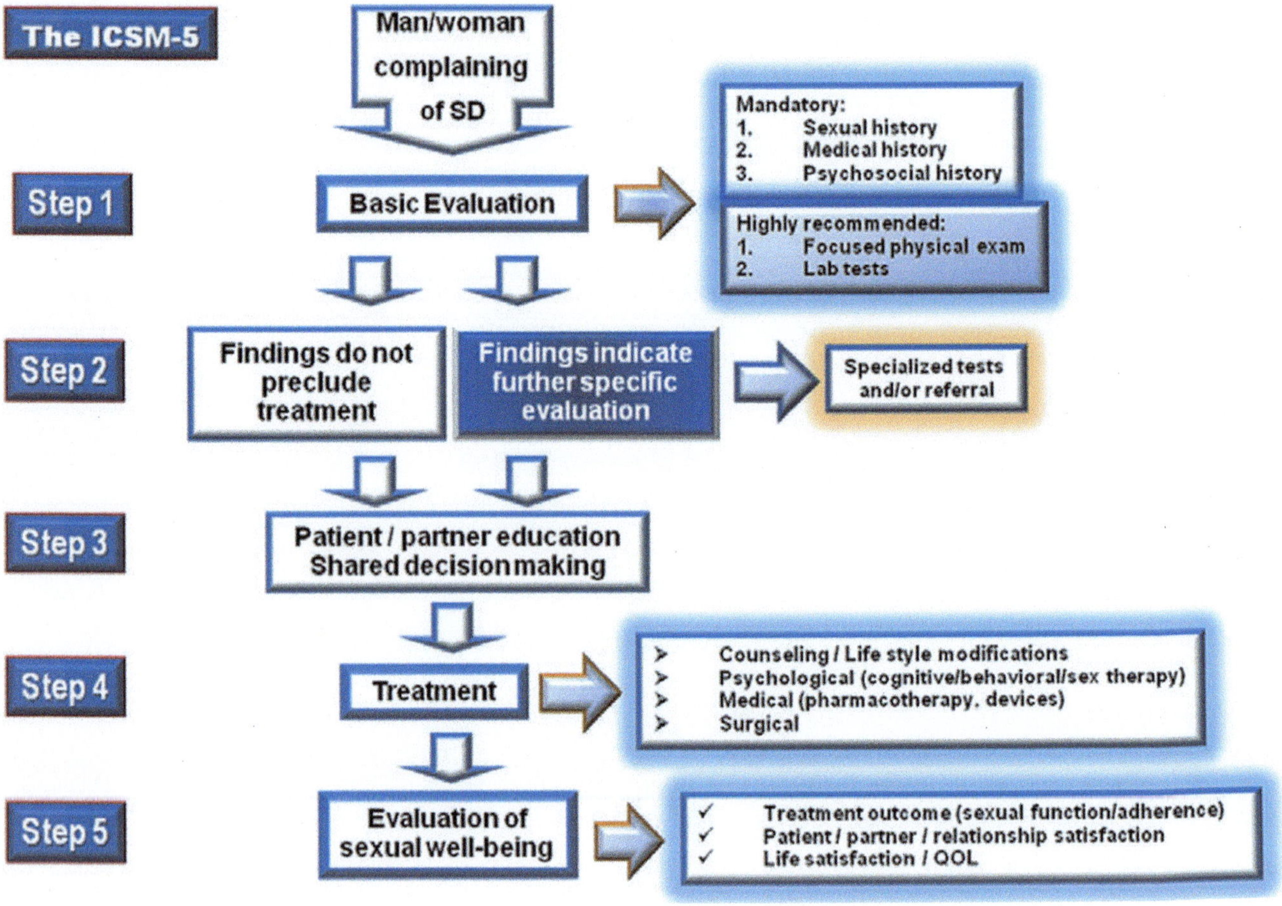

FIGURE 1. Diagnostic and treatment algorithm for sexual dysfunction in men and women by the International Consultation of Sexual Medicine (ICSM-5). [Reprinted from Montorsi F, Adaikan G, Becher E, Giuliano F, Khoury S, Lue TF, et al. Summary of the recommendations on sexual dysfunctions in men. J Sex Med. 2010;7(11): 3572–88 with permission from Elsevier].

Male Hypoactive Sexual Desire Disorder (HSDD)

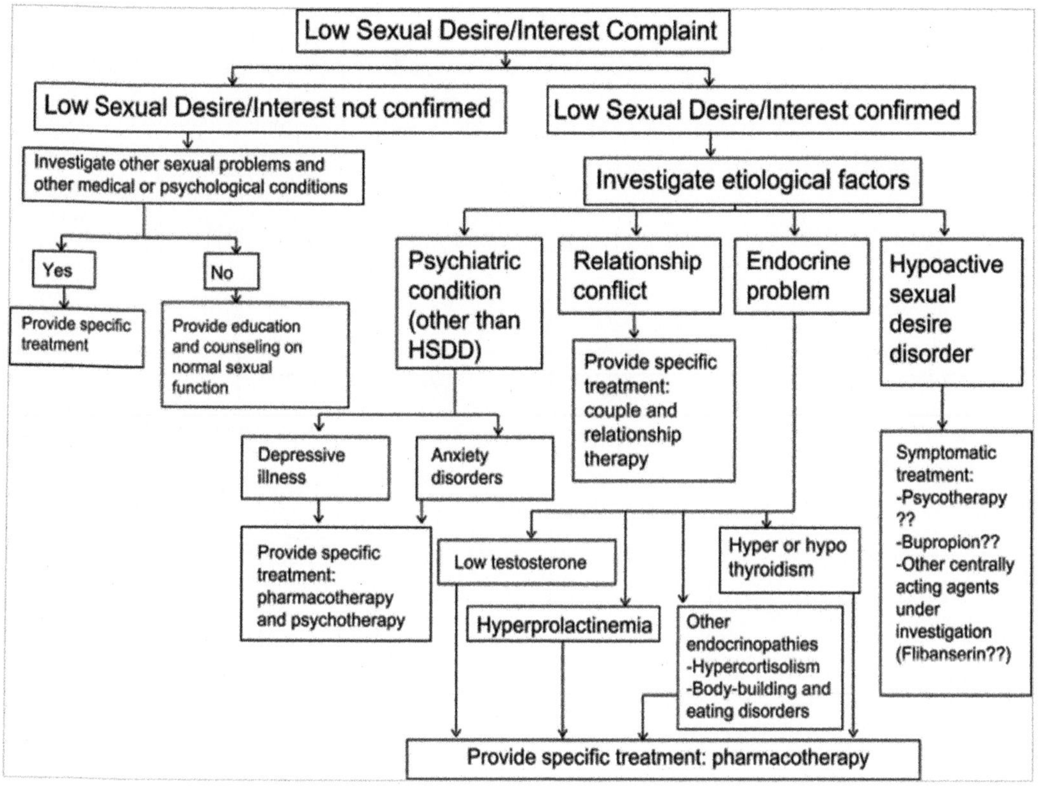

FIGURE 2. Male low sexual desire/interest. [Reprinted from Rubio-Aurioles E, Bivalacqua TJ. Standard operational procedures for low sexual desire in men. J Sex Med. 2013;10(1): 94–107 with permission from Elsevier].

Female Sexual Interest/Arousal Disorder

FIGURE 3. Women's circular sexual response cycle of overlapping phases of variable order by Rosemary Basson. [Reprinted from Basson R, Brotto LA, Laan E, Redmond G, Utian WH. Assessment and management of women's sexual dysfunctions: problematic desire and arousal. J Sex Med. 2005;2(3): 291–300 with permission from Elsevier].

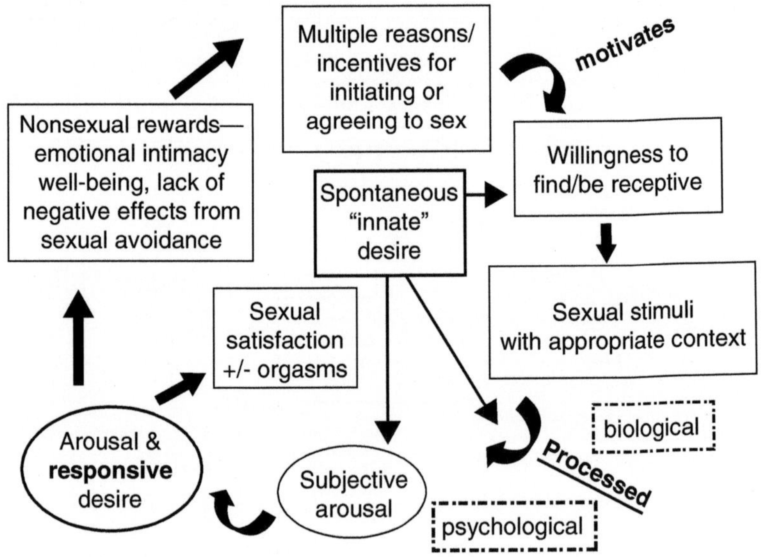

Erectile Disorder

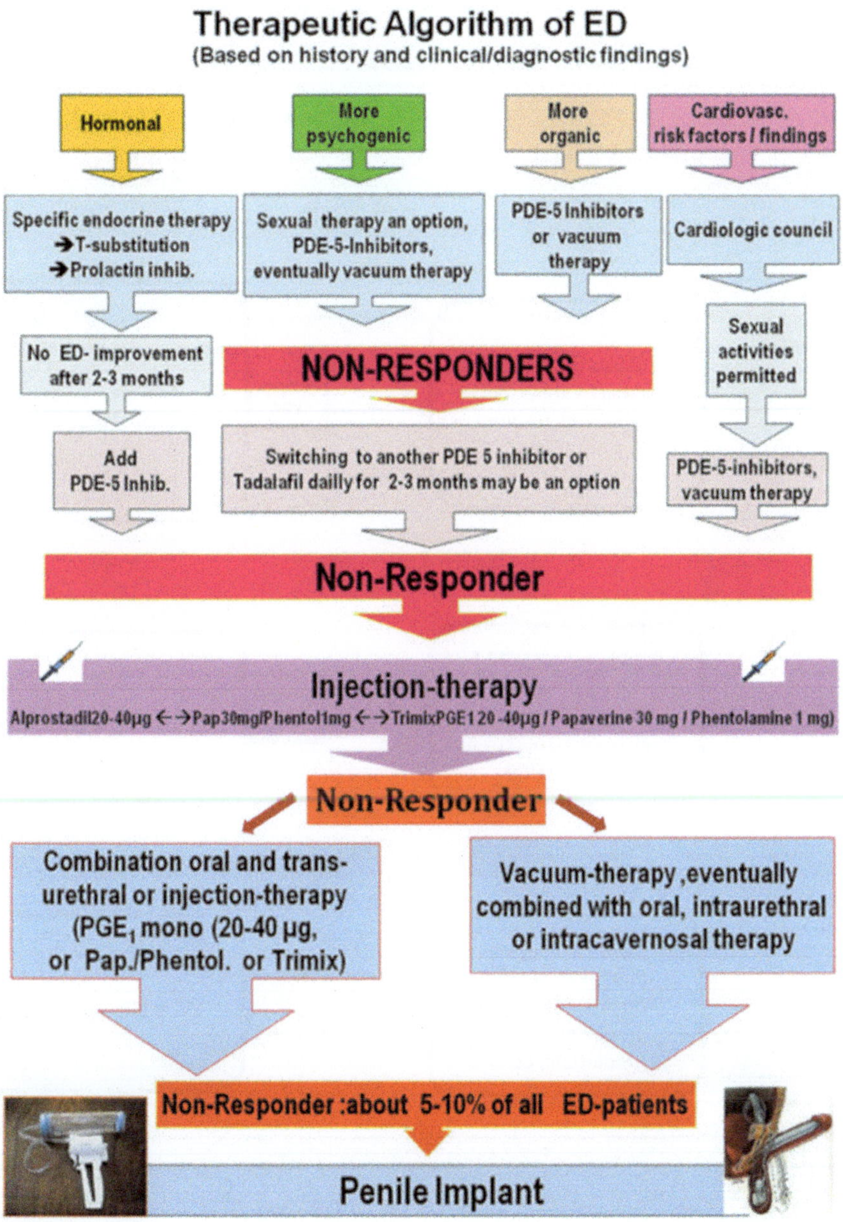

FIGURE 4. Treatment algorithm for erectile disorder. [Reprinted from Porst H, Burnett A, Brock G, Ghanem H, Giuliano F, Glina S, Hellstrom W, Martin-Morales A, Salonia A, Sharlip I; ISSM Standards Committee for Sexual Medicine. SOP conservative (medical and mechanical) treatment of erectile dysfunction. J Sex Med. 2013;10(1): 130–71 with permission from Elsevier].

Female Orgasmic Disorder (FOD)

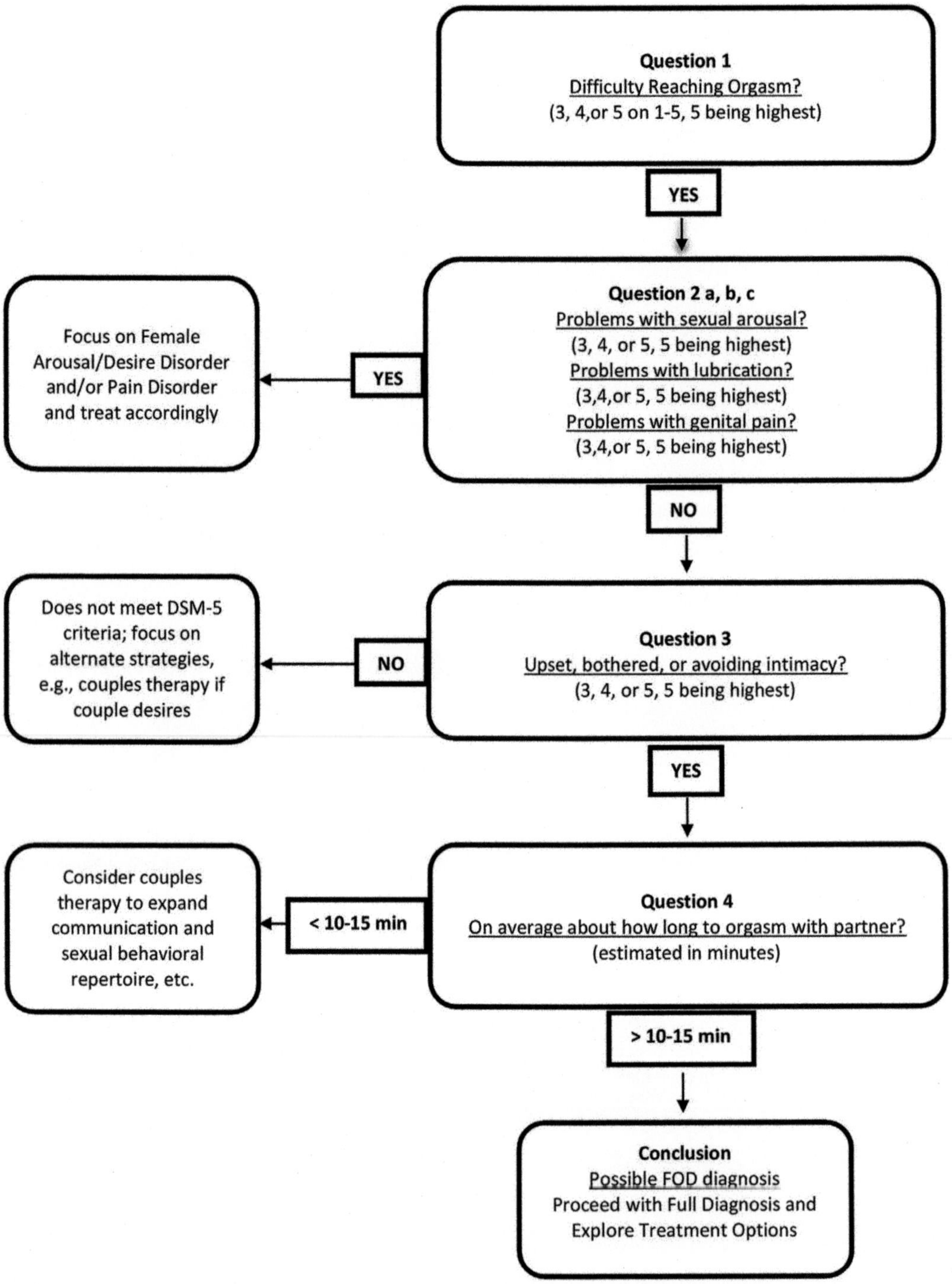

FIGURE 5. FOD and difficulty reaching orgasm in the context of partnered sex. [Reprinted from Rowland DL, Kolba TN. Understanding Orgasmic Difficulty in Women. J Sex Med. 2016;13(8): 1246–54 with permission from Elsevier].

Delayed Ejaculation (DE)

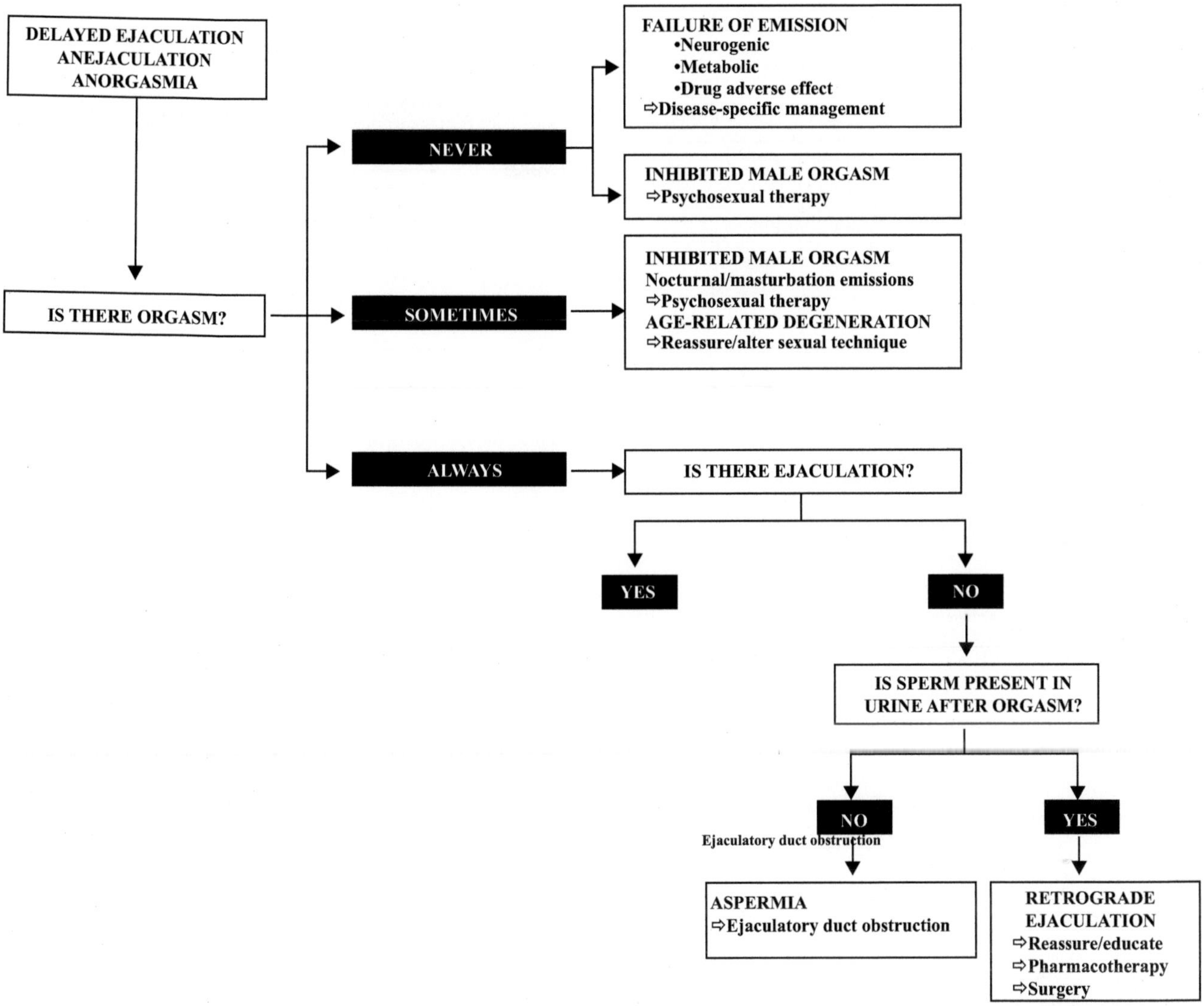

FIGURE 6. Evaluation and treatment algorithm in DE. [Reprinted from Montorsi F, Adaikan G, Becher E, Giuliano F, Khoury S, Lue TF, et al. Summary of the recommendations on sexual dysfunctions in men. J Sex Med. 2010;7(11): 3572–88 with permission from Elsevier].

Premature (Early) Ejaculation (PE)

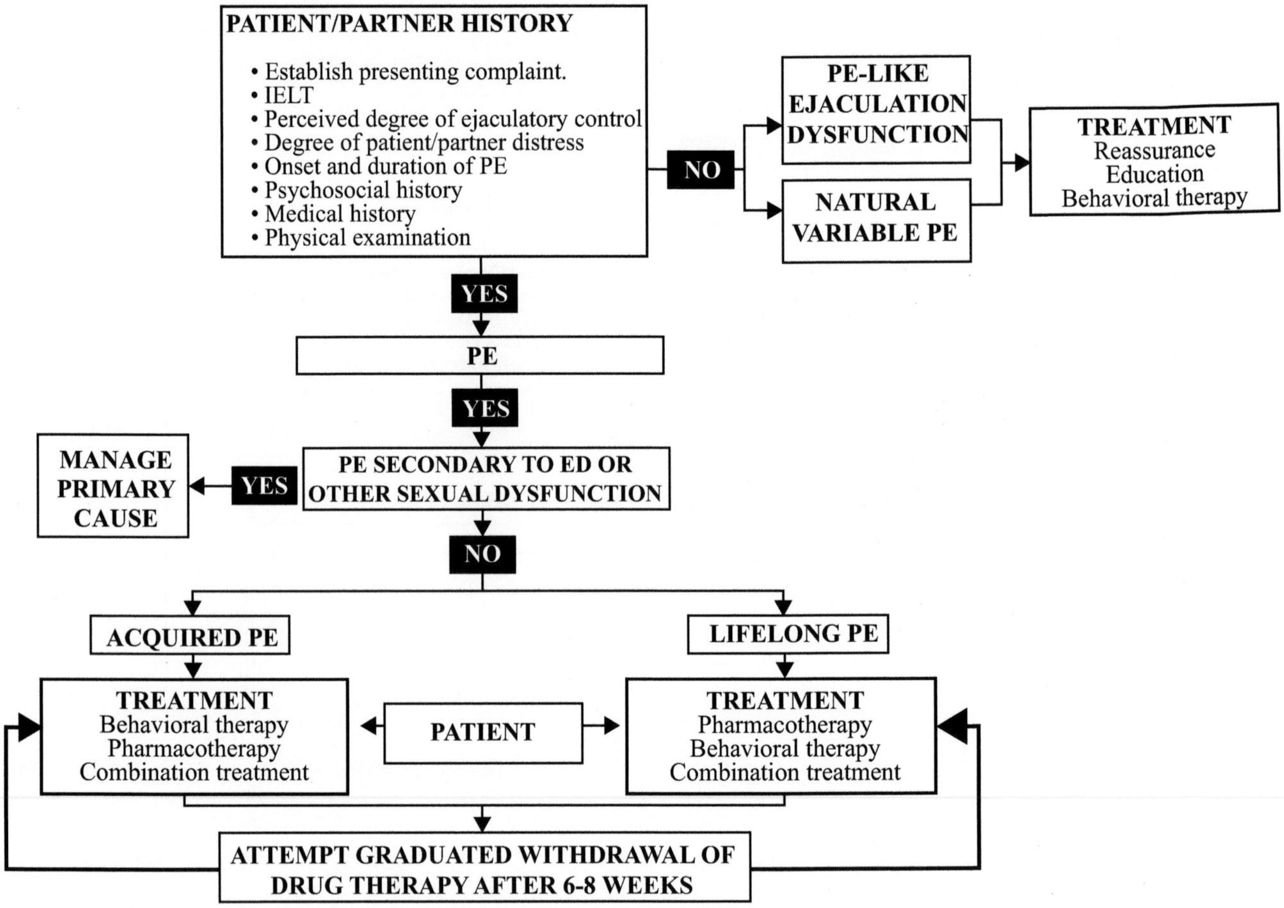

FIGURE 7. Evaluation and treatment algorithm in PE. [Reprinted from Montorsi F, Adaikan G, Becher E, Giuliano F, Khoury S, Lue TF, et al. Summary of the recommendations on sexual dysfunctions in men. J Sex Med. 2010;7(11): 3572–88 with permission from Elsevier].

Genito-Pelvic Pain/Penetration Disorder (GPPPD)

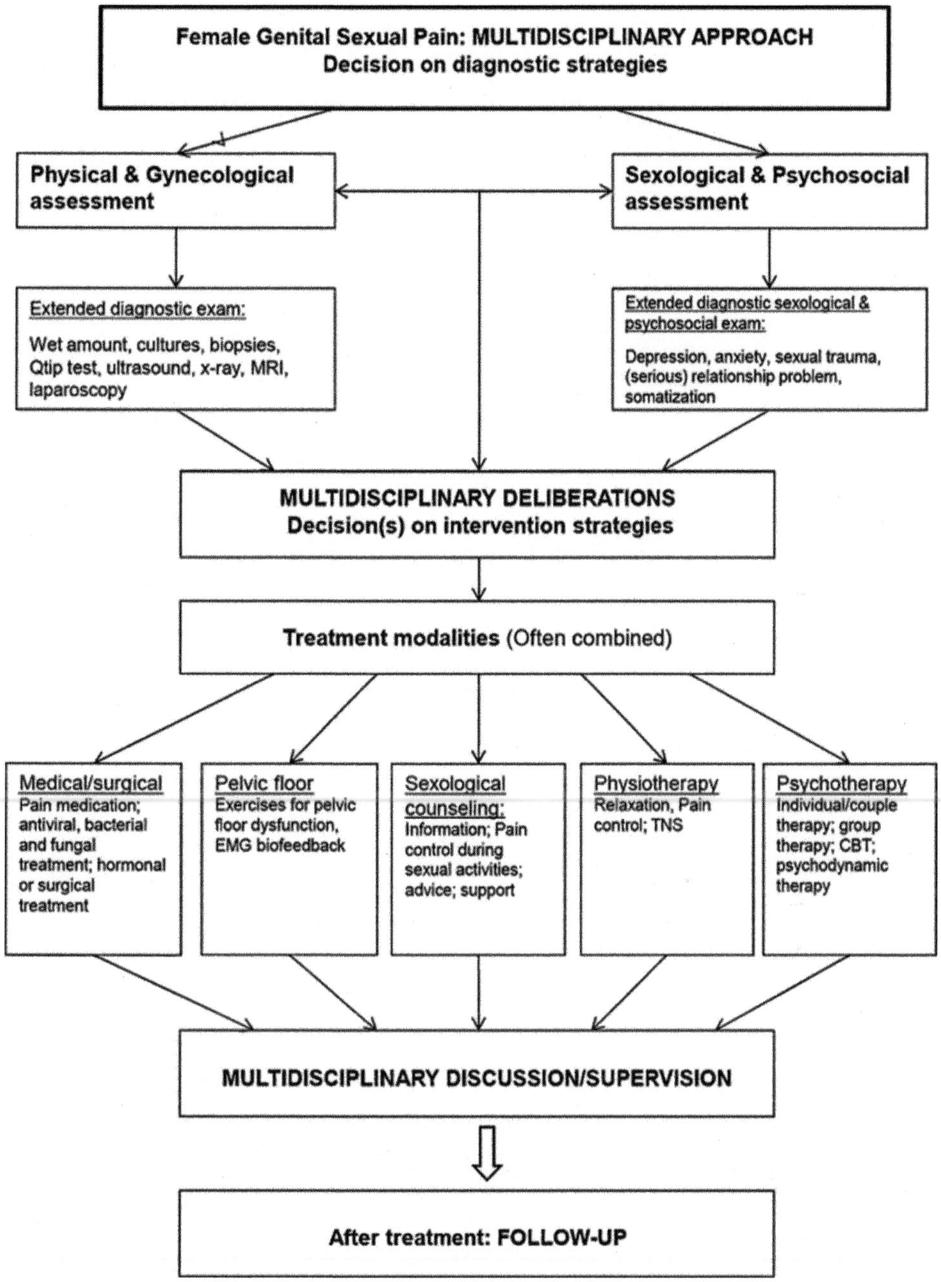

FIGURE 8. Evaluation and treatment algorithm in female genital sexual pain. [Reprinted from Fugl-Meyer KS, Bohm-Starke N, Damsted Petersen C, Fugl-Meyer A, Parish S, Giraldi A. Standard operating procedures for female genital sexual pain. J Sex Med. 2013;10(1): 83–93 with permission from Elsevier].

Index

W.W. IsHak (ed.), *The Textbook of Clinical Sexual Medicine*, DOI 10.1007/978-3-319-52539-6

D

F

G

CPI Antony Rowe
Chippenham, UK
2018-08-16 09:46